Electropharmacological Control of Cardiac Arrhythmias

To Delay Conduction or to Prolong Refractoriness?

Edited by

Bramah N. Singh, MD, DPhil, FRCP
Chief, Cardiology Section,
Veterans Affairs Medical Center
West Los Angeles, and
Professor of Medicine, UCLA School of Medicine,
Los Angeles, California

Hein J. J. Wellens, MD, FACC, FESC
Professor and Chairman, Department of Cardiology,
Academic Hospital Maastricht,
University of Limburg, The Netherlands

Masayasu Hiraoka, MD, PhD
Department of Cardiovascular Diseases,
Medical Research Institute,
Tokyo Medical and Dental University, Tokyo, Japan

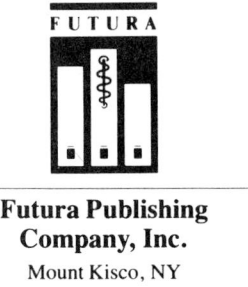

**Futura Publishing
Company, Inc.**
Mount Kisco, NY

Library of Congress Cataloging-in-Publication Data

Electropharmacologic control of cardiac arrhythmias : to delay
  conduction or to prolong refractoriness? / edited by B. N. Singh,
  Hein, J. J. Wellens, Masayasu Hiraoka.
        p.   cm.
    Includes bibliographical references and index.
    ISBN 0-87993-566-9
    1. Arrhythmia—Pathophysiology.   2. Arrhythmia—Chemotherapy.
3. Myocardial depressants.   4. Heart—Electric properties.   5. Anti-
Arrhythmia Agents—pharmacokinetics.   6. Electrophysiology.
I. Singh, B. N. (Bramah N.)   II. Wellens, H. J. J.   III. Hiraoka,
Masayasu, 1940–   .
    [DNLM: 1. Arrhythmia—physiopathology.   2 Arrhythmia—drug
therapy.   3. Anti-Arrhythmia Agents—therapeutic use.   DG 330 E382
1993]
RC685.A65E45   1993
616.1′28—dc20
DNLM/DLC
for Library of Congress   93-1874
                                                                     CIP

Copyright © 1994

Published by
Futura Publishing Company, Inc.
2 Bedford Ridge Road
Mount Kisco, New York 10549

LC #: 93-1874
ISBN #: 0-87993-566-9

Printed in the United States of America

Printed on acid-free paper.

To our wives
Roshni, Inez and Mari
For your love, understanding, and support

Acknowledgments

We are deeply indebted to all the contributors who provided their manuscripts in a timely fashion. Without them this monograph would not have been possible. Some of the work presented here was made possible by educational grants from Bristol-Myers-Squibb; Wyeth-Ayerst Laboratories; AB Hassle, Mitsui Toatsu Pharmaceuticals; Merck, Sharpe and Dohme Research Laboratories; G. B. Searle and Company; The Upjohn Company; Eisai Europe Ltd.; Pfizer Laboratories; Sanofi Pharma France; Berlax Laboratories; and Knoll AG.

We thank Susan Orrange, Diane Gerstchen, and Mary Schoenbaum for their administrative and secretarial assistance during all stages of the work leading to the completion of the book. They did this with alacrity and enthusiasm. We also would like to thank Steven Korn, Jacques Strauss, and Ann Kerr of Futura Publishing who made the steps to print smooth and uneventful.

The Editors

Contributors

Hitoshi Adaniya
Department of Cardiovascular Diseases, Medical Research Institute, Tokyo Medical and Dental University and Tsukuba Research Laboratories, Eisai Company, Ltd., Tokyo, Japan

M. J. Allen, MD
Pfizer Central Research, Department of Clinical Research, Sandwich, Kent, United Kingdom

Maurits A. Allessie, MD
Department of Physiology, University of Limburg, Maastricht, and the Department of Clinical and Experimental Cardiology, University of Amsterdam, and the Interuniversity Cardiology Institute, The Netherlands

Olle Almgren, MD, PhD
Clinical Research Laboratories, Astra Hassle AB, Molndal, Sweden

M. H. Anderson, MD
Department of Cardiological Sciences, St. George's Hospital Medical School, London, England

Takafumi Anno, MD
Department of Circulation, Research Institute of Environmental Medicine, Nagoya University, Nayoya City, Japan

Michael J. Antonaccio, PhD, FACC
Cardiovascular Diseases, Bristol-Myers Squibb Pharmaceutical Research Institute, Princeton, New Jersey

Takeo Awaji, MD
Department of Pharmacology, Yamanashi Medical College, Yamanashi, Japan

Y. Bashir, MD
Department of Cardiological Sciences, St. George's Hospital Medical School, London, United Kingdom

Mohamed Boutjdir, PhD
State University of New York Health Science Center and Senior Research Associate, Veterans Affairs Medical Centers, Brooklyn, New York

G. S. Butrous, MD, PhD
Pfizer Central Research, Department of Clinical Research, Sandwich, Kent, United Kingdom

A. John Camm, MD, FRCP
Department of Cardiological Sciences, St. George's Hospital Medical School, London, United Kingdom

Edward Carmeliet, MD, PhD
Laboratory of Physiology, University of Leuven, Leuven, Belgium

Dante R. Chialvo, MD
Computational Neuroscience, SUNY Health Science Center at Syracuse, Syracuse, New York

Craig D. Clark, MD
Department of Physiology, University of Nevada School of Medicine, Reno, Nevada

Thomas J. Colatsky, PhD
Division of Cardiovascular and Metabolic Disorders, Wyeth-Ayerst Research Laboratories, Princeton, New Jersey

Peter B. Corr, PhD
Departments of Medicine (Cardiology) and the Pharmacology and the Molecular Biology, Washington University School of Medicine, St. Louis, Missouri

Joëlle Courteix
Department de Biologie, Rhone Poulenc Rorer, Vitry-sur-Seine, France

Kenneth A. Courtney, PhD
Palo Alto Medical Foundation, Palo Alto, California and Professor, Palmer College of Chiropractic West, San Jose, California

James L. Cox, MD
Division of Cardiothoracic Surgery, Washington University School of Medicine, St. Louis, Missouri

W. W. Dalrymple, PhD
Pfizer Central Research, Department of Clinical Research, Sandwich, Kent, United Kingdom

John P. DiMarco, MD, PhD
Division of Cardiology, Department of Internal Medicine and Cardiology, University of Virginia Health Sciences Center, Charlottesville, Virginia

Paul C. Dolber, PhD
Department of Pediatrics, Duke University Medical Center, Durham, North Carolina

Nabil El-Sherif, MD
Department of Medicine, Physiology and Electrophysiology Program, State University of New York Health Science Center, and Cardiology Section, Veterans Administration Medical Center, Brooklyn, New York

Denis Escande
Laboratoire de Physiologie Cellulaire, Universite Paris, Paris, France

Gregory K. Feld, MD
Division of Cardiology, Department of Medicine, University of California, San Diego School of Medicine, San Diego, California

T. Bruce Ferguson, Jr, MD
Division of Cardiothoracic Surgery, Washington University School of Medicine, St. Louis, Missouri

Christopher H. Follmer, PhD
Division of Cardiology, VA Medical Center, West Los Angeles, and the Department of Medicine, and the UCLA School of Medicine, Los Angeles, California

Harry A. Fozzard, MD
Departments of Pharmacological and Physiological Sciences and Medicine, and the Committee on Cell Physiology, Department of Pharmacological and Physiological Sciences, The University of Chicago, Chicago, Illinois

J. Kenneth Gibson, PhD
The Upjohn Company, Kalamazoo, Michigan

Robert F. Gilmour, Jr., PhD
Department of Physiology, College of Veterinary Medicine, Cornell University, Ithaca, New York

William B. Gough, PhD
ANAQUEST, Murray Hill, New Jersey

Wolfram Grimm, MD
Department of Cardiology, Phillipps-Universitat, Marburg, Germany

Keitaro Hashimoto, MD
Department of Phamacology, Yamanashi Medical College, Yamanashi, Japan

Peter H. Held, MD, PhD
University of Göteborg, Department of Medicine, Section of Cardiology, Östra Hospital, Göteborg, Sweden

Bruce C. Hill, PhD
Research Institute, Palo Alto Medical Foundation, Palo Alto, California

Masayasu Hiraoka, MD, PhD
Department of Cardiovascular Diseases, Medical Research Institute, Tokyo Medical and Dental University, Tokyo, Japan

Joseph R. Hume, PhD
Department of Physicology, University of Nevada School of Medicine, Reno, Nevada

Jose Jalife, MD
Department of Pharmacology, SUNY Health Science Center at Syracuse, Syracuse, New York

Michiel J. Janse, MD
Department of Physiology, University of Limburg, Maastricht, and the Department of Clinical and Experimental Cardiology, University of Amsterdam, and the Interuniversity Cardiology Institute, The Netherlands

Mark E. Josephson, MD
Department of Medicine, Harvard Medical School, Harvard-Thorndike Electrophysiology Institute and Arrhythmia Service, Cardiovascular Division, Beth Israel Hospital, Boston, Massachusetts

Kaichiro Kamiya, MD
Department of Circulation, Research Institute of Environmental Medicine, Nagoya University, Nayoya City, Japan

Laurence S. Klein, MD
Indiana University School of Medicine, Indianapolis, Indiana

Itsuo Kodama, MD
Department of Circulation, Research Institute of Environmental Medicine, Nagoya University, Nayoya City, Japan

Michel Laville
Department de Biologie, Rhone Poulenc Rorer, Vitry-sur-Seine, France

Ralph Lazzara, MD
University of Oklahoma Health Sciences Center, Department of Medicine, Cardiovascular Section, *and* Veterans Administration Medical Center, Oklahoma City, Oklahoma

Sylvain Le Guern
Department de Biologie, Rhone Poulenc Rorer, Vitry-sur-Seine, France

Kai S. Lee, PhD
The Upjohn Company, Kalamazoo, Michigan

Paul C. Levesque, PhD
Department of Physiology, University of Nevada School of Medicine, Reno, Nevada

Benedict R. Lucchesi, PhD, MD
Department of Pharmacology, University of Michigan Medical School, Department of Pharmacology, Ann Arbor, Michigan

Jonathan C. Makielski, MD
Department of Medicine, Section of Cardiology, Department of Medicine, The University of Chicago Medical Center, Chicago, Illinois

Gabriella Malfatto, MD
Departimento di Medicina Interna, Universite di Pavia, Milan, Italy

William M. Miles, MD
Department of Medicine and Cardiology, Indiana University School of Medicine, Indianapolis, Indiana

Issam F. Moubarak, PhD
Division of Cardiovascular and Metabolic Disorders, Wyeth-Ayerst Research Laboratories, Princeton, New Jersey

Carlo Napolitano, MD
Centro di Fisiolgia Clinica e Ipertensione, Istito di Clinica Medica II, University of Milan, Milan, Italy

Stanley Nattel, MD
Montreal Heart Institute and McGill University, Montreal, Quebec

Junichi Nitta
Department of Cardiovascular Diseases, Medical Research Institute, Tokyo Medical and Dental University and Tsukuba Research Laboratories, Eisai Company, Ltd., Tokyo, Japan

Denis Noble, FRS, Hon MRCP
University of Oxford, University Laboratory of Physiology, Oxford, United Kingdom

Roderick W. Parsons, PhD
Division of Cardiovascular and Metabolic Disorders, Wyeth-Ayerst Research Laboratories, Princeton, New Jersey

Laurent Pradier
Department de Biologie, Rhone Poulenc Rorer, Vitry-sur-Seine, France

Silvia G. Priori, MD
Centro di Fisiolgia Clinica e Ipertensione, Istito di Clinica Medica II, University of Milan, Milan, Italy

H. S. Rasmussen, MD, PhD
Pfizer Central Research, Department of Clinical Research, Sandwich, Kent, United Kingdom

Flavia Ravelli, PhD
IRST, Trento, Via della Cascat, Povo, Italy

Mark Restivo, PhD
Assistant Professor of Medicine, State University of New York Health Science Center, and Senior Research Engineer, Veterans Administration Medical Centers, Brooklyn, New York

Dan M. Roden, MD
Professor of Medicine and Pharmacology, Director, Division of Clinical Pharmacology, Vanderbilt University, School of Medicine, Nashville, Tennessee

Michael R. Rosen, MD
Gustavus A. Pfeiffer Professor of Pharmacology, Professor of Pediatrics, Department of Pharmacology, College of Physicians and Surgeons of Columbia University, New York, New York

Philip T. Sager, MD
Department of Cardiology, Veterans Affairs Medical Center, West Los Angeles, Los Angeles, California, UCLA School of Medicine

Jonnalagedda S. M. Sarma, PhD
Division of Cardiology, Veterans Affairs Medical Center of West Los Angeles and City of Hope National Medical Center, Duarte, and the Department of Medicine, UCLA School of Medicine, Los Angeles, California

Kohei Sawada, PhD
Department of Cardiovascular Diseases, Medical Research Institute, Tokyo Medical and Dental University, Cardiovascular Research Section, and Tsukuba Research Laboratories, Eisai Company, Ltd., Tokyo, Japan

Melvin M. Scheinman, MD
Division of Electrophysiology and Electrocardiography, Department of Medicine and the Cardiovascular Research Institute, University of California, San Francisco, California

Peter J. Schwartz, MD
Department de Medicina Interna, Universita de Pavia and Istituto di Clinica Medica II, Universita di Milano, Milan, Italy

Bramah N. Singh, MD, DPhil, FRCP
Cardiology Section, VA Medical Center, West Los Angeles, and Professor of Medicine, UCLA School of Medicine, Los Angeles, California

Madison S. Spach, MD
Department of Pediatrics and Cell Biology, Duke University Medical Center, Durham, North Carolina

Walter Spinelli, PhD
Division of Cardiovascular and Metabolic Disorders, Wyeth-Ayerst Research Laboratories, Princeton, New Jersey

William G. Stevenson, MD
Division of Cardiology, UCLA School of Medicine, UCLA Medical Center, Los Angeles, California

Rachel A. J. Summers
Palo Alto Medical Foundation, Palo Alto, California

Koon K. Teo, MBBCh, PhD, FRCPC
Division of Cardiology, University of Alberta, Edmonton, Alberta, Canada

Junji Toyama, MD
Department of Circulation, Research Institute of Environmental Medicine, Nagoya University, Nayoya City, Japan

Andrew C. G. Uprichard, MD, MRCP
Cardiovascular Clinical Therapeutics, Parke-Davis Pharmaceutical Research Division, Warner-Lambert Company, Ann Arbor, Michigan

James T. VanderLugt, MD
The Upjohn Company, Kalamazoo, Michigan

Richard L. Verrier, PhD
Department of Pharmacology, Department of Pharmacology, Georgetown University School of Medicine, Washington, DC

Raymond L. Woosley, MD, PhD
Departments of Pharmacology and Medicine, Georgetown University Medical Center, Georgetown, Georgetown University School of Medicine, Washington, DC

Jianyi Wu, MD
Research Cardiovascular Division, Department of Medicine, Department of Molecular Biology and Pharmacology, Washington University School of Medicine, St. Louis, Missouri

Salim Yusuf, MBBS, FRCP, DPhil
Hamilton General Hospital, McMaster Clinic, Hamilton, Ontario, Canada

Sergey D. Zakharov, PhD
National Cardiology Research Center, Moscow, Russia

Antonio Zaza, MD
Universita di Milano, Dipartimento de Fisiolgia e Biochimica Generali, Milan, Italy

Zhi-hao Zhang, BBmed, Eng
Division of Cardiology and the Department of Medicine, and VA Medical Center, West Los Angeles, Los Angeles, California

Wu Zhenjiu, MD
Department of Pharmacology, Yamanashi Medical College, Yamanashi, Japan

Douglas P. Zipes, MD
Krannert Institute of Cardiology, Department of Medicine, Indiana University School of Medicine, and the Roudebush Veterans Administration Medical Center, Indianapolis, Indiana

Preface

The control of cardiac arrhythmias for the relief of symptoms, for an improvement in the quality of life, and for prolonged survival is a major component of contemporary cardiology. There have been striking changes in the field in the last decade. Some of these, in particular the development of implantable devices for arrhythmia termination and electrode catheter ablation of supraventricular arrhythmias, have been revolutionary. The changes that are occurring in drug therapy, which still remains the mainstay of arrhythmia treatment, are not only somewhat dramatic but also unsettling. The potential repercussions on clinical practice could be profound. The changes go against views and practices deeply entrenched for decades. There appears to be a need for the evolution of a newer perspective.

This comprehensive monograph compiles information from a variety of sources including clinicians and scientists engaged in bringing about changes in the manner in which arrhythmias should be treated on a rational basis. The material is presented in relation to the current ideas of cardiac electrophysiology, mechanisms of cardiac arrhythmias, how antiarrhythmic drugs work, and how their actions are modulated by the autonomic nervous system. The data from experimental and clinical studies, controlled clinical studies, and meta-analyses of randomized clinical trials are presented. The crucial significance of CAST and other trials that indicate the potential of sodium channel blockers to augment mortality in the course of treatment of cardiac arrhythmias have been given appropriate emphasis. The intent has been to indicate that it might be timely to shift to agents that fundamentally act by prolonging repolarization, especially to those that have the added property of autonomic modulation.

While the main focus of this book has been on the control of arrhythmias by drug therapy, several chapters on nonpharmacological approaches to rhythm control are included to indicate the growing importance of invasive modalities and their conjunctive use with antiarrhythmic agents. Thus, the monograph will be of interest to all physicians interested in caring for patients with rhythm disorders and experimental and clinical scientists who are involved in the development of safer and more effective antiarrhythmic and antifibrillatory compounds.

Bramah N. Singh
Hein J. J. Wellens
Masayasu Hiraoka

Guest Preface

Drugs have been, are, and will be the mainstay of antiarrhythmic management for the vast majority of patients troubled by cardiac arrhythmias, despite the popularity of nonpharmacological choices. Drugs are easier to use than radiofrequency catheter ablation or implantable cardioverter/defibrillators, are available to primary care physicians who treat most of the patients with arrhythmias, are easily started and stopped if necessary, and are cheaper initially than many other forms of treatment. Naturally, they do not eliminate the arrhythmia as ablation does, or reliably reduce the incidence of sudden cardiac death, as cardioverter/defibrillators do, and may be more expensive in the long run than either of these therapies if the arrhythmia is incompletely controlled or even exacerbated by the drug, requiring the patient to have repeated emergency room visits and hospitalizations.

Electropharmacological control of cardiac arrhythmias is an area of expertise required of every primary care specialist, internist, cardiologist, and of course, electrophysiologist. How to administer drugs knowledgeably, effective, and safely is the subject of this book. Since the chapters in the book are written for all of these doctors, whose level of expertise is wide-ranging, topics covered are also wide ranging. The book begins with five superb chapters on electrophysiological principles that are sure to appeal to the electrophysiologist. These chapters address the ionic basis of the heartbeat, excitability, conduction, and refractoriness, and how some of these properties are affected by drugs. Then come a wonderful series (even if I wrote one of them myself!) of nine chapters that addresses mechanism of a variety of arrhythmias, both in animal models and in humans. These chapters are certain to be of interest to the more clinically inclined who still like to keep abreast of basic mechanisms.

Next, we come to pharmacological considerations, an excellent discussion of antiarrhythmic drugs actions that includes sodium, potassium, and calcium channel blocking drugs, β adrenoceptor blockers, and Class III agents. This section also has chapters on drug action on atrial and ventricular arrhythmias, as well as proarrhythmic responses, and serves as a perfect lead in to five well-structured chapters on clinical therapeutics. These chapters deal with the use of programmed electrophysiological testing versus electrocardiographic monitoring to guide therapy, the significance of CAST, and summarize the impact of various drug treatments on mortality from cardiac arrhythmias. Finally, we have a very thorough discussion of controlling cardiac arrhythmias by prolonging ventricular repolarization with drugs such as sotalol and amiodarone. These drugs may exert unique antifibrillatory actions that improve survival in patients at risk for sudden cardiac death.

What's new on the horizon? The remaining chapters summarize new drugs coming down the "pipeline", put into perspective the nonpharmacological choices of surgery, catheter ablation, and implantable defibrillators, and finish with a look into the pharmacological crystal ball that considers the profibrillatory class action of sodium channel blockers, drug-specific versus technique-specific responses in the prediction of long-term therapy, and the need for a new conceptual model to determine pharmacological approaches for controlling ventricular arrhythmias.

Despite the advances summarized in these chapters, there are still major challenges for the basic scientist and the clinician. Many of the supraventricular and some of the ventricular tachycardias have fallen to the ablationists' catheter. Nothing beats a cure, sending the patient home *sans* tachycardia, drugs, and the need for a doctor. However, serious ventricular arrhythmias, especially those associated with coronary artery disease, continue to exert their horrendous toll in morbidity and mortality. And atrial fibrillation, an arrhythmia known since the birth of electrocardiography and considered to be fairly benign, has recently be recognized as a major cause of stroke and other forms of disability. While it may not kill as readily as ventricular tachycardia, it is a very troublesome arrhythmia to the patient and his physician. Conquering these two culprits represent the challenge of the next decade.

In summary, this is a super book, a sort of all-you-need-to-know about antiarrhythmic drugs and their use. It's for the basic scientist and the clinician, the former to understand how drugs work and the latter to learn how to use them safely and effectively . . . a partnership contributing to the benefit of patient care. I hope you enjoy reading this herculean effort.

Douglas P. Zipes, MD
Indianapolis, Indiana

Contents

Part 1. Electrophysiological Considerations

Part 2. Mechanism of Cardiac Arrhythmias

Part 3. Pharmacological Considerations

Part 7. Nonpharmacological Approaches to Cardiac Arrhythmias

Part 8. Future Perspectives

PART I

Electrophysiological Considerations

Chapter 1

The Ionic Basis of the Heartbeat and of Cardiac Arrhythmias

Denis Noble

The rhythm of the heart is generated by membrane proteins that control the flow of charged ions (principally sodium, potassium, calcium, and chloride) across the cell membrane. Some of these proteins act as voltage-sensitive gates that open channels that carry ions passively down their electrochemical gradients. Some are voltage-insensitive channels that generate a background (resting) level of membrane current. Others are highly specific co- or countertransporters that either use the energy of one gradient to move another ion against its gradient or that use the breakdown of adenosine triphosphate (ATP) to drive such a pumping action.

The first goal of this chapter is to show how the great wealth of information on these ionic channels and carrier mechanisms obtained since the introduction of the methods of isolated cells, patch clamping, and internal ion indicators has been incorporated into very detailed models of cardiac excitation and rhythm generation. The second goal is to use these models to reconstruct some of the cellu-

lar mechanisms of cardiac arrhythmias. Attention will also be called to several new approaches to drug therapy suggested by this work. (There is not space enough here to give the full experimental basis for the models described and used. For that, the reader is referred to the original papers listed at the end of the chapter.)

Ionic Mechanisms in the Normal Heartbeat

Figure 1 shows the general features of cardiac cells. In addition to the voltage-gated ionic channels used in older models of cardiac excitation, the new models also incorporate the activity of ionic pumps, and take into account internal and external ion concentration changes, including the mechanisms of buffering, sequestration, and release of calcium ions. Some of the models also include activation of contraction. The representation of ion concentration changes, particularly of internal

The original work reported in this chapter was supported by the British Heart Foundation and the Medical Research Council.
Note: All the cellular cardiac models described here are available in the OXSOFT HEART program. Information on the availability of this program in various parts of the world can be obtained from Oxsoft Ltd, 49 Old Road, Oxford OX3 7JZ, UK.

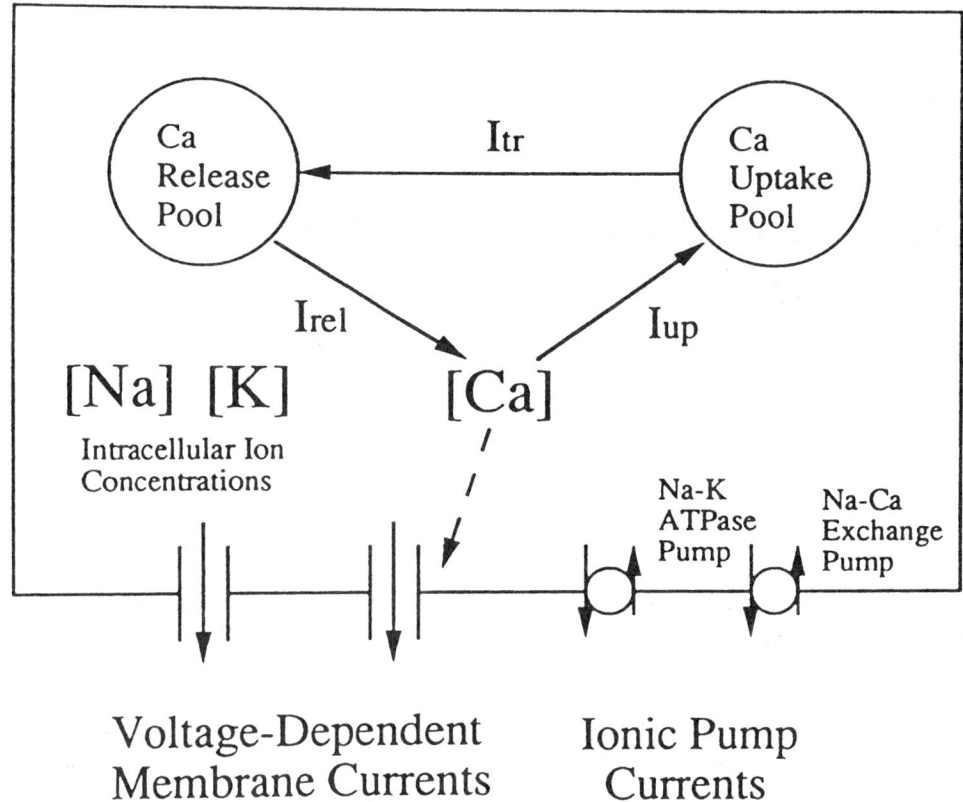

Figure 1. Generic type of cardiac cell model described in this chapter. In addition to voltage-dependent membrane currents (represented in previous models based on the Hodgin–Huxley-type of model), the models described also incorporate ionic pump and exchange currents, the variations of internal and external ion concentrations, the sequestration and buffering of internal calcium, the calcium release mechanism and, in some cases, contraction.

calcium and sodium and external potassium, and the possibility of feedback from the processes determining contraction to those determining excitation are of crucial importance in allowing this new generation of cardiac models to succeed in reconstructing many forms of cardiac arrhythmia.

The first pacemaker mechanism in the heart to be analyzed quantitatively was that of the Purkinje fiber conducting network. The analysis of this mechanism also illustrates some of the major changes in interpretation of cardiac ionic mechanisms that have occurred since 1980 (for a full review see Noble[1]). There are at least three major steps in this reinterpretation.

The first was the demonstration that sur-face membrane ionic currents depend strongly on intracellular processes, such as the calcium transient. The beginning of this understanding came from the important work of Lederer and Tsien[2] on the arrhythmogenic transient inward current (i_{TI}) that was shown to be activated by internal calcium changes rather than generating these changes. Later work showed that activation of inward current by calcium transients also occurs during normal beating as well as during arrhythmogenic conditions.[3] Therefore, there is feedback between the inotropic state of cardiac muscle and its excitation, which may produce stretch- or deformation-induced arrhythmias.[4–6]

Also relevant to work on arrhythmias was the demonstration that potassium channels exist in heart cells that open in response to low levels of intracellular ATP.[7] This mechanism is obviously important in ischemic conditions and, by greatly shortening the action potential duration, may be responsible for reentrant arrhythmias. Nichols and Lederer[8] have recently reconstructed this effect on the action potential.

The second major reinterpretation was the discovery that the pacemaker current in Purkinje fibers is an inward current, i_f, activated by hyperpolarization rather than an outward current activated by depolarization.[9,10] Therefore, this current directly generates the pacemaker depolarization. Previous models[11] relied entirely on decay of a potassium conductance unmasking a background inward current, $i_{b,Na}$. The identification of i_f was the basis of the Purkinje fiber model developed by DiFrancesco and Noble in 1985.[12] This model, illustrated in Figure 2, is the generic model from which those for other regions of the heart have subsequently been developed.

The third major advance underpinning these models is the discovery that a functionally important part of the slower phase of inward current in cardiac cells is attributable to calcium exit via sodium-calcium (Na-Ca) exchange, rather than to calcium entry via calcium channels. This idea, first proposed by Mullins,[13,14] has fundamentally changed our understanding of calcium balance in heart cells, which in mammalian cells is now known to be achieved almost entirely during the action potential itself with a phase of calcium efflux via Na-Ca exchange following and balancing a phase of calcium entry via calcium channels. This idea was incorporated into the DiFrancesco-Noble[12] model as a natural consequence of making the Na-Ca exchange electrogenic (DiFrancesco and Noble[12] found that a neutral exchange did not enable their model to achieve calcium balance). But the fullest expression of the idea occurred in the development of an atrial model[15] designed to reconstruct net calcium fluxes as revealed by measurements of fast extracellular calcium transients.[16]

As shown in Figure 3, this model succeeded in accurately reconstructing the calcium fluxes, and it did this by attributing the late plateau of the action potential entirely to inward current generated by calcium efflux through the exchange. Mitchell and colleagues[17,18] have already demonstrated experimentally that the late low plateau in the similarly shaped rat ventricular action potential is maintained by Na-Ca exchange. More recently, Earm, Ho, and So[19] have provided convincing experimental evidence in rabbit atrial cells.

The shape of the rat atrial and ventricular cell action potentials lends itself very easily to an analysis of this kind since the two phases of repolarization (rapid followed by slow) correspond neatly to the periods in which first the calcium current and then the Na-Ca exchange generate the major component of inward current. This neat separation cannot, however, be applied to the repolarization process of most ventricular cells, where the slow initial repolarization produces a high-level plateau that effectively masks the transition from net calcium entry to net calcium exit. It is then impossible to deduce when the transition occurs from the action potential alone.

There are two reasons why this 'masking' of the transition point is so effective. The first is that the high plateau voltage itself tends to switch off Na-Ca exchange or even reverse its direction since this process is highly voltage dependent and its reversal potential, for normal ion concentrations and internal calcium transients, is close to the plateau level. The exchange is therefore activated gradually, and may even change direction more than once, as repolarization slowly proceeds. A simple voltage time course, combined with a rapidly changing level of internal calcium may conceal a very complex time course for Na-Ca exchange. This is quite unlike the atrial action potential, where the inward exchange current is activated within 20–30 msec and rapidly reaches its peak at the beginning of the slow plateau.

The second reason is that it is possible to show, using the ventricular cell models that have now been constructed, that very similar

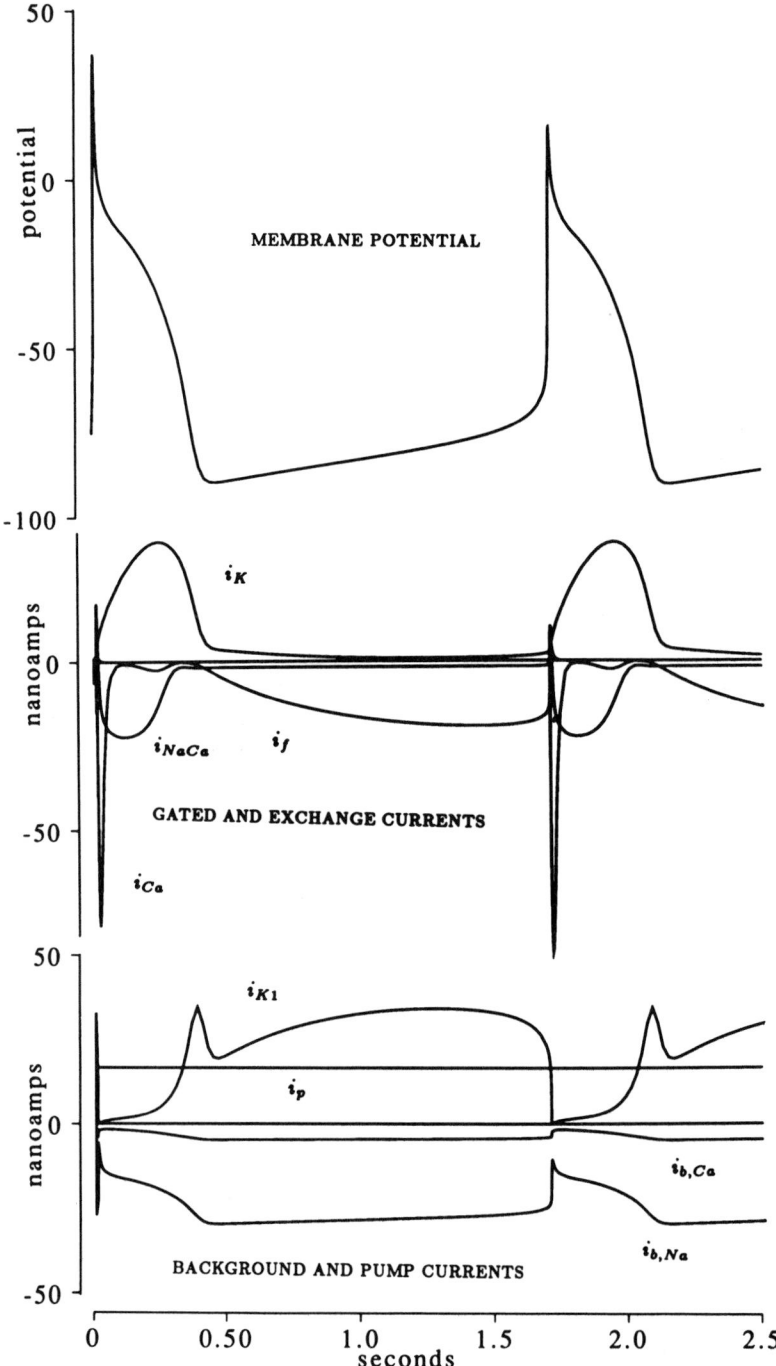

Figure 2. The Purkinje fiber model described by DiFrancesco and Noble.[12] Top: Variation in computed membrane potential showing the characteristic long plateau and the slow pacemaker depolarization. Middle: Computed variations in potassium and calcium channel currents, and in the pacemaker current, i_f, and the Na-Ca exchange current, i_{NaCa}. Bottom: Computed variations in sodium pump current, i_p, inward rectifier current, i_{K1} and the background currents, $i_{b,Na}$ and $i_{b,Ca}$.

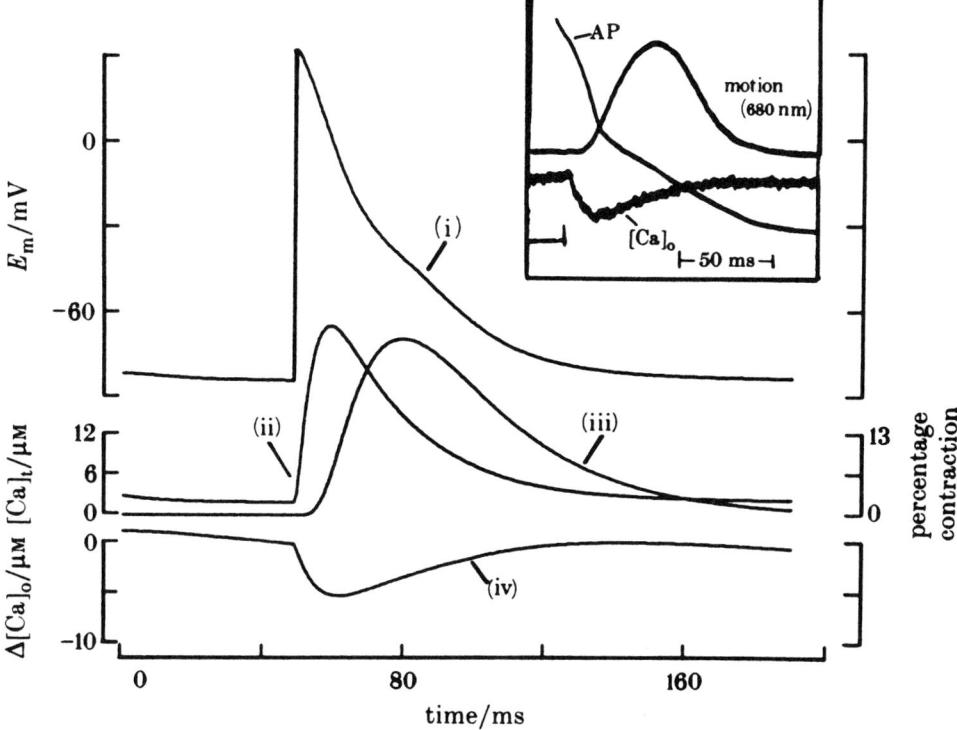

Figure 3. The rabbit atrial action potential model described by Hilgemann and Noble.[15] The main panel shows the computed action potential together with intracellular calcium (ii), contraction (iii), and extracellular calcium (iv). The top right panel shows experimental recordings of the action potential, contraction, and extracellular calcium. All three of these variables are closely reproduced by the model.

action potential shapes can be maintained either by very slow calcium current inactivation (which was the basis of the Beeler-Reuter[20] model) or by rapid calcium current inactivation followed by substantial flow of inward Na-Ca exchange current. The first type of action potential will occur in conditions where calcium release is small, so that very little activation of Na-Ca exchange current occurs and calcium-induced inactivation of the calcium current is minimized. The second type of response will occur when calcium release is very large, so that calcium current inactivation is speeded up and a large degree of activation of exchange current occurs. This fact also accounts for the otherwise puzzling observation that internal calcium buffering using patch electrodes allows perfectly normal-shaped ac-

tion potentials to occur despite the fact that the normal mechanisms achieving calcium balance on a beat-to-beat basis have been suppressed.

It has therefore been considerably more difficult to analyze the ionic currents during the typical and apparently much simpler, ventricular action potential and we must now view the situation as a dynamic one that depends as much on the inotropic state as on the identification of particular ionic current mechanisms.

Egan and co-workers[21] overcame some of these difficulties by using an interruption switch method to determine the activation of Na-Ca exchange current at different times during the ventricular action potential in guinea pigs. This data was used to develop the ven-

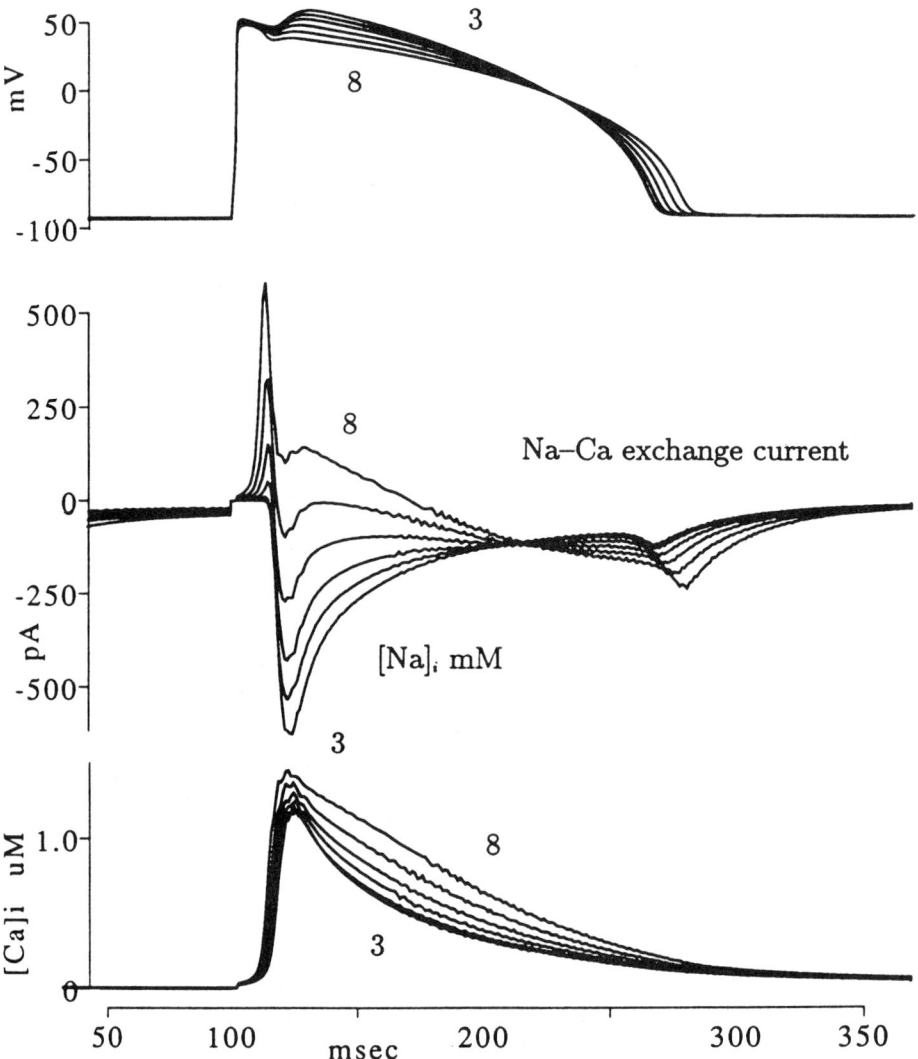

Figure 4. The guinea pig ventricular cell model described by Noble et al.[22] Top: Computed action potentials. Middle: Computed variations in Na-Ca exchange current at various levels of internal sodium from 3 to 8 mM. Note that the direction and amplitude of this current are both very strongly determined by internal sodium. Bottom: Computed variations in free calcium.

tricular action potential model illustrated in Figure 4.[22] In order to emphasize how the precise role of Na-Ca exchange can vary, Figure 4 shows reconstructions of exchange current for various levels of intracellular sodium. It can be seen that the shape, amplitude, and direction of the computed exchange current all vary markedly as sodium is varied from 3 mM (its lowest recorded value) to 8 mM (which is at the upper end of 'normal' recorded values for [Na]$_i$).

While this result is disappointing, inasmuch as it prevents us using the action potential shape to say very much about the exchange current, it is also functionally important since it shows that the Na-Ca exchanger has exactly the properties required to act as a very fine regulator of its own activity and to restore calcium balance following even very strong perturbations. Thus, high internal sodium will favor calcium entry and sodium extrusion, which will eventually enhance the internal calcium transient by loading the sarcoplasmic reticulum with calcium. The increased calcium transient will in turn eventually cause the exchange to pump calcium out, restoring calcium balance. Similarly, low internal sodium will favor calcium extrusion that will reduce the calcium transient progressively reducing the extrusion of calcium until once again, at a much lower inotropic level, calcium balance will occur. The possible significance of this self-regulation for new approaches to drug therapy will be discussed.

Although the pacemaker mechanism in Purkinje fibers was the first to be fully analyzed and reconstructed, the natural cardiac pacemaker is, of course, the sinoatrial node. The cells in this region are very small and it has taken longer to obtain reliable patch clamp information on their ionic mechanisms. Moreover, these differ very strikingly from those in other regions of the heart. For example, the sodium current plays a much smaller role. The sinus node continues to beat when g_{Na} is blocked by tetrodotoxin. The inward rectifier current, i_{K1} is also relatively weak in these cells, particularly at the center of the node, although there is significant contribution both from i_{K1} and from i_{Na} in peripheral cells.[23,24] The main ionic currents involved in rhythm generation in the natural pacemaker are therefore i_{Ca}, i_K, i_f, and $i_{b,Na}$. Figure 5 shows a recent reconstruction of rabbit sinus node pacemaker activity (for a valuable recent review of the electrophysiology of the sinus node see Irisawa et al.[25]).

Although relatively few ionic current mechanisms are involved, the sinus node nevertheless possesses two rhythmic mechanisms that are sufficient in themselves to generate pacemaker activity: the g_K decay process that acts by unmasking the flow of sodium through the background current channels, and the i_f (pacemaker current) mechanism

that can generate a pacemaker depolarization directly, as it does in Purkinje fibers. The result of this combination is to create an automatic rhythm that is very resilient. Any changes that weaken the role of one mechanism automatically produce voltage changes that increase the role of the other. This is in striking contrast to the situation in Purkinje fibers, where very moderate changes in $[K]_o$, for example, suffice to totally suppress the rhythm. The sinus node rhythm is very resistant to such changes.

This fact could be of great importance when information on the structure of the i_f channel becomes available since the development of a specific i_f blocker would provide a very useful form of therapy where a moderate (20–30%) slowing of heart rate is required. In principle, such a drug would be safe since even complete block of i_f would not arrest the sinus node. The clinical reason why such a drug might be attractive, particularly in combination with other forms of therapy, is that the most effective β-blockers used in combatting ischemic heart disease appear to be those that also have a significant cardiac slowing effect.

Abnormal Ionic Mechanisms: Cellular Basis of Arrhythmias

Hypokalemia and Hyperkalemia

It has been known since the earliest work on the inward rectifier current, i_{K1} that its unusual behavior in response to external potassium changes underlies two important electrophysiological characteristics of heart muscle. The first is that the action potential in ventricular and Purkinje cells greatly shortens as $[K]_o$ is increased. This is exactly the opposite effect to that which would be expected from the change in potassium gradient. The second is that automaticity in the Purkinje conducting system greatly increases in low $[K]_o$. Both these effects are well reproduced in the Purkinje fiber model (Figure 6).

These effects undoubtedly underlie some

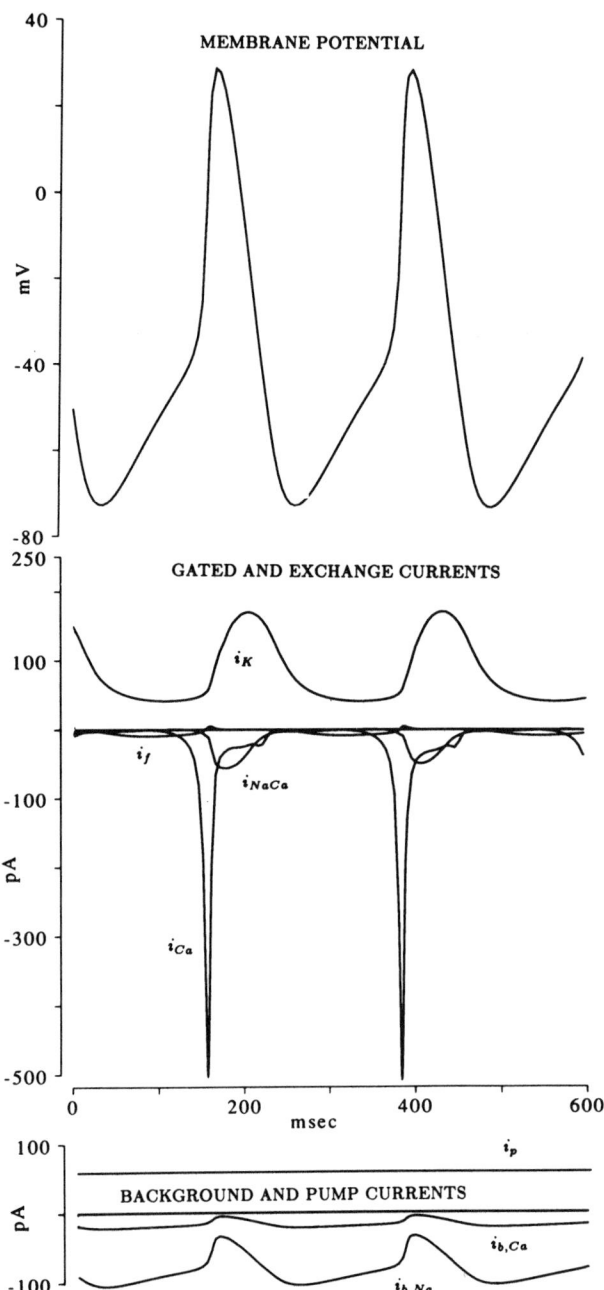

Figure 5. The single sinus node cell model described by Noble, DiFrancesco, and Denyer.[43]. Top: Computed variation in membrane potential. Middle: Computed variations in calcium, potassium and i_f channel currents, and in Na-Ca exchange current. Bottom: Computed variations in background and pump currents.

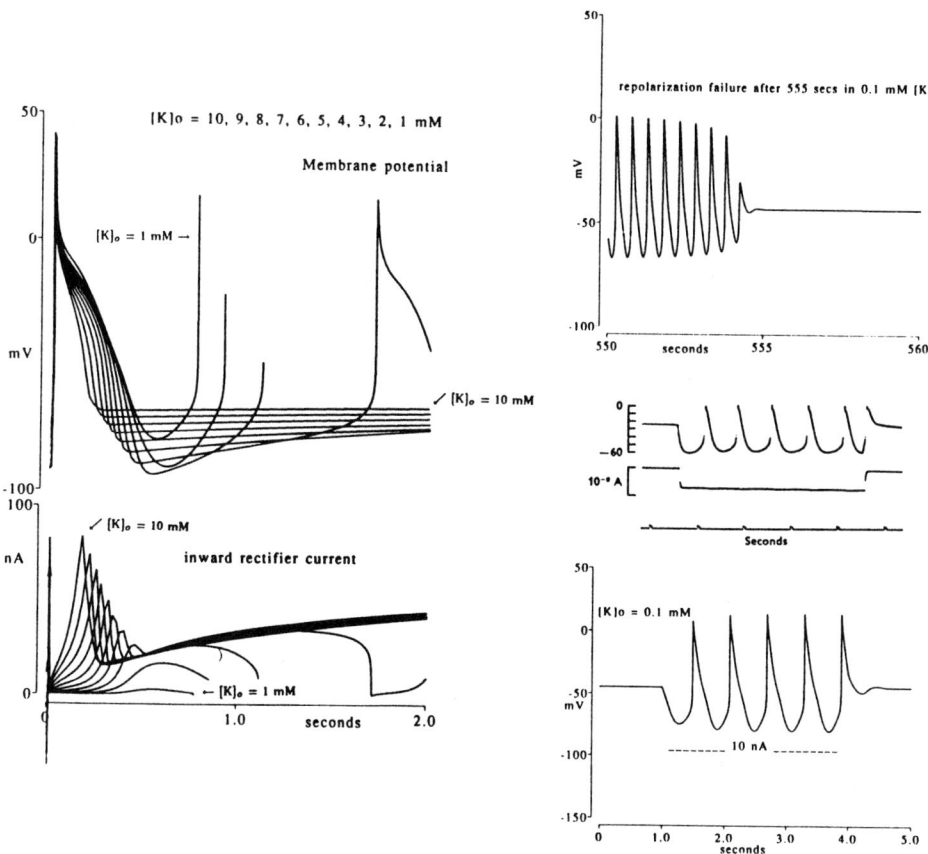

Figure 6. Left: Computed variations in membrane potential (top) and inward rectifier current (bottom) in the Purkinje fiber model at various levels of external potassium between 1 and 10 mM. Note that action potentials become longer and spontaneous activity becomes more prominent at the lower levels of [K]$_o$. Right: Result of calculation in which the Purkinje fiber model was run for hundreds of seconds with [K]$_o$ = 0.1 mM. The top record shows the sudden failure of repolarization at 554 msec. The middle record shows experimental recording of oscillatory activity induced by a small stimulus in such a depolarized Purkinje fiber. The bottom record shows a very similar response generated by the model in its "depolarized" state.

of the arrhythmic consequences of hypo- and hyperkalemia. The action potential shortening in high [K]$_o$ will favor reentrant arrhythmias by reducing the refractory period and favoring the establishment of reentrant circuits of activity. The increased automaticity at low [K]$_o$ may underlie the generation of ectopic beating in hypokalemia.

It is interesting to note that in the Di-Francesco-Noble model, repolarization succeeds even at the lowest values of [K]$_o$, whereas experimentally it is found that repolarization usually fails in Purkinje tissue at low

enough values of [K]$_o$. An explanation for this difference is that if the model behavior is examined over very long periods of time (corresponding to many minutes rather than seconds of real heart time) then failure of repolarization occurs in the model.[26] This failure is a secondary consequence of sodium pump inhibition at low values of [K]$_o$. The K$_m$ for activation of the sodium pump is approximately 1 mM, so the pump will only be half activated at this level of [K]$_o$. The right side of Figure 6 shows the results of a computation of 1,000 seconds of activity at 0.1 mM [K]$_o$. In this case, repolarization eventually fails after 550 seconds. It is in fact the case that the full effects of external potassium changes take several minutes to develop.[27]

Sodium Pump Inhibition

It is well known that pump inhibition itself, eg, in response to cardiac glycosides, is arrhythmogenic. This arrhythmic mechanism can now be totally reconstructed and represents a major achievement of integrative physiology, incorporating fundamental advances developed in many different laboratories. Some of the key advances include the original discovery of the transent inward current, i_{TI}, by Lederer and Tsien;[2] the demonstration that it is accompanied by intracellular calcium oscillations;[28] the discovery of calcium-induced release of calcium from the sarcoplasmic reticulum[29] that opened the way to understanding the nature of internal calcium oscillations as the response of a release mechanism with some degree of positive feedback at high levels of the driving variable, ie, calcium; the demonstration that Na-Ca exchange in heart cells is electrogenic and the determination of its current-voltage relation;[30] and the demonstration that the current-voltage relation of the transient inward current resembles that of Na-Ca exchange.[31] Many other steps in this work will be found in the proceedings of the first two international meetings on Na-Ca exchange.[32,33] Not all the transient inward current is attributable to Na-Ca exchange (calcium activated channels can also play a role in some circumstances), but it is clearly the major component as TI currents first develop in a ventricular or atrial cell.

Since all these experimental developments have been incorporated into computer models, it is an important check of their performance and usefulness to determine how well they reproduce the inotropic and arrhythmogenic features of cardiac glycoside action. Figure 7 shows the behavior of the atrial cell model in response to 90% inhibition of the sodium pump activity. The immediate ef-

fect is action potential prolongation as the outward pump current is suddenly reduced. Subsequently, as $[Na]_i$ increases, the action potential shortens. In the model, this is attributable to reduced inward current generated by Na-Ca exchange as the sodium gradient falls. Similar changes in duration are seen experimentally and the evidence that Na-Ca exchange is involved is good.[34] This does not, however, exclude the possibility that other mechanisms (such as sodium activated potassium channels) also play a role in these duration changes.

Subsequent to the rise in $[Na]_i$ and the consequent reduced efflux of calcium, internal calcium accumulates and more calcium is sequestered in the sarcoplasmic reticulum leading to larger releases of calcium during each beat. This is, of course, the basis of the increase in contractile response that develops over this period. Note that as in experimental work, the actual rise in basal calcium over this period of time is very small. Nearly all the increased sequestration of calcium occurs as a consequence of the fact that the balance between calcium pumping to the sarcoplasmic reticulum and surface calcium efflux via Na-Ca exchange shifts strongly toward the former as the latter weakens with the fall in sodium gradient that drives it. This is the reason that the peak inotropic effect is reached with only small changes in resting calcium (and resting contraction).

In fact, resting calcium and resting contraction only increase extensively once the peak inotropic effect has occurred. As the resting calcium then rises rapidly, the inotropic effect declines rapidly. These changes are connected, since once a certain level of resting calcium accumulation occurs, the calcium-induced calcium release process begins to operate even in the resting state. This is the point at which the process starts to become oscillatory and therefore arrhythmogenic. This is illustrated in Figure 8 (left), which shows the behavior of the atrial model at this time when the repetitive stimuli are stopped. The model generates trains of ectopic beats corresponding to each oscillation of internal calcium. The

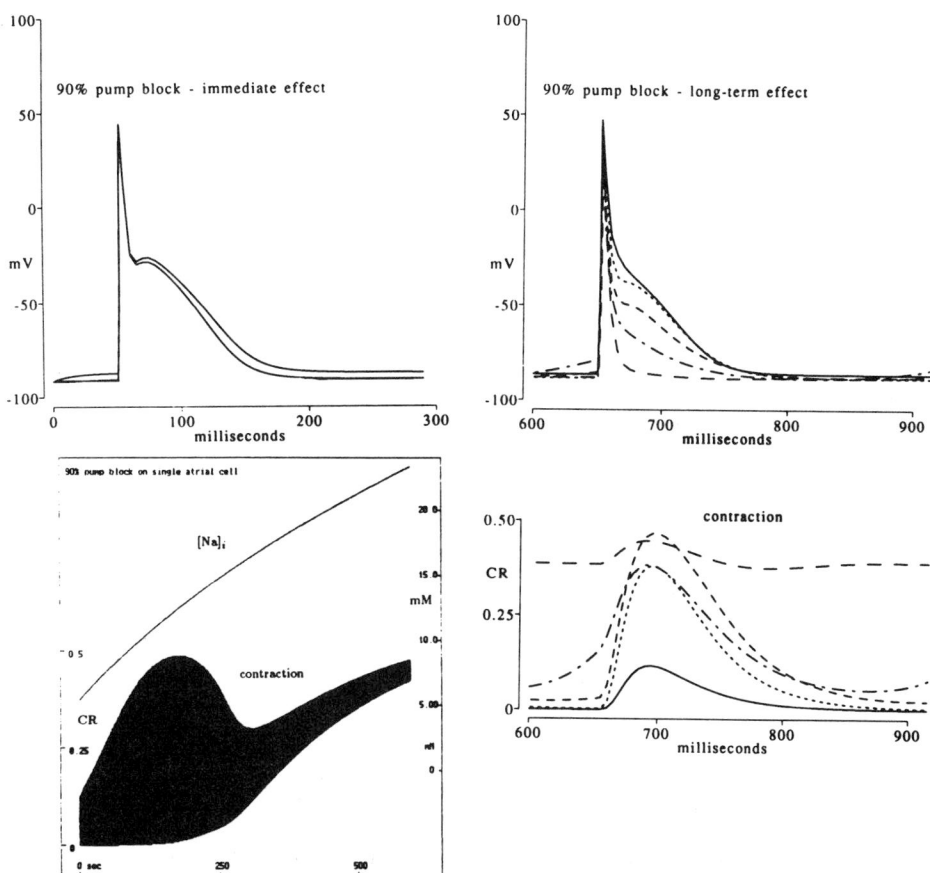

Figure 7. Reconstruction of the actions of cardiac glycosides using the Earm-Noble[44] model of the single rabbit atrial cell. Top left: Immediate effect of 90% sodium pump block is a small depolarization of the resting potential and a moderate lengthening of repolarization. Bottom left: Computed internal sodium and contractions (fraction of cross-bridge formations, CR) over a time scale of 600 seconds following 90% sodium pump block. Note the massive positive inotropic effect, which turns into a negative inotropic effect as the resting contraction starts to appear. Top right: Action potentials computed at the beginning (0 seconds, continuous line), 100 seconds (dotted line), 200 seconds (dashed line), 250 seconds (dot-dashed line), and 500 seconds (long dashed line). Bottom right: Corresponding computed contractions. Note that at 250 seconds there is oscillation of contraction (and thus of internal calcium). This is the transient inward current mechanism illustrated in later figures in this chapter. (Reproduced with permission from Reference 26.)

frequency of this beating and the form of the abnormal beat depend on the precise level of calcium reached and on the binding constant used to define the calcium induction of release (which is the actual parameter varied in Figure 8).

The right-hand side of Figure 8 shows the transient inward current oscillations, in this case generated by sodium overload of the sinus cell model—all the models generate this phenomenon because they all include the mechanisms responsible for it.

Early Afterdepolarizations

The transient inward current is a mechanism that generates what is called a *late* after-

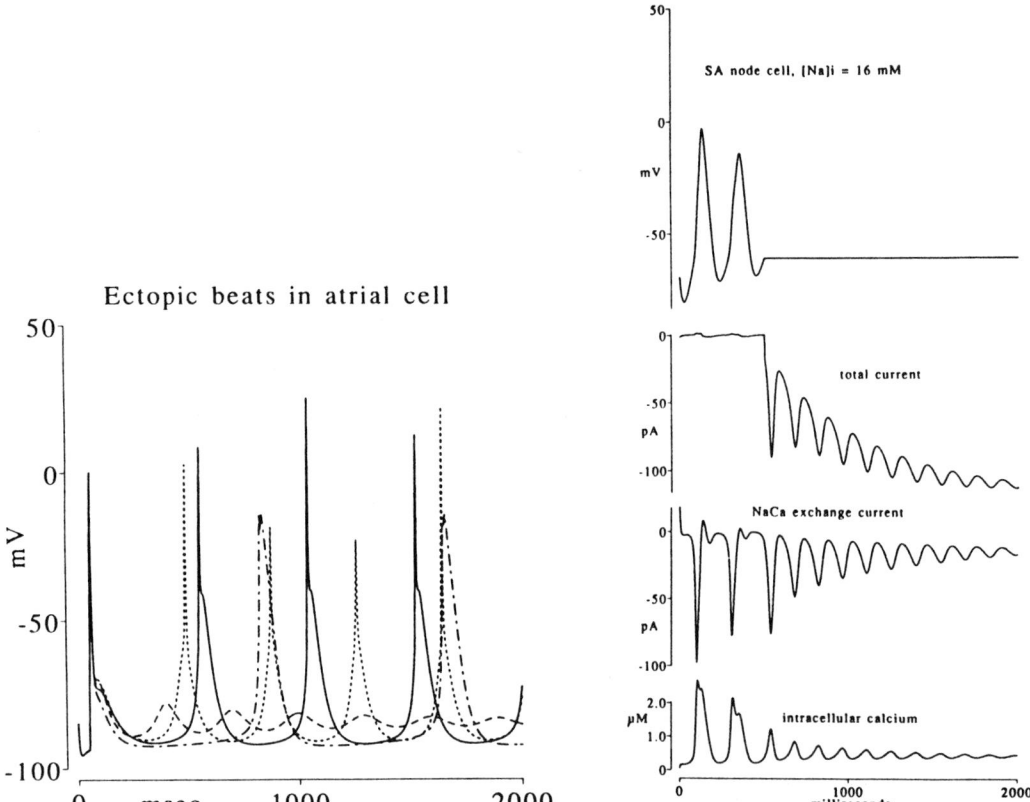

Figure 8. Left: Computed ectopic rhythmic activity in atrial cell model during calcium overload following 90% sodium pump inhibition as in Figure 7. Inhibition was maintained long enough for internal sodium to rise to 16.24 mM. This model is usually quiescent. The rhythmic activity computed here is therefore abnormal and is generated (as is the transient inward current and related ectopic beats in experimental situations) by oscillatory variations in internal calcium. The exact frequency and shape of action potential depend on the sensitivity assumed for the calcium-induced calcium release process, which is the variable that was changed between each of these computations. For the solid line a binding constant of 0.001 mM (ie, 1 μM) was assumed. The short dotted line gives the result for 0.0008 mM, the long dotted line (which shows only subthreshold oscillations after the initial beat) gives the result for 0.0006 mM, while the dot-dash line gives the result for 0.0015 mM. Right: Oscillatory transient inward currents generated in the sinus node cell model following calcium overload generated by sodium pump inhibition.

depolarization since there is a delay between the end of repolarization and the generation of the depolarization that may lead to an ectopic beat. Ectopic beats can also be generated as a consequence of *early* afterdepolarizations that occur during the repolarization phase itself.

Figure 9 shows the responses of the ventricular cell model to two types of ionic conductance change that can trigger early afterde-polarizations. The left-hand computations show the effect of varying the amplitude of the calcium channel permeability, PCa, thus mimicking the effect of calcium agonists. Initially, increase of PCa simply prolongs the action potential. At a certain level (PCa = 3 in this case) a single early afterdepolarization develops. A further increase converts this response into a high-frequency train of afterdepolarizations. The mechanism of this effect is

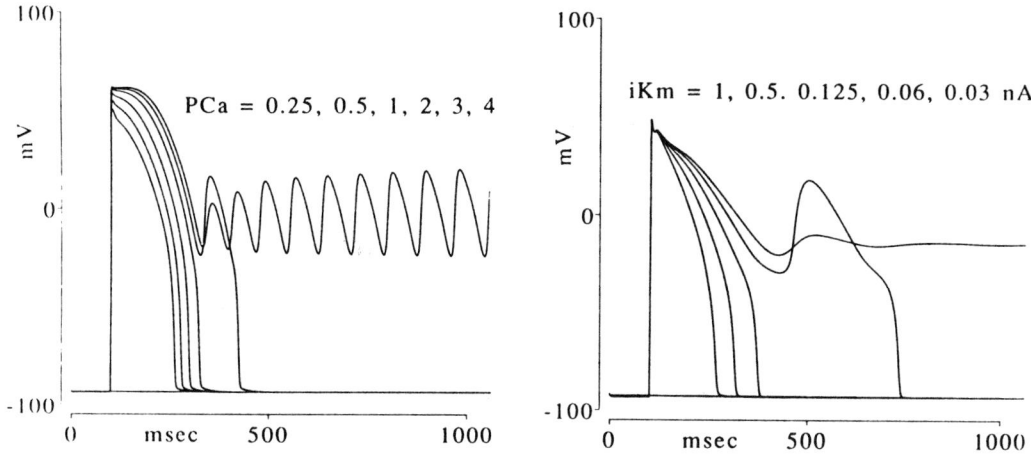

Figure 9. Left: Computed effect of increasing the calcium channel conductance on ventricular cell model. Small increases in calcium conductance simply prolong the action potential. Larger increases induce the appearance of single or multiple early afterdepolarizations. Right: Computed effect of block of delayed potassium current. The action potential is prolonged and, at nearly complete block, early afterdepolarizations or failure of repolarization occur.

that there is a range of potentials (called the calcium window) over which the activation aad inactivation curves for the calcium channel show significant overlap. As repolarization enters this range, it is a potential danger zone since calcium channels become reactivated and, if this effect is great enough, it can offset the repolarization process and reverse it. There is strong experimental evidence for this mechanism.[35] It is possible that repeated rapid reexcitation of this kind at a cellular level may contribute to rapid tachycardias such as torsades de pointes. Of course, the real situation will be much more complex than this since multicellular properties must also play a role. A later part of this chapter will indicate how these complexities are beginning to be addressed.

A similar result is obtained when repolarization is delayed by inhibition of the delayed potassium current. Figure 9 (right) shows computations done with various levels of i_K inhibition. It is interesting to note that, in this model at least, a very large degree of block (94%) is needed to induce an early afterdepolarization. Action potential prolongation using potassium channel blockers should therefore

be a relatively safe way of prolonging the refractory period.

Sodium-Calcium Exchange and Action Potential Duration

In view of the functional importance of the Na-Ca exchange reported in recent work it is natural to ask whether an alternative approach to drug therapy might be to develop agents that act on it. This is becoming possible now that the exchanger protein has been sequenced, allowing peptides with specific actions to be designed. For example, would activation or inhibition of the exchange be useful in modulating action potential duration? This question is explored in Figure 10. On the left the effects of sudden reduction in [Na]$_o$ during the computed action potential plateau are shown. The result is a very marked shortening of the action potential. This effect of sodium on the action potential has been known for a long time[36] and it has been recently observed in isolated cells subjected to sudden changes in [Na]$_o$. The effect was formerly thought to be evidence either for a role of the fast sodium current in the plateau (but in fact, TTX inhibition of g$_{Na}$ has very little action on the ventric-

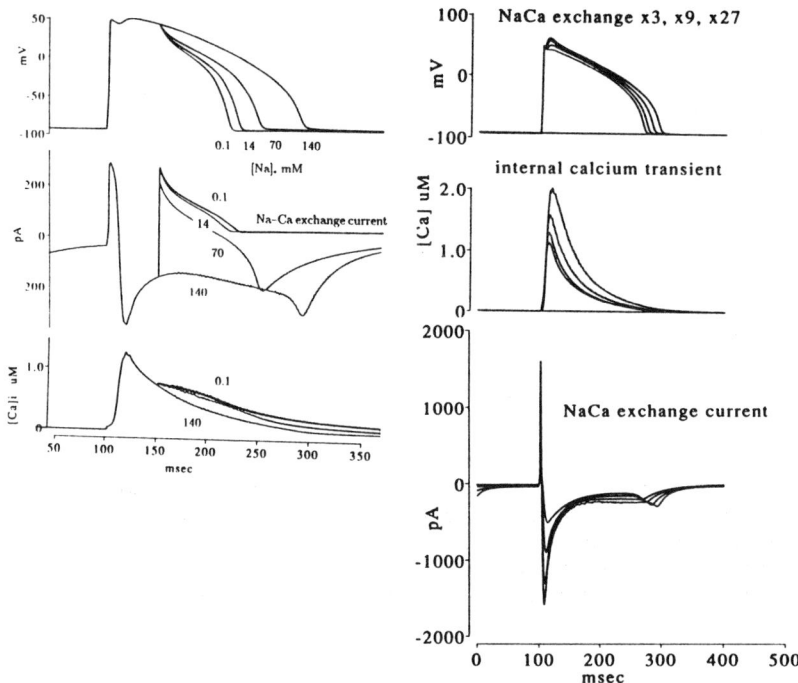

Figure 10. Left: Computed variations in action potential and Na-Ca exchange current following sudden changes in external sodium concentration during the action potential plateau. The large effect on action potential duration indicates a substantial contribution of the Na-Ca exchange current to delaying repolarization. Similar results are obtained experimentally (Bridge and Spitzer, personal communication). Right: Computed effects increasing the activity of the Na-Ca exchanger by factors of 3, 9, and 27. Despite the large immediate effects on action potential duration revealed in the computations on the left, a variation in the intrinsic level of activity of the exchanger has only a moderate net effect on action potential duration. This surprising result is attributable to a feedback mechanism, whereby variations in exchanger activity automatically change the internal calcium transient (middle computations) in a way that minimizes the net effect on exchange activity. (This computation was done with a version of the ventricular model of Noble et al.[22] that includes some compartmentation of internal calcium. A similar result is obtained with the original model. Note though that if HEART 3.5 or 3.6 is used via the screen menus, the boolean variable SPMIMIC must be switched off to obtain the original model.)

ular plateau) or for sodium transport through calcium channels.[37] In fact, it is now known that at normal calcium concentrations, sodium is excluded from the calcium channel. Therefore, it is clear that the greatest contribution of sodium to delaying repolarization in ventricular cells must be via the generation of inward current by Na-Ca exchange.

Could we therefore achieve a therapeutic effect with a specific Na-Ca exchange agonist? This question is explored on the right-hand side of Figure 10, where the effect of increas-

ing the activity of the exchange process is computed. The result is surprising. Only very moderate changes in action potential duration are predicted, even after massive changes in activity. Two questions arise. The first is how these results can possibly be consistent with those shown on the left-hand side of the figure. How can the exchange at one and the same time contribute so markedly to delaying repolarization and yet its overall activity should have such a small net effect on action potential duration?

The answer to this question lies in the timing of the activation or inhibition. The dramatic result of Figure 10 (left) is obtained by changing the activity of the exchange process after the calcium release has occurred, whereas the results on the right were obtained by altering the activity of the exchange throughout the action potential. This allows the activity of the exchange itself to influence the calcium transient that generates it, as is clear in the central panel of the figure, where the calcium transient becomes smaller as the exchange activity is increased. Moreover, since the exchange is the main process by which calcium balance is restored during each beat, this influence is very large. Recent experiments using combined recording of internal calcium and Na-Ca current show how strongly the exchange influences $[Ca]_i$.[38]

The result is a self-regulation of the exchange activity. If the exchange activity is enhanced, the internal calcium transient will be reduced, thus reducing the normal activator of the exchange. As the computations show, this effect could be large enough to nearly nullify the original intrinsic activation. An exchange agonist would therefore be expected to have a strong negative inotropic action.

The second question is whether this self-regulation means that an otherwise promising line of possible drug therapy relying on action potential duration changes is doomed to failure. Clearly, it is of great importance to check the predictions of Figure 10 experimentally. A model, after all, is only a model until it has an experimental back-up. All the other model results presented in this chapter do have extensive experimental back-up.

Assuming, however, that the prediction is correct, does this necessarily close this line of approach? The answer to this question depends on how effective it might be to use a combination of drug therapy. Conceivably, a combination of activation of the exchange, together with a positive inotropic drug to counter the negative inotropic action of an exchange agonist, might be effective since it ought then to be effective in prolonging action potential duration.

This is all very speculative, since the object is to ask fundamental questions about possible new directions in arrhythmia therapy given the spectacular failure of much of existing therapy. It does also, as an example, serve to stress another point. That is it may in any case be inappropriate to look for highly specific agents with only one class of action. Some of the best drugs currently available, after all, have several classes of action, and this may be their strength.

Multicellular Mechanisms

The heart is a connected network in which cellular interaction occurs not only with near neighbors, but also across the whole tissue.[39,40] It is therefore important not only to construct models of the individual cells in different regions of the heart, but also to incorporate these into massive network models. Until recently, such work was seriously inhibited by the computing power required. Thus, with the cellular models described above, with up to 30 simultaneous nonlinear differential equations to solve, several minutes are required to compute a few seconds of activity even on some of the fastest IBM machines. The computing time required for networks of anything more than a few cells then becomes prohibitive. Yet there are over 100,000 cells in the sinus node, several million in the atrium, and hundreds of millions in the ventricle. Of course, it may not be necessary to model on such a grand scale with the unit of modeling being a single cell. But it will certainly be necessary to model with at least tens of thousands of units, and preferably millions, if the multicellular mechanisms of arrhythmia and fibrillation are to be effectively addressed.

The requisite computing power is provided by the new generation of supercomputers, and very particularly by massively parallel computers. These are machines with up to tens of thousands of processors. An example is the Connection Machine® produced by Thinking Machines (Thinking Machines Corporation, Cambridge, MA). The first computations using cardiac cells to form networks using such a machine have now been done[41,42] and they are very encouraging. The work so far incorporates the models of the single rabbit sinus node cell and the atrial cell model into large-scale network models. These models are represented as N × N meshes with neighboring cells electrically coupled by resistors representing gap junctions. Regional variation of intrinsic cell properties (as seen in central, transitional, and peripheral cells) such as frequency, amplitudes of action potentials and maximum diastolic potentials, upstroke velocity, and sensitivity to external $[K^+]$ is included by adjusting the cell models to fit the data of Kodama and Boyett.[23] This information was obtained by segmenting a strip of the rabbit sinoatrial node running from its center to its periphery and then recording the electrophysiological characteristics in each isolated segment. By fine tuning the calcium and potassium conductances it is possible to reproduce Kodama and Boyett's data fairly accurately.

The first question was designed to determine the degree of cell-to-cell connection required to enable the sinus node to act as a synchronous unit and to send a coordinated signal to the atrium. To achieve this, 128 × 128 sinus cells were organized into a network on the Connection Machine assuming random distribution of intrinsic properties. The nexus conductance between cells was then progressively increased from 2 channels to 2,000 channels (of 50 pS each) between cell neighbors. The results[41] show that as few as 2 nexus channels connecting neighboring cells can achieve considerable frequency entrainment, while 20 channels achieve almost complete synchrony. These figures correspond to a very low density of gap junctions, which would occupy a very small fraction of the cell membrane surface. This result is consistent with the experimental observations[42] showing that in the central region of the sinus node nexus regions are indeed very sparse and occupy less than 0.2% of the cell surface.

The second question addressed with network modeling is how the wave of excitation propagates when the intrinsic single cell properties (fitted to the Kodama and Boyett data) are distributed between the node center and periphery in the way that was observed experimentally. With the same magnitude of cell-to-cell coupling as in the random network, the results show that an excitatory wave then starts in the peripheral regions of the node and propagates towards the center, ie, in the opposite direction to that in the normal heart. This result, is very encouraging since this is exactly what occurs experimentally when the rabbit sinus node is separated from the atrium.[39] Moreover, when the simulated sinus node is surrounded by an atrial network the site of origin of the impulse shifts toward the center of the node.[41] This effect is attributable to a large flow of current between the atrium and sinus: the electrical 'load' of the atrium on the sinus node thus strongly influences the pacemaker properties. This result has important implications for the way in which atrial tachycardias and fibrillation might propagate into the node. They should strongly influence and interfere with rhythmic activity in the periphery of the node, but as a consequence of the very sparse cell-to-cell connections in the sinus itself, the center should be relatively unaffected. This would explain why sinus rhythm reestablishes itself rapidly following such arrhythmias.

The network modeling is therefore already achieving significant results in line with experimental evidence. The future intention is to extend the modeling to arrhythmic mechanisms so that we can study the way in which the cellular and multicellular mechanisms of arrhythmia interact. The information so obtained could be of great value to those interested in developing new approaches to therapy for cardiac disease. With the parallel computer architecture planned for the future the possibility of Teraflop speed looms on the horizon and it becomes possible to envisage reconstruction of the electrical mechanism of a heart attack on a very grand scale indeed.

References

1. Noble D: The surprising heart: a review of recent progress in cardiac electrophysiology. *J Physiol* 353:1, 1984.

2. Lederer WJ, Tsien RW: Transient inward current underlying arrhythmogenic effects of cardiotonic steroids in Purkinje fibres. *J Physiol* 262:73, 1976.

3. Noble D, Powell T: Calcium currents and calcium-dependent inward current. In: J Parratt (ed): *Control and Manipulation of Calcium Movement*. New York: Raven Press, 1984, p. 29.

4. Lab MJ: Transient depolarization and action potential alterations following mechanical changes in isolated myocardium. *Cardiovasc Res* 14:624, 1980.

5. Lab MJ: Contraction-excitation feedback in myocardium. Physiological basis and clinical relevance. *Circ Res* 50:557, 1982.

6. Lab MJ, Allen DG, Orchard CH: The effects of shortening on myoplasmic calcium concentration and on the action potential in mammalian ventricular muscle. *Circ Res* 55:825, 1984.

7. Noma A: ATP-regulated K^+ channels in cardiac muscle. *Nature* 305:147, 1983.

8. Nichols CG, Lederer WJ: The regulation of ATP-sensitive K^+ channel activity in intact and permeabilized rat ventricular myocytes. *J Physiol* 423:91, 1990.

9. DiFrancesco D: A new interpretation of the pacemaker current, i_{K2} in Purkinje fibres. *J Physiol* 314:359, 1981.

10. DiFrancesco D: A study of the ionic nature of the pacemaker current in calf Purkinje fibres. *J Physiol* 314:377, 1981.

11. McAllister RE, Noble D, Tsien RW: Reconstruction of the electrical activity of cardiac Purkinje fibres. *J Physiol* 251:1, 1975.

12. DiFrancesco D, Noble D: A model of cardiac electrical activity incorporating ionic pumps and concentration changes. *Phil Trans R Soc B* 307:353, 1985.

13. Mullins LJ: A mechanism for Na/Ca transport. *J Gen Physiol* 70:681, 1977.

14. Mullins LJ: *Ion Transport in the Heart*. New York: Raven Press, 1981.

15. Hilgemann DW, Noble D: Excitation-contraction coupling and extracellular calcium transients in rabbit atrium: reconstruction of basic cellular mechanisms. *Proc R Soc B* 230:163, 1987.

16. Hilgemann DW: Extracellular calcium transients at single excitations in rabbit atrium. *J Gen Physiol* 87:707, 1986.

17. Mitchell MR, Powell T, Terrar DA, Twist VW: The effects of ryanodine, EGTA and low sodium on action potentials in rat and guinea-pig ventricular myocytes: evidence for two inward currents during the plateau. *Brit J Pharmacol* 81:543, 1984.

18. Mitchell MR, Powell T, Terrar DA, Twist VW: Calcium-activated inward current and contraction in rat and guinea-pig ventricular myocytes. *J Physiol* 391:545, 1987.

19. Earm YE, Ho WK, So IS: Inward current generated by sodium-calcium exchange during the action potential in single atrial cells of the rabbit. *Proc R Soc B* 240:61, 1990.

20. Beeler GW, Reuter H: Reconstruction of the action potential of ventricular myocardial fibres. *J Physiol* 268:177, 1977.

21. Egan TM, Noble D, Noble SJ, et al: Sodium-calcium exchange during the action potential in guinea-pig ventricular cells. *J Physiol* 411:639, 1989.

22. Noble D, Noble SJ, Bett GCL, et al: The role of sodium-calcium exchange during the cardiac action potential. *Ann NY Acad Sci* 639:334, 1991.

23. Kodama I, Boyett MR: Regional differences in the electrical activity of the rabbit sinus node. *Plügers Arch* 404:214, 1985.

24. Honjo H, Boyett MR: Correlation between action potential parameters and the size of single sino-atrial node cells isolated from rabbit heart. *J Physiol* 452:128P, 1992.

25. Irisawa H, Brown HF, Giles WR: Cardiac pacemaking in the sinoatrial node. *Physiol Rev* 73:197, 1993.

26. Noble D: Ionic mechanisms determining the timing of ventricular repolarization: significance for cardiac arrhythmias. *Ann NY Acad Sci* 644:1, 1991.

27. Noble D: Electrical properties of cardiac muscle attributable to inward-going (anomalous) rectification. *J Cell Comp Physiol* 66(Suppl 2):127, 1965.

28. Allen DG, Eisner DA, Orchard CA: Characteristics of oscillations of intracellular calcium concentration in ferret ventricular muscle. *J Physiol* 352:113, 1984.

29. Fabiato A: Calcium-induced release of calcium from the cardiac sarcoplasmic reticulum. *Am J Physiol* 245:C1, 1983.

30. Kimura J, Miyamae S, Noma A: Identification of sodium-calcium exchange current in single ventricular cells of guinea-pig. *J Physiol* 384:198, 1987.

31. Fedida D, Noble D, Rankin AC, Spindler AJ: The transient inward current, i_{TI} and related contraction in guinea-pig ventricular myocytes. *J Physiol* 392:523, 1987.

32. Allen TJA, Noble D, Reuter H: *Sodium-Calcium Exchange*. Oxford: Oxford University Press, 1989.

33. Blaustein MP, DiPolo R, Reeves JP (eds): *Proceedings of the Second International Meeting on Sodium-Calcium Exchange*. New York: Annals of the New York Academy of Sciences, 1991, volume 639.

34. Levi AJ: The effect of strophanthidin on action potential, calcium current and contraction in isolated guinea-pig ventricular myocytes. *J Physiol* 443:1, 1991.

35. January CT, Riddle JM: Early after-depolarizations: mechanism of induction and block. A role for L-type Ca^{2+} current. *Circ Res* 64:977, 1989.

36. Weidmann S: *Elektrophysiologie der Herzmuskelfaser.* Bern: Huber, 1956.

37. Reuter H, Scholz HA: A study of the ion selectivity and the kinetic properties of the calcium dependent slow inward current in mammalian cardiac muscle. *J Physiol* 264:17, 1977.

38. Noma A, Shioya T, Paver LFC, et al: Cytosolic free Ca^{2+} during operation of sodium-calcium exchange in guinea-pig heart cells. *J Physiol* 442:257, 1991.

39. Kirchhoff CJHJ, Bonke FIM, Allessie MA, Lammers WJEP: The influence of the atrial myocardium on impulse formation in the rabbit sinus node. *Pflügers Arch* 410:198, 1987.

40. Janse MJ, Wit AL: Electrophysiological mechanisms of ventricular arrhythmias resulting from myocardial ischemia and infarction. *Physiol Rev* 69:1049, 1989.

41. Winslow R, Kimball A, Varghese A, Noble D: Simulating cardiac sinus and atrial network dynamics on the Connection Machine. *Physica D* 64:281, 1993.

42. Masson-Pevet M, Bleeker WK, Mackaay AJC, Bouman LN: Sinus node and atrium cells from the rabbit heart: a quantitative electron microscopic description after electrophysiological localisation. *J Mol Cell Cardiol* 11:555, 1979.

43. Noble D, DiFrancesco D, Denyer J: Ionic mechanisms in normal and abnormal cardiac pacemaker activity. In: EW Jacklet (ed): *Cellular and Neuronal Oscillators.* New York: Marcel Dekker, 1989, p. 59.

44. Earm YE, Noble D: A model of the single atrial cell: relation between calcium current and calcium release. *Proc Roy Soc* 240:83, 1990.

Chapter 2

Cardiac Excitability and Myocardial Conduction

Jonathan C. Makielski
Harry A. Fozzard

This chapter discusses the underlying concepts of cardiac excitation and conduction and describes how these concepts operate and interact. (For in-depth discussions of these concepts, the reader is referred to reviews on conduction in the heart[1] and in excitable tissues in general.[2]) Some simple equations derived from cable theory are presented and used in this treatment; they are presented to complement the text and diagrams that describe current flow during a propagated action potential. Key membrane proteins involved in excitation and conduction (sodium [Na+] channels and gap junctions) are described first, followed by a description of excitation and conduction in the heart. As examples relevant to pathophysiological processes such as ischemia, and also relevant to the mechanism of action of antiarrhythmic drugs, the relationships between action potential upstroke velocity, conduction, Na+ current magnitude, and cell coupling will be discussed.

Ion Channels and Gap Junctions

The Na+ Channel

Sodium current (I_{Na}) is the excitatory current in atrial and ventricular muscle and in the specialized Purkinje conduction tissue. We will briefly summarize some features of the cardiac Na+ channel, and the reader is also referred to more comprehensive reviews by Fozzard et al.[3] and Fozzard and Hanck.[4]

The cardiac Na+ channel is a large (approximately 260 kD molecular weight) intrinsic membrane protein that forms a pore through the membrane allowing Na+ ions to pass through when the channel is open. Several useful ways to represent the Na+ channel regarding its structure and function are shown in Figure 1. One such representation is a "cartoon" of the Na+ channel showing the protein in the membrane bilayer with both structural and functional characteristics (Figure 1A). An-

From BN Singh, HJJ Wellens, M Hiraoka, (eds): *Electropharmacological Control of Cardiac Arrhythmias*. Mount Kisco, NY, Futura Publishing Company Inc., © 1994.

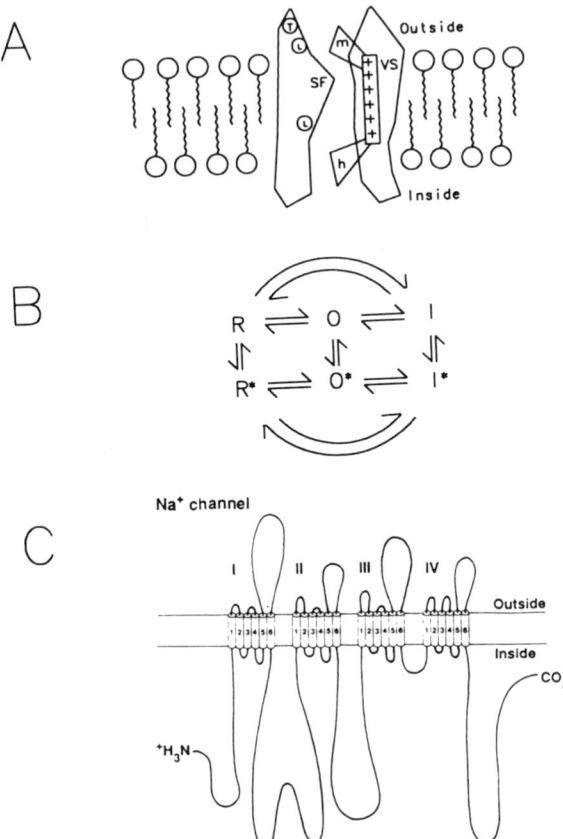

Figure 1. Representations of the Na$^+$ channel. (A) Illustration of structural and functional characteristics. (B) State diagram for gating kinetics with modulated receptor model for drug binding. (C) Proposed secondary structure of Na$^+$ channel based upon primary amino acid sequence. (Reproduced with permission from Reference 5.) See text for further explanation.

other such representaion (Figure 1B) is a state diagram for the Na$^+$ channel depicting the kinetic states the channel goes through with and without drugs bound, in this case depicting the modulated receptor model of drug binding. Finally, a topological diagram of the Na$^+$ channel (Figure 1C)[5] relates the known primary amino acid structure of the Na$^+$ channel to its secondary structure in the membrane.

The first representation (Figure 1A) depicts five essential characteristics. First, the

channel provides a path in the membrane through which ions can pass. Second, the channel is highly selective for Na$^+$ ions over K$^+$, calcium (Ca^{2+}), chloride (Cl$^-$), and other ions. The role of "selecting" Na$^+$ ions to pass is attributed to a selectivity filter (SF). Third, the Na$^+$ channel opens or activates in response to a depolarization and then closes or inactivates. This function is diagrammed as gates (m and h as in the Hodgkin-Huxley formulation). Next, the gates are controlled by a voltage sensor or sensors (VS). Finally, drug and toxin effects can be represented as binding at specific sites, such as the local anesthetic antiarrhythmic drug site(s) (L) and tetrodotoxin binding site (T). The location of these sites and functions on the diagram should be considered tentative. The most arbitrary assignment is the placement of the "m" or activation gate on the outside. The "h" or inactivation gate and the major local anesthetic binding site do appear to be to the inside of the channel, while the tetrodotoxin site has been shown to be on the outside.

The second representation of the Na$^+$ channel (Figure 1B) shows the kinetic states through which the channel passes during a cardiac cycle. The timing of these states with respect to the electrocardiogram and to an action potential is depicted in Figure 2. During diastole when the membrane potential is polarized or negative, Na$^+$ channels are in a closed "resting" state (state R in Figure 1B and Figure 2) from which the channel can open. When the membrane is depolarized in systole, Na$^+$ channels activate and open briefly (typically less than a millisecond, state O in Figure 1B and Figure 2) before they inactivate (state I in Figure 1B and Figure 2). The closed state I differs from the closed state R in that the channel will not open again, despite the fact that the membrane is depolarized. Before the channel can open again it must recover through state R, and this only happens after the membrane repolarizes in diastole. If the membrane is partially depolarized as occurs in ischemia, an increasing number of Na$^+$ channels become inactivated and incapable of opening. The three states (R, O, and I) de-

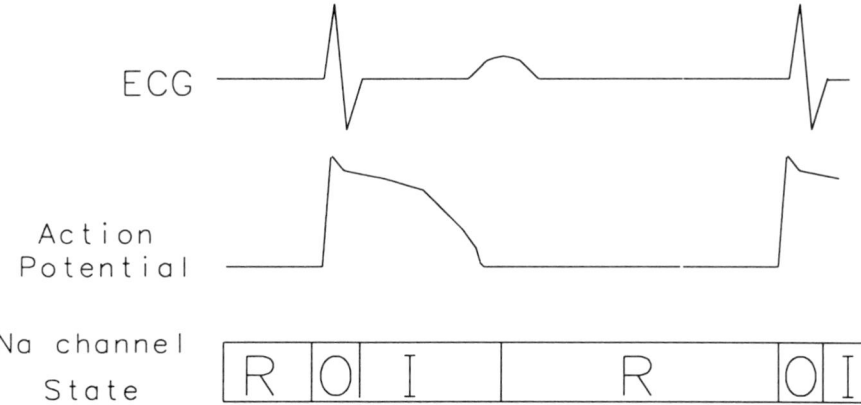

Figure 2. Time sequence of Na$^+$ channel kinetic states compared with an ECG signal and action potential. The Na$^+$ channel is in the resting state (R) during diastole, enters the open state (O) transiently during early systole before entering the inactivated state (I). Recovery to the resting state occurs during the subsequent diastole.

picted in the figures are actually a simplification. The classic Hodgkin and Huxley kinetic model[6] for the squid axon Na$^+$ channel calls for eight such states (1 open, 3 closed, 4 inactivated), and models for the cardiac Na$^+$ channel[7,8] call for five or more states. We often think of the three states depicted in the figure as "classes" of states because they can explain the salient kinetic behavior of the channel. Figure 1B also illustrates the complexities that can occur when antiarrhythmic drugs that bind to the Na$^+$ channel are added. According to the modulated receptor hypothesis[9,10] drugs can bind to the different kinetic states of the Na$^+$ channel with different affinities, and the drug-bound channels (asterisks in Figure 1B) have gating kinetics that are different from those not bound by drugs. This hypothesis can account for the use, frequency, and voltage dependence of antiarrhythmic drug block. The guarded receptor model[11] is an alternative and simplified model that does not postulate altered gating of drug-bound states, thus allowing quantitative rate constants of interaction of drugs with the channel to be calculated more easily.[12–15] Although the guarded receptor model is a useful simplification, it does not account for all aspects of block by some drugs.[16,17]

The amino acid structure of the Na$^+$

channel has been determined. Three brain Na$^+$ channels have been cloned and sequenced,[18,19] and recently a rat heart Na$^+$ channel has also been cloned, sequenced, and functionally expressed.[20,21] Although important differences exist, overall the heart Na$^+$ channel has a great deal of sequence homology with nonheart Na$^+$ channels. The diagram in Figure 1C is taken from Catterall[5] and represents a current model for the secondary structure of the Na$^+$ channel. The Na$^+$ channel sequence is divided into four repeats (labeled I–IV) based upon a similarity in the sequence of their amino acids, termed internal homology. Each repeat has six membrane-spanning segments labeled S_1–S_6. More recently it has been proposed[22] that the extracellular loops between S_5 and S_6 contain two short segments in each repeat that are folded into the membrane and make up at least part of the pore.

Although cardiac I_{Na} resembles I_{Na} reported in noncardiac tissues, important functional differences exist. For example, cardiac Na$^+$ channels are much less sensitive to block by tetrodotoxin[23] and divalents such as Cd^{2+}.[24,25] We know that the cardiac Na$^+$ channel has a unique structure,[21] so it is reasonable that it has unique functional properties. The availability of cloned Na$^+$ channels will permit detailed analysis of the structure-function of this channel and the differences between nerve and cardiac Na^+ current. The expression of these channels has been achieved and studies with channel mutants have begun. As structure and function are correlated to give more detailed molecular models, our understanding of cardiac Na^+ channels as distinct members of the Na^+ channel family will increase.

The magnitude of I_{Na} depends upon the density of Na^+ channels and upon the voltage- and time-dependent kinetics of opening and closing. The density of Na^+ channels is greatest in specialized conduction tissue, such as Purkinje cells, where it may be several hundred per square micron.[26] The channel density may be four- or fivefold less in atrial and ventricular cells. These estimates of density make many assumptions, which have been reviewed elsewhere.[4] The maximum I_{Na} achieved during an action potential depends not only upon the number of channels, but also upon the synchrony between opening and closing of the channels in the membrane.

Other Ion Channels

Although the Na^+ channel is the major provider of the current for excitation and conduction, other ion channels are important. Calcium current (I_{Ca}) is the principal excitatory current in the sinoatrial and atrioventricular nodes, and it can also generate an action potential in working myocardium when the I_{Na} current is suppressed.[27] This can occur because Ca^{2+} channels remain available for opening at partially depolarized potentials at which I_{Na} is inactivated. The I_{Ca} may also carry the charge in abnormal excitation such as early afterdepolarizations.[28] Because I_{Ca} inactivates more slowly than I_{Na}, it persists longer into the action potential and by sustaining the plateau, it may provide a current source for conduction to poorly coupled cells.[29]

Repolarizing currents are described in detail in Chapter 3. These currents can influence excitability and conduction directly and

indirectly. Potassium current (I_K) is responsible for maintaining the resting potential that keeps I_{Na} and I_{Ca} available for opening. Some I_K deactivates slowly after repolarization.[30] To the extent that I_K is "left over" from a previous action potential, this I_K would be a current "sink" that increases the inward current required to reach threshold for regenerative depolarizations, and slows the action potential, or even causes inexcitability (sometimes called postrepolarization refractoriness). Also, it is important to point out that repolarization can itself be a threshold phenomenon and can be conducted from cell to cell.

Finally, whereas I_{Na} is usually thought of in terms of its role on the upstroke of the action potential, I_{Na} also can play a role in repolarization. Some Na^+ channels open repeatedly[31] late in a depolarization leading to late or persistent Na^+ currents that have been called slowly inactivating currents.[32,33] Such currents, if augmented, would tend to lengthen the action potential, and if blocked would tend to shorten the action potential. Some experimental positively inotropic drugs such as DPI 201–601[34] prolong the action potential by this mechanism. Lysophosphatidylcholine, a metabolite that accumulates in ischemia, also produces persistent Na^+ channel openings.[35,36] Any drug that blocks or opens Na^+ channels may therefore affect refractoriness.

Gap Junctions

Cells are coupled together by gap junctions, which are ion pores that span the membranes of adjacent cells and the gap between them. Details of the structure and function of cardiac gap junctions have been recently reviewed by Page.[37] A gap junction is made up of two connexons, one in the membrane of each cell being coupled, and each connexon is itself made up of six subunits. Whether or not these subunits are identical, or whether or not other subunits are important in gap junction structure and function is controversial. The gap junction subunit from heart has been cloned[38] and sequenced; studies using expressed gap junctions should clarify the structure-function relationships of the cardiac gap junction.

The gap junction pore is larger than those of other ion channels, making it relatively non-selective and highly conductive. Gap junctions are not, however, a purely passive conduit from one cell to another. Gap junctional conductance can be studied in pairs of cardiac cells under voltage-clamp conditions[39] and it is decreased by H^+, Ca^{2+}, and Mg^{2+}. This suggests the possibility that cell coupling could change as Ca^{2+} levels rise and fall during the action potential. It may be, however, that the level of Ca^{2+}[40] and H^+[41] required to decrease gap junctional conductance is only found in situations where H^+ and Ca^{2+} are pathologically elevated, such as in ischemia. Low adenosine triphosphate levels also decrease gap junctional resistance[42] suggesting another mechanism for cellular uncoupling.

In addition to regulation of gap junctional conductance, the number and geometry of gap junctional connections is important in cellular coupling. Connections between cardiac cells tend to be most numerous at the ends of the cells and the connections from side to side are sparse. Thus, cells tend to be coupled better in the longitudinal direction rather than the transverse direction, a property called tissue anisotropy (see Chapter 7). No drug has been found that blocks gap junctions selectively. Heptanol will block cardiac gap junctions,[43] but it also blocks cardiac Na^+ channels,[44] although at some lower concentrations heptanol may be relatively selective for gap junctions. In addition to direct effects on gap junctions, drugs may influence cellular coupling indirectly through effects on internal pH or Ca^{2+}. Finally, the making and unmaking of connections in pathological states such as ischemia also surely plays a role in coupling and in altered excitability and conduction.[45,46]

Conceptual Approach to Conduction in the Heart

Much insight into conduction of the cardiac impulse was gained by applying the properties of an ideal cable to heart tissue. The assumptions of an ideal cable most closely apply to Purkinje fibers and perhaps papillary muscles, but all cardiac tissue deviates from an ideal cable because it consists of individual cells variably coupled by gap junctions in more complex geometries. Ventricular and atrial myocardium more closely resembles a two- or three-dimensional array of cells. A detailed and quantitative description of excitation and conduction in the heart requires mathematical modeling (see Chapter 1) that accounts both for the ionic currents involved in excitation and for the complex geometry leading to properties such as anisotropy (see Chapter 7). Considerations derived from conduction in a cable, however, can help to give an intuitive feel for how the action potential is generated and conducted in the heart. We confine our discussion to the excitation phase of the action potential; repolarization and refractoriness are covered in Chapter 3.

The ideas of a current sink and a current source will help in understanding the relationship of excitation to conduction. A current source is a cell or membrane element that supplies net excitatory current to the tissue, and a current sink is a cell or membrane element that drains off net excitatory current. An excitatory current is one that tends to depolarize a cell. Under standard conventions, an inward flow of positive ions (such as Na^+) is considered a negative current that tends to depolarize the cell or make the transmembrane potential more positive inside; an outward flow of positive ions (such as K^+) is considered a positive current that tends to repolarize the transmembrane potential to the resting potential, which is negative inside. The action potential is a regenerative depolarization and subsequent repolarization of the transmembrane potential, during which the membrane becomes a net current source by providing its own excitatory current. The transmembrane potential at which a cell or tissue becomes a net current source can be considered the threshold potential and the amount of current required to bring a cell or tissue to the threshold potential is the threshold current. A cell or tissue that is capable of having an action potential is said to be excitable. Conduction refers to the passing of an electrical impulse (usually depolarization) from one cell to a second cell. If the second cell reaches threshold and has an action potential, then the action potential has been conducted or propagated.

What then is the current source for excitation and conduction? The membrane channels open and close in response to transmembrane voltage changes, and currents flow in response to their electrochemical gradients. The channels can be represented as variable resistors in series with their electrochemical batteries (Figure 3). Na^+ and Ca^{2+} channels open in response to a depolarization, and allow Na^+ and Ca^{2+} ions to flow into the cell to provide a depolarizing current. Outward currents (eg, K^+ currents) and electrogenic pump current (such as Na^+-Ca^{2+} exchange and the Na^+-K^+ pump, not pictured) are generally overwhelmed during excitation (phase 0 of the action potential), but they may play important modulating roles under special conditions.

The excitatory current flowing into the cell (I_i for ionic current) flows into several sinks that slow the rate of depolarization. These sinks are also often called the "load." The first sink to be considered is the membrane capacity. The lipid bilayer of the membrane is a thin insulator surrounded by conducting electrolyte solutions, ie, a capacitor. A capacitor permits a change in potential in response to current flow as described by the equation:

$$I_c = C_m \, dV/dt \qquad (1)$$

where I_c is the current required to charge the capacitor C_m for a given rate of change in transmembrance potential (dV/dt). In the case of an isolated patch of membrane (Figure 3, top), the transmembrane ionic current $I_i = I_c$ because the current has nowhere else to flow. Excitation in a single membrane patch is called a membrane action potential and it is apparent that in this case the upstroke velocity of the action potential dV/dt is directly proportional to the net ionic current, which is dominated by I_{Na}. An electrical representation of a cell (Figure 3, middel panel) included multiple membrane patches connected by the cytoplasmic resistance to make a cable. In this simple case the membrane lining the T tubule is ignored, but it could be represented by an-

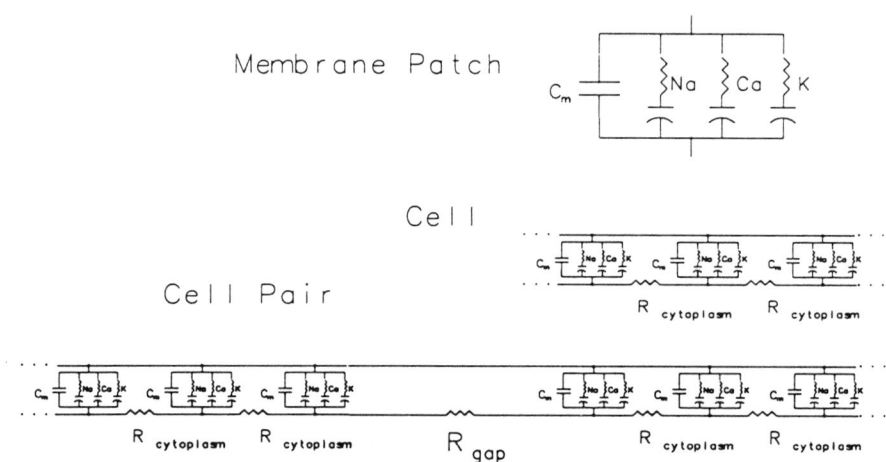

Figure 3. Equivalent electrical circuit diagrams for a cardiac membrane patch, a cardiac cell, and a cell pair. Membrane capacity (C_m), cytoplasmic resistance ($R_{cytoplasm}$), gap junctional resistance (R_{gap}), and ionic current generators (labeled Na, Ca, and K) are represented. See text for discussion.

other membrane element connected to the circuit through a distributed access resistance representing the T tubule lumens. For most purposes, this more complex geometry can be ignored and a cell can be considered a single unit. To begin to approximate myocardial tissue, cells are coupled together by gap junctions as diagrammed in Figure 3 (bottom panel). This cell pair model can be used to consider the new loading conditions that connecting a second cell imposes. The second cell is a sink for the current flowing through the membrane in the first cell. According to Kirchoff's law, the net current flowing into the cell must equal the current flowing out of the cell:

$$I_i = I_c + I_L \qquad (2)$$

where I_L is mainly the longitudinal current flow from one cell to another.

The second cell, therefore, acts as a current sink for the first cell until the second cell reaches threshold, generates its own inward current, and becomes a net current source. The second cell then becomes a source for a third cell, etc., and the action potential is thus conducted or propagated. The membrane action potential is just one element of a conducted action potential; the loading conditions for a conducted action potential are very different from that of a membrane action potential only. In myocardium and in Purkinje fibers, cells are connected in a complex way as described earlier. Another complexity not pictured in the diagram is the extracellular resistance of the clefts between cells. This feature could be represented in the diagram by a membrane patch with a series resistance representing the resistance caused by the clefts.[47]

Upstroke Velocity and Conduction

In experimental preparations the maximal upstroke velocity of the action potential ($\dot{V}_{max}$) has been used to measure excitability, and is often used as a means to characterize

I_{Na}. The use of $\dot{V}_{max}$ as a surrogate for I_{Na} as measured in a voltage clamp has a long and controversial history (see Sheets et al.[48] for discussion). Even in the simple case of a membrane action potential, the relationship between the voltage-clamp measurement of I_{Na} and $\dot{V}_{max}$ has not been shown to be strictly linear, and it deviates more with block of I_{Na}.[48] The relationship between $\dot{V}_{max}$ and activation of Na$^+$ channels can be even less directly correlated in the case of a conducted action potential where the loading conditions are more complex.

The way in which changes of cellular coupling affect $\dot{V}_{max}$ and conduction velocity can illustrate these complexities. Figure 4 demonstrates the current flow in an equivalent circuit representing three cells. The top panel represents the "control" situation where gap junctional resistance (R_{gap}) is normal. The first cell (on the left) has reached threshold and is generating I_{Na} as represented by the large downward arrow. This "source" current is split into two parts: a current filling the membrane capacity C_m of the first cell (upward arrow), which generates the upstroke velocity in that cell, and a current flowing into the middle cell to depolarize it (rightward arrow). The widths of the arrows were drawn to approximately equal the amount of current, so in the control example at the top approximately half of the current goes to fill the capacity and the other half flows into the middle cell. The current flowing into the middle cell is then split into two parts: a current to fill the capacitance of the middle cell (upward arrow) and a current flowing into the third cell (rightward arrow). It is not shown in Figure 4, but when the middle cell depolarizes sufficiently, I_{Na} will then be generated in the middle cell and it will become a net current source for action potential generation and conduction. What happens when the cells are more tightly coupled, that is, when the resistance (R_{gap}) between them is reduced as in the middle panel (Figure 4)? In this case more current flows into the adjacent cell because of the lower resistance, and less current is available to fill the membrane capacity. With less current to fill

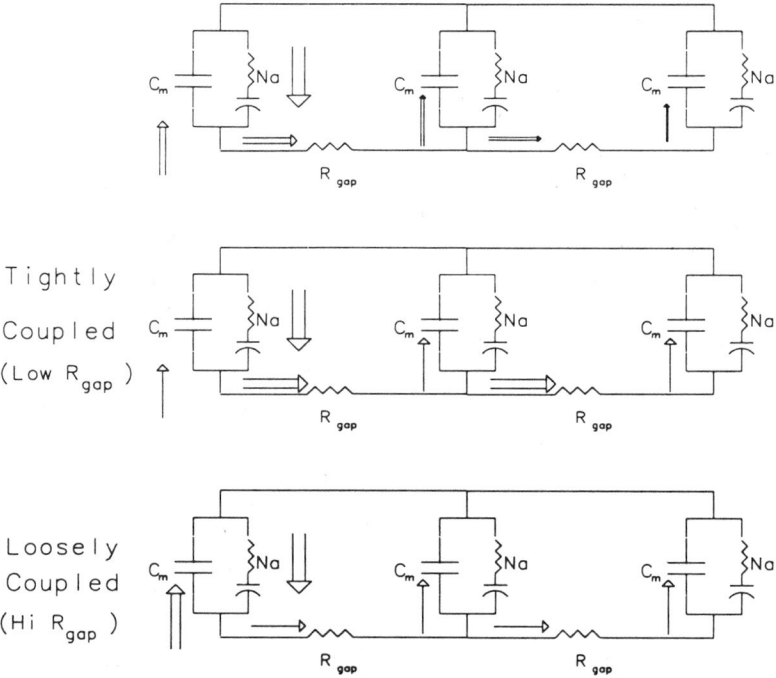

Figure 4. Current flow during excitation and conduction with normal cellular coupling (top), tight coupling (middle), and loose coupling (bottom). Arrows represent current flow with the width of the shaft corresponding to the amount of current flowing. See text for a discussion of the effects of coupling on current flow, upstroke velocity, and conduction velocity.

membrane capacity, $\dot{V}_{max}$ decreases. Note that $\dot{V}_{max}$ decreases despite the fact that I_{Na} has not changed, an instance where $\dot{V}_{max}$ is not a good indicator of I_{Na}. What happens to conduction velocity? Note that greater current flows longitudinally, so that more distal cells are provided with depolarizing current (middle panel of Figure 4). As long as this current is sufficient to bring those cells to threshold, conduction velocity will increase. If, however, coupling is too tight, the longitudinal current may be dissipated before adjacent cells are brought to threshold and conduction will fail.

When cells are more loosely coupled, that is the gap junctional resistance is increased (Figure 4, bottom panel), more current goes to fill the membrane capacity and less current flows longitudinally. More current discharging the capacity causes an increase in $\dot{V}_{max}$ without any change in I_{Na}. Once again $\dot{V}_{max}$ is not a good index of I_{Na}, but in

this case in the opposite direction. Because less current is flowing longitudinally, conduction velocity is slowed. Therefore, when a tissue is uncoupled without a change in I_{Na}, $\dot{V}_{max}$ can be expected to increase and conduction velocity to slow. This intuitive argument has been demonstrated in simple cable models of conduction (Figure 5) and in a model cable composed of multiple cells and also demonstrated experimentally in cardiac fibers.[49]

$\dot{V}_{max}$ and I_{Na} are often well correlated with the square of the conduction velocity.[50-52] This attests to the primary role of I_{Na} in determining upstroke velocity and conduction velocity under many conditions and experimental models of conduction. This has often caused the mistaken general notion that $\dot{V}_{max}$ changes if and only if I_{Na} changes and that conduction velocity always increases with increasing $\dot{V}_{max}$. The above example demonstrates that $\dot{V}_{max}$ (usually considered an "ac-

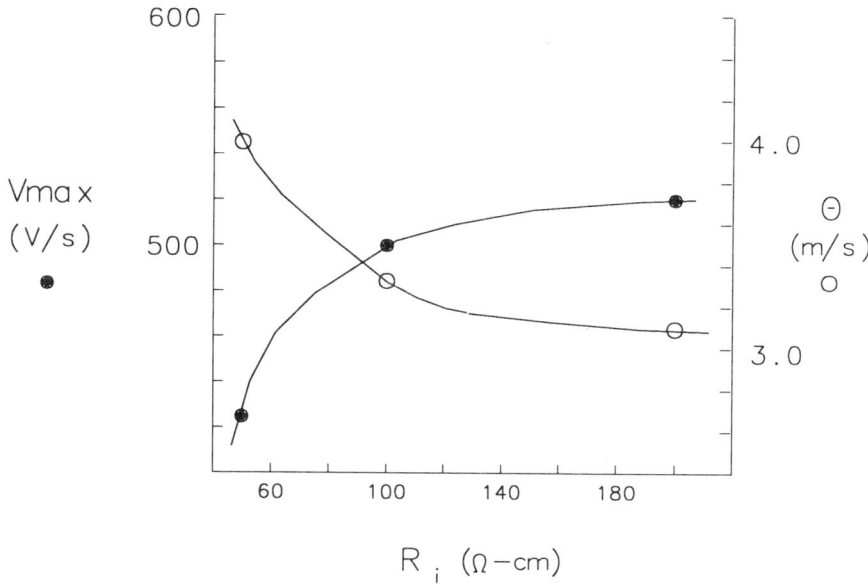

Figure 5. The effect of changes in internal longitudinal resistance (R_i) upon maximal upstroke velocity ($\dot{V}_{max}$) and conduction velocity (Θ) in a computer model of a conducted cardiac action potential. A model for the cardiac Purkinje cell action potential[53] was used in a model for action potential propagation in a cable.[54] Parameters of the runs included resting potential -78 mV, C_m, 4.3 $\mu F/cm^2$, and maximal Na^+ conductance 64.5 millisiemens/cm^2. As R_i was increased simulating cellular uncoupling, conduction velocity fell, but the upstroke velocity increased without a change in I_{Na}.

tive" property) changes when cell coupling is altered (usually considered a "passive" property). Change or lack of change in $\dot{V}_{max}$ must be interpreted with caution, especially when action potentials are allowed to conduct and when cell coupling or other components of the passive load might be changing. Such conditions often pertain to studies of conduction with ischemia and drugs.

References

1. Fozzard HA, Arnsdorf MF: Cardiac electrophysiology. In: HA Fozzard (ed): *The Heart and Cardiovascular System: Scientific Foundations.* 2nd ed. New York: Raven Press, 1991, p. 63.
2. Jack JJB, Noble D, Tsien RW: *Electric Current Flow in Excitable Cells.* Oxford: Clarendon Press, 1975.
3. Fozzard HA, January CT, Makielski JC: Brief reviews: new studies of the excitatory sodium currents in heart muscle. *Circ Res* 56:475, 1985.
4. Fozzard HA, Hanck DA: Sodium channels. In: HA Fozzard (ed): *The Heart and Cardiovascular System: Scientific Foundations.* 2nd ed. New York: Raven Press, 1991, p. 109.
5. Catterall WA: Structure and function of voltage-sensitive ion channels. *Science* 242:50, 1988.
6. Hodgkin AL, Huxley AF: A quantitative description of membrane current and its application to conduction and excitation in nerve. *J Physiol* 117:500, 1952.
7. Kunze DL, Lacerda AE, Wilson DL, et al: Cardiac Na currents and the inactivity, reopening, and waiting properties of single Na channels. *J Gen Physiol* 86:697, 1985.
8. Scanley BE, Hanck DA, Chay T, et al: Kinetic analysis of single sodium channels from canine cardiac Purkinje cells. *J Gen Physiol* 95:411, 1990.
9. Hondeghem LM, Katzung BG: Time- and voltage-dependent interaction of antiarrhythmic drugs with cardiac sodium channels. *Biochim Biophys Acta* 472:373, 1977.
10. Hille B: Local anesthetics: hydrophilic and hydrophobic pathways for the drug-receptor reaction. *J Gen Physiol* 69:497, 1977.
11. Starmer CF, Grant AO, Strauss HC: Mechanisms of use-dependent block of sodium channels in

excitable membranes by local anaesthetics. *Biophys J* 46:15, 1984.

12. Starmer CF, Grant AO: Phasic ion channel blockade: a kinetic model and parameter estimation procedure. *Mol Pharmacol* 28:348, 1985.

13. Starmer CF, Undrovinas AI, Scamps F, et al: Ethacizin blockade of calcium channels: a test of the guarded receptor hypothesis. *Am J Physiol* 257:H1693, 1989.

14. Makielski JC, Nesterenko VV, Nelson WL, et al: State dependence of ethacizin and ethmozin block of sodium current in voltage clamped and internally perfused cardiac Purkinje cells. *J Pharmacol Exp Ther* 253:1110, 1990.

15. Carmeliet E: Activation block and trapping of penticainide, a disopyramide analogue, in the Na^+ channel of rabbit cardiac Purkinje fibers. *Circ Res* 63:50, 1988.

16. Snyders DJ, Hondeghem LM: Effects of quinidine on the sodium current of guinea pig ventricular myocytes—evidence for a drug-associated rested state with altered kinetics. *Circ Res* 66:565, 1990.

17. Makielski JC, Hanck DA: Hyperpolarization enhances use and rest recovery of QX-222 blocked cardiac Na channels (abstract). *Circulation* 80:II-605, 1989.

18. Kayano T, Noda M, Flockerzi V, et al: Primary structure of rat brain sodium channel III deduced from the cDNA sequence. *FEBS Lett* 228:187, 1988.

19. Noda M, Shimizu S, Tanabe T, et al: Primary structure of *electrophorus electricus* sodium channel deduced from CDNA sequence. *Nature* 312:121, 1984.

20. Rogart RB, Cribbs LL, Muglia K, et al: Molecular cloning of a putative tetrodotoxin-resistant rat heart Na channel isoform. *Proc Natl Acad Sci U S A* 86:8170, 1989.

21. Cribbs LL, Satin J, Fozzard HA, et al: Functional expression of the rat heart-I Na^+ channel isoform—demonstration of properties characteristic of native cardiac Na^+ channels. *FEBS Lett* 275:195, 1990.

22. Guy HR, Conti F: Pursuing the structure and function of voltage-gated channels. *Trends Neurosci* 13:201, 1990.

23. Lombet A, Renaud J-F, Chicheportiche R, et al: A cardiac tetrodotoxin binding component: biochemical identification, characterization, and properties. *Biochemistry* 20:1279, 1981.

24. DiFrancesco D, Ferroni A, Visentin S, et al: Cadmium-induced blockade of the cardiac fast Na channels in calf Purkinje fibres. *Proc R Soc Lond Series B* 223:475, 1985.

25. Sheets MF, Hanck DA, Fozzard HA: Divalent block of sodium current in single canine cardiac Purkinje cells. *Biophys J* 53:535a, 1988.

26. Makielski JC, Sheets MF, Hanck DA, et al: Sodium current in voltage clamped internally perfused canine cardiac Purkinje cells. *Biophys J* 52:111, 1987.

27. Cranefield PF: *The Conduction of the Cardiac Impulse: The Slow Response and Cardiac Arrhythmias.* Mt Kisco, NY: Futura Publishing Company, Inc., 1975.

28. January CT, Riddle JM: Early afterdepolarizations: mechanism of induction and block. A role for L-type Ca^{++} current. *Circ Res* 64:977, 1989.

29. Sugiura H, Joyner RW: Calcium current modulates action potential conduction between cardiac ventricular cells. *Biophys J* 61:A340, 1992.

30. Delmar M, Michaels DC, Jalife J: Slow recovery of excitability and the Wenckebach phenomenon in the single guinea pig ventricular myocyte. *Circ Res* 65:761, 1989.

31. Patlak JB, Ortiz M: Two modes of gating during late Na^+ channel currents in frog sartorius muscle. *J Gen Physiol* 87:305, 1986.

32. Carmeliet E: Slow inactivation of the sodium current in rabbit cardiac Purkinje fibers. *J Physiol* 353:125P, 1984.

33. Fozzard HA, Hanck DA, Makielski JC, et al: Sodium channels in cardiac Purkinje cells. *Experientia* 43:1162, 1987.

34. Scholtysik G, Honerjager P, Markstein R, et al: Positive inotropic and electrophysiological effects of APP 201–533 can be explained by an increase of cardiac cyclic AMP. *J Cardiovasc Pharmacol* 7:597, 1985.

35. Burnashev NA, Undrovinas AI, Fleidervish IA, et al: Modulation of cardiac sodium channel gating by lysophosphatidylcholine. *J Mol Cell Cardiol* 23(Suppl I):23, 1991.

36. Burnashev NA, Undrovinas AI, Fleidervish IA, et al: Ischemic poison lysophosphatidylcholine modifies heart sodium channels gating inducing long-lasting bursts of openings. *Pflügers Arch* 415:124, 1989.

37. Page E: Cardiac gap junctions. In: HA Fozzard (ed): *The Heart and Cardiovascular System: Scientific Foundations.* 2nd ed. New York: Raven Press, 1991, p. 1003.

38. Beyer EC, Paul DL, Goodenough DA: Connexin 43: a protein from rat heart homologous to a gap junctional protein from liver. *J Cell Biol* 105:2621, 1987.

39. Spray DC, Harris AL, Bennett MVL: Equilibrium properties of a voltage-dependent junctional conductance. *J Gen Physiol* 77:77, 1981.

40. Maurer P, Weingart R: Cell pairs isolated from adult guinea pig and rat hearts: effects of $[Ca^{2+}]_i$ on nexal membrane resistance. *Pflügers Arch* 409:394, 1987.

41. Noma A, Tsuboi N: Dependence of junctional

conductance on proton, calcium and magnesium ions in cardiac paired cells of guinea-pig. *J Physiol* 382:193, 1987.

42. Sugiura H, Toyama J, Tsuboi N, et al: ATP directly affects junctional conductance between paired ventricular myocytes isolated from guinea pig heart. *Circ Res* 66:1095, 1990.

43. Rüdisüli A, Weingart R: Electrical properties of gap junction channels in guinea-pig ventricular cell pairs revealed by exposure to heptanol. *Pflügers Arch* 415:12, 1989.

44. Nelson WN, Makielski JC: Block of sodium current by heptanol in voltage-clamped canine cardiac Purkinje cells. *Circ Res* 68:977, 1991.

45. Hoyt RH, Cohen ML, Corr PB, et al: Alterations of intercellular junctions induced by hypoxia in canine myocardium. *Am J Physiol* 258:H1439, 1990.

46. Spear JF, Balke CW, Lesh MD, et al: Effect of cellular uncoupling by heptanol on conduction in infarcted myocardium. *Circ Res* 66:202, 1990.

47. Fozzard HA: Membrane capacity of the cardiac Purkinje fibre. *J Physiol* 182:255, 1966.

48. Sheets MF, Hanck DA, Fozzard HA: Nonlinear relation between $\dot{V}_{max}$ and I_{Na} in canine cardiac Purkinje cells. *Circ Res* 63:386, 1988.

49. Jalife J, Sicouri S, Delmar M, et al: Electrical uncoupling and impulse propagation in isolated sheep Purkinje fibers. *Am J Physiol* 257: H179, 1989.

50. Walton MK, Fozzard HA: The conducted action potential: models and comparison to experiments. *Biophys J* 44:9, 1983.

51. Walton MK, Fozzard HA: Experimental study of the conducted action potential in cardiac Purkinje strands. *Biophys J* 44:1, 1983.

52. Buchanan JWJ, Saito T, Gettes LS: The effects of antiarrhythmic drugs, stimulation frequency, and potassium-induced resting membrane potential changes on conductian velocity and dV/dt_{max} in guinea pig myocardium. *Circ Res* 56: 696, 1985.

53. McAllister RE, Noble D, Tsien RW: Reconstruction of the electrical activity of cardiac Purkinje fibres. *J Physiol* 251:1, 1975.

54. Cooley JW, Dodge FA Jr: Digital computer solutions for excitation and propagation of the nerve impulse. *Biophys J* 6:583, 1966.

Chapter 3

Action Potential Duration and Refractoriness

Edward Carmeliet

During the plateau, which is the main determinant of the action potential duration, a fine balance exists between inward and outward currents. The plateau is expressed differently in different parts of the heart, and even in the atrium or the ventricle a marked heterogeneity exists. A heterogeneity in currents corresponds to this heterogeneity in the configuration of the action potential plateau. A general and necessarily incomplete description is given of the interplay between different currents and their modulation with rate, metabolism, drugs, and development.

The sensitivity of the action potential duration to rate is because of the time dependency of the currents, which in turn is related to the activation and inactivation processes. Currents that only activate can undergo summation, currents that also inactivate may become less pronounced when the depolarization is repeated. Important changes in the configuration of the action potential occur with development and correlate with a change in the expression of different currents. The analysis of the underlying mechanisms is a challenge for molecular biologists and electrophysiologists. The plateau of the action potential is especially sensitive to metabolic

inhibition. The changes are different for ischemia and hypoxia and an explanation for the dramatic increase in extracellular K^+ in ischemia remains incomplete. Manipulation of the action potential duration by blocking outward K^+ currents is currently being studied as a therapeutic intervention to prolong refractoriness and thus to extinguish reentry arrhythmias. In order to be selective against tachyarrhythmias, these drugs should show use dependency and fulfill certain kinetic requirements for block development and recovery from block.

Repolarization in cardiac cells is usually described as consisting of three phases: phase 1 or initial rapid repolarization, phase 2 or plateau, and phase 3 or final repolarization.[1] The relative importance of these phases is different according to the cell type. A rather positive plateau is seen in the sinoatrial and auriculoventricular node cells and in the ventricle. In atrial cells the plateau is less expressed and repolarization in general is more rapid. In Purkinje fibers, a long, rather negative plateau follows the pronounced initial repolarization or spike potential. This superficial description is far from complete and heterogeneity is much more pronounced. In atrial tissue, for

From BN Singh, HJJ Wellens, M Hiraoka, (eds): *Electropharmacological Control of Cardiac Arrhythmias.* Mount Kisco, NY, Futura Publishing Company Inc., © 1994.

instance, marked differences have been described between cells in the roof, the pectinate muscle, the crista terminalis, and strands between trabecular muscles. More recently the existence of a marked heterogeneity in the ventricle has been emphasized.[2] Apart from the Purkinje system, different types of action potential have been differentiated in the endocardial, the epicardial, and the mid-region layers of the ventricular myocardium (Figure 1). Epicardial myocytes are characterized by an action potential with a prominent initial rapid repolarization followed by a secondary depolarization, resulting in a characteristic spike-dome appearance. In the mid-region these two phases are still prominent, but the secondary depolarization runs out in a much longer plateau; the rate of depolarization during phase 0 or upstroke is also much greater. To a certain extent, the action potential in the mid-region resembles the action potential in Purkinje fibers.

Heterogeneity of Ionic Currents

In their original analysis, Hodgkin and Huxley[3] described the nerve action potential in terms of two successive currents, ie, an inward current followed by an outward current.

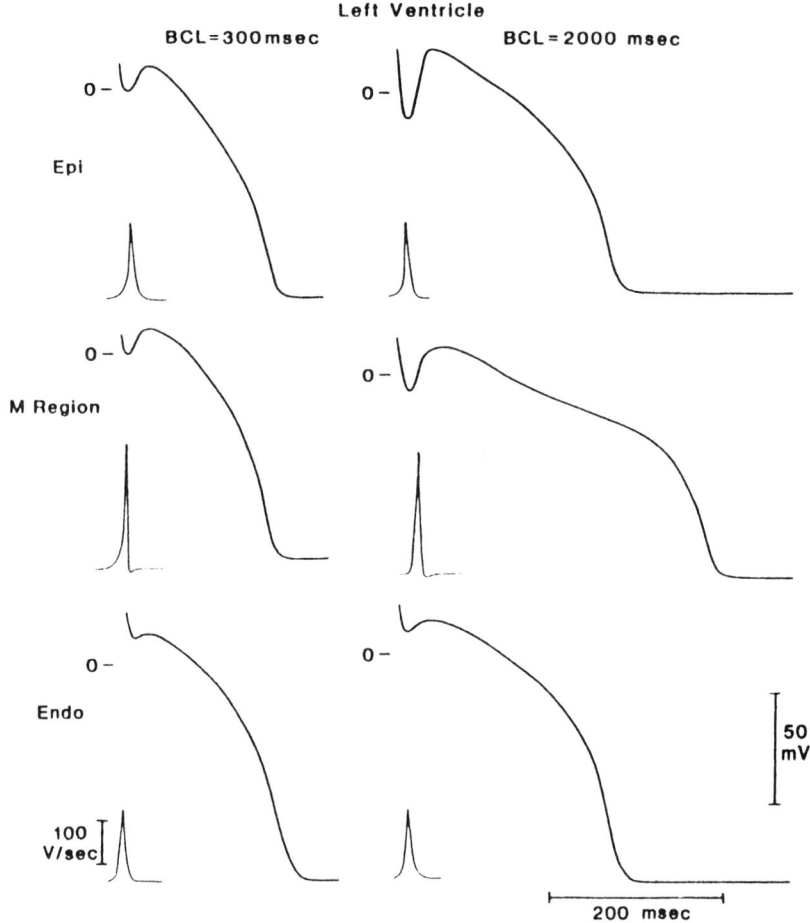

Figure 1. Action potential of epicardial (Epi), deep subepicardial (M Region), and endocardial (Endo) cells in the canine left ventricle at two basic cycle lengths of 0.3 and 2.0 seconds. (Reproduced with permission from Reference 2).

Since then, and especially following the development of the patch electrode,[4,5] electrophysiology has become more complex. Not only has the number of currents increased drastically but new mechanisms of activation have been described.[6] Actually, a distinction is made between voltage-operated, ligand-operated, and stretch-operated channels; important currents are also carried through exchanger and cotransporter molecules. In all these current systems the interaction between ions and transport molecules can be compared to enzymatic reactions, the difference is in the activation energy and the final outcome of the reaction. In contrast to classic enzymatic reactions, a channel or transporter does not transform a molecule, but translocates the ion across the membrane. For activation, energy is provided by a change in electrical gradient across the membrane (voltage-operated channels), by binding of a ligand (eg, acetylcholine, Ca^{2+} ions, adenosine triphosphate [ATP]), or by a mechanical deformation. In the case of exchangers and cotransporters, the situation resembles more closely the enzymatic reactions, and the ion movement is determined by the concentration gradient across the membrane.

Figure 2 illustrates the contribution of different ionic currents to the cardiac action potential and their time course. The typical configuration of the action potential in different parts of the heart depends on the relative density in which the channels and transporters are expressed. Attempts to quantify this information have been made and computer models are already available for the sinoatrial node action potential,[8,9] the Purkinje fiber,[10]

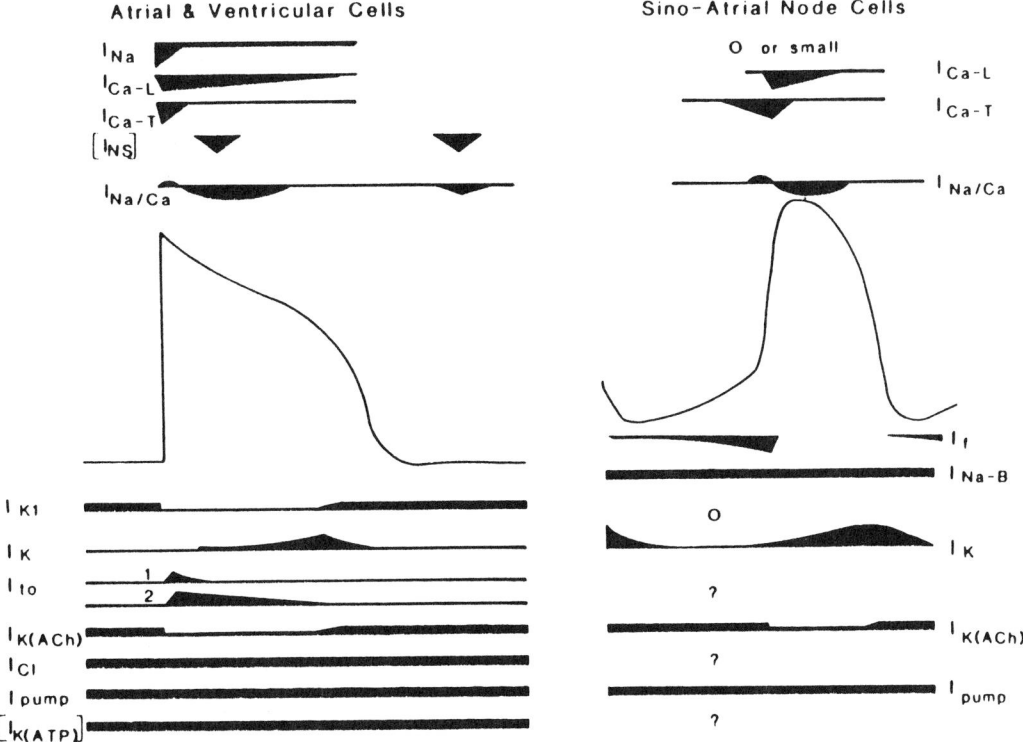

Figure 2. Schematic representation of currents involved in generating the resting and action potential in atrial and ventricular cells (left) and in sinoatrial cells (right). Above (inward currents) and below (outward currents) underlying the action potential. Only approximate time course and amplitudes are indicated. The relative contribution varies depending on the physiological condition, some currents (brackets) are only seen in pathological situations. (Reproduced with permission from Reference 7).

and the ventricular (endocardial) myocyte.[11,12] Such modeling is useful because it sets certain limits on the interpretation and makes it possible to propose new tests for future experiments. The actual picture however, is far from complete.

Modulation of the Action Potential Duration

Rate

By definition, time-dependent currents are sensitive to rate. The time dependence is related to the activation and inactivation processes. Currents that only activate undergo summation when the "diastolic" period is shorter than the time constant of deactivation. This can be the case for the delayed K^+ current in the range of elevated physiological frequencies. Conversely, currents that also inactivate become less pronounced when the diastolic period is too short to allow complete recovery from inactivation. This may be the case for Na^+ and Ca^{2+} currents and for the

transient outward current I_{to}. Furthermore, rate may affect currents by changing the intra- or extracellular concentration of ions (Na^+, K^+, Ca^{2+}). An increase in Na_i^+ stimulates the Na^+-K^+ pump and thus produces an outward current. Conversely, an increase in intracellular Ca^{2+} favors outward Ca^{2+} transport through the Na^+-Ca^{2+} exchanger and since 3 Na^+ ions move in for exchange of 1 Ca^{2+} ion it produces an inward current, especially at more negative potentials. The same increase in Ca^{2+}_i may, however, enhance the rate of Ca^{2+} current inactivation and decrease inward current at more depolarized levels. Extracellular accumulation of K^+, especially in multicellular preparations, stimulates the Na^+-K^+ pump, and modulates the inward rectifier channel. The inward rectifier channel indeed is very sensitive to K^+_e. In the absence of K^+_e the current is completely absent. A rise in K^+_e increases the current through the channel in such a way that the current-voltage relations cross each other. The current through this channel determines the resting membrane potential and also the "threshold" and rate for the final repolarization; at ele-

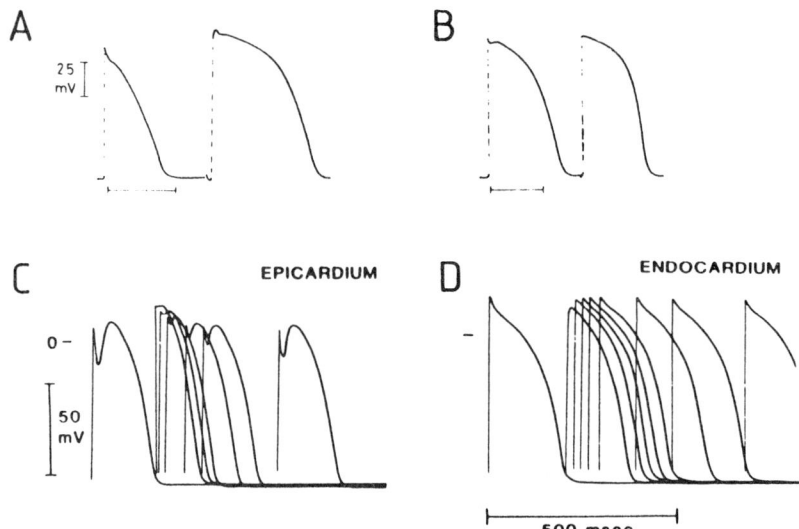

Figure 3. Changes in action potential configuration with premature stimulation. A and B are redrawn from Reference 13 (rabbit ventricle) and from Reference 14 (dog ventricle). Horizontal calibration is 0.1 seconds. C and D: Restitution of action potential parameters in epicardial and endocardial slices taken from the dog ventricle. (Reproduced with permission from Reference 15).

vated K^+_e concentration repolarization becomes shorter and faster.

In discussing the effect of rate it is necessary to distinguish between sudden changes in rhythm and changes in steady-state frequency. The action potential of an extrasystole can be shorter or longer (Figure 3), depending on whether activation of outward K^+ current, and inactivation of inward Na^+ or Ca^{2+} currents are more important than the inactivation of the transient outward current I_{to}. Inactivation of I_{to} is probably the reason for the prolongation and elevation of the plateau in the rabbit ventricular cell when the rate is suddenly increased. In most other species, how-

ever, an extrasystole is characterized by an overall shortening of the action potential duration that is accompanied by an elevation (epicardium) or a depression (endocardium) of the plateau level (Figure 3). Although inhibition of the transient outward current results in a slower repolarization, this effect is more than compensated by an increase in delayed K^+ current (due to the larger depolarization) and a decrease in inward Ca^{2+} current (more inactivation and smaller chemical gradient).

In steady state the action potential duration is shorter the greater the frequency, at least in the physiological range of frequencies (Figure 4). Cumulative effects in the activation

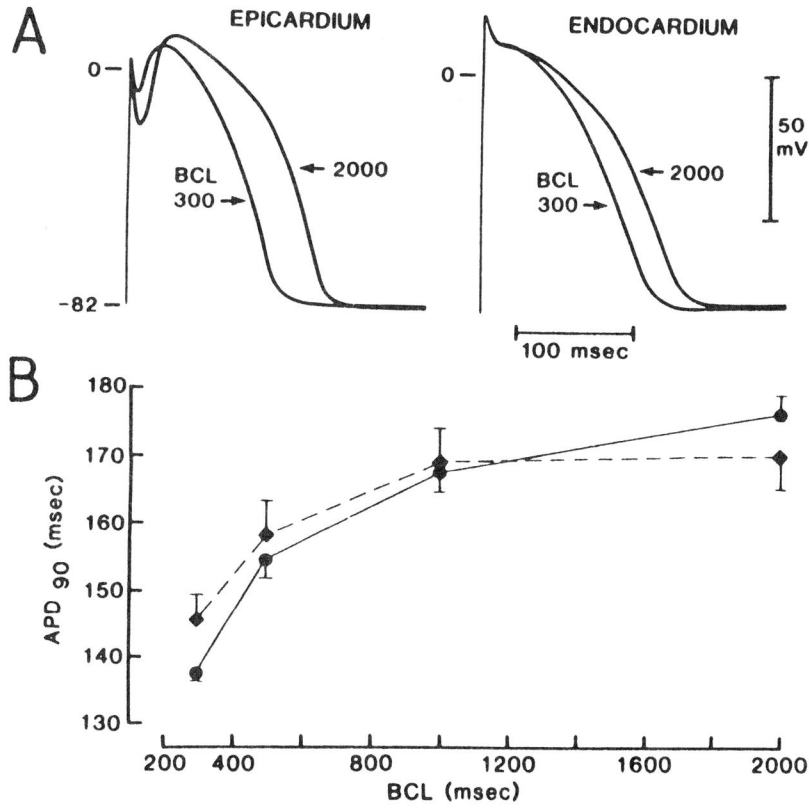

Figure 4. The effect of steady-state stimulation rate on transmembrane activity recorded from canine epicardial and endocardial ventricular preparations. A: Superimposed traces of action potentials recorded at basic cycle lengths (BCL) of 0.3 and 2.0 seconds. Epicardium, unlike endocardium, shows rate-dependent changes in the early phases of the action potential that contribute to the overall prolongation of the action potential following deceleration of the stimulation rate. B: Action potential duration measured at 90% repolarization (APD₉₀) plotted as a function of the BCL (steady-state conditions) for epicardial (circles) and endocardial (lozenges) preparations. (Reproduced with permission from Reference 15).

of i_K and inactivation of i_{Ca}, together with stimulatory effects of the Na^+-K^+ pump current and eventually K^+_e accumulation play an important role in causing this shortening of the action potential. But differences also exist between different parts of the heart and the shortening is more pronounced in the epicardium than in the endocardium (Figure 1 and Figure 4), resulting in specific changes of the T wave in the electrocardiogram.

Development

The change in action potential configuration and the accompanying change in ionic currents has best been analyzed in the rat ventricle. In the neonate, the action potential with a well-pronounced positive plateau changes to an action potential of a more complex nature: an initial spike-like repolarization is followed by a more or less pronounced plateau and finally by a much slower phase of repolarization at a more negative potential level (Figure 5). Voltage-clamp experiments have shown that the Na^+ current in the adult is increased in amplitude, an effect caused by a higher density of the channels; inactivation, however, occurs faster.[17] The change in Ca^{2+} current is quite different. Although the inactivation process is accelerated, the amplitude of the Ca^{2+} current (normalized to the surface of membrane) becomes smaller in the adult.[16] This decrease in Ca^{2+} current is accompanied by a greater development of the T tubular system and the sarcoplasmic reticulum, which is very dense in the adult rat ventricle even when compared to myocytes of other species. The morphological changes can be correlated with changes in sensitivity to ryanodine and in the excitation-contraction coupling process. For example, postextrasystolic potentiation is more pronounced in the adult. The faster inactivation of the Ca^{2+} current has been explained as caused by the pronounced increase in cytoplasmic Ca^{2+} following its release from the sarcoplasmic reticulum. A prominent Na^+-Ca^{2+} exchange current seems to be responsible for the final slow repolarization phase; it has been shown to be sensitive to external Na^+ and internal Ca^{2+}.[12,18] Conflicting results have been published on the inward rectifier K^+ channel. According to Kilborn and Fedida,[19] the i_{K1} current is decreased in magnitude, and this reduction explains the maturational slowing of repolarization during the final phase of the action potential. With development, there is

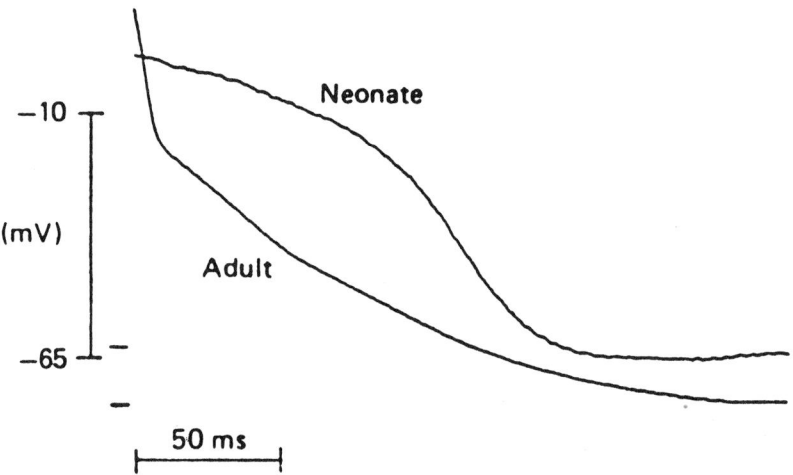

Figure 5. Action potentials in a single cultured neonatal and single adult ventricular myocyte from the rat ventricle. Stimulus rate: 0.5 Hz; temperature: 21–22°C. (Reproduced with permission from Reference 16).

an important increase in sensitivity to metabolic inhibition. This change can be correlated to a difference in the biochemical availability of enzymes necessary for anaerobic glycolysis, and probably to a greater density of the ATP-dependent K^+ channels.

Metabolism

Inhibition of metabolism has important consequences on the electrical activity of the cardiac cell. The changes depend on whether inhibition of metabolism is only due to a shortage of supply (hypoxia, absence of glucose) or is accompanied by a blockade of waste removal (ischemia). The electrical activity is changed during and following the metabolic insult.

During metabolic inhibition, the concentration of ATP drops, while that of H^+ increases.[20] A shift from aerobic metabolism towards anaerobic glycolysis is responsible for the less efficient production of ATP and the excess of protons. Both changes affect the behavior of ionic channels and transporters. In general, acidification is accompanied by an inhibition of the conductance and/or open probability of a number of channels, such as the i_{Ki}, i_{Ca}, and i_{Na}.[21] In some instances the effect is because of intracellular acidification, in others extracellular acidification. The fall in ATP concentration and changes in pH cause inhibition of active ion movement across the plasma membranes, which results in an increase of Na^+_i, Ca^{2+}_i, and a decrease in K^+_i. The fall in ATP, when of sufficient amplitude, may also activate the ATP-dependent K^+ channel that is abundantly present in cardiac cells. Activation requires very low ATP concentrations, which are unlikely if ATP is uniformly distributed in the cell cytoplasm. However, evidence indicates that microheterogeneity occurs in the distribution of a number of substances and even of ions in the cell cytoplasm (for a discussion, see Carmeliet[22]). In the case of ATP, the concentration near the cell membrane seems to be governed by local glycolysis, and activation of the ATP-dependent channel has been observed in inside-out patches following blockade of the glycolytic pathway.[23] The results suggest that the channels and enzymes of the glycolytic pathway form a functional unit. Activation of the ATP-dependent K^+ channel generates an outward current, favors repolarization, and shortens the action potential duration. This occurs in hypoxia or mild ischemia when washout of the extracellular space is still sufficient. It is interesting to note that shortening of the action potential by activation of the ATP-dependent K^+ channel is greater in the epicardial than in the endocardial fibers (Figure 6A). This effect is related to the ATP-dependent channel being more sensitive to ATP blockade in the endocardium.[24] A greater fall of ATP concentration is required to activate the channel (Figure 6B). It explains the so-called resistance to metabolic inhibition of the endocardial myocardium.

When washout of the extracellular space is insufficient (ischemia), K^+ accumulation occurs. The duration of the action potential is not markedly changed, but the cell depolarizes and finally inexcitability occurs (Figure 7). The increase in K^+_e can attain values of 10–15 mM.[26] The mechanisms involved are not well understood. It is clear that the ATP-dependent K^+ channel is activated under these conditions, but this alone is not sufficient to cause K^+ accumulation. There is a need for an inward leak current that causes the membrane potential to stay positive to the equilibrium potential for K^+ ions (E_K). It is not known whether the normal leak current that is responsible for the deviation between the resting membrane potential and E_K under nonischemic conditions is large enough or whether a leak current is generated under ischemic conditions. In this respect the transport of lactic acid to the extracellular medium has been considered.[27,28] Lactate efflux as an anion could balance the charge movement of K^+ ions. The following should be noted: (1) there is no direct experimental evidence for transport of lactate as a negative charge through the membrane; and (2) although the amount of lactic acid and K^+ may be of ap-

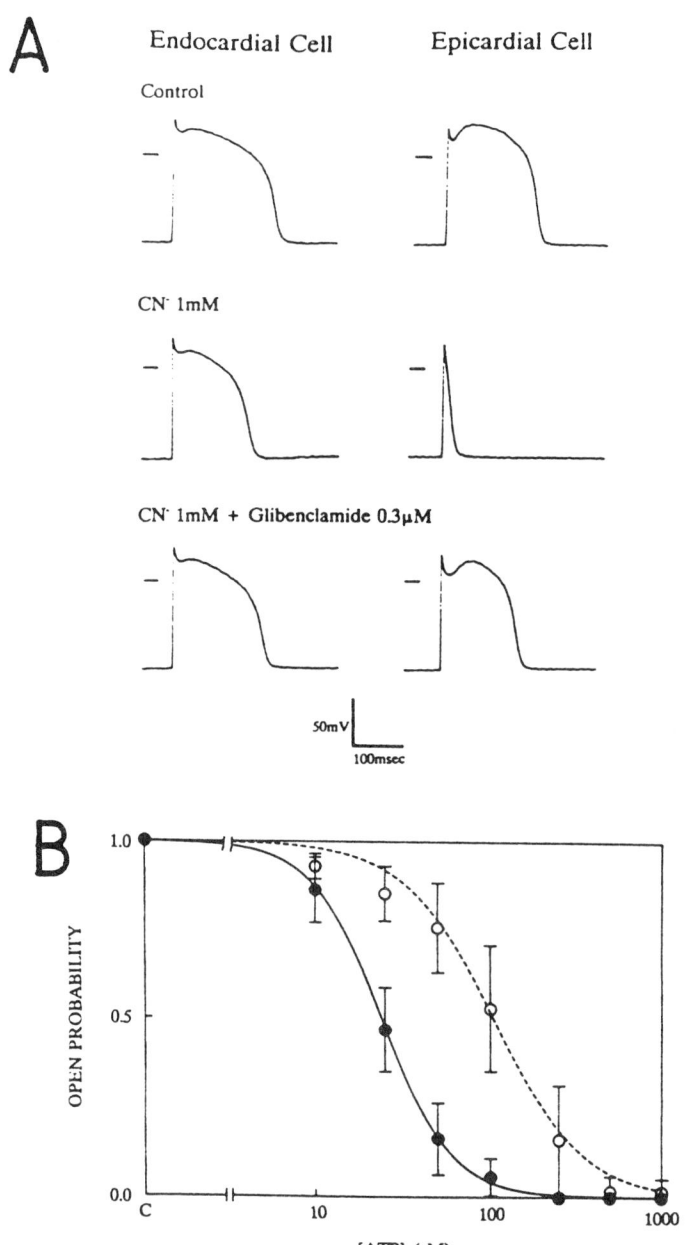

Figure 6. A: Recordings showing the effect of CN 1 mM and glibenclamide on the action potential in endocardial and epicardial ventricular cells from the cat. Stimulation rate 1 Hz. B: Plot showing dose-response relations between intracellular ATP concentration ([ATP]$_i$) and channel open state probability (expressed as a fraction of the value in the absence of ATP) for endocardial (filled circles, $n = 17$) and epicardial (open circles, $n = 14$) membrane patches. ATP concentration for half-maximal inhibition of channel activity was 23.6 ± 21.9 μM for endocardial cells and 97.6 ± 48.1 μM for epicardial cells ($p > 0.01$). (Reproduced with permission from Reference 24).

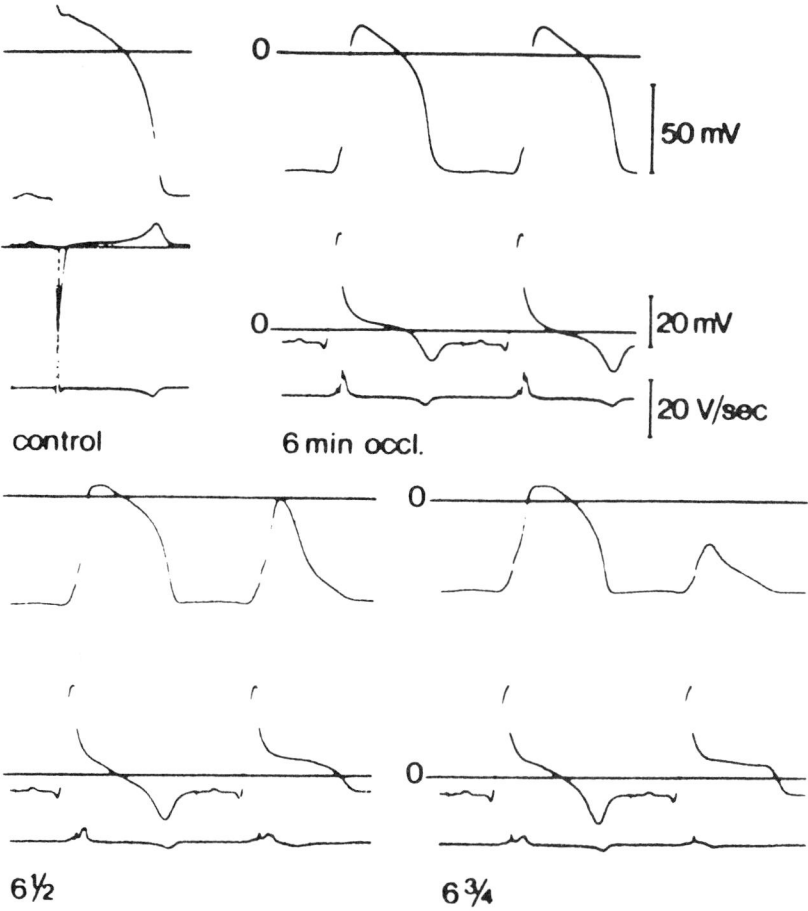

Figure 7. Transmembrane potentials (upper trace), local DC extracellular electrograms (middle trace), and dV/dt of transmembrane potential (lower trace) before and after coronary artery occlusion in an isolated, blood-perfused, porcine heart. (Reproduced with permission from Reference 25).

proximately the same magnitude, K^+ loss can occur in the presence of a block of lactic acid movement and even in the absence of permeant anions.[29] Therefore, the problem of which ion balances K^+ efflux remains unsolved.

On reperfusion the excess extracellular K^+ and H^+ is washed out, and an exchange of intracellular protons for extracellular Na^+ occurs. The increase in Na^+ may lead to a secondary rise in Ca^{2+}_i via the Na^+-Ca^{2+} exchanger; it also may activate Na^+-dependent K^+ channels. Restoration of the normal oxygen tension is further accompanied by the generation of large quantities of oxygen-free radicals. All these changes affect the electrical behavior of the cells and play a role in the generation of arrhythmias. Information on the electrical changes at the cellular level is only available from in vitro models in which oxygen-free radicals are generated by photoactivation of rose bengal[30,31] or superfusion with dihydroxyfumarate.[32] The effect on the action potential duration in these models is variable, although in most cases a prolongation was observed with development of early afterdepolarizations and eventually late afterdepolarizations following full repolarization (Figure 8A

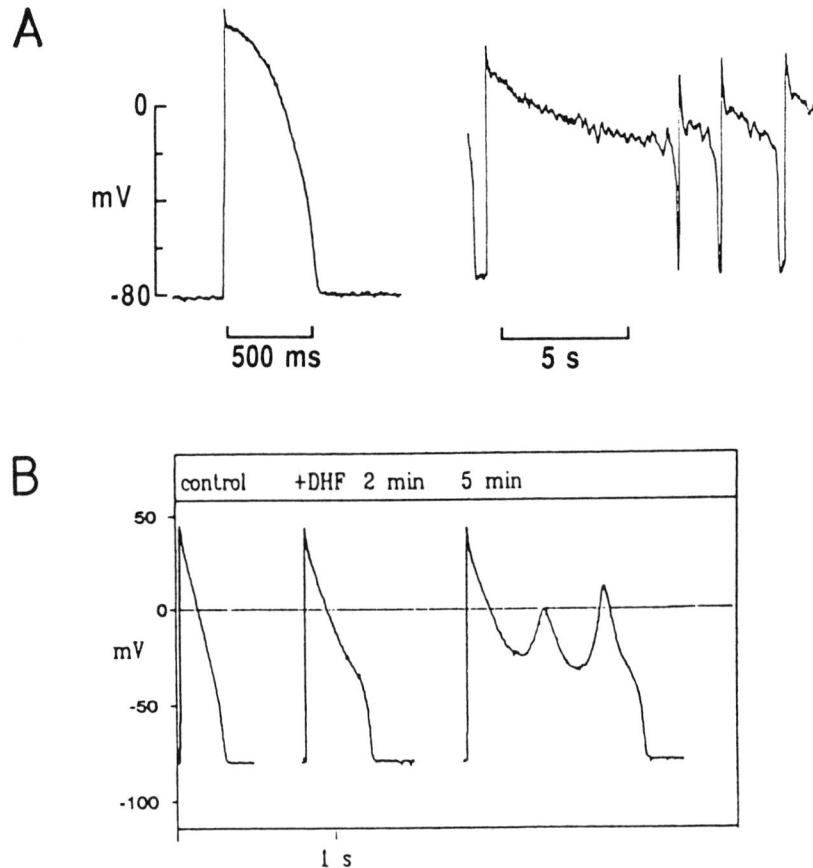

Figure 8. A: Action potentials recorded from an isolated rabbit ventricular myocyte before (left) and during exposure (right) to oxidant stress generated by the photoactivation of rose bengal (50 nmol/L) after 7-minute exposure. Recordings were made at a stimulation rate of 0.1-Hz via a wide-tipped patch pipette. (Reprinted with permission from Reference 30). B: Plot showing effects of oxygen radicals generated by dihydroxyfumarate (DHF) on action potential profile of isolated myocytes. (Reproduced with permission from Reference 32).

and 8B). The oscillations were shown to be correlated with a surcharge in intracellular Ca^{2+}, at the same time the Ca^{2+} current and the delayed K^+ current were inhibited.

Drugs

Manipulation, and more specifically prolongation, of the action potential duration by drugs is considered to be an important antiarrhythmic intervention. In reentry-type arrhythmias with a pathway containing a short excitable gap only a small increase in refractoriness is needed to block the arrhythmia. From a theoretical point of view, a prolongation of the action potential can be brought about by enhancing Na^+ and/or Ca^{2+} inward current or reducing K^+ outward current (Figure 9). It is noteworthy that for drugs acting on the inward Na^+ or Ca^{2+} current the increase in current is caused by one of the enantiomers, while the other exerts the opposite effect eventually at a higher concentration or at another voltage.[33,34] Enhancing Ca^{2+} influx could possibly produce Ca^{2+} overload and

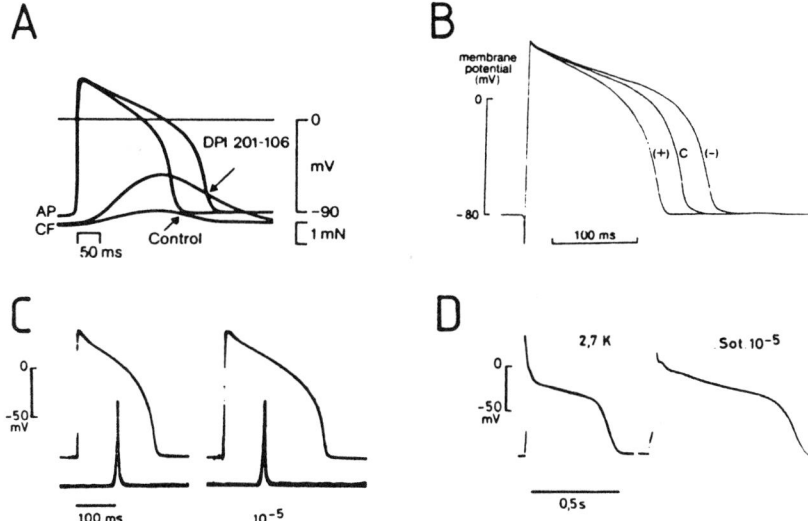

Figure 9. A: Superimposed action potentials and isometric contractions in guinea pig papillary muscles before (control) and during application of DPI 201–106 (10^{-6}M) (Reproduced with permission from Reference 33). B: Effect of Bay K 8644 enantiomers on action potential of guinea pig papillary muscles in control conditions (C), in the presence of 10^{-6}M (+)Bay K 8644(+) and in the presence of an additional concentration of 10^{-6}M (−) Bay K 8644 (−). The action potential duration increased to values higher than the control. (Reproduced with permission from Reference 34). C: Action potentials and upstroke velocities in guinea pig papillary muscle in control and in the presence of sotalol 10^{-5}M. (Reproduced with permission from Reference 35). D: Action potentials in a rabbit Purkinje fiber preparation in control and in the presence of 10^{-5}M sotalol. (Reproduced with permission from Reference 35).

trigger arrhythmias (delayed afterdepolarizations). DPI 201–106 increases the Na^+ current during the plateau by prolonging the inactivation process. If this effect is accompanied by an inhibition of the peak current (as is seen with the racemic mixture) the drug may act as an antiarrhythmic by reducing upstroke velocity and prolonging the refractory period. The absence of a marked change in total Na^+ inward movement explains the absence of a negative inotropic effect. Penticainide, a disopyramide analogue, also acts in a similar way.[36]

Block of outward current is an alternative mechanism to stop reentry arrhythmias. In the case of a block of the transient outward current the final result on the action potential duration is quite variable. In cells with a pronounced spike-dome configuration a small inhibition of I_{to} will be accompanied by a more positive early plateau, less activation of the

secondary depolarization, and paradoxically, a shortening of the action potential.[15] In cells with less secondary depolarization or less i_K, eg, rat ventrcular myocytes[37] or atrial cells in general, block of I_{to} will prolong the action potential.

The delayed K^+ current is a second target for substances blocking outward current and a number of newly developed drugs are being evaluated for their antiarrhythmic activity. Unfortunately, none of these drugs seem to fulfill the requirements of the "ideal" drug in the sense that they prolong the action potential preferentially at high frequencies of stimulation and minimally affect the duration at low frequencies.[38] In order to do so they should block the i_K channel during activation with a time constant greater than 1 second, and show a recovery from block during diastole with a time constant on the order of 100 msec. A drug that fulfills these requirements would show use and frequency dependency. A number of drugs under investigation show open channel and use-dependent block, but recovery from block is so slow that in steady state the frequency-dependent block is small or absent.[39–41] Quinidine allegedly blocks preferentially in the rested state, and unblocks during activation, a process that would lead to reverse use dependency.[42] More recent experiments have shown that the quinidine-induced change in current during depolarization in the guinea pig myocyte is not evidence for unblocking, but is due to the presence of two components, of which only one (ie, the rapid component) is sensitive to blockade.[43,44] More direct evidence for block during the open state has also been reported.[45,46] Actually there is no demonstration of reverse use dependency. This does not mean that there is no evidence for a "reverse" frequency dependency of the action potential duration. It should be emphasized, however, that the term reverse use dependency should not be used for the more pronounced lengthening of the action potential at low frequencies. Use dependency is a term that should be restricted to phenomena at the channel level. It should also be realized that the action potential duration depends on the interaction of many channels, and not only on the delayed K^+ current.

Action Potential Duration and Refractoriness

Under normal conditions a close relation exists between action potential duration and recovery of excitability. Excitability is determined by the current required to displace the membrane potential to a level where sufficient inward current is activated such that the membrane current becomes net inward. This starts the positive feedback cycle leading to a full-sized upstroke of the action potential. Following the upstroke of the action potential, the Na^+ channels remain inactivated during most of the plateau duration. It is only during the final repolarization phase that Na^+ channels recover from inactivation and may again

become activated. Recovery of the Na^+ channels is a potential-dependent phenomenon and very fast (10 msec or less) at negative membrane potentials. Under these conditions, action potential duration and refractoriness are closely connected. Any change or any difference in action potential duration is accompanied by a change or difference in refractoriness.

This close relationship, however, may be broken by other conditions such as ischemia, high extracellular K^+ concentration, or presence of drugs acting on the Na^+ channel. In the presence of high K^+_e, eg, the cell membrane depolarizes and part of the Na^+ channels become inactivated at rest. The remaining channels, when inactivated during the action potential, will recover more slowly because of the less negative resting potential. Refractoriness lags behind full repolarization. A similar situation is caused by the use of antiarrhythmic drugs acting on the Na^+ channels, especially those that block the channel in the inactivated state. A decrease in Na^+ current especially at depolarized levels will reduce excitability, prolong the time of recovery, and cause a dissociation between action potential duration and refractoriness. Antiarrhythmic drugs acting on the i_K current, however, will not exert this dissociating effect and any prolongation of the action potential will be accompanied by an equally important change in refractoriness without modification of the recovery phenomena during and after the final repolarization.

References

1. Hoffman BF, Cranefield PF: *Electrophysiology of the Heart.* New York: McGraw-Hill, 1960.
2. Sicouri S, Antzelevitch C: A subpopulation of cells with unique electrophysiological properties in the deep subepicardium of the canine ventricle. *Circ Res* 68:1729, 1991.
3. Hodgkin AL, Huxley AF: Currents carried by sodium and potassium ions through the membrane of the giant axon of Loligo. *J Physiol (Lond)* 116:449, 1952.
4. Neher E, Sakmann B: Single channel currents recorded from membrane of denervated frog muscle fibres. *Nature* 260:799, 1976.

5. Hamill OP, Marty A, Neher E, et al: Improved patch-clamp techniques for high-resolution current recordings from cells and cell-free membrane patches. *Pflügers Arch* 391:85, 1981.

6. Hille B: *Ionic Channels of Excitable Membranes*. Sunderland, MA: Sinauer Associates, 1992.

7. The Sicilian Gambit: Task force of the working group on arrhythmias of the European Society of Cardiology. A new approach to the classification of antiarrhythmic drugs based on their actions on arrhythmogenic mechanisms. *Circulation* 84:1831, 1990.

8. Noble D, Noble SJ: A model of sinoatrial node electrical activity using a modification of the DiFrancesco-Noble (1984) equations. *Proc R Soc Lond B Biol* 222:295, 1984.

9. Noble D, DiFrancesco D, Denyer JC: Ionic mechanisms in normal and abnormal cardiac pacemaker activity. In: JW Jacklet (ed): *Neonatal and Cellular Oscillators*. New York/Basel: Marcel Dekker, 1989, p. 59.

10. DiFrancesco D, Noble D: A model of cardiac electrical activity incorporating ionic pumps and concentration changes. *Philos Trans R Soc Lond B* 307:353, 1985.

11. Beeler GW Jr, Reuter H: Reconstruction of the action potential of ventricular myocardial fibres. *J Physiol (Lond)* 268:177, 1977.

12. Hilgemann DW, Noble D: Excitation-contraction and extracellular calcium transients in rabbit atrium: reconstruction of basic cellular mechansms. *Proc R Soc Lond B* 230:163, 1987.

13. Gibbs CL, Johnson EA: Effect of changes in frequency of stimulation upon rabbit ventricular action potential. *Circ Res* 9:165, 1961.

14. Hoffman BF, Suckling EE: Effect of heart rate on cardiac membrane potentials and the unipolar electrogram. *Am J Physiol* 179:123, 1954.

15. Antzelevitch C, Litovsky SH, Lukas A: Epicardium versus endocardium: electrophysiology and pharmacology. In: DP Zipes, J Jalife (eds): *Cardiac Electrophysiology. From Cell to Bedside*. Philadelphia, PA: W.B. Saunders Company, 1990, p. 386.

16. Cohen NM, Lederer WJ: Changes in the calcium current of rat heart ventricular myocytes during development. *J Physiol (Lond)* 406:115, 1988.

17. Conforti L, Tohse N, Sperelakis N: Developmental changes in fast sodium current of rat ventricular cardiomyocytes. *Biophys J* 61:A305, 1992.

18. Schouten VJA, ter Keurs HEDJ: The slow repolarization phase of the action potential in rat heart. *J Physiol (Lond)* 360:13, 1985.

19. Kilborn MJ, Fedida D: A study of the developmental changes in outward currents of rat ventricular myocytes. *J Physiol (Lond)* 430:37, 1990.

20. Gevers W: Generation of protons by metabolic processes in heart cells. *J Mol Cell Cardiol* 9:867, 1977.

21. Ito H, Vereecke J, Carmeliet E: Intracellular protons inhibits inward rectifier K^+ channel of guinea-pig ventricular cell membrane. *Pflügers Arch* 422:280, 1992.

22. Carmeliet E: A fuzzy subsarcolemmal space for intracellular Na^+ in cardiac cells? *Cardiovasc Res* 26:433, 1992.

23. Weiss JN, Lamp ST: Cardiac ATP-sensitive K^+ channels. Evidence for preferential regulation by glycolysis. *J Gen Physiol* 94:911, 1989.

24. Furukawa T, Kimura S, Furukawa N, et al: Role of cardiac ATP-regulated potassium channels in differential responses of endocardial and epicardial cells to ischemia. *Circ Res* 68:1693, 1991.

25. Janse MJ: Models of ischemia and mechanisms of arrhythmias. In: J Vereecke, PP van Bogaert, F Verdonck (eds): *Ionic Currents and Ischemia*. Leuven, Belgium: Leuven University Press, 1990, p. 145.

26. Hill JL, Gettes LS: Effect of acute coronary artery occlusion on local myocardial extracellular K^+ activity in swine. *Circulation* 61:768, 1980.

27. Kléber AG: Extracellullar K^+ accumulation in acute myocardial ischemia. *J Mol Cell Cardiol* 16:389, 1984.

28. Weiss JN, Lamp ST, Shine KI: Cellular K^+ loss and ion efflux during myocardial ischemia and metabolic inhibition. *Am J Physiol* 256:H1165, 1989.

29. Gasser RNA, Vaughan-Jones RD: Mechanism of potassium efflux and action potential shortening during ischaemia in isolated mammalian cardiac muscle. *J Physiol (Lond)* 431:713, 1990.

30. Shattock MJ, Hearse DJ, Matsuura H: Ionic currents underlying oxidant stress-induced arrhythmias. In: J Vereecke, PP van Bogaert, F Verdonck (eds): *Ionic Currents and Ischemia*. Leuven, Belgium: Leuven University Press, 1990, p. 165.

31. Matsuura H, Shattock MJ: Effects of oxidant stress on steady-state background currents in isolated ventricular cells of rabbit heart. *J Mol Cell Cardiol* 22(Suppl III):PW57, 1990.

32. Cerbai E, Ambrosio G, Porciatti F, et al: Cellular electrophysiological basis for oxygen radical-induced arrhythmias. A patch-clamp study in guinea pig ventricular myocytes. *Circulation* 84:1773, 1991.

33. Scholtysik G, Salzmann R, Berthold R, et al: DPI 201–106, a novel cardioactive agent. Combination of cAMP-independent positive inotropic, negative chronotropic, action potential prolonging and coronary dilatory properties. *Naunyn Schmiedebergs Arch Pharmacol* 329:316, 1985.

34. Franckowiak G, Bechem M, Schramm M, et al: The optical isomers of the 1.4-dihydropyridine Bay K 8644 show opposite effects on Ca channels. *Eur J Pharmacol* 114:223, 1985.

35. Carmeliet E: Electrophysiologic and voltage clamp analysis of the effects of sotalol on isolated cardiac muscle and Purkinje fibers. *J Pharmacol Exp Ther* 232:817, 1985.

36. Gruber R, Vereecke J, Carmeliet E: Dual effect of the local anaesthetic penticainide on the Na^+ current of guinea-pig ventricular myocytes. *J Physiol (Lond)* 435:65, 1991.

37. Dukes ID, Cleemann L, Morad M: Tedisamil blocks the transient and delayed rectifier K^+ currents in mammalian cardiac and glial cells. *J Pharmacol Exp Ther* 254:560, 1990.

38. Hondeghem LM, Snyders DJ: Class III antiarrhythmic agents have a lot of potential but a long way to go. Reduced effectiveness and dangers of reverse use-dependence. *Circulation* 81:686, 1990.

39. Carmeliet E: Block of the delayed K^+ current by Hässle 234/09 in rabbit cardiac myocytes. *J Mol Cell Cardiol* 23(Suppl I):P69, 1991.

40. Carmeliet E: Use-dependent block of the delayed K^+ current in cardiac cells. A comparison of different drugs with Class III activity (abstract). *J Mol Cell Cardiol* 24(Suppl I):S108, 1992.

41. Carmeliet E: Voltage- and time-dependent block of the delayed K^+ current in cardiac myocytes by dofetilide. *J Pharmacol Exp Ther* 262:809, 1992.

42. Roden DM, Bennett PB, Snyders DJ, et al: Quinidine delays I_K activation in guinea-pig ventricular myocytes. *Circ Res* 62:1055, 1988.

43. Sanguinetti MC, Jurkiewicz NK: Two components of cardiac delayed rectifier K^+ current: differential sensitivity to block by class III antiarrhythmic agents. *J Gen Physiol* 96:195, 1990.

44. Colatsky TJ, Follmer CH, Starmer CF: Channel specificity in antiarrhythmic drug action. Mechanism of potassium channel block and its role in suppressing and aggravating cardiac arrhythmias. *Circulation* 82:2235, 1990.

45. Furukawa T, Tsujimura Y, Kitamura K, et al: Time- and voltage-dependent block of the delayed K^+ current by quinidine in rabbit sinoatrial and atrioventricular nodes. *J Pharmacol Exp Ther* 251:756, 1989.

46. Snyders DJ, Knoth KM, Roberds SL, et al: Time-, and voltage-, and state-dependent block by quinidine of a cloned human cardiac potassium channel. *Mol Pharmacol* 41:322, 1992.

Chapter 4

Significance of Autonomically Regulated Chloride Channels for Antiarrhythmic Drug Action

Joseph R. Hume
Craig D. Clark
Sergey I. Zakharov
Paul C. Levesque

In the heart, adenosine $3',5'$-cyclic monophosphate (cAMP) is known to regulate a variety of membrane channels.[1] β-Adrenergic regulation of L-type Ca^{2+} channels[2–6] and delayed rectifier K^+ channels[7,8] involves the cAMP-dependent protein kinase (PKA) pathway (Figure 1) and modulation of these channels are believed to be largely responsible for the alterations of the cardiac action potential that are characteristic of β-adrenergic stimulation throughout the heart. Sympathetic modulation of the action potential duration is a complicated process that may result in action potential prolongation, shortening, or little change. This variability in response to sympathetic stimulation is due to activation of several ionic channels that may have mutually antagonistic effects on the action potential plateau and duration. In addition to modulation of myocardial Ca^{2+} and delayed rectifier K^+ channels, β-adrenergic stimulation of PKA has also been shown to regulate myocardial Na^+ channels,[9,10] the Na^+-K^+ pump[11] and the hyperpolarization-activated inward current, I_f,[12] which may contribute to the generation of the pacemaker potential in some cardiac cells. The recent discovery of a new class of ion channels, cAMP-dependent chloride channels $[I_{Cl(cAMP)}]$, which are also activated through PKA stimulation,[13,14] may prove to be an additional important mechanism for autonomic regulation of action potential duration. It is also clear that parasympathetic stimulation can also produce variable changes in the duration of the cardiac action potential by antagonizing β-adrenergic modulation of many of these channels through a guanine nucleotide protein inhibition (G_i protein) of adenylate cyclase activity,[1,7,15] although an additional effect of muscarinic stimulation on phosphodi-

Supported by NIH grant HL30143 (J.R.H.); a National Research Service Award Postdoctoral Fellowship (P.C.L); and the U.S.-U.S.S.R. Health Exchange Program in Sudden Cardiac Death (S.I.Z.).
From BN Singh, HJJ Wellens, M Hiraoka, (eds): *Electropharmacological Control of Cardiac Arrhythmias.* Mount Kisco, NY, Futura Publishing Company Inc., © 1994.

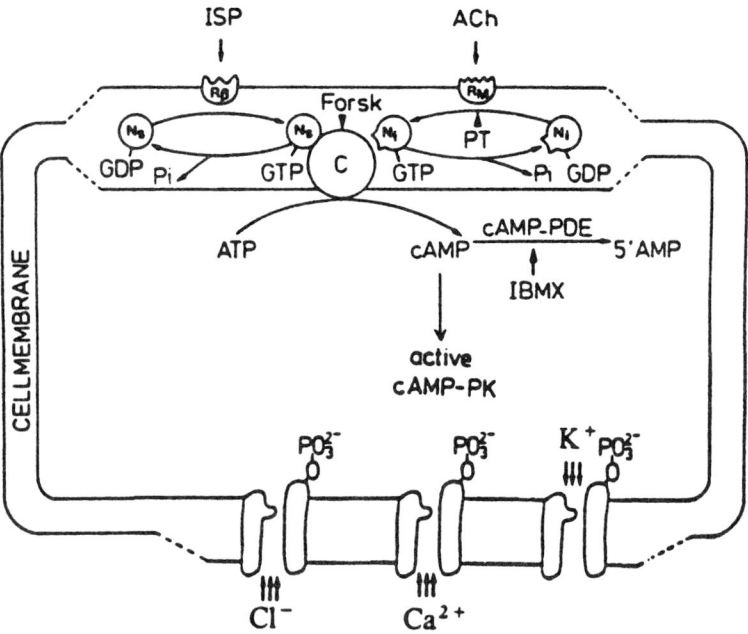

Figure 1. Simplified scheme of the β-adrenergic and muscarinic regulation of Ca^{2+}, K^+ and Cl^- channels in the heart. R_β: β-adrenergic receptor; R_M: muscarinic receptor; N_s: stimulatory guanine nucleotide proteins; N_i: inhibitory guanine nucleotide proteins; C: catalytic subunit of adenylate cyclase; cAMP-PDE: cAMP-dependent phosphodiesterase; cAMP-PK: cAMP-dependent protein kinase. (Modified with permission from Reference 15.)

esterase activity has also been reported.[16] Another complicating factor in understanding autonomic regulation of the cardiac action potential is the ability of norepinephrine to additionally act on myocardial α-adrenergic receptors, which have been reported to modulate K^+ currents[17,18] and possibly Ca^{2+} currents in the heart.[19,20]

The multitude of effectors that are modulated by autonomic stimulation makes it difficult to predict, under a given set of experimental or clinical conditions, which effects will prevail to alter the cardiac action potential plateau and duration. It is also obvious that cardiac cells have a number of mechanisms by which autonomic tone may alter the electrical response of cells to antiarrhythmic drugs that are designed to prolong action potential duration and refractoriness. This chapter focuses on the properties of the recently discovered cAMP-dependent Cl^- channels, their role in modulating the ventricular action potential,

and the potential usefulness of pharmacological antagonists of Cl^- channels as Class III antiarrhythmic agents.

Properties of cAMP-Dependent Cl^- Channels

The properties of anion channels in the heart has recently been reviewed.[21] Some of the properties of the cAMP-dependent Cl^- channels will be briefly summarized. These channels are activated by β-adrenergic stimulation that appears to involve a similar intracellular pathway that is also involved in regulating the activity of L-type Ca^{2+} channels and delayed rectifier K^+ channels. Involvement of this pathway is supported by the finding that the current can also be activated by forskolin, cAMP, phosphodiesterase inhibitors, and the catalytic subunit of PKA. Once the current is activated, it can be inhibited by β-adrenergic receptor antagonists, acetylcholine, and adenosine. The chloride current can also be activated by histamine acting on H_2 receptors in guinea pig ventricle.[22] These chloride channels have a relatively high permeability to chloride anions and exhibit rectification under conditions of an asymmetrical Cl^- gradient across the membrane.[23] The single channels responsible for $I_{Cl(cAMP)}$ exhibit a unitary conductance of approximately 8–13 picosiemens (pS).[24,25] Blockers of $I_{Cl(cAMP)}$ include relatively impermeant anions such as aspartate and glutamate, 9-anthracene carboxylic acid (9-AC), a blocker of skeletal muscle Cl^- channels, and the disulfonic stilbene derivatives, 4-acetamido-4′isothiocyanatostilbene-2,2′-disulphonic acid (SITS) and 4,4′-dinitrostilbene-2,2′-disulphonic acid (DNDS). All of these properties of $I_{Cl(cAMP)}$ in the heart are remarkably similar to the properties of Cl^- channels in airway epithelial cells,[26] the regulation of which may be altered in patients with cystic fibrosis.[27] Whether or not the cardiac Cl^- channel is structurally similar to the recently cloned protein, cystic fibrosis transmembrane regulator (CFTR), remains to be determined.

Figure 2 shows an example of $I_{Cl(cAMP)}$ activated by isoproterenol in an isolated guinea pig ventricular myocyte. In this experiment, Ca^{2+} channels were blocked using 1 μM nisoldipine and K^+ currents were blocked using cesium and TEA as impermeant cations (internal 120 mM cesium, 20 mM TEA; external 5.4 mM cesium). In control conditions (panel A), little membrane current was activated by voltage-clamp depolarizations over the range of -128 to $+42$ mV. However during exposure to isoproterenol (1 μM), it can be seen that time-independent outward and inward membrane currents were increased over this range of potentials. Panel B shows the current-voltage relationship of the isoproterenol-induced Cl^- current. This current exhibited a reversal potential near the predicted value of E_{Cl} of -33 mV. The transmembrane Cl^- gradient in this experiment ($[Cl^-]_o = 150$ mM, $[Cl^-]_i = 42$ mM) is close to that expected in situ.[28] This current-voltage relationship allows some predictions about the changes in the cardiac action potential that might be expected as a result of activation of $I_{Cl(cAMP)}$. Due to the outward rectification of the current, once activated it should provide outward membrane current during the plateau of the cardiac action potential, which would tend to accelerate repolarization and shorten action potential duration. A small inward Cl^- current is expected to be activated near the resting membrane potential, and some depolarization of the resting membrane is expected. However, this effect has been found to be small due to the normal dependence of the resting membrane potential on the inward rectifying K^+ current I_{K1}.

Role of Cl^- Channel in Adrenergic Modulation of Action Potential Duration

The ability of β-adrenergic stimulation to simultaneously activate L-type Ca^{2+} channels, delayed rectifier K^+ channels, and Cl^- channels means that β stimulation has the potential to prolong, shorten, or produce minimal changes in the action potential duration of ventricular myocardium. This is because the activation of several of these channels is expected to have opposing effects on the action potential plateau and duration. β Stimulation of L-type Ca^{2+} channels will elevate the plateau and prolong action potential duration, whereas stimulation of delayed rectifier K^+ channels will abbreviate the plateau and shorten action potential duration (Figure 3). Activation of Cl^- channels is expected to have similar effects as K^+ channel activation under conditions of a physiological Cl^- gradient. It is not known at this time whether all three channels respond to an elevation of cAMP with a similar sensitivity or whether effects on one of these types of channels may predominate. This issue is also complicated by the fact that the action potential plateau is characterized by very small net conductance changes,[29] so small changes in conductance to any of these

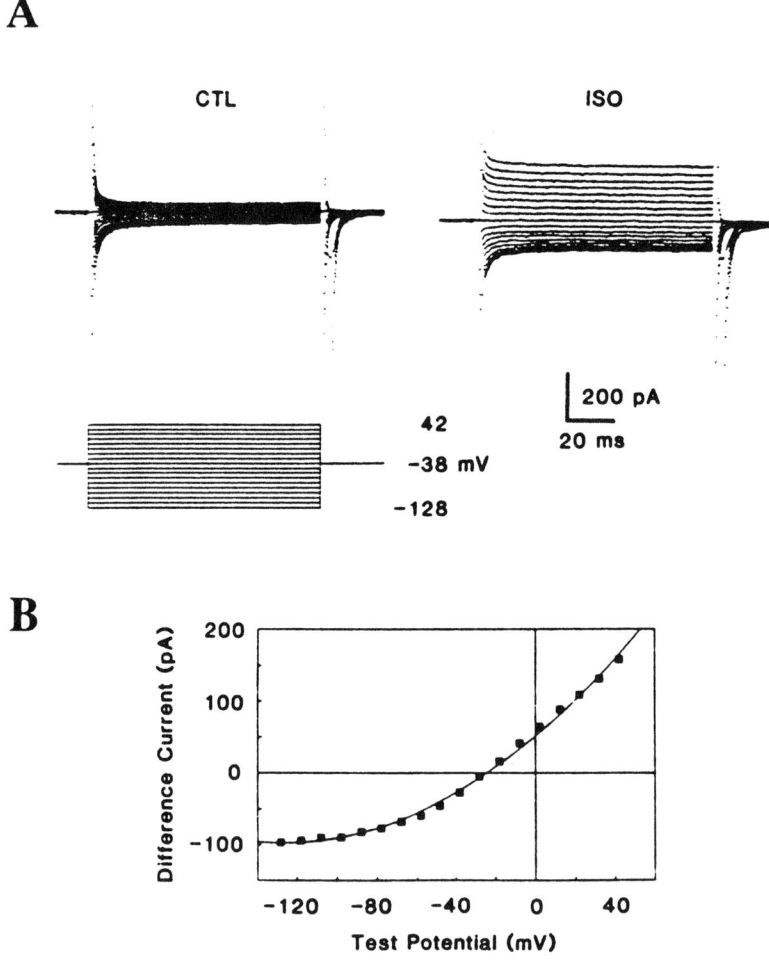

Figure 2. Isoproterenol-induced Cl^- currents in guinea pig ventricular cell under K^+-free conditions. A: Currents elicited during 100-msec voltage-clamp steps to membrane potentials between +42 and −128 mV from a holding potential of −38 mV before (CTL) and after exposure to 1 µM isoproterenol (ISO). B: Current-voltage relationship of the ISO-induced difference current. Intracellular K^+ was replaced with 120 mM Cs^+ and 20 mM TEA; extracellular K^+ was replaced with 5.4 mM Cs^+. Ca^{2+} current was blocked with 1 µM nisoldipine. Intracellular solution contained 42 mM Cl^- (ECl = −33 mV). (Reproduced with permission from Reference 22.)

ions may produce significant changes in action potential duration.

We have been interested in verifying that Cl^- channel activation plays a significant role in autonomic modulation of the ventricular action potential. We first tested whether in the absence of modulation of L-type Ca^{2+} channels and delayed rectifier K^+ channels, β stimulation might significantly alter action potential duration. To prevent gb modulation of

Ca^{2+} channels, cells were continuously exposed to the organic Ca^{2+} channel antagonist, nisoldipine using a dose (1 µM) nearly 100 times higher than the ED_{50} required for Ca^{2+} channel blockade, and experiments were carried out at 20°C. Low temperature has been reported to attenuate PKA modulation of delayed rectifier K^+ channels, but not to interfere with PKA modulation of Ca^{2+} or Cl^- channels.[8,23] Under these conditions, isopro-

Stimulation of Calcium Channels:

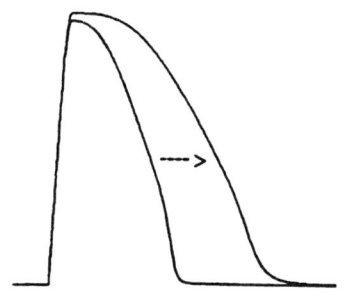

Stimulation of Potassium Channels

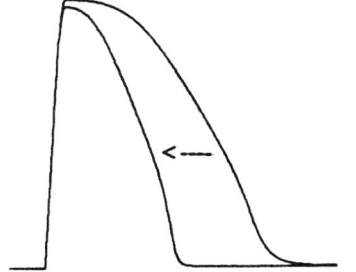

Stimulation of Chloride Channels

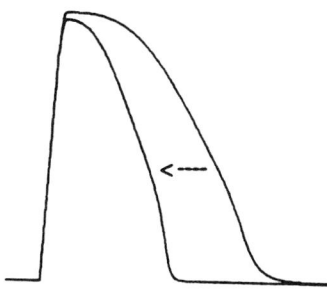

Figure 3. Predicted effects of β-adrenergic stimulation of different ion channels on action potential duration.

terenol produced a marked abbreviation of the plateau and duration of the guinea pig ventricular action potential (Figure 4A). In the continued presence of isoproterenol, exposure to acetylcholine effectively reversed these effects of isoproterenol. This ability of acetylcholine to reverse the effects of β stimulation is likely due to stimulation of an inhibitory G_i protein pathway.[1,15] These experiments suggest that in the absence of β-adrenergic modulation of L-type Ca^{2+} channels and delayed rectifier K^+ channels there remains a very potent mechanism for β-adrenergic modulation of the cardiac action potential. We next attempted to verify that such modulation might involve the cAMP-dependent Cl^- channels. Similar experimental conditions were used to minimize β-adrenergic modulation of Ca^{2+} and K^+ channels, and we tested the ability of a Cl^- channel antagonist, 9-AC, to reverse the effects of β stimulation under these conditions. We have previously shown in volt-

age-clamp studies[23] that 9-AC is an effective antagonist of cAMP-dependent Cl^- channels in guinea pig ventricular cells. Isoproterenol again significantly shortened action potential duration and 200 μM 9-AC was effective in reversing the effect (Figure 4B). This data is consistent with the idea that activation of cAMP-dependent Cl^- channels represents a new and potentially important mechanism for autonomic regulation of the cardiac action potential. Further studies are clearly needed to assess the specificity of this agent for myocardial Cl^- channels.

Cardiac Cl^- Channels: Potential Target for Class III Antiarrhythmic Drug Action

Activation of cAMP-dependent Cl^- channels may act normally to minimize the rather

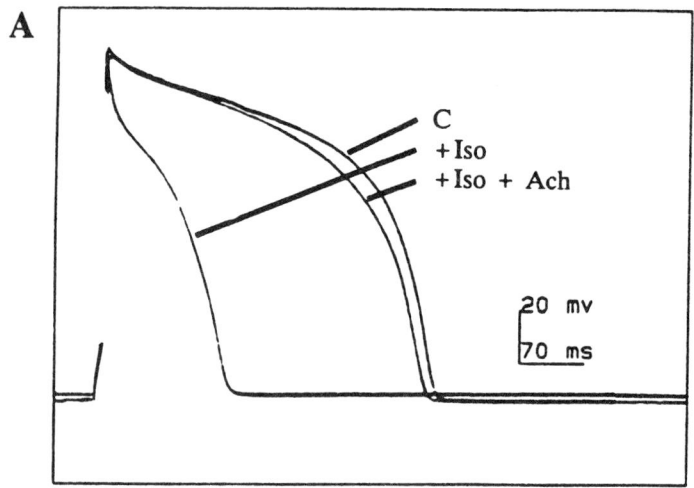

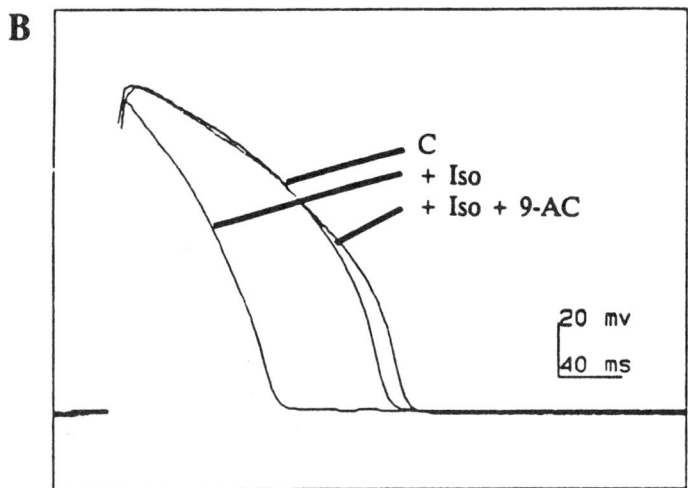

Figure 4. Isoproterenol-induced changes in guinea pig action potential in the absence of modulation of Ca^{2+} and K^+ channels. Ca^{2+} current modulation was minimized by using 1 μM nisoldipine and K^+ current modulation was minimized by carrying out experiments at 20°C (see text). A: Action potentials were elicited by intracellular current injection at a frequency of 0.25 Hz under control conditions (C), following exposure to 1 μM isoproterenol (Iso), and following exposure to isoproterenol and 10 μM acetylcholine (Iso + Ach). B: Action potentials elicited at 0.25 Hz under control conditions (C), following exposure to 1 μM isoproterenol (Iso), and following subsequent exposure to isoproterenol and 200 μM 9-AC (Iso + 9-AC).

significant action potential prolongation associated with β-adrenergic stimulation of Ca^{2+} channels, thus allowing β stimulation to produce large increases in Ca^{2+} entry into cardiac cells with minimal changes in action potential duration.[21] The demonstration that Cl^- channel activation can produce such profound changes in the cardiac action potential duration and refractoriness (Figure 4) raises the obvious possibility that agents that block these channels may have Class III antiarrhythmic efficacy. While this concept may have promise based upon theoretical considerations, rigorous tests of the effectiveness of such agents in animal arrhythmia models is required to establish their actual efficacy.

Class III antiarrhythmic agents are known to be effective in the treatment of self-sustaining reentrant arrhythmias. Considerable effort has been focused in recent years on the development of analogues of d-sotolol, a compound which can significantly prolong action potential refractoriness independent of its β-adrenergic blocking properties.[30] Many of these benzenesulfonamides have more potent Class III activity and less β-adrenergic blocking activity.[31-33] It is now known that d-sotolol and its derivative, E-4031, prolong action potential duration by blocking a specific component of the delayed rectifier K^+ current, I_{Kr},[34] which is a component of K^+ current distinct from I_{Ks}. I_{Ks}, but not I_{Kr}, is augmented by β-adrenergic stimulation.

The fact that these Class III agents and β-adrenergic stimulation have opposing effects on these two components of the delayed rectifier K^+ currents suggests that sympathetic influences may alter the responsiveness of cardiac cells to the action of these drugs. Indeed, it has recently been demonstrated that isoproterenol antagonizes the prolongation of refractory period by E-4031 in isolated guinea pig ventricular myocytes.[35] This study concluded that this antagonistic ability of isoproterenol was due to both augmentation of I_{Ks} and activation of cAMP-dependent Cl^- current, two effects that would promote earlier repolarization of the action potential.

It is not known at the present time if there are therapeutic consequences of this antagonistic interaction between Class III antiarrhythmic agents and β-agonists. We might speculate that sympathetic drive in the heart may reduce the effectiveness of this class of agents. Conversely, sympathetic influences may prevent excessive prolongation of refractoriness by these drugs and be beneficial. If the former case is true, then one might speculate that an agent that preferentially blocks cAMP-dependent Cl^- channels might improve the clinical efficacy of these Class III

agents. Related to these considerations, we recently examined whether 9-AC, an effective Cl^- channel antagonist,[36] could reverse the antagonistic effects of isoproterenol on action potential prolongation produced by the compound E-4031.[37]

Unlike previous experiments, these experiments were carried out at 35°C and in the absence of Ca^{2+} channel blocking agents to ensure the integrity of a full β-adrenergic response. Figure 5A illustrates that 5 μM E-4031 elicited the typical prolongation of action potential duration in an isolated guinea pig ventricular myocyte. In the continued presence of E-4031, 1 μM isoproterenol counteracted the effects of E-4031 and resulted in an action potential of shorter duration than observed in the control (Figure 5B). In the continued presence of E-4031 and isoproterenol, 200 μM 9-AC partially reversed the effects of isoproterenol, causing a prolongation of action potential duration back toward the duration observed in the presence of E-4031 alone. Experiments such as these suggest that Cl^- channel antagonists may prove to be useful agents capable of ameliorating the antagonistic effects of sympathetic stimulation on Class III activity.

Summary

β-Adrenergic stimulation can produce variable changes in the cardiac action potential due to the opposing effects of modulation of cardiac Ca^{2+}, K^+, and Cl^- channels on the action potential. Acetylcholine is capable of reversing the effects of β stimulation on each of these ion channels presumably through a G_i protein pathway that inhibits adenylate cyclase activity. The augmentation of K^+ and Cl^- channel activity by β-adrenergic stimulation will shorten action potential duration and will therefore, antagonize the ability of Class III antiarrhythmic agents to prolong action potential duration and refractoriness. Cl^- channel antagonists may represent a novel group of compounds with effective Class III properties when used alone or in combination with conventional Class III agents that specifically

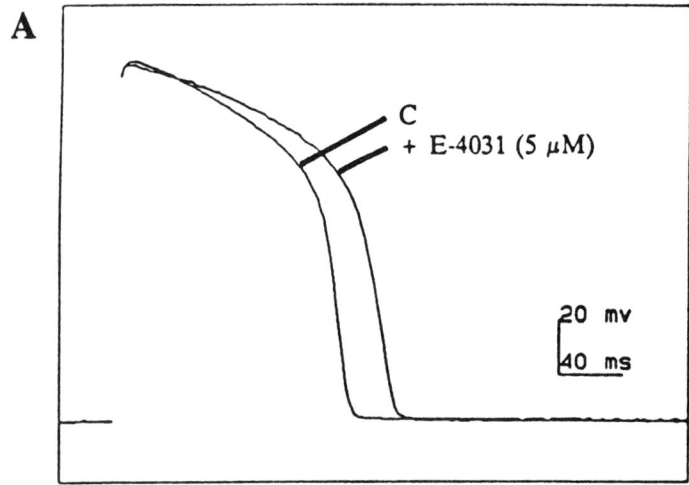

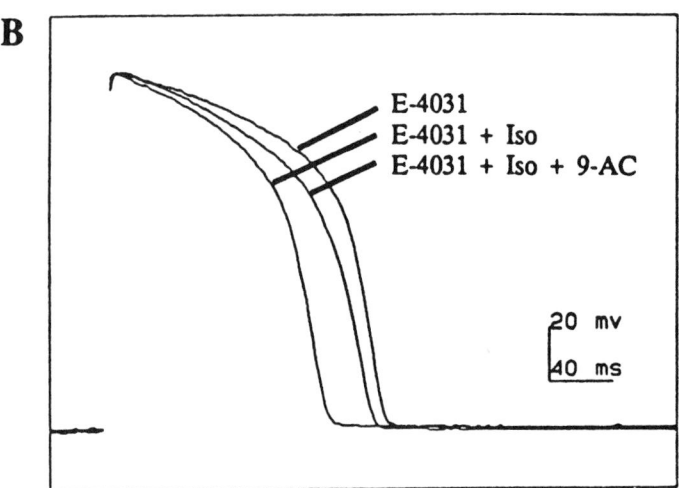

Figure 5. Modulation of action potentials by E-4031, isoproterenol, and 9-AC. Experiments carried out at 35°C in the absence of a Ca^{2+} channel blocker. A: Action potentials were elicited at 0.25 Hz under control conditions (C) and after exposure to 5 μM E-4031. B: In the continued presence of E-4031, the cell was exposed to 1 μM isoproterenol (Iso), and subsequently to isoproterenol and 200 μM 9-AC (Iso + 9-AC). (Reproduced with permission from Reference 37.)

inhibit myocardial K^+ channels. Recent molecular studies have provided evidence that the cAMP-dependent Cl^- channel in the heart is due to cardiac expression of a specific isoform of the epithelial CFTR Cl^- channel,[38,39] raising the possibility that future research efforts may provide cardiac specific antagonists of this channel protein. Finally, it is noteworthy that although under normal ionic conditions the major arrhythmogenic effects of activation of cAMP-dependent Cl^- channels can be attributed to changes in action potential duration and refractoriness, it has been demonstrated that during conditions of hypokalemia or decreased K^+ conductance, activation of this class of Cl^- channels may be arrhythmogenic due to induction of membrane depolarization and abnormal automaticity.[40]

References

1. Hartzell HC: Regulation of cardiac ion channels by catecholamines, acetylcholine and second messenger systems. *Prog Biophys Mol Biol* 52: 165, 1989.
2. Bean BP, Nowycky MC, Tsien RW: β-Adrenergic modulation of calcium channels in frog ventricular heart cells. *Nature (Lond)* 307:371, 1984.
3. Kameyama M, Hofmann F, Trautwein W: On the mechanism of β-adrenergic regulation of the Ca channel in the guinea-pig heart. *Pflügers Arch* 405:285, 1985.
4. Reuter H: Calcium channel modulation by neurotransmitters, enzymes and drugs. *Nature (Lond)* 301:569, 1983.
5. Trautwein W, Hescheler J: Regulation of cardiac L-type calcium current by phosphorylation and G-proteins. *Ann Rev Physiol* 52:257, 1990.
6. Tsien RW, Bean BP, Hess P, et al: Mechanisms of calcium channel modulation by beta-adrenergic agents and dihydropyridine calcium agonists. *J Mol Cell Cardiol* 18:691, 1986.
7. Harvey RD, Hume JR: Autonomic regulation of delayed rectifier K^+ current in mammalian heart involves G proteins. *Am J Physiol* 257: H818, 1989.
8. Walsh KB, Begenisich TB, Kass RS: β-Adrenergic modulation in the heart—independent regulation of K and Ca channels. *Pflügers Arch* 411: 232, 1988.
9. Ono K, Kiyosue T, Arita M: Isoproterenol, dbcAMP, and forskolin inhibit cardiac sodium current. *Am J Physiol* 256:C1131, 1989.
10. Schubert B, Vandongen AMJ, Kirsch GE, et al: Inhibition of cardiac Na^+ currents by isoproterenol. *Am J Physiol* 258:H977, 1990.
11. Desilets M, Baumgarten CM: Isoproterenol directly stimulates the Na^+-K^+ pump in isolated ventricular myocytes. *Am J Physiol* 251:H218, 1986.
12. DiFrancesco D: The cardiac hyperpolarizing-activated current, i_f. Origins and developments. *Prog Biophys Mol Biol* 46:163, 1985.
13. Bahinski A, Nairn AC, Greengard P, et al: Chloride conductance regulated by cyclic AMP-dependent protein kinase in cardiac myocytes. *Nature (Lond)* 340:718, 1989.
14. Harvey RD, Hume JR: Autonomic regulation of a chloride current in heart. *Science* 244:983, 1989.
15. Hescheler J, Kameyama M, Trautwein W: On the mechanism of muscarinic inhibition of the cardiac Ca current. *Pflügers Arch* 407:182, 1986.
16. Fischmeister R, Hartzell HC: Mechanism of action of acetylcholine on calcium current in single cells from frog ventricle. *J Physiol (Lond)* 376:183, 1986.
17. Apkon M, Nerbonne JM: α-Adrenergic agonists selectively suppress voltage-dependent K^+ currents in rat ventricular myocytes. *Proc Natl Acad Sci USA* 85:8756, 1988.
18. Fedida D, Shimoni Y, Giles WR: A novel effect of norepinephrine on cardiac cells is mediated by alpha₁-adrenoceptors. *Am J Physiol* 256: H1500, 1989.
19. Bruckner R, Scholz H: Effects of α-adrenoceptor stimulation with phenylephrine in the presence of propranolol on force of contraction, slow inward current and cyclic AMP content in bovine heart. *Br J Pharmacol* 82:223, 1984.
20. Hescheler J, Nawrath H, Tang M, et al: Adrenoceptor-mediated changes of excitation and contraction in ventricular muscle from guinea pigs and rabbits. *J Physiol (Lond)* 397:657, 1988.
21. Hume JR, Harvey RD: Chloride conductance pathways in heart. *Am J Physiol* 261:C399, 1991.
22. Harvey RD, Hume JR: Histamine activates the chloride current in cardiac ventricular myocytes. *J Cardiovasc Electrophysiol* 1:309, 1990.
23. Harvey RD, Clark CD, Hume JR: Chloride current in mammalian cardiac myocytes—novel mechanism for autonomic regulation of action potential duration and resting membrane potential. *J Gen Physiol* 95:1077, 1990.
24. Ehara T, Ishihara K: Anion channels activated by adrenaline in cardiac muscle. *Nature (Lond)* 347:284, 1990.
25. Nagel GA, Hwang T-C, Powe AC, et al: Chloride channels activated by protein kinase A in giant patches excised from guinea pig ventricular myocytes (abstract). *Biophy J* 61:A146, 1992.
26. Berger HA, Anderson MP, Gregory RJ, et al: Identification and regulation of the cystic fibrosis transmembrane conductance regulator-generated chloride channel. *J Clin Invest* 88: 1422, 1991.
27. Welsh MJ: Abnormal regulation of ion channels in cystic fibrosis epithelia. *FASEB J* 4:2718, 1990.
28. Walker JL: Intracellular inorganic ions in cardiac tissue. In: HA Fozzard (ed): *The Heart and Cardiovascular System.* New York: Raven Press, 1986, p. 561.
29. Weidmann S: Effect of current flow on the membrane potential of cardiac muscle. *J Physiol (Lond)* 115:227, 1951.
30. Carmeliet E: Electrophysiologic and voltage clamp analysis of the effects of sotolol on isolated cardiac muscle and Purkinje fibers. *J Pharmacol Exp Ther* 232:817, 1985.
31. Katoh H, Nomoto K, Sawada K, et al: Electrophysiologic, antiarrhythmic and hemodynamic effects of E-4031, a novel class III antiarrhyth-

mic agent in intact and infarcted dogs (abstract). *Eur Heart J* 9:232, 1988.

32. Gwilt M, Dalrymple HW, Burges RA, et al: UK-68,798 is a novel, potent and selective Class III antiarrhythmic drug (abstract). *J Mol Cell Cardiol* 21:S.11, 1989.

33. Gwilt M, Dalrymple HW, Blackburn KJ, et al: UK-66,914, a novel Class III antiarrhythmic agent which blocks potassium channels (abstract). *Circulation* 78(suppl II):II-150, 1988.

34. Sanguinetti MC, Jurkiewicz NK: Two components of cardiac delayed rectifier K^+ current: differential sensitivity to block by Class III antiarrhythmic agents. *J Gen Physiol* 96:194, 1990.

35. Sanguinetti MC, Jurkiewicz NK, Scott A, et al: Isoproterenol antagonizes prolongation of refractory period by the class III antiarrhythmic agent E-4031 in guinea pig myocytes. *Circ Res* 68:77, 1991.

36. Palade PT, Barchi RL: On the inhibition of muscle membrane chloride conductance by aromatic carboxylic acids. *J Gen Physiol* 69:879, 1977.

37. Levesque PC, Clark CD, Zakarov SI, et al: Anion and cation modulation of the guinea-pig ventricular action-potential during β-adrenoceptor stimulation. *Pflügers Arch* (in press).

38. Levesque PC, Hart PJ, Hume JR, et al: Expression of CFTR Cl^- channels in heart. *Circ Res* 71:1002, 1992.

39. Horowitz B, Tsung SS, Hart P, et al: Alternative splicing of CFTR Cl^- channels in heart. *Am J Physiol* (in press).

40. Yamawake N, Hirano Y, Sawanobori T, Hiraoka M: Arrhythmogenic effects of isoproterenol-activated Cl^- current in guinea-pig ventricular myocytes. *J Mol Cell Cardiol* 24:1047, 1992.

Chapter 5

Rate Dependence of Cardiac Repolarization: *Autonomic Modulation and Interference With Antiarrhythmic Drug Action*

Antonio Zaza
Gabriella Malfatto
Flavia Ravelli
Peter J. Schwartz

In most mammalians the cardiac action potential has a duration of hundreds of milliseconds and a distinct plateau phase. This has important physiological and pathophysiological implications. Indeed, action potential duration (APD) is relevant to many aspects of the normal cardiac excitation and electromechanical coupling, such as the uniform spread of the activation wave front and the transsarcolemmal influx of calcium ions, and it is also an important factor in arrhythmogenesis.

As the main determinant of refractoriness of Purkinje fibers and working myocardium, APD affects both the likelihood and the features of reentry;[1-3] early afterdepolarizations and the consequent triggered activity are invariably associated with a prolonged action potential which, at least in some cases, may be the causative factor.[4]

Action potential duration is highly rate dependent.[5] Since heart rate is an important factor in arrhythmogenesis, and arrhythmias generally imply a change in cycle length, this feature deserves careful consideration. Following a step change in heart rate between two constant values, APD changes gradually with a distinct time course, until it settles on a value appropriate for the new rate.[5] Thus, during the cycle length fluctuations that are intrinsic to sinus rhythm, the APD of each beat will be influenced by a sort of "weighed averages" of several preceding RR intervals, rather than by a single one. Accordingly we can recognize two aspects of APD rate dependence: the kinetics of the progressive change in APD toward its steady-state value, and the relationship between APD and cycle length at steady state. Both these aspects may be relevant to arrhythmogenesis. The former, which we will refer to as APD adaptation, defines how fast

From BN Singh, HJJ Wellens, M Hiraoka, (eds): *Electropharmacological Control of Cardiac Arrhythmias.* Mount Kisco, NY, Futura Publishing Company Inc., © 1994.

the refractoriness will shorten, for instance, after the onset of an ectopic tachycardia, and the latter will describe the entity of the final change in the refractory period. Thus, the steady-state value of APD will determine the cycle length of the reentrant circuit in the case of a functional reentry, or the size of the excitable gap of an anatomically determined pathway. No information is yet available on how differences in the kinetics of APD adaptation may impact on arrhythmogenesis. Nonetheless, it is possible to speculate that they might influence the ability of an ensuing reentrant circuit to become stable and sustained, as well as its tendency to evolve to the fractionated pattern peculiar to fibrillation. Regional differences in adaptation kinetics would be particularly significant in this regard.

As it will be discussed, rate dependence of APD corresponds to rate-dependent changes in the availability of the ionic currents determining repolarization. Accordingly, the effects of any intervention affecting APD by acting on these currents is expected to be rate dependent. Thus, autonomic and pharmacological modulation of APD are completely defined only if evaluated as changes in the action potential duration/cycle length (APD/CL) relationship, rather than as the effects observed at a single cycle length.

In this chapter we discuss some of our recent findings on two aspects of the rate dependence of APD relevant to the pathophysiology of cardiac arrhythmias: the autonomic modulation of the APD/CL relationship and the influence of APD on the use dependency of antiarrhythmic drug action. This will be preceded by a brief analysis of the ionic mechanisms involved.

Ionic Mechanisms of Action Potential Duration Rate Dependence

The ionic mechanisms of the rate dependence of APD have been extensively investigated and are still debated.[5] The superimposition of phenomena with substantially different kinetics is probably responsible for its various aspects. At a constant rate the duration of each action potential depends on the length of the preceding cycle, thus phenomena having a time course comparable to the diastolic interval (hundreds of milliseconds) would be enough to account for the steady-state APD/CL relationship. However, when the cycle length is abruptly changed, APD adaptation occurs with much slower kinetics (20–40 seconds) thus suggesting that APD is also determined by a factor that accumulates and dissipates over many cycles.[6]

The nature of the phenomena belonging to the faster class underlying the beat-to-beat control of APD, is tissue specific because the ionic currents responsible for the repolarization are different in Purkinje fibers than in working myocardium. Activation of a K^+ current, the delayed rectifier (I_K), dominates the repolarization process in Purkinje fibers.[5] Once activated by depolarization, this current deactivates at diastolic potentials with a time constant in the order of 200 msec in the cat;[7] if the diastolic interval is shorter than the 4–5 time constants required for complete I_K deactivation, this current will accumulate through subsequent beats, thus shortening their APD. In ventricular muscle, I_K is less prominent and the repolarization is mainly accounted for by inactivation of the Ca^{2+} current responsible for the action potential plateau (I_{CaL}). At diastolic potentials, recovery from inactivation of I_{CaL} requires several hundreds milliseconds,[8] thus at sufficiently short diastolic intervals the action potential plateau will be shortened because of incomplete recovery of the current supporting it. Besides incomplete recovery of membrane currents, phenomena related to fiber shortening may be involved in rate dependence of APD.[9,10]

Both I_K deactivation and I_{CaL} inactivation are far too fast to account for the time course of APD adaptation; other phenomena with a much slower time course are required. When heart rate is abruptly changed, K^+ concentration in the intercellular clefts changes with a time course closely comparable to that of APD adaptation.[11] Since fluctuations in extracellular K^+ concentrations within the range observed may affect APD through changes in K conductance, this phenomenon may contribute to adaptation. However, slow APD adaptation has also been observed in isolated ventricular myocytes, where intercellular clefts are absent and only a minor fraction of the extracellular space is restricted.[12] Therefore, although it may contribute, K^+ accumulation is not sufficient to account for adaptation. An increase in heart rate results in a transient elevation of intracellular Na^+ activity, due to augmented Na^+ influx per unit time; this is followed by activation of the electrogenic Na-K pump, which generates an outward repolarizing current. Boyett and Fedida[6] have shown that upon a step change in rate, intracellular Na^+ activity, Na-K pump current, and APD change with a parallel time course. Thus, activation of the Na-K pump is probably the main determinant of APD adaptation, and may account for this phenomenon both in Purkinje fibers and in ventricular muscle.

Autonomic Modulation of the Action Potential Duration/Cycle Length Relationship

In a recent study we evaluated the effects on the APD/CL relationship of selective sympathetic and parasympathetic denervations in the anesthetized cat.[13] Previous evidence[14,15] indicates that right and left sympathetic denervations affect ventricular electrophysiological properties differently, therefore, the effects of unilateral as well as bilateral stellate ganglionectomy were studied. Action potential duration was measured from monophasic action potentials recorded from the left ventricular endocardium by extracellular contact electrodes. The steady-state APD/CL relationship was evaluated by measuring APD after sustained pacing at 7–10 different cycle lengths. The rate of APD adaptation was determined by measuring APD from each beat after a step shortening of cycle length, until a steady state was achieved at the new cycle length. To quantitate the effects of autonomic interventions on the steady-state APD/CL relationship, APD values were plotted against cycle length and fitted by a hyperbolic function initially proposed by Elharrar et al.[16] for this purpose. This Michaelis-Menten type of equation is described by two parameters: APDmax, that is APD extrapolated at infinite cycle length; and CL_{50}, the cycle length at which 50% of APDmax is achieved. APDmax can be viewed as a measure of the intrinsic duration of the repolarization process, uninfluenced by the short-term effects of a previous activation. Validation of parameter estimates obtained with this function has been obtained in in vitro experiments. Action potential duration adaptation was best fitted by the sum of two exponentials described by the time constants T_{fast} and T_{slow}.

After measurements in the control situation (intact innervation), the animals were randomly assigned to two experimental groups. In the first group right stellectomy was followed by bilateral stellectomy; in the second group left stellectomy was the first intervention.

Right stellectomy, performed in the presence of intact left stellate ganglion (group 1), shortened APDmax to 80% and CL_{50} to 70% of their respective control values of 441 and 399 msec (Figure 1). This results in a decreased steepness of the steady-state APD/CL relationship (Figure 2A). Subsequent removal of the left stellate ganglion, resulting in bilateral stellectomy, reversed these changes prolonging APDmax to 111% and CL_{50} to 128% of control (Figure 1 and Figure 2B). Right and bilateral stellectomy had opposite effects on the kinetics of APD adaptation (Figures 3 and 4): right stellectomy accelerated the slow component of adaptation (T_{slow}: 51% of the control value of 66 beats), while bilateral stellectomy slowed it beyond the control values (T_{slow}: 260% of control). The shortening of APDmax induced by right stellectomy seems to contrast with the previous observation that this intervention prolongs the rate corrected QT interval (QTc; Bazett's formula) measured during sinus rhythm.[17] However, this discrepancy is only apparent because in our experi-

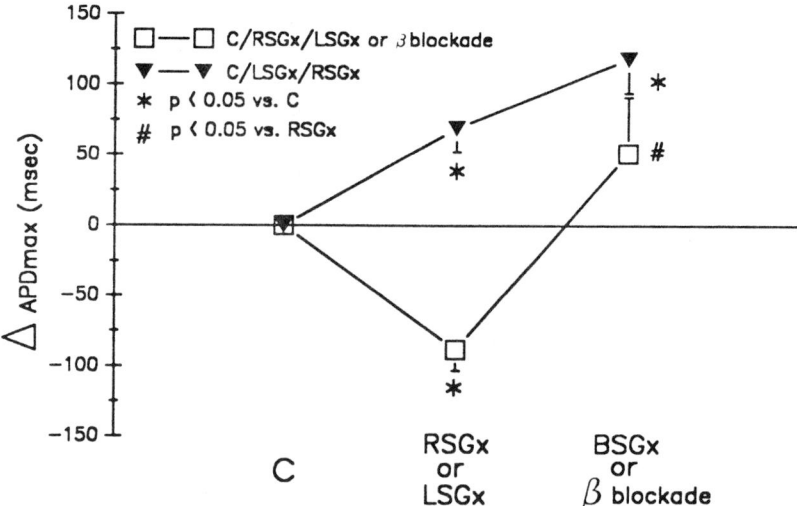

Figure 1. Changes of action potential duration (APD) at infinite cycle length (APDmax) with respect to control (C) values induced by unilateral and bilateral stellectomy. The opposite effects of right and left stellectomy (RSGx and LSGx, respectively) are clearly visible, together with the increase of APDmax induced by bilateral stellectomy (BSGx) or β-adrenergic blockade. (Reproduced with permission from Reference 13).

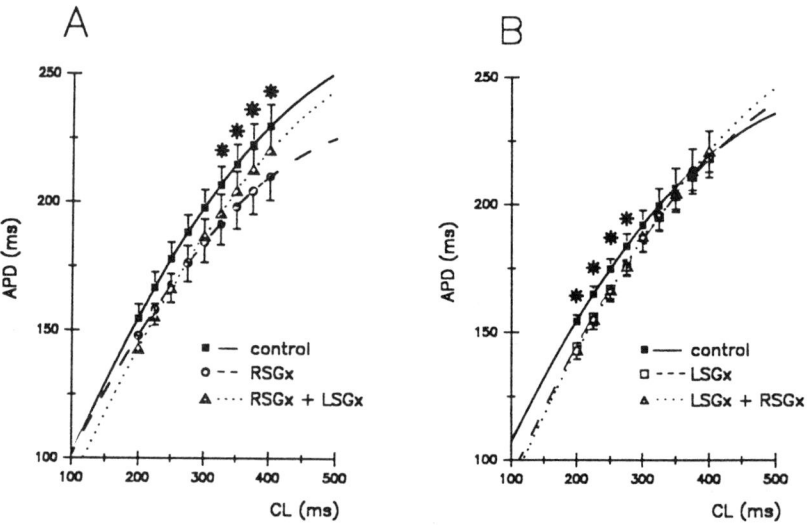

Figure 2. Changes in the shape of the steady-state APD/CL relation after unilateral and bilateral stellectomy. Panel A: group 1 experiments; Panel B: group 2 experiments. Points represent mean ± SEM of APDs computed in each experiment from individual APDmax and CL_{50} values. At each cycle length, APD in control and after unilateral and bilateral stellectomy were compared by analysis of variance. Note the opposite changes in the slope of the APD/CL relation induced by right versus left or bilateral stellectomy. *$p < 0.05$ of unilateral stellectomy versus control. Other symbols as in Figure 1. (Reproduced with permission from Reference 13.)

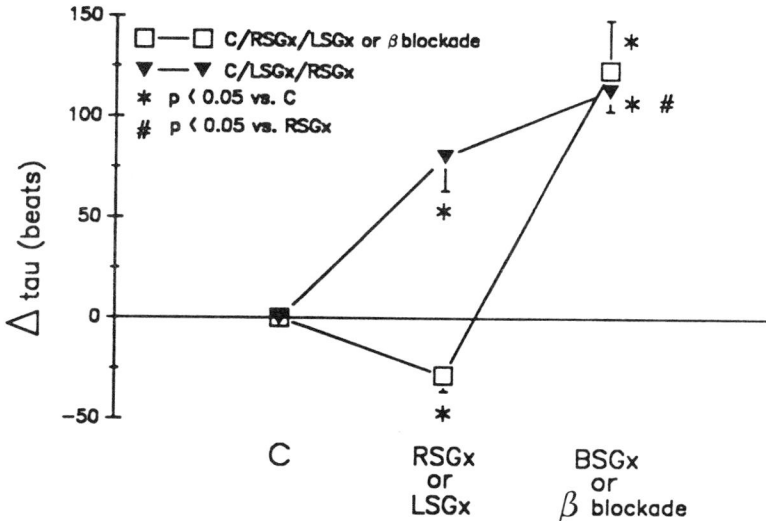

Figure 3. Changes induced with respect to control (C) values, by unilateral and bilateral stellectomy (BSGx) in the time constant of the slower component of action potential duration (APD) adaptation. Note the opposite effects of right and left stellectomy (RSGx and LSGx, respectively). (Reproduced with permission from Reference 13.)

ments QTc measured during sinus rhythm was prolonged by right stellectomy. However, when QT was measured during pacing at various rates and subjected to the same analysis as APD, right stellectomy shortened QTmax (the value of QT at infinite cycle length), exactly as it happened with APDmax. A possible interpretation of this puzzling observation is that, in Bazett's correction, QT is usually assumed to depend only on the RR interval immediately preceding the beat considered, thus ignoring the fact that APD adaptation is far from instantaneous. As a consequence, QTc may be influenced by changes in the kinetics of APD adaptation. When, as occurs after right stellectomy, APD adapts with a different time course, QTc becomes unreliable as a rate-independent index of the duration of ventricular repolarization.

Effects opposite to those of right stellectomy were exerted by left stellectomy (group 2). This intervention prolonged APDmax to 113% and CL_{50} to 133% of the respective control values. Subsequent bilateral stellectomy induced a further increase in both these parameters. The kinetics of APD adaptation was

slowed by left stellectomy (T_{slow}: 193% of the control value of 62 beats) and a further slowing occurred after subsequent removal of the contralateral sympathetic nerves.

Overall, left and bilateral stellectomy prolonged the intrinsic duration of the repolarization process; this effect was more prominent at slow pacing rates. Thus, the APD relation was "steeper" after these interventions. The rate dependence of sympathetic influence on APD may be accounted for by the different availability of the ionic currents modulated by catecholamines as a function of cycle length. For instance, two components of I_K have been described in mammalian ventricular myocytes:[18] a fast activating small conductance (I_{Kr}) that is catecholamine insensitive, and a large and slow one (I_{Ks}), increased by β-adrenergic receptor stimulation. Due to its slow activation kinetics I_{Ks} contribution to repolarization increases with increasing APD. Thus, by stimulating I_{Ks}, β-receptor agonists would shorten APD prevalently at slow heart rates, when APD is longer.[18] In ventricular myocytes of the cat, the species used in our experiments, only one I_K component is expressed, similar for magni-

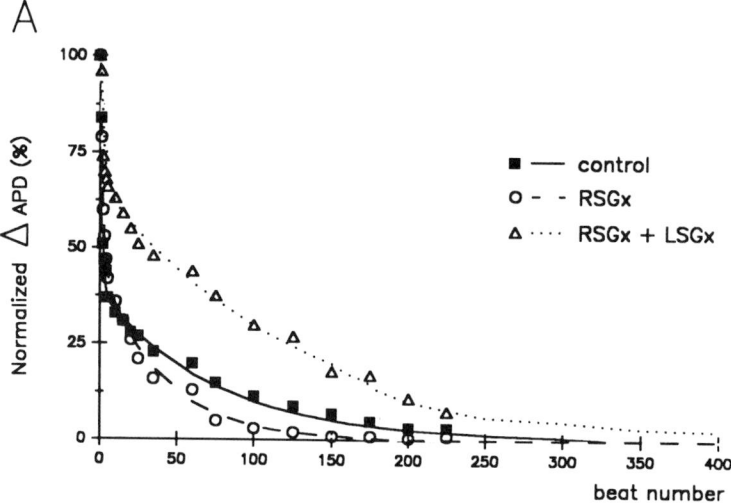

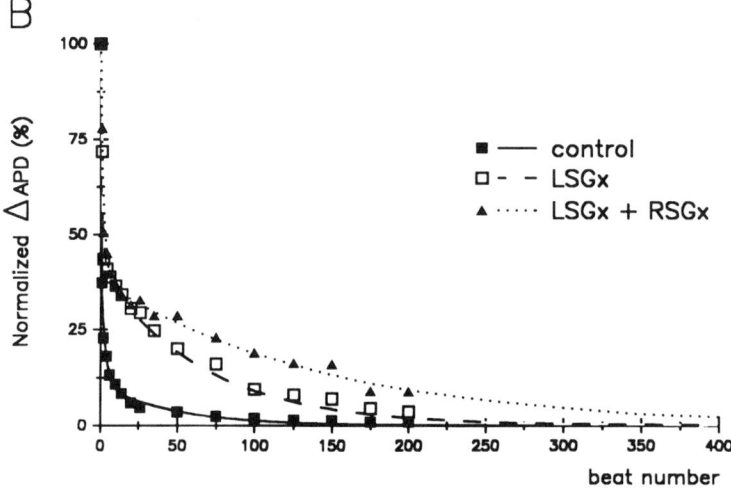

Figure 4. Examples of action potential duration (APD) adaptation after a step change in pacing cycle length in group 1 (panel A) and group 2 (panel B) experiments. The change in APD, as a percent of the total change occurring between the first beat and the steady state, is plotted against the sequential number of beats. Continuous lines are computed by fitting a double exponential through the points. Panel A: right stellectomy (RSGx) accelerated APD adaptation. This effect was reversed by subsequent left stellectomy (LSGx). Panel B: left stellectomy slowed APD adaptation, while subsequent right stellectomy did not result in further changes. (Reproduced with permission from Reference 13).

tude, ionic selectivity, and kinetics to I_{Ks} (time constant: 400–450 msec at plateau potentials at 37°C).[7] Recently, Taggart et al.,[19] have reported that infusion of adrenaline in the pig results in a steepening of the APD restitution curve at epicardial recording sites. Although APD restitution describes only one component of the steady-state APD/CL relation,[16] this finding is partly at variance with our results and with the effects of isoproterenol on Purkinje fibers reported by others.[16] This discrepancy probably reflects differences between epicardium and endocardium in terms of Purkinje fiber content, and of the currents determining repolarization in muscle fibers.[20–22]

Both β- and α-adrenergic stimulation increase Na-K pump activity;[23,24] thus, a removal of tonic sympathetic drive would decrease both the rate of Na^+ extrusion and the outward current generated by the Na-K exchange. According to the hypothesis discussed above,[6] this might explain the slower APD adaptation observed after left and bilateral stellectomy.

Right stellectomy exerted effects opposite those of left and bilateral denervation on both the kinetic and steady-state aspects of the APD/CL relationship. This observation is not completely unexpected, although not easily interpreted. An asymmetry in the cardiac effects of stellate ganglia ablation and stimulation has been previously reported and constitutes the basis for a model of the idiopathic form of the long QT syndrome.[17] The simplest hypothesis explaining this intriguing observation is that removal of the right stellate ganglion may increase the sympathetic output to the ventricles. This would occur if, in the presence of a quantitative prevalence of left-sided sympathetic influences on the heart, right stellectomy would reflexly increase activity through the contralateral nerves.[25] This idea is based on the fact that the effects of right stellectomy are reversed by removal of left-sided sympathetic nerves and by β blockade. Right stellectomy may increase activity in left-sided sympathetic nerves through baroreceptive reflexes or through the interruption of the neural input to central inhibitory pathways, as those supported by interneurons located in the vicinity of the intermediomedial nucleus in the spinal cord.[26]

A further substantial support of the hypothesis that the effects of right stellectomy may derive from an increased sympathetic drive to the ventricles, comes from another study in which we analyzed in the same experimental setting the changes induced on the steady-state APD/CL relationship by bilateral vagotomy.[27] To assess whether vagal influences on ventricular repolarization were "direct" rather than due to antagonism of the sympathetic component, we evaluated the effects of this intervention before and after bilateral stellectomy. In the presence of intact sympathetic innervation, vagotomy shortened APDmax and CL_{50} by 24% and 36%, respectively. Rather unexpectedly, these effects persisted when vagotomy was performed after sympathetic denervation. However, vagal modulation of APD disappeared when the action of circulating catecholamines was also eliminated by β-adrenergic blockade. These findings indicate that, at least in the cat, parasympathetic modulation of ventricular repolarization is indirect, ie, it is fully accounted for by antagonism of sympathetic action. The persistence of the effects of vagotomy after bilateral stellectomy, suggests that a quantitatively important sympatho-vagal interaction occurs in vivo at a site distal to β receptors, presumably at the level of adenylate cyclase modulation.[28]

From these observations, we concluded that both the steady-state and kinetic aspects of the dependence of APD on heart rate are under autonomic modulation. It seems logical to consider the possibility that such modulation may contribute to the arrhythmogenic effects of sympathetic activation[29] and to the antifibrillatory action of vagal influences.[30]

Influence of Action Potential Duration and its Rate Dependence on Antiarrhythmic Drug Action

The possibility that APD rate dependence and its modulation may influence the effects of antiarrhythmic drugs is another aspect of potential clinical relevance. In this section we present data recently obtained in our laboratory that suggests that such an interaction actually exists and that it may have considerable practical consequences.

Most antiarrhythmic agents acting as ion channel blockers show a major use-dependent component in their effect, which makes their action a steep function of heart rate.[31–33] Use dependency is a feature of remarkable practical importance, because a given concentration of drug may be effective at high, but not at low heart rates, or vice versa. A direct use dependency, ie, effects increasing with rate, may represent a favorable feature of the drug because doses that are effective at the high rates characteristic of repetitive ectopic rhythms would leave cardiac electrophysiological properties almost unchanged at resting sinus rate. This should result in an optimal balance between antiarrhythmic and undesired effects.[34] The opposite condition, reverse use dependency, can thus be considered undesirable.

Use dependency is currently interpreted as the result of a different probability of drug-channel interaction according to the "state" of the channel. This can be viewed either as a state depencence of the affinity of the drug binding site within the channel (modulated receptor model),[32] or as a change in the drug access to a constant affinity site due to site "guarding" by the channel gating mechanism (guarded receptor model).[35] During the membrane potential changes occurring in the cardiac cycle, membrane channels undergo voltage-dependent changes in their functional state, ie, they cycle through rested, activated and, for some of them, inactivated states. As a consequence, the rate of drug binding and unbinding to the channel varies in the different phases of the action potential. Given a set of "state specific" binding rates, the proportion of channels bound to the drug (ie, blocked channels) at steady state and the time course by which the steady state is achieved, both depend on the fraction of the cardiac cycle spent by the channel in the state of higher affinity (or higher accessibility) for the drug. If a drug binds preferentially to a state of the channel that persists during the entire permanence of the membrane at depolarized potentials such as the inactivated state, the amount and kinetics of use-dependent block should closely depend on APD. Since APD itself is a function of heart rate, this should result in rather complex patterns of use-dependent channel blockade. Steady-state APD should affect both the amount of use-dependent block present at each rate and the kinetics of block development during heart rate changes. Furthermore, the exponential time course of block development would be distorted by the progressive APD changes due to adaptation.

Although predicted by theory, the influence of APD on use dependency of local anesthetics has been generally assumed to be negligible, perhaps because the kinetics of block onset so far observed did not deviate markedly from the single exponential predicted by considering APD constant.[36-39]

During a study evaluating use dependency of propafenone and flecainide in canine Purkinje fibers,[40] we observed that the kinetic parameters measured for propafenone, at variance with those obtained for flecainide, did not accurately predict the dependence of its steady-state block on heart rate. A further analysis performed on a wider time scale[41] showed that the time course of block onset with propafenone consistently deviated from the simple exponential expected. Figure 5 shows the time course of $\dot{V}_{max}$ changes when stimulation (at cycle length = 450 msec) was initiated in a quiescent fiber in the presence of 1 μM propafenone. The bottom panel of this figure shows that after the beginning of stimulation, the maximum diastolic potential was reasonably constant, therefore, its changes could not account for the complex time course of block onset observed. This peculiar pattern was not evident with flecainide; with this drug the time course of block onset could still be fitted with a single exponential.

Based on the considerations presented, we tested the hypothesis that the distortion in the time course of propafenone block onset was due to a progressive change in APD, occurring as a consequence of the abrupt change in cycle length. For this purpose we performed experiments in which APD was measured from every beat during the protocols used to study the kinetics of block development. In the same fibers we also measured independently other parameters of use dependency, such as the rate of block dissipation. On the basis of the guarded receptor hy-

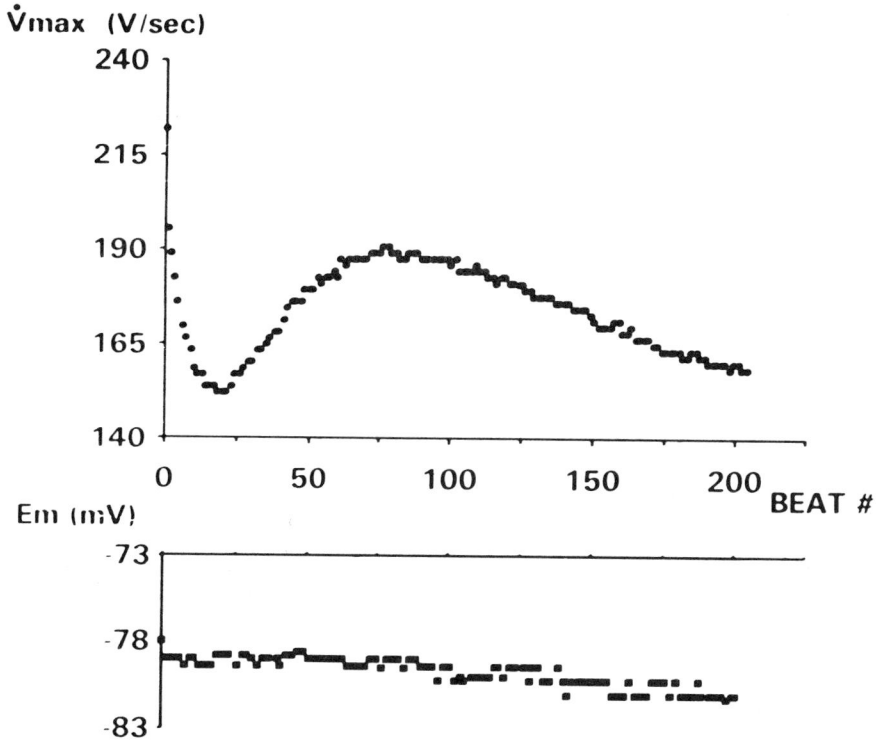

Figure 5. Upper panel: $\dot{V}_{max}$ changes after the onset of stimulation (CL = 0.45 seconds), during superfusion with propafenone 0.1 μM. $\dot{V}_{max}$ was measured from every beat for the first 200 beats (the *x* axis shows the sequential number of points from the onset of stimulation). Lower panel: changes of maximum diastolic potential measured from every beat during the same stimulation run. Note that the time course of $\dot{V}_{max}$ decay strongly deviates from a simple exponential. As shown in the bottom panel, such a deviation could not be accounted for by changes in the maximum diastolic potential.

pothesis,[35] we then developed model equations in which APD was allowed to change along an exponential function similar to that describing APD adaptation. Figure 6 shows that these equations accurately fitted the complex time course of propafenone block onset. A validation of the model could be obtained by comparing the parameters estimated by the fitting procedure to the same parameters directly measured in the same fiber through appropriate protocols. The parameters we used for this comparison were the time constant of recovery from block, and the time constant of APD adaptation. As shown in Figure 7 (A and B), mean estimated parameter values were not significantly different from measured ones. Moreover, a significant correlation was pres-

ent between individual values and their estimates (r > 0.8). From these data it is possible to conclude that the progressive change in the time spent by the membrane at depolarized potentials due to APD adaptation is adequate to explain the complex time course of block onset observed with propafenone.

Why was a distortion of the time course of block onset never observed in the numerous studies evaluating use dependency by action potential recordings? First, as already mentioned, the influence of APD changes will be significant only for drugs that bind preferentially to a persistent state of the channel such as the inactivated or rested states. Second, as illustrated in Figure 8 (A and B), the model we have developed predicts that a deviation

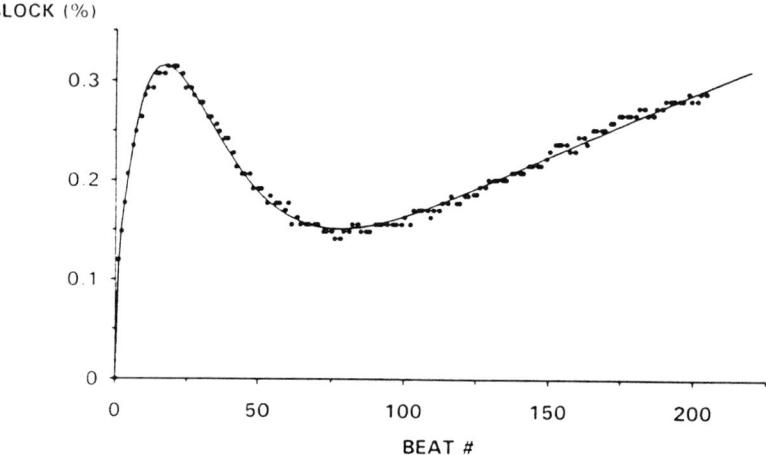

Figure 6. Development of use-dependent block in the same experiment as in Figure 5. *y* axis: percent of the block achieved at steady state. *x* axis: sequential number of points since the beginning of stimulation. The continuous line has been computed by fitting the points with the equations of the model taking into account action potential duration (APD) adaptation. Note that the model adequately fits the complex time course of block development.

from a simple exponential will be clearly visible on the steep portion of $\dot{V}_{max}$ decay only if time courses of APD adaptation and block onset critically overlap; if this is not the case, only minor deviations may be present within the time frame usually examined. These can be easily concealed by experimental noise, particularly if $\dot{V}_{max}$ is sampled at large intervals rather than measured from every beat. Thus, even if obvious distortions are absent from its early portion, the time course of block onset may still be influenced by APD adaptation. Finally, the influence of APD adaptation also depends on the total amount of APD shortening occurring after the change in rate. Since APD dependence on rate is steepest in the conduction system,[42] the consequences of adaptation should be larger in Purkinje fibers than in other cardiac tissues.

The finding that the kinetics of onset of block exerted by flecainide was closer to a simple exponential suggests that this drugs binds preferentially to a transient state of the channel, such as the activated one, whose duration is too short to be influenced by APD. This is consistent with previous more direct evidence indicating that flecainide binds pref-

erentially to activated Na^+ channels.[43] The block exerted by propafenone increases at depolarized resting membrane potentials, thus inducing an apparent shift in the inactivation curve of the Na^+ channel. This was assumed as an indication of a higher affinity of this drug for the inactivated state of the channel.[44] Recently, single channel experiments have shown that, when the inactivation mechanism is removed pharmacologically, propafenone binds to Na^+ channels in the open state. In light of this new finding, the sensitivity of propafenone block to steady membrane depolarizations has been attributed to the fact that a significant number of Na^+ channel openings may occur late during prolonged activating steps.[45] The sensitivity of propafenone effects to APD as observed in our study, implies that this drug binds preferentially to a persistent state assumed by the channel at depolarized membrane potentials, without discriminating between the activated or the inactivated ones.

A high sensitivity to APD of the use-dependent effects of a drug has several relevant consequences. In the case of propafenone, the most obvious is that drug potency will be maximal in tissues where APD is longest or within

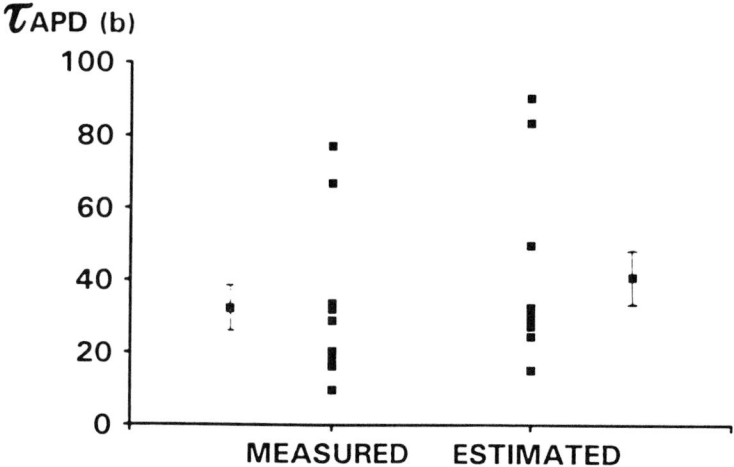

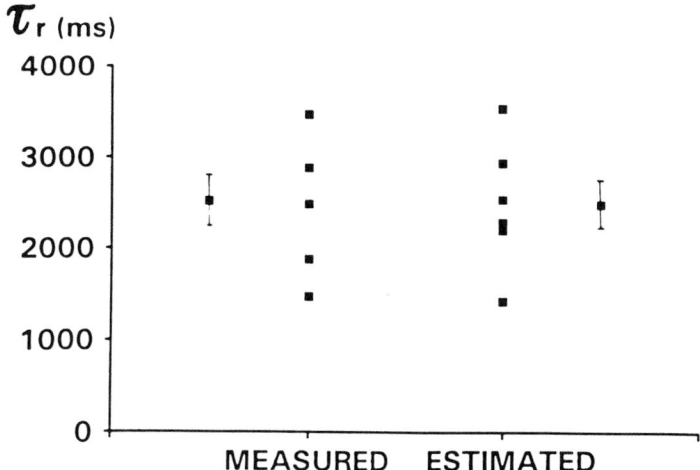

Figure 7. Measured time constants of recovery from block and of action potential duration (APD) adaptation are compared to the same parameters estimated by fitting the time course of block development with the model. Measured and estimated values do not differ significantly and are significantly correlated (r > 0.8; not shown).

the same tissue, in conditions of APD prolongation. This might explain why concentrations of propafenone sufficient to make Purkinje fibers almost inexcitable cause only a 50% depression in conduction velocity of ventricular muscle.[37,40,46] The relevance of tissue specificity in drug potency to antiarrhythmic or proarrhythmic actions of a drug is unknown.

Our findings also point out that APD prolongation, eg, by hypokalemia or pharmacological means, may potentiate the action of a local anesthetic and alter the kinetics of its use dependency. This represents a potentially important site of interaction between antiarrhythmic agents with different mechanisms of action such as Na^+ and K^+ channel blockers.

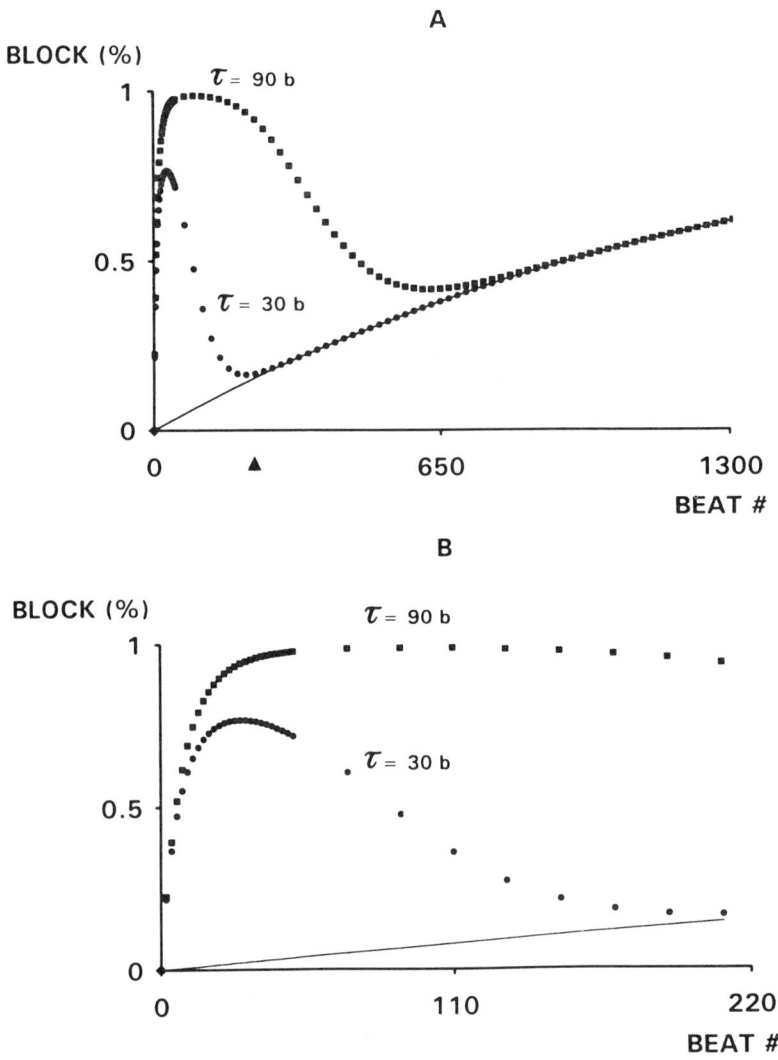

Figure 8. Panel A: effect of changing the rate of action potential duration (APD) adaptation on the kinetics of block development, according to predictions of the model. Squares and circles show block development with time constants of APD adaptation of 90 and 30 beats, respectively. The solid line represents the exponential blocking time course obtained by setting APD at its steady-state value throughout the stimulation; this simulates what would occur if APD changed instantaneously to its final value at the first beat of the run. The remaining parameters of the model where set at values similar to those found in propafenone experiments, and were the same in the three curves. Note how the change in APD adaptation kinetics modifies both the magnitude and the timing of the distortion in the kinetics of block. The early portion of panel A (from 0 to the arrow) is magnified in panel B. This shows that, if only the early steep portion of block onset were analyzed, the distortion in the time course present with τ = 90 beats would be easily overlooked.

Our findings also indicate that unless interference of APD adaptation is taken into account, estimation of use dependency kinetic parameters from action potential recordings may be misleading. Furthermore, kinetic parameters may be used to predict, through theoretical models, the rate dependence of drug effects. A new classification of antiarrhythmic agents according to patterns of rate dependence predicted according to the "guarded receptor hypothesis" has been recently proposed.[47] The practical utility of this interesting approach might be hampered, at least for what concerns some drugs, by the failure to consider the influence of APD changes on use-dependent drug effects.

Potential Autonomic Influences on Drug Action Occurring Through Modulation of Repolarization

The possibility that autonomic activation may interfere with antiarrhythmic drug action is supported by experimental and clinical observations[48,49] and is of remarkable practical importance. On the basis of the results presented so far, it is possible to speculate on how autonomic activation might affect drug use dependency through modulation of repolarization.

Catecholamines shorten APD in Purkinje fibers and have variable effects on ventricular muscle, according to the relative contribution of Ca^{2+} and K^+ currents to the repolarization process.[5,48] Sympathetic effects on APD are minimal at high heart rates, thus catecholamine-induced repolarization changes should affect use dependency predominantly at slow heart rates. Since adrenergic stimulation itself results in tachycardia, catecholamine-induced APD changes should have only a modest impact on drug effects. By contrast, modulation of the kinetics of APD adaptation by catecholamines may have potentially more substantial influences on drug action. By accelerating APD adaptation, sympathetic activation may change the degree of overlap between the time course of repolarization shortening and

of the onset of use-dependent block. Figure 8 shows that changing the time constant of APD adaptation from 90 (panel A) to 30 beats (panel B) reduces both the peak effect of the drug and the time during which it persists. Such a change, which is in the range of those produced by autonomic manipulations,[13] may determine whether conduction along a reentrant circuit will either be blocked, or only slowed by a given drug concentration.

References

1. Surawicz B: Dispersion of refractoriness in ventricular arrhythmias. In: DP Zipes, J Jalife (eds): *Cardiac Electrophysiology: From Cell to Bedside*. Philadelphia: W.B. Saunders Company, 1990, p. 377.
2. Allessie MA, Bonke FIM, Schopman FJG: Circus movement in rabbit atrial muscle as a mechanism of tachycardia. The "leading circle" concept: a new model of circus movement in cardiac tissue without the involvement of an anatomical obstacle. *Circ Res* 41:9, 1977.
3. Janse MJ: Reentry rhythms. In: HA Fozzard, RB Jennings, AM Katz, HE Morgan (eds): *The Heart and Cardiovascular System: Scientific Foundations*. New York: Raven Press, 1986, p. 1203.
4. January CT, Riddle JM: Early afterdepolarizations mechanism of induction and block. A role for L-type Ca^{2+} current. *Circ Res* 64:977, 1989.
5. Boyett MR, Jewell BR: Analysis of the effects of changes in rate and rhythm upon electrical activity in the heart. *Prog Biophys Mol Biol* 36:1, 1980.
6. Boyett MR, Fedida D: Changes in the electrical activity of dog cardiac Purkinje fibres at high heart rates. *J Physiol (Lond)* 350:361, 1984.
7. Kleiman RB, Houser SR: Outward currents in normal and hypertrophied feline ventricular myocytes. *Am J Physiol* 256:H1450, 1989.
8. Trautwein W, McDonald TF, Tripathi O: Calcium conductance and tension in mammalian ventricular muscle. *Pflügers Arch* 354:55, 1975.
9. Lab MJ: Contraction excitation feed back in myocardium: physiological basis and clinical relevance. *Circ Res* 50:757, 1982.
10. Lab MJ, Allen DG, Orchard CH: The effects of shortening on myoplasmic calcium concentration and on the action potential in mammalian ventricular muscle. *Circ Res* 55:824, 1984.
11. Kline RP, Kupersmith J: Effects of extracellular potassium accumulation and sodium pump activation on automatic canine Purkinje fibres. *J Physiol (Lond)* 324:507, 1982.

12. Robinson RB, Boyden PA, Hoffman BF, et al: Electrical restitution process in dispersed canine cardiac Purkinje and ventricular cells. *Am J Physiol* 253:H1018, 1987.

13. Zaza A, Malfatto G, Schwartz PJ: Sympathetic modulation of the relation between ventricular repolarization and cycle length. *Circ Res* 68: 1191, 1991.

14. Schwartz PJ, Snebold NG, Brown AM: Effects of unilateral cardiac sympathetic denervation on the ventricular fibrillation threshold. *Am J Cardiol* 37:1036, 1976.

15. Schwartz PJ, Verrier RL, Lown B: Effect of stellectomy and vagotomy on ventricular refractoriness in dogs. *Circ Res* 40:536, 1977.

16. Elharrar V, Atarashi H, Surawicz B: Cycle length-dependent action potential duration in canine cardiac Purkinje fibers. *Am J Physiol* 247: H936, 1984.

17. Schwartz PJ, Zaza A, Locati E, et al: Stress and sudden death. The case of the long QT syndrome. *Circulation* 83(Suppl II):71, 1991.

18. Sanguinetti MC, Jurkiewicz NK: Two components of cardiac delayed rectifier K^+ current. *J Gen Physiol* 96:195, 1990.

19. Taggart P, Sutton P, Lab M, et al: Interplay between adrenaline and interbeat interval on ventricular repolarization in intact heart in vivo. *Cardiovasc Res* 24:884, 1990.

20. Litovsky SH, Antzelevitch C: Differences in the electrophysiological response of canine ventricular subendocardium and subepicardium to acetylcholine and isoproterenol. *Circ Res* 67: 615, 1990.

21. Antzelevitch C, Sicouri S, Litovsky SH, et al: Heterogeneity within the ventricular wall. Electrophysiology and pharmacology of epicardial, endocardial, and M cells. *Circ Res* 69:1427, 1991.

22. Sicouri S, Antzelevitch C: A subpopulation of cells with unique electrophysiological properties in the deep subepicardium of the canine ventricle. The M cell. *Circ Res* 68:1729, 1991.

23. Zaza A, Kline RP, Rosen MR: Effects of alpha-adrenergic stimulation on intracellular sodium activity and automaticity in canine Purkinje fibers. *Circ Res* 66:416, 1990.

24. Desilets M, Baumgarten CM: Isoproterenol directly stimulates the Na^+-K^+ pump in isolated cardiac myocytes. *Am J Physiol* 251:H218, 1986.

25. Schwartz PJ: Sympathetic imbalance and cardiac arrhythmias. In: WC Randall (ed): *Nervous Control of Cardiovascular Function*. New York: Oxford University Press, 1984, p. 225.

26. McCall RB, Gebber GL, Barman SM: Spinal interneurons in the baroreceptor reflex arc. *Am J Physiol* 232:H657, 1977.

27. Malfatto G, Zaza A, Schwartz PJ: Parasympathetic control of cycle length dependence of

endocardial ventricular repolarization in the intact feline heart during steady state conditions. *Cardiovasc Res* 27:823, 1993.

28. Hartzell CH: Regulation of cardiac ion channels by catecholamines, acetylcholine and second messenger systems. *Prog Biophys Mol Biol* 52: 165, 1988.

29. Schwartz PJ, Priori SG: Sympathetic nervous system and cardiac arrhythmias. In: DP Zipes, J Jalife (eds): *Cardiac Electrophysiology. From Cell to Bedside*. Philadelphia: W.B. Saunders Company, 1990, p. 330.

30. Vanoli E, De Ferrari GM, Stramba-Badiale M, et al: Vagal stimulation and prevention of sudden death in conscious dogs with a healed myocardial infarction. *Circ Res* 68:1471, 1991.

31. Nattel S, Zeng FD: Frequency-dependent effects of antiarrhythmic drugs on action potential duration and refractoriness in canine cardiac Purkinje fibers. *J Pharmacol Exp Ther* 229:283, 1984.

32. Hondeghem LM, Katzung BG: Time- and voltage-dependent interactions of antiarrhythmic drugs with cardiac sodium channels. *Biochim Biophys Acta* 472:373, 1977.

33. McDonald TF, Pelzer D, Trautwein W: Cat ventricular muscle treated with D600: characteristics of calcium channel block and unblock. *J Physiol (Lond)* 352:217, 1984.

34. Hondeghem LM: Antiarrhythmic agents: modulated receptor applications. *Circulation* 75:514, 1987.

35. Starmer CF: Theoretical characterization of ion channel blockade: ligand binding to periodically accessible receptors. *J Theor Biol* 119:235, 1986.

36. Varro A, Elharrar V, Surawicz B: Frequency-dependent effects of several class I antiarrhythmic drugs on $\dot{V}_{max}$ of action potential upstroke in canine cardiac Purkinje fibers. *J Cardiovasc Pharmacol* 7:482, 1985.

37. Kolhardt M, Seifert C: Inhibition of $\dot{V}_{max}$ of the action potential by propafenone and its voltage-, time-, and pH-dependence in mammalian ventricular myocardium. *Naunyn Schmiedebergs Arch Pharmacol* 315:55, 1980.

38. Campbell TJ: Kinetics of onset of rate-dependent effects of Class I antiarrhythmic drugs are important in determining their effects on refractoriness in guinea-pig ventricle, and provide a theoretical basis for their subclassification. *Cardiovasc Res* 17:344, 1983.

39. Lee JH, Rosen MR: Use-dependent actions and effects on transmembrane action potentials of flecainide, encainide, and ethmozine in canine Purkinje fibers. *J Cardiovasc Pharmacol* 18: 285, 1991.

40. Zaza A, Malfatto G, Schwartz PJ: Different effects

of propafenone and flecainide in canine Purkinje fibers. *Eur Heart J* 13(suppl I):144, 1992.

41. Zaza A, Malfatto G, Ravelli F, Schwartz PJ: Action potential duration adaptation modulates use-dependent effects of propafenone. (submitted).

42. Elharrar V, Surawicz B: Cycle length effect on restitution of action potential duration in dog cardiac fibers. *Am J Physiol* 244:H782, 1983.

43. Anno T, Hondeghem LM: Interactions of flecainide with guinea pig cardiac sodium channels: importance of activation unblocking to the voltage dependence of recovery. *Circ Res* 66:789, 1990.

44. Kolhardt M, Seifert C: Tonic and phasic I_{Na} blockade by antiarrhythmics. Different properties of drug binding to fast sodium channels as judged from V_{max} studies with propafenone and derivatives in mammalian ventricular myocardium. *Pflügers Arch* 396:199, 1983.

45. Kolhardt M, Fichtner U, Frobe U, et al: On the mechanism of drug-induced blockade of Na^+ currents: interaction of antiarrhythmic drugs with DPI-modified single cardiac Na^+ channels. *Circ Res* 64:867, 1989.

46. Thompson KA, Iansmith DHS, Siddoway LA, et al: Potent electrophysiologic effects of the major metabolites of propafenone in canine Purkinje fibers. *J Pharmacol Exp Ther* 244:950, 1988.

47. Weirich J, Antoni H: Differential analysis of the frequency-dependent effects of class I antiarrhythmic drugs according to periodical ligand binding: implications on antiarrhythmic and proarrhythmic efficacy. *J Cardiovasc Pharmacol* 15:998, 1990.

48. Sanguinetti MC, Jurkiewicz NK, Scott A, et al: Isoproterenol antagonizes prolongation of refractory period by the class III antiarrhythmic agent E-4031 in guinea pig myocytes. Mechanism of action. *Circ Res* 68:77, 1991.

49. Myerburg RJ, Kessler KM, Cox MM, et al: Reversal of proarrhythmic effects of flecainide acetate and encainide hydrochloride by propranolol. *Circulation* 80:1571, 1989.

PART II

Mechanism of Cardiac Arrhythmias

Chapter 6

General Concepts in the Mechanisms of Cardiac Arrhythmias

Michael R. Rosen

Descriptions of irregular heartbeats are as old as the earliest written literature. In the Bible, Elihu says to Job, "At this my heart trembleth and is moved out of its place."[1] Was Elihu having bouts of paroxysmal tachycardia? In any event, as the practice of medicine evolved, irregularities of the pulse were noted to accompany disease. Scherf and Schott[2] quote the *Difficult Chapters of Medicine* by Pien Chio as documenting the importance of irregularities of the pulse in the sixth century B.C. Depending on the type of pulse intermittency, disease and death could be predicted, with a loss of every second beat suggesting the patient had only days to live. The concept that arrhythmias might have specific physiological causes did not evolve until the 19th century.[2] As technology advanced, first using photographic plates to record the motion of mechanically stimulated tissues and then rudimentary electrical recordings, the idea of the heart as a muscle that contained cellular elements having coordinated electrical activity that might—under a variety of circumstances—become disordered took hold.

Today, we understand mechanisms for arrhythmias as evolving from disorders of impulse initiation and impulse conduction, or combinations of the two. This formulation, although not recent, nonetheless remains convenient and will be used here. I will not dwell on the mechanisms for normal impulse initiation and conduction, as these are the province of earlier chapters. Similarly, I shall not consider arrhythmogenesis in a variety of specific experimental and clinical settings, as these will be found in subsequent chapters.

Abnormal Impulse Initiation

That focal sites of impulse initiation might be present in supraventricular or ventricular tissues has long been known. It was recognized, as early as the 17th century[2] that these sites might be "self-initiating" or automatic, and that automatic impulses could arise and compete with a primary pacemaker. Also demonstrated long before the microelectrode era but less readily accepted, was the fact that oscillations in membrane potential that are not automatic could give rise to focal arrhythmias.[3,4] At present, both automatic and oscilla-

Certain of the studies referred to were supported by USPHS-NHLBI grants HL-28958 and HL-43731.
From BN Singh, HJJ Wellens, M Hiraoka, (eds): *Electropharmacological Control of Cardiac Arrhythmias.* Mount Kisco, NY, Futura Publishing Company Inc., © 1994.

tory activity are recognized as contributing to arrhythmogenesis and both will be discussed.

Automaticity

Automaticity refers to the ability of a cell to initiate impulses de novo. This is the result of a pacemaker current, designated I_f,[5] which carries positive charge (Na^+) into the cell, depolarizing it from its resting level to a threshold potential at which a propagating action potential can be initiated. Inward current carried by Ca^{2+} may also contribute to membrane depolarization.[6] Counteracting the inward currents carried by sodium (Na) and calcium (Ca) are the effects of outward K currents[6] and the Na/K pump.[7]

Whereas all cells in the heart have the potential to generate pacemaker activity, the sinus node, which generates the most rapid pacemaker rate, fulfills this role in the normal heart. At such time that the sinus node is suppressed, then accessory pacemakers in the atrium or atrioventricular junction may take over, and at times of heart block, the same may occur with pacemakers in the His bundle and Purkinje system. The latter do not generate activity under normal circumstances as they are overdrive suppressed by the primary sinus node pacemaker (Figure 1). As detailed in Chapter 8 overdrive suppression depends on several factors, although perhaps chief among them is the stimulation of the Na/K pump as a result of Na entering the cell during the action potential.[7] The outward current generated by the pump in subsidiary pacemaker cells prevents them from generating spontaneous action potentials.[8]

If a subsidiary pacemaker site is "protected" from activation by the sinus node pacemaker by a site of conduction block (so-called entry block) then it will generate automatic impulses that may gain access to the rest of the heart and result in ectopic beats. Probably more important to arrhythmogenesis than this type of automatic activity is that which occurs when cardiac fibers (both specialized and myocardial) are depolarized to low levels of membrane potential (in the -40 to -60 mV range) as a result of ischemia or infarction (Figure 1). In this setting, the I_f pacemaker is inactivated (it activates on hyperpolarization).[5] However, inward currents carried by Ca^{2+} and Na^+ in the face of diminishing outward K currents do generate pacemaker activity that has two important characteristics: (1) it tends to initiate impulses at more rapid rates than the normal pacemaker current; and (2) because the fibers are depolarized to low membrane potentials there is little Na entry during the action potential, little stimulation of the Na/K pump, and minimal to no overdrive suppression. This type of automaticity, occurring at low levels of membrane potential, has been referred to as "abnormal automaticity," thereby distinguishing it from the "normal automaticity" that occurs in fully polarized fibers, and is overdrive suppressible.[9]

Afterdepolarizations and Triggered Activity

Afterdepolarizations are oscillations in membrane potential that do not occur spontaneously, but are induced by a preceding action potential. Afterdepolarizations may be early or delayed.[10] Early afterdepolarizations occur during phase 2 or 3 of repolarization (Figure 2). If they occur during the phase 2 plateau, a major component of inward current is supplied by Ca^{2+} entering via L-type Ca^{2+} channels (I_{CaL}).[11] Calcium channel agonists, like Bay K 8644, or catecholamines that activate the adenylate cyclase-cAMP second messenger system and phosphorylate calcium channels, can induce increases in I_{CaL} and induce early afterdepolarizations.[12] Early afterdepolarizations occurring later during phase 3 seem to depend more on a delay of repolarization resulting from decreased repolarizing K currents. Cesium ion and antiarrhythmic drugs having Class III effects can induce this type of behavior.[12,13]

Characteristic of early afterdepolarizations is the fact that they increase in amplitude at slow stimulation rates and, at sufficiently

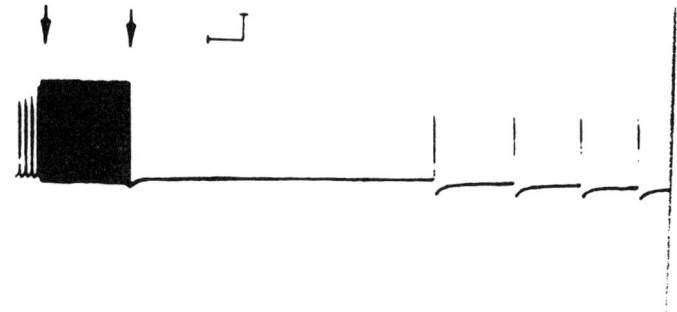

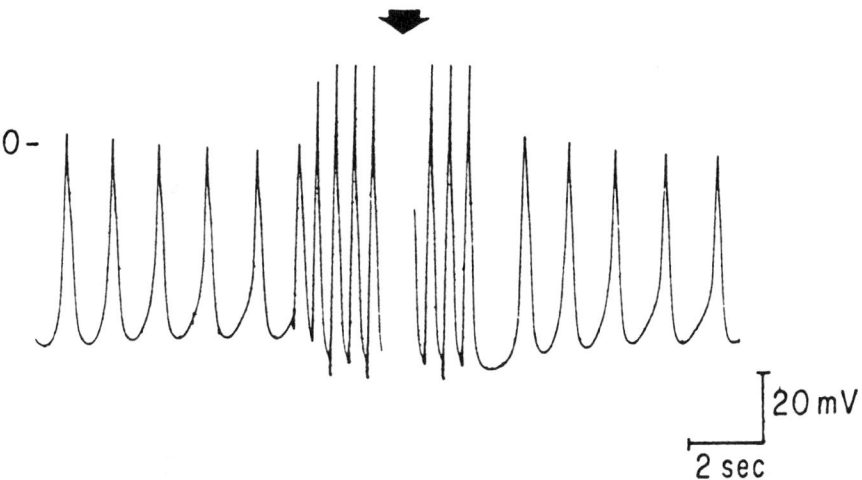

Figure 1. Top: A Purkinje fiber having a membrane potential of −90 mV is firing spontaneously (first three cycles) after which it is overdriven by an extrinsic pacemaker (onset and offset marked with arrows). Hyperpolarization of the fiber occurs. On cessation of overdrive, there is a long interval of quiescence followed by the onset and gradual acceleration of the automatic rhythm. (Modified with permission from Rosen M, Reder R: Does triggered activity have a role in the genesis of cardiac arrhythmias. *Ann Intern Med* 94:794, 1981.) Calibration = 30 mV and 6 msec. Bottom panel: A fiber having a low membrane potential is beating spontaneously. Following a period of overdrive pacing (arrow indicates 60 seconds) there is modest hyperpolarization but no suppression of the rhythm.

low rates, can reach threshold inducing single or multiple action potentials having a fixed coupling relationship to the initiating impulse.[14] They can also induce bursts of or sustained periods of tachyarrhythmias. When occurring at high membrane potentials, such bursts can be overdrive suppressed, much like automatic rhythms. In contrast, at low membrane potentials, overdrive suppression is often not possible. Interventions that suppress early afterdepolarizations include those that accelerate repolarization and/or speed stimulation rate.

Delayed afterdepolarizations are seen after full repolarization of the membrane (Figure 3). They are the result of an intracellular Ca^{2+} overload that may occur as the result of a variety of factors, eg, digitalis excess, cate-

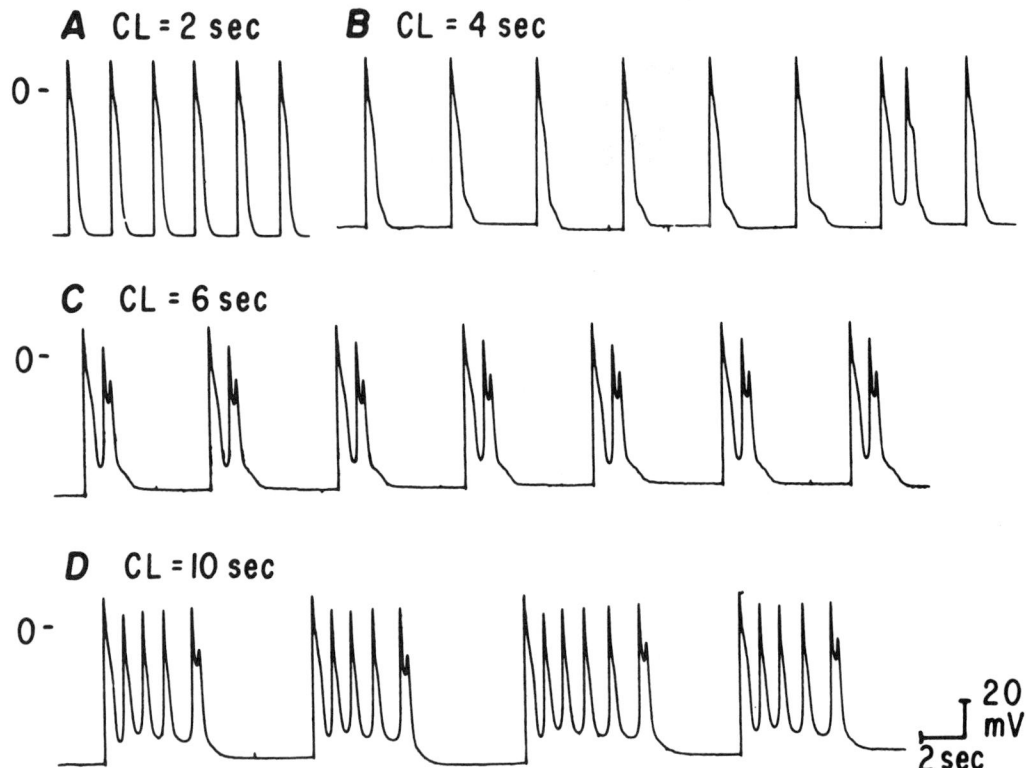

Figure 2. Cesium-induced early afterdepolarizations (EAD) and triggered activity in a Purkinje fiber. In (A), at a cycle length of 2 seconds, no EAD or triggered activity are seen. As drive cycle length is increased (B), EAD occur as a "shoulder" during phase 3 and there is one triggered beat. At a longer cycle length (C) the triggered beats manifest a bigeminal pattern and a second EAD is seen during the plateau of the coupled beat. At a cycle length of 10 seconds (D) each driven beat is followed by a burst of beats triggered by EAD. (Reprinted with permission from Reference 14.)

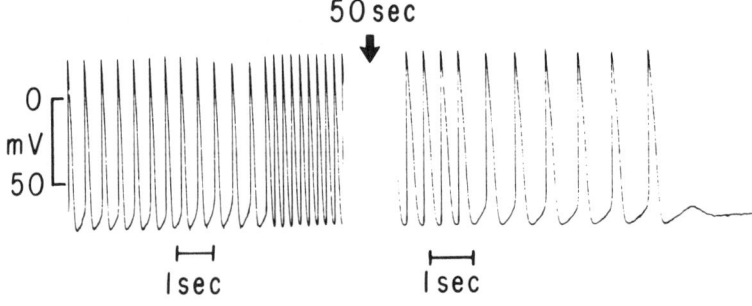

Figure 3. Delayed afterdepolarization (DAD)-induced triggered activity. A sustained rhythm is interrupted by a period of overdrive pacing. After the last four paced beats a burst of six beats occurs, followed by a subthreshold oscillation. The six beats are triggered and the oscillation is a DAD.

cholamines, ischemia, and reperfusion.[12] The Ca^{2+} overload induces an oscillatory transsarcolemmal current that may be contributed to by the Na/Ca exchanger. The major charge carrier for the current is Na$^+$.

In contrast to early afterdepolarizations, delayed afterdepolarizations increase in magnitude and show shortening in their coupling interval to the preceding action potential as drive rate increases.[15,16] When they attain threshold they induce coupled beats or bursts of tachyarrhythmias that, at least for the first triggered beat, bear a consistent relationship to the preceding drive period. That is, the faster the drive, the more rapid the triggered rhythm will be.[17] Interventions that slow drive rate or decrease inward current or enhance outward current during phase 4 will tend to suppress delayed afterdepolarizations and triggered activity.

Abnormal Conduction

Under normal circumstances, activation of the heart proceeds in an orderly fashion during each cardiac cycle. Studies done at the turn of the century in jellyfish and subsequently in vertebrates demonstrated that excitable tissues could, under certain circumstances develop sustained rhythms in which an impulse circulated, literally "following its tail" in a well-defined pathway.[18–20] The conditions needed to induce reentry are rigorous. As shown in Figure 4, a reentrant circuit has specific requisites. These include an area of conduction block and a path length sufficiently long and conduction velocity sufficiently low to permit an impulse propagating retrogradely through a depressed area to encounter tissues whose refractory periods have terminated, such that continued propagation is possible.

The normal sodium-dependent action potential in the Purkinje system propagates so rapidly ($\sim$ 2 M/sec) that its propagation in most circuits is too rapid for refractoriness to terminate such that reentry might occur. In contrast, fibers that are depolarized (as in the

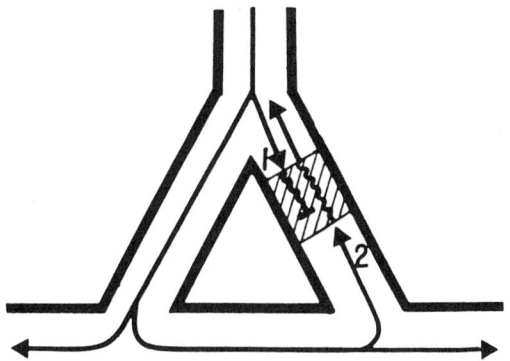

Figure 4. The Schmitt-Erlanger model of reentry. Depicted are a terminal portion of the Purkinje system with two fiber bundles linking to the myocardium. Under normal circumstances an impulse arising proximally would propagate through both limbs and activate the muscle. In this figure, a depressed segment exists in the right limb of the Purkinje system. Antegrade activation is blocked at site 1. The remainder of the system is activated via the remaining limb, and excitation enters the depressed segment retrogradely at site 2. It propagates slowly in the retrograde direction. If sufficient time has elapsed to permit refractoriness to terminate in the proximal tissues, activation will continue retrogradely, reenter the proximal conducting system, and reexcite the heart. (Reprinted with permission from Rosen M: Is the response to programmed electrical stimulation diagnostic of mechanisms for arrhythmias? *Circulation* 73:II-18, 1986.)

setting of an infarct) to the range of -50 mV no longer have a rapid inward Na$^+$ current. This current is inactivated at low levels of membrane potential. Nonetheless, action potentials can be generated that are the result of Ca^{2+} entry via L-type channels and that propagate with a velocity only 1/100th that of the Na-dependent action potential.[21] This is sufficiently slow to permit reentry to occur. The fact that specific conditions of conduction and refractoriness are required for reentry means that in any individual certain ranges of heart rates and rhythms will favor the initiation of a reentrant impulse. This requirement of specific rate characteristics has been used to develop the programmed electrical stimulation techniques that are used clinically to induce reentry.[22] Similarly, reentrant rhythms can be terminated if an extrasystole is induced in such a way that it invades the pathway at a site where it is excitable. This will render the site refractory to the continued propagation of the reentrant impulse. This characteristic has also been used to permit the termination of reentry by pacing techniques.[22] Pharmacological interventions can also modify reentry as long as they alter conduction or the duration of repolarization in such a way that the critical timing that is a requisite for the pathway is altered.

Other mechanisms permit reentry, even when no Ca^{2+}-dependent action potentials are occurring. For example, as detailed in Chapter 7, anisotropy may eventuate.[23] Propagation normally proceeds along the longitudinal axis of cardiac fibers, and depends on the presence of low-resistance gap junctions between adjacent cells. Gap junctional density is much lower on the transverse margins of cells, and as a result propagation transversely tends to be slow and discontinuous. In the event of conduction block longitudinally, conduction still may occur transversely, giving rise to slow conduction and facilitating reentry.

Reentry may occur not only in association with an anatomical conduction block, but as a result of functional block, a phenomenon referred to as leading circle reentry[24] (see Chapter 9). Moreover, rather than propagating around a circuit, an impulse may propagate back through a linear fiber bundle after encountering an area of block: a phenomenon referred to as reflection.[25]

Combined Abnormalities of Impulse Initiation and Conduction

The classic arrhythmia here is parasystole.[2] This depends on the presence of an automatic focus that is protected from depolarization by the dominant cardiac impulse because of the presence of a site of conduction block (so-called entry block). The focus can in turn propagate its own impulses to the rest of the heart, depending on the extent of exit block.

It is important to understand that the dominant cardiac impulse and the parasystolic impulse do not function independently of one another. Rather, depending on the extent of entry block, subthreshold impulses propagated from the dominant pacemaker can displace the membrane potential of the parasystolic focus and induce it to reach threshold earlier or later than might otherwise occur. This acceleration or delay are predictable.[26] As a result of this interdependency, parasystolic impulses may occur either independently of the dominant rhythm or may manifest a fixed relationship to the dominant pacemaker.

Conclusions

It is highly likely that the majority of cardiac arrhythmias of importance clinically are reentrant. However, all mechanisms mentioned have been demonstrated to play a role in experimental models and all are at least implicated in some clinical settings. The following chapters will provide further details concerning certain of these mechanisms as well as a consideration of their roles clinically.

References

1. *The Holy Scriptures*. Philadelphia: The Jewish Publication Society of America, 1951, p. 959.
2. Scherf D, Schott A: *Extrasystoles and Allied Arrhythmias*. 2nd edition. Chicago: Year Book Medical Publishers, 1973.
3. Segers M: Lebattement auto-entretenu du coeur. *Arch Int Pharmacodyn Ther* 75:144, 1947.
4. Bozler E: The initiation of impulses in cardiac muscle. *Am J Physiol* 138:273, 1943.
5. DiFrancesco D: The cardiac hyperpolarizing-activated current, I_f. Origins and developments. *Prog Biophys Mol Biol* 46:163, 1985.
6. Noble D: *The Initiation of the Heart Beat*. Oxford: Clarendon Press, 1975.
7. Eisner DA: The Na/K pump in cardiac muscle. In: H Fozzard, E Haber, R Jennings, et al. (eds): *The Heart and Cardiovascular System*. New York: Raven Press, 1986, p. 488.

8. Vassalle M: The relationship among cardiac pacemakers: overdrive suppression. *Circ Res* 41:269, 1977.

9. Dangman KH, Hoffman BF: Studies on overdrive stimulation of canine cardiac Purkinje fibers: maximal diastolic potential as a determinant of the response. *J Am Coll Cardiol* 6:1183, 1983.

10. Cranefield PF: Action potentials, afterpotentials and arrhythmias. *Circ Res* 41:415, 1977.

11. January CT, Riddle JM, Salata JJ: A model for early afterdepolarizations: induction with the Ca^{2+} channel agonist Bay K 8644. *Circ Res* 62:563, 1988.

12. Wit AL, Rosen MR: Afterdepolarizations and triggered activity. In: H Fozzard, E Haber, R Jennings, et al. (eds): *The Heart and Cardiovascular System*. New York: Raven Press, 1986, p. 1449.

13. Brachman J, Scherlag BJ, Rosenshtraukh LV, Lazzara R: Bradycardia-dependent triggered activity: relevance to drug-induced multiform ventricular tachycardia. *Circulation* 68:846, 1983.

14. Damiano BP, Rosen MR: Effects of pacing on triggered activity induced by early afterdepolarizations. *Circulation* 69:1013, 1984.

15. Ferrier GR, Saunders JH, Mendez C: A cellular mechanism for the generation of ventricular arrhythmias by acetylstrophanthidin. *Circ Res* 32:600, 1973.

16. Rosen MR, Gelband H, Merker C, Hoffman BF: Mechanisms of digitalis toxicity: effects of ouabain on phase 4 of canine Purkinje fiber transmembrane potentials. *Circulation* 47:681, 1973.

17. Johnson NJ, Rosen MR: The distinction between triggered activity and other cardiac arrhythmias. In: P Brugada, HJJ Wellens (eds): *Cardiac Arrhythmias: Where To Go From Here?* Mt.

Kisco, NY: Futura Publishing Company, Inc., 1987, p. 129.

18. Mayer AG: Rhythmical pulsation in Scyphomedusae. *Carnegie Inst Washington Publ* 47:115, 1906.

19. Mines GR: On circulating excitations in heart muscles and their possible relation to tachycardia and fibrillation. *Trans R Soc Can Inst* 8:43, 1914.

20. Schmitt FO, Erlanger J: Directional differences in the conduction of the impulse through the heart muscle and their possible relation to extrasystolic and fibrillary contractions. *Am J Physiol* 87:326, 1928.

21. Cranefield PF: *The Conduction of the Cardiac Impulse: The Slow Response and Cardiac Arrhythmias*. Mt. Kisco, NY: Futura Publishing Company, Inc., 1975.

22. Wellens HJJ: Value and limitations of programmed electrical stimulation of the heart in the study and treatment of tachycardias. *Circulation* 57:845, 1978.

23. Spach MS, Miller WT, Geselowitz DB, et al: The discontinuous nature of propagation in normal canine cardiac muscle: evidence for recurrent discontinuities of intracellular resistance that affect membrane currents. *Circ Res* 48:39, 1981.

24. Allessie MA, Bonke FIM, Schopman FJG: Circus movement in rabbit atrial muscle as a mechanism of tachycardia. III. The "leading circle" concept: a new model of circus movement in cardiac tissue without the involvement of an anatomical obstacle. *Circ Res* 41:9, 1977.

25. Antzelevitch C: Electrotonus and reflection. In: MR Rosen, MJ Janse, AL Wit (eds): *Cardiac Electrophysiology: A Textbook*. Mt. Kisco, NY: Futura Publishing Company, Inc., 1990, pp 491.

26. Jalife J, Moe GK: Effect of electrotonic potentials on pacemaker activity of canine Purkinje fibers in relation to parasystole. *Circ Res* 39:801, 1976.

Chapter 7

Abnormalities in Depolarization Mediating Arrhythmogenic Mechanisms: *Focus on Anisotropy and Reentry*

Madison S. Spach
Paul C. Dolber

The classic model of reentry involves the initiation of a premature impulse at a single site, following which the impulse conducts at a low velocity in one direction, while in another direction the impulse fails. Due to these directional differences in propagation, there is enough time for recovery of excitability to occur in the area of block, after which that area can sustain propagation when the slowly moving wave front arrives (reentry). The different types of reentrant circuits have been reviewed by Allessie et al.[1] Until recently the spatial inhomogeneities that are necessary to produce reentry within cardiac muscle were considered to be caused by regional differences in the kinetics of the sarcolemmal membrane ionic currents that control the time course of repolarization of the action potential. In turn, this produces spatial differences in the refractory period. From studies of directional differences of propagation in relation to the orientation of parallel oriented cardiac fibers, however, it became apparent a decade ago that the factors controlling conduction velocity and also the safety factors are determined by the anisotropic passive properties of the tissue due to the anisotropic nature of cardiac bundles and to associated microscopic discontinuities of resistance produced by the connections between cells.[2,3] Thus, it is now appreciated that the inhomogeneities necessary for reentry are produced either by properties of the membrane ionic currents or by anisotropic structure, or both. This chapter presents available evidence that complexities of anisotropic structure provide a new phenomenon underlying numerous conditions associated with reentrant atrial and ventricular reentrant tachyarrhythmias.

What is anisotropic propagation? Figure 1A illustrates the isochrone progression in a typical cardiac bundle in which excitation is initiated at a single site.[4] Fast conduction occurs along the long axis of the fibers (widely

Supported by U.S. Public Health Service Grants HL11307 and HL07063.
From BN Singh, HJJ Wellens, M Hiraoka, (eds): *Electropharmacological Control of Cardiac Arrhythmias.* Mount Kisco, NY, Futura Publishing Company Inc., © 1994.

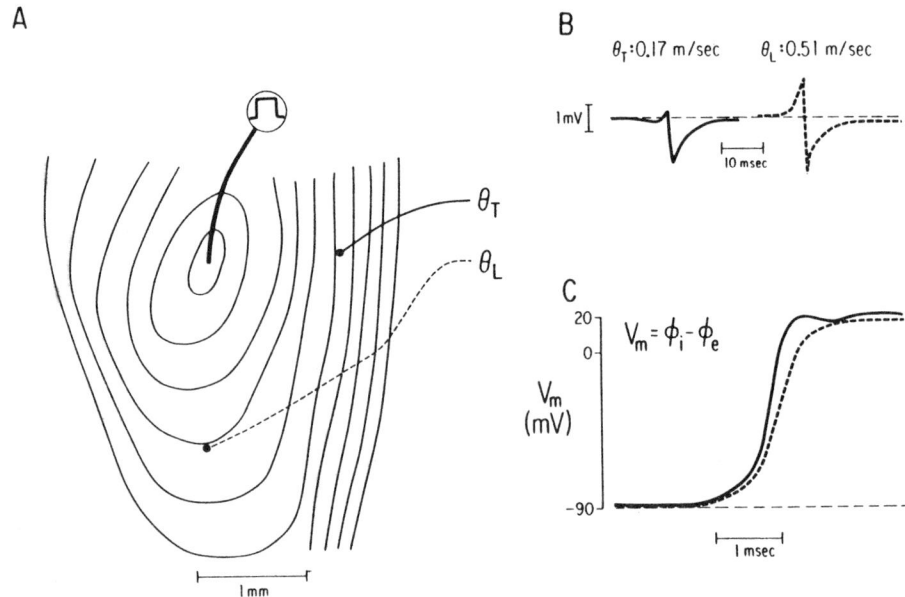

Figure 1. Anisotropic spread of excitation (A) and the extracellular and transmembrane potential waveforms (B) in uniform anisotropic ventricular muscle. The extracellular waveforms in panel B were recorded at the locations indicated by the solid dots in panel A. The velocity along the fast longitudinal axis of the fibers is represented by θ_L and θ_T represents the velocity in the transverse direction (propagation across fibers). In panel C, the transmembrane potential depolarization waveforms were obtained by measuring the extracellular potential ϕ_e and the intracellular potential ϕ_i at the same microelectrode impalement site. (Reproduced with permission from Reference 4.)

spaced isochrones) and slow conduction occurs across fibers (closely spaced isochrones). These differences in velocity are due to directional differences in the resistance to current flow produced by the internal structure of cells (eg, cytoplasm) and the number of gap junctions between cells along each axis of propagation. Although the distribution of the gap junctions is complex and irregular in two and three dimensions, in general there are fewer gap junctions per unit distance along the long axis of the fibers than across fibers. This results in a lower resistance along the long axis of the fibers than across the fibers in all cardiac bundles composed of parallel oriented fibers.

The above directional differences in velocity can be accounted for at a macroscopic level of 1 mm or greater by a structure that is continuous in nature, but with different resistances along different axes (anisotropy).[5,6]

Such a continuous medium produces extracellular potentials consistent with the experimentally measured extracellular waveforms shown in Figure 1B for longitudinal and transverse propagation. However, we found that the transmembrane action potentials recorded at a single site within an individual cell changed depolarization shape when the direction of propagation changed. Such a change in the time course of depolarization should not occur in a continuous medium, even if anisotropic. The maximum rate of rise (dV/dt_{max}) of the action potential was greater when slow conduction occurred across cells (transverse conduction) than it was when fast conduction occurred along the fibers.[2] This relationship between dV/dt_{max} is the opposite of that when the conduction velocity is altered by changes in the magnitude of the depolarizing sodium current, such as occurs with an early premature impulse. Subsequently, this directional difference in dV/dt_{max} as a single site within a cell was confirmed by numerous laboratories.[7,8] Based on these findings, we proposed that cardiac tissue cannot be modeled as a continuous syncytium and that the propagated action potential is greatly influenced by the microscopic structural properties of the tissue.[2,3]

Several explanations and theoretical models subsequently were put forward in an attempt to account for the directional differences in dV/dt_{max}. Suenson[9] considered that the lateral feed-off of current from the cells associated with longitudinal conduction ("drag" effect[10]) reduced dV/dt_{max} of longitudinal conduction sufficiently to account for the slower rate of depolarization than occurs with transverse conduction. The presence of a drag effect occurs only when wave fronts have a curvature similar to that of the wave fronts illustrated by the isochrones shown in Figure 1A for the typical anisotropic excitation spread that occurs following the initiation of propagation at single site. To test whether the drag effect was the cause of the direction differences in dV/dt_{max}, we stimulated at multiple sites along a line to produce a plane wave of conduction in the longitudinal direction of ventricular fibers and along another line to produce transverse plane wave conduction, similar to the experimental procedure used by Clerc.[5] The same prominent directional differences in dV/dt_{max} occurred with values 30–40 V/sec greater during transverse conduction, thus ruling out the drag effect as the primary mechanism (there is no drag effect with plane wave conduction). Knisley et al.[11] recently suggested another explanation—that the direction differences in the transmembrane potential are due to failure to adequately subtract the extracellular potential from the intracellular potential waveform when both are recorded in reference to a distant electrode. This is unlikely because our original demonstration of the directional differences in the rate of rise of the transmembrane potential emphasized the importance of subtracting the extracellular potential from the intracellular potential. Also, we have tested

this by recording the extracellular potential with the microelectrode at the membrane just before impalement occurred, and then subtracted the extracellular from the intracellular potential waveform. The higher values of dV/dt_{max} during transverse conduction persisted.

From the above we concluded that dV/dt_{max} is in fact greater during transverse than longitudinal conduction in cardiac bundles with parallel oriented fibers. The importance of this directional difference is that it implies that the safety factor of conduction is inherently greater during slow conduction across fibers rather than during fast conduction along the fibers. In the absence of any challenge to this original experimental finding of directional differences in dV/dt_{max}, we thought there should be considerable variations in the directional differences because of the considerable complexity of cardiac cellular structure. Recently, by using conventional microelectrodes positioned at a fixed site within a single cell, we confirmed that in most cases the above directional differences in dV/dt_{max} occur in both atrial and ventricular bundles. However, we found that dV/dt_{max} also changed when propagation remained constant along the longitudinal axis of the fibers and the direction of propagation was reversed 180°. The same phenomena occurred when propagation was maintained along the transverse axis, ie, although dV/dt_{max} in almost all impalements was greater than during longitudinal conduction (at the same site within a single cell), its value changed considerably when the direction was reversed 180°.

It is pertinent to note that one cannot invoke artifact, such as local injury, as having an effect on these results since each impalement site within a different cell serves as its own control for comparison of the differences in dV/dt_{max} for each of the four directions of conduction. On the other hand, we have emphasized that intracellular impalements at multiple sites within 200 μm result in injury and make that technique not applicable for mapping excitation spread at a cellular level (we usually create injury after three impalements within 100 μm along the long axis of the fibers).[12,13] The important procedure to follow is to use an associated extracellular measurement at the site of impalement, ie, changes in the extracellular waveform (or the lack thereof) provide a sensitive and accurate index of any injury that alters the local excitation events. When done carefully, as noted, we have made 10–20 single impalements at sites 500 μm to 1 mm apart along the long axis of fibers, allowing 3–5 minutes between impalements. This seemingly simple experimental technical feature is emphasized because the use of microelectrode impalements will likely be necessary in the future to obtain evidence about detailed events of conduction within a single cell located in a large multicellular preparation. Specifically, directional differences in the rate of rise of the action potential at the same site within a cell during four-way propagation indicate that conduction events within single cells cannot be ignored. For example, during propagation the transmembrane potential is not equipotential throughout a single cell (nor is the extracellular potential the same surrounding a single cell) and the parameters that affect conduction, such as dV/dt_{max} and the sodium current, are not the same within a single cell. The above evidence may be important in future considerations of variations in the density of sodium channels in myocytes as recently demonstrated by Makielski et al.[14]

Two Types of Conduction Properties of Cardiac Bundles: Normal Action Potentials

Figure 2 shows the most idealized type of anisotropic propagation properties of cardiac bundles. The isochrones and the extracellular waveforms with accompanying first derivatives are shown for an atrial bundle from a 2-year-old child. The excitation spread produces teardrop-shaped isochrones. The associated extracellular waveforms are, in general, smooth in contour with large biphasic deflections during longitudinal fast propagation and small deflections with slower transverse prop-

agation. Note, however, that the derivative of the extracellular waveform during transverse propagation (#3 in Figure 2) has small undulations, which are indicative of minor microscopic discontinuities of transverse conduction. The major interpretation of these propagating extracellular waveforms is that they indicate that there are many electrical connections between cardiac cells (tight electrical coupling) in all directions and that conduction is uniform throughout. Hence, we coined the term uniform anisotropy for bundles with this type of conduction of normal action potentials.

Figure 3 shows the second type of microscopic anisotropic propagation properties. These occur in bundles associated with chronic hypertrophy and with aging.[12] When propagation is initiated at a single site (the stimulating electrode is placed gently against the surface without injury) a very narrow zone (in this case 100 μm in width) of fast longitudinal conduction occurs along the long axis of the fibers and the transition to transverse propagation occurs quite abruptly (there are no teardrop-shaped isochrones). Also, transverse propagation is quite irregular. This is indicated by the irregular shapes of the low-amplitude extracellular waveforms that have multiple notches in both the original waveform and its derivative. These marked irregularities have only one explanation, there is a sparsity of electrical connections between fibers in a side-to-side direction. We applied the term nonuniform anisotropy to bundles with this type of conduction of normal action potentials. In such bundles, extracellular measurements with small-tipped metal microelectrodes indicated that propagation occurred in a zigzag manner as conduction progressed along the transverse axis.

A major consequence of these differences in propagation properties is that in both uniform and nonuniform anisotropic preparations, a low effective conduction velocity occurs when normal and abnormal action potentials propagate across fibers. In uniform anisotropic bundles with a plethora of side-to-side electrical connections between fibers, with

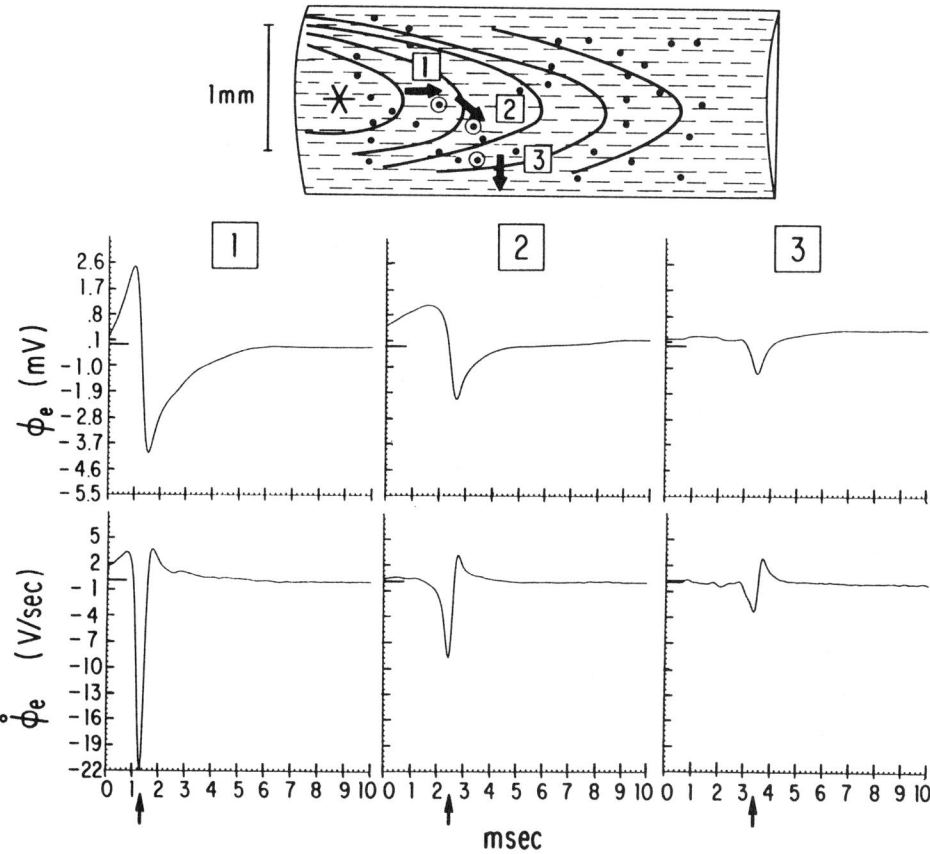

Figure 2. Excitation spread and extrace1lular potential waveforms and the associated derivatives in an atrial bundle with uniform anisotropic properties. Propagation was initiated at a point indicated by the asterisk. The points on the outline mark the sites where waveforms were measured to construct the isochrones. The encircled points indicate the locations where the depicted waveforms were recorded. The vertical arrows at the bottom mark the time of dV/dt_{max} of the intracellular action potential (not shown) to illustrate the close time relationship between the negative peak of the derivative of the extracellular waveform and dV/dt_{max} of the intracellular action potential. The preparation is from a 2-year-old male. (Reproduced with permission from Reference 12.)

normal action potentials the conduction velocity in the transverse direction generally is one third to one fourth the values of fast longitudinal conduction, eg, 0.14–0.22 m/sec transversely and 0.48–0.53 m/sec longitudinally. In the nonuniform anisotropic bundles with infrequent side-to-side connections between fibers, the conduction velocity of normal action potentials is reduced further to values that are in the range of those encountered in the atrioventricular node (0.03 m/sec).[12] Because of the low (and very low) effective conduction

velocities during propagation across fibers, in all reentrant circuits there must be slowing of conduction due to this anisotropic phenomenon in some parts of the circuit.

Considerations of the Topology of the Cell-to-Cell Connections: Gap Junctions

To highlight the topology of the electrical connections between cells, Figure 4 shows an

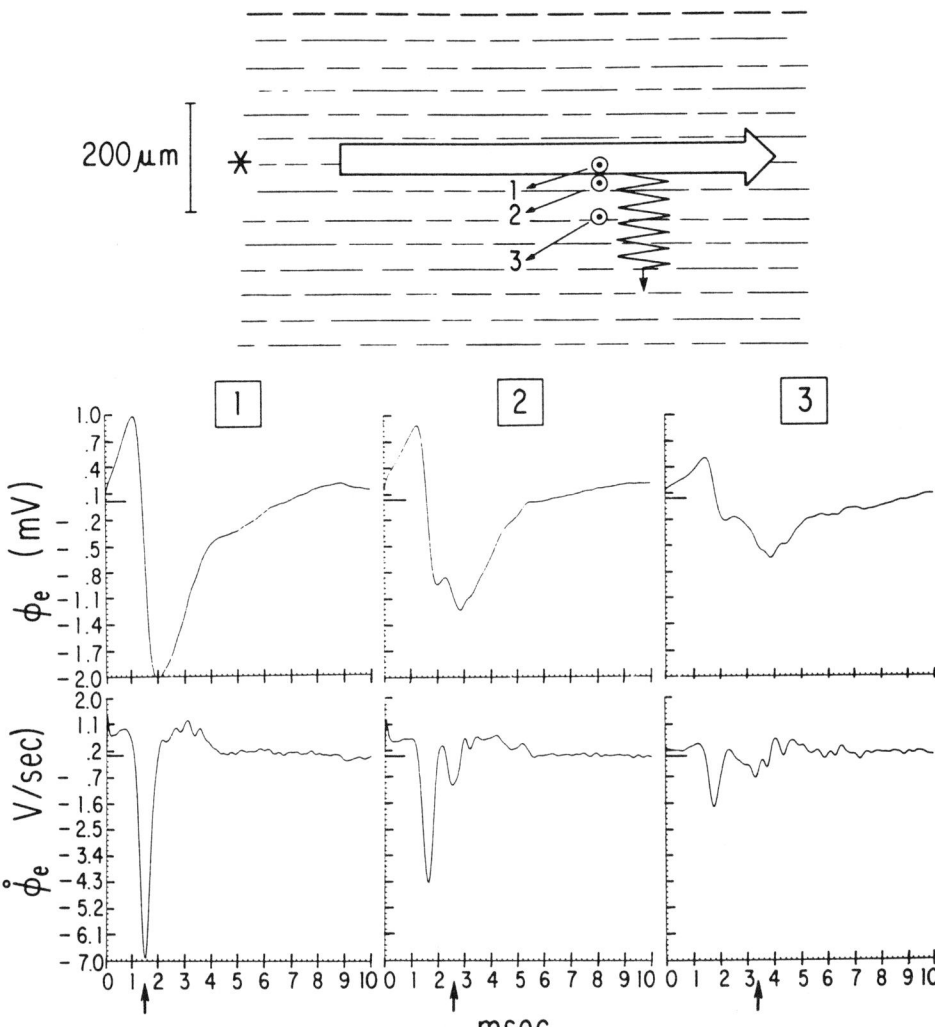

Figure 3. Excitation spread and extracellular potential waveforms and the associated derivatives in an atrial bundle with nonuniform anisotropic properties. In the drawing at the top, the prominent open arrow marks the narrow region of fast propagation along the long axis of the fibers. The "sawtooth" curve denotes the irregular zigzag course of propagation in the transverse direction (ie, propagation across fibers). The vertical arrows at the bottom mark the times of dV/dt$_{max}$ of the intracellular action potential (not shown). The preparation was from a 42-year-old male. (Reproduced with permission from Reference 12.)

example of the two-dimensional geometry of individual left ventricular myocytes placed together to form a multidimensional model of two hypothetical bundles of ventricular muscle. The geometry of each cell was measured from disaggregated isolated ventricular myocytes and each cell was placed in position as in a jigsaw puzzle. The final overall appearance can be seen to be quite similar to that of histologic sections. However, the array is shown to depict the locations of the connections between cells, which is quite difficult to do without actual three-dimensional reconstruction of multiple sections of the tissue.

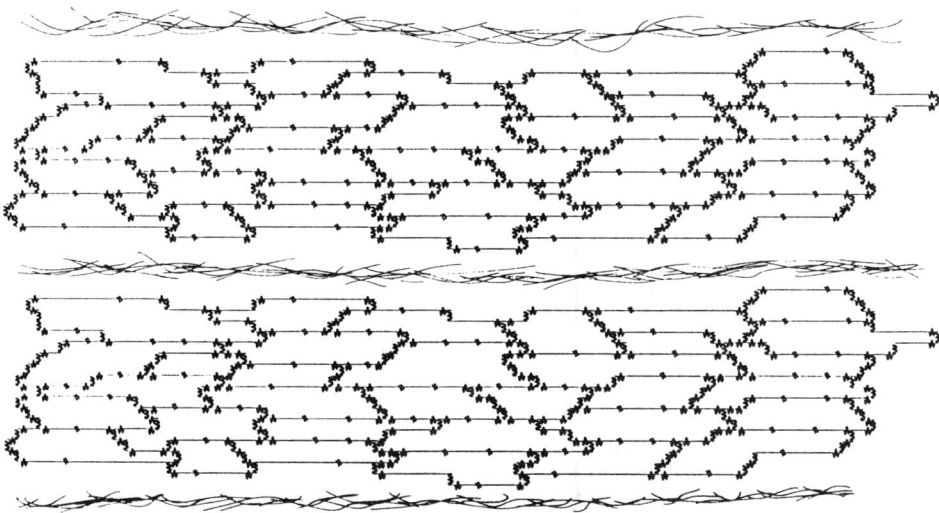

Figure 4. Two-dimensional representation of the individual ventricular myocytes and their associated intercalated disks within two bundles of ventricle muscle. The above is a hypothetical two-dimensional representation of the ventricular muscle constructed as a model from drawings of 33 isolated single disaggregated myocytes. The cells were placed to fit together as in a jigsaw puzzle, and the end result can be seen as similar to the familar picture of longitudinal sections of left ventricular muscle. The above two-dimensional reconstruction illustrates the irregular shapes of ventricular myocytes and the occurrence of "side-to-side" connections between myocytes due to interdigitating irregular shapes related to the plicate segments[15] (treads) of the intercalated disks (prominent curved lines at ends of segments of each myocyte). As shown by Hoyt et al.[15] the gap junctions are located within and adjacent to the plicate segments of the intercalated disks in canine ventricular muscle.

Two features of the topology of electrical connections between cells are illustrated: (1) Within each bundle, the geometry of each myocyte is complex, ie, cardiac cells are not shaped like bricks. Although the connections between cells (indicated by the bold curvature lines) occur primarily at the ends of the cells, the intercalated disks (prominent wavy lines) occur in a manner to produce quite irregular shapes of the myocytes and the intercalated disks at the end of some cells are connected to the middle part of adjacent cells. This staggered arrangement of the disks (the gap junctions are located within and adjacent to the intercalated disk) produces multiple step-like side-to-side connections between adjacent parallel oriented cells. This is noted because morphologically, the gap junction connections appear scattered over the surface of the myocytes, as identified by Hoyt et al.[15] (2)

The curvilinear horizontal lines are used to illustrate regions where connective tissue separates groups of fibers in a side-to-side manner in nonuniform anisotropic tissue. The irregular contours along the borders illustrate how intercalated disks (with which the gap junctions are associated) likely form the major areas of loss of side-to-side electrical connections when changes occur from uniform to nonuniform anisotropic properties. That is, isolated gap junctions connecting ventricular cells are rare and the functional side-to-side connections are produced by the irregularly located intercalated disks, ie, by identifying the location of the intercalated disks one is also localizing the sites where gap junctional membrane is located (within the plicate portion of the disk and the adjacent interplicate area).

These features of the topology of the connections between cells and the marked variations in the size and shape of ventricular myocytes are presented to emphasize that multidimensional consideration of conduction within myocytes likely will be required to account for the marked differences in dV/dt$_{max}$ that occur at a single point in a myocyte when the direction of conduction is altered. Similarly, the uptake and effect on conduction of sodium channel blocking drugs is likely to vary throughout the sarcolemmal membrane of individual myocytes.

Microreentry Depends on the Sparsity of Side-to-Side Electrical Connections Between Fibers

When premature stimuli are introduced at a single site in uniform anisotropic bundles, the universal response in our experience has been the following: as the premature interval is progressively decreased in the relatively refractory period of the tissue, there is an associated progressive decrease in conduction velocity in all directions and when the premature interval is shortened to the time of the absolute refractory period, conduction fails simultaneously in all directions with respect to fiber orientation. It should be mentioned at this point that reentry has been established in two-dimensional continuously uniform models[16] and in uniform anisotropic muscle[17] by an entirely different technique than in the classic reentry model that uses a single stimulus site for both the normal and premature impulses as described by Moe et al.[18] This technique uses a second stimulation site to initiate the premature action potentials distal to the site where normal action potentials are initiated. By initiating the premature impulse distal to the site of initiation of normal action potentials, spatial inhomogeneities of repolarization are established that result in reentry due to slow conduction in one direction and block in another area unrelated to fiber orientation. This "two-stimulus sites" method of in-

ducing reentry is emphasized as an experimental or functional way to create inhomogeneities of repolarization that are not inherent inhomogeneities of the tissue, and therefore these inhomogeneities will not be discussed here. Rather, matters related to the classic mode of establishing reentry from a single initiating site for normal and premature impulses, as done by Moe et al.[18] and Allessie et al.[1] will be adhered to for considerations of the role of anisotropy in reentry.

Figure 5 shows the typical events that occur when a premature impulse is initiated at progressively earlier premature intervals in bundles with sparse side-to-side electrical coupling between fibers, in this case a pectinate bundle from an older subject.[19] When the premature interval was reduced to 233 msec, longitudinal conduction block occurred (evidenced by small uniphasic positive deflection at site #5) while slow transverse propagation continued with marked discontinuities. With further reduction of the premature interval to 228 msec, slow transverse propagation continued, the area of longitudinal conduction block moved nearer the site of impulse initiation, and there was a reentrant impulse in the areas where longitudinal conduction block had occurred. This reentrant impulse was followed by three to four spontaneous reentrant beats (not shown). These events recurred repeatedly after a premature stimulus. This allowed us to map the area of the reentrant circuit, which was rectangular in shape and occupied 1.6 mm^2. Importantly, the conduction block in the longitudinal direction occurred in a region where the refractory periods were actually 3–5 msec shorter than at the stimulus site, ruling out the influence of a leading circle mechanism (the premature impulse blocking due to its encountering longer action potentials than at the site of initiation).

The effects of prolonging the refractory period on a microreentrant circuit are worth considering here. The time to traverse this microreentrant circuit was 90–100 m/sec and the basic background stimulus rate was 171 per minute. When the background rate was re-

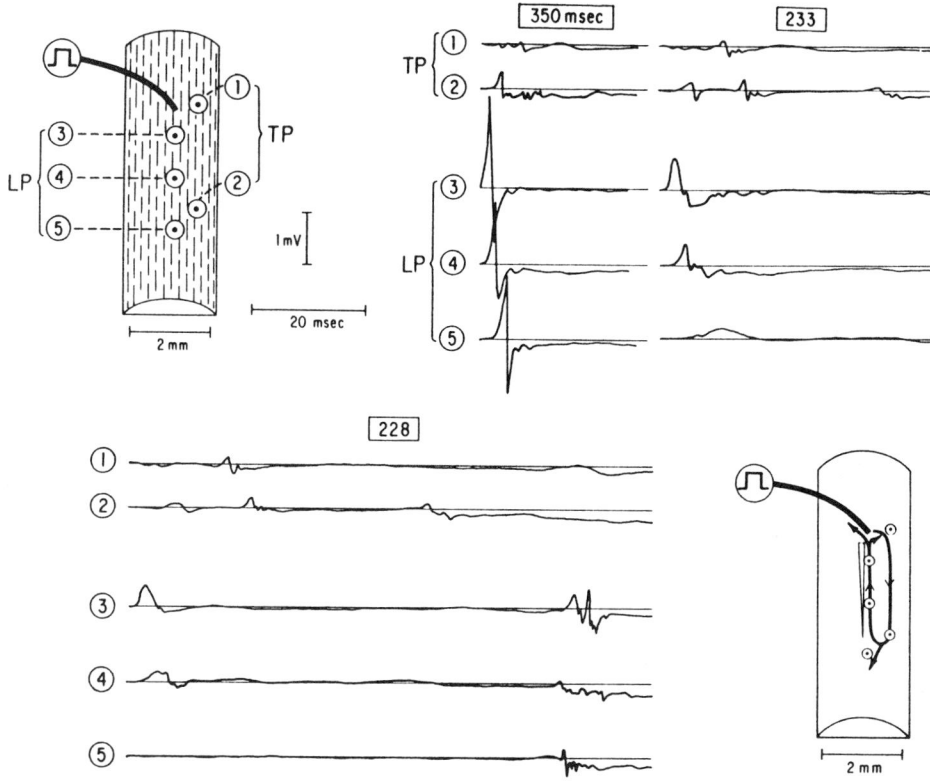

Figure 5. Microreentry of premature action potentials in nonuniform anisotropic bundle. The results were obtained at a basic stimulus rate of 171 per minute, and a premature stimulus was introduced after every 10th beat at the interval shown in the box above each group of waveforms. The schematic at the upper left shows sites where each waveform was recorded. The drawing at the lower right shows the reentrant circuit, indicated by the solid lines. The atrial preparation was from a 64-year-old patient with marked dilatation of the right atrium secondary to an atrial septal defect. (Reproduced with permission from Reference 19.)

duced to 60 per minute, microreentry did not occur although the initiating conduction events of very slow transverse conduction and longitudinal conduction block still occurred with premature stimulus. This can be accounted for by prolongation of the action potentials at the slow rate, which resulted in the central area of refractoriness increasing in size beyond the boundaries of the small pectinate muscle that contained the microreentrant circuit. Returning to a more rapid rate of 171 per minute resulted in reappearance of microreentry. Thus, relatively short refractory periods (short action potentials) are needed to produce microreentry due to anisotropy. In this type of reentrant circuit, Class III antiar-

rhythmic drugs that prolong the refractory period make reentry impossible within the limits of the single atrial bundle within such small areas. Thus, microreentrant circuits (ie, those within areas 1–2 mm²) are prime targets for investigation of potential major effects of disrupting "focal" reentry.

The effects on propagation secondary to exposure of cardiac bundles to Class I sodium channel blocking drugs is also dependent on the degree of side-to-side electrical coupling between fibers, ie, the presence of uniform versus nonuniform anisotropy.[19] Figure 6 shows the effects of quinidine within a single ventricular muscle bundle (dog papillary muscle) with uniform anisotropic properties.

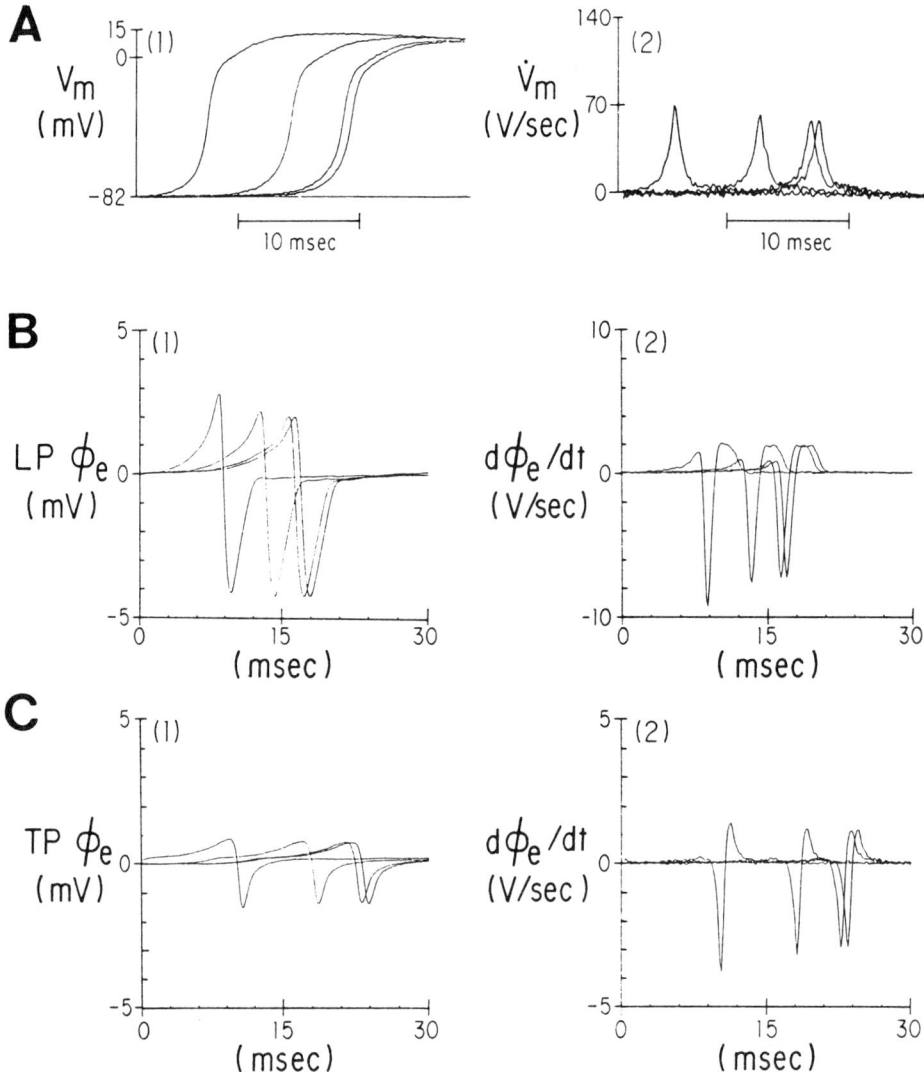

Figure 6. Wenckebach periodicity induced by quinidine within a single bundle with uniform anisotropic properties. The results shown were obtained after the stimulus rate was increased from 100 to 120 per minute during exposure to quinidine gluconate 10 μg/mL. Panel A shows the transmembrane potential (left) and its first time derivative (right). Panels B and C show the extracellular potential waveform (left) and their first-time derivatives (right) for longitudinal and transverse conduction (LP and TP, respectively). (Reproduced with permission from Reference 19.)

The maximum rate of rise changed with a periodicity that was similar to that of the Wenckebach phenomenon until block occurred simultaneously in all directions. With progressively greater block of the sodium channels, dV/dt_{max} decreased beat by beat in association with a similar change in the extracellular waveforms, which maintained the same general shape and remained smooth in contour for all directions of propagation. The extracellular waveforms, therefore, indicated that the general sequence of activation remained unchanged at a microscopic level, the major effect of quinidine being that of progressive slowing of conduction until block occurred simultaneously in all directions.

In nonuniform anisotropic bundles with sparse side-to-side electrical connections between fibers, however, use-dependent block of Class I antiarrhythmic agents produced a very different propagation response. With increasing sodium channel block, transverse propagation remained irregular in nature, similar to the conduction of normal action potentials in such tissues, although the effective velocity decreased in that direction. Conversely, longitudinal conduction changed remarkably as demonstrated in Figure 7. Dissociated longitudinal conduction at a microscopic level occurred as evidenced by the development of fragmented extracellular waveforms. We interpreted this to be caused by a shift from synchronized excitation of adjacent fibers to a zigzag course of microscopic propagation along the long axis of the fibers. The major functional consequence of the drug-induced type of anisotropic conduction response is that the disassociated longitudinal conduction resulted in a marked decrease in the effective conduction velocity to values considerably less than occur with premature action potentials in uniform anisotropic bundles, eg, to 0.28 that of the normal longitudinal conduction velocity (compared to a maximum reduction of longitudinal velocity to 0.46 in uniform tissue). This effect of sodium channel blocking antiarrhythmic agents would have a proarrhythmic effect in tissues with nonuniform anisotropic properties.[19] This is interesting in view of the widespread considerations

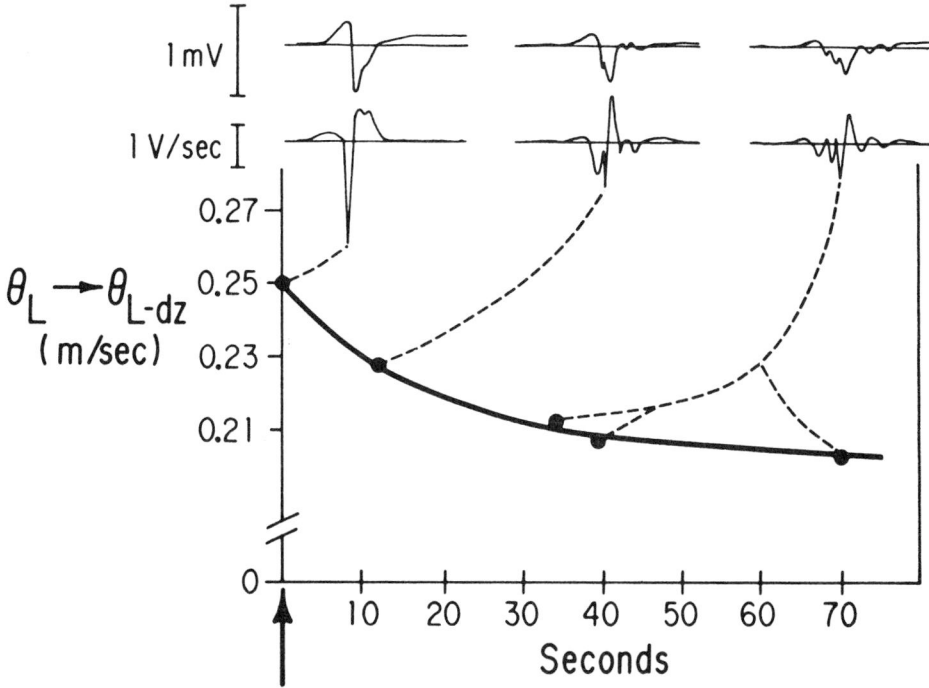

Figure 7. Quinidine-induced use-dependent microscopic dissociated longitudinal conduction in a nonuniform anisotropic bundle. The preparation was first allowed to achieve a steady-state condition during exposure to quinidine gluconate 10 μg/mL. The vertical arrow at the bottom indicates the time at which the stimulation rate was increased from 70 to 85 per minute. The progressive change from a single biphasic large deflection to one with multiple deflections in the original waveform and its derivative was characteristic of a change from normal longitudinal conduction to microscopic dissociated longitudinal conduction. The atrial preparation was from a 66-year-old patient. (Reproduced with permission from Reference 19.)

of the poor results of Class I agents in the CAST study in patients with healed infarcted tissue (tissue known to have regions of poor side-to-side electrical coupling[20]).

Relation of Loss of Side-to-Side Electrical Coupling Between Fibers and Microscopic Fibrosis

The major anisotropic electrical phenomenon underlying all of the above differences in the propagation response to an intervention is the dependence of the response of the degree of side-to-side electrical coupling between fibers. Figure 8 shows the histologic appearance of a human atrial bundle with nonuniform anisotropic propagation properties because of loss or sparsity of side-to-side connections between fibers. Such tissue oc-

curs in subjects of the geriatric age group and in older subjects with chronic atrial hypertrophy, eg, secondary to an atrial septal defect. In all of the tissues we have examined that demonstrate fragmented extracellular waveforms during conduction across fibers indicating sparse side-to-side electrical connections, there has been extensive collagenous septa in the interstitial spaces separating groups of fibers (perimysial collagenous septa) and often in the spaces separating individual fibers (prominent endomysial septa). In some areas small groups of fibers are surrounded by collagenous septa for distances of 1 mm. The electrophysiological significance of the collagenous septa is that side-to-side electrical connections (nexuses) between fibers cannot be present between fibers separated by the septa.

These combined electrophysiological and histologic results at a microscopic level are intriguing in view of the long known fact

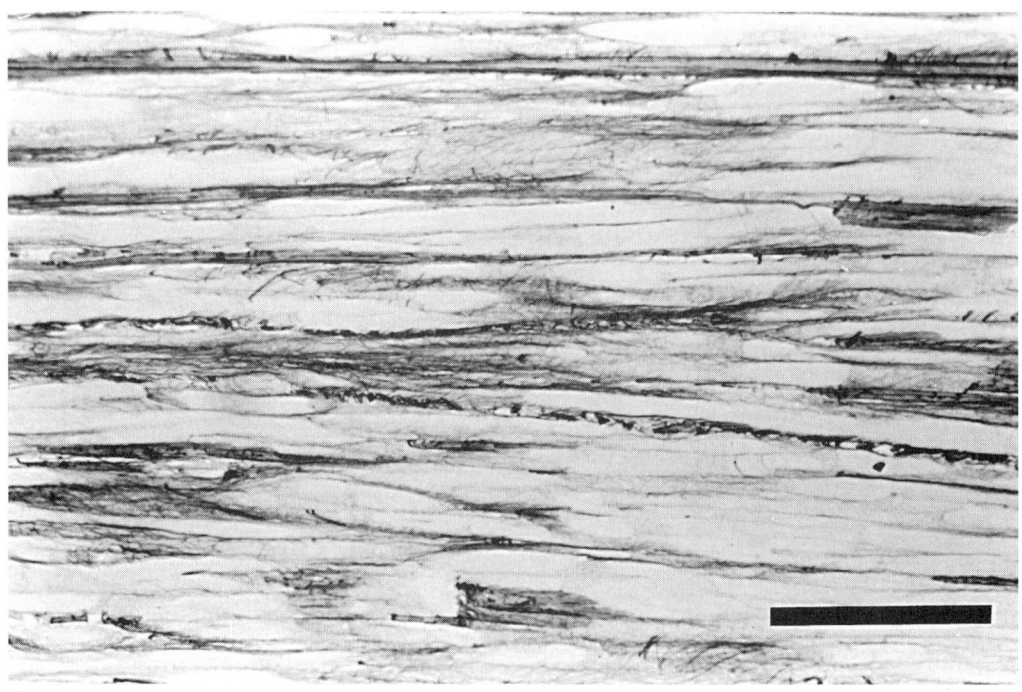

Figure 8. Collagenous septa in atrial bundle in which microreentry was induced as in Figure 5. Many of the collagenous septa (gray to black) in this longitudinal section are both thick and long and thus isolate adjacent fibers and groups of fibers (white). Bar: 200 μm. (Reproduced with permission from Reference 19.)

that increased cardiac fibrosis is associated with an increase in cardiac arrhythmias. In the past that association has involved visible regions of connective tissue that occur within enlarged chambers, the fibrotic areas being considered to provide barriers that enhance the development of reentry in large circuits with wavelengths of several centimeters (much greater wavelengths than that of the microreentry circuit shown in Figure 5).

The anisotropic conduction results presented in this chapter suggest a "new" structural mechanism for reentrant arrhythmias in subjects with cardiac fibrosis—the loss of side-to-side electrical connections between fibers that are associated with the development of microscopic fibrosis. These microscopic structural changes in the anisotropic distribution of the cellular connections that occur in association with enlarged and hypertrophied cardiac chambers may be the cause of the increased incidence of reentrant arrhythmias (especially chronic atrial tachyarrhythmias in elderly subjects) rather than the mechanism of gross anatomical enlargement.

Regional Differences in Anisotropic Propagation Properties

Thus far, the most "uniform" anisotropic tissue we have encountered has been the epicardial surface of the canine left ventricle. During transverse propagation, most waveforms are smooth in contour, similar to those shown in Figure 2. The one consistent exception is at the apex of the left ventricle where connective tissue septa occur on the epicardial surface in adult dogs and conduction across these visible connective tissue septa are associated with marked fragmentation of the extracellular waveforms.

The right ventricular epicardium is different from that of the left ventricle in that there are many areas that produce fragmented extracellular waveforms during conduction across fibers indicating nonuniform anisotropic conduction at a microscopic level. The

major functional consequence has been that premature stimuli given in all of the areas of the left ventricular epicardium (away from the apex) has resulted in the typical uniform anisotropic response of premature impulses with progressive slowing of the conduction until conduction block occurs simultaneously in all directions. In the normal right ventricular epicardium, however, we have frequently encountered unidirectional longitudinal conduction block and reentry. Figure 9 shows a typical result obtained using a linear microarray of extracellular electrodes to measure propagation at a cellular level in the region of reentry of a premature impulse. The premature impulse was initiated at the stimulus site following eight regular stimuli at a basic cycle length of 400 msec. When the premature interval was shortened to 200 msec, the reference extracellular electrode (Ref) demonstrated that unidirectional longitudinal conduction block occurred along the long axis of the fibers and this was followed by reentry in the region 3 mm distal to the stimulus electrode. The remaining waveforms illustrate transverse propagation occurring in the region of reentry with the progressive change in waveforms at the electrodes as numbered (each number representing an increment of 100 μm). It is important to emphasize that such measurements at a microscopic level with microarrays of electrodes with smooth surfaces are free from injury. For example, we have found that when the microarray is lowered to within 100–200 μm of the surface, slight irregularities appear in the waveforms during transverse conduction, even in uniform anisotropic preparations. Monitoring of the shapes of the waveforms to ensure that the slight irregularities persist allows the investigator to move the electrode tips up to the point of contact with the surface with assurance that the waveforms are not distorted and that there has been no development of local injury, which could affect propagation at a microscopic level.

Figure 10 (top) is a drawing that illustrates the considerable nonuniformities of the anisotropic properties that occur in the normal canine left and right ventricular epicardial

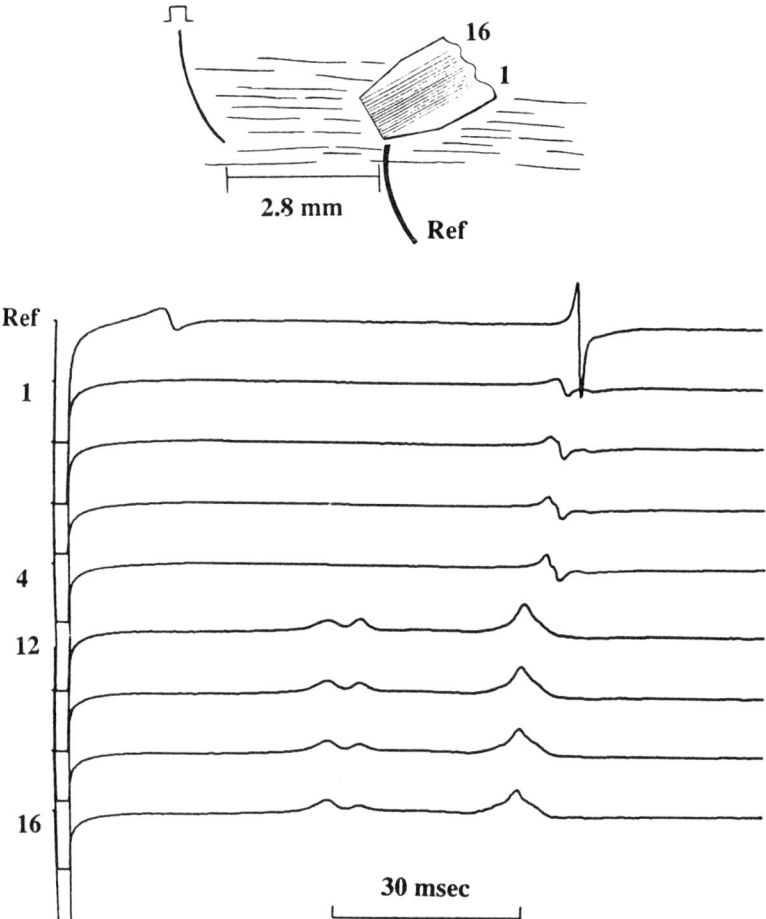

Figure 9. Reentry induced by a premature impulse in a right ventricular epicardial region of nonuniform anisotropy. The drawing at the top shows the stimulus site, the location of the reference extracellular electrode (ref) and the position of the linear microarray of 24 electrodes (each wire was 50 μm in diameter and the center-to-center spacing of the electrodes was 100 μm). The numbers beside the waveforms indicate the sequence of the electrode at which the waveform was recorded. The microarray of electrodes was oriented across the fibers. Note that the progressively later time of the deflections, which indicated that the wave front was conducting at a microscopic level in a direction across the fibers waveforms to that of the reentrant deflection of reference tracing.

surfaces. The prominent parallel lines on the right ventricular epicardial surface signify the markedly enhanced number of nonuniform anisotropic regions with sparse side-to-side electrical coupling compared to the thin parallel lines of the left ventricular epicardial surface which is comprised primarily of uniform anisotropic tissue. However, separation of parallel oriented bundles is found fre-quently in epicardial areas underneath the prominent blood vessels, regions known to be associated with the occurrence of prominent connective tissue septa. Finally, the easily visible epicardial connective tissue septa that emanate from a singular point at the apex of the left ventricle is intriguing with regard to the contraction patterns that can be visualized in the intact heart. The simple visual identifica-

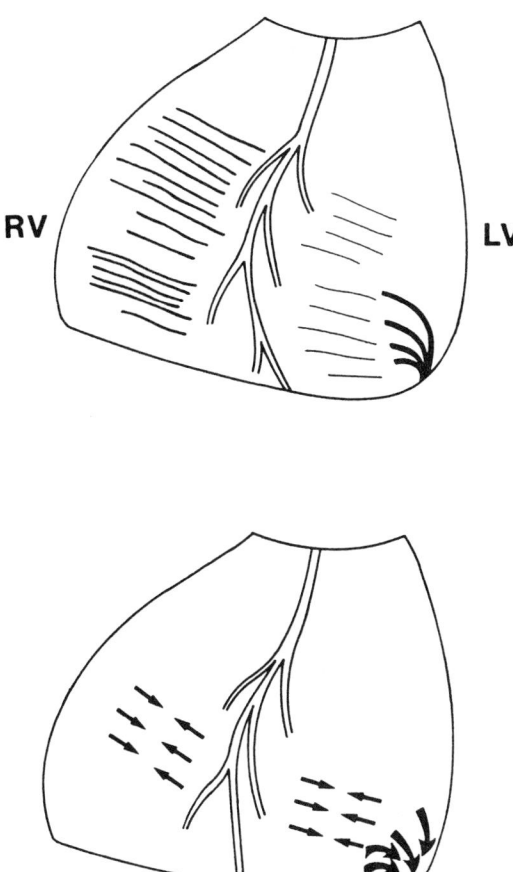

RV   LV

Figure 10. Schematic representation of the nonhomogeneous distribution of uniform and nonuniform anisotropic properties of the epicardial surface of the normal canine ventricle. At the top, the fine horizontal line of the left ventricular surface denote the sparsity of nonuniform anisotropic areas with connective tissue separating groups of fibers in a side-to-side manner. The more prominent lines on the right ventricular surface denote the considerably more frequently encountered areas of nonuniform anisotropy. The bold dark lines at the left ventricular apex represent prominent curvilinear connective tissue septa that converge at a point that is located at the left ventricular apex. In the bottom drawing, the arrow denote the easily visible movement of the epicardial muscle during systole in the in vivo beating canine heart.

tion of the epicardial contraction differences is schematized in the lower portion of Figure 10. The bulging of the anterior walls of both right and left ventricular surfaces appear to occur as a homogeneous phenomenon with bulging of the anterior surface during systole. At the apex of the left ventricle, however, the contraction pattern is different in that there is a twisting motion that is accompanied by a curvilinear course of multiple connective tissue septa that join at a point located at the ventricular apex.

The regional differences in the anisotropic properties (and connective tissue distribution) suggest that there may be important links between regional differences in contraction patterns of the ventricular fibers and the distribution of connective tissue septa and the associated anisotropic electrical properties of the tissue. Thus far, however, there is no information that relates the manner in which the loss of side-to-side connections between fibers occurs in association with the ingrowth of microscopic connective tissue between fibers. The implications extend to many states, including aging,[12] chronic hypertrophy, and marked loss of side-to-side connections in the subepicardial tissue that survives experimental infarction produced in dogs.[20]

Conclusions

1. The loss of side-to-side electrical connections between myocytes provides a new microscopic structural phenomenon underlying reentrant arrhythmias in many conditions, such as those that occur with hypertrophy, aging, and following healing of ventricular infarcted tissue.

2. Anisotropic conduction mechanisms appear to occur at a microscopic (cellular) level. This represents an area of investigation that at present is unexplored and that provides a much needed and challenging area of study.

3. Improved high-resolution and spatial and temporal measurement techniques will be needed to achieve the detection and delineation of the events at a microscopic level to understand mechanisms that enhance reentry.

4. Microreentrant circuits are enlarged by increasing the duration of the action potential; microreentrant circuits within small bundles can be enlarged to the point that the size of the circuit exceeds that of the boundaries of the bundle, thus resulting in the ablation of the microreentrant circuit. Thus, tachyarrhythmias secondary to microreentry within small bundles should be abated by Class III antiarrhythmic agents that prolong the refractory period.

5. Therapeutic challenges include: improved techniques for ablation of "nonuniform" anisotropic areas; selective pacemaker control of wave front movement with implantation of multiple pacemaker electrodes to control the direction of conduction at a microscopic level. For example, reentry does not occur when premature stimuli are initiated simultaneously at multiple sites located along the transverse axis of the fibers. (This prevents slow transverse propagation from establishing a microreentrant circuit); and pharmacological agents that have the end result of reducing microscopic "fibrosis," for example, enalapril has been shown to reduce ventricular arrhythmias in association with a decrease in connective tissue in hypertensive rats.[21]

References

1. Allessie MA, Lammers WJEP, Bonke IM, Hollen J: Intra-atrial reentry as a mechanism for atrial flutter induced by acetylcholine and rapid pacing in the dog. *Circulation* 70:123, 1984.
2. Spach MS, Miller WT III, Geselowitz DB, et al: The discontinuous nature of propagation in normal canine cardiac muscle. Evidence for recurrent discontinuities of intracellular resistance that affect the membrane currents. *Circ Res* 48:39, 1981.
3. Spach MS, Miller WT III, Dolber PC, et al: The functional role of structural complexities in the propagation of depolarization in the atrium of the dog. Cardiac conduction disturbances due to discontinuities of effective axial resistivity. *Circ Res* 50:175, 1982.
4. Spach MS, Dolber PC: The relation between discontinuous propagation in anisotropic cardiac muscle and the "vulnerable period" of reentry. In: DP Zipes, J Jalife (eds): *Cardiac Electrophysiology and Arrhythmias*. Orlando, FL: Grune & Stratton, 1985, p. 241.
5. Clerc L: Directional differences of impulse spread in trabecular muscle from mammalian heart. *J Physiol (Lond)* 255:335, 1976.
6. Spach MS, Miller WT III, Miller-Jones E, et al: Extracellular potentials related to intracellular action potentials during impulse conduction in anisotropic canine muscle. *Circ Res* 45:188, 1979.
7. Tsuboi N, Furta T, Kodama T, et al: Anisotropic conduction properties of canine ventricular muscles under high extracellular potassium concentration. *Environ Med* 26:95, 1982.
8. Delgado C, Steinhaus B, Delmar M, et al: Directional differences in excitability and margin of safety for propagation in sheep ventricular epicardial muscle. *Circ Res* 67:97, 1990.
9. Suenson M: Interaction between ventricular cells during the early part of excitation in the ferret heart. *Acta Physiol Scand* 125:81, 1985.
10. Leon LJ, Roberge FA: Directional characteristics of action potential propagation in cardiac muscle. *Circ Res* 69:378, 1991.
11. Knisley SB, Maruyama T, Buchanan JW Jr: Interstitial potential during propagation in bathed ventricular muscle. *Biophys J* 59:509, 1991.
12. Spach MS, Dolber PC: Relating extracellular potentials and their derivatives to anisotropic propagation at a microscopic level in human cardiac muscle. Evidence for electrical uncoupling of side-to-side fiber connections with increasing age. *Circ Res* 58:356, 1986.
13. Spach MS: High resolution of cardiac electrical sources. Use of the derivatives of extracellular potential waveforms. *J Electrocardiol* 22(Suppl):109, 1989.
14. Makielski JC, Sheets MF, Hanck DA, et al: Sodium current in voltage clamped internally perfused canine cardiac Purkinje cells. *Biophys J* 52:1, 1987.
15. Hoyt RH, Cohen ML, Saffitz JE: Distribution and three-dimensional structure of intercellular junctions in canine myocardium. *Circ Res* 64:563, 1989.
16. van Capelle FJL, Durrer D: Computer simulation of arrhythmias in a network of coupled excitable elements. *Circ Res* 47:454, 1980.
17. Ideker RE, Frazier DW, Krassowska W, et al: Experimental evidence for autowaves in the heart. *Annals NY Acad Sci* 591:208, 1990.
18. Moe GK, Pastelin G, Mendez R: Circus movement excitation of the atria. In: RC Little (ed): *Physiology of Atrial Pacemakers and Conductive Tissue*. Mount Kisco, NY: Futura Publishing Company, Inc., 1980, p. 207.
19. Spach MS, Dolber PC, Heidlage JF: Influence

of the passive anisotropic properties on directions differences in propagation following modification of the sodium conductance in human atrial muscle. A model of reentry based on anisotropic discontinuous propagation. *Circ Res* 62:811, 1988.

20. Dillon SM, Allessie MA, Ursell PC, Wit AL: Influences of anisotropic tissue structure on reentrant circuits in the epicardial border zone of subacute canine infarcts. *Circ Res* 63:182, 1988.

21. Pahor MIP, Bernabei R, Sgadari A, et al: Enalapril prevents cardiac fibrosis and arrhythmias in hypertensive rats. *Hypertension* 18:148, 1991.

Chapter 8

Prolongation of Repolarization: *Dispersion of Refractoriness or Afterdepolarizations*

Ralph Lazzara

The first student of reentry, Alfred G. Mayer, who recognized its existence and formulated its governing principles, also perceived the critical role of refractoriness.[1] The principle was enunciated that the refractory properties in the circuit determine the requisite minimum value for circuit time/length; therefore, prolongation of refractoriness opposes reentry.

> *"This single wave going constantly in one direction around the circuit may maintain itself for days, travelling at a uniform rate. The circuit must, however, be long enough to allow each point to rest for an appreciable interval of time before the return of the wave."*

The influence of refractoriness on reentry has received quantitative expression in the concept of wavelength, the product of the conduction velocity and the refractory period, which has the dimension of length.[2] The wavelength is the distance the excitation wave (impulse) travels during one refractory period and it defines the minimum length of a reentry circuit. A strong indirect relationship between the measured wavelength and the probability of reentrant atrial arrhythmias has been demonstrated in atrial myocardium of dogs under conditions in which conduction velocity and refractory period varied widely.[3,4] In these experiments the measured wavelength was relatively uniform throughout the atrial myocardium. A similar relationship was not demonstrated for ischemic ventricular myocardium,[5] possibly because the variability of the electrophysiological properties in acutely ischemic myocardium both in space and in time, especially with varying cycle length, makes the wavelength a variable and labile entity elusive of accurate estimation.

Initially, it was also appreciated that not only brevity of refractoriness but also disparity of refractoriness fosters reentry. This idea originated from observations of the primal model of reentry, circling excitation in a simple ring of tissue. It was recognized that the site of the longest duration of refractory periods within the ring could be the site of unidirectional block that allowed the circuit to form.[6]

> *"In such a preparation a single stimulus applied to any point in the ring starts a wave in each direction. Waves meet on the opposite*

From BN Singh, HJJ Wellens, M Hiraoka, (eds): *Electropharmacological Control of Cardiac Arrhythmias.* Mount Kisco, NY, Futura Publishing Company Inc., © 1994.

side of the ring and die out, but by the application of several stimuli in succession it is sometimes possible to start a wave in one direction only while the tisse on the other side of the point stimulated is still refractory. Such a wave moves around the ring sufficiently slowly for the refractory phase to have passed off in each part of the ring when the wave approaches it."

These remarkable comments by Mines first identified the potent action of premature excitation to activate reentrant circuits, now an axiom of the workplace of reentrant arrhythmias, and identified critical effects of premature excitation for the induction of reentry: (1) slow conduction (reduced wavelength); and (2) increased dispersion of refractoriness. The abbreviated refractoriness of the premature impulse also contributes to the reduced wavelength.

Garrey championed the hypothesis that fibrillation is a chaotic manifestation within the cardiac syncytium of the circus movement phenomenon in simple rings of tissue, in which multiple simultaneous wave fronts continually shift in ever changing directions seeking receding refractoriness.[7]

"Finally, we see the wildest turmoil of fibrillation involving the whole auricle in a process which is anything but a simple circuit. In this last mentioned process, the impulse is diverted into different paths, weaving and inter-weaving through the tissue mass, crossing and recrossing old paths again to course over them or to stop short as it impinges on some barrier of refractory tissue."

The term reentry is not applicable literally because the moving wave of activation does not return with regularity to the same sites. The migrations are chaotic. Nonetheless, it was recognized that the process is fundamentally akin to reentry in rings, that refractoriness is a critical determinant of the process, and the heterogeneity of this property favors the induction and maintenance of fibrillation. Prolonged refractoriness was considered antifibrillatory just as it was antireentry in the simple ring circuits.[7]

"In auricular fibrillation, a slow wave front is maintained by the presence of multiple blocks which cause a sinuous path or actual shuttling

of the impulse. The refractory period may be shortened to one-fifth or one-sixth of the normal, although vagus action is a necessary accompaniment of such high-grade shortening. This change makes rapid reexcitation possible and the formation of circuits having diameters of but a few millimeters. Since the refractory phase does not occur simultaneously in all fibers, the circuits must be formed in different and shifting locations. All such circuits have an open, excitable stretch which makes a continuous circuit possible, and the object of therapy is to close the ring, to render the entire circuit, if only momentarily, inexcitable. One method of accomplishing this would be to lengthen the refractory period and this at present seems to be accomplished best by the administration of quinidine."

The introduction of the recording of intracellular potentials of cardiac cells verified that refractoriness is tightly linked in cardiac cells to repolarization[8,9] and that repolarization has greatly different time courses and durations among different types of cardiac cells and among cells in different locations.[10,11] Therefore, there is a natural heterogeneity in repolarization that results in a "dispersion of refractoriness" in normal cardiac tissue (Figure 1). This dispersion is modified in terms of recovery times in the tissue mass by differences in activation times that may augment or diminish the dispersion of recovery times.[12]

In certain cardiac tissues, notably the atrioventricular (AV) and sinoatrial (SA) nodes, refractoriness outlasts repolarization by significant periods, so-called "postrepolarization refractoriness."[13,14] This phenomenon may be prominent in certain pathological states such as ischemic injury[14] and it amplifies the heterogeneity in recovery times due to disparity of repolarization and differing activation times (Figure 1). This phenomenon in the nodes is due to slow recovery from inactivation of calcium current, but in abnormal tissues it is poorly understood. It may be due to slow recovery of abnormally functioning sodium channels.[15,16] This heterogeneity of repolarization and dispersion of recovery times is greatly influenced by physiological and pathological states.[17–19] Figure 2 illustrates a diverse array of action potentials

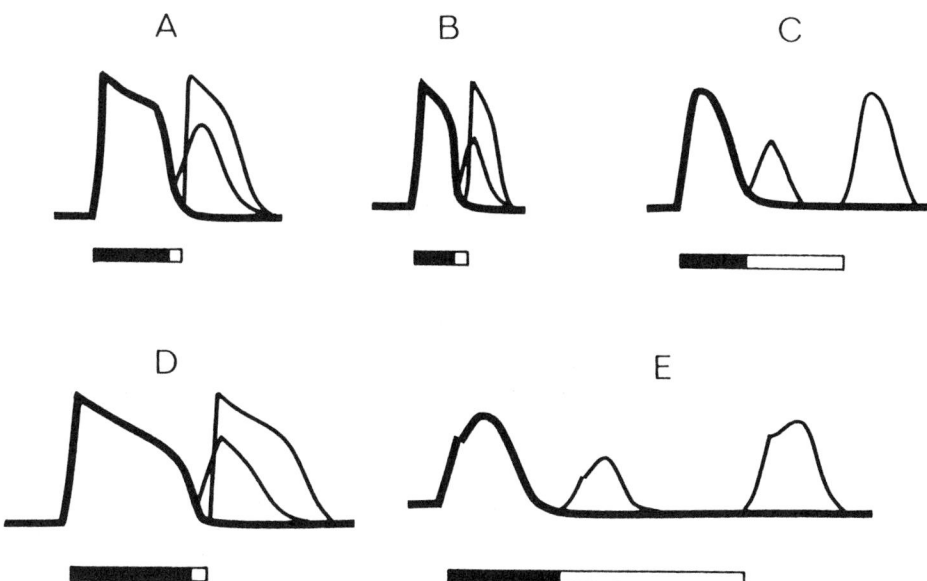

Figure 1. The relationships of absolute (solid bars) and relative (open bars) refractory periods to action potentials in relatively normal cells with differing time courses of repolarization (A and D) and abnormal cells with (C and E) and without (B) postrepolarization refractoriness. In B, the cell is mildly depolarized and has a shortened action potential as might been seen in early ischemia, and in C and E the cells show more depolarization and lesser (C) and greater (E) postrepolarization refractoriness with prolonged relative refractory periods when conduction is more impaired.

recorded from a canine heart 24 hours after coronary occlusion.

There have been many attempts to quantify the magnitude of differences in refractoriness by determining refractory periods, recording electrograms with activation and repolarization potentials, recording monophasic action potentials (injury potentials), and recording QT intervals from the body surface at various sites.[19] In general, all methods tend to underestimate the true magnitude of the absolute differences of refractory periods throughout the heart because of a general problem of undersampling. Another difficulty is that the important and relevant differences may occur at specific sites where reentry circuits form. Global differences as usually estimated may relate more to vulnerability to ventricular fibrillation than to the formation of local reentry circuits. This point will be discussed later.

Many observations under a variety of conditions have generated the concept that prolongation of repolarization is proreentry rather than antireentry when the prolongation is heterogeneous and dispersion of refractoriness is significantly enhanced. Well-known experimental examples include the facilitation of reentry by local cooling of regions of ventricular myocardium[20,21] and the enhanced vulnerability to fibrillation provoked by electrical stimulation when repolarization is prolonged at slow heart rates.[22] There is a widespread perception that increased heterogeneity of refractoriness usually accompanies a global prolongation of repolarization.[19]

"Prolonged repolarization may be expected to increase the asynchrony of repolarization within the ventricular myocardium, between the ventricular myocardium and the Purkinje fibers, or both. In many conditions associated with prolonged QT interval, the presence of

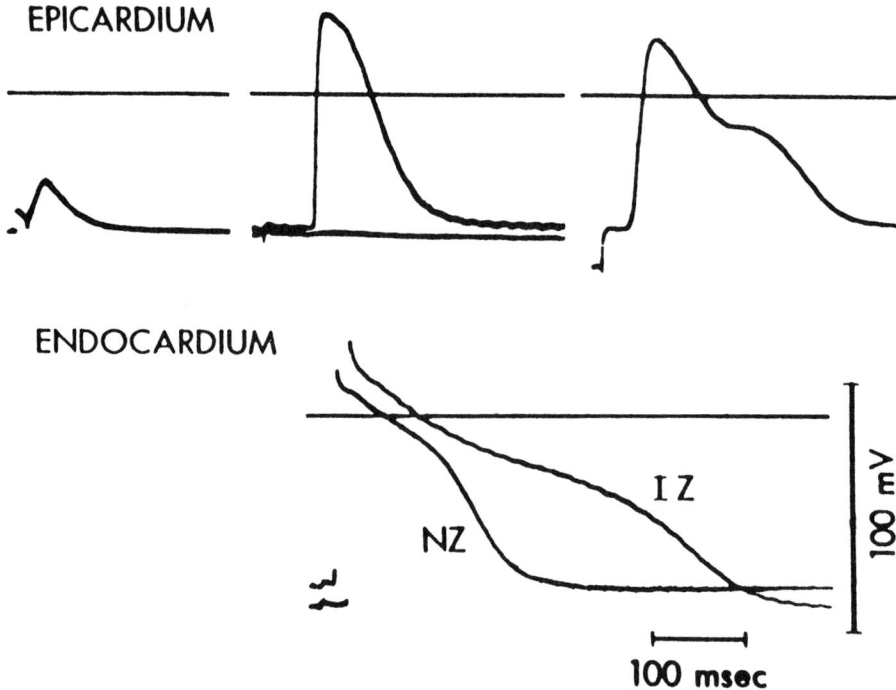

EPICARDIUM

ENDOCARDIUM

I Z

NZ

100 mV

100 msec

Figure 2. Marked diversity of action potentials and repolarization demonstrated in intracellular recordings from various sites of the canine left ventricle 24 hours after occlusion of the left anterior descending coronary artery. The recordings from the epicardium were from surviving myocardial cells overlying the infarction. Recordings from the endocardium are from the Purkinje network in the normal zone (NZ) and ischemic zone (IZ). There is a wide variation in the time course and duration of repolarization, and some cells show poor responses or resting potentials with no responses.

large dispersion of repolarization can be deduced from the occurrence of premature ventricular complexes interrupting the T wave.

Another factor of importance in the genesis of ventricular arrhythmias is the increase duration of the terminal repolarization slope, i.e. the interval from the onset of recovery of excitability to the end of repolarization. Prolongation of this interval, e.g. by hypokalemia or quinidine-like drugs, means prolonged relative refractory period, i.e the period during which the excitability and the conduction remain non-homogeneous."

The clinical entities usually offered as epitomes of this rule are the long QT syndromes, congenital (adrenergic dependent), and acquired (pause dependent).[19,23] It has been postulated that the prolonged and abnormal T-U waves represent marked and heterogeneous prolongation of repolarization throughout the ventricles and that reentrant arrhythmias are generally facilitated in this milieu. However, this concept has been challenged in recent years by the hypothesis that the tachyarrhythmias of the long QT syndromes are derived primarily from early afterdepolarizations (EADs) and triggered firing.[23–26]

The point was made earlier that the fundamentals of reentry were perceived and articulated very soon after the discovery of the phenomenon, but important embellishments of the conceptual framework have appeared in recent years. The demonstration by Allessie and co-workers[27–29] of the formation of a regularly circulating wave front in the myocardial syncytium in the absence of a nonconducting obstacle was a signal advance. This type of cir-

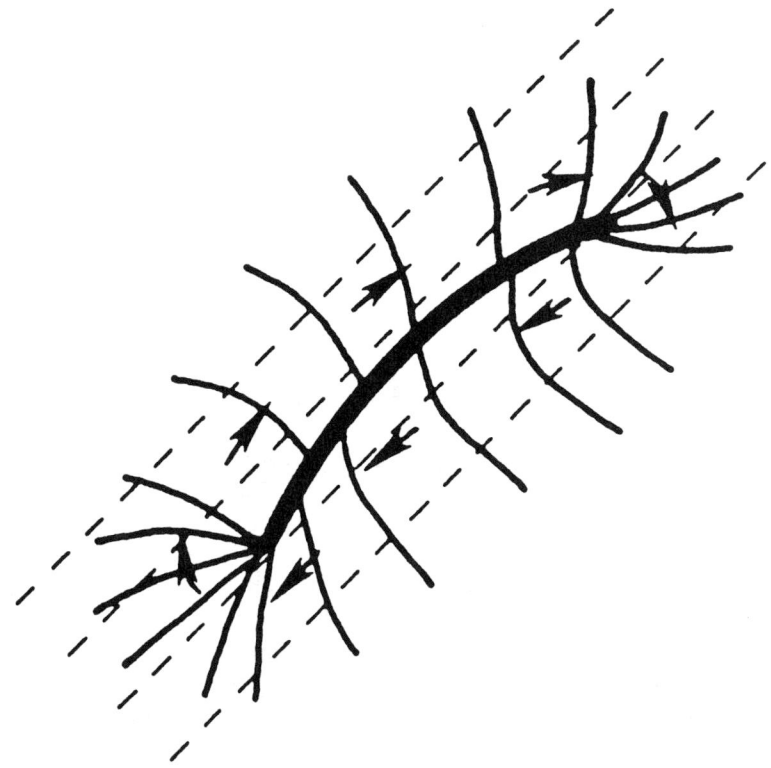

Figure 3. Schematic depiction of a reentrant circuit of the "leading circle" type in which the interface of block (heavy bar) is aligned along the long axis of the fibers (broken lines) and the wave front at the turning point proceeds slowly (isochromes closer together) transverse to the long axis of the fibers. Greater slowing of conduction at the turning points due to higher intercellular coupling resistance and reduced excitatory current in the transverse direction of the circuit allows full recovery of cells in the limbs parallel to the interface of block with faster conduction (isochrones farther apart) and the possibility of an excitatory gap in those regions.

cuit, illustrated in Figure 3, depends on refractoriness not only for the development of the initiating unidirectional block, as in the ring model, but also for the functional interface of block around which the wave front circles. These circuits form most readily when an early activation wave proceeds from a region of lesser refractoriness toward a region of steeply increasing refractoriness, and encounters an interface of block of sufficient extent. The study of this kind of circuit and its variant the "figure-of-eight" circuit described by El-Sherif and co-workers[30] and Wit and co-workers[31] has brought to light the concept that dispersion of refractoriness operates not just by absolute differences in refractory periods throughout the myocardium, but according to spatial patterns of distribution of the refractory periods.[32] The spatial gradient of change in refractoriness is important, as is the spatial extent of the prolonged refractoriness around which a circuit might form.

In circuits without an inert obstacle, anisotropic conduction may be important in regulating conduction around the circuit. When circuits are oriented so that the interface of block is aligned along the long axis of the fibers, slow transverse conduction takes place as activation proceeds around the edges of the interface of block (Figure 3).[33] Thus, conduction decelerates as the turn is made around the edges and accelerates as the wave front returns to the direction parallel to the interface of block and the long axis of the fibers.[33,34]

Because these circuits do not have inert barriers, significant electrotonic interactions occur between contiguous electrically coupled cells that affect the operation of the circuit and the refractory properties. Cells at the interface of block remain at depolarized potentials for longer periods because of the electrotonic influence of the activation of cells on either side of the interface.[34] As a consequence the cells on the interface function more effectively as a refractory barrier. Also cells at the turning points of transverse conduction have action potentials prolonged by step potentials preceding the upstrokes.[34] The transverse slow conduction at the turning points is thought to allow the formation of a partially excitable gap in other portions of the circuit.

These circuits can have circulation times prolonged by agents that prolong refractoriness but do not directly affect excitatory current. For example sotalol, an agent that does not affect sodium current directly, can slow the rate of ventricular tachycardia.[35] Prolongation of the relative refractory period could indirectly reduce excitatory current and conduction velocity in portions of the circuit where activation of incompletely repolarized cells occurs. Also, since activation of these circuits follows receding refractoriness, longer refractory periods in the circuit could cause larger interfaces of block, ie, circuits of greater dimensions. Even if conduction were not slowed the greater dimensions would entail longer circuit times and slower rates.

To capitalize on heterogeneity of refractoriness to initiate reentry, premature stimulation is required. However a single premature stimulus may not be sufficient as was noted by Mines[6] many years ago. Repetitive premature stimulation may be necessary because each premature excitation serves to further abbreviate refractoriness and enhance the differences in refractoriness in normal tissues.[36,37] These differences may be exaggerated when abnormal tissues are involved because abnormal tissues may respond differently to shorter cycle lengths: refractoriness may not shorten to the same degree or it may even be lengthened.[14] In addition, the prolonged repolarization occurring after a long cycle length increases the dispersion of recovery times in normal tissues.[22] Therefore, the introduction of premature stimuli after a relatively longer cycle may facilitate the induction of reentry, a point emphasized by Denker and associates.[38]

While the importance of refractoriness and repolarization in reentry has been appreciated and examined for a long time, in the past decade attention has been increasingly directed to another arrhythmogenic mechanism associated with repolarization: EADs and triggered firing. Though these phenomena were observed more than half a century ago[39] (Figure 4), there was little interest until evidence was presented that EADs are the cellular electrophysiological phenomena that underlie the long QT syndromes and the attendant ventricular tachycardias called torsades de pointes.[23–26] The first intimations of this concept came from two sources. Bonatti and co-workers[26] reported monophasic action potential (MAP) recordings in patients with the

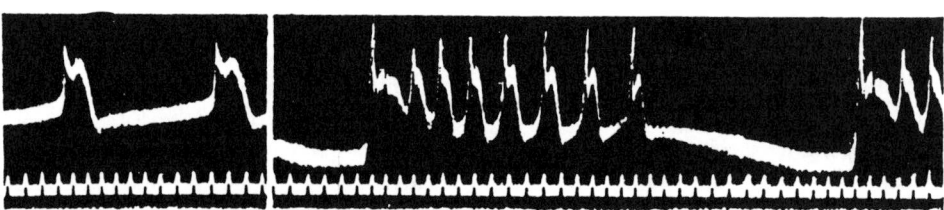

Figure 4. Injury potentials reported by Goldenberg and Rothberger in 1936[39] illustrating early afterdepolarization in Purkinje fibers exposed to veratrine.

long QT syndromes that demonstrated waveforms resembling EAD. At about the same time Brachmann and co-workers[24] prolonged repolarization in dogs by blocking potassium channels with cesium and observed ECG changes and arrhythmias indistinguishable from the long QT syndromes in humans. When they recorded intracellular potentials from cesium-treated Purkinje fibers they observed bradycardia-dependent EAD. They suggested that the EAD recorded in vitro were responsible for the long QT syndrome produced by cesium in intact dogs. It was later demonstrated that MAPs in vivo from cesium-treated dogs also showed waveforms compatible with EAD (Figure 5).[40,41] Early afterdepolarizations have been produced under numerous and diverse conditions that prolong repolarization by reduction of outward currents or by enhancement of long-lasting inward currents.[42,43] It is not clear that all means for prolonging repolarization are capable of inducing EAD nor has a quantitative relationship between the prolongation of repolarization and the generation of EAD been established. For example, reduced extracellular calcium delays repolarization, but EADs have not been observed in cells directly exposed to low extracellular calcium. The prolongation of the QT interval in patients with hypocalcemia has not been associated with torsades de pointes except for one recent case report.[44]

The ionic currents directly responsible for EAD have not been completely elucidated. By comparison with delayed afterdepolarizations (DADs), EADs by phenomenological ap-

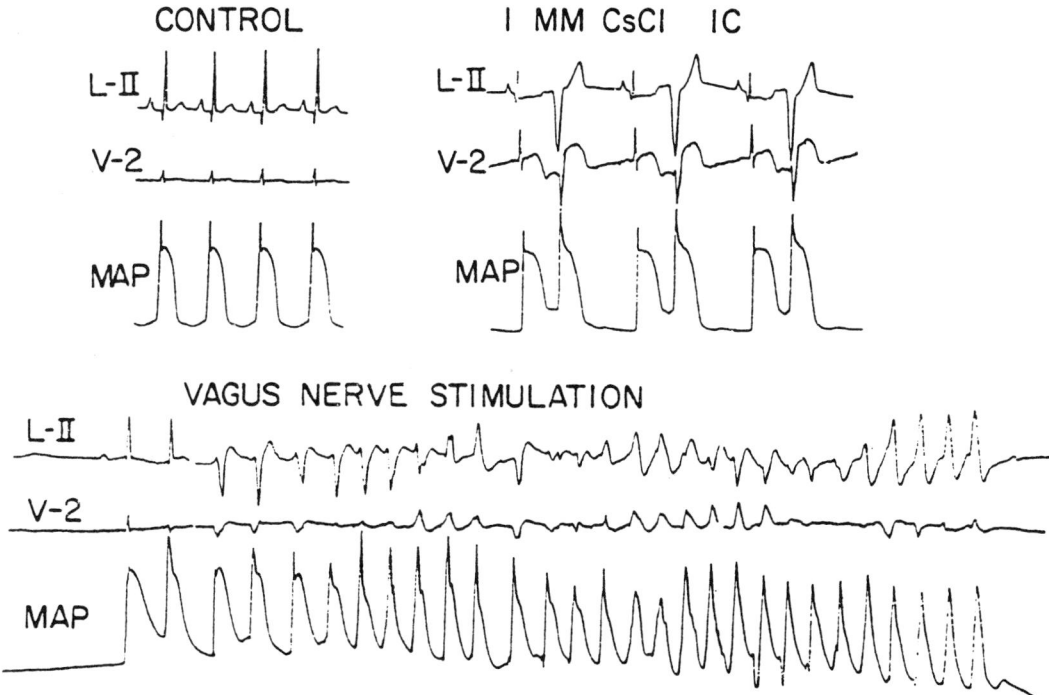

Figure 5. Torsades de pointes and early afterdepolarizations (EAD) generated in a dog treated with cesium intracoronary (IC). ECG leads 2 (L-II), and V$_2$ and endocardial injury recordings with a Franz electrode (MAP). The injection of cesium led to bigeminal ectopic ventricular complexes associated with the appearance of EADs on the MAP are shown. With slowing of the heart rate by vagal stimulation torsades de pointes appeared and the MAP recording illustrated EADs and triggered firing from depolarized levels of membrane potential. (Figure provided by Eugene Patterson.)

pearance are more complex, defying simple description or classification. They may occur at widely different times and voltages during repolarization and appear in varying forms, even if the same intervention, for example, cesium is used to induce them as illustrated in Figure 6. This diversity is amplified among the numerous interventions that cause EADs. The multiplicity of forms of EAD suggests that there is not a common and universal current generator for EADs under all conditions. It is useful to distinguish between currents involved in EAD from those involved in upstrokes triggered by EAD (Figure 7), but this distinction may be difficult when EAD demonstrate a slow positive upturn of potential at relatively depolarized levels of membrane potential in the plateau range (Figure 6E). In general, at more negative levels of membrane potential during repolarization, EAD manifest as a retardation of the rate of repolarization and the upstroke is easily distinguishable as a separate phenomenon.

Study of EAD induced by cesium in isolated ferret myocytes led to the conclusion that abnormal release of calcium by the sarcoplasmic reticulum (SR) was not involved in the induction of the inward currents responsible for EAD.[45] This conclusion contrasted with the demonstrated role of SR release in the induction of DADs. It was proposed that EADs result from a shift in dominance between outward and inward currents flowing through sarcolemmal ion channels so that inward currents, notably I_{CaL} dominate. This hypothesis fits with the well-established therapeutic efficacy of β blockers in adrenergic-dependent long QT syndromes and with the recently recognized efficacy of calcium channel blockers and magnesium (also a calcium channel blocker) in the long QT syndromes.[46] I_{CaL} has also been implicated as the primary current in EAD induced by Bay K 8644[47,48] and quinidine.[49] Conversely, I_{Na} has been suggested as the primary agent of charge transfer for EAD induced by agents that enhance long-lasting sodium currents such as aconitine, veratridine, and anthopleurin A.[42]

In clinical practice the agents that induce EAD most commonly appear to do so by

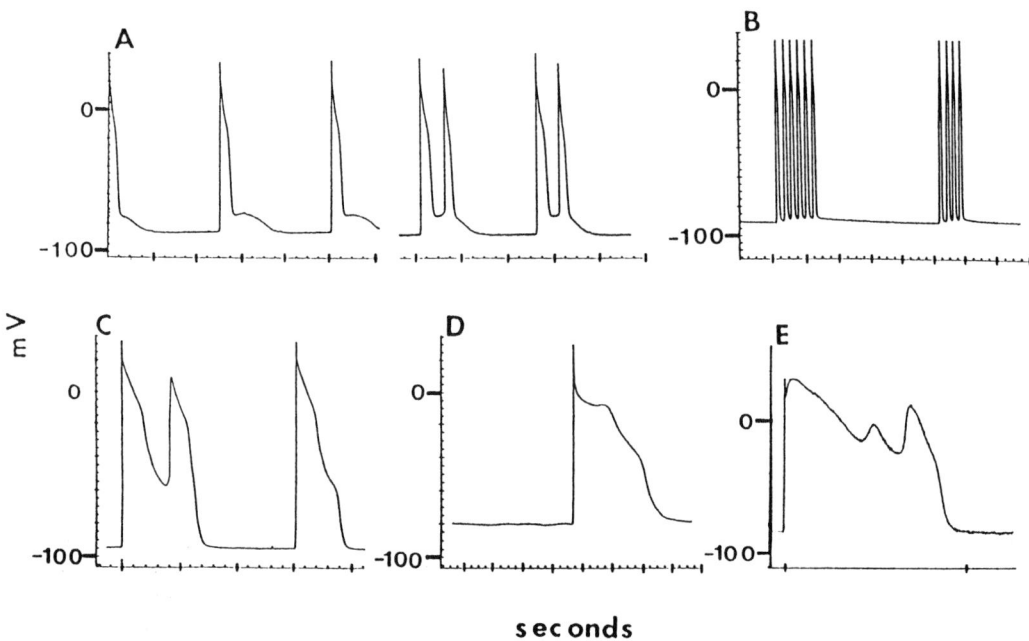

Figure 6. Diverse array of early afterdepolarizations induced in Purkinje fibers and myocytes by cesium under various conditions of exposure and concentration.

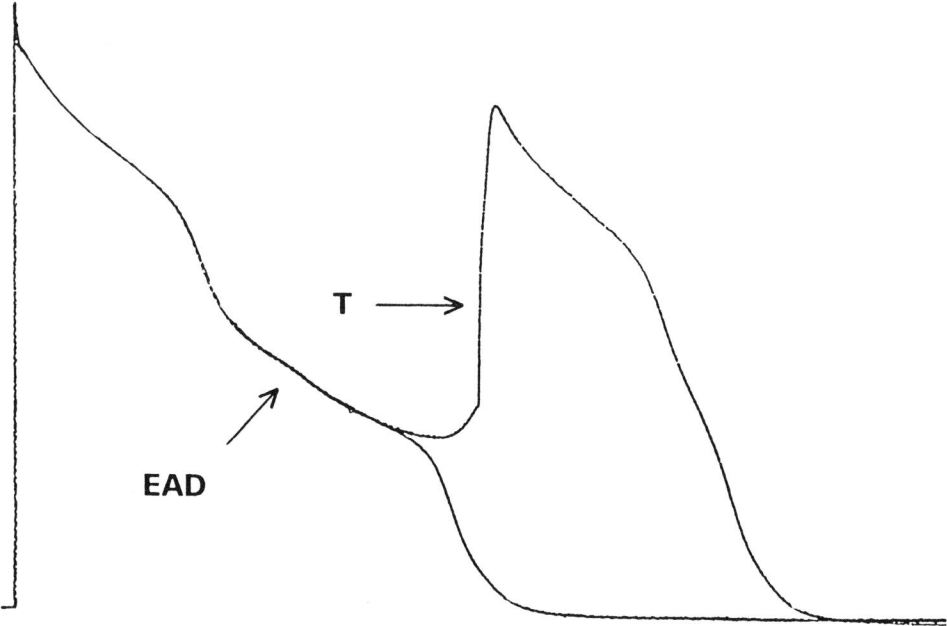

Figure 7. Action potentials recorded from cesium-treated Purkinje fiber showing early afterdepolarizations (EAD) and EAD with triggering (T). The ionic mechanisms for EAD may not be the same as the ionic mechanism for the triggered upstroke. (Figure provided by Bela Szabo.)

blocking potassium channels. The current vigorous initiative to develop new antiarrhythmic agents that prolong repolarization (Class III) consists primarily, but not exclusively of the formulation of new agents that block one or more of the potassium channels. Therefore, elucidation of the ionic mechanisms of EAD occurring when potassium currents are blocked is of great practical importance. Our observations suggest that when potassium currents are blocked in canine myocytes, the cells become loaded with calcium and the Na-Ca exchanger may play a dominant role in the generation of EADs.[50]

The sites of generation of EADs may depend on the mode of induction. There is a general perception that EADs occur more readily in Purkinje cells than myocardial cells because Purkinje cells normally have the longest repolarization.[42,43] However, this observation may be a result of the isolation of tissue preparations in which the myocardial cells are less well sustained and perhaps exposed to higher extracellular potassium levels. M cells in the interior of the canine myocardium, which have action potentials of longer durations, have been shown to be more susceptible to EADs induction than other myocardial cells with action potentials of lesser durations.[51] Therefore, agents acting relatively uniformly throughout the heart such as drugs delivered to the normal heart during systemic distribution, may generate EADs heterogeneously, favoring tissues with longer repolarization. This situation is further complicated by heterogeneous abnormal conditions, for example ischemia or hypertrophy of one chamber and not the others. It has been shown that ischemically injured Purkinje fibers and hypertrophied myocardial cells, which have delayed repolarization, are more susceptible to EADs generation than normal myocardium.[52,53] The possible heterogeneity of EADs generation raises the question of propagation of triggered upstrokes from sites of EADs generation to adjoining tissue. There have been demonstrations in preparations in vitro of triggered upstrokes that fail to propagate to neighboring tissue.[42,54,55] The more positive the membrane potential at which triggered upstrokes originate, the lower their amplitudes and the less likely their propagation.

The arrhythmogenic role of EADs in clinical arrhythmias is best supported for the long QT syndromes. The evidence for their involvement is abundant and derived from diverse sources. Many agents and alterations known to cause the long QT syndrome have been shown to produce EAD, for example low extracellular potassium, bradycardia, catecholamine stimulation, quinidine, NAPA, and sotalol.[23,42,43] Conversely, agents known to be efficacious against the long QT syndromes have been shown to suppress EADs and/or triggered firing, for example increasing heart rate, adrenergic blockade or withdrawal, calcium channel blockade, and magnesium.[23,42,43] Electrocardiographic changes and torsades de pointes can be generated in dogs by agents that induce EADs and the EADs generation has been conclusively linked to the manifestations. Finally, multiple investigators, beginning with the seminal observations of Bonatti and co-workers[26] have shown deflections strongly resembling EADs in recordings of MAPs (injury potentials) by both suction and pressure techniques from hearts of patients with the long QT syndrome.[46] Notwithstanding the uneasiness concerning movement artifact that might mimic EADs in such recordings, the responses of these deflections to rate and interventions, and their correlation with body surface recordings of T-U waves leaves little doubt that they reflect EADs at least in some cases.[46,56] The enhancement after a pause of an apparent EADs on an MAP reading is shown in Figure 8.

Early afterdepolarizations are very likely the initiating mechanism of the first beats of tachyarrhythmia in the long QT syndromes, but their role in the continuing tachyarrhythmia is less clear. Dispersion of repolarization is exaggerated in the long QT syndromes[19] and it is probably amplified by EADs occurring heterogeneously. Therefore, reentry should be facilitated. The common clinical observation that the sustained arrhythmias can be terminated by countershock is an observation in keeping with reentry, but not proof of it. The electrophysiological basis for the characteristic twisting pattern of the mean QRS vector is not clarified.

The observation that EADs can occur with hypoxia and acidosis,[57,58] conditions in vitro simulating reperfusion,[59] and with exposure to oxygen free radicals[60–62] suggests a role for them in ischemia, infarction, and reperfusion. Monophasic action potential recordings from the ischemic zones of cats during reperfusion showed EAD.[63] Detailed global mapping of arrhythmias during acute ischemia[64] demonstrated predominantly reentrant excitation, but sometimes focal excitation, which could be triggering. Evidence has been presented that hypertrophied myocytes, which manifest longer action potentials than normal myocytes, are more susceptible to EADs generation.[53] It has been proposed that the increased incidence of life-threatening ventricular arrhythmias observed in clinical conditions associated with hypertrophy,[53] most notably hypertrophic cardiomyopathy is due in part to generation of afterdepolarizations and triggered firing.

The sundry conditions that spawn EADs in the laboratory prompt the speculation that there may be a variety of pathophysiological conditions in which they operate to generate arrhythmias. The conditions for which there is positive evidence of their operation, the long QT syndromes and ischemia-reperfusion, represent environments in which triggering and reentry are likely to coexist. Early afterdepolarizations exaggerate heterogeneity of refractoriness and create an environment in which reentry thrives.

Manipulating the factors that create reentry, the scientist and clinician encounter a troubling paradox in the case of conduction and refractoriness. The pharmacotherapy of reentrant arrhythmias has always relied strongly upon the depression of conduction within the circuit to terminate the circulating wave front. However, depression of conduction is a fundamental condition for reentrant excitation. Consequently, potential harm has

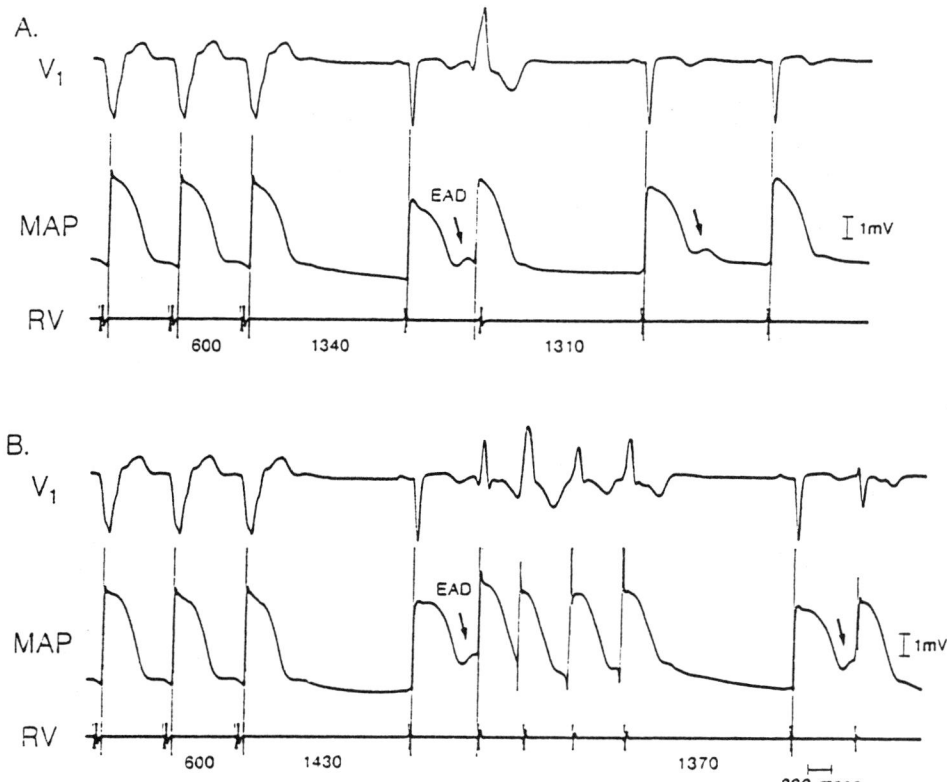

Figure 8. Relationship between pause length and early afterdepolarization (EAD) amplitude on monophasic action potential (MAP) recording in a 65-year-old man with an idiopathic, nonfamilial, pause- and adrenergic-dependent long QT syndrome. Tracings are ECG lead V_1, MAP recording from the right ventricular outflow tract, and a bipolar electrogram from the right ventricular apex (RV). Both panels begin with the last three complexes of a train of eight complexes of right ventricular pacing at cycle length 600 msec. Panel A: a postpacing pause of 1340 msec results in a prominent postpause EAD in the MAP electrogram (left arrow) and a single triggered ventricular extrasystole. Panel B: a longer pause of 1430 msec results in a larger EAD (left arrow) and a four-beat episode of ventricular tachycardia. The patient was not receiving any medications known to prolong repolarization and serum electrolytes were normal. (Reproduced with permission from Reference 46.)

always shadowed benefit in the treatment of reentry with agents that depress excitatory current. Similarly, we have seen that prolongation of refractoriness, a powerful inhibitor of reentry, carries the potential to exacerbate reentrant excitation by the enhancement of heterogeneity of refractoriness. In addition, more recently there has surfaced the disturbing realization that prolongation of repolarization brings a risk of induction of EADs and triggered firing. To fully exploit the antiarrhythmic effect of prolongation of refractori-

ness the challenge of the future is to eliminate the risk of proarrhythmia by minimizing heterogeneity and by elucidating the mechanisms for EADs so as to avoid them.

References

1. Mayer AG: Nerve conduction and other reactions in cassiopea. *Am J Physiol* 39:375, 1916.
2. Wiener N, Rosenblueth A: The mathematical formulation of the problem of conduction of impulses in a network of connected excitable

elements, specifically in cardiac muscle. *Arch Inst Cardiol Mex* 16:205, 1946.

3. Smeets JLRM, Allessie MA, Lammers WJEP, et al: The wavelength of the cardiac impulse and reentrant arrhythmias in isolated rabbit atrium. *Circ Res* 58:96, 1986.

4. Rensma PL, Allessie MA, Lammers WJEP, et al: Length of excitation wave and susceptibility to reentrant atrial arrhythmias in normal conscious dogs. *Circ Res* 62:395, 1988.

5. Opthof T, Coronel R, Shander GS, et al: Electrophysiologic changes and ventricular fibrillation in acute regional ischemia in the porcine heart: the concept of wavelength. *J Cardiovasc Electrophysiol* 3:128, 1992.

6. Mines GR: On dynamic equilibrium in the heart. *J Physiol (Lond)* 46:349, 1966.

7. Garrey WE: Auricular fibrillation. *Physiol Rev* 4:215, 1924.

8. Weidmann S: Effect of current flow on the membrane potential of cardiac muscle. *J Physiol (Lond)* 115:227, 1951.

9. Weidmann S: The effect of the cardiac membrane potential on the rapid availability of the sodium carrying system. *J Physiol (Lond)* 127:213, 1955.

10. Brooks CMcC, Hoffman BF, Suckling EE, Orias O: The heart cell—transmembrane potentials of cardiac muscle. In: CMcC Brooks, BF Hoffman, EE Suckling O Orias: *Excitability of the Heart*. New York/London: Grune & Stratton, 1955, p. 98.

11. Antzelevitch C, Sicouri S, Litovsky SH, et al: Heterogeneity within the ventricular wall: electrophysiology and pharmacology of epicardial, endocardial, and M cells. *Circ Res* 69:1427, 1991.

12. Franz MR, Bargheer K, Costard-Jackle A, et al: Human ventricular repolarization and T wave genesis. *Prog Cardiovasc Dis* 33:369, 1991.

13. Hoffman BF, Cranefield PF: *Electrophysiology of the Heart*. New York: McGraw-Hill, 1960, p. 120.

14. Lazzara R, El-Sherif N, Hope RR, Scherlag BJ: Ventricular arrhythmias and electrophysiological consequences of myocardial ischemia and infarction. *Circ Res* 42:740, 1978.

15. Lue WM, Boyden PA: Abnormal electrical properties of myocytes from chronically infarcted canine heart: alterations in $\dot{V}_{max}$ and the transient outward current. *Circulation* 85:1175, 1992.

16. Patterson E, Scherlag BJ, Lazzara R: Rapid inward current in ischemically injured subepicardial myocytes bordering myocardial infarction. *J Cardiovasc Electrophysiol* 4:9, 1993.

17. Han J, Goel BG: Electrophysiologic precursors of ventricular tachyarrhythmias. *Arch Intern Med* 129:749, 1972.

18. Surawicz B: Dispersion of refractoriness in ventricular arrhythmias. In: D Zipes, J Jalife (eds): *Cardiac Electroohysiology: From Cell to Bedside*. Philadelphia, PA: W.B. Saunders Company, 1990, p. 377.

19. Surawicz B: The QT interval and cardiac arrhythmias. *Ann Rev Med* 38:81, 1987.

20. Kuo CS, Munakata K, Reddy CP, Surawicz B: Characteristics and possible mechanism of ventricular arrhythmia dependent on the dispersion of action potential durations. *Circulation* 67:1356, 1983.

21. Wallace AG, Mignone RJ: Physiologic evidence concerning the re-entry hypothesis for ectopic beats. *Am Heart J* 72:60, 1966.

22. Han J, Millet HJ, Chizzonitti B, Moe GK: Temporal dispersion of recovery of excitability in atrium and ventricle as a function of heart rate. *Am Heart J* 71:481, 1966.

23. Jackman WM, Friday KJ, Anderson JL, et al: The long QT syndromes: a critical review, new clinical observations and a unifying hypothesis. *Prog Cardiovasc Dis* 31:115, 1988.

24. Brachmann J, Scherlag BJ, Rosenshtraukh LV, Lazzara R: Bradycardia-dependent triggered activity: relevance to drug-induced multiform ventricular tachycardia. *Circulation* 68:846, 1983.

25. Schechter E, Freeman C, Lazzara R: Afterdepolarizations as a mechanism for the long QT syndrome: electrophysiologic studies of a case. *J Am Coll Cardiol* 3:1556, 1984.

26. Bonatti V, Finardi A, Botti G: Enregistrement des potentiels d'action monophasiques du ventricule droit dans un cos de QT long et alternance solee de l'onde U. *Arch Mal Coeur* 72:1180, 1979.

27. Allessie MA, Bonke FLM, Schopman FJG: Circus movement in rabbit atrial muscle as a mechanism of tachycardia. *Circ Res* 33:54, 1973.

28. Allessie MA, Bonke FIM, Schopman FJG: Circus movement in rabbit atrial muscle as a mechanism of tachycardia. II. The role of non-uniform recovery of excitability in the occurrence of unidirectional block as studied with multiple microelectrodes. *Circ Res* 39:168, 1976.

29. Allessie MA, Bonke FIM, Schopman FJG: Circus movement in rabbit atrial muscle as a mechanism of tachycardia. III. The "leading circle" concept: a new model of circus movement in cardiac tissue without the involvement of an anatomical obstacle. *Circ Res* 41:9, 1977.

30. El-Sherif N, Smith RA, Evans K: Canine ventricular arrhythmias in the late myocardial infarction period. 8. Epicardial mapping of reentrant circuits. *Circ Res* 49:255, 1981.

31. Wit AL, Allessie MA, Bonke FIM, et al: Electrophysiologic mapping to determine the mecha-

nisms of experimental ventricular tachycardia initiated by premature impulses. *Am J Cardiol* 49:166, 1982.

32. Gough WB, Mehra R, Restivo M, et al: Reentrant ventricular arrhythmia in the late myocardial infarction period in the dog. 13. Correlation of activation and refractory maps. *Circ Res* 57:432, 1985.

33. Dillon SM, Allessie MA, Ursell PC, Wit AL: Influence of anisotropic tissue structure on reentrant circuits in the subepicardial border zone of subacute canine infarcts. *Circ Res* 63:182, 1988.

34. Van Capelle FJL, Allessie MA: Computer simulation of anisotropic impulse propagation: characteristics of action potentials during re-entrant arrhythmias. In: *Cell to Cell Signalling: From Experiments to Theoretical Models.* London/San Diego: Academic Press Limited, 1989, p. 577.

35. Senges J, Lengfelder W, Jauernig R, et al: Electrophysiologic testing in assessment of therapy with sotalol for sustained ventricular tachycardia. *Circulation* 69:577, 1984.

36. Kuo CS, Amlie JP, Munakata K: Dispersion of monophasic action potential durations and activation times during atrial pacing, ventricular pacing, and ventricular premature stimulation in canine ventricles. *Cardiovasc Res* 17:152, 1983.

37. Kuo CS, Atarashi H, Reddy CP: Dispersion of ventricular repolarization and arrhythmia: study of two consecutive ventricular premature impulses. *Circulation* 72:370, 1985.

38. Denker S, Lehman M, Mahmud R, et al: Facilitation of macroreentry within the His-Purkinje system with abrupt changes in cycle length. *Circulation* 69:26, 1984.

39. Goldenberg M, Rothberger CJ: Uber die wirkung von veratrin auf den Purkinjefaden. *Pflügers Arch* 238:137, 1936.

40. Levine JH, Spear JF, Guarnieri T, et al: Cesium chloride-induced long QT syndrome: demonstration of afterdepolarizations and triggered activity in vivo. *Circulation* 72:1092, 1985.

41. Patterson E, Szabo B, Scherlag BJ, et al: Early and delayed afterdepolarizations associated with cesium chloride-induced arrhythmias in the dog. *J Cardiovasc Pharmacol* 15:323, 1990.

42. El-Sherif N, Craelius W, Boutjdir M, Gough WB: Early afterdepolarizations and arrhythmogenesis. *J Cardiovasc Electrophysiol* 1:145, 1990.

43. Wit AL, Rosen RM: Afterdepolarizations and triggered activity: distinction from automaticity as an arrhythmogenic mechanism. In HA Fozzard, E Haber, RB Jennings, et al. (eds): *The Heart and Cardiovascular System.* 2nd edition. New York: Raven Press, 1991, p. 2113.

44. Akiyama T, Batchelder J, Worsman J, et al: Hypocalcemic torsades de pointes. *J Electrocardiol* 22:89, 1989.

45. Marban E, Tsien RW: Enhancement of calcium current during digitalis inotropy in mammalian heart: positive feedback regulation by intracellular Ca? *J Physiol* 329:589, 1982.

46. Jackman WM, Szabo B, Friday KJ, et al: Ventricular tachyarrhythmias related to early afterdepolarizations and triggered firing: relationship to QT interval prolongation and potential therapeutic role for calcium channel blocking agents. *J Cardiovasc Electrophysiol* 1:170, 1990.

47. January CT, Riddle MJ: Early afterdepolarizations: mechanism of induction and block: a role for L-type Ca^{++} current. *Circ Res* 64:977, 1989.

48. January CT, Riddle MJ, Salata JJ: A model for early afterdepolarizations: induction with the Ca^{2+} channel agonist Bay K 8644. *Circ Res* 62:563, 1988.

49. Nattel S, Quantz MA: Pharmacological response of quinidine induced early afterdepolarizations in canine Purkinje fibers: insights into underlying ionic mechanisms. *Cardiovasc Res* 22:808, 1988.

50. Szabo B, Sweidan R, Patterson E, et al: Increased intracellular Ca^{++} may be important also for early afterdepolarizations (abstract). *J Am Coll Cardiol* 9:210A, 1987.

51. Sicouri S, Antzelevitch C: Afterdepolarizations and triggered activity develop in a select population of cells (M cells) in canine ventricular myocardium: the effects of acetylstrophanthidin and Bay K 8644. *PACE* 14:1714, 1991.

52. Gough WB, El-Sherif N: The differential response of normal and ischaemic Purkinje fibres to clofilium D-sotalol and bretylium. *Cardiovasc Res* 23:554, 1989.

53. Aronson RS: Mechanisms of arrhythmias in ventricular hypertrophy. *J Cardiovasc Electrophysiol* 2:249, 1991.

54. Mendez C, Delmar M: Triggered activity: its possible role in cardiac arrhythmias. In: DP Zipes, J Jalife (eds): *Cardiac Electrophysiology and Arrhythmias.* Orlando, FL: Grune & Stratton, 1985, p. 311.

55. Kupersmith J, Hoff P: Occurrence and transmission of localized repolarization abnormalities in vitro. *J Am Coll Cardiol* 6:152, 1985.

56. El-Sherif N, Bekheit S, Henkin R: Quinidine-induced long QTU interval and torsade de pointes: role of bradycardia-dependent early afterdepolarizations. *J Am Coll Cardiol* 14:252, 1989.

57. Adamantidis MM, Caron JF, Dupuis BA: Triggered activity induced by combined mild hypoxia and acidosis in guinea pig Purkinje fibers. *J Mol Cell Cardiol* 18:1287, 1986.

58. Kupersmith J, Hoff P, Duo GS: In vitro characteristics of repolarization abnormality—a possible cause of arrhythmias. *J Electrocardiol* 19: 361, 1986.

59. Rozanski GJ, Witt RC: Early afterdepolarizations and triggered activity in rabbit cardiac Purkinje fibers recovering from ischemic-like conditions: role of acidosis. *Circulation* 83:1352, 1991.

60. Barrington PL, Meyer CF Jr, Weglicki WB: Abnormal electrical activity induced by free radical generating systems in isolated cardiocytes. *J Mol Cell Cardiol* 20:1163, 1988.

61. Tarr M, Valenzeno DP: Modification of cardiac action potential by photosensitizer-generated reactive oxygen. *J Mol Cell Cardiol* 21:539, 1989.

62. Cerbai E, Ambrosio G, Porciatti F, et al: Cellular electrophysiological basis for oxygen radical-induced arrhythmias: a patch-clamp study in guinea pig ventricular myocytes. *Circulation* 84:1773, 1991.

63. Priori SG, Mantica M, Napolitano C, Schwartz PJ: Early afterdepolarizations induced in vivo by reperfusion of ischemic myocardium: a possible mechanism for reperfusion arrhythmias. *Circulation* 81:1911, 1990.

64. Pogwizd SM, Corr PB: Electrophysiologic mechanisms underlying arrhythmias due to reperfusion of ischemic myocardium. *Circulation* 72:404, 1987.

Chapter 9

Mechanisms of Atrial Arrhythmias

Maurits A. Allessie
Michiel J. Janse

The elucidation of arrhythmia mechanisms has been dependent both on the analysis of activation patterns of the heart and on insights in cellular electrophysiology. Microelectrode recordings from isolated cardiac preparations obtained from patients during cardiac surgery have provided important data on abnormalities in transmembrane potentials in diseased tissue. The technical advances during the last decade have been instrumental in the detailed analysis of excitation patterns during arrhythmias, mainly because they offered the possibility of recording extracellular potentials simultaneously at many sites in the heart. The purpose of this chapter is to describe both mapping experiments and other electrophysiological studies aimed at elucidating mechanisms of atrial arrhythmias, particularly atrial fibrillation and flutter. A distinction will be made between reentrant and nonreentrant mechanisms.

Reentrant Arrhythmias

Atrial Fibrillation

Experimental atrial fibrillation can be induced in various ways. Rapid stimulation of

the atrium, especially when combined with vagal stimulation, and local application of aconitine produce atrial fibrillation with the same characteristics as far as rate and irregularity are concerned.[1-3] Yet the underlying mechanisms of both arrhythmias are completely different. When atrial fibrillation is induced by rapidly stimulating an atrial appendage and the appendage is clamped off, fibrillation ceases in the appendage but continues in the rest of the atria.[1,3] When, after application of aconitine to an appendage, this structure is clamped off, sinus rhythm is restored in the rest of the atria while the clamped-off appendage shows a fast regular tachycardia.[3] In this case, the arrhythmia is due to a focus that discharges so rapidly that uniform excitation of the atria is no longer possible. This kind of fibrillation is best described as fibrillatory conduction, where at multiple and varying sites rate-dependent arcs of conduction block develop.[4] To explain the mechanism of the other type, best called true fibrillation, Moe and Abildskov[3] formulated the multiple wavelet hypothesis. The key element of this hypothesis is that the "wave front becomes fractionated as it divides about islets or strands of refractory tissue, and each of the daughter

From BN Singh, HJJ Wellens, M Hiraoka, (eds): *Electropharmacological Control of Cardiac Arrhythmias.* Mount Kisco, NY, Futura Publishing Company Inc., © 1994.

wavelets may now be considered as independent offspring. Such a wavelet may accelerate or decelerate as it encounters tissue in a more or less advanced state of recovery. It may divide again or combine with a neighbor; it may be expected to fluctuate in size and change in direction. Its course, though determined by the excitability or refractoriness of surrounding tissue, would appear to be as random as Brownian motion. Fully developed fibrillation would then be a state in which many such randomly wandering wavelets coexist. The likelihood of persistence of this process should depend upon the number of wavelets present. If the number is large, there is little chance that all elements will fall into phase (i.e., be refractory or excitable simultaneously), but if the number is small, there is a considerable probability that they may fuse and permit resumption of sinus rhythm. The average number, in turn, will depend upon the atrial mass, the mean duration of the refractory period, and the mean conduction velocity."

At the time this hypothesis was formulated, simultaneous recording from a sufficient number of sites in the atria to document the complex excitation pattern was impossible, and Moe wrote that "direct test of the hypothesis is difficult, if not impossible in living tissue."[5] Moe and associates[6] developed a computer model, with a nonhomogeneous distribution of refractory periods as a key feature to simulate atrial fibrillation. Premature stimulation of sites with short refractory periods initiated a rapid, irregular rhythm, which was sustained by "irregular drifting eddies which varied in position and size." The number of wavelets varied between 23 and 40. The arrhythmia could be terminated by prolonging the refractory period.

Some 25 years later, when equipment became available to simultaneously record from multiple atrial sites, Moe's hypothesis could be tested directly.[4] To this end, two solid egg-shaped multi-electrodes were inserted into the cavities of right and left atria of isolated, Langendorff-perfused dog hearts. Each egg electrode contained 480 recording electrodes equally spaced on the surface at interelectrode distances of 3 mm. At the side of the interatrial septum, the eggs were flattened to better fit the shape of the atrial cavities. Simultaneous recordings could be made from 192 electrodes. Atrial fibrillation was induced by a single premature stimulus while acetylcholine (0.3 mg/L) was being continuously infused into the perfusion fluid. Detailed analysis of the activation patterns during atrial fibrillation revealed the following characteristics:

(1) In this model, fibrillation is indeed caused by multiple wavelet reentry.

(2) Although circulating excitation of the leading circle type can occur, it is exceptional that an impulse follows the same circular route more than once. Rather, reentry as the basis for fibrillation means reexcitation of a given area that had already been excited by another wave front. This has been called random reentry.

(3) Conduction velocity of the wavelets varies between 20 and 90 cm/sec.

(4) Wavelets can be as narrow as a few millimeters, but broad wave fronts propagating uniformly over large segments of atrial tissue occur as well.

(5) Each wavelet exists for only a short time, not longer than a few hundred milliseconds. Extinction of a wavelet can be caused by fusion or collision with another wavelet, by reaching the border of the atria, or by meeting refractory tissue. New wavelets can be formed by fusion of a wave at a local area of conduction block, or by an offspring of a wave traveling toward the other atrium.

(6) The critical number of wandering wavelets for perpetuation of fibrillation is between three and six. In any chamber, an average of three wavelets is present with a maximum of four and a minimum of zero. With an average of three simultaneously present wavelets the chance for all wavelets ceasing to exist is rather high, but with an average of six (three in each atrium), fibrillation did not spontaneously terminate. When the concentration of acetylcholine in the perfusion medium was

reduced resulting in a prolongation of refractoriness and a prolongation of the wavelength (vide infra), the number of wavelengths gradually decreased to three or less and the arrhythmia terminated.

Figure 1 shows a series of "snapshots," each representing a time window of 10 msec,

where the various wave fronts during stable fibrillation are shown in the right atrium. The 30 frames represent 0.3 seconds of fibrillation. In this example, the average number of wavelets present in the right atrium was three, with a maximum of four (frames 7, 8, and 28) and a minimum of zero wavelets (frames 18 and 19). The latter observation indicates that in

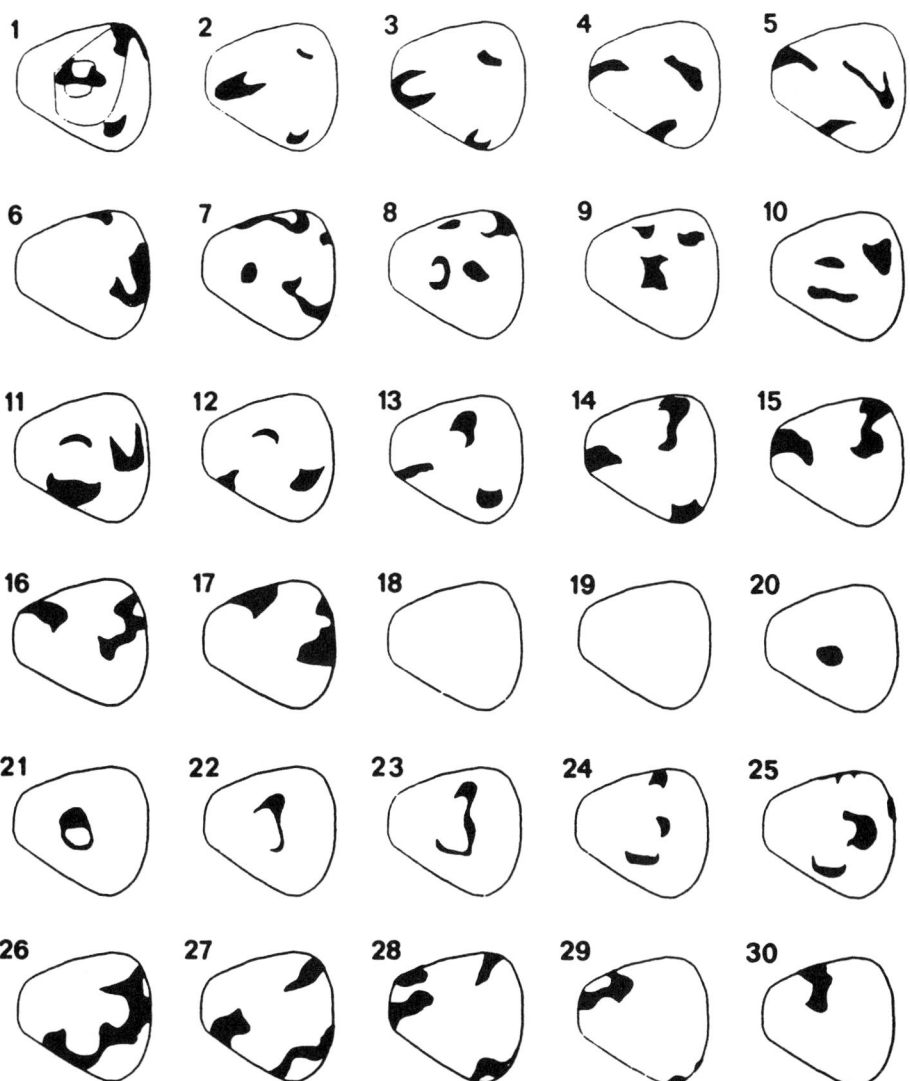

Figure 1. Thirty consecutive "snapshots" of electrical activity of the right atrium during stable fibrillation. Each panel represents a time window of 10 msec; the black zones indicate areas activated during that window. Note absence of electrical activity in frames 18 and 19, indicating that the chance of cancellation of wave fronts is rather high when only three wavelets are present. (Reproduced with permission from Reference 4.)

the presence of three wavelets the chance for cancellation of all wavelets is rather high. Fibrillation in the right atrium alone would not have been sustained.

In patients with Wolff-Parkinson-White (WPW) syndrome who underwent cardic surgery, atrial fibrillation was induced by programmed electrical stimulation and epicardial mapping was performed using a multiple electrode containing 240 unipolar terminals at 2.5 mm distance.[7] In essence, the findings were similar to those obtained in the canine heart. It was not, however, possible to determine the minimal number of simultaneously present wavelets necessary to sustain fibrillation. In view of the larger size of the atria in humans, this number may be larger than in dogs.

Whereas experiments such as described above clearly provided evidence that random reentry causes atrial fibrillation, it must be emphasized that various other mechanisms could, in principle, also give rise to the electrocardiographic pattern of fibrillation. The definition of fibrillation is a descriptive one based on the electrocardiogram, and usually includes characteristics as rapid, irregular, and the inability to distinguish individual QRS complexes (ventricular fibrillation) or P waves (atrial fibrillation). Electrophysiological mechanisms that could produce such ECG characteristics other than random reentry are: (1) A single wandering reentrant circuit. In the ventricles, this has been shown to occur in acutely ischemic myocardium where a single reentrant circuit that changed size and location from beat to beat produced extracellular potentials that were indistinguishable from fibrillation caused by random reentry.[8] In the atria, this possibility is also suggested by maps made from canine and human atria during atrial fibrillation;[9] (2) A single rapid focus (automatic, triggered, or microreentrant) with fibrillatory conduction, where because of inhomogeneities in refractoriness not all parts of the tissue are able to follow the rapid rate, and rate-dependent arcs of conduction block develop that change in size and location; (3) Two independent foci at fixed sites with different intrinsic rates of discharge (parasystolic fibrillation); and (4) Combination of a single focus and a single reentrant circuit.

The Wavelength Concept

For sustained reentry, all cells in the reentrant circuit must have recovered their excitability before being reexcited. This can only occur if the pathlength of the reentrant circuit is greater than the wavelength of the propagating impulse, which is given by the product of conduction velocity and refractory period. If wavelength is short, because of a short refractory period, slow conduction or both, more reentrant wavelets can be present in a given tissue mass and therefore the likelihood for fibrillation will be increased. In the normal dog, there is a close relationship between wavelength and the occurrence of induced atrial arrhythmias.[10] In conscious dogs in which multiple electrodes for stimulation and recording had been attached to both atria, refractory periods and conduction velocity were measured. To change wavelength, a number of agents (acetylcholine, propafenone, lidocaine, ouabain, quinidine, and sotalol) were administered and refractory period duration, conduction velocity, and their product were correlated with the induction of atrial arrhythmias by single premature stimuli. In all 19 dogs, atrial arrhythmias, including atrial fibrillation could be induced. Although at shorter refractory periods, a relatively high incidence of atrial fibrillation was observed, prolongation of the refractory period did not always prevent atrial fibrillation. In fact, the predictive value of refractory period duration alone, or conduction velocity alone, for induction of arrhythmias was poor. Figure 2 shows the correlation between the induction of atrial fibrillation (and the instances when no arrhythmias could be induced) and refractory period, conduction velocity and wavelength of the provoking premature impulse. The critical wavelength where atrial arrhythmias (repetitive responses or atrial flutter) started to be induced was 12 cm; the critical wavelength

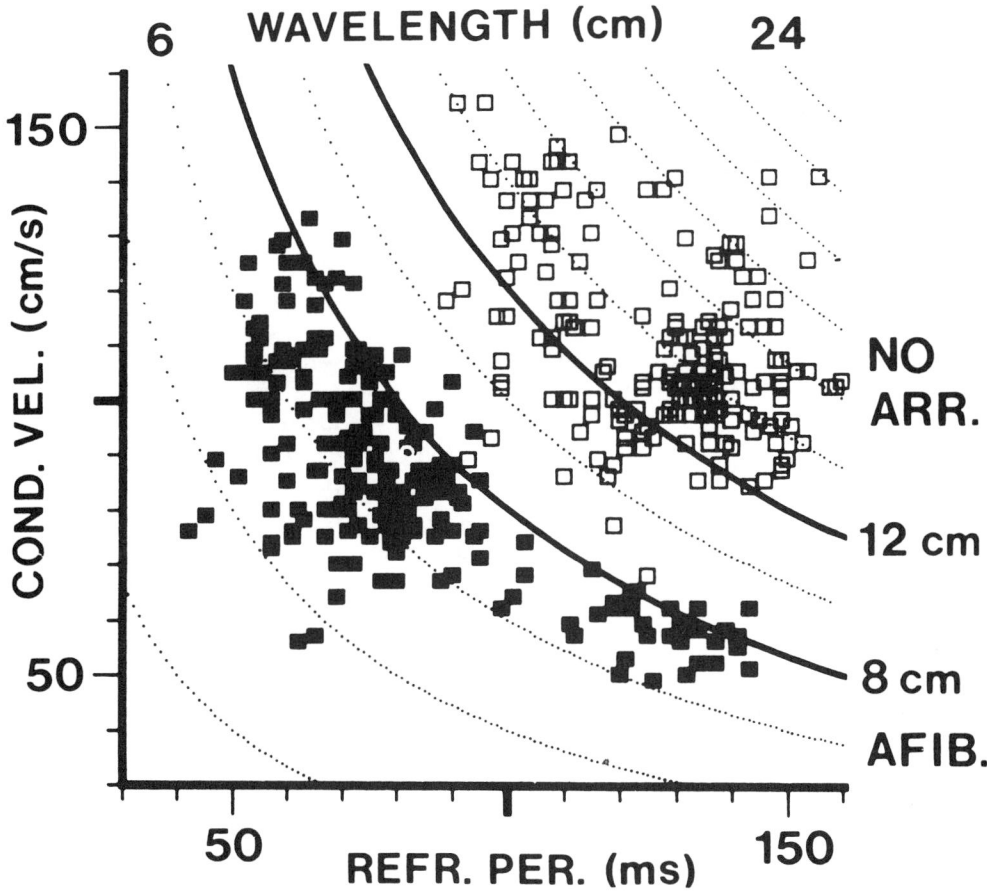

Figure 2. Relation between induction of atrial fibrillation and refractory period, conduction velocity and wavelength of the initiating premature beat. Because wavelength is the product of refractory period and wavelength, "iso-wavelength" curves are drawn at 8 cm and 12 cm. Because of the effects of a wide variety of administered drugs, a wide range of refractory periods and conduction velocities was achieved. Different responses to premature stimulation, ie, either no arrhythmias or atrial fibrillation, were obtained over a wide range of conduction velocities and refractory periods. However, wavelength discriminated well between the two types of response.

for atrial fibrillation was 8 cm. Because of the variety of drugs administered, values for conduction velocity and refractory period varied widely. Atrial fibrillation could be induced over a wide range of refractory periods (50 to 150 msec) and conduction velocities (50 to 140 cm/sec). For each of these parameters there is a wide overlap between the population of "no arrhythmias" and atrial fibrillation. However, when wavelength was used as a criterion, there was a clear separation between both populations.

These findings suggest that it might be useful to describe part of the properties of antiarrhythmic drugs in terms of wavelength. It must be emphasized, however, that these results are valid for normal dog atria, in which it may be supposed that electrophysiological characteristics are fairly homogeneous throughout the atrial tissue. In diseased atria, with possibly an inhomogeneous distribution of refractory periods and conduction velocity, there may not be a single wavelength, but varying wavelengths at different sites. In such atria, it may not be as easy to demonstrate a similar relationship between wavelength and arrhythmogenesis.

Electrophysiological Abnormalities of Atria Prone to Fibrillation

Several electrophysiological abnormalities have been reported to be associated with atrial fibrillation. Transmembrane potentials have been recorded from tissue obtained from fibrillating human atria, and it was found that resting membrane potential levels were significantly reduced compared to resting membrane potentials of cells from nonfibrillating atria.[11] This would imply that because of the reduced upstroke velocity of the action potential as a consequence of the low resting membrane potential level, conduction velocity would be decreased, which as discussed above, would promote reentry by decreasing wavelength. It is not known whether resting membrane potential varies in different parts of fibrillating atria.

Attuel and associates[12] were the first to describe an intriguing abnormality in patients vulnerable to atrial fibrillation. In these patients there was no, or hardly any adaptation of the atrial refractory period to changes in heart rate. At the most rapid rates investigated (cycle lengths in the order of 350 to 400 msec) the range of refractory periods was similar to that of normal patients (approximately from 160 to 250 msec). Upon slowing of the heart rate, however, no prolongation of the refractory period was observed, so that at cycle lengths between 800 and 1,000 msec the refractory periods of the patients prone to atrial fibrillation were much shorter than those of normal patients. These findings were largely confirmed in a later study in which action potentials were recorded from isolated pieces of atrial tissue at different pacing rates.[13] Importantly, dispersion of action potential duration was much greater in the atrial fibrillation group than in the control group, indicating that in atria prone to fibrillate dispersion in recovery of excitability is increased.

The classic method to determine refractory period duration is to deliver a premature stimulus S_2 after every eighth or tenth basic stimulus S_1 during a regularly driven rhythm and to vary the coupling interval until the shortest S_1S_2 is found at which S_2 results in a propagated response. To determine refractory periods at multiple sites is a very time consuming procedure. The average interval between local activations during both atrial fibrillation[14] and ventricular fibrillation[15] has been used as an index for local refractoriness. This is based on the concept, supported by microelectrode recordings, that during fibrillation cells are reexcited as soon as their refractory period ends by one of the many wandering wavelets. Recording local electrograms simultaneously at many sites during fibrillation allows assessment of spatial dispersion in refractoriness in a very short time. The correlation between fibrillation interval at various sites and refractory period duration measured after defibrillation at the same sites by the classic S_1S_2 method was very good, both for atrial and ventricular fibrillation.[14,15] A difference between shortest and longest fibrillation interval of some 15 msec corresponded to a difference in refractory period duration at a regularly driven rhythm (cycle length 350 msec) of 35 to 40 msec. The fibrillation interval should be regarded as an index of the shortest possible refractory period.

In patients undergoing cardiac surgery, atrial fibrillation was induced by premature stimulation in a group of patients who never had atrial fibrillation, and in a group of patients with paroxysmal atrial fibrillation, and fibrillation intervals were determined at up to 40 atrial sites in each patient. In the atrial fibrillation group, the average fibrillation interval was 25 msec shorter than in the control group, and the spatial dispersion in fibrillation intervals was three times larger.[16] An example is shown in Figure 3, where the atrial fibrillation intervals at 37 sites are plotted in a control patient and in a patient with paroxysmal atrial fibrillation. These findings support those of earlier studies, and indicate that as far as refractoriness is concerned, atria of patients with

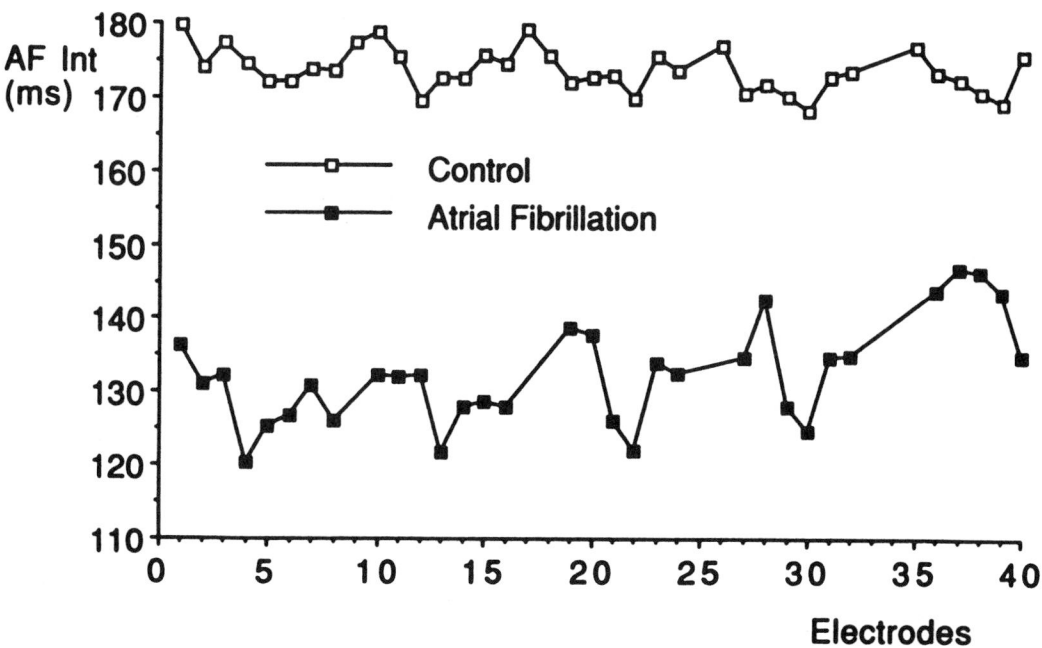

Figure 3. Plot of atrial fibrillation intervals, determined from simultaneous recordings from 37 atrial sites in a control patient and in a patient with paroxysmal atrial fibrillation. Note marked spatial inhomogeneity in fibrillation intervals in the patient with spontaneous atrial fibrillation, indicating a large dispersion in refractoriness. In addition, the fibrillation intervals are much shorter than in the control patients, indicating that the average refractory period is much shorter. (Reproduced with permission from Reference 16.)

spontaneous atrial fibrillation are inhomogeneous. The wavelength concept is still valid, but there is no single value for wavelength in such atria.

In summary, the experimental evidence obtained from both animal and human studies indicates that atrial fibrillation is generally due to random reentry caused by multiple reentrant wavelets. Other mechanisms, however, such as a single wandering reentrant circuit or a focal mechanism, may cause atrial fibrillation as well. Electrophysiological abnormalities of atria prone to fibrillation include short refractory periods, failure to adapt the refractory period duration to changes in heart rate, low resting potentials, and a large dispersion in action potential duration and refractoriness. Short wavelengths predispose to atrial fibrillation, but in inhomogeneous tissue it is difficult to determine the critical wavelength.

Atrial Flutter

Atrial flutter was the first arrhythmia in which mapping experiments supported the concept of circus movement reentry.[17] The early experiments indicated that the arrhythmia was caused by a large circus movement around an anatomical obstacle, provided by the orifices of the caval veins.[17–19] This would imply that the reentrant circuit has an excitable gap so that premature stimuli applied during flutter might entrain or terminate the arrhythmia. Clinically, two types of atrial flutter have been distinguished[20]: type I, with an atrial rate of 240 to 338 per minute, which can be entrained by atrial pacing; and type II, with an atrial rate of 340 to 433 per minute in which atrial pacing is without effect. The latter type may be expected to have no, or a very short, excitable gap. Evidence for a leading circle

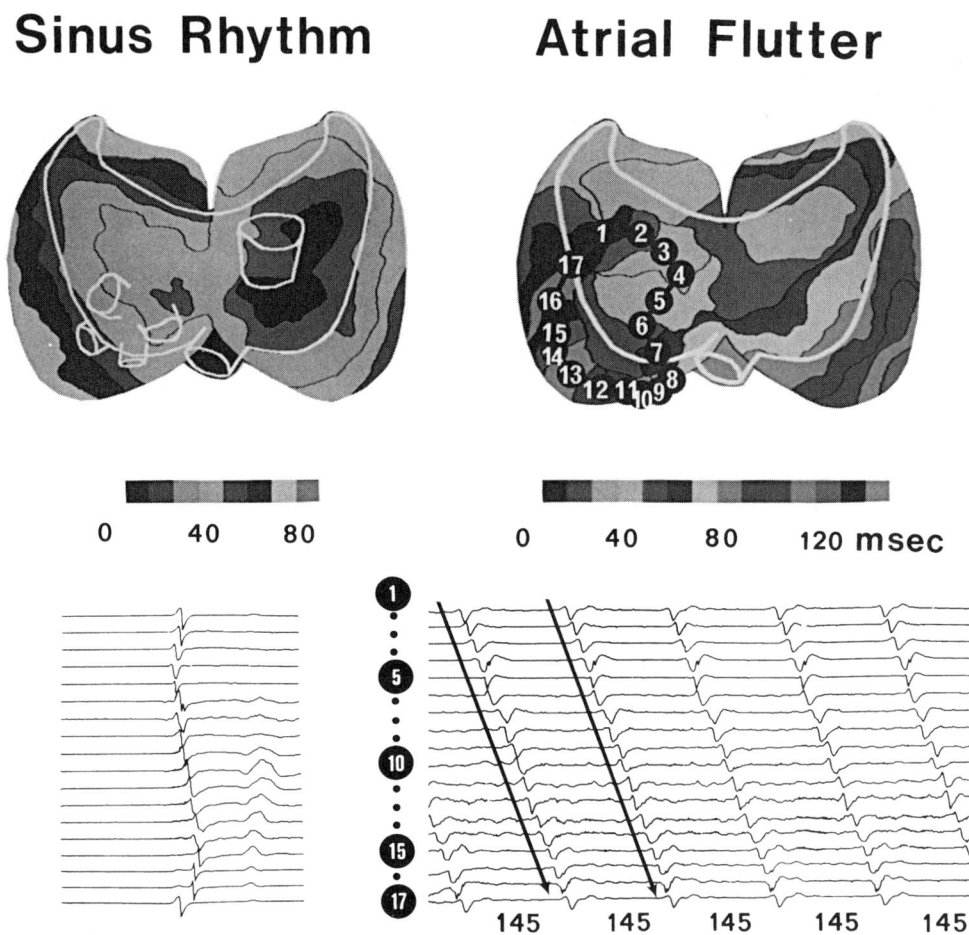

Figure 4. Activation maps of right and left atrium of the dog heart during sinus rhythm and during atrial flutter. During flutter a functional reentry circuit of the leading circle type is present. (Reproduced with permission from Reference 21.)

type of reentry, in which the crest of the reentrant wave front encroaches upon its own relative refractory tail and the vortex of the reentrant circuit consists of refractory tissue has been provided by mapping experiments in isolated dog hearts.[21] Cycle lengths of flutter induced by premature stimulation in the presence of acetylcholine, varied from 65 to 145 msec, and the lengths of the reentrant circuits varied from 5 to 10 cm. No site of special preference was found; the circuits could be anywhere in the left or right atrium. An example is shown in Figure 4, where 17 unipolar electrograms, selected from the total of 960 recorded electrograms, are shown during sinus rhythm and during flutter. During flutter, the activation times of these 17 electrodes bridged the entire flutter cycle of 145 msec, whereas during sinus rhythm the greatest difference in activation times was 40 msec.

Nonreentrant Mechanisms

A number of atrial arrhythmias appear to be caused by nonreentrant mechanisms. Most of these are caused by enhanced or abnormal automaticity, and are characterized by a gradual rather than an abrupt increase in atrial rate. In automatic atrial tachycardia, atrial rates gradually accelerate to reach rates between 125 and 200 per minute. The P wave morphology is different from that during sinus rhythm, and overdrive pacing usually captures the focus. Upon cessation of pacing, some overdrive suppression is usually seen. The most likely cause is abnormal automaticity, ie, automaticity occurring at a partially depolarized level of membrane potential.[22] Rossi and Matturri[23] described a case of automatic atrial tachycardia, where after surgical removal of the arrhythmia focus, the tissue was placed in a tissue bath and microelectrode recordings were performed. Abnormal automaticity was found in histologically normal atrial cells. In another case report[24] of an atrial tachycardia, which resembled reentrant tachycardia because the arrhythmia could be initiated and terminated by premature stimuli, microelectrode recordings from the arrhythmogenic area revealed that the arrhythmia was due to triggered activity based on delayed afterdepolarizations. Thus, although the great majority of atrial arrhythmias are reentrant in nature, focal mechanisms must be considered as well.

Conclusions

The ability to record extracellular potentials simultaneously from multiple atrial sites provided the basis for mapping studies in both experimental animals and humans during atrial flutter and fibrillation. These studies leave little doubt that both types of arrhythmias may be caused by reentry. Experimental studies in which changes in both conduction velocity and refractory period duration were induced provided data supporting the concept that interventions that shorten the wavelength (the product of conduction velocity and refractory period duration) are proarrhythmic. Studies in patients prone to atrial fibrillation indicated that refractory periods are not only short, but also inhomogeneously distributed throughout the atria. Thus, in such patients wavelength may differ from site to site.

Even though the case for reentry being a dominant mechanism in atrial arrhythmias is strong, it must be recognized that nonreentrant mechanisms cannot be excluded. Focal activity, be it abnormal automaticity or triggered activity due to afterdepolarization, may initiate reentrant arrhythmias, play a role in the maintenance of such arrhythmias, or be the sole arrhythmogenic mechanism for certain atrial tachycardias.

References

1. Garrey WE: The nature of fibrillary contraction of the heart. Its relation to tissue mass and form. *Am J Physiol* 33:397, 1914.
2. Scherf D: Studies on auricular tachycardia caused by aconitine administration. *Proc Soc Exp Biol Med* 64:233, 1947.
3. Moe GK, Abildskov JA: Atrial fibrillation as a self-sustaining arrhythmia independent of focal discharge. *Am Heart J* 58:59, 1959.
4. Allessie MA, Lammers WJEP, Bonke FIM, Hollen J: Experimental evaluation of Moe's multiple wavelet hypothesis of atrial fibrillation. In: DP Zipes, J Jalife, (eds): *Cardiac Electrophysiology and Arrhythmias*. Orlando, FL: Grune and Stratton, 1985, p. 265.
5. Moe GK: On the multiple wavelet hypothesis of atrial fibrillation. *Arch Int Pharmacodyn Ther* 140:183, 1962.
6. Moe GK, Rheinboldt WC, Abildskov JA: A computer model of atrial fibrillation. *Am Heart J* 67:200, 1964.
7. Allessie MA, Brugada J, Boersma L, et al: Mapping of atrial fibrillation in man (abstract). *Eur Heart J* 11(suppl 5):28, 1990.
8. Janse MJ, van Capelle FJL, Morsink H, et al: Flow of "injury" current and pattern of excitation during early ventricular arrhythmias in acute regional myocardial ischemia in isolated porcine and canine hearts. *Circ Res* 47:151, 1980.
9. Cox JL, Canavan TE, Schuessler RB, et al: The surgical treatment of atrial fibrillation. II. Intraoperative electrophysiologic mapping and description of the electrophysiologic basis of atrial flutter and fibrillation. *J Thorac Cardiovasc Surg* 101:406, 1991.
10. Rensma PL, Allessie MA, Lammers WJEP, et al: Length of excitation wave and susceptibility to reentrant atrial arrhythmias in normal conscious dogs. *Circ Res* 62:395, 1988.
11. Rosen MR, Bowman FO, Mary-Rabine L: Atrial fibrillation: the relationship between cellular electrophysiologic and clinical data. In: HE

Kulbertus, SB Olsson, M Schlepper (eds): *Atrial Fibrillation*. Mölndal: AB Hässle, 1982, p. 62.

12. Attuel P, Childers R, Cauchemez B, et al: Failure in rate adaptation of the atrial refractory period: its relationship to vulnerability. *Int J Cardiol* 2: 179, 1982.

13. Le Heuzey JY, Boutjdir M, Gagey S, et al: Cellular aspects of atrial vulnerability. In: P Attuel, P Coumel, MJ Janse (eds): *The Atrium in Health and Disease*. Mount Kisco, NY: Futura Publishing Company, Inc., 1989, p. 81.

14. Lammers WJEP, Allessie MA, Rensma PL, Schalij MJ: The use of fibrillation cycle length to determine spatial dispersion in electrophysiological properties and to characterize the underlying mechanism of fibrillation. *New Trends Arrhythmias* 2:109, 1986.

15. Opthof T, Ramdat Misier AR, Coronel R, et al: Dispersion in refractoriness in canine ventricular myocardium: effects of sympathetic stimulation. *Circ Res* 68:1204, 1991.

16. Ramdat Misier AR, Opthof T, van Hemel NM, et al: Increased dispersion in "refractoriness" in patients with idiopathic paroxysmal atrial fibrillation. *J Am Coll Cardiol* 19:1531, 1992.

17. Lewis T, Feil S, Stroud WD: Observations upon flutter and fibrillation. II. The nature of auricular flutter. *Heart* 7:291, 1920.

18. Rosenblueth A, García Ramos J: Studies on flutter and fibrillation. II. The influence of artificial obstacles on experimental auricular flutter. *Am Heart J* 33:677, 1947.

19. Hayden WG, Hurley EJ, Rytand DA: The mechanism of canine atrial flutter. *Circ Res* 20:496, 1967.

20. Wells JL, MacLean WAH, James TW, Waldo AL: Characterization of atrial flutter. Studies in man after open heart surgery using fixed atrial electrodes. *Circulation* 60:665, 1979.

21. Allessie MA, Lammers WJEP, Bonke FIM, et al: Intra-atrial reentry as a mechanism for atrial flutter induced by acetylcholine and rapid pacing in the dog. *Circulation* 70:123, 1984.

22. Gillette PG, Crawford FC, Zeigler VL: Mechanisms of atrial tachycardias. In: DP Zipes, J Jalife (eds): *Cardiac Electrophysiology. From Cell to Bedside*. Philadelphia: W.B. Saunders, Co., 1990, p. 559.

23. Rossi L, Matturri L: *Clinicopathological Approach to Cardiac Arrhythmias*. Torino: Centro Scientifica Torinese Editore, 1990, p. 176.

24. Wyndham LRC, Arnsdorf MF, Levitsky S, et al: Successful surgical excision of focal paroxysmal atrial tachycardia. Observations in vivo and in vitro. *Circulation* 62:1365, 1980.

Chapter 10

Arrhythmia Mechanisms During Acute Ischemia

Michiel J. Janse

Sudden cardiac death occurs most often in patients with coronary artery disease and may either be due to an acute ischemic event or to arrhythmias occurring in a heart with a healing or healed infarct.[1,2] The percentage of patients suffering a cardiac arrest unrelated to an acute ischemic event varies in different clinical reports from 22% to 64%.[3,4] Davies et al.[2] found that 73% of individuals who died suddenly from ischemic heart disease had an acute coronary vascular lesion. Thus, although acute myocardial ischemia is not the only cause of sudden death, it does seem to play a major role in causing lethal arrhythmias.

Since the mechanisms underlying fatal arrhythmias are not easily studied in patients, animal models have been developed that approach as much as possible the clinical situation. Because of the variety of experimental models used, it is impossible to provide precise figures on the incidence of ventricular arrhythmias caused by acute myocardial ischemia. To give just one example, when coronary artery occlusion was performed in a series of dogs in different laboratories, the incidence of ventricular fibrillation varied from 0% to 70%. Only when a series of 100 dogs was used, stable values were reached, the

range for incidence of fibrillation being 14% to 36%.[5]

Many factors determine whether, and how frequently arrhythmias occur following coronary artery occlusion. These factors include size of the ischemic area, size of the heart, presence of preexisting collaterals, use of anesthetics, stress in conscious animals, activity of the autonomic nervous system, heart rate, presence of a previous infarction, presence of cardiac hypertrophy, mode of coronary artery occlusion, and whether or not reperfusion is allowed.[6]

Thus, experimental studies of interventions that alter the incidence of ischemia-induced arrhythmias must be interpreted with caution. When the major factors that determine the occurrence of arrhythmias such as size of the ischemic zone, the extent of collateral circulation and heart rate are not controlled or unknown, only very large series can provide reliable data.

In order to understand the mechanism underlying ischemia-induced arrhythmias, it is useful to first describe the changes in cellular electrical activity, and the changes in transmembrane ionic gradients that occur during arrest of coronary flow.

From BN Singh, HJJ Wellens, M Hiraoka, (eds): *Electropharmacological Control of Cardiac Arrhythmias*. Mount Kisco, NY, Futura Publishing Company Inc., © 1994.

Changes in Transmembrane Potential

Application of the microelectrode technique to intact hearts has enabled the recording of transmembrane potentials during ischemia. Although the extent and the time course of changes varies with the location of the recording site, the basic changes of the transmembrane potential are consistent and have been observed in a variety of animal models, such as the pig,[7] dog,[8] guinea pig,[9] rabbit,[10] and humans.[11]

Figure 1 shows the changes in transmembrane potential as well as those in the local

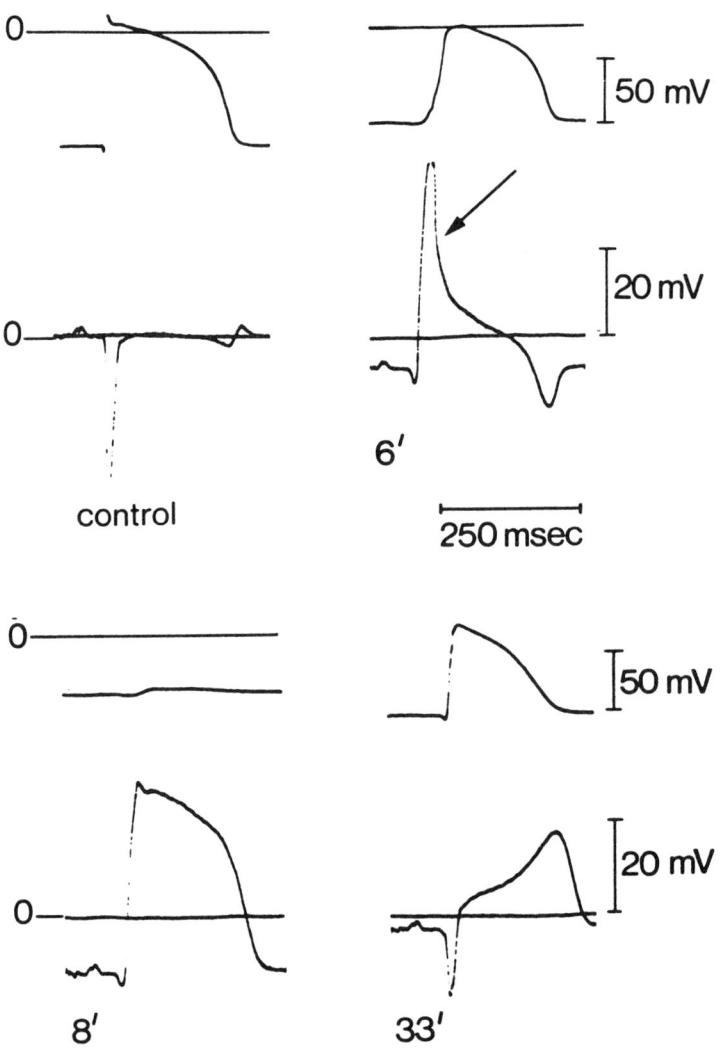

Figure 1. Transmembrane potentials (top traces) and local direct current extracellular electrograms (lower traces) from an intact pig heart before (control) and 6, 8, and 33 minutes after occlusion of the left anterior descending coronary artery. Note loss of resting membrane potential; slowing of action potential upstroke resulting in a delayed intrinsic deflection in the electrogram (arrow in upper right panel); inexcitability at resting membrane potential of about −50 mV (lower left panel); and restoration of excitability after 33 minutes (lower right panel).

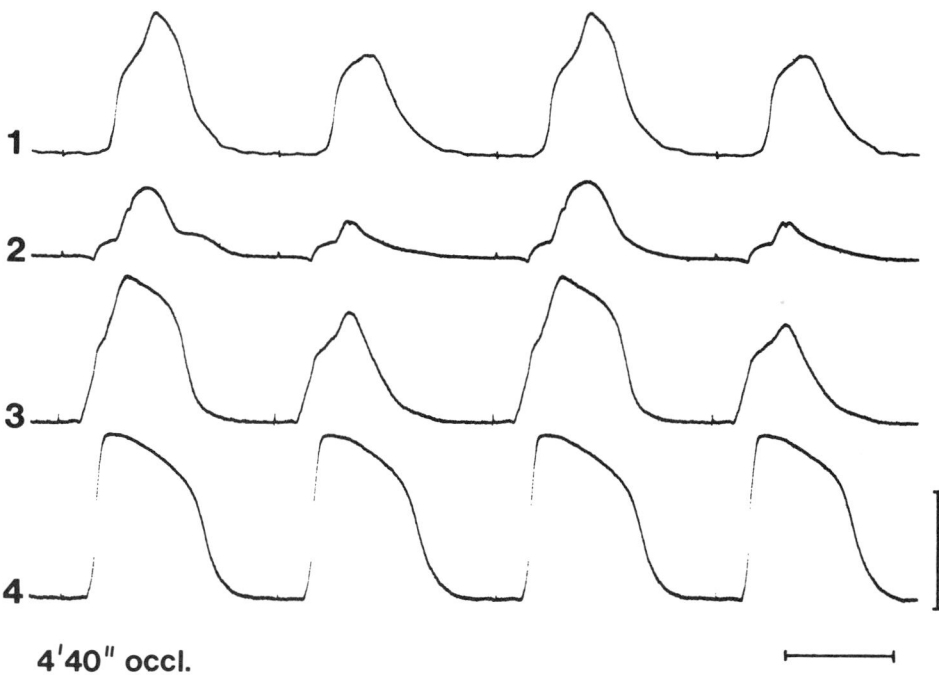

4'40" occl.

Figure 2. Four simultaneously recorded transmembrane potentials, 4 minutes and 40 seconds after coronary occlusion. Note alternation and inhomogeneity in action potential configuration throughout the ischemic zone.

direct current extracellular electrogram following coronary artery occlusion. The decrease in resting membrane potential is reflected in the extracellular complex by the depression of the TQ segment. The decrease in action potential amplitude and upstroke velocity results in a delayed intrinsic deflection in the electrogram (arrow). The extracellular complex becomes monophasic when the ischemic cell has become inexcitable at resting membrane potentials of −50 to −60 mV. With maintained occlusion, previously inexcitable cells regain excitability after approximately 30 minutes. These changes are not homogeneous at any given time throughout the ischemic zone, as shown in Figure 2. Here, the characteristic alternation in action potential duration and amplitude is also shown, which often heralds the onset of arrhythmias.[7] The most important factor causing the decrease in resting membrane potential is the

net loss of K^+ ions from ischemic cells and their accumulation in the extracellular space.[9] The decrease in action potential amplitude and upstroke velocity cannot be attributed solely to the increase in extracellular K^+ concentration. When porcine hearts are regionally perfused with normoxic high K^+ solutions, action potentials have larger amplitudes and faster upstrokes than action potentials at the same sites during ischemia even when resting membrane potential levels are the same.[12] Action potentials with the same configuration as those during ischemia can be obtained by exposing myocardium to hypoxic, acidotic, high K^+ solutions, either in the intact heart by regional perfusion of a coronary artery or in vitro by superfusion.[13] In addition to hypoxia, high K^+ and a low pH, other components of ischemia, such as lysophosphoglycerides and catecholamines also play a role.

Inhomogeneity in Recovery of Excitability

Figure 3 shows in a schematic fashion the effect of varying K^+ concentrations in a severely hypoxic and acidotic milieu on action potential configuration and recovery of excitability. At a K^+ concentration of 5 mm, hypoxia caused a marked shortening of the action potential, but the recovery of excitability, measured as the return of maximal upstroke velocity of premature action potentials induced by electrical stimulation at varying intervals following complete repolarization to control values, is similar to that during control conditions. When extracellular K^+ is increased, marked postrepolarization refractoriness occurs. It can intuitively be appreciated that a premature beat occurring at a certain coupling interval may be conducted at normal velocity in ischemic cells with a K^+ of 5 mM, slowly in zones with a K^+ of 10 mM, and will be blocked in areas where K^+ has risen to 12 mM. Studies using K^+-sensitive electrodes have shown distinct spatial inhomogeneity in extracellular K^+ in hearts with regional ischemia.[14,15] In a zone of 1 cm extending from the border between normal and ischemic myocardium toward the central ischemic zone, differences in extracellular K^+ at different recording sites in the order of 8 mM were found.[14] Thus, cells within this zone have different degrees of postrepolarization refractoriness. The fact that action potential characteristics are cycle length dependent has several important consequences: (1) During regular rhythms that are relatively fast, full recovery time may exceed the basic cycle length. This results in alternation (Figure 2), Wenckebach-type of block, 2:1 block, or even higher degrees of block; and (2) The degree of postrepolarization refractoriness is very sensitive to small changes of resting membrane potentials caused by relatively small changes in extracellular K^+ (Figure 3). Thus, a mere increase in sinus rate or a single premature beat may unmask the inhomogeneity in recovery of excitability and produce conduction block and reentry at sites which are conducting homogeneously at longer cycle lengths. An example is shown in Figure 4. It is of interest that the only drugs that have been shown to reduce the incidence of sudden death are β-adrener-

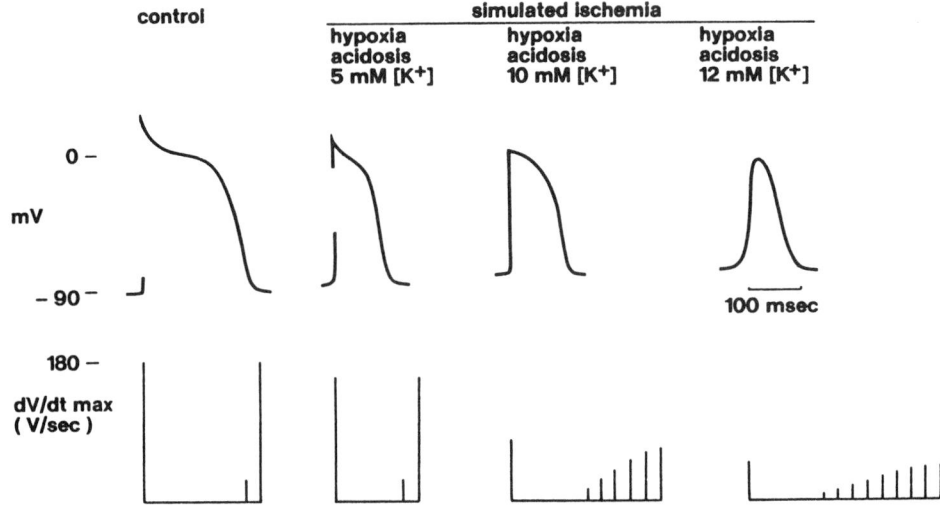

Figure 3. Schematic illustration of the changes in transmembrane potential (upper panels) and the recovery of maximal upstroke velocity dV/dt$_{max}$ of premature impulses following an action potential in normal ventricular myocardium (control) and in three different conditions of simulated ischemia.

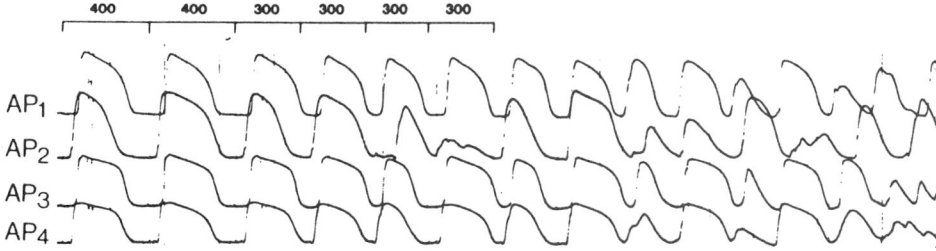

Figure 4. Increase in heart rate unmasks inhomogeneity in recovery of excitability and induces fibrillation. Four action potentials were recorded simultaneously from acute ischemic myocardium. The atria were paced at a cycle length of 400 msec. At this driving rate, the four cells are activated rather synchronously. The synchronicity is lost when the pacing cycle is reduced to 300 msec. Cell 2 becomes activated with delay (beat 5) and shows conduction block (beat 6) because of a greater degree of postrepolarization refractoriness than the other cells. This sets the stage for unidirectional block and reentry.

gic blocking agents, particularly those that reduce heart rate.[16]

Changes in Conduction Velocity

During the first 2 minutes after onset of ischemia, conduction velocity remains fairly constant to decrease rapidly thereafter. For conduction velocity along the longitudinal axis of myocardial fibers, the following values have been measured: control situation to 2 minutes after coronary artery occlusion: 50 cm/sec; after 3 minutes of ischemia: 40 cm/sec; and after 4 to 5 minutes: 30 cm/sec. After 5 minutes of ischemia conduction velocity could no longer be accurately determined because of the development of regional conduction block, shortly followed by inexcitability.[17] The major reason for the early decrease in conduction velocity is the decrease in action potential amplitude and upstroke velocity. Passive electrical properties, particularly changes in extracellular and intracellular longitudinal resistance, have been measured in isolated, arterially-perfused papillary muscle placed in a H_2O-saturated gaseous environment.[18] In such a preparation, arrest of coronary flow in addition to changing the gaseous environment to 94% N_2 and 6% CO_2 resulted in an immediate increase in extracellular resistance (related to loss of intravascular volume) followed by a secondary slower increase, most likely caused by osmotic cell swelling. Intracellular resistance remained constant during the first 10 to 15 minutes. Thereafter, ischemic cells rapidly uncoupled and intracellular longitudinal resistance increased by 400% within 5 minutes. Thus, during the first 10 minutes of ischemia, electrical uncoupling is unlikely to play any role in the slowing of conduction. However, in a later period, 15 to 20 minutes after coronary occlusion, electrical uncoupling may cause slow and inhomogeneous conduction, and thus may be an arrhythmogenic factor for arrhythmias occurring at that time.

Arrhythmias

During the first 30 minutes of ischemia, ventricular arrhythmias occur in two distinct phases. The first phase (phase 1a) occurs between 2 and 10 minutes, the second phase (phase 1b) approximately between 12 and 30 minutes. Sinus rhythm is present between the two phases.[19] In guinea pig hearts, phase 1b arrhythmias were always preceded by spontaneous improvement of action potential characteristics (Figure 1) and this improvement appeared related to release of endogenous catecholamines.[20] Since phase 1b arrhythmias often occur in the absence of delayed epicardial conduction, it has been suggested that

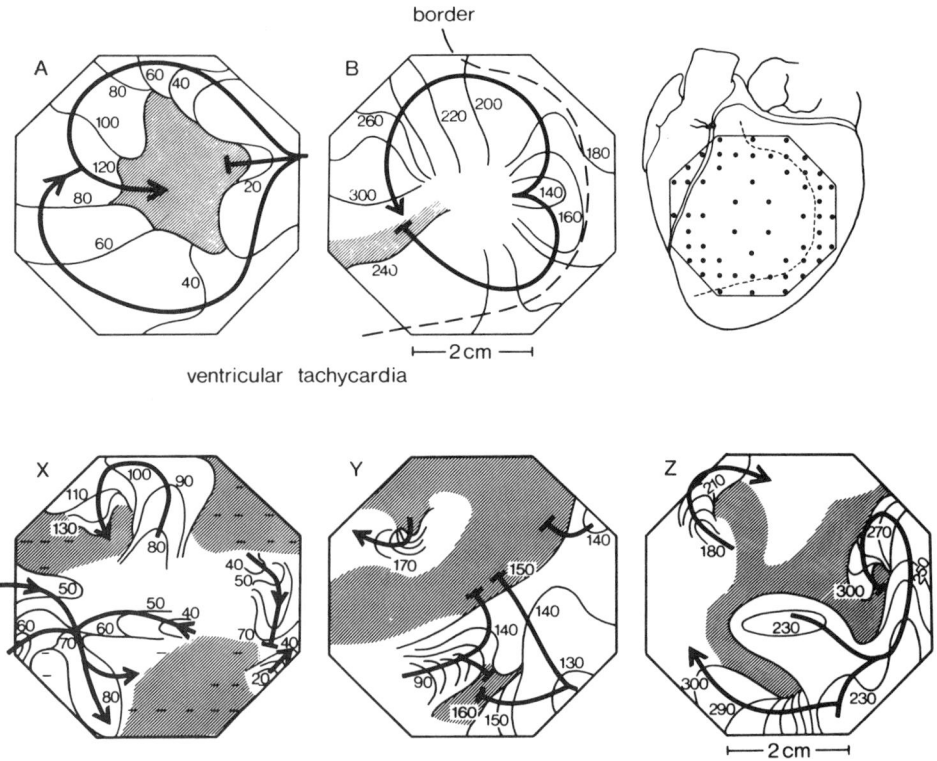

border

ventricular tachycardia

├── 2 cm ──┤

ventricular fibrillation

├── 2 cm ──┤

Figure 5. Upper panels: pattern of excitation of the first two beats of a spontaneous ventricular tachycardia after 4 minutes of ischemia. In the right panel the electrode configuration is shown: each dot is a recording terminal; the broken line is the border between ischemic and normal tissue. Isochronic lines are drawn in 20-msec increments. Thick lines with arrows depict general spread of excitation. Shaded areas are zones of block. Lower panels show pattern of activation of three successive "beats" when the tachycardia above had degenerated into ventricular fibrillation. See text for discussion.

mechanisms other than reentry (such as abnormal automaticity) might be the cause of phase 1b arrhythmias.[19] Further experiments are needed to substantiate this suggestion. As for phase 1a arrhythmias, there is abundant evidence that reentry is the dominant mechanism, although nonreentrant mechanisms may often be the trigger for sustained reentry.

Figure 5 shows patterns of ventricular activation during spontaneously occurring tachycardia and fibrillation, some 5 minutes after occlusion of the left anterior descending coronary artery in an isolated, Langendorff-perfused pig heart. The upper right panel shows the configuration of the multielectrode

with which 64 electrograms were simultaneously recorded.[21] Panel A depicts the activation sequence of a spontaneous premature ventricular beat that triggered a run of ventricular tachycardia that degenerated into ventricular fibrillation. Earliest ectopic activity occurred on the nonischemic side of the border (indicated by dotted line in upper right panel), and no activity bridging the latest activated site during the preceding sinus beat and earliest activated ectopic site could be detected. The premature wave front was blocked in the central ischemic zone (shaded area in panel A) and propagated slowly around this zone of block. The two semicircular wave fronts merged after 120 msec, retrogradely invaded the zone of unidirectional block to reexcite the tissue proximal to the block at 140 msec (panel B). Again, two semicircular wave fronts were set up, one of which was blocked after 240 msec, the other continuing until 300 msec. Because at this point the recording ended, it is not certain how this arrhythmia continued. Several seconds later, the activation sequence depicted in the lower panels X, Y, and Z was recorded. Instead of a figure-of-eight–type of reentrant circuit, the pattern of excitation now had the characteristics of multiple wavelet reentry, where at any time window several independent wavelets are present. These wavelets can extinguish because of collision or because they meet refractory tissue. They can merge with other wavelets and reexcite tissue that previously had been excited by another wavelet. Only rarely is a reentrant circuit completed; an example is the wave in the upper part of panels X, Y, and Z, which follows a pretzel-like route.

In our initial studies, the accuracy of the reconstruction of activation patterns during spontaneous arrhythmias was hampered by the fact that simultaneous recordings could only be made from 64 sites. Later experiments, using 128 simultaneous recordings confirmed our early results and also provided evidence for intramural reentry. Pogwizd and Corr[22] recorded simultaneously from 232 intramural sites in the cat heart. They found that about 75% of all ventricular premature beats occurred through intramural reentry where a sinus beat was delayed in mid-mural and subendocardial areas, giving rise to reexcitation in the subendocardium. In the other 25%, premature beats or the first beats of ventricular tachycardia were caused by a nonreentrant mechanism. This observation was in agreement with our findings.[21,23] We proposed that injury current flowing between ischemic and nonischemic myocardium could initiate premature beats, either by directly stimulating the nonischemic myocardium at the end of the refractory period, or by enhancing automaticity in the Purkinje system.[21,23]

The Injury Current as a Trigger for Reentrant Arrhythmias

In 1950, Harris[24] suggested that "the injury potential can be regarded as a probable contributing factor in ectopic excitation after coronary occlusion." Later, he wrote: "excitation of cells situated within the boundary of a local region of ischemia, with thresholds reduced by elevated local potassium concentration, has been postulated to be induced by 'injury' current that results from the potassium gradient across the boundary."[25] Harris was correct in many, but not in all aspects. Recent studies have demonstrated that at the boundary, both ischemic areas (with mildly elevated extracellular K^+ concentrations) and nonischemic areas (with an unchanged extracellular K^+ concentration) have reduced diastolic thresholds for excitation.[26] However, the diastolic injury current is not strong enough to excite cells at the boundary, it merely reduces stimulation threshold. Ectopic premature excitation by injury current may, however, arise in a different way.

In diastole, the potential difference between the intracellular compartments of ischemic cells (about -70 mV) and that of normal cells (-90 mV) is such that an intracellular current flows from ischemic to normal cells, tending to depolarize the latter. By diminishing the potential difference between actual membrane potential and threshold potential, diastolic excitability is increased in normal cells adjacent to the border. When activation of ischemic cells is delayed, and ischemic cells are still depolarized at the time normal cells have already repolarized, the potential difference between ischemic and normal cells is in the same direction as during diastole, but its magnitude is 5 to 10 times greater. Figure 6 depicts in a schematic fashion the flow of injury current at that particular moment of the cardiac cycle. In the diagram, ischemic cells that are activated with considerable delay are separated from normal cells by a group of ischemic cells that are inexcitable. At the moment indicated by the dotted line,

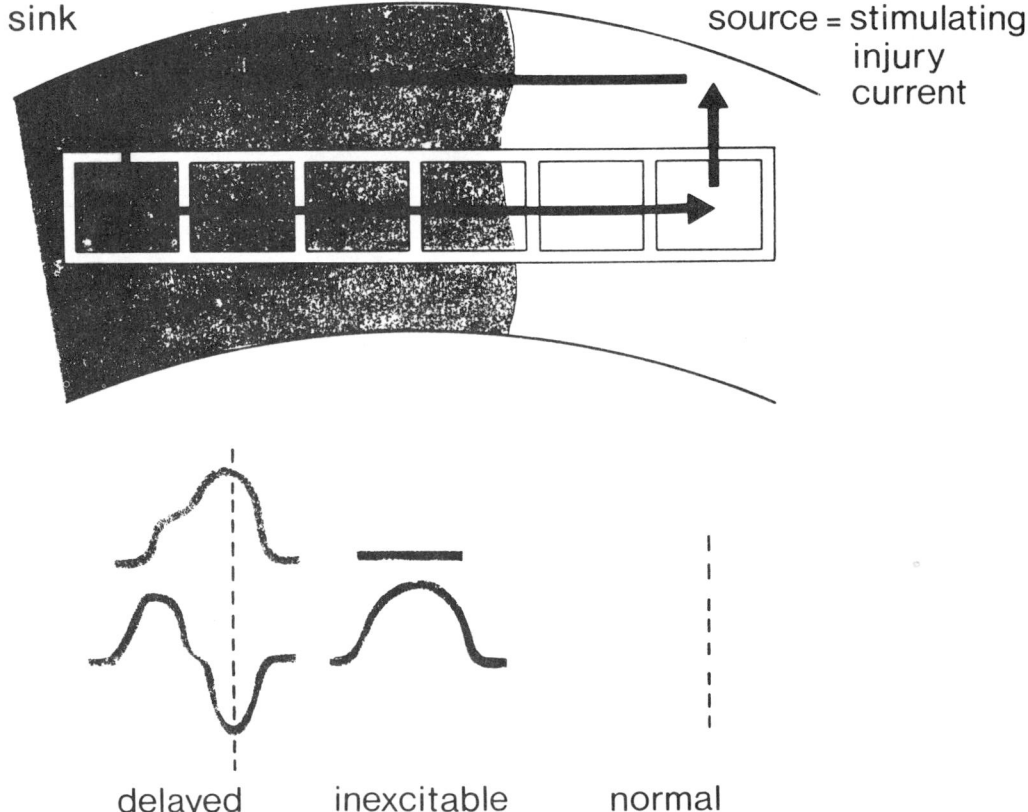

Figure 6. Schematic representation of flow of injury current across the ischemic border during that part of the cardiac cycle indicated in the schematic recordings in the lower part by a dotted line. The recordings are transmembrane potentials (upper tracings) and extracellular electrograms (lower tracings) from ischemic sites activated with delay, ischemic sites that are inexcitable, and from nonischemic tissue close to the border. Note that the local current circuit produces current "sources" in the normal tissue, which exert a depolarizing effect on that tissue.

the injury current flowing across the ischemic border via the inexcitable cells, which act as a purely passive resistor, depolarizes the normal cells just after they have repolarized. This current may indeed be strong enough to bring these cells to threshold.[21,23]

References

1. Meissner M, Akhtar M, Lehmann MH: Nonischemic sudden tachyarrhythmic death in atherosclerotic heart disease. *Circulation* 84:905, 1991.
2. Davies MJ, Bland JM, Hangartner JRW, et al: Factors influencing the presence or absence of acute coronary artery thrombi in sudden ischemic death. *Eur Heart J* 10:203, 1989.
3. Goldstein S, Landis JR, Leighton R, et al: Characteristics of the resuscitated out-of-hospital cardiac arrest victim with coronary heart disease. *Circulation* 64:977, 1981.
4. Myerburg RJ, Conde CA, Sung HJ, et al: Clinical, electrophysiological and hemodynamic profile of patients resuscitated from prehospital cardiac arrest. *Am J Med* 68:568, 1980.
5. Trolese-Mongheal Y, Duchenne-Marulluz P, Trolese JF, et al: Sudden death and experimental acute myocardial infarction. *Am J Cardiol* 56:677, 1985.
6. Janse MJ, Wit AL: Electrophysiological mecha-

nisms of ventricular arrhythmias resulting from myocardial ischemia and infarction. *Physiol Rev* 69:1049, 1989.

7. Downar E, Janse MJ, Durrer D: The effect of acute coronary artery occlusion on subepicardial transmembrane potentials in the intact porcine heart. *Circulation* 56:217, 1977.

8. Kléber AG, Janse MJ, Downar E, et al: Die Veränderung der TQ und ST/T-Segmente in Elektrokardiogramm und deren Beziehung zu den ventrikulären Rhythmusstörungen während der akuten transmuralen Ischämie. *Schweiz Med Wsch* 107:1700, 1978.

9. Kléber AG: Resting membrane potential, extracellular potassium activity, and intracellular sodium activity during acute global ischemia in isolated perfused guinea pig heart. *Circ Res* 52: 442, 1983.

10. Weiss J, Shine KI: K^+ accumulation and electrophysiological alterations during early myocardial ischemia. *Am J Physiol* 243:H318, 1982.

11. Janse MJ, Kléber AG: Electrophysiological changes and ventricular arrhythmias in the early phase of regional myocardial ischemia. *Circ Res* 49:1069, 1981.

12. Moréna H, Janse MJ, Fiolet JWT, et al: Comparison of the effects of regional ischemia, hypoxia, hyperkalemia and acidosis on intracellular and extracellular potentials and metabolism in the isolated porcine heart. *Circ Res* 46:634, 1980.

13. Kodama I, Wilde AAM, Janse MJ, et al: Combined effects of hypoxia, hyperkalemia and acidosis on membrane action potential and recovery of excitability of guinea pig ventricular muscle. *J Mol Cell Cardiol* 16:246, 1984.

14. Coronel R, Fiolet JWT, Wilms-Schopman FJG, et al: Distribution of extracellular potassium and its relation to electrophysiologic changes during acute myocardial ischemia in the isolated perfused porcine heart. *Circulation* 77: 1125, 1988.

15. Hill JL, Gettes LS: Effect of acute coronary artery occlusion on local myocardial extracellular K^+ activity in swine. *Circulation* 61:768, 1980.

16. Kjekshus JK: Importance of heart rate in determining beta-blocker efficacy in acute and long-term acute myocardial infarction intervention trials. *Am J Cardiol* 57:43F, 1986.

17. Kléber AG, Janse MJ, Wilms-Schopman FJG, et al: Changes in conduction velocity during acute ischemia in ventricular myocardium in the isolated porcine heart. *Circulation* 73:189, 1986.

18. Kléber AG, Riegger CB, Janse MJ: Electrical uncoupling and increase of extracellular resistance after induction of ischemia in isolated, arterially perfused rabbit papillary muscle. *Circ Res* 61:271, 1987.

19. Kaplinsky E, Ogawa S, Balke CW, et al: Two periods of early ventricular arrhythmias in the canine acute infarction model. *Circulation* 60: 397, 1979.

20. Penny WJ: The deleterious effects of myocardial catecholamines on cellular electrophysiology and arrhythmias during ischemia and reperfusion. *Eur Heart J* 5:960, 1984.

21. Janse MJ, van Capelle FJL, Morsink H, et al: Flow of "injury" current and patterns of excitation during early ventricular arrhythmias in acute regional myocardial ischemia in isolated porcine and canine hearts: evidence for two different arrhythmogenic mechanisms. *Circ Res* 47: 151, 1980.

22. Pogwizd S, Corr PB: Reentrant and nonreentrant mechanisms contribute to arrhythmogenesis during early myocardial ischemia: results using three-dimensional mapping. *Circ Res* 61: 352, 1987.

23. Janse MJ, van Capelle FJL: Electrotonic interaction across an inexcitable region as a cause of ectopic activity in acute regional myocardial ischemia. A study in intact porcine and canine hearts and computer models. *Circ Res* 50:527, 1982.

24. Harris AS: Delayed development of ventricular ectopic rhythms following experimental coronary occlusion. *Circulation* 1:1318, 1950.

25. Harris AS, Otero H, Bocagte AJ: The induction of arrhythmias by sympathetic activity before and after occlusion of a coronary artery in the canine heart. *J Electrocardiol* 4:34, 1971.

26. Coronel R, Wilms-Schopman FJG, Opthof T, et al: Injury current and gradients of diastolic stimulation threshold, TQ potential, and extracellular potassium concentration during acute regional ischemia in the isolated perfused pig heart. *Circ Res* 68:1241, 1991.

Chapter 11

Autonomic Control of Cardiac Arrhythmias

Richard L. Verrier

The main goal of this chapter is to highlight new themes that have emerged in the study of neural control of cardiac rhythm. The first is that neural factors act not only directly through effects of neurotransmitters on the myocardium and its specialized conducting system, but also through influences on myocardial perfusion. These latter effects may result from changes in coronary vascular tone and/or enhanced platelet aggregability. This concept, which is illustrated in Figure 1, pervades the discussion and will not be presented separately. The second major area of progress is the application of computerized analysis of the T wave alternans to quantify the influence of neural activity on cardiac electrical stability. T wave alternans has been shown to exhibit a high degree of correlation with the ventricular fibrillation (VF) threshold and the occurrence of spontaneous VF under diverse autonomic interventions. Recently, the predictive value of T wave alternans has been demonstrated clinically using programmed cardiac electrical stimulation. The third motif is the role of behavioral factors in triggering ischemia and arrhythmias. This relationship has been exten-

sively documented and defined experimentally and clinically. Finally, some thoughts will be presented regarding the diagnostic and therapeutic potential of the field of neurocardiac investigation.

Tracking Neurally Induced Cardiac Vulnerability by Analysis of T Wave Alternans

Renewed interest in this clinically prevalent phenomenon[1-9] has been stimulated by several studies indicating that computerized analysis of T wave alternans may provide a quantitative, noninvasive means for assessing susceptibility to VF.[10-14] Adam and co-workers[10] and Smith and colleagues[11] demonstrated a statistically significant correlation between fluctuations in overall energy of the T wave and the VF threshold during coronary artery occlusion and hypothermia in dogs. Furthermore, it was shown in humans that there is a close relationship between the magnitude of T wave alternans and the inducibility

Supported by Grant HL-33567 from the National Heart, Lung, and Blood Institute of the National Institutes of Health, Bethesda, Maryland.

From BN Singh, HJJ Wellens, M Hiraoka, (eds): *Electropharmacological Control of Cardiac Arrhythmias*. Mount Kisco, NY, Futura Publishing Company Inc., © 1994.

135

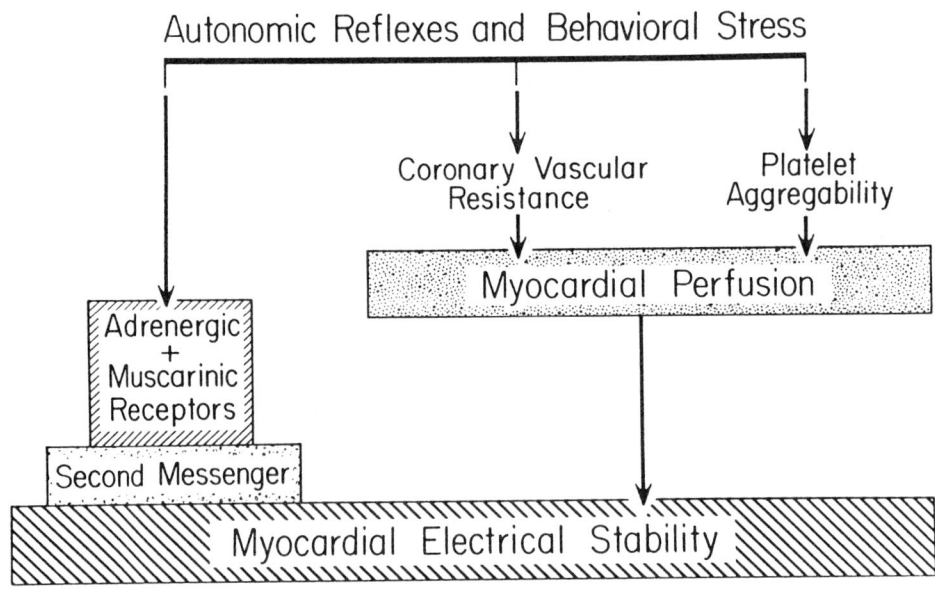

Figure 1. Summary of the mechanisms mediating the effects of the autonomic nervous system on ventricular electrical stability. (Reproduced with permission from Reference 86.)

of arrhythmias using programmed electrical stimulation.[11,14]

Recently, we applied the analytical technique of complex demodulation of the T wave to track cardiac vulnerability dynamically during both myocardial ischemia and reperfusion.[12] This method was selected because of its relative insensitivity to changes in stationarity of the data and because it provides a rapid estimate of physiological events with a time course as brief as 30 seconds.[13] The experiments were carried out in chloralose-anesthetized dogs during fixed-rate atrial pacing at 150 beats per minute. The ECG was recorded from a catheter positioned in the apex of the left ventricle.

Left anterior descending (LAD) coronary artery occlusion and reperfusion resulted in marked increases in the magnitude of beat-to-beat alternation in T wave amplitude (Figure 2). The increase in alternans was manifest within 2 to 3 minutes of occlusion and progressed until the occlusion was abruptly terminated at 8 minutes (Figure 3). Upon release of the occlusion, there was a rapid increase

in alternans that lasted less than 1 minute. A remarkable feature of the alternans pattern was that during reperfusion, the T waves alternated bidirectionally, with waveforms above and below the isoelectric line. It is especially significant that the time course of appearance and disappearance of T wave alternans during the occlusion/release sequence corresponded precisely with the spontaneous emergence of malignant tachyarrhythmias including VF.[15] The observation that the alternation pattern during occlusion and reperfusion differ is consistent with the well-established concept that differing mechanisms are responsible for ischemia versus reperfusion-induced arrhythmias.[16,17]

Measuring Sympathetic Nervous System Influences by T Wave Alternans Analysis

Our studies also demonstrated that the influence of the sympathetic nervous system

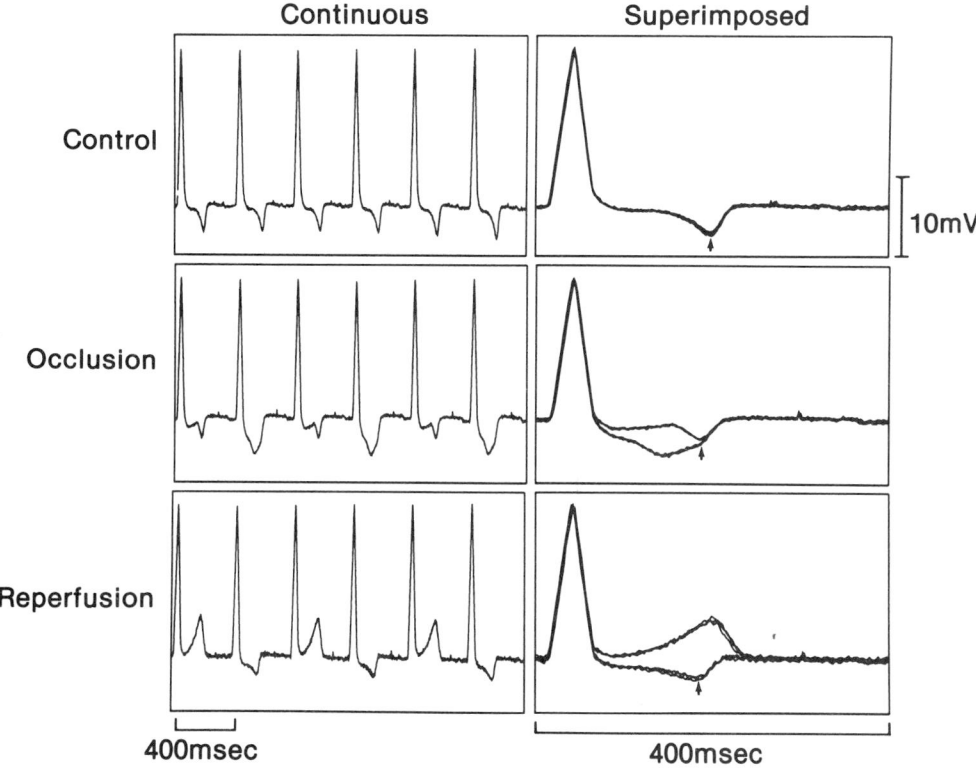

Figure 2. Electrocardiogram recorded within the left ventricle before, during, and after coronary artery occlusion in a single representative animal. Right panels show superimposition of six successive beats. Prior to occlusion (top tracing), the T waves of each succeeding beat are uniform (arrow designates apex of T wave). After 4 minutes of coronary artery occlusion (middle tracing), there is marked alternation of the first half of the T wave, coinciding with the vulnerable period of the cardiac cycle. The second half of the T wave remains uniform. After release of the occlusion (bottom tracing), alternans is bidirectional, with T waves alternately inscribed above and below the isoelectric line. (Reproduced with permission from Reference 12.)

on vulnerability in the normal and ischemic heart can be detected with precision. It was found that stellectomy reduced alternans during occlusion but enhanced its magnitude during reperfusion (Figure 4).[4,18] This effect is consistent with the fact that extra-adrenergic factors appear to be decisive during this phase of vulnerability.[16,19,20]

During stellate ganglion stimulation, there was a moderate increase in T wave alternans before occlusion and a major effect during acute ischemia. These findings are likewise consistent with a number of published reports indicating that sympathetic activation is highly arrhythmogenic during coronary artery occlusion.[4,16,18] Moreover, our recent data indicate that β-receptor activation appears to be the key factor in sympathetically induced T wave alternans. Eventually T wave alternans detection could prove useful in the context of the long QT syndrome, wherein major changes in alternans level can be elicited by diverse adrenergic stimuli such as fear and exercise, and abolished by anti-adrenergic interventions such as β blockade and stellectomy.[4,5]

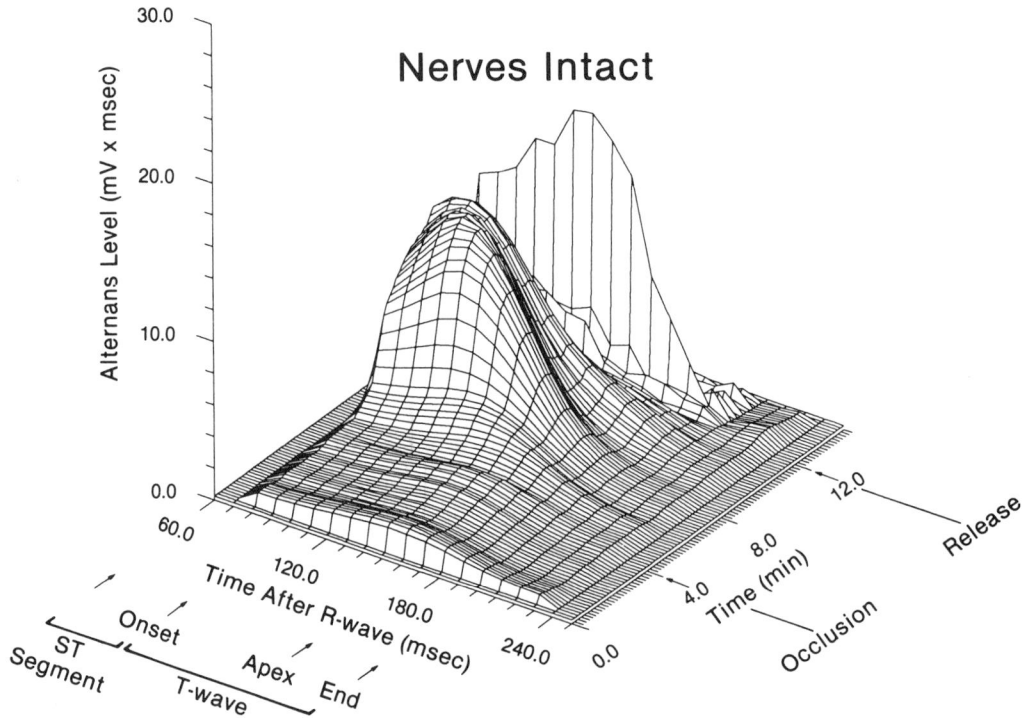

Figure 3. Surface plot display derived by complex demodulation of the T wave of the electro-cardiogram before, during, and after coronary artery occlusion in eight dogs with intact cardiac innervation. (Reproduced with permission from Reference 12.)

Quantifying Parasympathetic Nervous System Influences by T Wave Alternans Analysis

Vagus nerve stimulation has also been shown to exert a significant effect on T wave alternans in the occlusion-release model.[21] Specifically, we found that the surge in T wave alternans that occurs during acute LAD coronary artery occlusion can be markedly suppressed by electrical stimulation of the left vagus nerve. However, vagus nerve excitation was ineffectual in preventing alternans during reperfusion. These findings concur with reports from several laboratories indicating an important antifibrillatory effect of vagus nerve stimulation during acute myocardial ischemia.[22–26] Vagus nerve activation was not effective against reperfusion arrhythmias

when heart rate was kept constant, as in our study.

The likely basis for these differing effects of vagal activity on alternans during occlusion and reperfusion is that the antifibrillatory influence of this pathway is dependent on accentuated antagonism of adrenergic activity (Table 1). Thus, during coronary occlusion, the profibrillatory surge in sympathetic discharge to the heart is opposed by presynaptic inhibition of the release of catecholamines and by an opposition at the receptor level due to muscarinic stimulation.[27,28] Cyclic nucleotides appear to be responsible for the adrenergic/muscarinic receptor interaction.[27] The failure of vagal stimulation to protect during reperfusion is probably due to the fact that release of ischemic byproducts rather than adrenergic factors appears to play a critical role in reperfusion-induced arrhythmogenesis.[15,24]

An observation from the clinical literature suggests that vagal activation may suppress T wave alternans and consequently reduce susceptibility to ventricular tachyarrhythmias. Navarro-Lopez et al.[29] reported the case of a 60-year-old woman with acute gastroenteritis who experienced recurring ventricular tachyarrhythmias. During bilateral carotid sinus massage, she exhibited momentary interruption of chronic T wave alternans. Since this maneuver is known to elicit profound vagotonia, these observations provide an enticing suggestion of a correspondence between animal and human studies.

Electrophysiological Basis for T Wave Alternans

It is likely that multiple mechanisms underlie T wave alternans.[30-32] Therefore, the electrophysiological basis can only be identified in the context of the specific physiological and pathophysiological conditions under which alternans arises. For example, there appears to be strong evidence that T wave alternans during pericardial tamponade is due to a mechano-electrical interaction attributable to the swinging action of the heart in the chest.[8] However, in the context of myocardial ischemia and concomitant changes in autonomic tone, the factors are probably far more complex. While it is not possible to discuss all of these mechanisms in detail, we would like to highlight a few concepts that have recurred in the literature.

The first possibility is that alternans represents increased dispersion of repolarization. In their initial article on the subject, Smith and Cohen[33] proposed that alternation may be due to summation of electrical activity

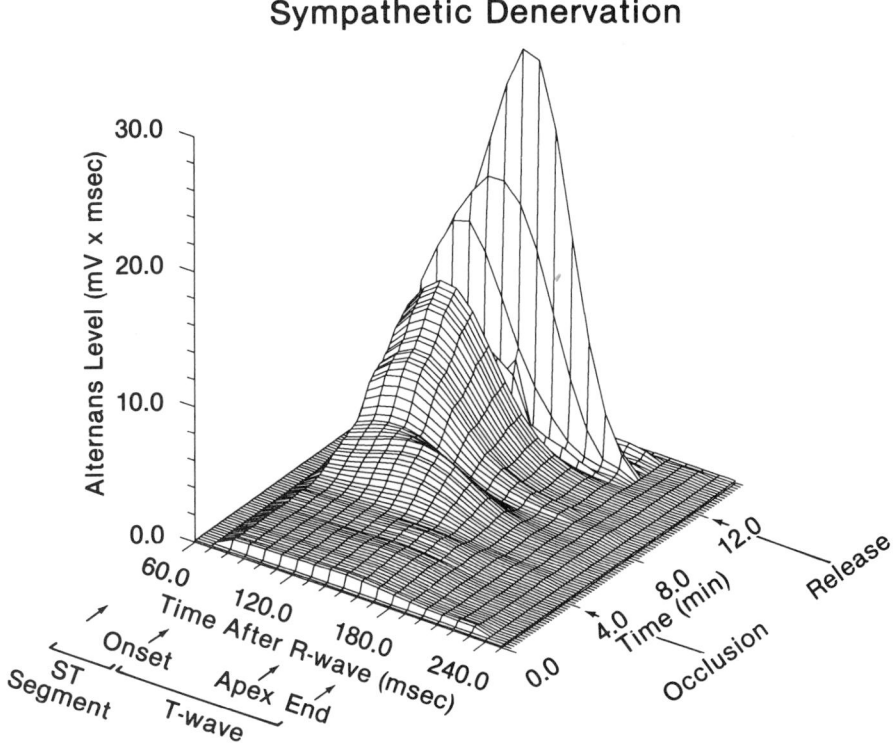

Sympathetic Denervation

Figure 4. Surface plot display derived by complex demodulation of the T wave of the electrocardiogram before, during, and after coronary artery occlusion following bilateral stellectomy in six dogs. (Reproduced with permission from Reference 12.)

Table 1
Sympathetic-Parasympathetic Interactions
and Myocardial Electrical Stability

Vagal tone increases myocardial electrical stability and protects against ventricular fibrillation during myocardial ischemia.

Vagally induced reduction in heart rate plays an important role during both myocardial ischemia and reperfusion because it increases diastolic perfusion time and reduces cardiac metabolic demand.

Enhanced vagal activity has an additional antifibrillatory effect due to antagonism of adrenergic influences.

The bases for sympathetic-parasympathetic interactions are:
- Inhibition of norepinephrine release from nerve endings
- Attenuation of response to catecholamines at receptor sites

Beneficial effects of vagal activity may be vitiated if profound bradycardia and hypotension ensue.

Myocardial infarction may alter autonomic influences by damaging neural fibers.

Adapted from Reference 87.

of subpopulations of myocardial cells that generate action potentials only on alternate beats. Our results also point to an important link between dispersion of repolarization and alternans, as there is a close temporal correspondence between these two electrophysiological entities.[34]

Another recurring theme is that alternans is due to alternation in action potential morphology of individual cells.[35] Consistent with this suggestion are the observations in a number of laboratories of alternating patterns of action potential morphology.[35–38] Antzelevitch and colleagues[36] have suggested that alternation in the appearance and disappearance of the dome portion of the epicardial action potential, which occurs during simulated ischemia in isolated tissues, may account for such alternating T wave patterns.[36] The activation map studies of Carson and co-workers[37] provide cogent evidence that a change in activation sequence is not the basis for T wave alternation phenomenon during myocardial ischemia.

Priori and co-workers[39] have provided evidence that early afterdepolarizations (EADs) may conduct 2:1 upon reperfusion and that this alternating pattern may be responsible for oscillation in T wave magnitude. This notion is further supported by the work of El-Sherif and co-workers,[40] who have reported summation of repolarization activity due to EADs in animals treated with the inotropic agent anthopleurin A.

Studies by Hashimoto and colleagues[41,42] and ourselves[43] have demonstrated that ionized calcium may represent a final common pathway for ischemia- and reperfusion-induced T wave alternans. Specifically, it has been shown that calcium channel blockade with either verapamil or diltiazem is capable of preventing alternans during coronary artery occlusion and release reperfusion. Electrical alternans can be suppressed by this means without concomitant prevention of mechanical alternans. The precise electrophysiological basis whereby ionized calcium can provoke alternans remains to be determined, along with the intracellular compartment from which alternans is elicited.[44]

Finally, the alternation pattern itself provides a compelling suggestion that this behavior represents a prechaotic state, because bifurcative behavior is the hallmark of chaos. Recent studies by Chialvo and others indicate that myocardial cells can exhibit chaotic dynamics.[45–48] To establish with certainty that T wave alternans represents prechaotic behavior requires demonstration of multupling just in advance of fibrillation. Although Ritzenberg and colleagues[49] observed T wave multupling during infusion of high concentrations of norepinephrine, the progression to lethal arrhythmia remains to be demonstrated. Definitive proof may be elusive because higher order bifurcations represent extremely unstable, transitory states.

Behavioral Studies of Neurocardiac Interactions

The diversity of neural patterning that attends changes in behavioral state has provided a rich source of insights into our understanding of neural control of heart rhythm. Among the most clinically relevant states to be studied have been anger, fear, and sleep. Experimental models of these states have provided a unique opportunity to study clinically prevalent, but poorly understood pathophysiological phenomena such as poststress arrhythmogenesis and nocturnal angina. In this chapter we focus on two extremes of the behavioral spectrum, namely, anger and sleep.

Anger

Effects on Cardiac Electrical Stability

This state can be elicited in experimental animals using a relatively simple paradigm that involves placing a dish of food in front of a leashed, instrumented dog. When a second leashed dog was allowed to consume the food, the instrumented animal exhibited an intense, anger-like state, as evidenced by growling and baring its teeth. The behavioral response was accompanied by sinus tachycardia, hypertension, and marked elevation in plasma catecholamines. There was a marked decrease in the repetitive extrasystole threshold, indicating enhanced cardiac electrical instability, even in the normal heart.[50,51] It is reasonable to assume, although it has not yet been established, that in the damaged myocardium, major arrhythmias would be precipitated.

Poststress Ischemia and Arrhythmias

Using the anger model, we made a serendipitous observation regarding the effects of the poststress state on myocardial perfusion.[50] Specifically, in dogs with coronary stenosis we observed a severe large vessel coronary constriction that developed within 2 to 3 minutes after cessation of anger. The vasoconstriction lasted well after heart rate and arterial blood pressure had returned to normal. In some animals the response was so intense as to obstruct flow in the affected vessel completely. The presence of myocardial ischemia was in-

dicated by significant regional ST segment changes in the territory supplied by the stenosed circumflex coronary artery (Figure 5). An additional consideration is that persistently elevated levels of myocardial catecholamines contributed to the repolarization abnormalities observed.

This phenomenon of poststress ischemia is closely akin to clinical experience in which myocardial perfusion deficits and repolarization abnormalities have been reported to occur within a few minutes after cessation of emotional arousal or exercise.[52,53] Particularly significant in terms of electrophysiology is the fact that postexercise stress ischemia in humans can result in T wave alternation (Figure 6).[6]

Mechanisms and Clinical Implications of Poststress Ischemia

Our working hypothesis is that delayed myocardial ischemia results from an interplay between adrenergic and hemodynamic factors and that this interaction is the likely basis for the delayed nature of the ischemic response. The following hypothesis is proposed to account for the available data.[50,54–56] During activation of the sympathetic nervous system, arterial blood pressure increases in response to either behavioral stress or direct excitation of the stellate ganglia, thereby opposing the vasoconstrictor influence of α-adrenergic receptor stimulation on vascular smooth muscle. The net result is that coronary vascular resistance remains unaltered. However, during the postexcitation phase, systemic pressure returns abruptly to the control level, thereby lessening distending pressure within the coronary vessel. We hypothesize that the dissipation of catecholamines is delayed and thus the active adrenergic vasoconstriction influence predominates over the passive distending force. The imbalance leads to a decrease in coronary diameter and to an increase in vascular resistance. This formulation is analogous to that proposed by Masuda and Levy[57] to account for a delayed recovery of

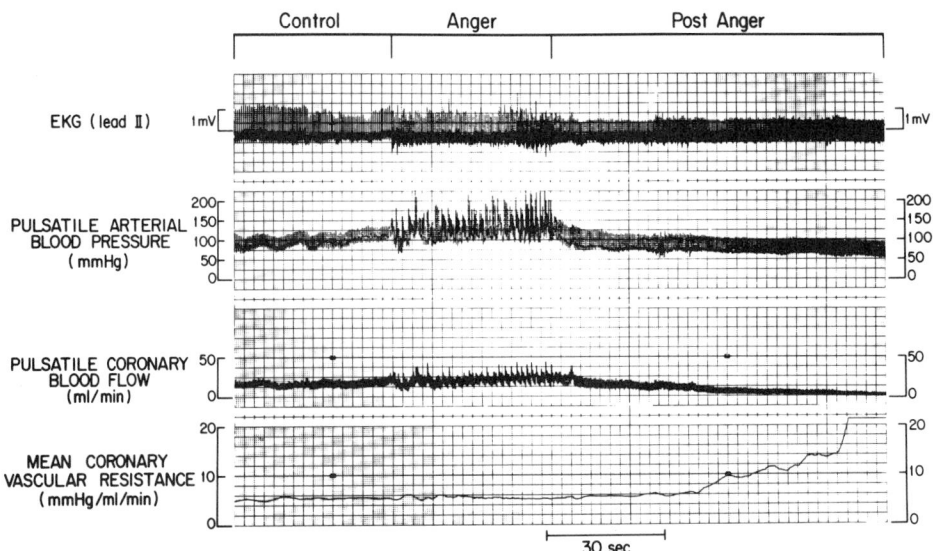

Figure 5. Recordings of effects on coronary hemodynamic function of inducing an anger-like state in a dog with coronary artery stenosis. During stress state, coronary arterial blood flow increased substantially and coronary vascular resistance decreased (left side). However, during poststress recovery phase (right side), a pronounced coronary vasoconstriction is evidenced by a decrease in coronary arterial blood flow and an increase in coronary vascular resistance. These changes occurred when heart rate and arterial blood pressure returned to prestress levels, suggesting primary coronary vasoconstriction. ECG: electrocardiogram. (Reproduced with permission from Reference 50.)

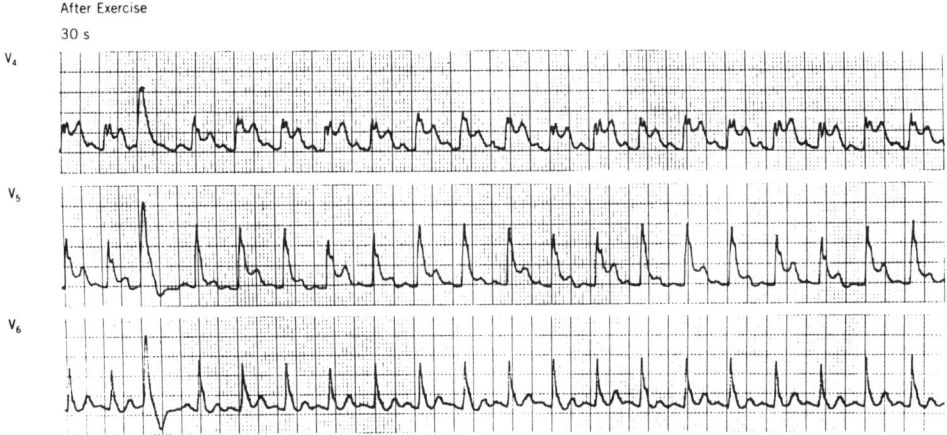

Figure 6. Immediate postexercise tracing, leads V_4 to V_6. ST segment elevation and ST-T alternans, best seen in lead V_5 became most prominent at 30 seconds after exercise, and isolated ventricular premature beats appeared (third complex from left). (Reproduced with permission from Reference 6.)

Table 2
Mechanisms Responsible for Delayed
Myocardial Ischemia

1. The ischemic state ensues 2 to 3 minutes following provocation of stress.
2. Delayed ischemia can be prevented by stellectomy and induced by sympathetic stimulation. The latter effect can be blocked by α_1-adrenergic blockade.
3. The interaction between coronary distending pressure and adrenergic factors appears to be responsible for the delayed nature of the response.
4. These findings carry important clinical implications as they may help to explain the occurrence of myocardial ischemia in hemorrhage and heart failure. Under such conditions, the neurally induced rise in intravascular pressure may not be adequate to offset the coronary vasoconstrictor influence.

Adapted from Reference 86.

heart rate and contractility following cessation of sympathetic nerve stimulation.

Our findings, summarized in Table 2, indicate that several characteristics of the poststress state are conducive to myocardial ischemia and arrhythmias. They include relatively elevated catecholamine levels and reduced coronary distending pressure in the face of lingering neurohumorally mediated vasoconstrictor drive. These factors may be responsible for the delayed onset of ischemia following cessation of exercise or intense emotional arousal. This hazardous coexistence of enhanced neurogenic activity and inadequate coronary distending pressure may also occur under conditions such as heart failure or hemorrhage. Schwartz et al.[58] have postulated that the markedly elevated sympathetic tone and concomitantly low coronary distending pressure may be responsible for the occurrence of coronary insufficiency and myocardial ischemia during hemorrhage.[59] It is clear that experimental modeling of these conditions and those associated with the poststress state could lead to important new insights into the pathophysiology of coronary artery disease.

Sleep

Impact of Sleep on Myocardial Perfusion and Arrhythmias

It is well established clinically that ischemic events occur during the nocturnal period.[60–63] These have been documented in patients with advanced coronary disease[60] and Prinzmetal's variant angina.[61] The available evidence suggests that the rapid eye movement (REM) phase of sleep is especially conducive to ST segment changes and perfusion abnormalities.[60,61] It has been estimated that 8% to 10% of ischemic attacks occur during sleep.[64,65] An important new clinical observation is the high incidence of ischemic events associated with arousal from sleep.[66] This phenomenon may be due in part to increased platelet aggregation that is exacerbated by assumption of the upright posture.[67,68] However, other factors regulating coronary vascular tone must be considered.[69–71]

Recent experimental studies have shed light on the fundamental mechanisms involved in sleep-induced changes in myocardial perfusion and arrhythmogenesis.[72–75] Namely, it has been shown that both REM and slow wave sleep significantly increase the effective refractory period of the ventricles.[76] This effect is independent of alterations in heart rate, as it occurs during fixed-rate pacing. The changes in the excitable properties of the heart are not influenced by bilateral stellectomy but are abolished by muscarinic blockade with atropine methylnitrate, indicating that the sleep-induced changes in cardiac excitability are largely mediated by increases in cardiac vagal tone. Furthermore, even low-intensity electrical scanning of the cardiac cycle induced VF during REM but not slow wave sleep.

Subsequent investigations reveal that there are periodic surges in sympathetic activity during REM sleep that could destabilize the heart electrophysiologically.[72,73] The experiments involved chronically instrumented dogs in which heart rate, arterial blood pressure, coronary arterial blood flow, and electroencephalographic data were recorded simultaneously. Coronary stenosis was set to reduce baseline flow by 60%. During REM sleep, there were transient increases in heart rate with concomitant reductions in coronary flow (Figure 7). Because the basic surge phenomenon is abolished by bilateral stellectomy, it is assumed that increased adrenergic discharge is responsible for the flow deficit. Our current studies indicate that the heart rate surges occur predominantly during those periods of REM sleep marked by intensely phasic activity.[74] It remains to be determined whether this is a direct effect of α-adrenergic stimulation and/or a decrease in diastolic perfusion time secondary to the accompanying sinus tachycardia. The link between REM sleep-induced changes in heart rate and coronary insufficiency appears to be consistent with clinical reports of patients with advanced ischemic heart disease. In particular, Nowlin and co-workers[60] found in patients with advanced coronary artery disease that attacks of nocturnal angina occurred predominantly (32 of 39 episodes in 4 patients) during REM sleep and were associated with heart rate acceleration (Figure 8).

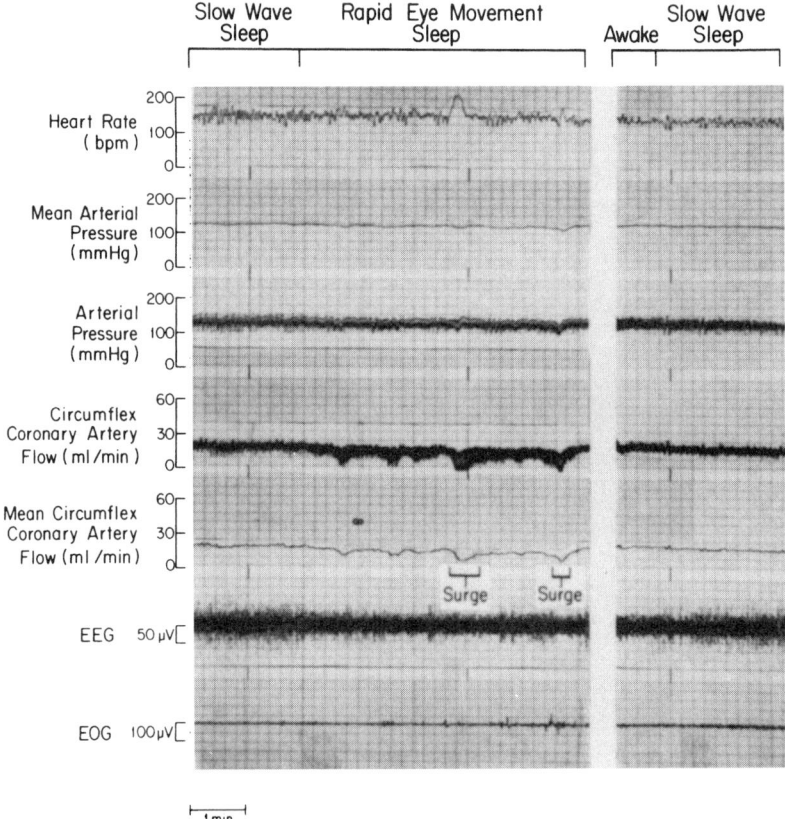

Figure 7. Recordings of effects of sleep stage on heart rate, mean and phasic arterial pressures, and mean and phasic circumflex coronary artery flows in a representative experiment during stenosis. Note phasic decreases in coronary flow occurring during heart rate surges while the dog is in rapid eye movement sleep. EEG: electroencephalogram; EOG: electrooculogram. (Reproduced with permission from Reference 73.)

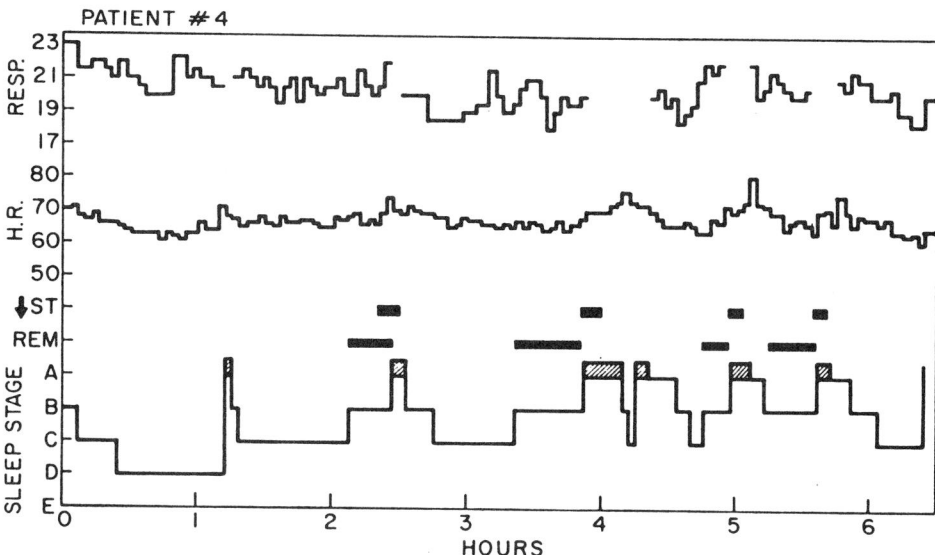

Figure 8. Composite graph of a night of sleep in a patient with nocturnal angina pectoris. Note association between rapid eye movement (REM)-related surges in heart rate and occurrence of ST segment changes. Resp: respirations; H.R: heart rate; ST: periods of significant ST segment depression on electrocardiogram. (Reproduced with permission from Reference 60.)

Heart Rhythm Pauses and Arrhythmogenesis During Sleep

We have recently observed in chronically instrumented dogs prolonged pauses in heart rhythm during transitions from slow wave sleep to periods marked by desynchronized electroencephalographic rhythms.[77,78] These pauses persist from 1 to 8 seconds and are followed by dramatic increases in coronary blood flow averaging 30% and ranging up to 84%. The postpause surges in coronary blood flow do not appear to be mediated by local metabolic factors since the heart rate-blood pressure product indicates no change in cardiac metabolic activity. An intense burst of vagal activity appears to produce the phenomenon, since the pauses develop against a background of marked respiratory sinus arrhythmia, varying degrees of heart block with nonconducted P waves, and low heart rate. Furthermore, the phenomenon, including the postpause surge in coronary flow, can be emulated by electrical stimulation of the vagus nerve.

These observations carry important implications for diagnosing and treating neurogenically induced ischemia and arrhythmias. Nocturnal asystolic events have been reported in both young adults[79] and individuals with obstructive sleep apnea.[80,81] Pauses in heart rhythm could set the stage for triggered activity, as abrupt changes in cycle length are conducive to early and late afterdepolarizations. An intriguing possibility is that in individuals who may be sensitized by proarrhythmic medications, sleep-induced pauses may initiate severe arrhythmias such as torsades de pointes.

Conclusions

For the past few years, the term neurocardiology has been bantered about.[82,83] Are we ready to regard this area of study as a bona fide discipline? If neurocardiology is to be identified as a distinct field, several criteria must be met. These include establishment of a sizeable, cohesive body of information, proven diagnostic utility, and therapeutic effi-

Table 3
Current Approaches for Containment of
Neural Triggers for Malignant Ventricular
Arrhythmias

Approach	Method
Central nervous system	Decreasing cardiac sympathetic tone
	Neurochemical agents[88-92]
	Increasing vagal tone
	Digitalis drugs[93]
	Opioid agents[94-96]
	Modification of baroreceptor sensitivity by exercise conditioning[84,97]
Peripheral nervous system	Adrenergic receptor blockade[98-101]
	Stellectomy[102-105]
	Calcium channel blockade[20,106-111]

cacy. We believe that the first criterion has been met and that potential for diagnostic utility has been demonstrated. This assertion is supported by increased interest in baroreceptor testing in the context of myocardial infarction and the use of power spectrum analysis of interbeat variability to evaluate neurocardiac interactions in diverse clinical conditions.[84,85] In the future, T wave alternans analysis may be used to determine the influence of neural activity on cardiac electrical stability. In terms of therapy, a substantial armamentarium of neurocardiac medications has been developed (Table 3). While we cannot yet answer definitively whether neurocardiology has arrived as a discipline, it is safe to say that the neurocardiac approach continues to hold great promise.

Acknowledgment

The author thanks Sandra S. Verrier for her editorial contributions.

References

1. Lewis T: Notes upon alternation of the heart. *Q J Med* 4:141, 1911.

2. Wellens HJJ: Isolated electrical alternans of the T wave. *Chest* 62:319, 1972.

3. Rozanski JJ, Kleinfeld M: Alternans of the ST segment and T wave. A sign of electrical instability in Prinzmetal's angina. *PACE* 5:359, 1982.

4. Schwartz PJ, Malliani A: Electrical alternation of the T wave: clinical and experimental evidence of its relationship with the sympathetic nervous system and with the long Q-T syndrome. *Am Heart J* 89:45, 1975.

5. Schwartz PJ: Idiopathic long QT syndrome: progress and questions. *Am Heart J* 109:399, 1985.

6. Belic N, Gardin JM: ECG manifestations of myocardial ischemia. *Arch Intern Med* 140:1162, 1980.

7. Raeder EA, Rosenbaum DS, Bhasin R, et al: Alternating morphology of the QRST complex preceding sudden death. *N Engl J Med* 326:271, 1992.

8. Goldberger AL, Shabetai R, Bhargava V, et al: Nonlinear dynamics, electrical alternans, and pericardial tamponade. *Am Heart J* 107:1297, 1984.

9. Joyal M, Feldman RL, Pepine CJ: ST-segment alternans during percutaneous transluminal coronary angioplasty. *Am J Cardiol* 54:915, 1984.

10. Adam DR, Smith JM, Akselrod S, et al: Fluctuations in T-wave morphology and susceptibility to ventricular fibrillation. *J Electrocardiol* 17:209, 1984.

11. Smith JM, Clancy EA, Valeri CR, et al: Electrical alternans and cardiac electrical instability. *Circulation* 77:110, 1988.

12. Nearing BD, Huang AH, Verrier RL: Dynamic tracking of cardiac vulnerability by complex demodulation of the T wave. *Science* 252:437, 1991.

13. Nearing BD, Verrier RL: Personal computer system for tracking cardiac vulnerability by complex demodulation of the T wave. *J Appl Physiol* 74:2606, 1993.

14. Rosenbaum DS, Jackson L, Leigh A, et al: Repolarization alternans: an electrocardiographic marker of arrhythmia vulnerability in man (abstract). *Circulation* 84:II-J, 1991.

15. Lown B, Verrier RL: Neural activity and ventricular fibrillation. *N Engl J Med* 294:1165, 1976.

16. Corr PB, Yamada KA, Witkowski FX: Mechanisms controlling cardiac autonomic function and their relation to arrhythmogenesis. In: HA Fozzard, et al (eds): *The Heart and Cardiovascular System*. New York: Raven Press, 1986, p. 1343.

17. Janse MJ: Electrical activity immediately following myocardial infarction. In: MR Rosen,

MJ Janse, AL Wit (eds): *Cardiac Electrophysiology: A Textbook*. Mt. Kisco, NY: Futura Publishing Company, Inc., 1990, p. 739.

18. Lombardi F, Verrier RL, Lown B: Relationship between sympathetic neural activity, coronary dynamics, and vulnerability to ventricular fibrillation during myocardial ischemia and reperfusion. *Am Heart J* 105:958, 1983.

19. Corbalan R, Verrier RL, Lown B: Differing mechanisms for ventricular vulnerability during coronary artery occlusion and release. *Am Heart J* 92:223, 1976.

20. Verrier RL, Hagestad EL: Mechanisms involved in reperfusion arrhythmias. *Eur Heart J* 7(Suppl A):13, 1986.

21. Nearing BD, Verrier RL: Evaluation of antifibrillatory interventions by complex demodulation of the T-wave (abstract). *Circulation* 84:II-499, 1991.

22. Kent KM, Smith ER, Redwood DR, et al: Electrical stability of acutely ischemic myocardium. Influences of heart rate and vagal stimulation. *Circulation* 47:291, 1973.

23. Kolman BS, Verrier RL, Lown B: The effect of vagus nerve stimulation upon vulnerability of the canine ventricle: role of sympathetic-parasympathetic interactions. *Circulation* 52:578, 1975.

24. Verrier RL: Neurogenic aspects of cardiac arrhythmias. In: N El-Sherif, P Samet (eds): *Cardiac Pacing and Electrophysiology*. Philadelphia: WB Saunders, 1991, p. 77.

25. Zuanetti G, De Ferrari GM, Priori SG, et al: Protective effect of vagal stimulation on reperfusion arrhythmias in cats. *Circ Res* 61:429, 1987.

26. Zipes DP, Miyazaki T: The autonomic nervous system and the heart: basis for understanding interactions and effects on arrhythmia development. In: DP Zipes, J Jalife (eds): *Cardiac Electrophysiology: From Cell to Bedside*. Philadelphia: WB Saunders, 1990, p. 312.

27. Levy MN, Warner MR: Autonomic interactions in cardiac control: role of neuropeptides. In: DP Zipes, J Jalife (eds): *Cardiac Electrophysiology: From Cell to Bedside*. Philadelphia: WB Saunders, 1990, p. 305.

28. Levy MN, Blattberg B: Effect of vagal stimulation on the overflow of norepinephrine into the coronary sinus during cardiac sympathetic nerve stimulation in the dog. *Circ Res* 38:81, 1976.

29. Navarro-Lopez F, Cinca J, Sanz G, et al: Isolated T wave alternans. *Am Heart J* 95:369, 1978.

30. Rosenbaum MB, Acunzo RS: Pseudo 2:1 atrioventricular block and T wave alternans in the long QT syndromes. *J Am Coll Cardiol* 18:1363, 1991.

31. Surawicz B: The pathogenesis and clinical significance of primary T wave abnormalities. In: RC Schlant, JW Hurst (eds): *Advances in Electrocardiography*. New York: Grune & Stratton, 1972, p. 377.

32. Sutton PM, Taggart P, Lab M, et al: Alternans of epicardial repolarization as a localized phenomenon in man. *Eur Heart J* 12:70, 1991.

33. Smith JM, Cohen RJ: Simple finite-element model accounts for wide range of ventricular dysrhythmias. *Proc Natl Acad Sci USA* 81:233, 1984.

34. Verrier RL, Nearing BD, Huang AH: Method for assessing dispersion of repolarization during acute myocardial ischemia without cardiac electrical testing (abstract). *Circulation* 82:III-450, 1990.

35. Kléber AG, Janse MJ, van Capelle FJL, et al: Mechanism and time course of ST and TQ segment changes during acute regional ischemia in the pig heart determined by extracellular and intracellular recordings. *Circ Res* 42:603, 1978.

36. Antzelevitch C, Sicouri S, Litovsky SH, et al: Heterogeneity within the ventricular wall: electrophysiology and pharmacology of epicardial, endocardial, and M cells. *Circ Res* 69:1427, 1991.

37. Carson DL, Cardinal R, Savard P, et al: Characterisation of unipolar waveform alternation in acutely ischaemic porcine myocardium. *Cardiovasc Res* 20:521, 1986.

38. Russell DC, Smith HJ, Oliver MF: Transmembrane potential changes and ventricular fibrillation during repetitive myocardial ischaemia in the dog. *Br Heart J* 42:88, 1979.

39. Priori SG, Mantica M, Napolitano C, et al: Early afterdepolarizations induced in vivo by reperfusion of ischemic myocardium: a possible mechanism for reperfusion arrhythmias. *Circulation* 81:1911, 1990.

40. El-Sherif N, Zeiler RH, Craelius W, et al: QTU prolongation and polymorphic ventricular tachyarrhythmias due to bradycardia-dependent early afterdepolarizations: afterdepolarizations and ventricular arrhythmias. *Circ Res* 63:286, 1988.

41. Hashimoto H, Suzuki K, Miyake S, et al: Effects of calcium antagonists on the electrical alternans of the ST segment and on associated mechanical alternans during acute coronary occlusion in dogs. *Circulation* 68:667, 1983.

42. Hashimoto H, Nakashima M: Evidence for a link between mechanical and electrical alternans in acutely ischaemic myocardium of anesthetized dogs. *Acta Physiol Scand* 141:63, 1991.

43. Nearing BD, Verrier RL: Diltiazem reduces T-

wave alternation and vulnerability to fibrillation during both coronary artery occlusion and reperfusion (abstract). *J Am Coll Cardiol* 19:346A, 1992.

44. Saitoh H, Bailey JC, Surawicz B: Action potential duration alternans in dog Purkinje and ventricular muscle fibers: further evidence in support of two different mechanisms. *Circulation* 80:1421, 1989.

45. Chialvo DR, Jalife J: Non-linear dynamics of cardiac excitation and impulse propagation. *Nature* 330:749, 1987.

46. Chialvo DR, Michaels DC, Jalife J: Supernormal excitability as a mechanism of chaotic dynamics of activation in cardiac Purkinje fibers. *Circ Res* 66:525, 1990.

47. Smith JM, Kaplan DT, Cohen RJ: The physics of reentry and fibrillation. In: DP Zipes, J Jalife (eds): *Cardiac Electrophysiology: From Cell to Bedside*. Philadelphia: WB Saunders, 1990, p. 215.

48. Guevara MR, Glass L, Shrier A: Phase locking, period doubling bifurcations, and irregular dynamics. *Science* 214:1350, 1981.

49. Ritzenberg A, Adam DR, Cohen RJ: Period multupling—evidence for nonlinear behaviour of the canine heart. *Nature* 307:159, 1984.

50. Verrier RL, Hagestad EL, Lown B: Delayed myocardial ischemia induced by anger. *Circulation* 75:249, 1987.

51. Verrier RL, Dickerson LW: Autonomic nervous system and coronary blood flow changes related to emotional activation and sleep. *Circulation* 83(suppl II):II-81, 1991.

52. McLaughlin PR, Doherty PW, Martin RP, et al: Myocardial imaging in a patient with reproducible variant angina. *Am J Cardiol* 39:126, 1977.

53. Lahiri A, Subramanian B, Millar-Craig M, et al: Exercise-induced ST-segment elevation in variant angina. *Am J Cardiol* 45:887, 1980.

54. Hagestad EL, Verrier RL: Delayed myocardial ischemia following the cessation of sympathetic stimulation. *Am Heart J* 115:45, 1988.

55. Verrier RL, Kirby DA, Papageorgiou P: Plasma catecholamines and anger-induced delayed myocardial ischemia (abstract). *Circulation* 78:II-555, 1988.

56. Papageorgiou P, Hagestad EL, Verrier RL: Coronary distending pressure and delayed myocardial ischemia. *Am Heart J* 116:59, 1988.

57. Masuda Y, Levy MN: Heart rate modulates the disposition of neurally released norepinephrine in cardiac tissues. *Circ Res* 57:19, 1985.

58. Schwartz JS, Carlyle PF, Cohen JN: Effect of coronary arterial pressure on coronary stenosis resistance. *Circulation* 61:70, 1980.

59. Master AM, Dack S, Horn H, et al: Acute coronary insufficiency due to acute hemorrhage: an analysis of one hundred and three cases. *Circulation* 1:1302, 1950.

60. Nowlin JB, Troyer WG Jr, Collins WS, et al: The association of nocturnal angina pectoris with dreaming. *Ann Intern Med* 63:1040, 1965.

61. King MJ, Zir LM, Kaltman AJ, et al: Variant angina associated with angiographically demonstrated coronary artery spasm and REM sleep. *Am J Med Sci* 265:419, 1973.

62. Murao S, Harumi K, Katayama S, et al: All-night polygraphic studies of nocturnal angina pectoris. *Jpn Heart J* 13:295, 1972.

63. Quyyumi AA, Wright CA, Mockus LJ, et al: Mechanisms of nocturnal angina pectoris: importance of increased myocardial oxygen demand in patients with severe coronary artery disease. *Lancet* 1:1207, 1984.

64. Barry J, Selwyn AP, Nabel EG, et al: Frequency of ST-segment depression produced by mental stress in stable angina pectoris from coronary artery disease. *Am J Cardiol* 61:989, 1988.

65. Campbell S, Barry J, Rebecca GS, et al: Active transient myocardial ischemia during daily life in asymptomatic patients with positive exercise tests and coronary artery disease. *Am J Cardiol* 57:1010, 1986.

66. Barry J, Campbell S, Yeung AC, et al: Waking and rising at night as a trigger of myocardial ischemia. *Am J Cardiol* 67:1067, 1991.

67. Muller JE, Stone PH, Turi ZG, et al: Circadian variation in the frequency of onset of acute myocardial infarction. *N Engl J Med* 313:1313, 1985.

68. Brezinski DA, Tofler GH, Muller JE, et al: Morning increase in platelet aggregability: association with assumption of the upright posture. *Circulation* 78:35, 1988.

69. Yasue H, Ogawa H, Okumura K: Coronary artery spasm in the genesis of myocardial ischemia. *Am J Cardiol* 63:29E, 1989.

70. Ludmer PL, Selwyn AP, Shook TL, et al: Paradoxical vasoconstriction induced by acetylcholine in atherosclerotic coronary arteries. *N Engl J Med* 315:1046, 1986.

71. Maseri A, L'Abbate A, Ballestra AM: Significance of spasm in the pathogenesis of ischemic heart disease. *Am J Cardiol* 44:788, 1979.

72. Kirby DA, Verrier RL: Differential effects of sleep stage on coronary hemodynamic function. *Am J Physiol* 256(Heart Circ Physiol 25): H1378, 1989.

73. Kirby DA, Verrier RL: Differential effects of sleep stage on coronary hemodynamic function during stenosis. *Physiol Behav* 45:1017, 1989.

74. Dickerson LW, Huang AH, Thurnher MM, et al: Relationship between coronary hemodynamic changes and the phasic events of rapid eye movement sleep in dogs *Sleep* (in press).

75. Verrier RL: Behavioral state and cardiac arrhythmias. In: R Lydic, JF Biebuyck (eds): *Clinical Physiology of Sleep*. Bethesda: American Physiological Society, 1988, p. 31.

76. Francis GC, Hagestad EL, Verrier RL: Influence of sleep stage on ventricular refractoriness (abstract). *Physiologist* 29:163, 1986.

77. Dickerson LW, Huang AH, Nearing BD, et al: Primary coronary vasodilation associated with pauses in heart rhythm during sleep. *Am J Physiol* 264:R186, 1993.

78. Dickerson LW, Verrier RL: Asystole linked to EEG desynchronization during sleep: is the initiating event of CNS or cardiovascular origin? (abstract) *Sleep Res* 20A:83, 1991.

79. Guilleminault CP, Pool P, Motta J, et al: Sinus arrest during REM sleep in young adults. *N Engl J Med* 311:1006, 1984.

80. Guilleminault C, Connolly SJ, Winkle RA: Cardiac arrhythmia and conduction disturbances during sleep in 400 patients with sleep apnea syndrome. *Am J Cardiol* 52:490, 1983.

81. Shaw TRD, Corrall RJM, Craib IA: Cardiac and respiratory standstill during sleep. *Br Heart J* 40:1055, 1978.

82. Natelson BH: Neurocardiology: an interdisciplinary area for the 80s. *Arch Neurol* 42:178, 1985.

83. Kulbertus HE, Franck G (eds): *Neurocardiology*. Mount Kisco, NY: Futura Publishing Company, Inc., 1988.

84. LaRovere MT, Specchia G, Mortara A, et al: Baroreflex sensitivity, clinical correlates and cardiovascular mortality among patients with a first myocardial infarction. A prospective study. *Circulation* 78:816, 1988.

85. Bigger JT, Fleiss JL, Steinman RC, et al: Frequency domain measures of heart period variability and mortality after myocardial infarction. *Circulation* 85:164, 1992.

86. Verrier RL: Central nervous system modulation of cardiac rhythm. In: MR Rosen, Y Palti (eds): *Lethal Arrhythmias Resulting from Myocardial Ischemia and Infarction*. Boston, MA: Kluwer Academic Publishers, 1988, p. 149.

87. Verrier RL: Autonomic substrates for arrhythmias. *Prog Cardiol* 1:65, 1988.

88. Falk RH, DeSilva RA, Lown B: Reduction in vulnerability to ventricular fibrillation by bromocriptine, a dopamine agonist. *Cardiovasc Res* 15:175, 1981.

89. Gillis RA: Neurotransmitters involved in the central nervous system control of cardiovascular function. In: OA Smith, RA Galosy, SM Weiss (eds): *Circulation, Neurobiology, and Behavior*. New York: Elsevier Science Publishing, 1982, p. 41.

90. Rabinowitz SH, Lown B: Central neurochemical factors related to serotonin metabolism and cardiac ventricular vulnerability for repetitive electrical activity. *Am J Cardiol* 41:516, 1978.

91. Wurtman RJ, Fernstrom JD: Control of brain neurotransmitter synthesis by precursor availability and nutritional state. *Biochem Pharmacol* 25:1691, 1976.

92. Verrier RL: Neurochemical approaches to the prevention of ventricular fibrillation. *Fed Proc* 45:2191, 1986.

93. Brooks WW, Verrier RL, Lown B: Digitalis drugs and vulnerability to ventricular fibrillation. *Eur J Pharmacol* 57:69, 1979.

94. Carr DB, Saini V, Verrier RL: Opioids and cardiovascular function: neuromodulation of ventricular ectopy. In: HE Kulbertus, G Franck (eds): *Neurocardiology*. Mt. Kisco, NY: Futura Publishing Company, Inc., 1987, p. 223.

95. Saini V, Carr DB, Hagestad EL, et al: Antifibrillatory action of the narcotic agonist fentanyl. *Am Heart J* 115:598, 1988.

96. Verrier RL, Carr DB: Stress-specific influences of opioids on cardiac electrical stability. *J Cardiovasc Electrophysiol* 2(Suppl):S124, 1991.

97. Billman GE, Schwartz PJ, Stone HL: The effects of daily exercise on susceptibility to sudden cardiac death. *Circulation* 69:1182, 1984.

98. Beta-Blocker Heart Attack Study Group: The beta-blocker heart attack trial. *JAMA* 246:2073, 1981.

99. Corr PB, Sharma AD: Alpha- versus beta-adrenergic influences on dysrhythmias induced by myocardial ischemia and reperfusion. In: A Zanchetti (ed): *Advances in Beta-Blocker Therapy II*. Amsterdam: Excerpta Medica, 1982, p. 163.

100. Hjalmarson A, Elmfeldt D, Herlizt J, et al: Effect on mortality of metoprolol in acute myocardial infarction. *Lancet* 2:823, 1981.

101. Norwegian Multicenter Study Group: The timolol-induced reduction in mortality and reinfarction in patients surviving acute myocardial infarction. *N Engl J Med* 304:801, 1981.

102. Schwartz PJ: The rationale and role of left stellectomy for the prevention of malignant arrhythmias. *Ann NY Acad Sci* 427:199, 1984.

103. Schwartz PJ, Motolese M, Pollavini G, et al: Prevention of sudden cardiac death after a first myocardial infarction by pharmacologic or surgical antiadrenergic interventions. *J Cardiovasc Electrophysiol* 3:2, 1992.

104. Schwartz PJ, Snebold NG, Brown AM: Effects of unilateral cardiac sympathetic denervation

on the ventricular fibrillation threshold. *Am J Cardiol* 37:1034, 1976.

105. Schwartz PJ, Stone HL, Brown AM: Effects of unilateral stellate ganglion blockade on the arrhythmias associated with coronary occlusion. *Am Heart J* 92:589, 1976.

106. Stone PH, Antman EM (eds): *Calcium Channel Blocking Agents in the Treatment of Cardiovascular Disorders.* Mt. Kisco, NY: Futura Publishing Company, Inc., 1983.

107. Singh BN for the Bepridil Collaborative Study Group: Comparative efficacy and safety of bepridil and diltiazem in chronic stable angina pectoris refractory to diltiazem. *Am J Cardiol* 68:306, 1991.

108. Schwartz PJ, Priori SG, Vanoli E, et al: Efficacy of diltiazem in two experimental feline models of sudden cardiac death. *J Am Coll Cardiol* 8:661, 1986.

109. Multicenter Diltiazem Postinfarction Trial Research Group: The effect of diltiazem on mortality and reinfarction after myocardial infarction. *N Engl J Med* 319:385, 1988.

110. Danish Study Group on Verapamil in Myocardial Infarction: Effect of verapamil on mortality and major events after acute myocardial infarction (The Danish verapamil infarction trial II—DAVIT II). *Am J Cardiol* 66:779, 1990.

111. Clusin WT, Bristow MR, Baim DS, et al: The effects of diltiazem and reduced serum ionized calcium on ischemic ventricular fibrillation in the dog. *Circ Res* 50:518, 1982.

Chapter 12

The Role of Slow Conduction in the Genesis of Ventricular Tachycardia After Myocardial Infarction

William G. Stevenson

After coronary thrombosis the infarcted myocardium is gradually replaced with fibrous scar tissue. In some patients, however, strands of ventricular myocytes survive within the scar, becoming encased in fibrous tissue.[1-3] This is the pathological substrate for reentrant ventricular tachycardia late after infarction. In many of these regions conduction velocity is slowed, ranging from 0.06 to 0.7 m/sec.[3] Microelectrode studies of these surviving myocytes have demonstrated that some have depressed excitability, and/or slow action potential upstrokes, which may lead to conduction slowing.[3-6] Many, however, have relatively normal action potentials. The cause of slow conduction in the latter case is not entirely clear, but there are several possible factors involved. Intracellular resistance may be increased possibly due to the increase in collagen surrounding the myocytes, slowing propagation.[7,8] Insulating bands of fibrous tissue may in some cases create a circuitous route for impulse propagation.[9] Thus, conduction velocity on the cellular level may be normal but at the multicellular, macroscopic level, the excitation wave front may take a prolonged time to traverse the abnormal area.

The geometry of the myocyte bundles in the scar may also play an important role. Propagation of an excitation wave front slows as a wave front moves from a narrow path to a larger mass of tissue due to impedance mismatch.[10] Theoretically, a winding path also slows the propagation of an excitation wave front due to the effects of tissue geometry on the curvature of the excitation wave front.[11] In addition, some surviving myocytes in areas of scar tissue have markedly prolonged action potential duration and recovery times such that seconds are required before another stimulus can again depolarize the cell. If these cells exist adjacent to more normal myocytes in narrow conduction paths they could theoretically slow conduction by serving as a current sink.[11] In summary, slow conduction in infarct scars may result from abnormal membrane properties of surviving myocytes, increased intracellular resistance, the geometrical arrangement of the surviving cells, or a combination of these factors.

From BN Singh, HJJ Wellens, M Hiraoka, (eds): *Electropharmacological Control of Cardiac Arrhythmias.* Mount Kisco, NY, Futura Publishing Company Inc., © 1994.

Slow Conduction
Facilitates Reentry

The conduction velocity and length of the reentry path determine the revolution time through a reentry circuit. Hence, the slower the conduction velocity in the circuit, the slower the tachycardia cycle length. The slower the tachycardia, the more time is available for each point in the reentry circuit to recover before arrival of the next tachycardia excitation wave front. Hence, slow conduction makes a reentry circuit more stable by allowing a greater "safety margin" for tissue to recover during each cycle through the circuit. At any point in the reentry circuit, the difference between the refractory period and the tachycardia cycle length creates an "excitable gap" in the circuit. Following recovery of the site, but before arrival of the next excitation wave

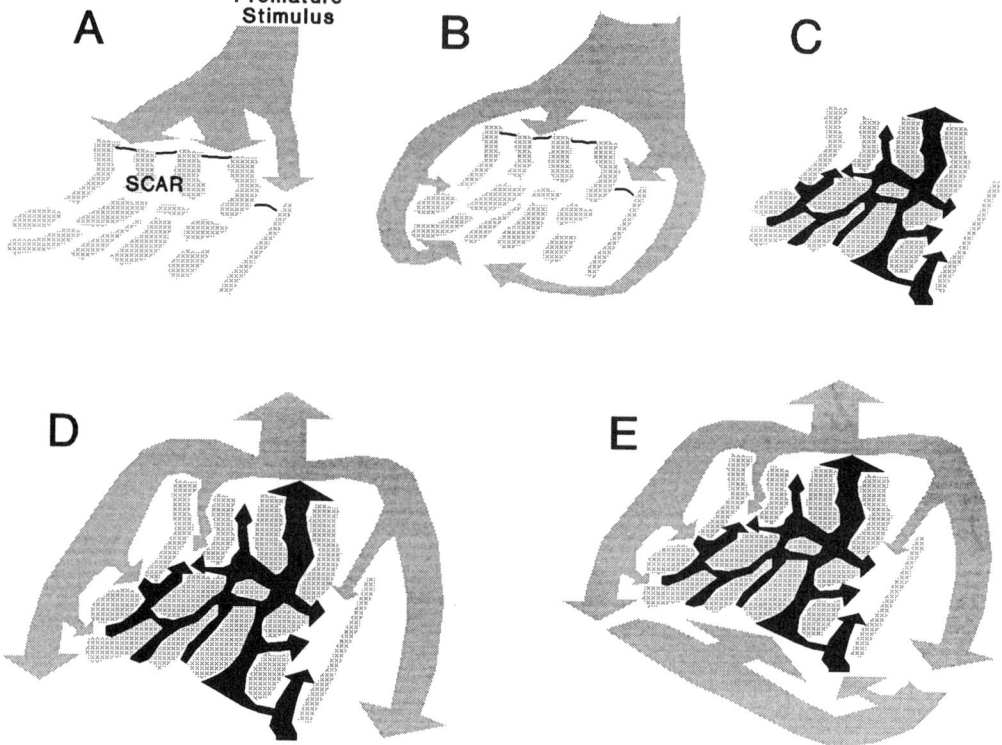

Figure 1. Initiation of reentrant ventricular tachycardia arising from a theoretical reentry circuit incorporating a region of scar is shown. The area of scar contains branching pathways for conduction surrounded by inexcitable fibrous tissue (hatched areas). Excitation wave fronts outside the scar are shown as gray arrows. Excitation waves propagating through the scar are shown as black arrows. In panel A a premature stimulus produces an excitation wave front (gray arrows) that propagates to the superior border of the scar. Tissue in this region has not yet recovered from the preceding depolarization and the premature wave front is blocked from entering the scar as indicated by the thin black lines. In panel B, the wave front propagates along the border of the scar until it encounters pathways into the scar that are able to allow wave front propagation, in the inferior and leftward regions of the scar. In panel C the excitation wave front propagates through the scar, toward the superior border of the scar. If the conduction time is sufficiently slow to allow recovery of the initial sites of block in the superior border of the scar, the excitation wave front emerges from the scar to reexcite the surrounding myocardium (panel D). Panel E shows the complete reentry circuit. Excitation wave fronts travel clockwise and counterclockwise around the margin of the scar and propagate slowly through the central region of the scar, giving the circuit figure-of-eight configuration.

front, a premature stimulus can depolarize the site. The existence of an excitable gap is the basis for entrainment and resetting of ventricular tachycardia by programmed stimulation that has been used to help elucidate mechanisms of ventricular tachycardia in humans. The slower conduction is in the circuit relative to the refractory period, the longer the excitable gap.

Slow conduction also facilitates initiation of reentry.[12] This is illustrated for formation of a theoretical reentry circuit (Figure 1). An excitation wave front propagates toward an area of scar tissue, and encounters tissue in the border of the scar that has not yet recovered excitability due to heterogeneous recovery properties of tissue in the scar (panel A). The excitation wave front propagates along the margin of the scar until it reaches an entrance to the scar where the tissue is excitable (panel B). The wave front then propagates through the scar toward the region at the superior margin of the scar where the excitation wave front had initially encountered refractory tissue (panel C). If conduction through the scar is rapid, the excitation wave front reaches the superior border of the scar before that region has recovered and the excitation wave front is extinguished. If conduction is sufficiently slow, allowing time for the tissue at the initial regions of conduction block to recover, the wave front will propagate

through this area, reentering the tissue outside the scar (panel D). In the example shown this produces a figure-of-eight–type of reentry circuit with propagation of two excitation wave fronts around regions of conduction block maintained by collision of the wave fronts propagating from the center of the scar toward its periphery with wave fronts propagating along the outer border of the scar. Although other configurations of reentry circuits occur, this configuration has been observed in animal models[8,13–16] and humans[9,17–20] and will subsequently be used to illustrate some of the features of reentry.

Detection of Slow Conduction in Human Infarct Scars

Fractionated Electrograms

Slow conduction in infarct scars is detectable in several ways. Slow conduction leads to asynchronous activation of adjacent myocyte bundles. Gardner et al.[21] demonstrated that depolarization of adjacent muscle bundles separated in time produces multiple rapid deflections giving the electrogram recorded at that site a fractionated appearance with multiple rapid components (Figure 2). During catheter mapping fractionated electrograms are

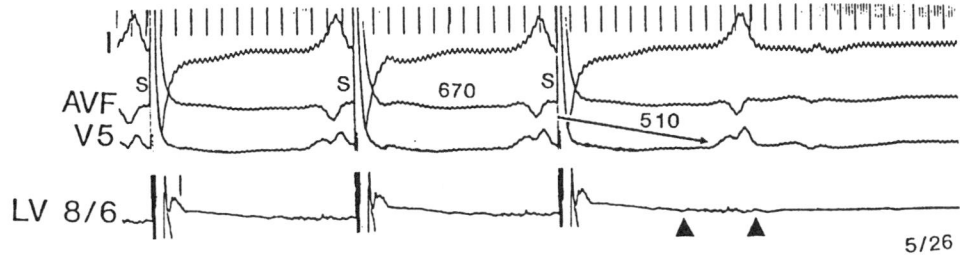

Figure 2. Pacing during sinus rhythm at a site in an inferior wall infarct scar in a patient with recurrent, slow ventricular tachycardia. From the top the time lines are in 50-msec increments, surface electrocardiogram leads I, aVF, and V_5, and an intracardiac recording (filtered at 30 to 500 Hz) from the left ventricular (LV) pacing site (LV 8/6). The LV electrogram (delineated by the two arrows for the last paced beat) is low amplitude, has a long duration, and is markedly fractionated. During pacing at a cycle length of 670 msec, the QRS complex follows the paced stimulus by 510 msec. This is consistent with markedly slow conduction from the pacing site in the ventricular scar to the border of the scar. All times are in milliseconds.

commonly recorded from areas in and around the infarct scar.[22-24] Further evidence that these electrograms are associated with slow conduction in humans comes from a study of pacing at these sites during catheter mapping.[25] During pacing at sites with normal electrograms, the duration from the stimulus to the paced QRS onset is less than 40 msec due to rapid propagation of the excitation wave front away from the pacing site. In contrast, at approximately half of the sites with fractionated electrograms, there is a discrete delay between the pacing stimulus and the QRS onset, consistent with slow conduction from the pacing site to the distant myocardium (Figure 2).

Fractionated electrograms are more common in patients with ventricular tachycardia after infarction than in those without ventricular tachycardia after infarction.[26] Surgical resection of areas from which fractionated electrograms are recorded is often associated with cure of ventricular tachycardia, supporting that they are associated with ventricular tachycardia circuits.[23]

The amplitude of signals generated from areas of slow conduction is not sufficient enough to be detected from the standard electrocardiogram recorded from the body surface. Signal averaging to reduce noise followed by amplification and filtering, however, allows detection of this high-frequency electrical activity when it extends beyond the end of the QRS complex.[27-30] These low-amplitude potentials are known as late potentials. Late potentials are associated with inducible and spontaneous ventricular tachycardia after myocardial infarction.[28-31] Dennis and co-workers[31] found sustained ventricular tachycardia was inducible in 41% of patients with late potentials present 7 to 28 days after myocardial infarction. In contrast, ventricular tachycardia was inducible in only 13% of patients who did not have late potentials on the signal-averaged electrocardiogram.

In summary, studies of sinus rhythm ventricular mapping and signal-averaged electrocardiograms have shown that fractionated, high-frequency ventricular electrical activity is associated with ventricular tachycardia late after myocardial infarction. There is strong evidence that this electrical activity is due to slow conduction through areas of scar.

Activation Mapping

Evidence supporting the direct participation of slow conduction areas in human ventricular reentry circuits comes from the intraoperative mapping studies of de Bakker,[3,17] Downar,[19,20] Littman and Svenson,[32,33] and Kaltenbrunner[34] and their co-workers. Intraoperative mapping frequently identifies regions of slow propagation in apparent reentry circuits. This has been further confirmed in studies of human hearts explanted at the time of cardiac transplantation by de Bakker and co-workers.[9] Conduction velocity can be as slow as 0.06 to 0.04 m/sec through areas of chronic infarction.[3,9]

These studies assess conduction velocity from measurement of activation times at multiple sites and interpolating activation times at intervening sites. In areas of scar the excitation waves may travel serpiginous routes and the wave fronts constructed from multipoint mapping are therefore subject to some error.[9,17,35,36] Nonetheless, there is strong evidence for the existence of regions of slow conduction in the reentry circuit.

Endocardial catheter activation mapping during ventricular tachycardia also suggests the presence of slow conduction areas.[37-46] During ventricular tachycardia, fractionated electrograms can frequently be recorded from areas in and around the scar (Figure 3). In some cases, the fractionated potentials recorded during tachycardia initiation, termination, and resetting or entrainment by pacing at a distance from the presumed tachycardia circuit showed a consistent relation to the tachycardia QRS complexes. The inability to dissociate the abnormal electrograms recorded from the tachycardia and the success of catheter ablation in abolishing tachycardia in a few cases suggested that the site was involved in the tachycardia circuit.[37,38,42-47]

Figure 3 shows tracings recorded during

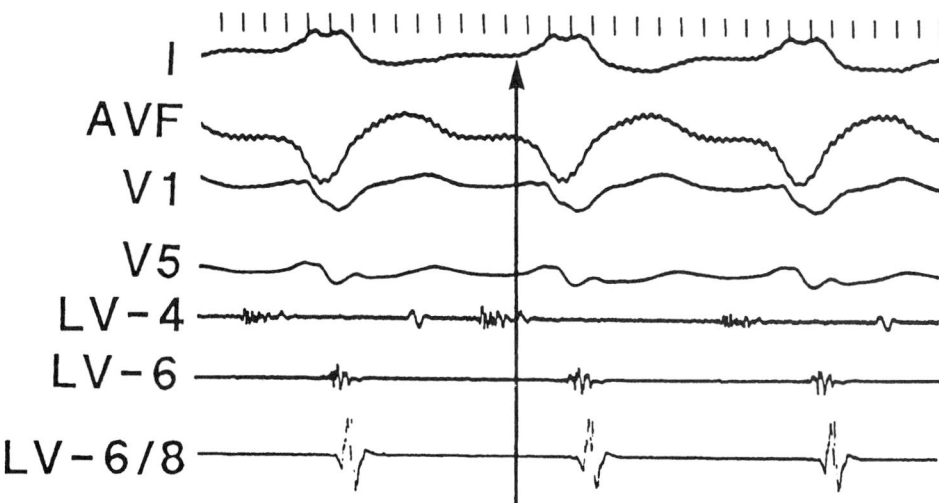

Figure 3. Tracings recorded during monomorphic ventricular tachycardia arising from an inferior wall infarct scar are shown. From the top the time lines are in 50-msec increments, surface electrocardiogram leads I, aVF, V_1, V_5, and bipolar, intracardiac recordings filtered at 30 to 500 Hz from three left ventricular sites (LV-4, LV-6, and LV-6/8). The QRS onset is indicated by the vertical arrow. During tachycardia, fractionated long duration electrograms are recorded from sites LV-4 and LV-6/8. Atrial activity is present in the LV-4 tracing, evident as slower potentials after the first and third beat. Programmed stimulation at sites LV-4 and LV-6 are shown in Figures 4 and 5.

catheter mapping of sustained monomorphic ventricular tachycardia in a patient with a previous inferior myocardial infarction. The electrograms recorded from sites LV-4 and LV-6 are fractionated, consistent with an area of slow conduction. In contrast the electrogram recorded from site LV-6/8 is narrower and lacks the multiple high-frequency components seen at the other two sites, suggesting that this is outside the area of slow conduction.

Programmed Stimulation During Ventricular Tachycardia

Further evidence of slow conduction in the reentry circuit comes from studies of programmed stimulation during mapping of ventricular tachycardia.[32,43,48–55] In reentry circuits, which give rise to ventricular tachycardia late after myocardial infarction, the tachycardia cycle length usually exceeds the time required for recovery of each site in the circuit, creating excitable gaps. A premature stimulus or excitation wave front that depolarizes a site in the circuit prior to arrival of the next tachycardia excitation wave front will propagate through the circuit, advancing or resetting the tachycardia. Entrainment is the continual resetting of a tachycardia by a train of stimuli in a manner that provides strong evidence for reentry.[54–57] This is illustrated schematically in Figures 4 and 5.

Figure 4 shows entrainment of the sustained ventricular tachycardia shown in Figure 3. The stimulation site (LV-6/8) is adjacent to the scar. The tachycardia cycle length is 570 msec. A stimulus train at a cycle length of 470 msec continually resets the tachycardia. Immediately following each stimulus, the QRS morphology is altered by the stimulated excitation wave front. These QRS complexes represent fusion of the stimulated wave front with the excitation wave fronts exiting the tachycardia circuit. Following the last stimulus the next QRS occurs at the pacing cycle length of 470 msec, but is not fused. The mechanism for

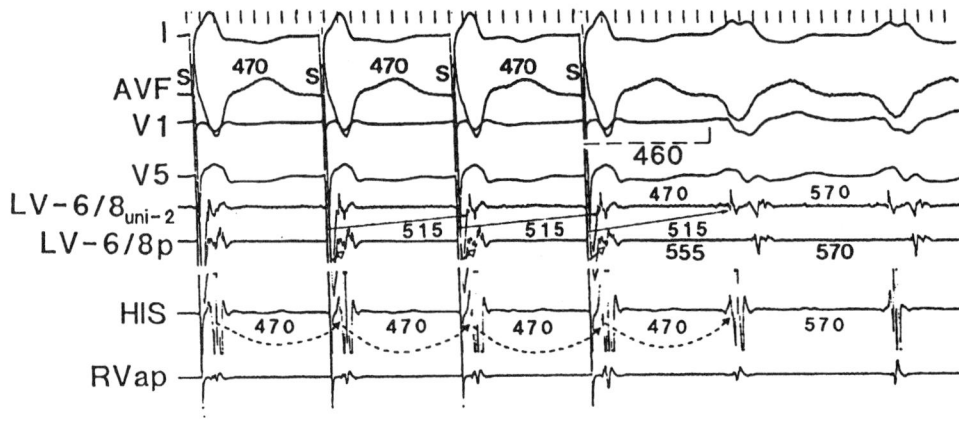

527

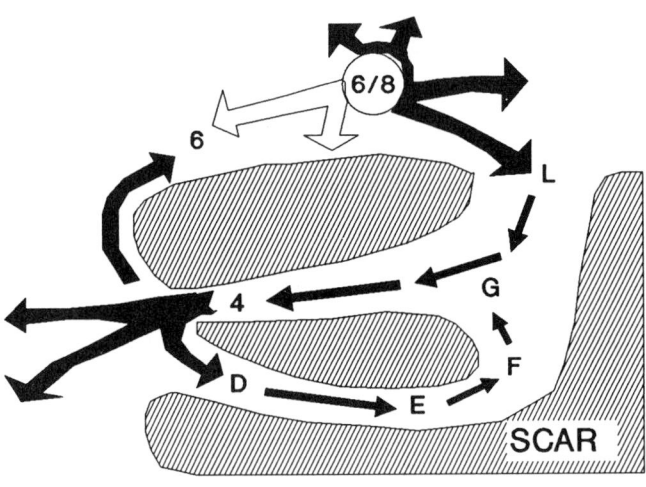

Figure 4. The top tracing shows classical entrainment of the same ventricular tachycardia shown in Figure 3. From the top the time lines are in 50-msec increments, surface electrocardiogram leads I, aVF, V₁, V₅, a unipolar recording from electrode 2 of the mapping catheter (LV-6/8uni-2), and bipolar recordings from the proximal electrode pair at site 6/8 (LV-6/8p), the His-bundle position (HIS), and the right ventricular apex (RVap). Sustained monomorphic ventricular tachycardia having a cycle length of 570 msec is present. The last four stimuli (S) of a train with a cycle length of 470 msec at LV site 6/8 is shown. Immediately following the stimulus the QRS morphology is altered. The final entrained QRS occurs 470 msec after the last QRS (460 msec after the last stimulus), and is identical in morphology to the tachycardia QRS (last QRS shown). The likely mechanism of this finding is shown in the schematic at the bottom of the tracing for a theoretical figure-of-eight reentry circuit. Hatched areas are regions of inexcitable scar or conduction block. Orthodromic wave fronts are shown as black arrows and antidromic stimulated excitation wave fronts are shown as open arrows. The reentry circuit consists of two wave fronts propagating from site 4, around an outer loop to sites 6, 6/8, and L, and a wave front that propagates through an inner loop from site 4 to sites D, E, and F. Both wave fronts share a common central slow conduction zone extending from site G to site 4. The QRS onset occurs when the excitation wave front exits from the scar distal to site 4, and propagates out to the surrounding myocardium. The stimulation site at 6/8 is circled. During tachycardia, pacing at this site produces orthodromic and antidromic wave fronts. The antidromic wave fronts collide near site 6 with an orthodromic wave front exiting from the common slow conduction zone. The antidromic wave fronts alter the sequence of ventricular

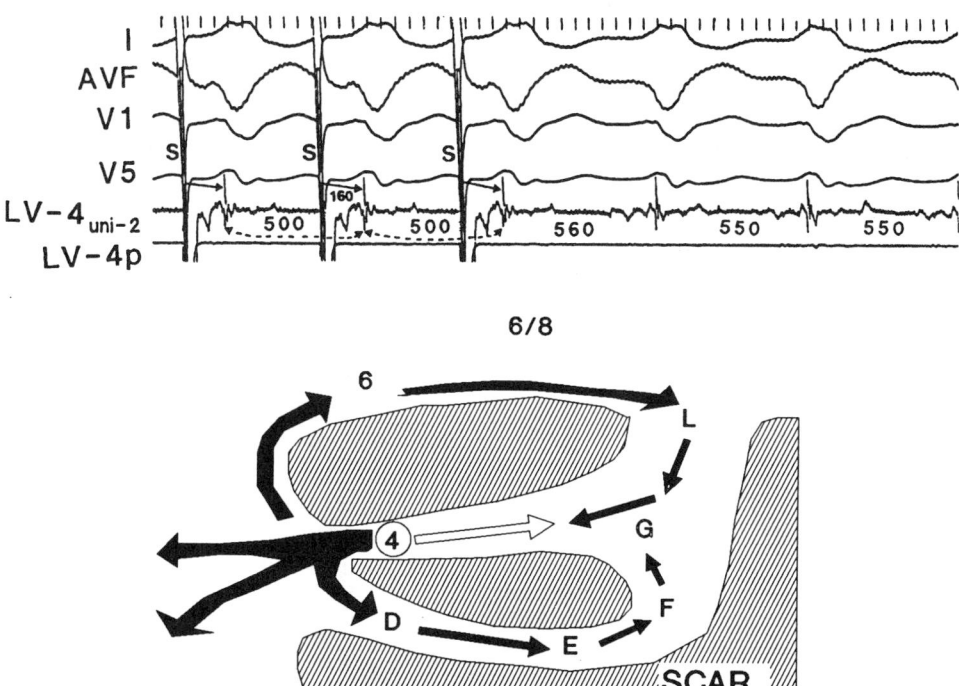

Figure 5. The top tracing shows entrainment with concealed fusion during pacing at left ventricular (LV) site 4 during the same ventricular tachycardia shown in Figures 3 and 4. From the top the time lines are in 50-msec increments, surface electrocardiogram leads I, aVF, V_1, V_5, a unipolar recording from electrode 2 of the mapping catheter (LV-4/uni-2), and a bipolar recording the proximal electrode pair at site 4 (LV-4p). Sustained monomorphic ventricular tachycardia (last 2 QRS complexes) has a cycle length of 550 msec. The last 4 stimuli (S) of a train with a cycle length of 500 msec at LV site 4 is shown. The tachycardia is accelerated to the pacing cycle length. Each stimulus is followed after 100 msec by a QRS complex similar in morphology to the tachycardia QRS complexes. The likely mechanism of this finding is shown in the schematic in the bottom panel illustrating the theoretical figure-of-eight reentry circuit shown in Figure 4. Site 4 is in the distal end of the common slow conduction zone. During tachycardia, pacing at site 4 produces orthodromic (black arrows) and antidromic (open arrows) wave fronts. The antidromic wave fronts collide between site 4 and site G with a returning orthodromic wave front and is extinguished within the scar. Thus, the antidromic wave front does not reach the myocardium outside the scar and does not alter the QRS complex. The stimulated orthodromic wave front propagates from site 4 out of the scar from the same point as the tachycardia wave fronts, resetting the tachycardia with little or no alteration in QRS morphology. The stimulus to QRS interval of 100 msec reflects the conduction time from the pacing site to the exit from the scar. Direct current shock catheter ablation at this site abolished ventricular tachycardia. See text for discussion.

---

activation outside the scar, producing QRS complexes that reflect fusion between the stimulated wave fronts and the orthodromic wave front that has exited from the scar distal to site 4. Because the pacing site is on the edge of the scar, there is little or no delay between the stimulus and the altered QRS. The last stimulated orthodromic wave front propagates through the scar reaching the exit 460 msec after the stimulus, and propagates into the surrounding myocardium where it does not collide with an antidromic wave front. Hence, the last paced beat is entrained but not fused. See text for discussion.

these findings is shown schematically below the tracings using a theoretical figure-of-eight–type of reentry circuit for purposes of illustration. In this figure-of-eight circuit, the excitation wave fronts (dark arrows) propagate around two areas of block sharing a common central area of slow conduction from site G to site 4. This circuit contains an outer loop in which the excitation wave front propagates out of the scar from site 4 to site 6 and back into the scar at site L. An "inner loop" is contained within the scar from site 4 to sites D, E, and F. The excitation wave fronts from the two loops enter the common slow conduction zone at site G. Depolarization of myocytes in the scar generates low-amplitude electrical activity that is not detected from the body surface. The onset of the QRS complex occurs when the excitation wave front propagates out of the scar away from site 4. Stimulation at site 6/8 produces antidromic wave fronts (clear arrows) and orthodromic wave fronts (dark arrows). The antidromic wave front alters the ventricular activation sequence distant from the scar, and collides near site 6 with the wave front that is exiting from the tachycardia circuit. The fusion QRS complexes are due to activation of the myocardium outside the scar by these two excitation wave fronts. The stimulated orthodromic wave front propagates to site L, into the scar and continues through the common slow conduction zone, resetting the tachycardia circuit. This wave front then exits from the slow conduction zone distal to site 4, continuing the tachycardia. The conduction time from the stimulus site, to site L, through the common slow conduction zone to the QRS onset site is the stimulus to QRS interval of 460 msec in the upper panel. This long stimulus to QRS interval of the last entrained (but not fused) beat is consistent with slow conduction in the reentry circuit. This is the classic type of entrainment that was initially described by Waldo and co-workers.[54,56–59] The stimulus site is outside the slow conduction region. There is constant QRS fusion during pacing because after the first few beats of the stimulus train, the stimulated antidromic wave fronts and orthodromic wave fronts consistently collide in the same locations.[59,60]

Figure 5 shows the effects of stimulation at a site probably within a region of slow conduction in the reentry circuit of the same ventricular tachycardia shown in Figures 2 and 4. A train of stimuli at a cycle length of 500 msec advances each beat to the pacing cycle length. In contrast to stimulation distant from the circuit, all QRS complexes are similar to the nonpaced QRS complexes of the ventricular tachycardia that has a cycle length of 550 msec. The stimulus to QRS interval is 100 msec. This is consistent with stimulation within the reentry circuit, close to the "exit" from the slow conduction zone as shown schematically below the tracings. The stimulus at site 4 produces an orthodromic excitation wave front (dark arrows) and an antidromic wave front (clear arrows). The orthodromic wave front propagates out of the scar from the same site as the tachycardia excitation waves. Thus the tachycardia is advanced and the QRS morphology is the same as that of the nonpaced tachycardia beats. The antidromic wave front collides with a returning orthodromic wave front and is confined within the scar. The antidromic wave front does not propagate out from the scar to the surrounding myocardium, does not alter the sequence of ventricular activation distant from the scar, and therefore does not alter the QRS morphology. Endocardial catheter ablation with a direct current electrical shock abolished this ventricular tachycardia, rendering this patient free of inducible or spontaneous ventricular tachycardia over a follow-up of over 2 years, supporting the participation of this site in the tachycardia circuit.

Ventricular tachycardia arising after remote myocardial infarction has been intensively studied with programmed electrical stimulation. If pacing is performed from multiple sites entrainment can be demonstrated for almost all hemodynamically tolerated chronic ventricular tachycardias.[59,60] In our experience, an area of slow conduction that appears to be participating in the ventricular tachycardia circuit can be identified with endocardial stimulation in two thirds of patients. Comparisons of computer simulations of reentry circuits with observations during programmed stimulation at suspected slow conduction areas further support that some of these areas participate in the reentry circuit.[51,62]

In up to one third of patients, intraoperative mapping studies have found reentry circuits in the subepicardium.[32–34] Programmed stimulation at sites in these circuits entrains the tachycardia with concealed fusion and long stimulus to QRS delays consistent with slow conduction.[32] Laser ablation of epicardial tissue at some of these sites is successful in abolishing reentry.

Bystander Slow Conduction Areas

It is important to recognize that not all areas of slow conduction participate in ventricular reentry circuits.[37,38,63–66] Some areas give rise to low-amplitude fractionated electrograms, but can be dissociated from the ventricular tachycardia circuit by pacing at the site. In other areas variable conduction can occur with 2:1 or Wenckebach-like conduction intermittently depolarizing an area of slow conduction. In these bystander areas impulse propagation may be too tenuous to support a reentry circuit. These slow conduction "bystanders" further complicate mapping and ablation attempts because they generate low-amplitude fractionated electrical activity, and in some cases pacing at the bystander can entrain ventricular tachycardia with concealed fusion and long stimulus to QRS delays.[52] Analysis of electrogram timing, stimulus to QRS intervals and stimulus to next electrogram interval (postpacing interval) during entrainment may allow bystander sites to be distinguished from slow conduction sites in the reentry circuit.[62,67] Multiple morphologies of monomorphic ventricular tachycardia in the same patient are common, however, and may arise from either different reentry circuits, or multiple "exits" from one circuit.[18,19,37,68] It is possible that a bystander slow conduction area for one reentry circuit may participate in another reentry circuit in some patients.

In summary, intraoperative and catheter mapping demonstrate areas of slow conduction in and adjacent to ventricular reentry circuits in the majority of patients with ventricular tachycardia late after myocardial infarction. Surgical and catheter ablation procedures that target these areas have been able to abolish ventricular tachycardia, but the number of patients studied is relatively small.

Does Slow Conduction Determine the Clinical Presentation of Ventricular Tachycardia?

Dennis et al.[31] performed programmed electrical stimulation in 403 consecutive myocardial infarction survivors. Sustained ventricular tachycardia was inducible in 20% of patients, and late potentials were detectable in 26% of patients. At 2 years of follow-up, 20% of patients with inducible ventricular tachycardia or late potentials had suffered a spontaneous episode of sustained ventricular tachycardia or died suddenly as compared to fewer than 5% of patients who did not have inducible ventricular tachycardia. Further analysis revealed that the rate of the induced ventricular tachycardia had prognostic importance. Patients with induced ventricular tachycardia cycle lengths slower than 230 msec were more likely to suffer a spontaneous arrhythmia than patients with faster tachycardias. The relation of slow conduction in the reentry circuit to the clinical presentation is further supported by the findings of Brugada and co-workers[69] in patients presenting with a variety of ventricular arrhythmias late after myocardial infarction. The cycle length of inducible ventricular tachycardia in patients who presented with sustained monomorphic ventricular tachycardia was 315 msec. The mean cycle length of inducible sustained monomorphic ventricular tachycardia in patients who presented with ventricular fibrillation was 274 msec. In patients who had not suffered a spontaneous sustained arrhythmia, the mean cycle length of inducible sustained monomorphic ventricular

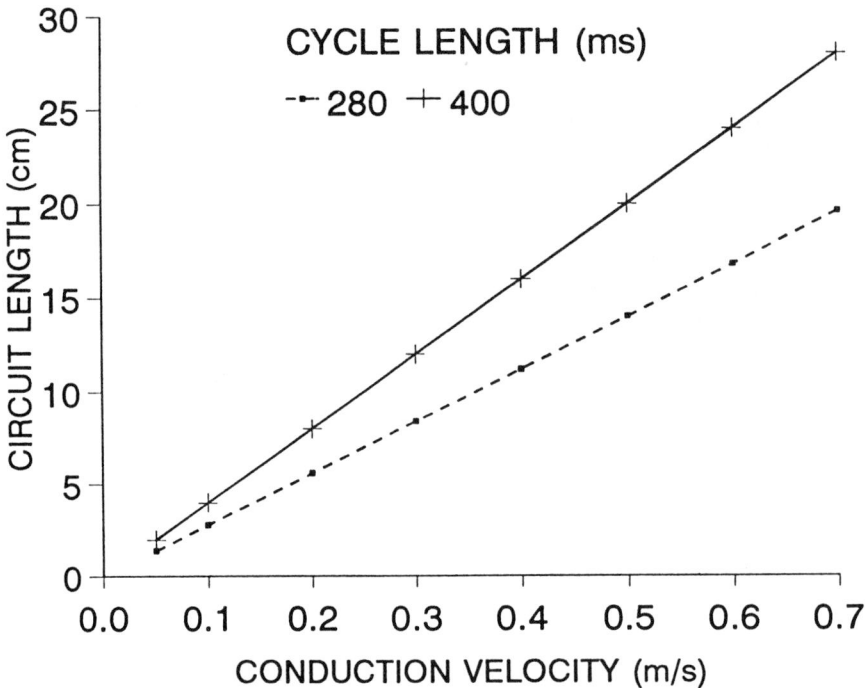

Figure 6. A plot of average conduction velocity in a reentry circuit (*x* axis) versus circuit length (*y* axis) for a tachycardia with a cycle length of 280 msec (215 beats per minute) and a tachycardia with a cycle length of 400 msec (150 beats per minute) is shown. If conduction velocity is relatively rapid (eg, 0.5 m/sec), the circuit length must exceed 12 cm. Thus, the larger the infarct scar, and the slower the conduction velocity, the more likely that a conduction path of sufficient length to sustain a reentry circuit exists.

tachycardia was 214 to 232 msec. During programmed electrical stimulation rapid ventricular tachycardias are generally more difficult to initiate, requiring a greater number of premature stimuli, than slower tachycardias.[69–71] This is consistent with the facilitation of reentry by slow conduction discussed above. Thus reentry circuits with short cycle lengths may be initiated less frequently by mechanisms which occur spontaneously. A rapid tachycardia is more likely, however, to lead to cardiac arrest and ventricular fibrillation than slow ventricular tachycardia.[69,72,73] Reentry circuits with short revolution times, producing rapid tachycardias may be less likely to cause a spontaneous arrhythmia, but more likely to produce cardiac arrest if a tachycardia does occur.

The tachycardia cycle length is determined by the length of the reentry path and the conduction velocities throughout the circuit. Both factors are likely to be important in determining the characteristics of tachycardia. In animal models, infarct scars giving rise to sustained monomorphic ventricular tachycardia have fractionated electrograms recorded over a larger area and have longer QRS durations on signal-averaged electrocardiograms than those giving rise to ventricular fibrillation.[74,75]

Infarct Size, Infarct Reperfusion, and Slow Conduction

Inducible ventricular tachycardia and late potentials are relatively infrequent after small infarcts, when the left ventricular ejection fraction remains greater than 40%. The incidence increases markedly as infarct size increases.[76,77] Although the reasons for this are not known, a possible explanation is suggested by the theoretical considerations shown in Figure 6 that graphs the relation between the average conduction velocity in a theoretical reentry circuit versus the length of the reentry path required to produce a tachycardia with a cycle length of either 400 msec (150 beats per minute) or 280 msec (215 beats per minute). If conduction velocity in the circuit is near normal (eg, greater than 0.5 m/sec) the length of the reentry path exceeds 12 cm. As the average conduction velocity diminishes the length of the reentry path diminishes to less than 4 cm when conduction velocity is markedly depressed. A large infarction may be more likely to have slow conduction areas of sufficient length to sustain reentry, while in a small reentry circuit conduction velocity would have to be quite slow for sustained ventricular tachycardia with a cycle length within this relatively common range. Successful reperfusion during the acute infarction decreases the incidence of inducible ventricular tachycardia and late potentials on the signal-averaged electrocardiogram.[78,79] Whether reperfusion prevents reentry circuits by preventing development of slow conduction areas, reducing the length of the slow conduction areas and reentry paths, or by a combination of these or other mechanisms is unknown.

Clinical Implications for Antiarrhythmic Drug Therapy

From these considerations, it can be appreciated that a potential reentry circuit that is too small to sustain reentry may be able to produce an arrhythmia in the presence of an antiarrhythmic drug that slows conduction velocity without prolonging refractoriness. Slowing conduction may also facilitate initiation of reentry as discussed above. Slowing of conduction in the reentry circuit is a likely cause of increased frequency or new occurrence of ventricular tachycardia occasionally produced by antiarrhythmic drugs.[80–82] Consistent with this hypothesis is the observation that proarrhythmia is more frequent with Class IC drugs that prominently slow conduction, than with Class III drugs that predominantly prolong refractoriness.[80]

References

1. Fenoglio JJ, Pham TD, Harken AH, et al: Recurrent sustained ventricular tachycardia: structure and ultrastructure of subendocardial regions in which tachycardia originates. *Circulation* 68:518, 1983.
2. Bolick DR, Hackel DB, Reimer KA, Ideker RE: Quantitative analysis of myocardial infarct structure in patients with ventricular tachycardia. *Circulation* 74:1266, 1986.
3. de Bakker JM, van Capelle FJL, Janse MJ, et al: Reentry as a cause of ventricular tachycardia in patients with chronic ischemic heart disease: electrophysiologic and anatomic correlation. *Circulation* 77:589, 1988.
4. Ursell PC, Gardner PI, Albala A, et al: Structural and electrophysiologic changes in the epicardial border zone of canine myocardial infarcts during infarct healing. *Circ Res* 56:436, 1985.
5. Gilmour RF, Heger JJ, Prystowsky EN, Zipes DP: Cellular electrophysiologic abnormalities of diseased human ventricular myocardium. *Am J Cardiol* 51:137, 1983.
6. Spear JF, Horowitz LN, Hodess AB, et al: Cellular electrophysiology of human myocardial infarction. 1. Abnormalities of cellular activation. *Circulation* 59:247, 1979.
7. Spach MS, Miller WT, Geselowitz DB, et al: The discontinuous nature of propagation in normal canine cardiac muscle: evidence for recurrent discontinuities of intracellular resistance that affect the membrane currents. *Circ Res* 48:39, 1981.
8. Dillon SM, Allessie MA, Ursell PC, Wit AL: Influence of anisotropic tissue structure on reentrant circuits in the epicardial border zone of subacute canine infarcts. *Circ Res* 63:182, 1988.
9. de Bakker JMT, Coronel R, Tasseron S, et al: Ventricular tachycardia in the infarcted, Langendorff-perfused human heart: role of the arrangement of surviving cardiac fibers. *J Am Coll Cardiol* 15:1594, 1990.
10. de la Fuente D, Sasyniuk B, Moe GK: Conduction through a narrow isthmus in isolated canine atrial tissue: a model of the WPW syndrome. *Circulation* 14:803, 1971.

11. Kogan B, Karpul W, Billett B, Stevenson WG: Excitation wave propagation within narrow pathways: geometric configurations facilitating unidirectional block and reentry. *Phys D* 59:275, 1992.

12. Stevenson WG, Weiss JN, Wiener I, Nademanee K: Slow conduction in the infarct scar: relevance to the occurrence, detection, and ablation of ventricular reentry circuits resulting from myocardial infarction. *Am Heart J* 117:452, 1989.

13. Mehra R, Zeiler RH, Gough WB, El-Sherif N: Reentrant ventricular arrhythmias in the late myocardial infarction period. 9. Electrophysiologic-anatomic correlation of reentrant circuits. *Circulation* 67:11, 1983.

14. El-Sherif N, Mehra R, Gough WB, Zeiler RH: Reentrant ventricular arrhythmias in the late myocardial infarction period. Interruption of reentrant circuits by cryothermal techniques. *Circulation* 68:644, 1983.

15. Garan H, Fallon JT, Rosenthal S, Ruskin JN: Endocardial, intramural amd epicardial activation patterns during sustained monomorphic ventricular tachycardia in late canine myocardial infarction. *Circ Res* 60:887, 1987.

16. Cardinal R, Vermeulen M, Shenasa M, et al: Anisotropic conduction and functional dissociation of ischemic tissue during reentrant VT in canine myocardial infarction. *Circulation* 77:1162, 1988.

17. de Bakker JMT, van Capelle FJL, Janse MJ, et al: Macroreentry in the infarcted human heart: mechanism of ventricular tachycardias with a focal activation pattern. *J Am Coll Cardiol* 18:1005, 1991.

18. Kaltenbrunner W, Cardinal R, Dubuc M, et al: Epicardial and endocardial mapping of ventricular tachycardia in patients with myocardial infarction. Is the origin of the tachycardia always subendocardially localized? *Circulation* 84:1058, 1991.

19. Downar E, Harris L, Mickleborough LL, et al: Endocardial mapping of ventricular tachycardia in the intact human ventricle: evidence of reentrant mechanisms. *J Am Coll Cardiol* 11:783, 1988.

20. Harris L, Downar E, Mickleborough L, et al: Activation sequence of ventricular tachycardia: endocardial and epicardial mapping studies in the human ventricle. *J Am Coll Cardiol* 10:1040, 1987.

21. Gardner PI, Ursell PC, Fenoglio JJ, Wit AL: Electrophysiologic and anatomic basis for fractionated electrograms recorded from healed myocardial infarcts. *Circulation* 72:596, 1985.

22. Wiener I, Mindich B, Pitchon R: Determinants of ventricular tachycardia in patients with ventricular aneurysms: results of intraoperative epicardial and endocardial mapping. *Circulation* 65:856, 1982.

23. Wiener I, Mindich B, Pitchon R: Fragmented endocardial electrical activity in patients with ventricular tachycardia: a new guide to surgical thrapy. *Am Heart J* 107:86, 1984.

24. Kienzle MG, Miller J, Falcone RA, et al: Intraoperative endocardial mapping during sinus rhythm: relationship to site of origin of ventricular tachycardia. *Circulation* 70:957, 1984.

25. Stevenson WG, Weiss JN, Wiener I, et al: Fractionated endocardial electrograms are associated with slow conduction in humans: evidence from pace-mapping. *J Am Coll Cardiol* 13:369, 1989.

26. Cassidy DM, Vassallo JA, Miller JM, et al: Endocardial catheter mapping in patients in sinus rhythm: relationship to underlying heart disease and ventricular arrhythmias. *Circulation* 73:645, 1986.

27. Simson MB, Euler D, Michelson EL, et al: Detection of delayed ventricular activation on the body surface in dogs. *Am J Physiol* 241:H363, 1981.

28. Simson MB: Use of signals in the terminal QRS complex to identify patients with ventricular tachycardia after myocardial infarction. *Circulation* 64:235, 1981.

29. Simson MB, Untereker WJ, Spielman SR, et al: Relation of late potential to site of origin of ventricular tachycardia associated with coronary heart disease. *Am J Cardiol* 55:985, 1985.

30. Denes P, Uretz E, Santarelli P: Determinants of arrhythmogenic ventricular activity detected on the body surface QRS in patients with coronary artery disease. *Am J Cardiol* 53:1519, 1984.

31. Denniss AR, Richards DA, Cody DV, et al: Prognostic significance of ventricular tachycardia and fibrillation induced at programmed stimulation and delayed potentials detected on the signal-averaged electrocardiogram of survivors of acute myocardial infarction. *Circulation* 74:731, 1986.

32. Littman L, Svenson RH, Gallagller JJ, et al: Functional role of the epicardium in post-infarction ventricular tachycardia. Observations derived from computerized epicardial activation mapping, entrainment and epicardial laser photoablation. *Circulation* 83:1577, 1991.

33. Svenson RH, Littmann L, Colavita PG, et al: Laser photoablation of ventricular tachycardia: correlation of diastolic activation times and photoablation effects on cycle length and termination-observations supporting a macroreentrant mechanism. *J Am Coll Cardiol* 19:607, 1992.

34. Kaltenbrunner W, Cardinal R, Dubuc M, et al: Epicardial and endocardial mapping of ventric-

ular tachycardia in patients with myocardial infarction: is the origin of the tachycardia always subendocardially localized? *Circulation* 84: 1058, 1991.

35. Ideker RE, Smith WM, Blanchard SM, et al: The assumption of isochronal cardiac mapping. *PACE* 12:456, 1989.

36. Kadish A, Shinnar M, Moored EN, et al: Interaction of fiber orientation and direction of impulse propagation with anatomic barriers in anisotropic canine myocardium. *Circulation* 78:1478, 1988.

37. Fitzgerald D, Friday KJ, Yeung-Lai-Wah J, et al: Myocardial regions of slow conduction participating in the reentrant circuit of multiple ventricular tachycardia: report on ten patients. *J Cardiovasc Electrophysiol* 2:193, 1991.

38. Fitzgerald DM, Friday KJ, Wah JAYL, et al: Electrogram patterns predicting successful catheter ablation of ventricular tachycardia. *Circulation* 77:806, 1988.

39. Josephson ME, Wit AL: Fractionated electrical activity and continuous electrical activity: fact or artifact. *Circulation* 70:529, 1984.

40. Josephson ME, Horowitz LN, Farshidi A: Continuous local electrical activity. A mechansim of recurrent ventricular tachycardia. *Circulation* 57;659, 1978.

41. Josephson ME, Wit AL: Fractionated electrical activity and continuous electrical activity: fact or artifact? *Circulation* 70:529, 1984.

42. Trappe HJ, Klein H, Auricchio A, et al: Catheter ablation of ventricular tachycardia: role of the underlying etiology and the site of energy delivery. *PACE* 15:411, 1992.

43. Kuck KH, Schluter M, Geiger M, Siebles J: Successful catheter ablation of human ventricular tachycardia with radiofrequency current guided by an endocardial map of the area of slow conduction. *PACE* 14:1060, 1991.

44. Borggrefe M, Breithardt G, Podczeck A, et al: Catheter ablation of ventricular tachycardia using defibrillator pulses: electrophysiological findings and long-term results. *Eur Heart J* 10: 591, 1989.

45. Hauer RNW, de Medina EOR, Kuijer PJ, Westerhof PW: Electrode catheter ablation for ventricular tachycardia: efficacy of single cathodal shock. *Br Heart J* 61:38, 1989.

46. Garan H, Kuchar D, Freeman C, et al: Early assessment of the effect of map-guided transcatheter intracardiac electrical shock on sustained ventricular tachycardia secondary to coronary artery disease. *Am J Cardiol* 61:1018, 1988.

47. Morady F, Scheinman MM, Di Carlo L, et al: Catheter ablation of ventricular tachycardia with intracardiac shocks: results in 33 patients. *Circulation* 75:1037, 1987.

48. Stevenson WG, Weiss JN, Wiener I, et al: Localization of slow conduction in a ventricular tachycardia circuit by entrainment: implications for catheter ablation. *Am Heart J* 114: 1253, 1987.

49. Stevenson WG, Weiss JN, Weiner T, et al: Resetting of VT: implications for localizing the area of slow conduction. *J Am Coll Cardiol* 11:522, 1988.

50. Morady F, Frank R, Kou WH, et al: Identification and catheter ablation of a zone of slow conduction in the reentrant circuit of ventricular tachycardia in humans. *J Am Coll Cardiol* 11:775, 1988.

51. Stevenson WG, Nademanee K, Weiss JN, et al: Programmed electrical stimulation at sites in ventricular reentry circuits: comparison of predictions from computer simulations with observations in humans. *Circulation* 80:793, 1989.

52. Morady F, Kadish A, Rosenheck S, et al: Concealed entrainment as a guide for catheter ablation of ventricular tachycardia in patients with prior myocardial infarction. *J Am Coll Cardiol* 17:678, 1991.

53. Frank R, Tonet JL, Kounde S, et al: Localization of the area of slow conduction during ventricular tachycardia. In: P Brugada, HJJ Wellens (eds): *Cardiac Arrhythmias: Where to Go From Here.* Mt Kisco, NY: Futura Publishing Company, Inc., 1987, p. 191.

54. Kay GN, Epstein AE, Plumb VJ: Resetting of ventricular tachycardia by single extrastimuli. Relation to slow conduction within the reentrant circuit. *Circulation* 81:1507, 1990.

55. Okumura K, Olshansky B, Henthorn RW, et al: Demonstration of the presence of slow conduction during sustained ventricular tachycardia in man: use of transient entrainment of the tachycardia. *Circulation* 75:369, 1987.

56. Okumura K, Henthorn RW, Epstein AE, et al: Further observations on transient entrainment: importance of pacing site and properties of the components of the reentry circuit. *Circulation* 72:1293, 1987.

57. Waldo AL, Olshansky B, Okumura K, Henthorn RW: Current perspectives on entrainment of tachyarrhythmias. In: P Brugada, HJJ Wellens (eds): *Cardiac Arrhythmias: Where to Go From Here.* Mt. Kisco, NY: Futura Publishing Company, Inc., 1987, p. 171.

58. Waldo AL, Henthorn RW, Plumb VJ, MacLean WAH: Demonstration of the mechanism of transient entrainment and interruption of ventricular tachycardia with rapid atrial pacing. *J Am Coll Cardiol* 3:422, 1984.

59. Henthorn RW, Okumura K, Olshansky B, et al: A fourth criterion for transient entrainment: the electrogram equivilant of progressive fusion. *Circulation* 77:1003, 1988.

60. Stevenson WG, Woo MA: Determinants of antidromic wave front propagation during entrainment of reentrant arrhythmias. *J Cardiovasc Electrophysiol* 2:215, 1991.

61. Kay GN, Epstein AE, Plumb VJ: Incidence of reentry with an excitable gap in ventricular tachycardia: a prospective evaluation utilizing transient entrainment. *J Am Coll Cardiol* 11:530, 1988.

62. Stevenson WG, Khan H, Sager P, et al: Identification of reentry circuit sites during catheter mapping and radiofrequency ablation of ventricular tachycardia late after myocardial infarction. *Circulation* (in press).

63. Brugada P, Abdollah H, Wellens HJJ: Continuous electrical activity during sustained monomorphic ventricular tachycardia. Observations on its dynamic behavior during the arrhythmia. *Am J Cardiol* 55:402, 1985.

64. Miller JM, Vassallo JA, Hargrove WC, Josephson ME: Intermittent failure of local conduction during VT. *Circulation* 72:1286, 1985.

65. Gallagher JD, Del Rossi AJ, Fernandez J, et al: Cryothermal mapping of recurrent ventricular tachycardia in man. *Circulation* 71:733, 1985.

66. Gessman LJ, Endo T, Egan J, et al: Dissociation of the site of origin from the site of cryo-termination of ventricular tachycardia. *PACE* 6:1293, 1983.

67. Fontaine G, Frank R, Tonet J, Grosgogeat Y: Identification of a zone of slow conduction appropriate for VT ablation: theoretical considerations. *PACE* 12:262, 1989.

68. Kavanagh KM, Kabas JS, Rollins DL, et al: High-current stimuli to the spared epicardium of a large infarct induced ventricular tachycardia. *Circulation* 85:680, 1992.

69. Brugada P, Waldecker B, Kersschot Y, et al: Ventricular arrhythmias initiated by programmed stimulation in four groups of patients with healed myocardial infarction. *J Am Coll Cardiol* 8:1035, 1986.

70. Doherty JU, Kienzle MG, Waxman HL, et al: Relation of mode of induction and cycle length of ventricular tachycardia: analysis of 104 patients. *Am J Cardiol* 52:60, 1983.

71. Buxton AE, Waxman HL, Marchlinski FE, et al: Role of triple extrastimuli during electrophysiologic study of patients with documented sustained ventricular tachyarrhythmias. *Circulation* 69:532, 1983.

72. Stevenson WG, Brugada P, Waldecker B, et al: Clinical, angiographic and electrophysiologic findings in patients with aborted sudden death as compared with patients with sustained ventricular tachycardia after myocardial infarction. *Circulation* 71:1146, 1985.

73. Adhar GC, Larson LW, Bardy GH, Greene HL: Sustained ventricular arrhythmias: differences between survivors of cardiac arrest and patients with recurrent sustained ventricular tachycardia. *J Am Coll Cardiol* 12:159, 1988.

74. Denniss RA, Richards DA, Waywood JA, et al: Electrophysiologic and anatomic differences between canine hearts with inducible ventricular tachycardia and fibrillation associated with chronic myocardial infarction. *Circ Res* 64:155, 1989.

75. Kuchar DL, Rosenbaum DS, Ruskin J, Garan H. Late potentials on the signal-averaged electrocardiogram after canine myocardial infarction: correlation with induced ventricular arrhythmias during the healing phase. *J Am Coll Cardiol* 15:1365, 1990.

76. Richards DA, Byth K, Ross DL, Uther JB: What is the best predictor of spontaneous ventricular tachycardia and sudden death after myocardial infarction? *Circulation* 83:756, 1991.

77. Bourke JP, Richards DAB, Ross DL, et al: Routine programmed electrical stimulation in survivors of acute myocardial infarction for prediction of spontaneous ventricular tachyarrhythmias during follow-up results, optimal stimulation protocol and cost-effective screening. *J Am Coll Cardiol* 18:780, 1991.

78. Kersschot IE, Brugada P, Ramentol M, et al: Effects of early reperfusion in acute myocardial infarction on arrhythmias induced by programmed stimulation: a prospective randomized study. *J Am Coll Cardiol* 7:1234, 1986.

79. Gang ES, Lew AS, Hong M, et al: Decreased incidence of ventricular late potentials after successful thrombolytic therapy for acute myocardial infarction. *N Engl J Med* 321:712, 1989.

80. Stanton MS, Prystowsky EN, Fineberg NS, et al: Arrhythmogenic effects of antiarrhythmic drugs: a study of 506 patients treated for ventricular tachycardia or fibrillation. *J Am Coll Cardiol* 14:209, 1989.

81. Morganroth J, Horowitz LN: Flecainide: its proarrhythmic effect and expected changes in the surface electrocardiogram. *Am J Cardiol* 58:89B, 1984.

82. Falk RH: Flecainide-induced ventricular tachycardia and fibrillation in patients treated for atrial fibrillation. *Ann Intern Med* 11:107, 1989.

Chapter 13

Mechanisms of Clinically Occurring Cardiac Arrhythmias

Douglas P. Zipes
William M. Miles
Laurence S. Klein

The mechanisms responsible for producing cardiac arrhythmias are generally divided into categories of disorders of impulse formation, disorders of impulse conduction, or combinations of both (Table 1).[1-5] Unequivocal determination of the electrophysiological mechanisms responsible for many clinically occurring arrhythmias is difficult. Particularly, it is often very difficult to separate reentry occurring in a small area from automaticity. Furthermore, one mechanism can start a tachyarrhythmia that is then perpetuated by another mechanism.[6] For example, a premature ventricular depolarization due to reentry may then initiate a sustained tachycardia due to triggered activity, or a premature complex caused by abnormal automaticity may start a tachycardia maintained by reentry. Despite these obstacles, several clinically occurring arrhythmias can be definitely ascribed to one mechanism or another.

Disorders of Impulse Formation

Automaticity

Inappropriate discharge rate of the sinus node, for example, sinus rates too fast or too slow for the physiological needs of the patient, or automatic discharge from an ectopic pacemaker constitutes a disorder of impulse formation. Latent or subsidiary pacemakers located at ectopic sites can control the cardiac rhythm in two ways. First, slowing of the normal sinus rate can allow the ectopic focus to escape at its normal automatic rate. This may occur when a junctional escape beat or rhythm results during a sinus bradycardia. Second, if the discharge rate from the latent pacemaker speeds, it can wrest control of the cardiac rhythm from the sinus node. This may occur during a premature complex or a tachycardia from an ectopic site, atrial, junctional, or ventricular.

Supported in part by the Herman C. Krannert Fund; grants HL-42370 and HL-07182 from the National Heart, Lung, and Blood Institute of the National Institutes of Health, US Public Health Service; and by the American Heart Association, Indiana Affiliate, Inc.

From BN Singh, HJJ Wellens, M Hiraoka, (eds): *Electropharmacological Control of Cardiac Arrhythmias.* Mount Kisco, NY, Futura Publishing Company Inc., © 1994.

Table 1
Mechanisms of Arrhythmogenesis

I. Disorders of Impulse Formation
  A. Automaticity
    1. Normal automaticity
       a. Experimental examples—Normal in vivo or in vitro sinus node, Purkinje fibers, others.
       b. Clinical examples—Sinus tachycardia or bradycardia inappropriate for the clinical situation; possibly ventricular parasystole.
    2. Abnormal automaticity
       a. Experimental example—Depolarization-induced automaticity in Purkinje fibers or ventricular muscle.
       b. Clinical example—Possibly accelerated ventricular rhythms after myocardial infarction.
  B. Triggered Activity
    1. Early afterdepolarizations (EADs)
       a. Experimental examples—EADs produced by barium, hypoxia, high concentrations of catecholamines, drugs such as sotalol, N-acetylprocainamide, cesium.
       b. Clinical examples—Possibly idiopathic and acquired long Q–T syndromes and associated ventricular arrhythmias
    2. Delayed afterdepolarizations (DADs)
       a. Experimental example—DADs produced in Purkinje fibers by digitalis
       b. Clinical example—Possibly some digitalis-induced arrhythmias

II. Disorders of Impulse Conduction
  A. Block
    1. Bidirectional or unidirectional without reentry
       a. Experimental example—SA, AV, bundle branch, Purkinje-muscle, others.
       b. Clinical example—SA, AV, bundle branch, others
    2. Unidirectional block with reentry
       a. Experimental examples—AV node, Purkinje-muscle junction, infarcted myocardium, others
       b. Clinical examples—Reciprocating tachycardia in WPW syndrome, AV nodal reentry, VT due to bundle branch reentry, others
    3. Reflection
       a. Experimental example—Purkinje fiber with area of inexcitability
       b. Clinical example—Unknown

III. Combined Disorders
  A. Interactions between automatic foci
    1. Experimental examples—Depolarizing or hyperpolarizing subthreshold stimuli speed or slow automatic discharge rate
    2. Clinical examples—Modulated parasystole
  B. Interactions between automaticity and conduction
    1. Experimental examples—Deceleration-dependent block, overdrive suppression of conduction, entrance and exit block
    2. Clinical examples—Similar to experimental

Examples of automatic discharge as described may be due to normal or abnormal ionic mechanisms. Clinically, we can only infer which may be operative. For example, the patient with inappropriate sinus discharge rates may have normal ionic mechanisms responsible for sinus node discharge, although the kinetics or magnitude of the currents may be altered. In contrast, abnormal ionic mechanisms may be responsible for some ventricular tachycardias that result during acute myocardial infarction.[7,8]

Triggered Activity

A second major category of impulse formation is triggered activity.[9] Triggered activity is pacemaker activity that results consequent to a preceding impulse or series of impulses, without which electrical quiescence occurs. While automaticity is the property of a fiber that initiates an impulse spontaneously without need for prior stimulation, triggered activity must be initiated by a depolarizing impulse that results in an early afterdepolarization or a delayed afterdepolarization. Early afterdepolarizations are depolarizing potentials that arise from a reduced level of membrane potential during phases 2 and 3 of the cardiac action potential, while late or delayed afterdepolarizations occur after completion of repolarization (phase 4) generally at more negative membrane potentials than that from which early afterdepolarizations arise. If the afterdepolarization reaches threshold potential and produces a propagated response, it can trigger another afterdepolarization and thus, self-perpetuate.

A variety of interventions can produce early afterdepolarizations (Table 1), including many drugs, high concentrations of catecholamines, and reperfusion.[10,11] Clinically, early afterdepolarizations may be responsible for both the acquired and idiopathic congenital long QT syndrome and torsades de pointes.[12–15]

Delayed afterdepolarizations have been demonstrated in many different cardiac tissues than are thought responsible for some digitalis-induced arrhythmias.[16,17] The drug flunarizine appears to selectively eliminate arrhythmias due to delayed afterdepolarizations.[18]

Disorders of Impulse Conduction

Conduction delay and block can result in bradyarrhythmias or tachyarrhythmias, the former when the propagating impulse blocks and is followed by asystole or a slow escape rhythm, and the latter when the delay and block produce reentrant excitation. Normally, electrical activity during each cardiac cycle continues until the entire heart has been activated, and the cardiac impulse dies out when all fibers have been discharged and are completely refractory. If, however, a group of fibers not activated during the initial wave of depolarization recovers excitability in time to be discharged before the original impulse dies out, they may serve as a link to reexcite areas that were just discharged and have now recovered from the initial depolarization. Such a process results in reentry.[19] Reentry can occur over pathways that are separated anatomically, over pathways that are distinct because of functional electrophysiological differences or because anisotropic structural features create variations in conduction velocity and time course of repolarization.[20]

Clinical Tachycardias Due to Reentry

Reentry is probably the cause of many tachyarrhythmias, including various kinds of supraventricular and ventricular tachycardias, flutter, and fibrillation. However, in large pieces of tissue it is often difficult to prove unequivocally that reentry exists. Initiation or termination of tachycardia by pacing stimuli, the demonstration of electrical activity bridging diastole, fixed coupling, and a variety of other clinically used techniques such as entrainment and resetting curves, while consistent with reentry, do not constitute unequivocal proof of its existence.

Atrial and Ventricular Fibrillation

A critical mass of myocardium, either atrial or ventricular, is required to maintain fibrillation. Moe and Abildskov[21] advanced the hypothesis that multiple wavelets of reentry, influenced by the mass of tissue, refractory periods and conduction velocity, maintains fibrillation. These factors influence the number of wavelets present, which determines the likelihood of fibrillation to continue. Recent mapping studies have supported conclusively the multiple wavelet concept.[22]

Atrial Flutter

Reentry is the most likely cause of atrial flutter, with the wave front traveling a pathway established by atrial anatomy, distribution of refractoriness, and conduction delay.[23]

During atrial flutter, zones of slow fragmented conduction occur mainly in the lower and posterior portion of the right atrium near the coronary sinus os, and less commonly in the middle posteroseptal region between the two venae cavae. Ablation of atrial tissue in the area of slow conduction can eliminate the flutter.

Sinus Reentry

Reentry in parts of the atrium has been reported to occur in several experimental models as well as in humans.[24] The sinus node shares similar electrophysiological features with the atrioventricular (AV) node, particu-

larly the capacity for dissociation of conduction. A premature impulse can conduct in some sinus nodal fibers, but not in others. This capacity allows for the development of reentrant circuits that can be located entirely within the sinus node or use part of the sinus node and atrium (Figure 1).

Atrial Reentry

Reentry within the atrium, unrelated to the sinus node, has been shown experimentally in several animal species and is a cause of supraventricular tachycardias in humans.[25] Differentiating atrial tachycardia due to automaticity from atrial tachycardia sustained by reentry over small areas is quite difficult.

Atrioventricular Nodal Reentry

Longitudinal dissociation of the AV node into two or more pathways remains a plausible mechanism of AV node reentry, based on multiple studies in isolated rabbit AV nodal preparations. However, more recent observations in patients undergoing AV nodal modifi-

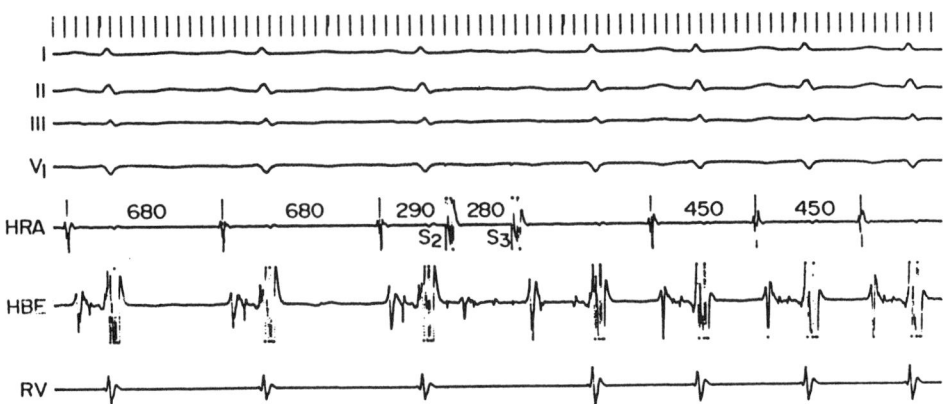

Figure 1. Sinus nodal reentry. Scalar leads I, II, III, and V_1 are shown. HRA: high right atrial electrograms; HBE: His bundle electrogram; RV: right ventricular apical electrogram. S_2, S_3: premature stimuli delivered to the high right atrial site. Numbers in milliseconds. Following S_3 a sustained tachycardia at a cycle length of 450 msec is initiated. The high-low atrial activation sequence and P wave morphology are consistent with origin of the supraventricular tachycardia at a site near or within the sinus node. Large time lines 50 msec.

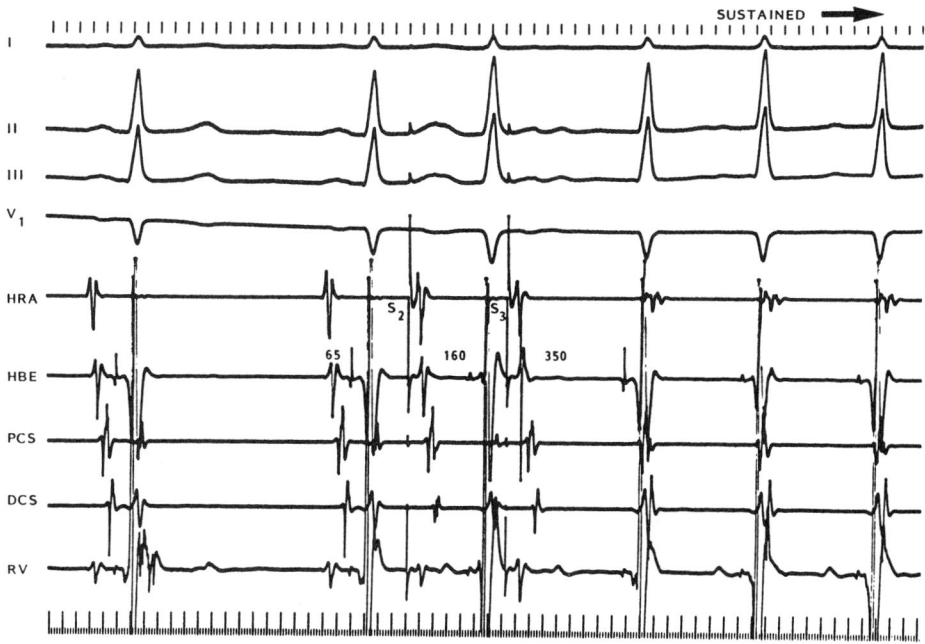

Figure 2. Precipitation of atrioventricular (AV) nodal reentry. Two premature stimuli are delivered to the high right atrial site. The first (S_2) conducts with delay (from 65 to 160 msec) over the AV nodal fast pathway. S_3 finds the fast pathway refractory and conducts to the His bundle over the slow pathway with a marked increase (350 msec) in the AV nodal conduction time. The impulse then returns to reexcite the atrium over the previously blocked fast pathway. The retrograde P wave is lost within the QRS complex and the atria are excited in a low-high activation sequence. Conventions as in Figure 1. PCS: proximal coronary sinus electrogram; DCS: distal coronary sinus electogram.

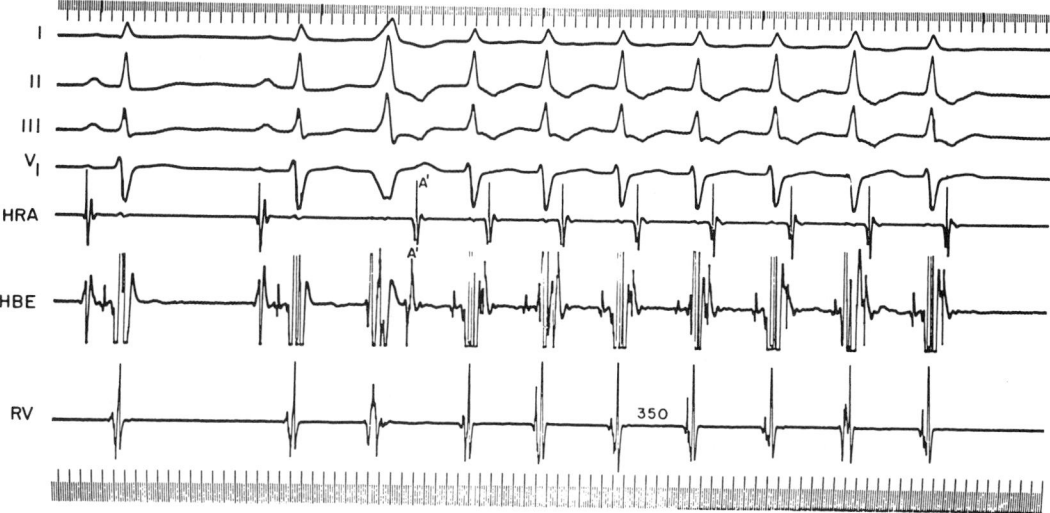

Figure 3. Spontaneous onset of atrioventricular (AV) nodal reentry following a premature ventricular complex. A premature ventricular complex (third QRS complex) conducts retrogradely to the atrium, presumably over the fast AV nodal pathway and returns to the ventricle over the slow AV nodal pathway, thus initiating a short run of AV nodal reentry at a cycle length of 350 msec. Note that the retrograde P wave occurs early in the ST segment and could be confused with AV reentrant tachycardia using a posteroseptal accessory pathway.

cation using radiofrequency ablation have demonstrated that the two pathways participating in AV nodal reentry, so-called fast and slow AV nodal pathways, are anatomically distinct, with the fast AV nodal pathway lying anteriorly near the His bundle and representing the usual anterograde conduction route during sinus rhythm and the putative retrograde route during AV nodal reentry. The slow AV nodal pathway, usually representing the anterograde conduction pathway during AV nodal reentry, inserts into the atrium in a more posterior location, near the coronary sinus os.[26]

A premature atrial stimulus that blocks anterogradely in the fast AV nodal pathway (which typically has a longer refractory period than the slow AV nodal pathway) and propa-

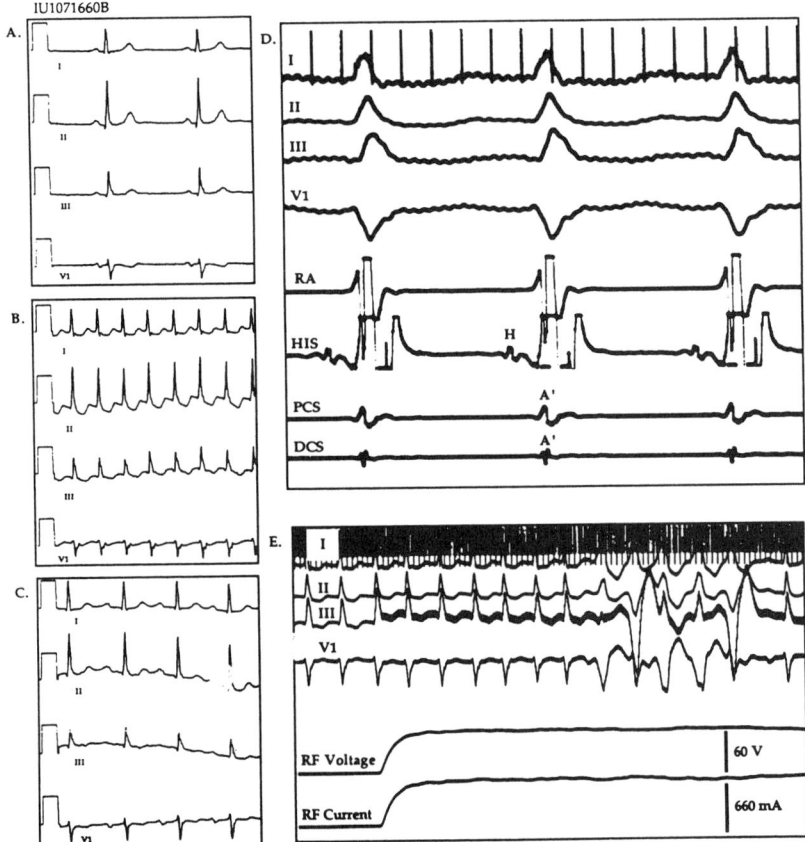

Figure 4. Radiofrequency atrioventricular (AV) nodal modification for AV nodal reentrant tachycardia. Panel A: Normal sinus rhythm. Panel B: AV nodal reentrant tachycardia. Panel C: Normal sinus rhythm following AV nodal ablation. Note prolonged PR interval. Panel D: AV nodal reentrant tachycardia with intracavitary recordings. Note virtual simultaneous activation of atria and ventricles, consistent with AV nodal reentrant tachycardia. Panel E: Radiofrequency ablation with catheter placed in the anterior region of the AV node producing selective ablation of the anterogradely conducting fast pathway. Vertical bars: calibration for radiofrequency voltage and current. (Reproduced with permission from Zipes DP: Management of cardiac arrhythmias: pharmacological, electrical and surgical techniques. In: E Braunwald (ed): *Heart Disease. A Textbook of Cardiovascular Medicine*. 4th edition. Philadelphia, PA: WB Saunders, 1992, p. 654.

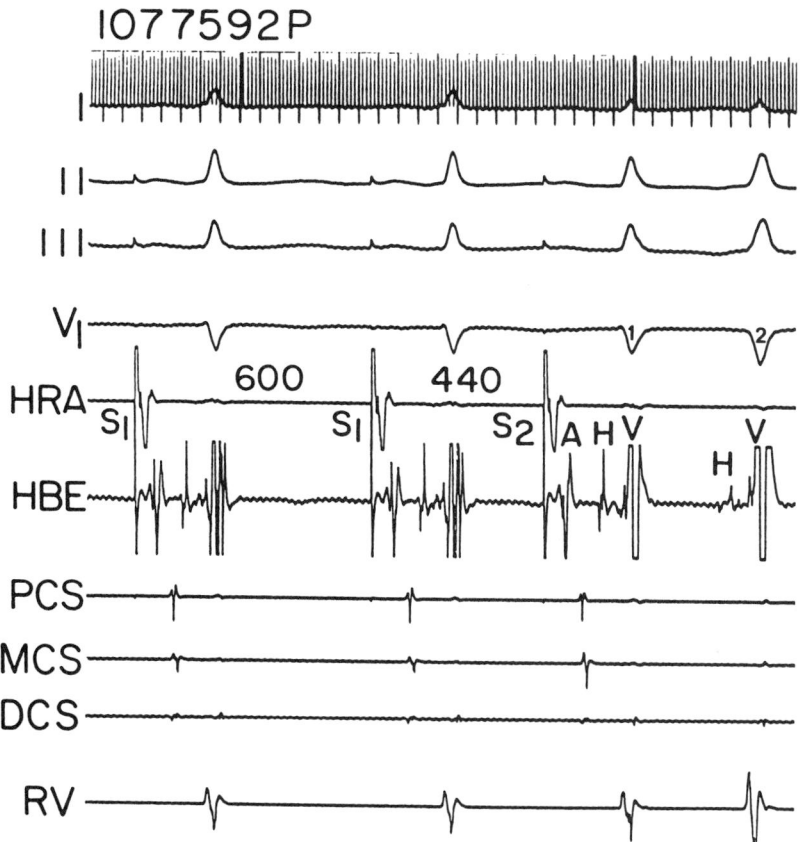

Figure 5. Two QRS complexes in response to a single premature atrial complex. Following a basic train of S_1 stimuli at 600 msec, an S_2 at 440 msec is introduced. The first QRS complex in response to S_2 occurs following a short (95 msec) atrio-His interval due to anterograde conduction over the fast atrioventricular (AV) nodal pathway. The first QRS complex is labeled number 1 in V_1. The second QRS complex in response to the S_2 stimulus (labeled number 2) follows a long AH interval (430 msec) due to anterograde conduction over the slow AV nodal pathway. (Reproduced with permission from Zipes DP: Specific arrhythmias: diagnosis and treatment. In: E Braunwald (ed): *Heart Disease: A Textbook of Cardiovascular Medicine*. 4th edition. Philadelphia, PA: WB Saunders, 1992, p. 689.)

gates anterogradely to the His bundle over the slow AV nodal pathway is the usual method of initiating AV nodal reentry (Figures 2 and 3). The impulse is then capable of returning to the atrium retrogradely over the fast AV nodal pathway. Less commonly the reentrant pathway occurs in an opposite direction, anterogradely over the fast AV nodal pathway and retrogradely over the slow AV nodal pathway. It is very likely that some patients have multiple slow AV nodal pathways that may sustain tachycardia. In most patients, the atrium probably plays an obligatory role in the reentry pathway. Selective ablation of either the slow or fast pathway with elimination of AV nodal reentrant tachycardia provides the most definitive proof of reentry (Figure 4), while two QRS complexes in response to one P wave (Figure 5) and atrial preexcitation by premature ventricular stimulation during tachycardia (Figure 6) offer corroborative evidence.[27,28]

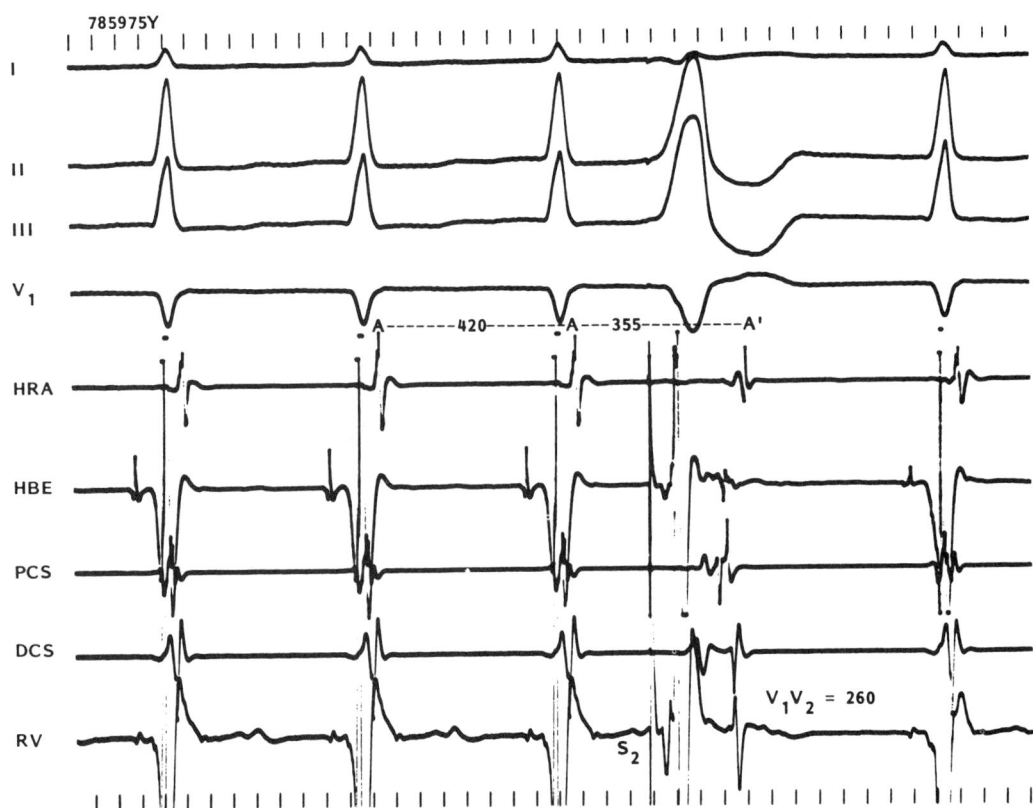

Figure 6. Atrial preexcitation during atrioventricular (AV) nodal reentry. AV nodal reentrant tachycardia is present with a cycle length of 420 msec. A premature ventricular complex (S₂) from the right ventricular outflow tract with a coupling interval of 260 msec is introduced during the tachycardia before the His bundle is activated anterogradely and penetrates the AV node retrogradely to shorten the AA interval to 355 msec. Dual AV nodal pathways best explain how two impulses can travel in opposite directions in the AV node (ie, the impulse from the tachycardia traveling anterogradely and the impulse from the premature ventricular stimulation traveling retrogradely) and not collide.

Preexcitation Syndrome

Patients with the Wolff-Parkinson-White syndrome have reciprocating tachycardias due to reentry over the normal and accessory pathways.[29] In most patients, the accessory pathway conducts more rapidly than does the normal AV node but takes a longer time to recover excitability, ie, the anterograde refractory period of the accessory pathway exceeds that of the AV node at long cycles. Consequently, a premature atrial complex that occurs sufficiently early blocks anterogradely in the accessory pathway and continues to the

ventricle over the normal AV node and His bundle. After the ventricles have been excited, the impulse is able to enter the accessory pathway retrogradely and return to the atrium. A continuous conduction loop of this kind establishes the circuit for the tachycardia. It produces a normal QRS complex tachycardia and is called orthodromic atrioventricular reciprocating tachycardia (AVRT) (Figures 7 and 8). Occasionally, the activation wave travels in a reverse (antidromic) direction, reaching the ventricles over the accessory pathway and traveling retrogradely in the His bundle-AV node to the atria. Two accessory pathways may form the circuit for antidromic AVRT in some patients. As in AV nodal reentry, definitive proof of reentry comes from eliminating tachycardia by interrupting conduction in either the AV node-His bundle or the accessory pathway.[30,31] Ancillary proof is provided by a single atrial complex initiating two QRS complexes (Figure 9) and by atrial preexcitation during tachycardia (Figure 10).

In some patients, the accessory pathway may only conduct retrogradely and therefore the manifestations of overt Wolff-Parkinson-White syndrome, ie, short PR interval, delta wave and abnormal QRS complex, are not present in the scalar ECG. Nevertheless, the accessory pathway can participate in an orthodromic AVRT and the reentrant pathway is the same as that described above. The only difference is that patients with this form of Wolff-Parkinson-White syndrome, so-called concealed Wolff-Parkinson-White, are not at risk

of developing rapid ventricular rates during atrial fibrillation since anterograde conduction must use the AV node.

There are several variants to the reentrant pathways described above for the typical patient with Wolff-Parkinson-White syndrome. In one group of patients, the accessory pathway conducts exceedingly slowly and rarely manifests anterograde conduction to the ventricle. Tachycardia in these patients is almost incessant and the term, permanent form of AV junctional reciprocating tachycardia (PJRT), has been applied (Figures 11 and 12). Importantly, in these patients, the QRS complex during tachycardia is normal because of anterograde conduction over the normal pathway and the retrograde P wave occurs at a very long RP (short PR) interval. This distinguishes them from the usual patient with orthodromic AVRT in whom the RP interval is short and the PR interval is long.

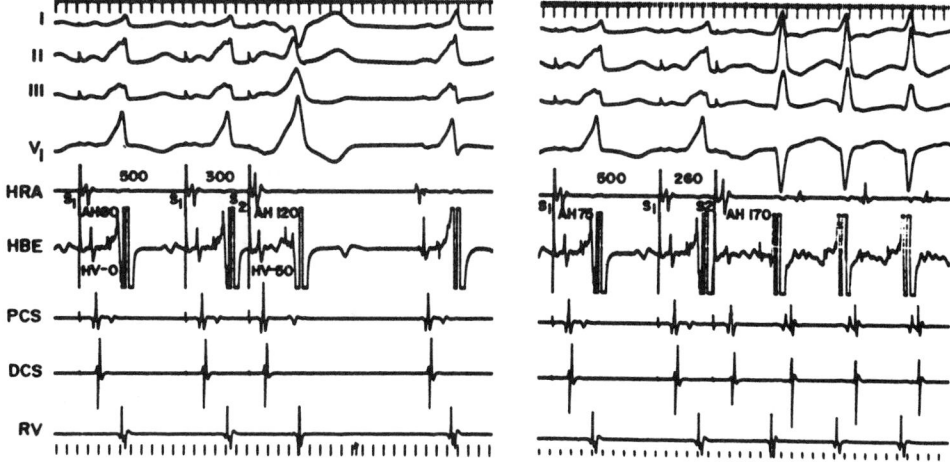

Figure 7. Initiation of orthodromic atrioventricular (AV) reciprocating tachycardia in a patient with a left free wall accessory pathway. In the left panel, the atria are driven at a basic cycle length of 500 msec. The AH interval is 80 msec and His-bundle activation occurs simultaneously with ventricular activation. A premature atrial stimulus at an S_1-S_2 interval of 300 msec prolongs AV nodal conduction time and His-bundle activation now occurs 50 msec after the onset of the QRS complex, since the AV interval does not prolong due to the accessory pathway. In the panel on the right, the S_1-S_2 interval is shortened to 260 msec and anterograde propagation in the accessory pathway fails. The resultant QRS complex has a normal contour due to activation over the normal AV node-His Purkinje system. The AH interval is 170 msec and the HV interval is 40 msec. Following anterograde block over the accessory pathway, the impulse is able to return retrogradely in the previously blocked accessory pathway and reexcite the atrium to initiate a sustained orthodromic AV reciprocating tachycardia.

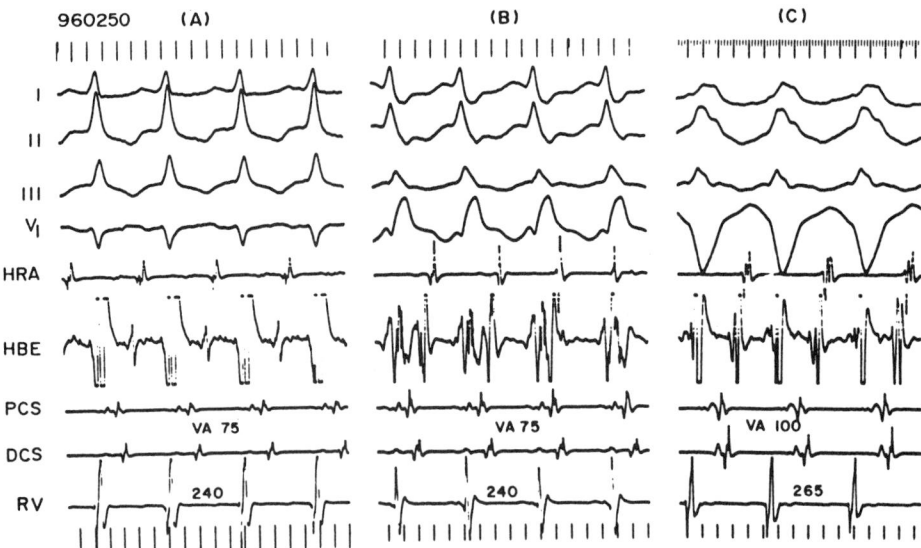

Figure 8. Orthodromic atrioventricular reciprocating tachycardia (AVRT), with and without functional bundle branch block. In panel A, typical orthodromic AVRT occurs due to antero-grade conduction over the normal pathway and retrograde conduction over a left posterolat-eral accessory pathway. In panel B, functional right bundle branch block occurs. No change in tachycardia cycle length or ventriculoatrial (VA) interval results because the functional bundle branch block is contralateral to the site of the accessory pathway. In panel C, functional left bundle branch block occurs and results in a 25-msec increase of the VA interval and tachycar-dia cycle length. This occurs because the functional bundle branch block is ipsilateral to the site of the accessory pathway and therefore the anterograde impulse has to travel over the right bundle branch, across the septum, and to the left ventricle before it can enter the acces-sory pathway and continue the reentrant loop.

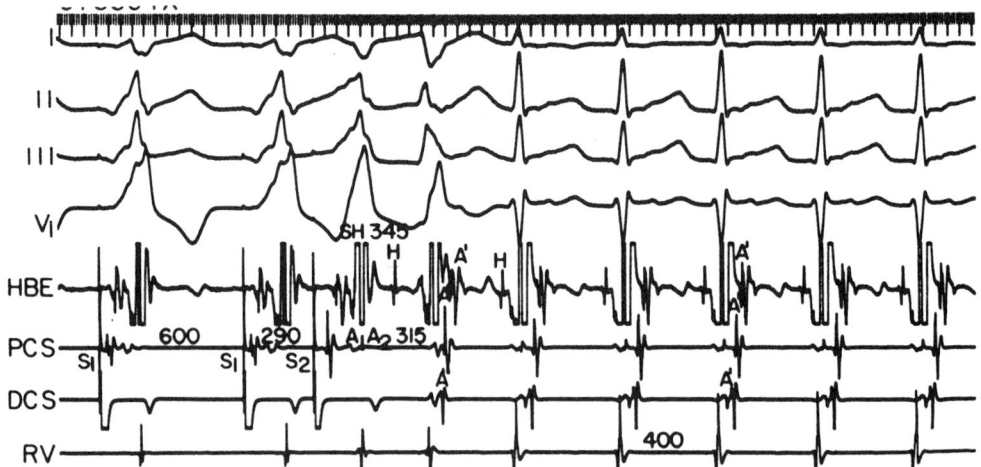

Figure 9. Two QRS complexes in response to a single premature atrial stimulus. During coro-nary sinus pacing at a cycle length of 600 msec, a premature stimulus (S₂) at 290 msec results in a premature atrial response at 315 msec. The premature atrial response propagates to the ventricle over the accessory pathway (third QRS complex), as well as to the ventricles over the normal atrioventricular (AV) node-His bundle pathway (fourth QRS complex), with His-Purkinje conduction delay and functional left bundle branch block and probable posterior fascicular block. Following this, the impulse invades the accessory pathway retrogradely, re-turns to the atrium (A') and initiates sustained orthodromic atrioventricular reciprocating tachycardia (AVRT) at a cycle length of 400 msec over a left free wall accessory pathway.

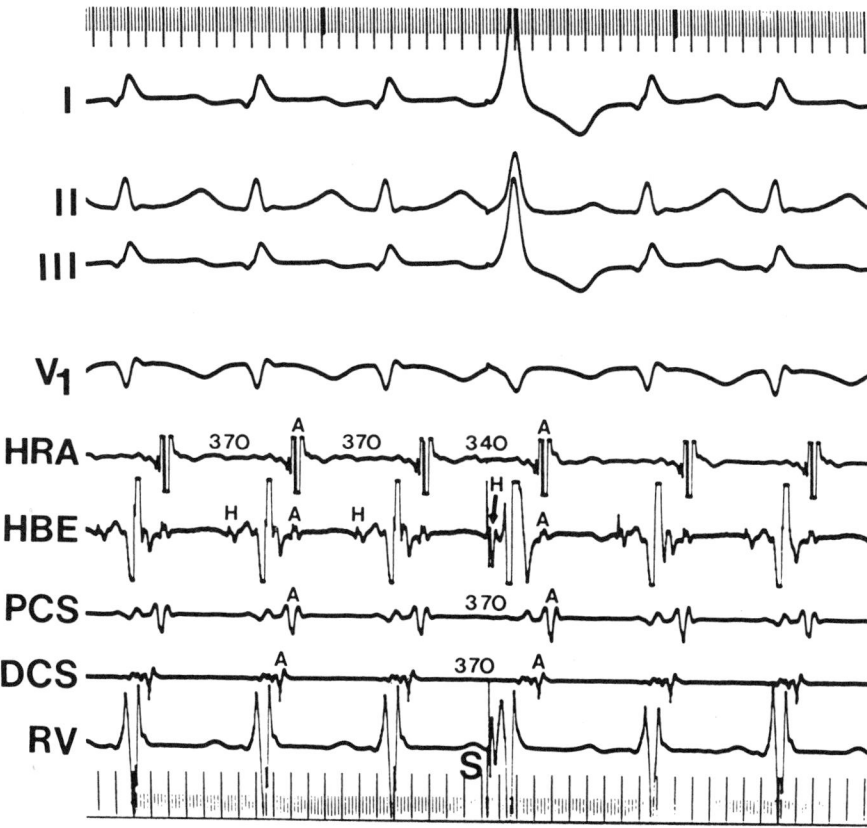

Figure 10. Atrial preexcitation during tachycardia when His bundle is refractory. A sustained orthodromic atrioventricular reciprocating tachycardia (AVRT) is present, with anterograde conduction over the normal pathway and retrograde conduction over a left ventricular free wall accessory pathway (note that atrial excitation recorded in the distal coronary sinus lead precedes atrial excitation at all other recording sites). During tachycardia, when the His bundle is refractory, a premature stimulus is delivered to the right ventricular apex (S). The AA interval recorded in the His bundle and high right atrial leads shortens from 370 to 340 msec. There is no shortening in the atrial cycle recorded from the coronary sinus. Thus, the ventricular stimulus, despite His bundle refractoriness, still reaches the atrium. The only way this can be explained is via excitation over a retrogradely conducting accessory pathway. Note also that the atrial activation sequence changes following S so that atrial activity in HRA and HBE occur slightly earlier than atrial activity in distal coronary sinus electrogram (DCS) or proximal coronary sinus electrogram (PCS). The patient has two accessory pathways, a left lateral accessory pathway and a right posteroseptal accessory pathway. During orthodromic AVRT, the impulses travel retrogradely over the left lateral accessory pathway. However, in response to the premature ventricular stimulus, retrograde conduction occurs over the right posteroseptal accessory pathway as well as over the left free wall accessory pathway.

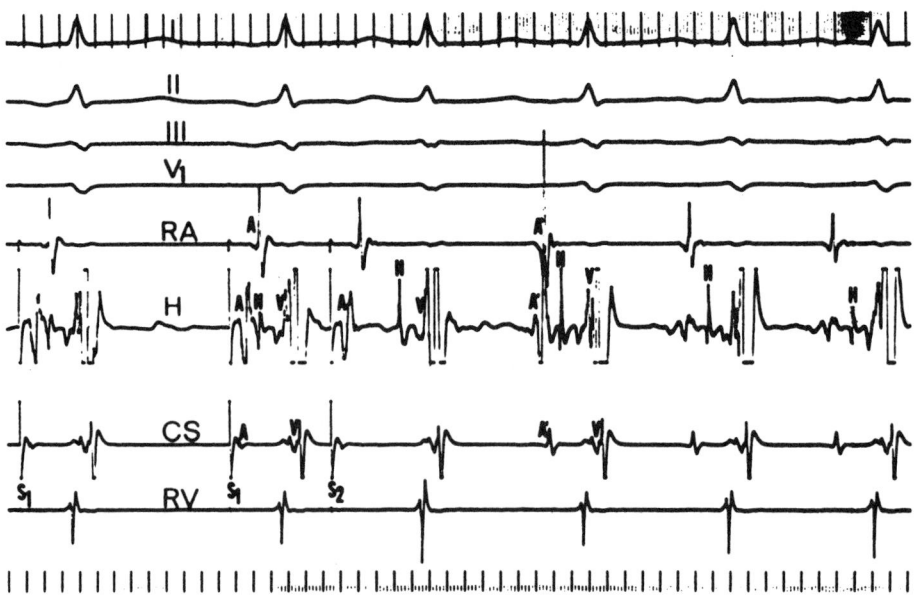

Figure 11. Permanent form of atrioventricular (AV) junctional reciprocating tachycardia (PJRT). During coronary sinus pacing (S₁) conduction travels anterogradely over the normal AV node-His bundle pathway. Following a premature stimulus (S₂) the impulse delays over the normal AV node and conducts retrogradely over the accessory pathway to reach the atrium (A'), producing a low-high atrial activation sequence. Recording from the distal coronary sinus (CS) shows late atrial activation. Note the long RP-short PR interval consistent with this type of tachycardia and quite in contrast to that which occurs during AV nodal reentry and orthodromic AVRT. Note the negative P waves in leads II, III, and aVF, consistent with a posterior insertion of the accessory pathway near the coronary sinus os.

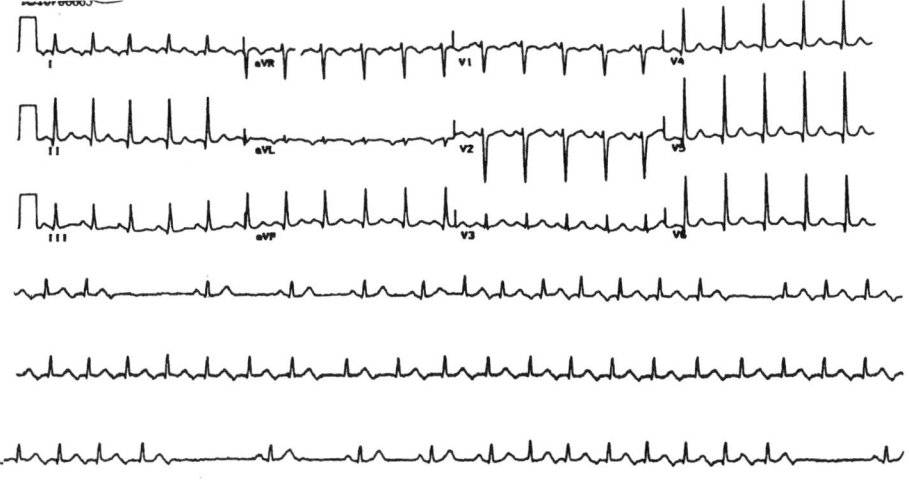

Figure 12. Permanent form of atrioventricular junctional reciprocating tachycardia (PJRT) in a patient with a left-sided accessory pathway. The 12-lead ECG demonstrates a long RP interval-short PR interval tachycardia, which, in contrast to the usual form of PJRT, exhibits negative P waves in leads I and aVL. The rhythm strips below (lead I) indicate that whenever a nonconducted P wave occurs, the tachycardia always terminates, only to begin again after several beats. At times, tachycardia begins with a negative P wave. This is in marked contrast to patients who have atrial tachycardias in which the tachycardia continues despite nonconducted P waves. It is important to recognize this tachycardia, since it is virtually incessant and can cause a cardiomyopathy. It can be cured by radiofrequency catheter ablation, as was the case in this patient.

Another group of patients have atriofascicular pathways, accessory pathways that connect the atrium to the bundle branches, generally the distal portion of the right bundle branch. In these patients, anterograde conduction over the accessory pathway is relatively slow. Tachycardia results from anterograde conduction over the atriofascicular accessory pathway and retrograde conduction over the normal pathway, giving rise to a tachycardia with a left bundle branch block contour.

Patients with a short PR interval and normal QRS complex who also exhibit tachycardia have been reported and have been called the Lown-Ganong-Levine syndrome. The short PR interval and normal QRS complex has been ascribed to so-called James fibers that connect the atrium to the distal portion of the AV node and His bundle. No functional evidence has been published to support that conduction actually occurs over these James fibers and the general perception is that the Lown-Ganong-Levine syndrome does not exist. Nevertheless, a rare patient with an unusual atrio-His connection, distinct from the James fibers, and tachycardia has been described. However, this appears to be an unusual entity.

Ventricular Reentry

Many animal and clinical studies support reentry in the ventricle as a cause of sustained ventricular tachycardia. While bundle branch reentry has been demonstrated in dogs and humans, reentry in ventricular muscle, with or without contribution from specialized tissue, is responsible for many or most ventricular tachycardias in patients with ischemic heart disease. Surviving myocardial tissue separated by fibrous connective tissue provides serpentine routes of activation that can establish reentry pathways. Both figure-of-eight and single circle reentrant loops have been described, circulating around an area of functional block or conducting slowly across an apparent area of block created by anisotropy. Structural discontinuities that separate muscle bundles, owing to naturally occurring myocardial fiber orientation and anisotropic conduction, as well as to collagen matrices formed from the fibrosis after a myocardial infarction, establish the basis for slowed conduction, fragmented electrograms, and continuous electrical activity that can lead to reentry. After the infarction, action potential recordings from surviving cells return to normal, suggesting that depressed activity in these cells does not account for the slowed conduction. During acute ischemia, however, a variety of factors, including elevated extracellular potassium concentration and reduced pH, combine to create depressed action potentials in ischemic cells that retard conduction and can lead to reentry. In many patients with coronary artery disease, it is likely that the origin of the tachycardia, part of its reentrant loop, or a necessary pathway for exit to the rest of the ventricle resides in the endocardium after myocardial infarction.

Ventricular tachycardia can be associated with a variety of disease states and in most instances, the electrophysiological mechanisms responsible are unclear or likely involve more than one possibility. For most patients who have recurrent ventricular tachycardia associated with chronic coronary artery disease, usually after myocardial infarction, the most likely mechanism responsible for the ventricular tachycardia is reentry. However, during acute myocardial ischemia/infarction, normal or abnormal automaticity, triggered activity and reentry can play a role. In patients with dilated cardiomyopathy, bundle branch reentry is a common cause, while in patients with the long QT syndrome, early afterdepolarizations or sympathetic imbalance may be the basis. Patients following surgical repair of congenital heart disease may develop ventricular tachycardia at the site of the myocardial scar due to reentry. Autonomic dysfunction has been implicated in the genesis of some ventricular tachycardias associated with mitral valve prolapse, but the precise mechanisms are unclear. For the remaining disease states (Table 2), the specific mechanisms are not clear.

Table 2
Ventricular Tachycardia

Disease States
   Coronary artery disease
   Dilated cardiomyopathy
   Right ventricular dysplasia
   Hypertrophic cardiomyopathy
   Structurally normal hearts
   Long QT syndrome
   Sudden cardiac death
   Mitral valve prolapse
   Postoperative surgery for congenital heart disease
   Congestive heart failure
Specific Type
   Bundle branch reentry
   Torsades de pointes
   Triggered
   Verapamil sensitive
   Adenosine sensitive
   Accelerated idioventricular

Bundle Branch Reentry

In the normal ventricle, sustained reentry over the bundle branches generally is not possible because the rapid conduction makes the pathway too short to perpetuate the reentrant excitation. When the ventricle dilates, the pathway may lengthen and sustained ventricular tachycardia due to bundle branch reentry is possible. Retrograde conduction over the left bundle branch system and anterograde conduction over the right bundle branch is the usual route, and creates a QRS complex with a left bundle branch block contour and a normal or leftward frontal plane axis characteristic of bundle branch reentry (Figure 13). Less commonly, conduction in the opposite direction produces a right bundle branch block contour. Bundle branch reentry has been clearly demonstrated to occur in animals and in humans (Figure 14), with sustained ventricular tachycardia appearing to be more prevalent in patients with dilated cardiomyopathy.[32] Therapeutically, creation of bundle branch block interrupts the reentry circuit and eliminates the tachycardia.[33]

Torsades de Pointes

Electrophysiological mechanisms responsible for torsades de pointes (Figure 15) are not completely understood. Intraventricular reentry caused by dispersion of repolarization has been suggested. Against that mechanism is the fact that torsades de pointes is usually difficult to initiate by premature stimulation. More recent data suggests that early afterdepolarizations may be responsible for both the long QT interval and the torsades de pointes.[34]

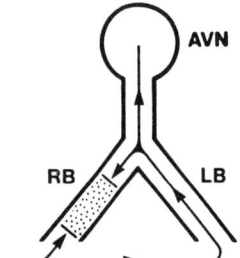 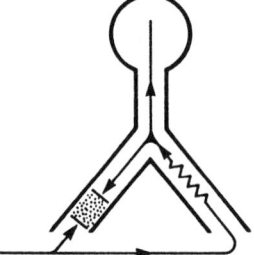 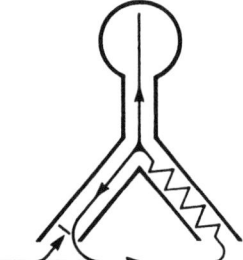

Figure 13. Diagrammatic representation of the proposed mechanism of bundle branch reentry. Stimuli introduced with increasing prematurity blocked retrogradely in the right bundle branch and encountered increased conduction delay in the left bundle branch, until finally the delay is long enough for the right bundle branch to have recovered excitability. It is then able to conduct the impulse in an anterograde direction to complete the circuit. (Reproduced with permission from Lloyd EA, Zipes DP, Heger JJ, et al: Sustained ventricular tachycardia due to bundle branch reentry. *Am Heart J* 104:1095, 1982.)

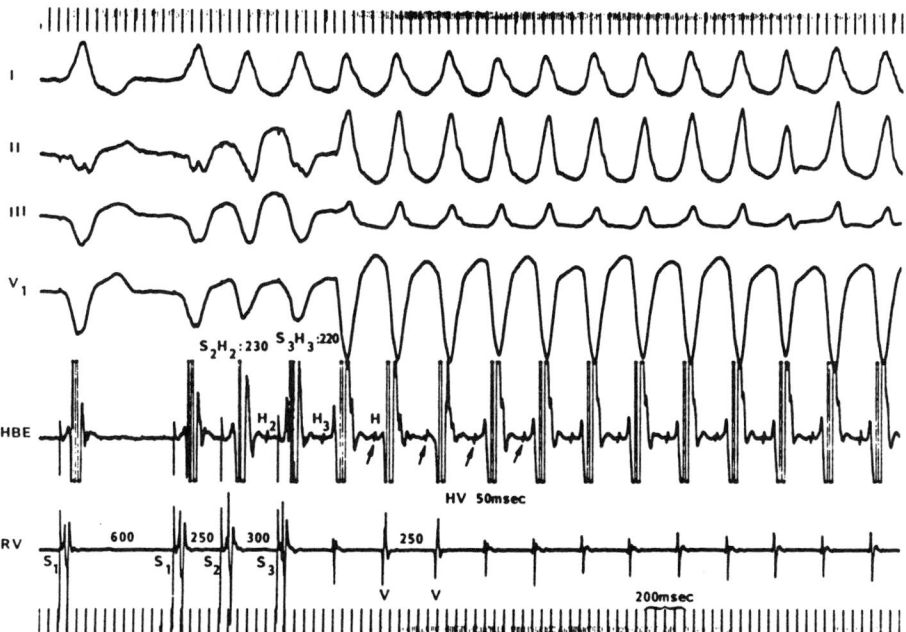

Figure 14. Induction of sustained ventricular tachycardia due to bundle branch reentry. Note the His potential before each ventricular complex with an HV interval of 50 msec that was comparable to the HV interval during normal sinus rhythm. (Reproduced with permission from Lloyd EA, Zipes DP, Heger JJ, et al: Sustained ventricular tachycardia due to bundle branch reentry. *Am Heart J* 104:1095, 1982.)

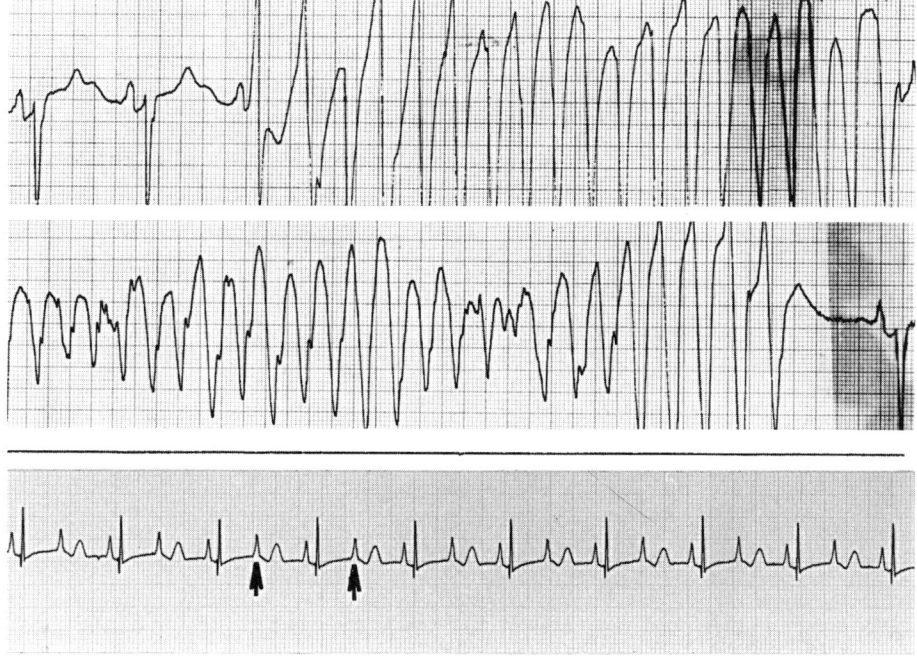

Figure 15. Torsades de pointes and long QT syndrome. The top example illustrates a patient with an acquired long QTU syndrome due to amiodarone with the onset of a polymorphic ventricular tachycardia beginning at a very late coupling interval and alternating polarity, consistent with torsades de pointes. The tachycardia is nonsustained. In the lower panel, the ECG of an infant with congenital long QT syndrome is illustrated. The arrows point to P waves. A 2:1 block is present and the nonconducted P wave occurs prior to the T wave of the preceding QRS complex.

Ventricular Tachycardia in Patients With Structurally Normal Hearts

Patients with normal hearts can have ventricular tachycardia (Figure 16), often arising from the outflow tract of the right ventricle and producing a left bundle branch block morphology with an inferior axis. In other patients, a right bundle branch block-left axis deviation morphology occurs with a probable left ventricular origin. Ventricular tachycardias from the right ventricular outflow tract are often sensitive to adenosine (Figure 16), while ventricular tachycardias with right bundle branch block and left axis deviation can be suppressed by verapamil. Endomyocardial biopsy in some of these patients is abnormal, indicating that at least a percentage of those with apparently primary electrical disease do have histologic abnormalities of the myocardium. Metaiodobenzylguanidine scanning is often abnormal as well, providing evidence for sympathetic denervation.[35] It is likely that the ventricular tachycardia is originating from the endocardium since it can be eliminated by radiofrequency ablation in a high percentage of patients (Figure 17).[36]

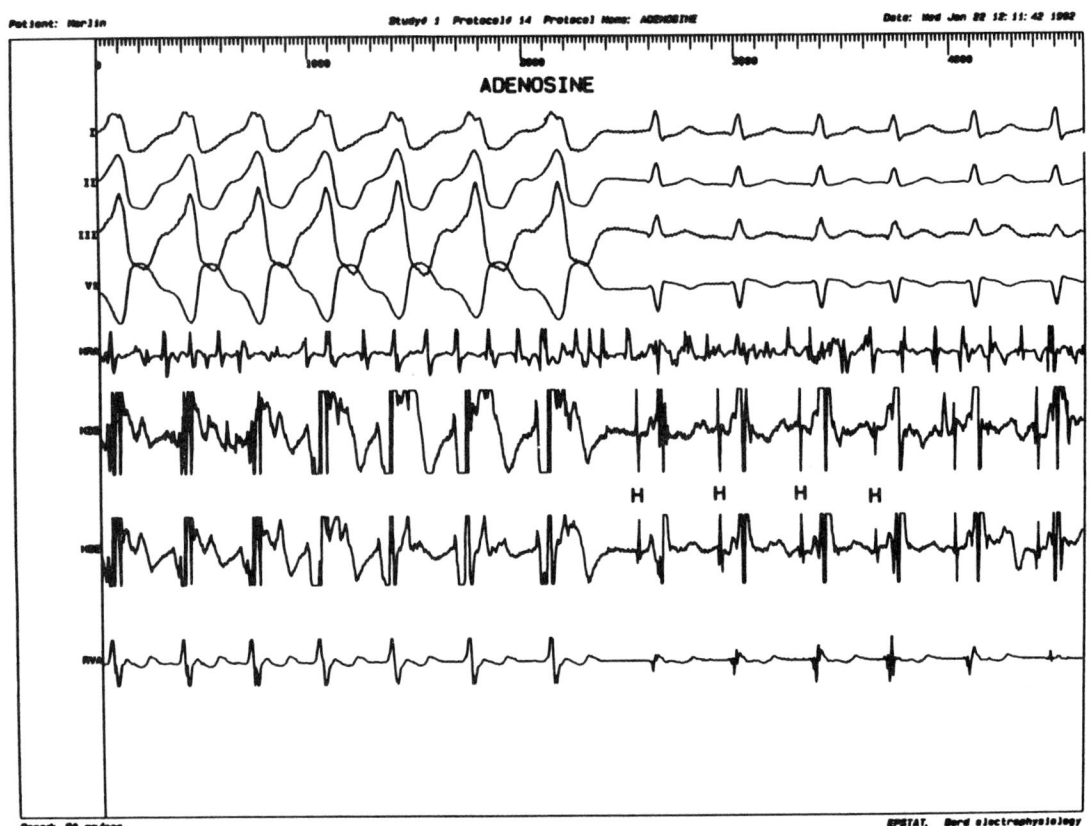

Figure 16. Termination of ventricular tachycardia with adenosine. Ventricular tachycardia arising from the right ventricular outflow tract was initiated in this patient. Adenosine, 12 mg intravenously, terminated the ventricular tachycardia. Atrial fibrillation is present. Note His bundle activation preceding each of the normal QRS complexes but none of the wide QRS complexes. Scalar leads I, II, III, and V₁, and electrograms from the high right atrium, His bundle (2), and right ventricular apex are shown.

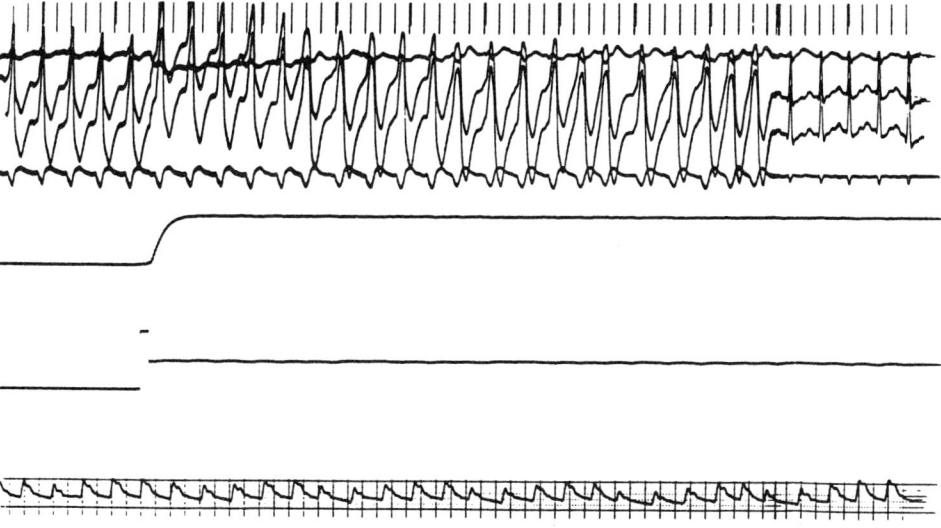

Figure 17. Radiofrequency ablation of the ventricular tachycardia in Figure 16. Voltage and current delivered during radiofrequency ablation, and systemic arterial blood pressure are shown.

References

1. Zipes DP, Jalife J (eds): *Cardiac Electrophysiology. From Cell to Bedside*. Philadelphia, PA: WB Saunders Company, 1990.
2. Brugada P, Wellens HJJ (eds): *Cardiac Arrhythmias: Where Do We Go From Here?* Mt. Kisco, NY: Futura Publishing Company, Inc., 1987.
3. Ward DE, Camm AJ: *Clinical Electrophysiology of the Heart*. New York: Edward Arnold Publishers, 1987.
4. Rosen MR: Mechanisms for arrhythmias. *Am J Cardiol* 61:2a, 1988.
5. Akhtar M, Tchou PJ, Jazayeri M: Mechanisms of clinical tachycardias. *Am J Cardiol* 61:9a, 1988.
6. Pogwizd SM, Corr PB: Reentrant and nonreentrant mechanisms contribute to arrhythmogenesis during early myocardial ischemia: results using three-dimensional mapping. *Circ Res* 61:352, 1987.
7. Kimura S, Bassett AL, Kohya T, et al: Automaticity, triggered activity, and responses to adrenergic stimulation in cat subendocardial Purkinje fibers after healing of myocardial infarction. *Circulation* 75:651, 1987.
8. Dangman KH, Dresdner KP Jr, Zaim S: Automatic and triggered impulse initiation in canine subepicardial ventricular muscle cells from border zones of 24-hour transmural infarcts. New mechanisms for malignant cardiac arrhythmias? *Circulation* 78:1020, 1988.
9. Cranefield PF, Aronson RS: *Cardiac Arrhythmias: The Role of Triggered Activity and Other Mechanisms*. Mt. Kisco, NY: Futura Publishing Company, Inc., 1988.
10. January CT, Shorofsky S: Early afterdepolarizations: newer insights into cellular mechanisms. *J Cardiovasc Electrophysiol* 1:161, 1990.
11. El-Sherif N, Craelius W, Boutjdir M, et al: Early afterdepolarizations and arrhythmogenesis. *J Cardiovasc Electrophysiol* 1:145, 1990.
12. Jackman WM, Szabo B, Friday KJ, et al: Ventricular tachyarrhythmias related to early afterdepolarizations and triggered firing: relationship to QT interval prolongation and potential therapeutic role for calcium channel blocking agents. *J Cardiovasc Electrophysiol* 1:170, 1990.
13. El-Sherif N, Bekheit S, Henkin R: Quinidine-induced long QTU interval and torsades de pointes: role of bradycardiac-dependent early afterdepolarizations. *J Am Coll Cardiol* 14:252, 1989.
14. Zipes DP: Monophasic action potentials in the diagnosis of triggered arrhythmias. *Prog Cardiovasc Dis* 33:385, 1991.
15. Ben-David J, Zipes DP: Alpha adrenoceptor stimulation and blockade modulated cesium-induced early afterdepolarizations and ventricular tachyarrhythmias in dogs. *Circulation* 82:225, 1990.
16. Boutjdir M, El-Sherif N, Gough WB: Effects of caffeine and ryanodine on delayed afterdepolarizations and sustained rhythmic activity in 1-day-old myocardial infarction in the dog. *Circulation* 81:1393, 1990.

17. Wit AL, Tseng G, Henning B, et al: Arrhythmogenic effects of quinidine on catecholamine-induced delayed afterdepolarizations in canine atrial fibers. *J Cardiovasc Electrophysiol* 1:15, 1990.

18. Park JK, Danilo P, Rosen M: Effects of flunarizine on impulse initiation in canine Purkinje fibers. *J Cardiovasc Electrophysiol* (in press).

19. Boyden PA, Frame LH, Hoffman BF: Activation mapping of reentry around an anatomic barrier in the canine atrium. Observations during entrainment and termination. *Circulation* 79:406, 1989.

20. Wit AL, Dillon SM: Anisotropic reentry. In: DP Zipes, J Jalife (eds): *Cardiac Electrophysiology. From Cell to Bedside.* Philadelphia, PA: WB Saunders Company, 1990, p. 353.

21. Moe GK, Abildskov JA: Atrial fibrillation as a self sustaining arrhythmia independent of focal discharge. *Am Heart J* 58:59, 1959.

22. Allessie MA, Rensma PL, Brugada PL, et al: Pathophysiology of atrial fibrillaiton. In: DP Zipes, J Jalife (eds): *Cardiac Electrophysiology. From Cell to Bedside.* Philadelphia, PA: WB Saunders Company, 1990, p. 548.

23. Waldo AL, Carlson MD, Henthorn RW: Atrial flutter: transient entrainment and related phenomena. In: DP Zipes, J Jalife (eds): *Cardiac Electrophysiology. From Cell to Bedside.* Philadelphia, PA: WB Saunders Company, 1990, p. 530.

24. Bonke FIM, Kirchhof CJHS, Allessie MA: Sinus node reentry. In: DP Zipes, J Jalife (eds): *Cardiac Electrophysiology. From Cell to Bedside.* Philadelphia, PA: WB Saunders Company, 1990, p. 526.

25. Haines DE, DiMarco JP: Sustained intraatrial reentrant tachycardia: clinical, electrocardiographic and electrophysiologic characteristics and long-term follow-up. *J Am Coll Cardiol* 15: 1345, 1990.

26. Sung RJ, Huycke EC, Keung EC, et al: Atrioventricular node reentry: evidence of reentry and functional properties of fast and slow pathways In: DP Zipes, J Jalife (eds): *Cardiac Electrophysiology: From Cell to Bedside.* Philadelphia, PA: WB Saunders Company, 1990, p. 513.

27. Jackman WM, Beckman KJ, McClelland JH: Treatment of supraventricular tachycardia due to atrioventricular nodal reentry by radiofrequency catheter ablation of slow pathway conduction. *N Engl J Med* 327:313, 1992.

28. Mitrani R, Klein LS, Hackett K, et al: Radiofrequency ablation for atrioventricular nodal reentrant tachycardia: comparison between fast (anterior) versus slow (posterior) pathway ablation. *J Am Coll Cardiol* 21:432, 1992.

29. Wellens HJJ, Brugada PC, Penn OC, et al: Preexcitation syndromes. In: DP Zipes, J Jalife (eds): *Cardiac Electrophysiology: From Cell to Bedside.* Philadelphia, PA: WB Saunders Company, 1990, p. 691.

30. Jackman WM, Wang X, Friday KJ, et al: Catheterization of accessory atrioventricular pathways (Wolff-Parkinson-White syndrome) by radiofrequency ablation. *N Engl J Med* 324:1605, 1991.

31. Calkins H, Sousa J, El-Atassi R, et al: Diagnosis and cure of the Wolff-Parkinson-White syndrome or paroxysmal supraventricular tachycardias during a simple electrophysiologic test. *N Engl J Med* 324:1612, 1991.

32. Caceres J, Jazayeri M, McKinnie J, et al: Sustained bundle branch reentry as a mechanism of clinical tachycardia. *Circulation* 79:256, 1989.

33. Tchou P, Jazayeri M, Denker S, et al: Transcatheter electrical ablation of right bundle branch. A method of treating macroreentrant ventricular tachycardia attributed to bundle branch reentry. *Circulation* 78:246, 1988.

34. Kadish AH, Morady F: Torsades de pointes. In: DP Zipes, J Jalife (eds): *Cardiac Electrophysiology: From Cell to Bedside.* Philadelphia, PA: WB Saunders Company, 1990, p. 605.

35. Mitrani R, Klein LS, Miles WM, et al: Regional cardiac sympathetic denervation in patients with ventricular tachycardia in the absence of coronary artery disease. *PACE* 15:535, 1992.

36. Klein LS, Hackett K, Zipes DP, Miles WM: Radiofrequency catheter ablation of ventricular tachycardia in patients without structural heart disease. *Circulation* 85:1666, 1992.

Chapter 14

Evolving Concepts in the Long QT Syndrome

Silvia G. Priori
Carlo Napolitano
Peter J. Schwartz

Despite much progress, idiopathic long QT syndrome (LQTS) remains a mystery, a "unique example of non-coronary neurally mediated sudden cardiac death".[1] This definition points to one critical aspect of the disease, ie, the striking link between the sympathetic nervous system and the development of lethal arrhythmias. However, the most remarkable and qualifying feature of LQTS is the prolongation of the QT interval on the surface electrocardiogram (ECG). Accordingly, LQTS is correctly regarded as a congenital abnormality of ventricular repolarization. As synthesized by Moss and Schwartz[2] in 1979, "LQTS seems to provide a mechanistic link between the central nervous system, a delayed repolarization in the heart and sudden death." Indeed, LQTS has been repeatedly compared to the Rosetta stone[3] because of its intriguing secret and because, once fully elucidated, LQTS has the potential to allow an understanding of how the link between duration of ventricular repolarization, sympathetic activity, and life-threatening arrhythmias operates.

The clinical presentation, epidemiology, and management of LQTS have been thoroughly discussed elsewhere.[4–7] In consideration of the major thrust of this volume, it seems appropriate to focus on some electrophysiological aspects, including the potential role of specific ionic mechanisms and their relationship with adrenergic activation. First, we briefly review the ionic basis for ventricular repolarization, and then discuss the two leading hypotheses for LQTS. We conclude with an overview on the electrophysiological mechanisms involved in the arrhythmias that so often lead to the sudden death of many patients affected by the LQTS.

Ionic Basis of Ventricular Repolarization

In this section we briefly identify the major players involved in cardiac repolarization. For a more extensive review of this subject the readers are referred to Chapters 1 and 3. This short overview will serve as introduction to one of the two leading hypotheses put

From BN Singh, HJJ Wellens, M Hiraoka, (eds): *Electropharmacological Control of Cardiac Arrhythmias.* Mount Kisco, NY, Futura Publishing Company Inc., © 1994.

forward to explain the prolonged repolarization in LQTS: "the intracardiac abnormality hypothesis."[8,9]

Action potential duration (APD) in ventricular myocytes of most mammals depends on the duration of the phase 2 repolarization, ie, the so-called plateau. This component of the action potential is characterized by a fine balance of inward and outward currents, and even a small change in ionic conductance can dramatically alter APD. At the depolarized level at which the plateau develops most ionic channels actively conduct positive (Na^+, Ca^{2+}, K^+) and negative charges (Cl^-). This situation is summarized in Figure 1.

During phase 1 of the action potential, at

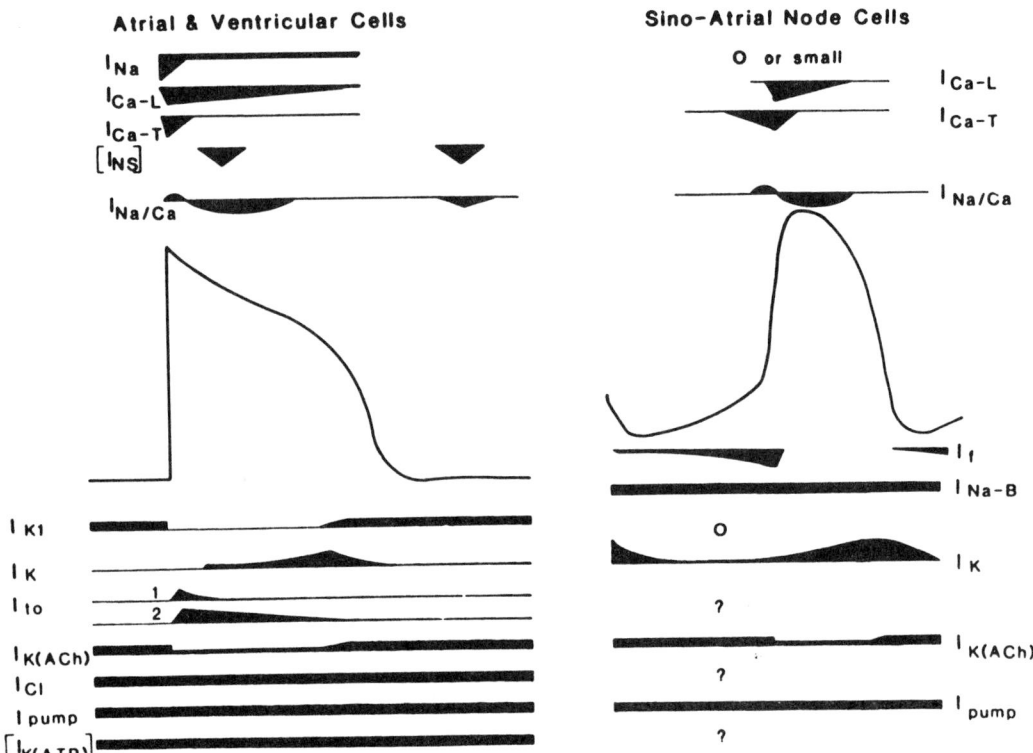

Figure 1. Currents and channels involved in generating the resting and action potential. The time course of a stylized action potential of atrial and ventricular cells is shown on the left and sinoatrial node cells on the right. Above and below are the various channels and pumps that contribute the currents underlying the electrical events. Where possible, the approximate time courses of the currents associated with the channels or pumps are shown symbolically without effort to represent their magnitudes relative to each other. The heavy bars for I_{Cl}, I_{pump}, and $I_{K(ATP)}$ only indicate the presence of these channels or pump without implying magnitude of currents since that would vary with physiological and pathophysiological conditions. The channels identified by brackets [I_{NS} and $I_{K(ATP)}$] imply that they are active only under pathological conditions. For the sinoatrial node cells, I_{Na} and I_{K1} are small or absent. Question marks indicate that experimental evidence is not yet available to determine the presence of these channels in sinoatrial cell membranes. Although it is likely that other ionic current mechanisms exist, they are shown here because their roles in electrogenesis are not sufficiently well defined. (Reproduced with permission from The Sicilian gambit: A new approach to the classification of antiarrhythmic drugs based on their actions on arrhythmogenic mechanisms. Task Force of the Working Group on Arrhythmias of the European Society of Cardiology. *Circulation* 84:1831, 1991.)

the time in which sodium conductance decreases sharply, a small repolarization occurs that brings the intracellular potential to more negative values. This repolarization process has been related to the potassium current I_{to}. Phase 1 repolarization is actually not a constant feature of ventricular myocytes throughout the ventricular wall. Sicouri and Antzelevitch[10] have extensively characterized the different behavior of ventricular myocytes in respect to the presence of I_{to}, and have shown that I_{to} is more prominent at subepicardial level and that its presence is indicated by a characteristic "spike-and-dome" morphology.

The early concept that a chloride current is implicated in the early phase of repolarization has been recently questioned,[11] but new evidence focuses on the role of chloride that is now considered, at least in some animal species, as a component of I_{to}.[12]

The plateau or phase 2 of the action potential is a very complex transition in which many small currents become operant. As it appears in Figure 1, the major determinant of the plateau is the slow inward current mediated by the flow of calcium ions. However, this is by no means the only inward current active at this time. Among the many currents that have been implicated, one should also mention the Na "window" current, a slowly inactivating Na^+ current, possibly a Ca^{2+} "window" current, and the electrogenic Na-Ca^{2+} exchanger.

Despite the fact that many inward currents are involved in the regulation of repolarization, when this critical component of the action potential is discussed most people make an almost automatic association with the outward currents and particularly with the many K^+ currents. This direct association between repolarization and potassium currents may partially depend on the fact that there are several K^+ currents implicated in the control of return of membrane potential to the resting value (the most important are I_k, I_{kl}, I_{to}, I_{k-ATP}). Additionally, the pharmacological tools aimed at modifying the APD are active on potassium currents, as extensively discussed in this book.

On this basis it is rather logical that for the idiopathic LQTS, an abnormality in the control of the potassium currents has been suggested as a possible hereditary defect responsible for creating the substrate of a prolonged action potential.[8,9] More vaguely, but along the same lines, this concept had been previously proposed by Jervell[13] and by James.[14]

The Cardiac Abnormality Hypothesis

The hypothesis that an undefined alteration in the regulation of K^+ channels or currents may create the substrate on which catecholamines act as a trigger for the induction of tachyarrhythmias in the LQTS has progressively attracted growing consensus. This makes sense because the possibility of a genetically transmitted defect in one specific channel or current is intellectually very attractive.

Since it was proposed by Moss and Schwartz in 1986,[8,9] this elegant hypothesis has been more extensively discussed by Schwartz et al.[6] and by Vincent et al.[15] However, it is fair to remember that already in 1975 Schwartz et al.[4] wrote: "The possibility cannot be ruled out that some local myocardial abnormality might also be involved in the pathogenesis of the disease. In such a case, the sympathetic interventions would only trigger the syncopal episodes." This concept was more explicitly presented by Schwartz in 1985[5] "... leaves open the possibility that the basic defect in LQTS is an unknown intracardiac abnormality that decreases electrical stability and makes the myocardium more vulnerable to the effect of sympathetic discharges. In this case the sympathetic nervous system, acting mostly through the quantitatively dominant left stellate ganglion, would merely represent the trigger for the ventricular arrhythmias that lead to death the patients with LQTS." Thus, concepts that to some appear as new have already been presented years ago.

From a theoretical standpoint it is clear that many features of LQTS could be accounted for by an abnormal function of potassium channels and that several arrhythmogenic mechanisms could be potentiated. As an example, a decrease in I_k conductance may prolong APD, thus favoring the development of early afterdepolarizations (EADs), as occurs in the experimental setting when cesium is used to block I_k,[16] thus inducing EADs,[17] which are markedly enhanced by sympathetic stimulation.[18]

A reduction in potassium currents may also facilitate reentry by enhancing dispersion of repolarization. In fact, since the APD of Purkinje fibers is more strictly dependent on K^+ conductance[19] as opposed to the APD of ventricular myocytes that mainly rely upon fading of inward currents,[20] a decrease in I_k may selectively prolong APD in Purkinje fibers more than in muscle. This would increase the discrepancy in refractoriness among the two tissues. Inhomogeneity in refractoriness between adjacent tissues may become an ideal substrate for the establishment of reentrant circuits.[21] Finally, a reduction of potassium background current may result in an increase of input resistance of myocardial cells, which means that a smaller amount of inward current as provided by electrotonic propagation or by delayed afterdepolarizations (DADs) may trigger a larger depolarization of the cells and bring them to threshold.[22]

Direct evidence for the implication of an abnormal function of potassium channels in LQTS is not yet available. However, new insights are being provided by significant genetic studies that have recently shed more light on the abnormality that may be present in the LQTS. A linkage analysis performed by Keating et al.[23,24] in a large family affected by LQTS has provided data that are quite likely to represent a major breakthrough. Indeed, a DNA marker at the Harvey ras-1 locus, located on the short arm of chromosome 11, was found to be linked to LQTS. The current hypothesis as shown in Figure 2, is that ras proteins likely to be involved in signal transduction, exist in an equilibrium between an inactive conformation (p21-GDP) and an active conformation (p21-GTP), which in turn can form a complex with a GTPase-activating protein (GAP) and then becomes able to interact with its target molecule(s).[25] The relation between ras proteins and G proteins has led to speculations about the possibility that this locus might be involved in the regulation of potassium channels. However, the situation may be more complex than what may appear at first glance. Indeed, Yatani et al.[26] have demonstrated that ras p21-GTP complexed with GAP blocks the current Ik(ACh), which is the potassium current affecting repolarization in the atria. Conversely, no evidence is yet available on the potential effects of p21 GTP-GAP on the potassium currents involved with ventricular repolarization, such as I_k or I_{kl} or I_{to}. The recent proposal that ras p21 causes a conformational change in GAP that relieves a negative constraint that normally prevents GAP interacting with its target has already been discussed in relation to the LQTS.[27] Further complexities become also apparent as more LQTS families are tested for linkage on chromosome 11. Although Keating et al.[28] confirmed their original observations in another group of five families, Towbin et al.[29] were able to confirm it in 7 of 11 LQTS families; this finding can be interpreted to suggest that LQTS is linked to the Harvey ras 1 locus in the majority of families, but also that genetic heterogeneity does exist.

At this time the intracardiac abnormality hypothesis is receiving a lot of attention. It is fair to keep in mind that, despite its intellectual appeal, it is not yet clear if it could satisfactorily explain the diverse and bizarre clinical manifestations of LQTS, eg, low heart rate, T wave alternans, abnormal movement of the left posterior wall, and so on. If proven correct, there would be several advantages from both a scientific as well as a clinical standpoint. As far as therapy is concerned, however, in 1975[4] and again in 1985[5] it has been clearly indicated that in this case also the syncopal episodes would depend on hyperactivity of cardiac sympathetic nerves with a special role for the quantitatively dominant left ones. Thus, therapy would still rest primarily on β-adrenergic blockade and/or left cardiac sympathetic denervation.

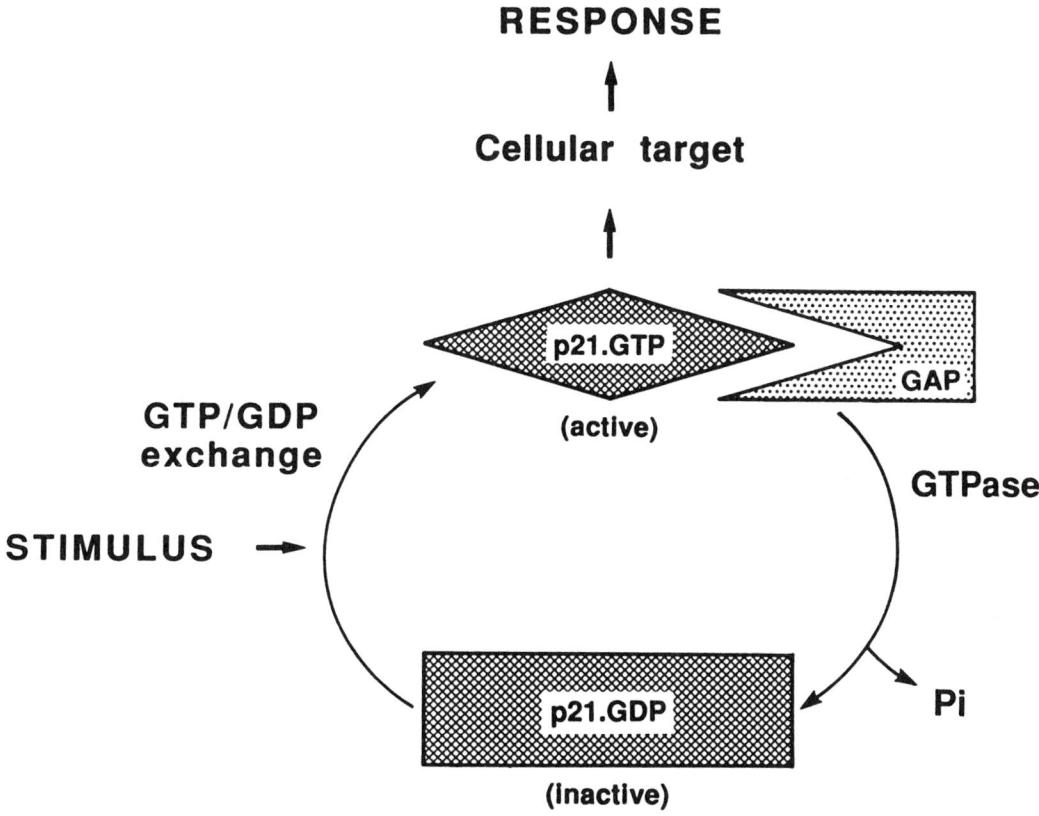

Figure 2. Biochemical model of ras function. See text for details. (Modified with permission from Reference 25.)

Modulation of Repolarization by the Sympathetic Nervous System

Clinical evidence has indicated that sympathetic activity plays a major role in triggering the onset of the arrhythmias of LQTS. Accordingly, there is considerable interest in the influence of adrenergic stimulation on ventricular repolarization which, as matter of fact, has been extensively investigated.

β-Adrenergic stimulation has been shown by several investigators to modify APD. However, since different cardiac tissues and various concentrations of β-adrenergic agonists have been used, some uncertainty still remains regarding the effect of catecholamines on APD under physiological conditions.

An example is represented by the fact that β-adrenergic stimulation can either prolong or shorten APD. Giotti et al.[30] reported in 1973 that isoproterenol reduces APD in Purkinje fibers in a dose-dependent manner. Belardinelli and Isenberg[31] reported instead that exposure of isolated myocytes to low (10^{-9} mol/L) concentrations of isoproterenol prolonged APD, and Reuter[32] observed a prolongation of APD at high concentrations of isoproterenol (10^{-6} mol/L) in a multicellular ventricular preparation. Quadbeck and Reuter[33] reported a biphasic effect consisting of a transient prolongation of APD followed by a shortening. They suggested that the initial prolongation depends on the enhancement of calcium conductance, while the shortening that follows was attributed to an indirect mechanism dependent on the effect of intracellular calcium

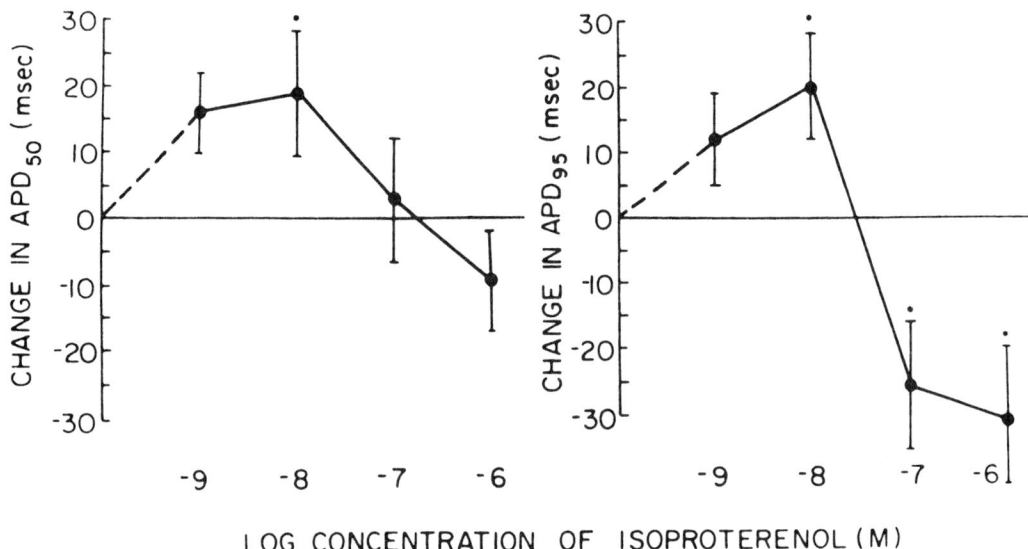

Figure 3. Changes in action potential duration (APD) at 50% of full repolarization (APD$_{50}$, left) and 95% of full repolarization (APD$_{95}$, right) induced by increasing concentrations of isoproterenol (10^{-9} mol/L, $n = 3$; 10^{-8} mol/L, $n = 5$; 10^{-7} mol/L, $n = 5$; 10^{-6} mol/L, $n = 5$). Values are mean $\pm$ SD. *$p < 0.05$ versus control. (Reproduced with permission from Reference 34.)

concentration on g$_K$. Priori and Corr[34] more recently found that canine ventricular myocytes present a dose-related biphasic response to isoproterenol; they observed a prolongation of APD at low concentrations (10^{-8} mol/L and 10^{-9} mol/L) and a shortening at high concentrations (10^{-7} mol/L and 10^{-6} mol/L) (Figure 3). The effect of α-adrenergic stimulation on the APD has been more consistent and it has concordantly been shown[34] that α-adrenergic agonists induce a prolongation of the APD.

It is fair to note that in vivo, during activation of the sympathetic nervous system, both α- and β-adrenergic receptors activation coexist and that the overall effect on APD may be difficult to predict. Priori et al.[35] recorded monophasic action potentials in cats and observed shortening during maximal stimulation of the left stellate ganglion; this suggests that a shortening of APD may be the predominant steady-state response to adrenergic activation in vivo.

In order to understand how such a diversity of effects can be induced by sympathetic stimulation on the APD, we briefly analyze the effect of α- or β-adrenergic stimulation on the major ionic currents that influence APD.

Effect of Adrenergic Stimulation on I$_{Ca-L}$

The concept that β-adrenergic activation increases calcium current dates back to the 1960s, when Reuter[32] and Rougier et al.[36] made their initial observation, subsequently confirmed by several investigators. In the early 1970s it was discovered that the mediator of the effect of β-adrenergic agonists was indeed the second messenger cAMP,[37] which activates a cAMP-dependent kinase that in turn phosphorylates the calcium channel: when the channel is phosphorylated the influx of calcium in the cell is potentiated. More recently it has been shown that β-adrenergic stimulation increases I$_{Ca-L}$ by altering the gating properties of the channel[38] so that an increased number of channels are activated by depolarization while the conductance of the single channel is not altered.[39] Is this relevant to LQTS? Perhaps, because this increase of calcium inward current mediated by catecholamines may favor prolongation of the action potential, particularly in ventricular myocytes whose plateau is largely influenced by inward currents. It has also been suggested that an increase in g_{Ca}, especially if associated with a reduced K^+ conductance might result in EAD.[40] This arrhythmogenic mechanism may be operant in LQTS if one postulates the existence of an intrinsic abnormality of K^+ channels (substrate) on which adrenergic activation may act as a trigger that enhances calcium conductance.

α-Adrenergic stimulation has been implicated in the activation of calcium currents,[41-43] however, at present a direct role of α receptor in the modulation of I_{Ca-L} seems unlikely.[44] It is still under debate whether activation of these receptors may increase intracellular calcium by activating phospholipase C, which in turns activates the IP3 pathway.[45,46]

Effects of β-Adrenergic Stimulation on the Delayed Rectifier I_k

Although several studies have shown that β-adrenergic agonists increase the amplitude of I_k, the regulation of the delayed rectifier is not as well understood as the regulation of I_{Ca-L}. Part of this incomplete understanding is a result of the difficulty in discriminating between a direct activation of I_k by catecholamines and an indirect activation induced by intracellular calcium that would increase I_k, or alternatively, by the activation of Na^+/K^+ pump that can change the K^+ driving force.[47,48] However, considerable evidence has proven that cAMP-dependent phosphorylation regulates also I_k[49] and it has also been shown that the concentration response curves for I_{Ca} and I_k are very similar[50] suggesting that augmentation of the two currents is likely to be simultaneous.

Effects of Adrenergic Stimulation on Transient Outward Current I_{to}

The transient outward current has been identified in many cardiac preparations and at least two conductances that may or may not coexist in the same preparation have been identified, one of which is Ca^{2+} dependent and the other that is sensitive to 4-aminopyridine.[51] I_{to} is thought to play a role in frequency-dependent changes in APD.[52] It has also been suggested that a component of I_{to} may be represented by a chloride current[53] that is regulated by intracellular cAMP.[11] This hypothesis would suggest that catecholamines may also control APD by acting through the modulation of chloride permeability.

If a relatively tight association has been suggested for catecholamines and the chloride component of I_{to}, little is known about the regulation of its K^+ component. It has recently been reported that at least the calcium-insensitive component is significantly increased by norepinephrine[54]; the effects of norepinephrine appear to be mediated by β-adrenergic receptors. In fact, as it has been suggested by Apkon and Nerbonne,[44] $α_1$-adrenergic receptors activation indeed reduces I_{to}; an analogous finding has also been reported by Fedida et al.[55] Such an effect on I_{to} has been used to explain the prolongation of APD observed during α-adrenergic stimulation. This prolongation of APD may favor the development of EAD and triggered arrhythmias and may also increase intracellular calcium accumulation and facilitate the development of DADs.

We have analyzed the effects of adrenergic activation on the major ionic determinants of repolarization. It seems clear that no simplistic conclusion can be drawn to predict whether in a given condition sympathetic stimulation will shorten or prolong APD. In fact, many effects occur simultaneously: depolarizing and repolarizing currents are activated by the same second messengers, α- and β-adrenergic receptors are concomitantly stimulated and they often produce opposite effects. It is therefore impossible to predict which effects will predominate at any point in time. This picture is even more complicated by the fact that APD depends on heart rate, and therefore, it adapts constantly to the driving frequency. The kinetics of this adaptation of APD to heart rate is strongly influenced by the sympathetic nervous system, with major differences between right and left cardiac sympathetic activity.[56] Additionally, our analysis has been substantially simplified by the fact that we did not take into consideration the influences of autonomic modulation on ionic pumps and exchangers and factors such as the voltage level of the plateau and dynamic interactions among the various currents.

These limitations notwithstanding, the analysis of the effects of sympathetic stimulation at the level of ionic channels may help to single out the several arrhythmogenic mechanisms that may become operant during adrenergic activation.

The Sympathetic Imbalance Hypothesis

The role of the activation of the sympathetic nervous system in the development of the lethal arrhythmias in the LQTS has been extensively demonstrated together with the therapeutic effectiveness of anti-adrenergic interventions.[5,57,58] What remains unsettled is whether an abnormality in sympathetic innervation of the heart is also a contributing cause to LQTS.

In 1975, Schwartz et al.[4] proposed for the first time as the primary abnormality in LQTS a lower than normal right cardiac sympathetic activity that would reflexively result in a higher than normal activity of the quantitatively dominant[59] left cardiac sympathetic nerves. This hypothesis has been tested in the laboratory by observing the changes that follow the creation of a sympathetic imbalance obtained by removing the right stellate ganglion and also by stimulating the left stellate ganglion. The results of these experimental studies are generally consistent with the possibility of a sympathetic imbalance in LQTS. Re-

markable is the fact that most, if not all, of the clinical features of LQTS are reproduced by this specific type of sympathetic imbalance. In this section we list some of the characteristics of LQTS and discuss how they may relate to a lower than normal right cardiac sympathetic activity.

QT Interval Prolongation

In 1966, Yanowitz and co-workers[60] showed that removal of the right stellate ganglion prolongs ventricular repolarization, as can be seen by the increase in duration of the QT interval. This original observation has been confirmed in several animal species and in humans as well.[61] The mechanism by which an imbalance in cardiac sympathetic innervation, characterized by left dominance, can prolong repolarization remains undefined.

An inhomogeneous release of catecholamines to ventricular cells, as would occur in the presence of a lower than normal right cardiac sympathetic innervation, could create discrepancies in APD in a way similar to what has been suggested to be the case when local denervation is caused by myocardial infarction. Dispersion of APD in LQTS has already been shown by Gavrilescu and Luca[62] and by Bonatti et al.[63] who used monophasic action potential recordings.

A more direct link between cardiac sympathetic innervation and the QT interval duration comes from a recent analysis[58] of the patients enrolled in the LQTS International Registry who underwent left cardiac sympathetic denervation because β-adrenergic blockade was ineffective in preventing syncope or cardiac arrest. For the first time it was demonstrated that, at variance with what previously thought, this selective denervation reduces the duration of QT interval (mean QTc shortens from 548 ± 81 to 507 ± 84, $p < 0.005$; the data and changes are similar for the uncorrected QT). It was also shown in the same study that although the degree of shortening is independent of the initial length, there is a correlation with outcome. The patients who

EFFECT OF LCSD ON QTc AND CARDIAC EVENTS

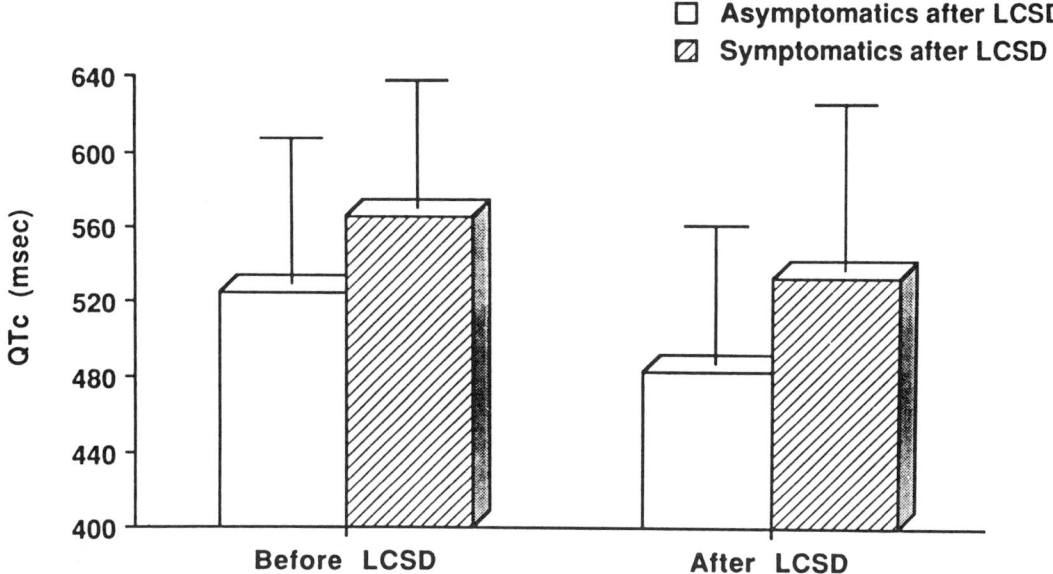

Figure 4. QTc of long QT syndrome (LQTS) patients who, after left cardiac sympathetic denervation (LCSD), became completely asymptomatic (*n* = 45) or still have one or more cardiac events (symptomatics, *n* = 37). It is evident that: (1) before surgery the QTc was already less prolonged among those patients destined to become asymptomatic; (2) that after LCSD, QTc shortened to a similar extent in both groups; and (3) because of the different starting points, the QTc of the patients who became asymptomatic is definitely closer to the upper limit of normal values (440 msec). (Reproduced with permission from Reference 61.)

became fully asymptomatic after denervation were those who had a relatively shorter QTc prior to surgery and who, because of the ensuing shortening, ended up with a QTc closer to normal values (Figure 4).

Heart Rate

A lower than normal heart rate is often observed in LQTS patients, particularly in the young ones and also during exercise, as it was originally described by Schwartz et al. in 1975[4] and later confirmed by Vincent in a comparative study.[64] It is remarkable that no intrinsic abnormality of sinus node function has been identified in LQTS patients. The attention has therefore turned toward the sympathetic innervation of the sinus node. As the sympathetic control of sinus node activity depends

primarily on the nerves originating from the right stellate ganglion,[65,66] the clinical observation of a lower than normal heart rate is just what one would expect with a lower than normal right sympathetic activity. Indeed, conscious dogs without the right stellate ganglion have significantly lower heart rates both at rest and during exercise.[66]

T Wave Alternans

Alternation of the T wave is a striking feature of LQTS, as first reported and discussed in 1975 by Schwartz and Malliani.[67] In addition to their clinical observation, they were able to reproduce T wave alternans in cats by electrical stimulation of the left stellate ganglion (Figure 5). The same phenomenon has been observed in LQTS patients either after right

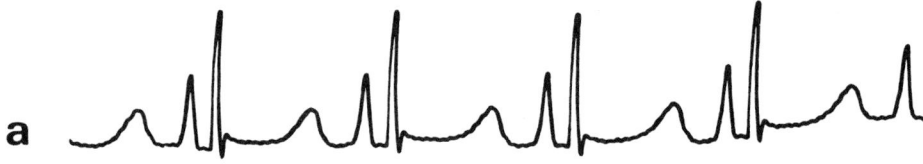

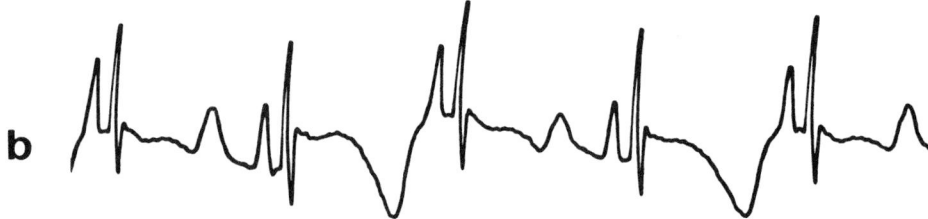

Figure 5. Anesthetized cat: ECG (D2). (a): control and (b): 5 seconds after the cessation of a 30-second electrical stimulation of both stellate ganglia (left ganglion: 20 V, 2 msec, and 20 Hz; right ganglion: 10 V, 2 msec, and 20 Hz). Alternation in polarity of the T wave is evident. (Reproduced with permission from Reference 67.)

stellate ganglion blockade[68] or after stimulation of the left stellate ganglion.[69] These data are clearly consistent with the sympathetic imbalance hypothesis.

Echocardiographic Abnormality

A recent case control study[70] performed in 42 LQTS patients and in 42 healthy controls carefully matched for several variables, has demonstrated the frequent occurrence of an unusual and specific ventricular wall motion abnormality in LQTS, and its association with history of syncope or cardiac arrest. Two new measurements were developed to assess quantitatively the abnormalities observed. The first is an index of the rapidity of the early contraction phase and the second is an index of the presence of a slow movement in the late thickening phase with a plateau morphology. The study showed that LQTS patients reach half-maximal systolic contraction more rapidly than controls, and then spend much more time at a very low thickening rate just prior to the fast relaxation (Figure 6). These abnormalities were found in 55% of LQTS and in 5% of the controls ($p < 0.005$). Also important is the fact that they occur much more frequently among the LQTS patients with syncope or cardiac arrest (77% versus 19%, $p < 0.005$). It is relevant to note that the same alterations were produced by right stellectomy in 9 of 9 dogs. Once more, the sympathetic imbalance has reproduced the clinical feature.

Dispersion of Repolarization

As previously discussed, a nonhomogeneous duration of action potentials may determine the prolongation of QT interval observed in LQTS. Additionally, as it will be discussed, dispersion of repolarization may create the substrate for the development of ventricular tachyarrhythmias by reentry.

The existence of anomalous patterns of repolarization in LQTS has been demonstrated and quantified by the analysis of the body surface distribution of electrocardio-

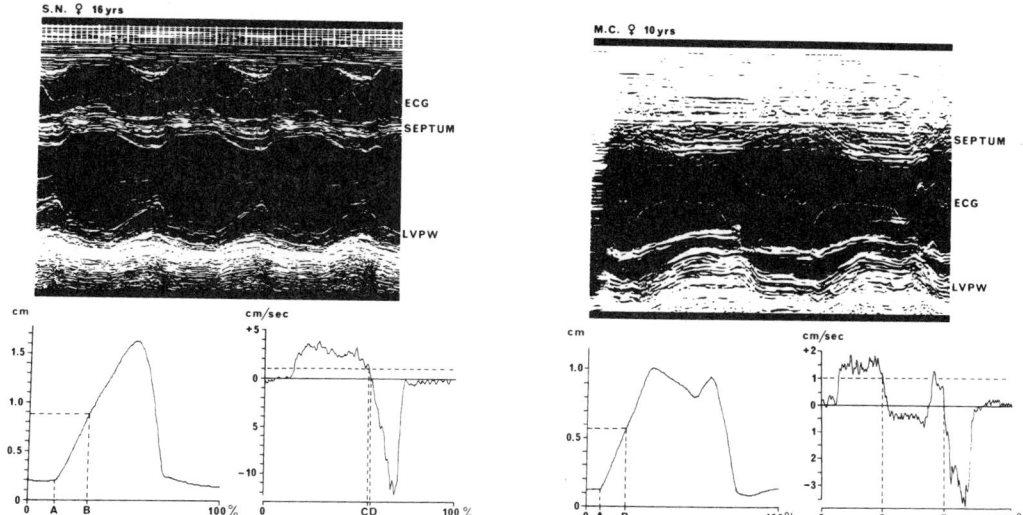

Figure 6. Left panel: control subject, M-mode examination from the long-axis parasternal view. Upper panel shows the echocardiographic tracing and the ECG at a speed of 100 mm/sec. Lower left panel reproduces the endocardial contour of the movement of the left ventricular posterior wall. Lower right panel shows the first derivative of wall thickening. Segment A–B indicates the time to reach half of maximal systolic contraction as percent of cardiac cycle (Th1/2). Segment C–D indicates the time spent during the late thickening phase, before rapid relaxation, at a rate smaller than 1 cm/sec (TSTh). LVPW: left ventricular posterior wall. **Right panel:** LQTS patient, M-mode examination from the long-axis parasternal view. In this case, the main abnormality is represented by a major prolongation of the time spent in the late thickening phase and especially by the occurrence of a dip followed by a second anterior movement of the endocardium, resulting in a double peak morphology. (Modified with permission from Reference 70.)

graphic potentials in LQTS patients as assessed by body surface mapping studies. The original observation by Abildskov et al.[71] was confirmed and extended by De Ambroggi et al.[72] who found a larger than normal area of negative values in the anterior chest that was interpreted as a delayed repolarization of the anterior ventricular wall. This is consistent with the concept of a lower than normal right cardiac sympathetic activity, which is preferentially distributed to the anterior ventricular wall. The other critical finding was that a complex multipolar distribution is observed in 15% of 48 LQTS patients and in none of the controls. This aspect suggests regional electrical disparities in the recovery process (Figure 7). In a subsequent study involving 40 LQTS patients, a group almost entirely different from the previous one, and 30 controls, a simi-

larity index was computed by applying a principal component analysis, which represents (in percent) to what extent one fundamental pattern of ST-T reproduces all the recorded waveforms.[73] It was found that the mean value of the similarity index was significantly lower in LQTS patients than in control subjects (49 ± 10 versus 77 ± 8%, $p < 0.0001$), as illustrated in Figure 8. A value less than 61% (corresponding to 2 standard deviations below the mean value for controls) was found in 35 of 40 patients and in only one control (sensitivity 87%, specificity 96%). The low value of the similarity index found in patients with LQTS indicates a large variety of ST-T waveforms, suggesting a high degree of dispersion of ventricular recovery times.

In consideration of the logistic limitations contingent on the use of body surface

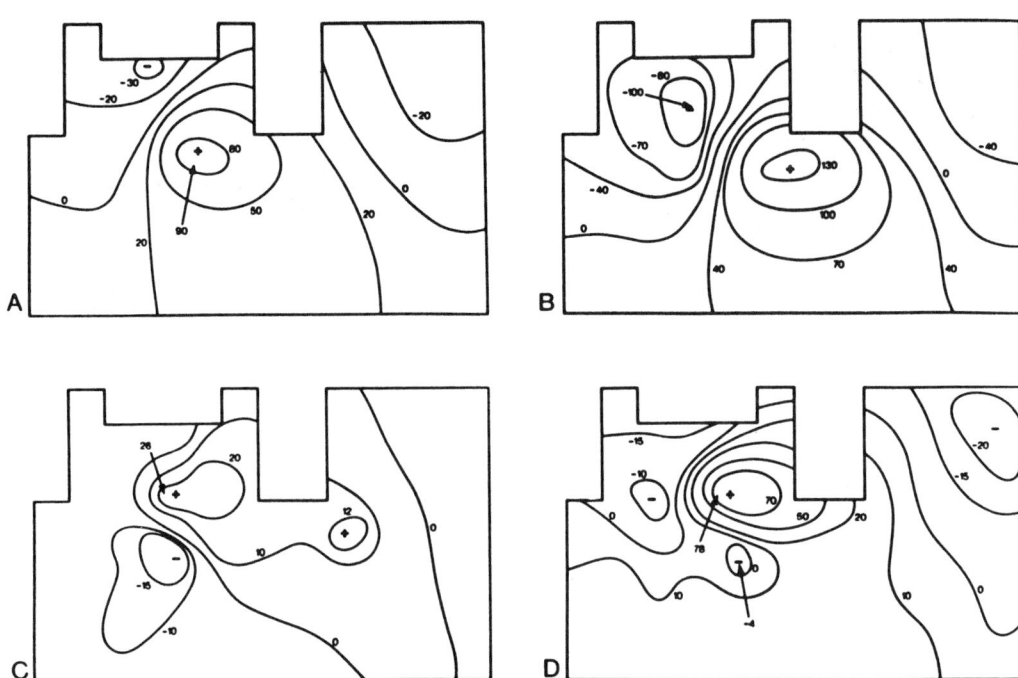

Figure 7. Body surface potential maps illustrating mean isointegral maps of ST-T (in each diagram, the left side represents anterior chest from the right midaxillary line, and the right side, the posterior chest to the left midaxillary line). A: Control subject, negative area in the right clavicular area extending to the posterior chest and positive area on the right anterior chest. B: 36-year-old female LQTS patient, large negative area on the anterior chest. C: 14-year-old female LQTS patient, multipolarity with two positive peaks. D: 13-year-old female LQTS patient, complex multipeak distribution. (Modified with permission from Reference 72.)

mapping, we have considered the applicability of simpler forms of analysis that would be available everywhere. Accordingly, we have evaluated dispersion of repolarization in LQTS[74] using the surface ECG in order to explore whether a quantification of repolarization dishomogeneity by 12-lead ECG may become a clinical tool. We used dispersion of the QT interval measured at surface ECG as an index of dishomogeneous repolarization. Dispersion has been measured by multiple parameters to avoid the limitations inherent in a single approach. We used as a first index of dispersion the algebraic difference between the maximal and the minimal QT interval measured on the 12-lead ECG (QT_{max}-QT_{min}) as suggested by Day et al.[75] This approach is limited by the fact that it relies entirely on two leads to extrapolate the behavior

of the entire heart. Therefore, we also calculated the coefficient of dispersion (SD/mean × 100) of the QT interval, which is the averaged deviation of the QT interval in each lead from the mean duration of repolarization. We also calculated both parameters for the QT interval corrected for the heart rate according to the Bazett formula. Using this multiple approach we measured dispersion of repolarization in LQTS patients refractory to β-blocking therapy who required left cardiac sympathetic denervation (LCSD) to control their arrhythmias and in a group of age-matched controls (Figure 9). The study showed that LQTS patients have a higher dispersion of repolarization (171 ± 40 msec) as compared to controls (70 ± 20 msec, $p < 0.005$) and that in this subgroup of patients β blockade did not prevent cardiac arrhythmias and at the same time

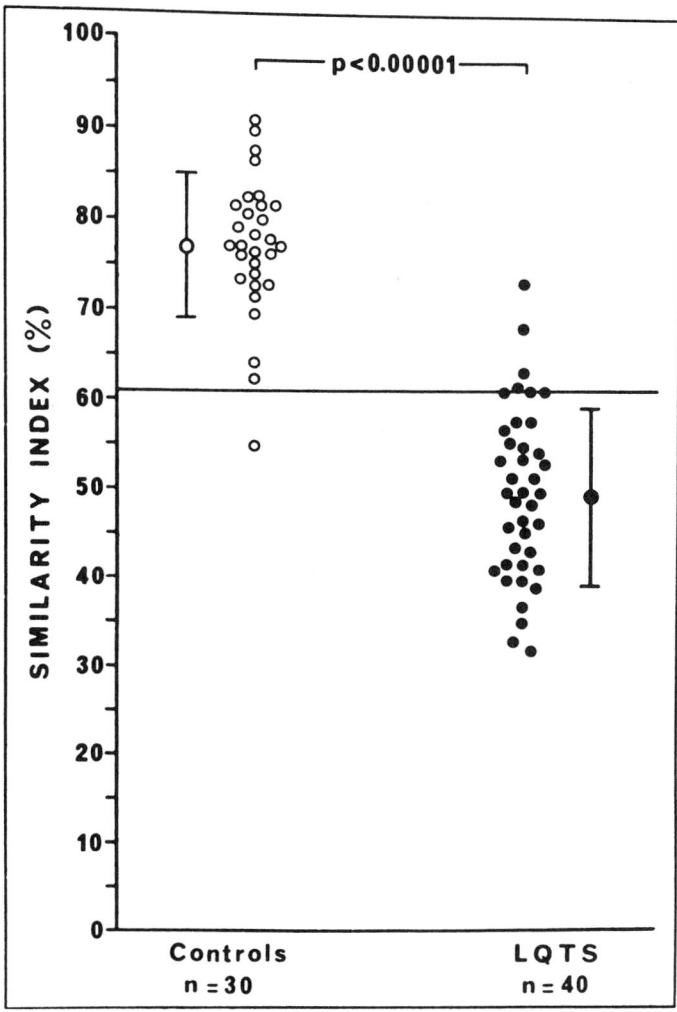

Figure 8. Individual values of the similarity index of the control and long QT syndrome (LQTS) groups. Mean and 1 SD is indicated by a vertical bar for each group. A cutoff value corresponding to the mean of the control group − 2 SD is indicated by the horizontal line. (Reproduced with permission from Reference 73.)

failed to normalize dispersion of repolarization. On the contrary, LCSD was not only able to prevent recurrence of syncope/cardiac arrest, but also reduced dispersion of repolarization to values comparable to those observed in the control group. This study provides the first evidence that LCSD plays an important role in enhancing homogeneity of ventricular repolarization and it also suggests that this action is correlated to its antifibrillatory effect.[76]

Other than the well-known effects of

right stellectomy on T wave morphology,[60,77] we are not aware of quantitative studies either supporting or denying a role of sympathetic imbalance in increasing dispersion of repolarization.

It is objectively remarkable that not a single clinical feature of LQTS is in contrast with the sympathetic imbalance hypothesis. The fact that these characteristic and often unique clinical aspects are so impressively mimicked by right stellectomy, undoubtedly constitutes

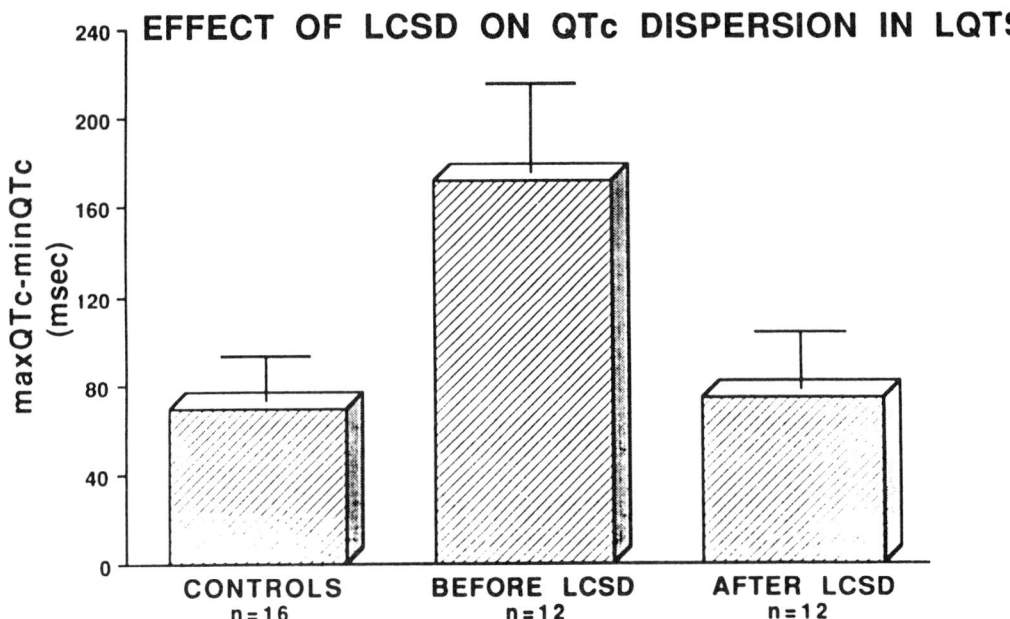

Figure 9. QTc$_{max}$-QTc$_{min}$ is one of the possible indexes of dispersion of repolarization. The subgroup of long QT syndrome (LQTS) patients refractory to β-blocker therapy shows a greater dispersion of repolarization (171 ± 40 msec) compared to controls (70 ± 20 msec). After left cardiac sympathetic denervation (LCSD), besides a complete control of the arrhythmic events, a reduced dispersion or repolarization to values close to the control (80 ± 20) becomes evident.

a "tough act to follow" for any other hypothesis. However, as we have consistently stated during the last 17 years,[4-6] this does not prove at all that a sympathetic imbalance is indeed the primary defect in LQTS. The quantitative dominance of left-sided cardiac sympathetic nerves[59] is sufficient to explain the therapeutic efficacy of antiadrenergic interventions in the case of an intracardiac abnormality that sensitizes the heart to the arrhythmogenic effects of catecholamines.[78]

At a time when based on major genetic findings the consensus goes to the cardiac abnormality hypothesis, it is important to not lose track of the correct scientific methodology. The validity of any hypothesis should undergo careful and unbiased scrutiny. In the present case, the basic requirement is that the mechanism proposed should be in agreement with the several well-documented clinical characteristics of LQTS.

Mechanisms for Arrhythmias in Long QT Syndrome

As we have seen so far, none of the proposed hypotheses as the basic defect in LQTS has been proven conclusively. An additional area of intense research that has not yet provided definitive answers is the one dealing with the electrophysiological mechanism(s) underlying the ventricular tachyarrhythmias typical of LQTS.

The most common arrhythmias in LQTS is one of the most intriguing forms of ventricular tachycardia, namely torsades de pointes. For a more detailed discussion on torsades de pointes, the reader is referred to one of several extensive reviews on the subject.[79,80] Torsades de pointes consists of a polymorphic ventricular tachycardia in which the QRS complex morphology is twisting around an imaginary baseline. The basis for the peculiar shape of this tachycardia is not fully understood. The most popular theory relates it to different automatic foci that in turn take the lead and activate the ventricle from different areas, thus creating the polymorphic morphology of the tachycardia.[81,82] However, a definitive explanation has not been provided and therefore the shape of the tachycardia is of modest value for inferring the arrhythmogenic mechanisms.

Reentry

Reentry was among the first mechanisms proposed to account for arrhythmias in LQTS.[83] In fact, great consideration has been given to the dispersion of refractoriness hypothesis, which suggests that different durations in APD create a vulnerable substrate on which a reentrant circuit can develop.[21] Among the clinical evidences in favor of this theory are the observations of very different APD durations made by recording monophasic action potential in LQTS patients, the nonhomogeneous recovery process assessed by body surface mapping, and the measurement of an excessive dispersion of repolarization measured at surface ECG. More recently, another piece of evidence has been found that seems to support the theory of reentry, ie, the identification of fragmented activation in LQTS patients. According to the study by Napolitano et al.[84] if high-amplification ECG is recorded in LQTS patients and in normal age-matched controls, a prolongation of low-amplitude signals is found in the group of patients. The identification of late potentials, which are considered the classic substrate for reentry may become one of the major points in favor of a reentrant origin for arrhythmias.

The major argument raised against reentry is the lack of inducibility at electrophysiological study of LQTS patients.[85,86] However, this argument is not entirely satisfactory because at variance with myocardial infarction where reentry is generated by the presence of an anatomical substrate, in LQTS the transient

prolongation of repolarization may prolong refractoriness, thus delaying activation, as it is seen in the high-amplification ECG. However, in order for reentry to occur, it may be required that a critical amount of dispersion is generated, and this may well occur during adrenergic activation, but probably not during an electrophysiological study.

On the basis of these considerations and recent studies that still require confirmation, the role of reentry on LQTS may be less forcibly excluded than in the past.

Triggered Activity

Currently, the leading hypothesis for the development of arrhythmias in LQTS is still correctly represented by triggered activity. It has been proposed that both EADs and DADs may play a role in LQTS[85,87] and a rationale indeed exists to account for the development of both types of afterdepolarizations.

Early Afterdepolarizations

Early afterdepolarizations (EADs) are favored by a prolonged repolarization and by a low heart rate: both factors are present in LQTS. Any event occurring during repolarization that is capable of reducing repolarizing currents or of enhancing the depolarizing ones may induce EADs. In fact, in the laboratory, EADs are induced by blockade of K^+ channels with cesium[16,17] and by enhancing Ca^{2+} inward current with the calcium agonist BAY K 8644.[40] In LQTS, an intrinsic abnormality of the K^+ channels that would reduce K^+ conductance, would obviously favor the development of EAD. Also, an augmented sympathetic discharge would favor the development of EADs as it has been demonstrated by Priori and co-worker[34] in isolated myocytes in which EADs were induced by isoproterenol.

A remarkable characteristic of adrenergic-dependent EADs is their inducibility at frequencies higher than is generally the case with cesium chloride.[34] The fact that adrenergic-mediated EADs can develop at physiological frequencies[34] represents a strong argument in favor of their role in LQTS. Although EADs may reach the threshold for the development of arrhythmias, it should be remembered that they also represent one of the major causes for regional APD prolongation. It is indeed possible that, as shown by the monophasic action potential studies by Gavrilescu and Luca[62] and by Bonatti et al.,[63] EADs may develop only in a few areas of the myocardium and may therefore become arrhythmogenic before reaching the threshold for the development of triggered beats.

Delayed Afterdepolarizations

Delayed afterdepolarizations (DADs) can be induced by adrenergic stimulation even in normal cardiac tissue, as was demonstrated both in vitro[34,88] and in vivo preparations (Figure 10).[35] It is therefore logical to consider

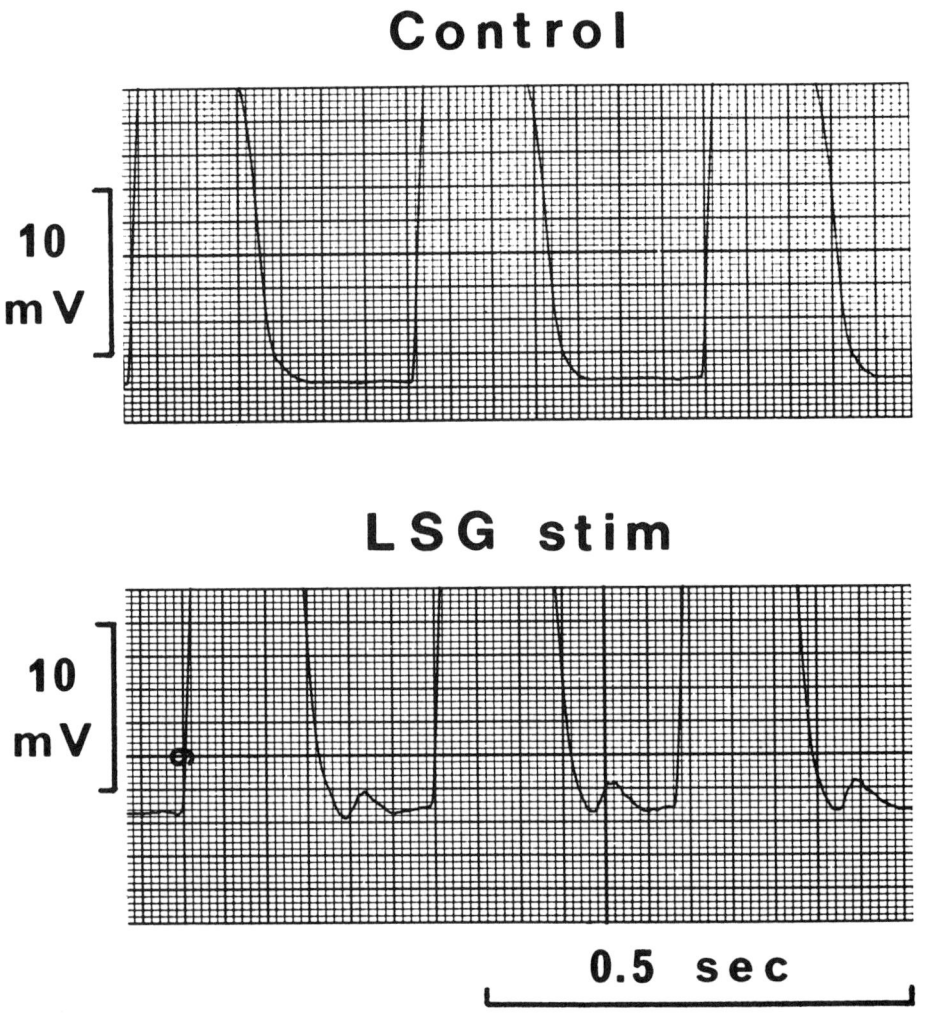

Figure 10. Monophasic action potential recording at high amplification in control conditions and after left stellate ganglion stimulation (LSG stim) when delayed afterdepolarizations (DADs) are present. (Reproduced with permission from Reference 35.)

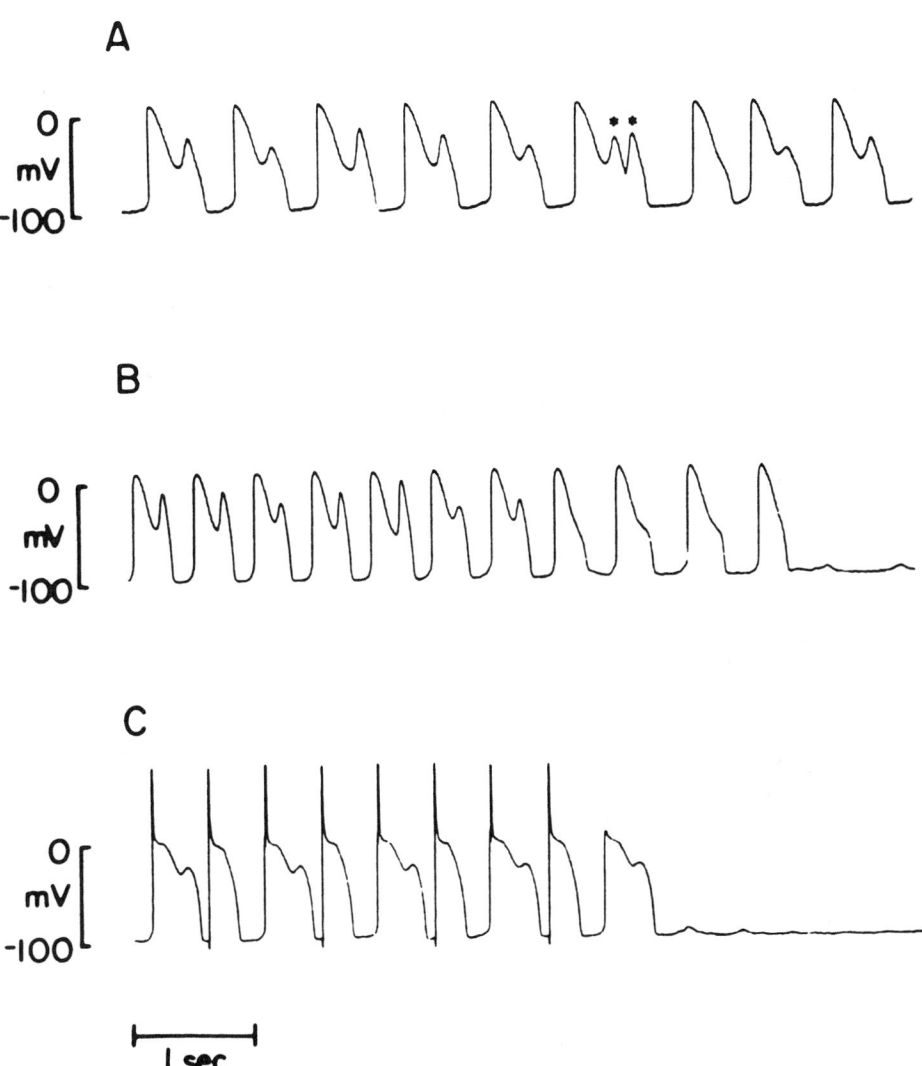

Figure 11. Characteristics of early afterdepolarizations (EADs) induced by isoproterenol in ventricular myocytes. A: Example of a triggered rhythm induced by a delayed afterdepolarization (DAD). Pacing was discontinued several minutes earlier and two sustained triggered rhythms developed. Early afterdepolarizations (EADs) are also present, and in one case (asterisk) multiple EADs developed on the same action potential. B: Example of spontaneous termination with progressive slowing (from 500 to 650 msec of cycle length) in rate of triggered rhythm induced by DADs. Pacing was discontinued here minutes before (not shown) and resulted in the sustained triggered activity. Early afterdepolarizations are simultaneously present. Note that termination of triggered rhythm is paralleled by a higher activation voltage for EADs and finally by their disappearance. C: Example of EADs present on alternate beats during pacing. After last paced beat, a triggered action potential develops followed by two DADs. (Reproduced with permission from Reference 34.)

their potential role in this most typical clinical example of adrenergic-dependent arrhythmias. As it has been suggested that both EADs and DADs could play a role in LQTS,[85,87] this hypothesis would be in agreement by the evidence obtained in vitro by Priori and co-worker[34] that activation of β-adrenergic receptors may simultaneously induce EADs and DADs (Figure 11). In an unusual case report, Malfatto et al.[87] also provided presumptive evidence for the simultaneous presence of EADs and DADs in several Holter recordings from one LQTS patient. They suggested that the notches observed on the T wave, which were potentiated by long pauses, might be the electrocardiographic counterpart of EADs, and that the pause-dependent premature ventricular beats could be triggered by the attainment of the activation threshold of these EADs. However, not all the arrhythmic episodes observed on the Holter recordings fit the characteristics of the EADs; on the contrary, some runs of ventricular tachycardia were triggered by increased heart rate as would be expected by arrhythmias triggered by DADs.

It is likely that the identification of the electrophysiological mechanism for the arrhythmias in LQTS remains difficult because indeed more than one mechanism is implicated. As already mentioned, not only may EADs and DADs be simultaneously present, but EADs may prolong repolarization and therefore favor development of reentrant circuits. The presence of EADs may be required for refractoriness to be prolonged to the point at which reentry may be established. Alternatively, premature ventricular beats triggered by EADs or DADs may be the initiating mechanism, but then reentry may be the cause that makes the tachyarrhythmia a sustained one.

The same complexity applies to the identification of the basic defect that causes LQTS. So far, both leading hypotheses (sympathetic imbalance and cardiac abnormality), remain unproven. However, they could also coexist, and a basic defect during embryonic development of cardiac innervation might affect the development of regulatory proteins that control ionic channels. This possibility has been proposed by Malfatto et al.[89] in a study performed in neonatal rats treated with antiserum against nerve growth factor, which resulted in a reduced synthesis of a 41-kD GTP regulatory protein apparently also involved in the control of potassium channels.

Conclusions

The picture of LQTS remains a complex one, despite considerable progress. The most advanced techniques from the fields of molecular biology and electrophysiology, always coupled with careful clinical observations and studies, are likely to provide new insights in this puzzling and so often lethal disease. The understanding of mechanisms involved in LQTS will result in a much better understanding of repolarization and of its regulation and a more thorough appreciation for the potential arrhythmogenic role of sympathetic activation.

References

1. Crampton RS, Schwartz PJ: Some aspects of sudden cardiac death. In: PJ Schwartz, AM Brown, A Malliani, A Zanchetti (eds): *Neural Mechanisms in Cardiac Arrhythmias*. New York: Raven Press, 1978, p. 1.
2. Moss AJ, Schwartz PJ: Sudden death and the idiopathic long QT syndrome. *Am J Med* 66:6, 1979.
3. Zipes DP: The long QT interval syndrome: a Rosetta Stone for sympathetic related ventricular tachyarrhythmias. *Circulation* 84:1414, 1991.
4. Schwartz PJ, Periti M, Malliani A: The long QT syndrome. *Am Heart J* 89:378, 1975.
5. Schwartz PJ: The idiopathic long QT syndrome: progress and questions. *Am Heart J* 109:399, 1985.
6. Schwartz PJ, Locati E, Priori SG, Zaza A: The idiopathic long QT syndrome. In: DP Zipes, J Jalife (eds): *Cardiac Electrophysiology. From Cell to Bedside*. Philadelphia, PA: W.B. Saunders Co., 1990, p. 589.
7. Moss AJ, Schwartz PJ, Crampton RS, et al: The long QT syndrome: prospective longitudinal study of 328 families. *Circulation* 84:1136, 1991.

8. Moss AJ: Prolonged QT interval syndrome. *JAMA* 256:2985, 1986.

9. Schwartz PJ: Prevention of the arrhythmias in the long QT syndrome. In: HE Kulbertus (ed): *Medical Management of Cardiac Arrhythmias*. Edinburgh: Churchill Livingstone, 1986, p. 153.

10. Sicouri S, Antzelevitch C: A subpopulation of cells with unique electrophysiological properties in the deep subepicardium of the canine ventricle. The M cell. *Circ Res* 68:1729, 1991.

11. Hume JR, Harvey RD: Chloride conductance pathways in heart. *Am J Physiol* 261:C399, 1991.

12. Zygmunt AC, Gibbons WR: Calcium-activated chloride current in rabbit ventricular myocytes. *Circ Res* 68:424, 1991.

13. Jervell A: Surdocardiac and related syndromes in children. *Adv Intern Med* 17:425, 1971.

14. James TN: Congenital deafness and cardiac arrhythmias. *Am J Cardiol* 19:627, 1967.

15. Vincent GM: Hypothesis for the molecular physiology of the Romano-Ward long QT syndrome. *J Am Coll Cardiol* 30:500, 1992.

16. Isenberg G: Cardiac Purkinje fibers: cesium as a tool to block inward rectifying potassium currents. *Pflügers Arch* 365:99, 1976.

17. Brachmann J, Scherlag BJ, Rosenshtraukh LV, et al: Bradycardia-dependent triggered activity: relevance to drug induced multiform ventricular tachycardia. *Circulation* 68:846, 1983.

18. Ben-David J, Zipes DP: Differential response to right and left ansae subclaviae stimulation of early afterdepolarizations and ventricular tachycardia induced by cesium in dogs. *Circulation* 78:1241, 1988.

19. Hauswirth O, Noble D, Tsien RW: The dependence of plateau currents in cardiac Purkinje fibers on the interval between action potentials. *J Physiol* 222:27, 1972.

20. Giebisch G, Weidman S: Membrane currents in mammalian ventricular heart muscle fibers using a voltage clamp technique. *J Gen Physiol* 57:290, 1971.

21. Han J, Moe GK: Nonuniform recovery of excitability in ventricular muscle. *Circ Res* 14:44, 1964.

22. Arnsdorf MF, Sawicki GJ: Effects of quinidine sulfate on the balance among active and passive cellular properties that comprise the electrophysiologic matrix and determine excitability in sheep Purkinje fibers. *Circ Res* 61:244, 1987.

23. Keating M, Atkinson D, Dunn C, et al: Linkage of a cardiac arrhythmia, the long QT syndrome, and the Harvey ras-1 gene. *Science* 252:704, 1991.

24. Keating MA: Linkage analysis and long QT syndrome. *Circulation* 85:1973, 1992.

25. Santos E, Nebreda AR: Structural and functional properties of ras proteins. *FASEB J* 3:2151, 1989.

26. Yatani A, Okabe K, Polakis P, et al: Ras p21 and GAP inhibit coupling of muscarinic receptors to atrial K^+ channels. *Cell* 61:769, 1990.

27. Martin GA, Yatani A, Clark R, et al: Gap domains responsible for ras p21-dependent inhibition of muscarinic atrial K^+ channel currents. *Science* 255:192, 1992.

28. Keating MA, Atkinson D, Dunn C, et al: Linkage of the long QT syndrome to the Harvey ras-1 locus on chromosome 11. *Am J Hum Genet* 49:1335, 1991.

29. Towbin JA, Pagotto L, Siu B, et al: Romano-Ward long QT syndrome (RWLQTS): evidence of genetic heterogeneity (abstract). *Pediatr Res* 31:23A, 1992.

30. Giotti A, Ledda F, Mannaioni PF: Effects of noradrenaline and isoprenaline, in combination with alpha and beta receptor blocking substances, on the action potential of cardiac Purkinje fibers. *J Physiol (Lond)* 229:99, 1973.

31. Belardinelli L, Isenberg G: Actions of adenosine and isoproterenol on isolated mammalian ventricular myocytes. *Circ Res* 53:287, 1983.

32. Reuter H: Localization of beta-adrenergic receptors, and effects of noradrenaline and cyclic nucleotides on action potentials, ionic currents and tension in mammalian cardiac muscle. *J Physiol (Lond)* 242:429, 1974.

33. Quadbeck J, Reuter M: Adrenoceptors in cardiac ventricular muscle and changes in duration of action potential caused by noradrenaline and isoprenaline. *Naunyn-Schmiedeberg's Arch Pharmacol* 288:403, 1975.

34. Priori SG, Corr PB: Mechanisms underlying early and delayed afterdepolarizations induced by catecholamines. *Am J Physiol* 258:H1796, 1990.

35. Priori SG, Mantica M, Schwartz PJ: Delayed afterdepolarizations elicited in vivo by left stellate ganglion stimulation. *Circulation* 78:178, 1988.

36. Rougier O, Vassort G, Stampfli R: Voltage clamp experiments on frog atrial heart muscle fibers with the sucrose gap technique. *Pflügers Arch* 301:91, 1968.

37. Tsien RW: Cyclic AMP and contractile activity in heart. *Adv Cyclic Nucleotide Res* 8:363, 1977.

38. Tsien RW, Fox AP, Hirning LD, et al: Calcium channels, calcium stores and norepinephrine release in sympathetic neurons. In: NA Thorn, M Treiman, OH Peterson (eds): *Molecular Mechanisms in Secretion*. Copenhagen: Munksgaard, 1988, p. 66.

39. Bean BP, Nowycky MC, Tsien RW: Beta-adrenergic modulation of calcium channels in frog ventricular heart cells. *Nature* 307:371, 1984.

40. January CT, Riddle JM: Mechanisms of early afterdepolarizations comparison of Bay K 8644

and Cs models (abstract). *Circulation* 78(Suppl II):II-123, 1988.

41. Miura Y, Inui J, Imamura H: Alpha-adrenoceptor-mediated restoration of calcium dependent potential in the partially depolarized rabbit papillary muscle. *Naunyn-Schmiedeberg's Arch Pharmacol* 301:201, 1978.

42. Ledda F, Mantelli L, Mugelli A: Alpha-sympathomimetic amines and calcium-mediated action potentials in guinea-pig ventricular muscle. *Br J Pharmacol* 69:565, 1980.

43. Inui J, Brodde OE, Schuman HJ: Influence of acetylcholine on the positive inotropic effect evoked by alpha- or beta-adrenoceptor stimulation in the rabbit heart. *Naunyn-Schmiedeberg's Arch Pharmacol* 320:152, 1982.

44. Apkon M, Nerbonne JM: Alpha-adrenergic agonists selectively suppress voltage-dependent K^+ currents in rat ventricular myocytes. *Proc Natl Acad Sci USA* 85:8756, 1988.

45. Lacerda AE, Rampe D, Brown AM: Effect of protein kinase C activators on cardiac Ca^{++} channels. *Nature (Lond)* 335:249, 1988.

46. Walsh KB, Kass RS: Regulation of a heart potassium channel by protein kinase A and C. *Science* 242:67, 1988.

47. Hume JR: Do catecholamines directly modulate the delayed plateau potassium current in frog atrium? *J Mol Cell Cardiol* 17:813, 1985.

48. Desilets M, Baumgarten CM: Isoproterenol, intracellular Na^+ activity and the Na^+/K^+ pump in isolated ventricular myocytes. In: WR Giles (ed): *Recent Studies of Ion Transport and Impulse Propagation in Cardiac Muscle*. New York: Alan R. Liss, 1988.

49. Tsien RW, Giles W, Greengard P: Cyclic AMP mediates the effect of adrenaline on cardiac Purkinje fibers. *Nature* 240:181, 1972.

50. Kass RS, Wiegers SE: The ionic basis of concentration-related effects of noradrenaline on the action potential of cardiac Purkinje fibers. *J Physiol (Lond)* 322:541, 1982.

51. Coraboeuf E, Carmeliet E: Existence of two transient outward currents in sheep cardiac Purkinje fibers. *Pflügers Arch* 392:352, 1982.

52. Fozzard HA, Hiraoka M: The positive dynamic current and its inactivation properties in cardiac Purkinje fibers. *J Physiol* 234:569, 1973.

53. Bouron A, Potreatu D, Raymond G: Possible involvement of a chloride conductance in the transient outward current on the whole cell voltage clamped ferret ventricular myocytes. *Pflügers Arch* 419:534, 1991.

54. Nakayama T, Fozzard HA: Adrenergic modulation of the transient outward current in isolated canine Purkinje cells. *Circ Res* 62:162, 1988.

55. Fedida D, Shimoni Y, Giles WR: Alpha-adrenergic agonists reduce a transient outward current in single cells from rabbit atrium. *Biophysics* 55:294a, 1989.

56. Zaza A, Malfatto G, Schwartz PJ: Sympathetic modulation of the relationship between ventricular repolarization and cycle length. *Circ Res* 68:1191, 1991.

57. Schwartz PJ, Locati E: The idiopathic long QT syndrome. Pathogenetic mechanisms and therapy. *Eur Heart J* 6(Suppl D):103, 1985.

58. Schwartz PJ, Locati E, Moss AJ, et al: Left cardiac sympathetic denervation in the therapy of the congenital long QT syndrome: a world-wide report. *Circulation* 84:503, 1991.

59. Schwartz PJ: Sympathetic imbalance and cardiac arrhythmias. In: WC Randall (ed): *Nervous Control of Cardiovascular Function*. New York: Oxford University Press, 1984, p. 225.

60. Yanowitz R, Preston JB, Abildskov JA: Functional distribution of right and left stellate innervation to the ventricles: production of neurogenic electrocardiographic changes by unilateral alteration of sympathetic tone. *Circ Res* 18:416, 1966.

61. Schwartz PJ, Bonazzi O, Locati E, et al: Pathogenesis and therapy of the idiopathic long QT syndrome. *Ann NY Acad Sci* 644:112, 1992.

62. Gavrilescu S, Luca C: Right ventricular monophasic action potential in patients with long QT syndrome. *Br Heart J* 40:1014, 1978.

63. Bonatti V, Rolli A, Botti G: Recording of monophasic action potentials of the right ventricle in long QT syndromes complicated by severe ventricular arrhythmias. *Eur Heart J* 4:168, 1983.

64. Vincent GM: The heart of Romano-Ward syndrome patients. *Am Heart J* 112:61, 1986.

65. Langley JN: On the origin from the spinal cord of the cervical and upper thoracic sympathetic fibers, with some observations on white and grey rami communicantes. *Phil Trans R Soc Lond* 107:85, 1892.

66. Schwartz PJ, Stone HL: Effects of unilateral stellectomy upon cardiac performance during exercise in dogs. *Circ Res* 44:637, 1979.

67. Schwartz PJ, Malliani A: Electrical alternation of the T wave. Clinical and experimental evidence of its relationship with the sympathetic nervous system and with the long QT syndrome. *Am Heart J* 89:45, 1975.

68. Moss AJ, McDonald J: Unilateral cervicothoracic sympathetic ganglionectomy for the treatment of long QT interval syndrome. *N Engl J Med* 285:903, 1970.

69. Crampton RS: Preeminence of left stellate ganglion in the long QT syndrome. *Circulation* 59:769, 1979.

70. Nador F, Beria G, De Ferrari GM, et al: Unsuspected echocardiographic abnormality in the

long Q-T syndrome: diagnostic, prognostic, and pathogenetic implications. *Circulation* 84: 1530, 1991.

71. Abildskov JA, Vincent GM, Evan AK, et al: Distribution of body surface potentials in familial QT interval prolongation. *Am J Cardiol* 47:480, 1981.

72. De Ambroggi L, Bertoni T, Locati E, et al: Mapping of body surface potentials in patients with idiopathic long QT syndrome. *Circulation* 74: 1334, 1986.

73. De Ambroggi L, Negroni MS, Monza E, et al: Dispersion of ventricular repolarization in the long QT syndrome. *Am J Cardiol* 68:614, 1991.

74. Napolitano C, Diehl L, Bonazzi O, et al: Dispersion of repolarization: a marker of successful therapy in long QT syndrome patients (abstract). *Eur Heart J* 13:365, 1992.

75. Day CP, Comb JM, Campbell RWF: QT dispersion: an indication of arrhythmia risk in patients with long QT intervals. *Br Heart J* 63:342, 1990.

76. Schwartz PJ: The rationale and the role of left stellectomy for the prevention of malignant arrhythmias. *Ann NY Acad Sci* 427:199, 1984.

77. Rothberger J, Winterberg H: Uber die Beziehungen der Herznerven zur Form des Elektrokardiogramms. *Plügers Arch Ges Physiol* 135: 506, 1910.

78. Schwartz PJ, Priori SG: Sympathetic nervous system and cardiac arrhythmias. In: DP Zipes, J Jalife (eds): *Cardiac Electrophysiology. From Cell to Bedside.* Philadelphia, PA: WB Saunders Co, 1990, p. 330.

79. Surawicz B: Electrophysiologic substrate of torsade de pointes. Dispersion of repolarization or early afterdepolarizations? *J Am Coll Cardiol* 14:172, 1989.

80. Priori SG, Napolitano C, Schwartz PJ: Electrophysiologic mechanisms involved in the development of torsade de pointes. *Cardiovasc Drugs Ther* 5:203, 1991.

81. Dessertenne F: La tachycardie ventriculaire a deux foyers opposes variables. *Arch Mal Coeur* 59:263, 1966.

82. Bardy GH, Ungerleider RM, Smith WM, et al: A mechanism of torsades de pointes in a canine model. *Circulation* 67:52, 1983.

83. Ratshin RA, Hunt D, Russell RO Jr, et al: QT-interval prolongation, paroxysmal ventricular arrhythmias, and convulsive syncope. *Ann Intern Med* 75:919, 1971.

84. Napolitano C, Bonazzi O, Locati EH, et al: Late potentials in the long QT syndrome. *J Amb Monit* 5(Abstr Suppl):20, 1992.

85. Jackman WM, Friday KJ, Anderson JL, et al: The long QT syndromes: a critical review, new clinical observations and a unifying hypothesis. *Prog Cardiovasc Dis* 2:115, 1988.

86. Bhandari AK, Shapiro WA, Morady F, et al: Electrophysiologic testing in patients with the long QT syndrome. *Circulation* 71:63, 1985.

87. Malfatto G, Rosen MR, Foresti A, Schwartz PJ: Idiopathic long QT syndrome exacerbated by beta adrenergic blockade and responsive to left cardiac sympathetic denervation. Implications regarding electrophysiologic substrate and adrenergic modulation. *J Cardiovasc Electrophysiol* 3:295, 1992.

88. Schechter E, Freeman CC, Lazzara R: Afterdepolarizations as a mechanism for the long QT syndrome. Electrophysiologic study of a case. *J Am Coll Cardiol* 3:1556, 1984.

89. Malfatto G, Rosen TS, Steinberg SF, et al: Sympathetic neural modulation of cardiac impulse initiation and repolarization in the newborn rat. *Circ Res* 66:427, 1990.

PART III

Pharmacological Considerations

Chapter 15

Comparative Mechanisms of Action of Antiarrhythmic Drugs

Stanley Nattel
Bramah N. Singh

Since 1918 when quinidine was first introduced in clinical therapeutics, antiarrhythmic drugs have been increasingly used for controlling irregularities of cardiac rhythm. A great deal has been learned about how antiarrhythmic compounds work, especially in the last 20 years. Our understanding of their actions has evolved parallel with our knowledge of basic electrophysiology and mechanisms of cardiac arrhythmias.[1] Changes in two electrophysiological parameters—conduction and refractoriness and how they are modified by autonomic transmitters in health and disease—have become topics of investigative focus. Other chapters in this volume deal specifically with arrhythmia mechanisms (Chapters 6–10), with rationale and principles of pharmacological therapy of cardiac arrhythmias in certain subsets of patients (see Chapter 47), and with specific groups of antiarrhythmic drugs (see Chapters 16–19). This chapter deals in a general way with mechanisms of antiarrhythmic drug action and with the classification of antiarrhythmic agents.

Mechanisms of Antiarrhythmic Drug Action

The mechanism of antiarrhythmic drug action can be discussed at a variety of levels. These include actions at a subcellular level (eg, ionic currents, pump and exchange mechanisms, membrane receptors, etc.). Alternatively, drug effects on the action potential, reflecting changes at the cellular level, can be considered. Finally, drug-induced changes in macroscopic electrical properties such as conduction, refractoriness, and patterns of impulse propagation can be evaluated.

Cellular and Subcellular Mechanisms of Action

Many antiarrhythmic drugs act by blocking specific ion currents. Sodium channel blockers suppress the entry of sodium ions during phase 0 of the cardiac action potential

From BN Singh, HJJ Wellens, M Hiraoka, (eds): *Electropharmacological Control of Cardiac Arrhythmias.* Mount Kisco, NY, Futura Publishing Company Inc., © 1994.

Table 1
Classical Electrophysiological Effects Associated With Various Classes of Antiarrhythmic Drug Action

	Sodium channel blockade	Sympathetic antagonism†	Action potential prolongation (class III)	Calcium channel blockade
Macroscopic electrical properties:				
Automaticity—SA node	0	↓	0	↓
—atrial, ventricular specialized fibers	↓	sl. ↓	0	0
Conduction velocity—AV node	0	↓	0	↓
—atrium, ventricle	↓	0	0	0
Refractory period—AV node	0	↑	0	↑
—atrium, ventricle	0	sl. ↑	↑	0
Electrocardiographic/electrophysiological properties:				
ECG intervals:　　RR	0	↑	0	0 (↓ ↑)*
PR	0	↑	0	↑ (0 ↓)*
QRS	↑	0	0	0
QT	0	0	↑	0
Conduction intervals: AH	0	↑	0	↑ (0 ↓)*
HV	↑	0	0	0

All effects shown are those expected for a drug that is specific for the action indicated, ie, devoid of actions from all other classes.
* Major effect shown is the one most commonly seen. The net effect of a calcium channel blocker depends on the balance between direct actions (suppress calcium entry-dependent electrophysiological properties) and reflex autonomic effects (increase calcium entry-dependent properties).
† Effects shown are those most commonly observed clinically. The magnitude of the effect of a sympathetic antagonist (eg, β-blocker) will depend on the extent of background sympathetic tone and the degree to which the latter alters the electrophysiological variable of interest.

that are responsible for conduction in working cardiac muscle and the His-Purkinje system. Their major electrophysiological effects are summarized in Table 1 and include depression of automaticity and slowing of conduction in fast channel tissue. The degree to which such effects are manifest under specific conditions will depend on the associated extent of sodium channel blockade. Various sodium channel blocking drugs have characteristic dissociation rates from the sodium channel at diastolic potentials,[2,3] as discussed in detail in Chapter 16. A sodium channel blocking antiarrhythmic drug that rapidly dissociates from the sodium channel (eg, lidocaine, mexiletine) will produce little change in cardiac conduction at normal heart rates, but may slow conduction during very rapid

tachyarrhythmias. Because of their typical voltage-dependent action such agents will progressively reduce sodium current during phase 4 diastolic depolarization in spontaneously automatic tissue, and thereby suppress automaticity in fast channel tissues. In addition, they may suppress or block conduction in diseased, depolarized zones.

Calcium channel blocking drugs inhibit voltage-dependent calcium entry. As discussed in Chapter 19, these agents, like sodium channel blockers, exhibit time-dependent dissociation from calcium channels at negative potentials that results in use-dependent calcium channel blockade.[2,4] Their characteristic electrophysiological properties are to slow conduction and prolong refractoriness in zones such as the sinus node and atrioventricular (AV) node that are activated by calcium inward current. In addition, calcium antagonists tend to suppress sinus node automaticity. All calcium channel blockers produce peripheral vasodilation. This results in reflex sympathetic enhancement and vagal withdrawal that antagonizes direct drug effects.[5] The electrophysiological effects of a calcium antagonist will depend on the balance between its direct effects and autonomic responses. Agents that have stronger peripheral vasodilating actions than direct cardiac actions (characteristic of the dihydropyridines) result in reflex responses that are stronger than direct cardiac effects and can cause net increases in heart rate or AV nodal conduction velocity.

A wide variety of agents are capable of blocking cardiac potassium channels. These compounds are discussed in Chapter 18. Typically, potassium channel blocking drugs increase action potential duration in fast channel tissue. Consequently, they increase the refractory period and tend to suppress reentrant cardiac arrhythmias.[6] Conversely, by preventing repolarization they can cause excessive action potential prolongation and early afterdepolarizations (EADs) due to plateau calcium or sodium inward currents.[7–10]

Other antiarrhythmic drugs act by interacting with the autonomic nervous system. β-Adrenergic receptor stimulation plays an important part in the genesis of a variety of supraventricular and ventricular arrhythmias (see Chapter 11). Indirect evidence (see Chapters 17, 30, and 47) suggests that β-adrenergic receptor stimulation may play an important role in sudden cardiac death.[1] A variety of agents inhibit cardiac arrhythmias by diminishing the level of β-adrenergic receptor stimulation. The most widely used compounds in this class are competitive β-adrenergic receptor antagonists, which are discussed in more detail in Chapters 17 and 33. Other drugs, such as amiodarone, noncompetitively inhibit the effects of β-adrenergic receptor stimulation[11,12] by decreasing receptor number[13] or interfering with hormonal modulation of sympathetic actions[14–17] (see Chapters 31, 35, and 48). Still other agents, such as bretylium, block adren-

ergic neurotransmission by depleting noradrenaline stores.[18] In numerous studies, decreasing the level of β-adrenergic receptor stimulation has been shown to prevent sudden cardiac death probably due to ventricular fibrillation in survivors of acute myocardial infarction.[19] Because β-adrenergic receptor stimulation accelerates AV nodal conduction and shortens the AV node refractory period, β-adrenergic receptor antagonists can be useful in the treatment of a variety of supraventricular arrhythmias whose occurrence and manifestations depend on AV node function.[20]

Drugs that enhance vagal effects on the heart are also capable of suppressing AV node impulse propagation. They are potentially useful in the treatment of reentrant tachycardias involving the AV node, and can reduce the ventricular response rate to atrial fibrillation. The major beneficial electrophysiological action of digitalis is mediated by an enhancement of vagal effects on the heart.[21] Acetylcholinesterase inhibitors also enhance vagal effects on the heart, and have been used in the emergency treatment of paroxysmal reentrant tachycardias.[22] The latter compounds have been largely supplanted by calcium antagonists and adenosine, which are more reliably effective.

Adenosine affects the heart by stimulating a specific purinergic receptor (of the A_1 subtype).[23–26] Other compounds, such as adenosine triphosphate (ATP), also act via this mechanism.[25,26] Purinergic receptor stimulation activates an outward potassium conductance, much like vagal influences, and suppresses AV node conduction.[24] The depressant effect of purinergic agonists on human AV nodal conduction is strong, and because of their rapid breakdown and cellular uptake their action is fleeting. They are widely used as first-line drugs to terminate AV node reentrant tachycardia.

A variety of compounds are considered to possess potential antiarrhythmic activity by interacting with ion channels and receptors in a fashion different from those described. Alinidine inhibits I_f, a cardiac current that is believed to play a role in spontaneous automaticity.[27] A variety of compounds inhibit α-adrenergic receptor stimulation. A new series of compounds has been identified that act by stimulating potassium currents, thereby accelerating repolarization. While there is experimental evidence suggesting potential antiarrhythmic activity of all of these agents,[27] there is as yet no specific clinical indication for their use in the treatment of cardiac arrhythmias.

Mechanisms of Action on Arrhythmias

The underlying mechanisms of cardiac arrhythmias are discussed extensively in Chapters 6 through 13. We will limit ourselves to a discussion of the ways in which antiarrhythmic drugs can interact with specific cardiac arrhythmia mechanisms. Evidence has accrued to implicate enhanced automaticity, triggered activity (due to early or delayed afterdepolarizations), and reentry in specific clinical cardiac arrhythmias, examples of which are provided in Table 2. Mechanisms of clinically-occurring arrhythmias have been discussed at length in Chapter 13.

Enhanced Automaticity

Automaticity involves gradual diastolic depolarization during phase 4 of the action potential. When the membrane potential

Table 2
Examples of Clinical Tachyarrhythmias, Their Mechanism, and Antiarrhythmic Drug Therapy That Can Suppress Them

Arrhythmia	Mechanism	Effective drugs
Ectopic atrial and ventricular tachycardias	Enhanced automaticity Triggered activity	Sodium channel blockers Sodium, calcium channel blockers
AV node reentrant tachycardia	Reentry	Calcium channel blockers, vagotonic agents, sympathetic antagonists, adenosine
AV reentrant tachycardia using accessory pathway	Reentry	Calcium channel blockers, vagotonic agents, sympathetic antagonists, adenosine, drugs that block accessory pathway conduction (eg, sodium channel blockers)
Atrial flutter	Reentry	Drugs that increase atrial refractory period
Atrial fibrillation	Reentry	Drugs that increase atrial refractory period
Ventricular tachycardia 6–24 hr post-acute MI	Abnormal automaticity	Sodium channel blockers
Ventricular tachycardia in chronic ischemic heart disease	Reentry	Drugs that increase ventricular refractory period
Acquired long QT syndrome	EADs	Drugs that increase heart rate, calcium antagonists, magnesium
Digitalis-toxic arrhythmias	DADs	Sodium, calcium channel blockers

AV: atrioventricular; MI: myocardial infarction; EADs: early afterdepolarizations; DADs: delayed afterdepolarizations.

reaches threshold, spontaneous activation occurs. Enhanced or abnormal automaticity can thus cause premature excitation and ectopic beats. The level of transmembrane potential depends on the relative magnitude of inward (depolarizing) and outward (repolarizing) currents. Spontaneous phase 4 depolarization is due to an increase in total inward current relative to outward current during diastole. Antiarrhythmic agents could suppress automaticity either by inhibiting an inward current responsible for depolarization (eg, alinidine, which inhibits I_f) or by enhancing diastolic outward potassium current (eg, muscarinic enhancers, adenosine). Alternatively, drugs that inhibit phase 0 inward current (such as calcium channel blockers in the sinus or AV node and sodium channel blockers in the His-Purkinje system) make the threshold voltage for activation more positive and therefore also suppress automaticity. In addition to the latter effect, such agents decrease the recruitment of voltage-dependent inward current during spontaneous depolarization, and therefore contribute to a reduction in the slope of phase 4, particularly during the second half of the diastolic interval.

Triggered Activity

Triggered activity may be due to EADs or to delayed afterdepolarizations (DADs). Early afterdepolarizations are due to delayed repolarization and can result from factors that increase plateau inward current or suppress plateau outward current.[10] Potassium channel blocking antiarrhythmic drugs that prolong action potential duration are notorious for causing EADs in vitro and related arrhythmias (torsade de pointes) in humans.[7,8] Agents that enhance potassium current will accelerate repolarization and terminate arrhythmias related to EADs.[28-30]

Delayed afterdepolarizations are associated with calcium overload. Arrhythmias due to DADs can be caused by agents that, like digitalis, increase total cellular calcium.[31-33] They can be suppressed either by inhibiting

calcium entry (by calcium channel blockade) or by blocking sodium current, which makes the threshold for activation more positive and prevents the DADs from reaching threshold.[34] In addition, as in the case of enhanced automaticity, sodium channel blockade inhibits the recruitment of sodium current, which contributes to the amplitude of DADs as the cell depolarizes into a voltage range in which sodium current is activated.

Reentry

Reentry depends on a functional or anatomical circuit in which electrical activity can continuously travel, exciting all points in the circuit consecutively in a repetitive fashion. The key factor permitting reentry to maintain itself is the presence of excitable tissue in front of the propagating wave front at all times. This, in turn, depends on a critical relationship between propagation velocity and refractory period. In general, slowing of conduction favors reentry and prolongation of refractoriness makes it less likely. Agents that block the inward current mechanism responsible for propagation tend, therefore, to facilitate the occurrence of reentry. For example, potent sodium channel blockers are capable of favoring the occurrence of reentrant ventricular arrhythmias.[35-37] Agents that have as a sole action the prolongation of refractoriness, such as pure potassium channel blockers, tend to be particularly effective in suppressing reentrant arrhythmias in fast channel tissue.[19]

In slow channel tissue, conductivity and refractoriness are intimately linked and the safety factor for propagation is limited. Therefore, compounds that potently suppress conduction in slow channel tissue, such as calcium antagonists and adenosine, effectively terminate reentrant arrhythmias in such tissues by impairing propagation to the point of complete block. Of course, the latter action is only desirable if it is manifest selectively during tachycardia. If such compounds produced complete AV block of significant duration, they would be very difficult to use. Fortunately, a variety of drugs are capable of selectively depressing AV nodal conduction at rapid rates, resulting in the possibility of blocking conduction during conduction reentrant tachycardia with limited effects when sinus rhythm resumes. Sympathetic antagonists reverse the conduction-facilitating effects of adrenergic stimulation, but do not directly suppress AV node conduction. Unless background adrenergic effects are strong, such compounds (like β-blockers) have a limited ability to terminate reentrant arrhythmias involving the AV node.

Reflection and Modulated Parasystole

Other arrhythmia mechanisms have been identified, but their clinical importance remains uncertain. Reflection is an arrhythmia mechanism closely related to reentry, involving electrotonic spread across a zone of reduced excitability rather than direct reentrant propagation.[38] Modulated parasystole is a related mechanism that involves enhanced automaticity whose manifestations are determined by interaction with the dominant pacemaker.[39]

Importance of Heart Rate as a Modulator of Antiarrhythmic Drug Action

Recent work has shown that activation rate plays an important role in modulating the actions of many antiarrhythmic drugs. The action of sodium and calcium channel blocking drugs shows use-dependence, ie, is enhanced by more frequent channel activation.[2,3,40–46] Therefore, the more frequently a target tissue is activated, the greater the depression of sodium or calcium current. This tachycardia-dependent blocking action amplifies the effect of a calcium channel blocker during arrhythmia, contributing to its efficacy in terminating reentrant arrhythmias involving the AV node[47] and

in controlling the ventricular response rate during atrial fibrillation.[48] Conversely, rate-dependent depression of conduction may result in the facilitation of important reentrant arrhythmias by sodium channel blocking compounds.[35,40].

Enhancement of drug action at faster rates is not only a property of channel blocking drugs. The AV node is unique among cardiac tissues in the rate dependence of its conduction properties, a feature that contributes to its important filtering function during supraventricular arrhythmias. A variety of interventions, including vagal activation,[49] β-adrenergic receptor blockade,[50] and purinergic activation[51] alter the intrinsic rate-dependent properties of the AV node so as to exaggerate the slowing in AV nodal conduction that results from increased activation rate. This type of modulation may play a significant role in the ability of such interventions to suppress reentrant arrhythmias involving the AV node.

Drugs that prolong action potential duration frequently manifest this action to a greater extent as rate slows.[52–54] This property, termed "reverse use dependence," facilitates the production of EADs, along with excess QT interval prolongation and ventricular tachyarrhythmias. The mechanism of reverse use dependence is unknown, although some investigators have suggested that it is due to accentuation of potassium channel blocking action at slower rates.[55–56] Some drugs increase action potential duration to a greater extent at faster rates in certain tissues.[57] This action is theoretically highly desirable, because it could lead to preferential action during tachycardia with reduced risk of toxicity during resting sinus rhythm.

Because heart rate can strongly modulate drug action, any understanding of mechanisms and classification must include an appreciation for the effect of interest at clinically relevant heart rates. For example, the beneficial effects of flecainide in atrial fibrillation appear paradoxical unless the ability of this drug to increase atrial action potential duration at rapid rates is kept in mind.

Antiarrhythmic Drug Classifications

The practice of classifying antiarrhythmic drugs began with the introduction of lidocaine and phenytoin as antiarrhythmic agents in the 1960s. These compounds were found to have electrophysiological actions different from those of the previously developed agents, quinidine and procainamide. Unlike the latter compounds, which prominently slow conduction, prolong refractoriness, and increase the QT interval, lidocaine and phenytoin had little effect on these variables. Corresponding differences were noted in cellular electrophysiological effects. Quinidine and procainamide increase action potential duration and refractory period, while decreasing $\dot{V}_{max}$ (an index of phase 0 sodium current).[58–60] In contrast, phenytoin and lidocaine decreased action potential duration without altering $\dot{V}_{max}$.[61–63] At about the same time, β-adrenergic receptor blockers were noted to have antiarrhythmic properties. Two classification systems for antiarrhythmic drugs were developed in the early 1970s. These classifications, one developed by Hoffman and Bigger and the other proposed by Singh and Vaughan Williams, formed the basis for discussion of antiarrhythmic drugs in the 1970s and 1980s. The classification presently in clinical use is based on the Singh-Vaughan Williams system (Figure 1), although the entire ap-

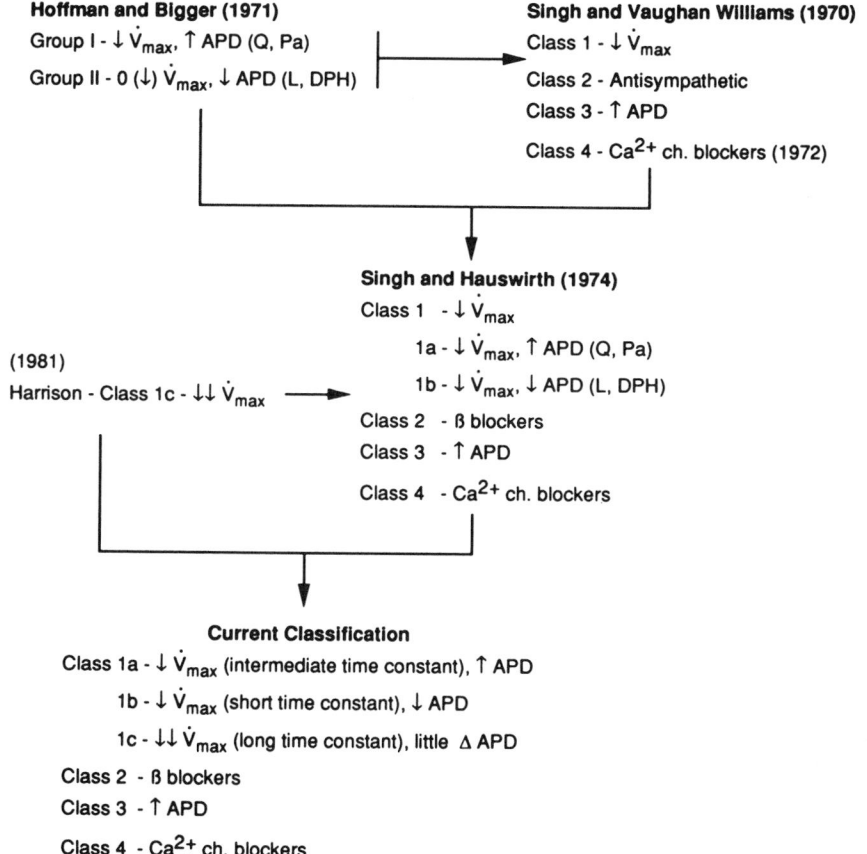

Figure 1. Evolution of the current classification of antiarrhythmic drugs. Titles of classification systems are shown in bold. Q: quinidine; Pa: procainamide; L: lidocaine; DPH: diphenylhydantoin.

proach to classification has recently been subjected to serious scrutiny.[27]

The Hoffman-Bigger Classification

In 1971, Hoffman and Bigger proposed a classification of antiarrhythmic drugs in *Drill's Pharmacology in Medicine*.[64] Drugs were divided into two sets of compounds based on their effects on the cardiac action potential. Quinidine, procainamide, and propranolol were classified as group I drugs, with the characteristic properties of reducing myocardial excitability and phase 0 sodium current. Lidocaine and phenytoin, on the other hand, were classified as group II agents. The latter were considered to be devoid of sodium channel blocking properties and either to leave conduction unchanged or even to improve it. In addition, group I drugs characteristically increase action potential duration (with the exception of propranolol, which shortens it), while group II drugs shorten action potential duration. Group I drugs were thought to suppress reentry by causing bidirectional block in a potential reentry circuit, while group II agents were believed to abolish unidirectional block by improving conduction.

The Singh-Vaughan Williams Classification

In contrast to Hoffman and Bigger, Singh and Vaughan Williams grouped all local anesthetic antiarrhythmic drugs (ie, agents that reduce $\dot{V}_{max}$ of the action potential), including quinidine, procainamide, lidocaine, and phenytoin, into a single drug group, and distinguished the local anesthetics from drugs that act by reducing adrenergic effects on the heart (Figure 1). They added an additional class of antiarrhythmic action, action potential prolongation, to describe the antiarrhythmic properties of amiodarone and sotalol.[65,66] In subsequent work, they identified a "fourth class of anti-dysrhythmic action," exhibited by calcium channel blocking compounds.[67]

Initially, the Hoffman-Bigger classification was more widely used because it accounted for clinically important differences between actions of local anesthetic antiarrhythmic drugs. Specifically, the propensity of quinidine and procainamide to slow ventricular conduction, prolong the QT interval, increase refractoriness and suppress reentrant arrhythmias[68–71] was well explained by their placement in a single antiarrhythmic drug group, as in the Hoffman-Bigger classification. Lidocaine and phenytoin, in contrast, do not alter ventricular conduction velocity in normal tissue, change the QT interval significantly, alter refractoriness, or terminate reentrant arrhythmias.[72–73] With time, however, several important weaknesses of the Hoffman-Bigger classification became evident. First, while propranolol does have local anesthetic properties, these occur at plasma concentrations that are at the upper limit of the clinically relevant range, and are not responsible for many of the drug's antiarrhythmic actions. Moreover, a whole range of β-blocking drugs were developed that had significant antiarrhythmic properties, but did not act as local anesthetics. In addition, under certain conditions the group II compounds lidocaine and phenytoin were found to have clear sodium channel blocking properties.[74] A third deficiency was the absence of a category in which to place drugs that acted by prolonging action potential duration like bretylium, which came into extensive use in the 1970s.[75,76] At about the same time, interest increased in the antiarrhythmic capabilities of amiodarone, a drug thought to act predominantly by increasing action potential duration.[77,78] Finally, the calcium channel blockers, an important group of drugs used to treat supraventricular arrhythmias, was not considered in the Hoffman-Bigger classification.

Evolution of the Currently Used Classification System

Given the respective advantages of the Hoffman-Bigger and Singh-Vaughan Williams classifications, it was logical to develop a hybrid system that would combine the advantages of both classifications. In 1974, Singh and Hauswirth modified the Singh-Vaughan Williams classification to include quinidine, procainamide, and disopyramide (Hoffman-Bigger group I agents), as Class Ia, and phenytoin and lidocaine (Hoffman-Bigger group II), as Class Ib agents.[79] As in the original Singh-Vaughan Williams classification, Class II drugs were agents acting by sympathetic antagonism (including the β-blockers such as propranolol). Class III drugs acted by prolonging action potential duration in fast channel tissue, and Class IV referred to the calcium antagonists.

During the 1970s, several compounds were identified that acted via potent sodium channel blockade.[80–82] These agents were different in electrophysiological actions from the classes of drugs described by Singh and Hauswirth, and were designated Class Ic compounds by Harrison.[83] The latter emphasized the important local anesthetic actions of these drugs (including flecainide, encainide, and lorcainide), while separating them from typical Class Ia and Ib compounds. This classification, shown in Figure 1, has constituted the basis for antiarrhythmic drug classification since the 1980s.

Values and Limitations of the Current Classification

To be useful, a classification should assign drugs to a specific and limited number of categories. These categories should provide useful information about the mechanisms of drug action, electrophysiological effects, clinical indications and potential adverse drug reactions. The mode of category assignment should be clear, and ideally it should be consistent.

Effects on Electrophysiological Properties

The first question to address is whether drugs within a given class segregate homogeneously with respect to electrophysiological descriptors. Figures 2 and 3 show the effects of a variety of antiarrhythmic drugs of various classes on electrocardiographic and electrophysiological variables, based on an analysis of extensive data from the literature.[19] In general, Class Ia drugs moderately increase indices of ventricular conduction (QRS and HV intervals), as well as reflectors of action potential duration (QTc, AERP, VERP). Class Ib drugs have no significant effect on these variables. Class Ic drugs tend to prolong conduction indices (PR, QRS, AH, and HV intervals) more than Class Ia drugs. This effect is particularly noteworthy for increases in AH and HV intervals. Conversely, Class Ic drugs produce modest increases in QTc, AERP, and VERP. Overall, each subclass behaves more or less homogeneously. The differences between class Ib compounds and the other two groups of local anesthetic agents are clear, but there is some overlap between the properties of Class Ia and Ic compounds. The mechanism by which Class Ic drugs increase the AH and PR intervals is uncertain. These changes are most likely due to strong conduction slowing in fast channel tissue within the AV node complex, but slow channel blockade cannot be completely excluded. In general, the electrophysiological and electrocardiographic properties of Class I compounds are consistent with their classification, with Class Ia agents increasing atrial and ventricular refractoriness and slowing ventricular conduction moderately, Class Ib agents having little effect on either conduction or refractoriness in normal tissue, and Ic agents slowing conduction more potently than Ia compounds. While Class Ic agents are frequently assumed to have no effect on repolarization, this is probably incorrect as the consistent, albeit modest, increases in QTc (Figure 2), AERP and VERP (Figure 3) indicate.

The Class II compound, nadolol, increases RR, PR, and AH intervals, as expected from the effects of a β-blocker. Data for pure Class III compounds are limited. The results of amiodarone therapy indicate conduction slowing in both fast and slow channel tissues, as well as bradycardic actions. While these are

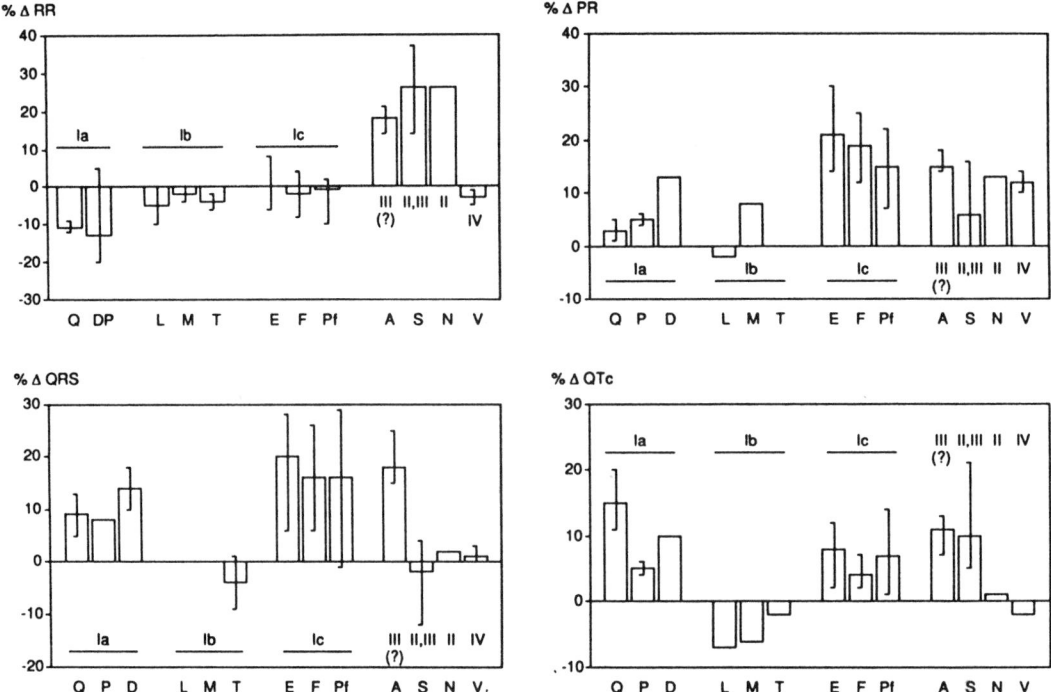

Figure 2. Effects of drugs of various classes on electrocardiographic variables, based on a recent meta-analysis.[19] For each drug, vertical bars indicate average of mean effects in a number of trials; vertical range indicator shows the range of mean effects across available trials. Q: quinidine; P: procainamide; D: disopyramide; L: lidocaine M: mexiletine; T: tocainide; E: encainide; F: flecainide; Pf: propafenone; A: amiodarone; S: sotalol; N: nadolol; V: verapamil.

not necessarily consistent with expectations for a Class III compound, amiodarone has been well shown to possess properties of Classes I,[84] II,[11–13] and IV,[85,86] as well as of Class III. Sotalol possesses no Class I or IV drug action, and this is well reflected by its electrophysiological properties, some of which resemble those of nadolol (RR, PR, and AH prolongation), while others are typical Class III actions (QTc, AERP, and VERP prolongation). Verapamil produces the PR prolongation and AH prolongation expected from a drug that blocks slow channel-dependent conduction in the AV node. The lack of sinus slowing by the drug is consistent with the autonomic reflexes elicited by its vasodilating action.

Overall, the electrocardiographic and electrophysiological effects of various drugs

agree with predictions from the current classification. Problems lie in greater overlap between compounds than might be expected, as well as agents, such as amiodarone and sotalol, possessing properties of more than one class of drugs.

Effects on Cardiac Arrhythmias

Figure 4 shows the effects of a variety of antiarrhythmic drugs on ventricular tachycardia induction as determined by an analysis of available clinical trials.[19] The graph shows mean percent efficacy in the treatment of ventricular tachycardia obtained from the average of a series of clinical trials for each compound. The first point to note is that no single com-

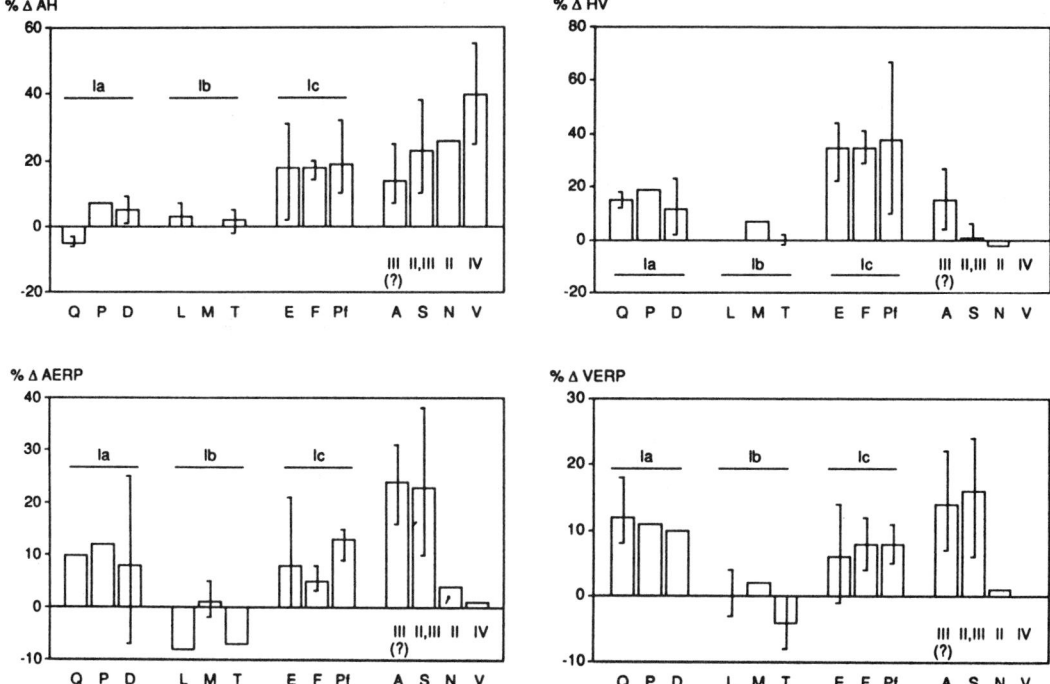

Figure 3. Effects of drugs of various classes on electrophysiological variables, based on a recent meta-analysis.[19] For each drug, vertical bars indicate average of mean effects in a number of trials; vertical range indicator shows the range of mean effects across available trials. Q: quinidine; P: procainamide; D: disopyramide; L: lidocaine; M: mexiletine; T: tocainide; E: encainide; F: flecainide; Pf: propafenone; A: amiodarone; S: sotalol; N: nadolol; V: verapamil.

pound is terribly efficacious. However, Class Ia and Ic compounds have modest efficacy (in the range of 20%), consistent with their mixed effects on conduction and refractoriness. Class Ib, II, and IV compounds appear to be less effective. Amiodarone has similar efficacy to Class Ia and Ic compounds, consistent with its electrophysiological actions on indices of conduction and refractoriness (Figures 2 and 3). Sotalol, however, appears to be more effective than the other agents. This probably reflects its ability to prolong ventricular refractoriness without slowing conduction (Figure 3), a Class III type of action on fast channel tissue. Overall, while no single compound is very effective against sustained ventricular tachycardia induction, drug actions are consistent with expectations from the classification system, based on the idea that the greater the

prolongation of refractoriness and the less the slowing of conduction caused by a given compound, the greater will be its efficacy against sustained ventricular tachycardia.

Effects on Sudden Cardiac Death

Figure 5 shows the effects of various classes of antiarrhythmic drugs on the incidence of sudden cardiac death, based on a meta-analysis by Yusuf and Teo.[87] Assuming that acute myocardial ischemia plays a major role in sudden cardiac death, for which there is a great deal of circumstantial clinical evidence,[1] the results of clinical trials are consistent with expectations based on the classification system. Class I compounds tend to have a

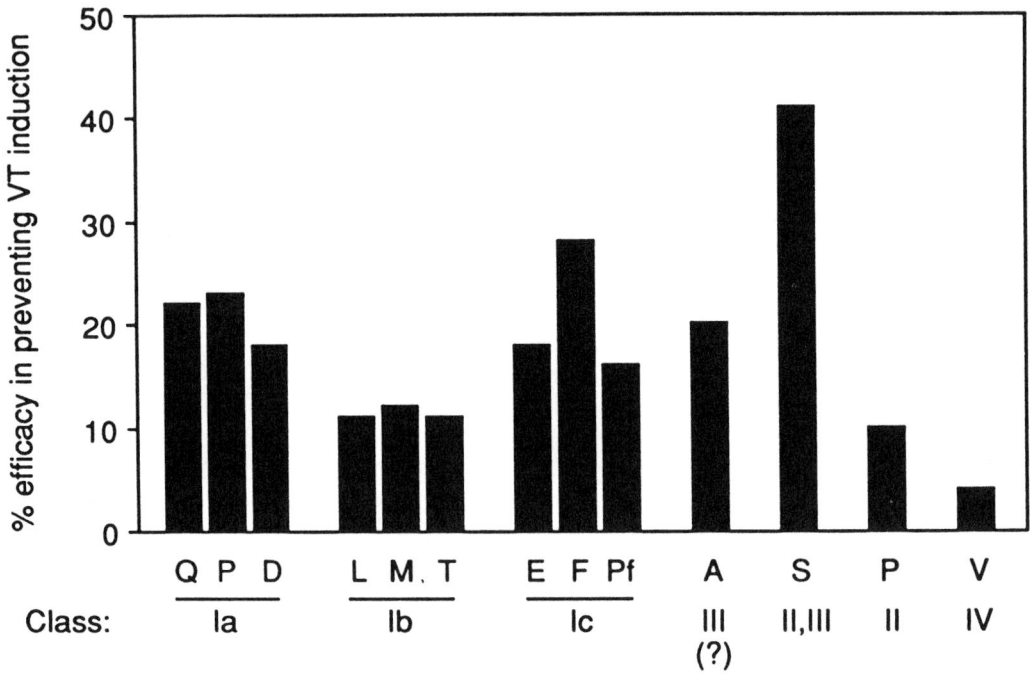

Figure 4. Percent efficacy in preventing induction of monomorphic VT, based on a meta-analysis of available clinical trials.[19] Results are averages of mean efficacies in individual studies. Q: quinidine; P: procainamide; D: disopyramide; L: lidocaine; M: mexiletine; T: tocainide; E: encainide; F: flecainide; Pf: propafenone; A: amiodarone; S: sotalol; P: propranolol; V: verapamil.

deleterious effect on the prevalence of sudden cardiac death, consistent with their actions in experimental animal models of acute ischemic ventricular fibrillation.[88–90] Furthermore, the most potent Class I agents, the Class Ic compounds, appear to have the greatest potentially deleterious actions. Class II drugs, known to have important anti-ischemic properties, are consistently effective in preventing sudden cardiac death, as demonstrated in a substantial number of clinical trials. The data on Class III agents are limited by the small number of patients studied (see Chapter 35 through 43), but Class IV compounds do not appear to reduce the prevalence of sudden cardiac death. This is somewhat surprising, given the efficacy of such compounds in preventing ischemic ventricular fibrillation[91,92] in animal models, and points to potential deficiencies in our understanding of the mechanisms of sudden cardiac death. However, vera-

pamil and diltiazem seem to behave similarly in post-infarction trials, again suggesting the overall homogeneous behavior of various drug classes.

Ventricular Proarrhythmic Actions

Ventricular antiarrhythmic drugs are capable of causing de novo ventricular tachyarrhythmias. Two specific patterns have been identified. Paroxysmal, generally nonsustained polymorphic ventricular tachycardia associated with QT prolongation is caused by drugs that prolong action potential duration.[7,8] This complication is most frequently noted with Class Ia and Class III compounds, and occurs rarely, if at all, as a result of Class Ib, Ic, II, or IV drug therapy. However, sustained ventricular tachyarrhythmias, often

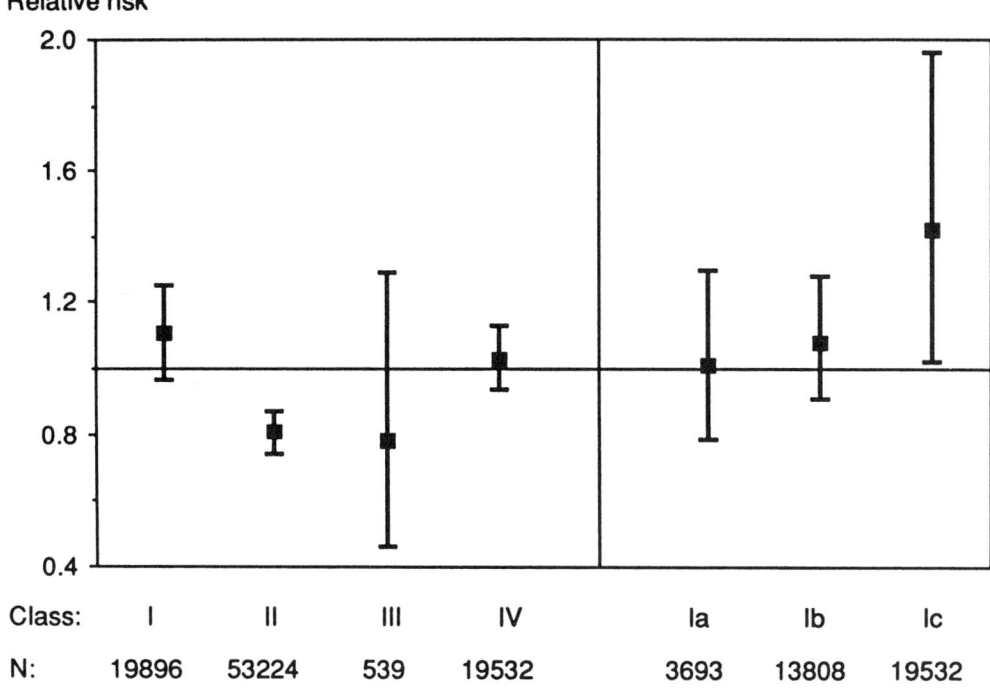

Figure 5. Relative risk compared to placebo therapy (mean and 95% confidence interval) of death during therapy with various classes of antiarrhythmic drugs. Results are based on a preliminary meta-analysis of randomized, controlled clinical trials by Teo et al.[19]

with excess ventricular conduction slowing, are typically produced by Class Ic compounds.[36,37] Once again, there seems to be a fair degree of consistency of behavior within an antiarrhythmic drug class.

Drugs That Don't Fit

The major deficiencies of the current classification relate to drugs that don't fit, either because there is no class to which to assign them or because they belong to multiple drug classes. The examples of amiodarone and sotalol have already been discussed. Other agents, such as bepridil (a Class III and Class IV drug), bretylium (with Class II and Class III properties), and propafenone (with weak Class II properties in addition to Class Ic actions) exist. Some newer compounds that prolong action potential duration are considered to have Class III properties, but are classi-

fied as having additional Class Ia or Ib action.[93,94]

There is no category into which digitalis can be placed, and digitalis compounds are very commonly used to treat cardiac arrhythmias. Similarly, there is no category for purinergic agonists, muscarinic agonists, magnesium and α-adrenergic receptor antagonists.

The Sicilian Gambit

A Task Force of the working group on arrhythmias of the European Society of Cardiology recently published an extensive analysis of antiarrhythmic drug classifications. They reviewed in detail the potential mechanisms of drug action on voltage-dependent channels, background currents, pumps, and exchange mechanisms. The various mechanisms of cardiac arrhythmia were discussed, along with the ways that they might be modified by altering electrophysiological properties. The working group proposed an approach using a series of tables and figures, with classification based on arrhythmogenic mechanisms and the identification of vulnerable parameters. Their concluding remarks suggest that they considered their work as a basis for discussion and the evolution of a better approach to antiarrhythmic drug classification, rather than a definitive classification per se.[27] Table 4 of their manuscript lists representative drugs used to improve specific arrhythmias by altering a critical vulnerable parameter. Of the 27 drug groups listed, 22 correspond to classes of the current antiarrhythmic drug classification. Of the rest, two are muscarinic agonists, which are rarely used to treat clinical arrhythmias. β-Agonist and vagolytic agents, two other listings, are used to increase heart rate, and while they are an important component of the approach to treating torsade de pointes arrhythmias, they cannot be considered antiarrhythmic agents per se. Magnesium and adenosine are listed, and would require modification of the current classification to be included. A significant proportion of magnesium's antiarrhythmic properties may, however, be due to antagonism of calcium currents.[95] Adenosine activates a potassium current very similar to I_{KAch}, and may therefore be considered to be part of a group of drugs that act by enhancing G-protein coupled potassium current. Other limitations of the Sicilian gambit have been discussed elsewhere.[96]

Thus, while the working group considers the current classification to be inadequate, the information listed in their Table 4 suggests that, on the contrary, the classification is in fact still quite useful for identifying specific types of drugs that are effective in treating arrhythmias of specific mechanisms.

Prospects for the Future

Antiarrhythmic drug classifications have been used since the number of antiarrhythmic drugs increased beyond two. Given the likelihood that the number of available antiarrhythmic agents will if anything increase, there will always be a need to consider antiarrhythmic drugs in groups with similar mechanisms of pharmacological action. A recent review[19] suggests that many of the difficulties with the current classification can be diminished by returning to the original concept of Singh and Vaughan Williams of classes of drug action, rather than classes of drugs per se. This would allow for greater flexibility, while preserving the important mechanistic information contained in the current classification system. Some additions are certainly necessary, to include important compounds such as adenosine, and digitalis.

Table 3 suggests a revised approach to dividing drugs according to their class actions. Digitalis, adenosine, and agents that increase M_2-muscarinic receptor stimulation could be included in a single new class of compounds that act by increasing G-protein coupled potassium channel activity. Existing compounds combining actions of various classes could be so identified, eg, quinidine is a drug with Class III and moderate Class I actions; amiodarone has actions of all four drug classes; lidocaine has a moderate voltage- and rate-dependent Class I action, etc. This approach would deal with some of the limitations of the current classification, while allowing new compounds to be added and increasing flexibility.

Table 3
Divide Drugs According to Class Actions

Class 1 — Sodium channel blockade
Class 2 — Sympathetic antagonism
Class 3 — Action potential prolongation (or potassium channel blockade)
Class 4 — Calcium channel blockade
Class 5 — Activators of muscarinic-purinergic potassium channels

References

1. Nattel S, Waters D: What is an antiarrhythmic drug? From clinical trials to fundamental concepts. *Am J Cardiol* 66:96, 1990.

2. Hondeghem LM, Katzung BG: Antiarrhythmic agents: the modulated receptor mechanism of action of sodium and calcium channel-blocking drugs. *Ann Rev Pharmacol Toxicol* 24:387, 1984.

3. Grant AO, Starmer CF, Strauss HC: Antiarrhythmic drug action: blockade of the inward sodium current. *Circ Res* 55:427, 1984.

4. Uehara A, Hume JR: Interactions of organic calcium channel antagonists with calcium channels in single frog atrial cells. *J Gen Physiol* 85:621, 1985.

5. Nayebpour M, Talajic M, Jing W, Nattel S: Autonomic modulation of the frequency-dependent electrophysiologic and antiarrhythmic actions of diltiazem in anesthetized dogs. *J Pharmacol Exp Ther* 253:353, 1990.

6. Colatsky TJ, Follmer CH, Starmer CF: Channel specificity in antiarrhythmic drug action: mechanism of potassium channel block and its role in suppressing and aggravating cardiac arrhythmias. *Circulation* 82:2235, 1990.

7. Jackman WM, Friday KJ, Anderson JL, et al: The long syndromes: a crtical review in new clinical observations and a unifying hypothesis. *Prog Cardiovasc Dis* 31:115, 1988.

8. Roden DM, Thompson KA, Hoffman, BF, Woosley RL: Clinical features and basic mechanisms of quinidine-induced arrhthmias. *J Am Coll Cardiol* 8:73A, 1986.

9. January CT, Riddle JM, Salata JJ: A model for early afterdepolarizations: induction with the Ca^{2+} channel agonist Bay K 8644. *Circ Res* 62:563, 1988.

10. Nattel S, Quantz MA: Pharmacological response of quinidine induced early afterdepolarization in canine cardiac Purkinje fibers: insights into underlying ionic mechanisms. *Cardiovasc Res* 22:808, 1988.

11. Charlier F: Cardiac actions in the dog of a new antagonist of adrenergic excitation which doess not produce competitive blockade of adrenoreceptors. *Br J Pharmacol* 39:668. 1970.

12. Polster P, Broekhuysen J: The adrenergic antagonism of amiodarone. *Biochem Pharmacol* 25:131, 1976.

13. Nokin P, Clinet M, Schoenfeld P: Cardiac beta-adrenoceptor modulati8on by amiodarone. *Biochem Pharmacol* 32:2473, 1983.

14. Venkatesh N, Padbury JF, Singh BN: Effects of amiodarone and desethyl-amiodarone on rabbit myocardial β-adrenoceptors and serum thyroid hormones. Absence of relationship to serum and myocardial drug concentrations. *J Cardiovasc Pharmacol* 8:989, 1986.

15. Franklyn JA, Davis JR, Gammage MD, et al: Amiodarone and thyroid hormone action. *Clin Endocrin* 22:257, 1985.

16. Latham KR, Sellitti OF, Goldstein RE: Interaction of amiodarone and desethylamiodarone with solubilized nuclear thyroid hormone receptors. *J Am Coll Cardiol* 9:872, 1987.

17. Talajic M, Nattel S, Davies M, McCans J: Attenuation of class 3 and sinus node effects of amiodarone by experimental hypothyroidism. *J Cardiovasc Pharmacol* 13:447, 1989.

18. Kniffen FJ, Lomas TE, Counsell RE, Lucchesi BR: The antiarrhythmic and antifibrillatory actions of bretylium and its o-iodobenzyl trimethylammonium analog, UM-360. *J Pharmacol Exp Ther* 192:120, 1975.

19. Nattel S: Antiarrhythmic drug classifications. A critical appraisal of theirhistory, present status, and clinical relevance. *Drugs* 41:672, 1991.

20. Sung RJ, Tai DY, Svinarich JT: Beta-adrenoceptor blockade: electrophysiology and antiarrhythmic mechanisms. *Am Heart J* 108:1115, 1984.

21. Schaal SF, Sugimoto T, Wallace AG, Sealy WC: Effects of digitalis on the functional refractory period of the AV node: studies in awake dogs with and without cardiac denervation. *Cardiovasc Res* 4:356, 1968.

22. Cantwell JD, Dawson JE, Fletcher GF: Supraventricular tachyarrhythmias: treatment with edrophonium. *Arch Intem Med* 130:221, 1972.

23. Belardinelli L, Shryock J, West A, et al: Effects of adenosine and adenine nucleotides on the atrioventricular node of isolated guinea pig hearts. *Circulation* 70:1083, 1989.

24. Ragazzl E, Wu SN, Shryock J, Belardinelli L: Electrophysiological and receptor binding studies to assess activation of the cardiac adenosine receptor by adenine nucleotides. *Circ Res* 68:1035, 1991.

25. Belhassen B, Pelleg A: Electrophysiologic effects of adenosine triphosphate and adenosine on the mammalian heart: clinical and experimental aspects. *J Am Coll Cardiol* 4:414, 1984.

26. Pelleg A: Cardiac cellular electrophysiologic actions of adenosine and adenosine triphosphate. *Am Heart J* 110:688, 1985.

27. The Sicilian Gambit. A new approach to the classification of antiarrhythmic drugs based on their actions on arrhythmogenic mechanisms. *Circulation* 84:1831, 1991.

28. Fish FA, Prakash C, Roden DM: Suppression of repolarization-related arrhythmias in vitro and in vivo by low-dose potassium channel activator. *Circulation* 82:1362, 1990.

29. Spinelli W, Sorota S, Siegal M, Hoffman BF: Antiarrhythmic actions of the ATP-regulated $^+$ activated by pinacidil. *Circ Res* 68:1127, 1991.

30. Carlsson L, Abrahamsson C, Drews L, Duker G: Antiarrhythmic effects of potassium channel openers in rhythm abnormalities related to de-

layed repolarization. *Circulation* 85:1491, 1992.

31. Kass RS, Lederer WJ, Tsien RW, Weingart R: Role of calcium ions in transient inward currents and aftercontractions induced by strophantidin in cardiac Purkinje fibers. *J Physiol* 281:187, 1987.

32. Rosen MR, Gelband HB, Hoffman BF: Correlation between effects of ouabain on the canine electrocardiogram and transmembrane potentials of isolated Purkinje fibers. *Circulation* 47:65, 1973.

33. Ferrier GR, Saunders JH, Mendez C: A cellular mechanism for the generation of ventricular arrhythmias by acetylstrophanthidin. *Circ Res* 32:600, 1973.

34. Rosen MR, Danilo P Jr: Effects of tetrodotoxin, lidocaine, verapamil and AHR-2666 on ouabain-induced delayed afterdepolarizations in canine Purkinje fibers. *Circ Res* 46:117, 1980.

35. Ranger S, Talajic M, Lemery R, et al: Amplification of flecainide-induced ventricular conduction slowing by exercise: a potentially significant clinical consequence of use-dependent sodium channel blockade. *Circulation* 79:1000, 1989.

36. Levine JH, Morganroth J, Kadish AH: Mechanisms and risk factors for proarrhythmia with type 1a compared with Ic antiarrhythmic drug therapy. *Circulation* 80:1063, 1989.

37. Winkle RA, Mason JW, Griffin JC, Ross D: Malignant ventricular tachyarrhythmias associated with the use of encainide. *Am Heart J* 102:857, 1981.

38. Davidenko JM, Antzelevitch C: The effect of milrinone on conduction, reflection and automaticity in canine Purkinje fibers. *Circulation* 69:1026, 1984.

39. Jalife J, Moe GK: Effect of electrotonic potentials on pacemaker activity of canine Purkinje fibers in relation to parasystole. *Circ Res* 39:801, 1976.

40. Nattel S: Frequency-dependent effects of amitriptyline on ventricular conduction and cardiac rhythm in dogs. *Circulation* 72:898, 1985.

41. Nattel S: Relationship between use-dependent effects of antiarrhythmic drugs on conduction and $\dot{V}_{max}$ in canine cardiac Purkinje fibers. *J Pharmacol Exp Ther* 241:282, 1987.

42. Nattel S, Jing W: Rate-dependent changes in intraventricular conduction produced by procainamide in anesthetized dogs. A quantitative analysis based on the relation between phase 0 inward current and conduction velocity. *Circ Res* 65:1485, 1989.

43. Villemaire C, Savard P, Talajic M, Nattel S: A quantitative analysis of use-dependent ventricular conduction slowing by procainamide in anesthetized dogs. *Circulation* 85:2255, 1992.

44. Ranger S, Talajic M, Lemery R, et al: Kinetics of use-dependent ventricular conduction slowing by antiarrhythmic drugs in humans. *Circulation* 83:1987, 1991.

45. Talajic M, Nattel S: Frequency-dependent effects of calcium antagonists on atrioventricular conduction and refractoriness: demonstration and characterization in anesthetized dogs. *Circulation* 74:1156, 1986.

46. Talajic M, Lemery R, Roy D, et al: The rate-dependent effects of diltiazem on human atrioventricular nodal properties. *Circulation* 86:870, 1992.

47. Talajic M, Papadatos D, Villemaire C, et al: Antiarrhythmic actions of diltiazem during experimental atrioventricular reentrant tachycardias. Importance of use-dependent calcium channel-blocking properties. *Circulation* 81:334, 1990.

48. Talajic M, Nayebpour M, Jing W, Nattel S: Frequency-dependent effects of diltiazem on the atrioventricular node during experimental atrial fibrillation. *Circulation* 80:380, 1989.

49. Nayebpour M, Talajic M, Villemaire C, Nattel S: Vagal modulation of the rate-dependent properties of the atrioventricular node. *Circ Res* 67:1152, 1990.

50. Nayebpour M, Talajic M, Nattel S: Effects of β-adrenergic receptor stimulation and blockade on rate-dependent atrioventricular nodal properties. *Circ Res* 70:902, 1992.

51. Nayebpour M, Billette J, Amellal F, Nattel S: Adenosine suppresses AV reentrant tachycardia by causing rate-dependent increases in wavelength. *J Am Coll Cardiol* 19(Suppl A):346A, 1992.

52. Nattel S, Zeng F-D: Frequency dependent effects of antiarrhythmic drugs on action potential duration and refractoriness. *J Pharmacol Exp Ther* 229:283, 1984.

53. Roden DM, Hoffman BF: Action potential prolongation and induction of abnormal automaticity by low quinidine concentrations in canine Purkinje fibers. Relationship to potassium and cycle length. *Circ Res* 56:857, 1985.

54. Hondeghem LM, Snyders DJ: Class III antiarrhythmic agents have a lot of potential but a long way to go: reduced effectiveness and dangers of reverse-use dependence. *Circulation* 81:686, 1990.

55. Roden DM, Bennett PB, Snyders DJ, et al: Quinidine delays I, activation in guinea pig ventricular myocytes. *Circ Res* 62:1055, 1988.

56. Balser JR, Bennett PB, Hondeghem LM, Roden DM: Suppression of time-dependent outward current in guinea pig ventricular myocytes. Actions of quinidine and amiodarone. *Circ Res* 69:519, 1991.

57. Wang Z, Pelletier LC, Talajic M, Nattel S: The effects of flecainide and quinidine on human atrial action potentials. *Circulation* 82:274, 1990.

58. Johnson EA: The effects of quinidine, procaine amide and pyrilamine on the membrane resting and action potential of guinea pig ventricular muscle fibers. *J Pharmacol Exp Ther* 108:237, 1956.

59. Vaughan Williams EM: The mode of action of quinidine on isolated rabbit atria interpreted from intracellular potential records. *Br J Pharmacol* 13:276, 1958.

60. Weidmann S: Effects of calcium ions and local anesthetics on electrical properties of Purkinje fibers. *J Physiol* 129:568, 1955.

61. Bigger JT Jr, Mandel WJ: Effect of lidocaine on conduction in canine Purkinje fibers and at the ventricular muscle-Purkinje fiber junction. *J Pharmacol Exp Ther* 172:239, 1970.

62. Bigger JT Jr, Mandel WJ: Effect of lidocaine on the electrophysiological properties of ventricular muscle and Purkinje fibers. *J Clin Invest* 49:563, 1970.

63. Bigger JT Jr, Bassett AL, Hoffman BF: Electrophysiological effects of diphenylhydantoin on canine Purkinje fibers. *Circ Res* 22:221, 1968.

64. Hoffman BF, Bigger JT Jr: Antiarrhythmic drugs. In: JR DiPalma (ed): *Drill's Pharmacology in Medicine*. 4th edition. New York: McGraw-Hill Book Company, 1971, p. 824.

65. Singh BN, Vaughan Williams EM: The effect of amiodarone, a new anti-anginal drug on cardiac muscle. *Br J Pharmacol* 39:657, 1970.

66. Singh BN, Vaughan Williams EM: A third class of anti-arrhythmic action: effects on atrial and ventricular intracellular potentials and other pharmacological actions on cardiac muscle of MJ 1999 and AH 3474. *Br J Pharmacol* 39:675, 1970.

67. Singh BN, Vaughan Williams EM: A fourth class of anti-dysrhythmic action? Effect of verapamil on ouabain toxicity, on atrial and ventricular intracellular potentials, and on other features of cardiac function. *Cardiovasc Res* 6:109, 1972.

68. Josephson ME, Caracta AR, Ricciutti MA, et al: Electrophysiologic properties of procainamide in man. *Am J Cardiol* 33:596, 1974.

69. Josephson ME, Seides SF, Batsford WP, et al: The electrophysiological effects of intramuscular quinidine on the atrioventricular conduction system in man. *Am Heart J* 87:55, 1974.

70. Giardina EGV, Bigger JT Jr: Procaine amide against re-entrant ventricular arrhythmias. *Circulation* 48:959, 1973.

71. Heissenbuttel RH, Bigger JT Jr: The effect of oral quinidine on intraventricular conduction in man: correlation of plasma quinidine with changes in QRS duration. *Am Heart J* 80:453, 1970.

72. Bekheit S, Muragh JG, Morton P, Fletcher E: Effect of lignocaine on conducting system of human heart. *Br Heart J* 35:305, 1973.

73. Damato AN, Berkowitz WD, Patton RD, Lau SH: The effect of diphenylhydantoin on atrioventricular and intraventricular conduction in man. *Am Heart J* 79:51, 1970.

74. Singh BN, Vaughan Williams EM: Effect of altering potassium concentration on the action of lidocaine and diphenylhydantoin on rabbit atrial and ventricular muscle. *Circ Res* 29:286, 1971.

75. Holder DA, Sniderman AD, Fraser G, Fallen EL: Experience with bretylium tosylate by a hospital cardiac arrest team. *Circulation* 55:541, 1977.

76. Heissenbuttel RH, Bigger JT Jr: Bretylium tosylate: a newly available antiarrhythmic drug for ventricular arrhythmias. *Ann Intern Med* 91:229, 1979.

77. Rosenbaum MB, Chiale PA, Halpern MS, et al: Clinical efficacy of amiodarone as an antiarrhythmic agent. *Am J Cardiol* 38:934, 1976.

78. Singh BN: Amiodarone: Historical development and pharmacologic profile. *Am Heart J* 106:788, 1983.

79. Singh BN, Hauswirth O: Comparative mechanisms of action of antiarrhythmic drugs. *Am Heart J* 87:367, 1974.

80. Carmeliet E, Janssen PAJ, Marsboom R, et al: Antiarrhythmic, electrophysiological and hemodynamic effects of lorcainide. *Arch Int Pharmacodyn Ther* 231:104, 1978.

81. Carmeliet E: Electrophysiological effects of encainide on isolated cardiac muscle and Purkinje fibers and on the Langendorff-perfused guinea-pig heart. *Eur J Pharmacol* 61:247, 1980.

82. Cowan JC, Vaughan Williams EM: Characterization of a new oral antiarrhythmic drug, flecainide (R818). *Eur J Pharmacol* 73:333, 1981.

83. Harrison DC, Winkle RA, Sami M, Mason JW: Encainide: a new and potent antiarrhythmic agent. In: DC Harrison, JW Mason, HA Miller, RA Winkle (eds): *Cardiac Arrhythmia: A Decade of Progress*. Boston, MA: GK Hall Medical Publishers, Boston, MA: 1981, p. 315.

84. Mason JW, Hondeghem LM, Katzung BG: Block of inactivated sodium channels and of depolarization-induced automaticity in guinea pig papillary muscle by amiodarone. *Circ Res* 55:277, 1984.

85. Nattel S, Talajic M, Quantz M, DeRoode M: Frequency-dependent effects of amiodarone on atrioventricular nodal function and slow-channel action potentials: evidence for calcium

channel-blocking activity. *Circulation* 76:442, 1987.

86. Nishimura M, Follmer CH, Singer DH: Amiodarone blocks calcium current in single guinea pig ventricular myocytes. *J Pharmacol Exp Ther* 251:650, 1989.

87. Yusuf S, Teo KK: Approaches to prevention of sudden death: need for fundamental re-evaluation. *J Cardiovasc Electrophysiol* 2:5233, 1991.

88. Elharrar V, Gaum WE, Zipes DP: Effect of drugs on conduction delay and incidence of ventricular arrhythmias induced by acute coronary occlusion in dogs. *Am J Cardiol* 39:544, 1977.

89. Nattel S, Pedersen DH, Zipes DP: Alterations in regional myocardial distribution and arrhythmogenic effects of aprindine produced by coronary artery occlusion in the dog. *Cardiovasc Res* 15:80, 1981.

90. Lederman SN, Wenger TL, Boslter DE, Strauss HC: Effects of flecainide on occlusion and reperfusion arrhythmias in dogs. *J Cardiovasc Pharmacol* 13:541, 1989.

91. Kaumann AJ, Aramendia P: Prevention of ventricular fibrillation induced by coronary ligation. *J Pharmacol Exp Ther* 164:326, 1968.

92. Clusin Wr, Bristow MR, Baim DS, et al: The effects of diltiazem and reduced serum ionized calcium on ischemic ventricular fibrillation in the dog. *Circ Res* 50:518, 1982.

93. Frederick LG, McDonald SJ, Garthwaite SM: Cardiovascular profile of a new anti-arrhythmic agent, SC-40230. *Cardiovasc Res* 23:897, 1989.

94. Toyama J, Kodama I, Honjo H, Kamiya K: Electrophysiological effects of OPC-881 17, a new antiarrhythmic agent on papillary muscles and single ventricular myocytes isolated from guinea-pig hearts. *Br J Pharmacol* 98:177, 1989.

95. Nattel S, Turmel N, MacLeod R, Solymoss BC: Actions of intravenous magnesium on ventricular arrhythmias caused by acute myocardial infarction. *J Pharmacol Exp Ther* 259:939, 1991.

96. Ahmed R, Singh BN: Antiarrhythmic drugs. *Curr Opinion Cardiol* 8:10, 1993.

Chapter 16

Modes of Sodium Channel Blocking Action of Class I Drugs

Junji Toyama
Itsuo Kodama
Kaichiro Kamyia
Takafumi Anno

Class I drugs, which are most frequently used in the treatment of both ventricular and supraventricular arrhythmias, have been subclassified into Class Ia, Ib, and Ic according to the actions of these drugs on the action potential duration (APD) or QT interval.[1-4] This classification has been widely recognized for 20 years relative to the experimental findings. It has also been used as a basis for the choice of antiarrhythmic agents in the treatment of certain clinical cardiac arrhythmias.

However, the classification and subclassification of drug mechanisms by this approach is not always cognizant of the fact that some of the agents produce divergent results such as shortening or lengthening of the APD relative to the species of animals used for evaluating drug effects. For example, propafenone, which is usually classified as a Class Ic agent, prolongs the APD of the guinea pig ventricular muscle at concentrations lower than 0.5 μM and then shortens it dose dependently at higher concentrations as shown in Figure 1.[5]

Such a biphasic effect is observed more or less in almost all the Class Ia and Ic drugs.[6]

Another issue is that modification of the APD by sodium channel blockers is related more intimately to their blocking actions on the potassium channels (I_{to}, I_k, and I_{K1}) than those on the sodium channel.[7] Therefore, it might be preferable to devise a new classification of sodium channel blockers that take into consideration the differences in the mode of sodium channel blocking actions of these drugs.

Recent developments in our knowledge of cardiac electropharmacology have provided us with further insight into the interaction of Class I drugs with the sodium channel.[8,9] In particular, the modulated receptor hypothesis appears to be the most plausible theory that explains the mechanisms of sodium channel block on the basis of kinetics of drug binding to the channel, and may permit a more comprehensive characterization of the profiles of Class I drugs. Against this background, we tried to reexamine the profiles

From BN Singh, HJJ Wellens, M Hiraoka, (eds): *Electropharmacological Control of Cardiac Arrhythmias.* Mount Kisco, NY, Futura Publishing Company Inc., © 1994.

225

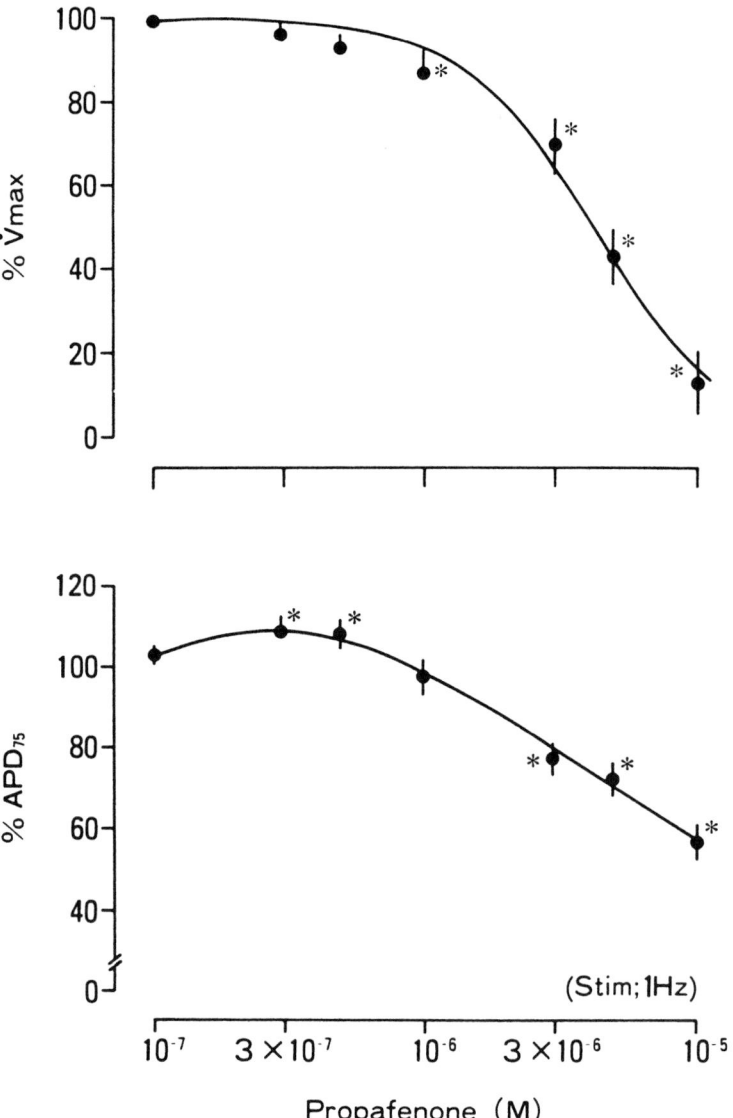

Figure 1. Concentration-dependent effects of propafenone on $\dot{V}_{max}$ and APD_{75}. Values are indicated as mean with SE by vertical line (n = 5). *Significantly different from the reference values at $p < 0.05$. (Reproduced with permission from Reference 5.)

of Class I drugs from the standpoint of the modulated receptor hypothesis.[10]

State Dependency of the Drug Binding to the Sodium Channel

According to the modulated receptor hypothesis, the drug affinity to sodium channel is modulated by the state of the channel. The sodium channel has three states: the activated, the inactivated, and the resting state. Generally speaking, the drug binds to the activated and/or inactivated state channel with higher affinities and unbinds from the resting channel because the drug affinity to the channel is reduced in the resting state.

Figure 2 is a diagrammatic illustration of

the correlation between drug binding and unbinding kinetics and the action potential configuration in ventricular muscle. To examine such state dependency of drug binding to the sodium channel in detail, we applied a depolarizing prepulse that makes the channel activated and then inactivated, and measured the amplitude of $\dot{V}_{max}$ of the action potential that was excited 100 msec after the prepulse.[10] The 100-msec interval between the prepulse and the ensuing excitation is then long enough for the recovery process of the drug-unbound channel from the inactivated state, but too short for the dissociation of the drug from the drug-bound channel. Figure 3 illustrates the difference in the reduction of the width of the prepulse on the $\dot{V}_{max}$ between the separate treatments of the inactivated state channel blocker (ICB) and activated state channel blocker (ACB). In the presence of the drug that binds only to the inactivated channel, the

$\dot{V}_{max}$ of the action potential induced after the prepulse will decrease its amplitude in a time-dependent fashion as the duration of the pulse is prolonged from 10 to 1,000 msec, because the drug binding to the channel is reported to proceed with a half-time of several hundred milliseconds during the inactivated state. However, in the presence of the ACB the $\dot{V}_{max}$ reduction is almost completed by the 10-msec pulse and no additional reduction of $\dot{V}_{max}$ is observed with a further prolongation of the pulse duration.

Figure 4 illustrates the relationship between the duration of the prepulse and $\dot{V}_{max}$ in the presence of mexiletine or disopyramide. $\dot{V}_{max}$ is reduced markedly by the former drug and an equilibrium is reached as the pulse duration is prolonged to 300 msec, but $\dot{V}_{max}$ reduction appears to be completed at the 10-msec pulse by the latter drug. From these results it is considered that mexiletine acts on

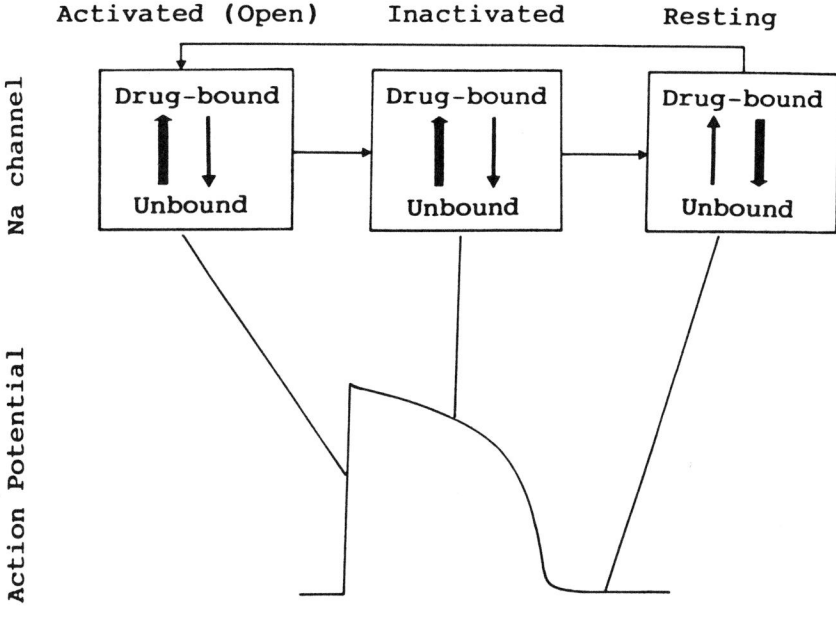

Figure 2. Diagram of the interaction between Class I drug and the sodium channel depicted on the basis of the modulated receptor hypothesis. Inactivated state blocker reduces $\dot{V}_{max}$ more markedly as the prepulse is lengthened toward 1,000 msec, because the drug binding to the inactivated channel proceeds slowly (with a half time of several hundreds milliseconds). In the presence of activated state blocker (ACB), the width of the prepulse does not affect $\dot{V}_{max}$ because the drug binding is completed at the upstroke phase of the prepulse.

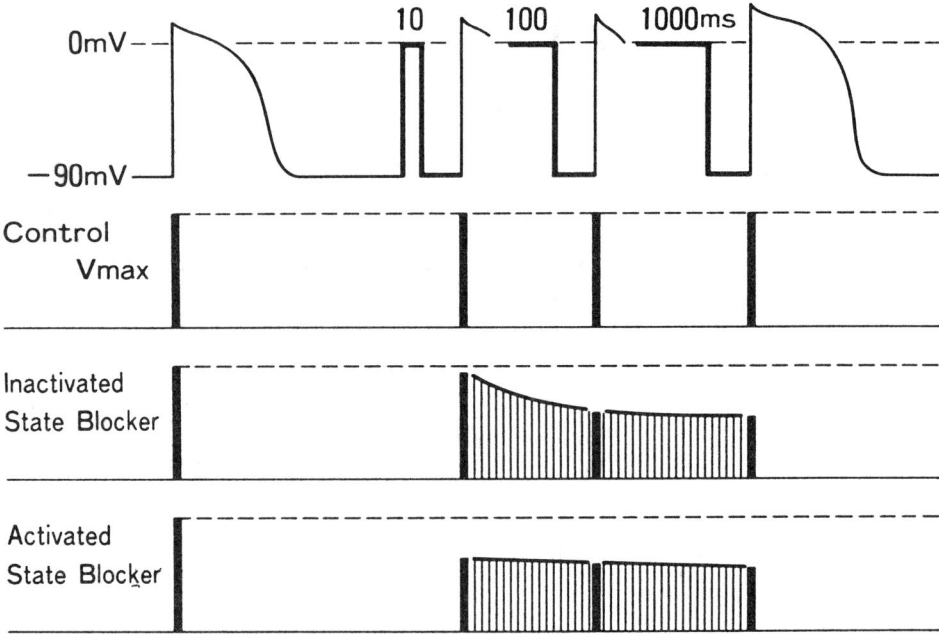

Figure 3. A diagram illustrating effects of the width of the depolarizing prepulse on the $\dot{V}_{max}$ reduction in the presence of inactivated (ICB) and activated state channel blockers (ACB). In the control, any $\dot{V}_{max}$ reduction is not induced by the prepulse of 10- to 1,000-msec wide that is applied 100 msec before the action potential.

the sodium channel mainly in an ICB. However, there is small but definite $\dot{V}_{max}$ reduction at the 10-msec pulse in the presence of mexiletine, indicating that this drug has also the feature of a weak ACB as well.

We estimated state dependency of the channel blocking actions of Class I drugs[11,12] by taking the ratio of the ICB to the ACB, which is obtained by dividing the $\dot{V}_{max}$ reduction into the two fractions as shown in the lower panel of Figure 5. It is of interest that all Class Ib drugs have a high ratio in comparison to Class Ia drugs tested (quinidine and disopyramide). This finding may explain the reason why Class Ib drugs are empirically used in the treatment of ventricular rather than supraventricular arrhythmias, because these drugs block the sodium channel of the ventricular muscle during their long plateau phase more significantly than that of the atrial muscle that has almost no plateau phase.

The Drug Unbinding from the Resting Sodium Channel

Kinetics of unbinding of the Class I drugs from the resting sodium channel have been evaluated by measuring the time constant of $\dot{V}_{max}$ recovery from the use-dependent block that is induced by rapid pacing[10,13,14] (Table 1). Table 1 compares the recovery time constant of $\dot{V}_{max}$ from the use-dependent block among the Class I drugs tested. It is noteworthy that all Class Ib compounds except aprindine have short recovery time constants (within 1 second) compared with Class Ia and Ic drugs.[15] As for aprindine, this drug has an intermediate recovery time constant (5 to 9 seconds) similar to that of quinidine or propafenone.

Cibenzoline has a long recovery time constant (around 30 seconds) similar to those

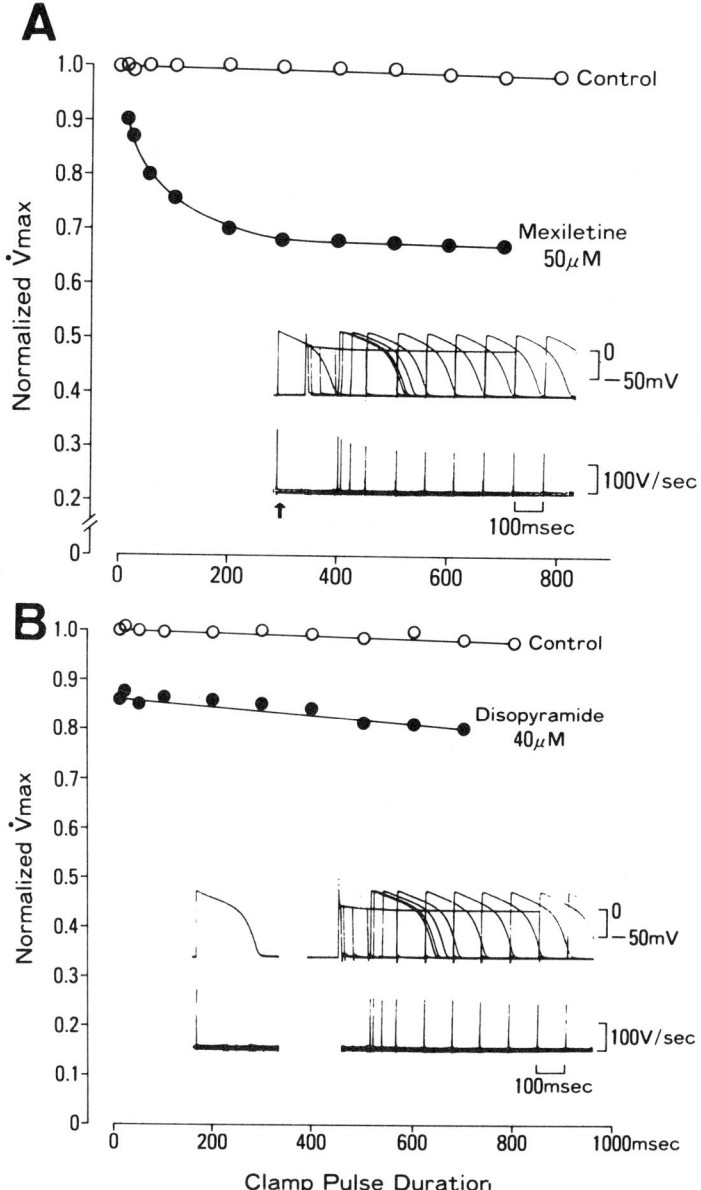

Figure 4. Effects of width of prepulse on $\dot{V}_{max}$ in the presence of mexiletine (A) and disopyramide (B). The inset of each panel is an example of the actual recordings. The recordings in the left end of the inset are controls, and the series of tracings are those obtained after prepulses of various durations. See text for details.

with flecainide and SUN1165, which are grouped into Class Ic. As for disopyramide, the reported data varies widely from several seconds to several tens of seconds.[10,14,16] This variation may be explained by the experimen-

tal result that the recovery time constant is markedly affected by a change in the resting potential level of the cardiac muscle exposed to this drug.

Figure 6 compares the dependency of the

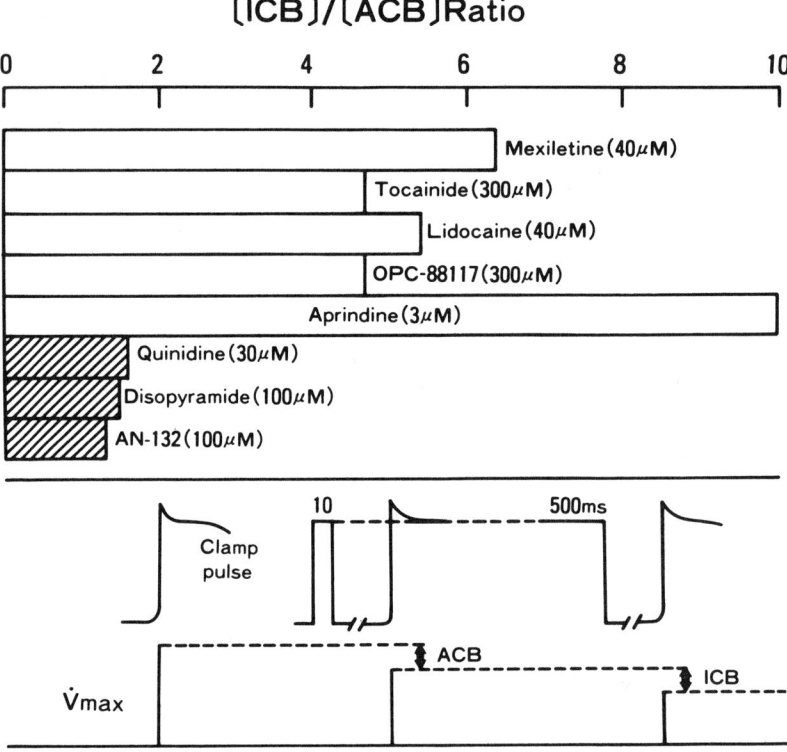

Figure 5. Dependency of blocking action of Class I drugs on the channel state. Reduction of $\dot{V}_{max}$ induced by the 10-msec prepulse and the further $\dot{V}_{max}$ reduction by lengthening the prepulse to 500 msec are defined as ICB and ACB as illustrated the lower diagram. The ratios of (ICB)/(ACB) calculated for Class I drugs. See text for details.

recovery time constant on the resting potential level of the isolated guinea pig ventricular myocyte. In the presence of disopyramide, a long recovery time constant (43 ± 1 second, mean $\pm$ SE; n = 5) was obtained under the resting potential of -90 mV but they were shortened to around 10 seconds when the membrane was depolarized by 15 to 20 mV (see the right graph of Figure 6). A similar tendency was observed in the case of penticainide. This dependency of the $\dot{V}_{max}$ recovery process on the resting potential level can be explained by assuming a process of drug unbinding from the activated state channel in addition to the unbinding process of the drug from the resting channel as is suggested by Carmeliet.[17] On the contrary, such a dependency was not observed among the drugs examined in the figure on the left, indicating

that these drugs unbind not from the activated channel but mainly from the resting channel.

To test whether or not disopyramide may unbind from the activated channel, we stimulated the ventricular myocyte of guinea pig in the presence of disopyramide 100 µM with the pulse protocols that are similar to those proposed by Anno and co-worker[18] (Figure 7).

(1) Fifty beats of depolarizing pulses (10 msec wide) from the holding potential of -75 mV to 0 mV were applied at an interval of 50 msec to accumulate the drug-bound inactivated fraction of the sodium channel (see protocol 1, and the dotted lines in Figure 7).

(2) An asystolic pause with the holding potential of -110 mV was allowed with various intervals before protocol 3, to promote the

Table 1
Recovery Time Constant
of Use-Dependent Block

Recovery of use-dependent block

Drug (μM)	MW	Recovery time constant (sec)
Lidocaine (20)	234	0.19
Mexiletine (20)	216	0.35
Tocainide (100)	192	0.46
Phenytoin (100)	252	0.52
Aprindine (3)	322	5.1
Quinidine (10)	324	6.8
Propafenone (3)	378	8.6
Flecainide (3)	439	29
Cibenzoline (10)	262	35
SUN-1165 (30)	317	37
Disopyramide (30)	309	6–43

(guinea pig papillary muscle)

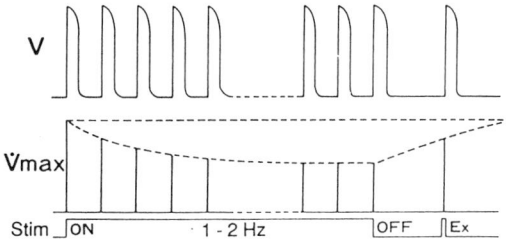

accumulation of the drug-bound resting fraction (see protocol 2 and a shaded lines), and

(3) A train of the depolarizing pulses was applied at a frequency of 5 Hz in order to enhance the drug unbinding from activated channel (see protocol 3 and dense solid lines).

The tracings in the inset of Figure 8 illustrates a typical example of $\dot{V}_{max}$ changes in response to the above stated stimulation protocols. The significant use-dependent reduction of $\dot{V}_{max}$, which is induced by the rapid depolarizing pulses indicates that the fraction of the drug-bound inactivated channel accumulates beat by beat, resulting in a progressive reduction of the drug-unbound channel. After the attainment of the steady-state level as indicated by the solid arrow in the inset, the membrane was hyperpolarized to the level of

−110 mV for 1 second, and was excited by the pulse train. The spike indicated by an open arrow is the $\dot{V}_{max}$ of the first beat that responded to the pulse train. The difference in the amplitude between the traces of $\dot{V}_{max}$ indicated by the solid and open arrow is consistent with a marked increase in the sodium channel activation through the ID-RD-AD-A process that is illustrated in the lower panel of Figure 7. The graph in Figure 8 shows the effects preceding pause on $\dot{V}_{max}$ of the first beat of the pulse train. As the pause was lengthened from 0.1 to 2 seconds, the two components of the $\dot{V}_{max}$ recovery were observed: the rapid component (75% of the final recovery) that was attained within 0.1 seconds, and the other slow one (the remaining 25%) that increased with a time constant of 25 seconds. Thus, the first rapid $\dot{V}_{max}$ recovery corresponds to the fraction of channel activation through the above stated process of ID-RD-AD-A, and the second slow recovery of $\dot{V}_{max}$ does to the channel activation through RD-R-A. Therefore, it is concluded that the drug binding and unbinding kinetics with the activated channel may mainly determine the sodium channel blocking action of disopyramide.

Profiles of Binding and Unbinding Kinetics for Class I Drugs

Table 2 shows a summary of our observations on the binding and unbinding kinetics for Class I drugs. All the Class Ib drugs except aprindine have the common profiles characterized as follows: they bind to the inactivated channel preferentially, and unbind from the resting channel with a fast rate. Aprindine has the same interaction to sodium channel as the other Class Ib drugs, but it unbinds from the channel with a slower time constant. As for Class Ia drugs, quinidine and disopyramide bind mainly to the activated channel, and unbind from the activated channel as well as the resting channel. In particular, the activated state unblocking is very important for disopyr-

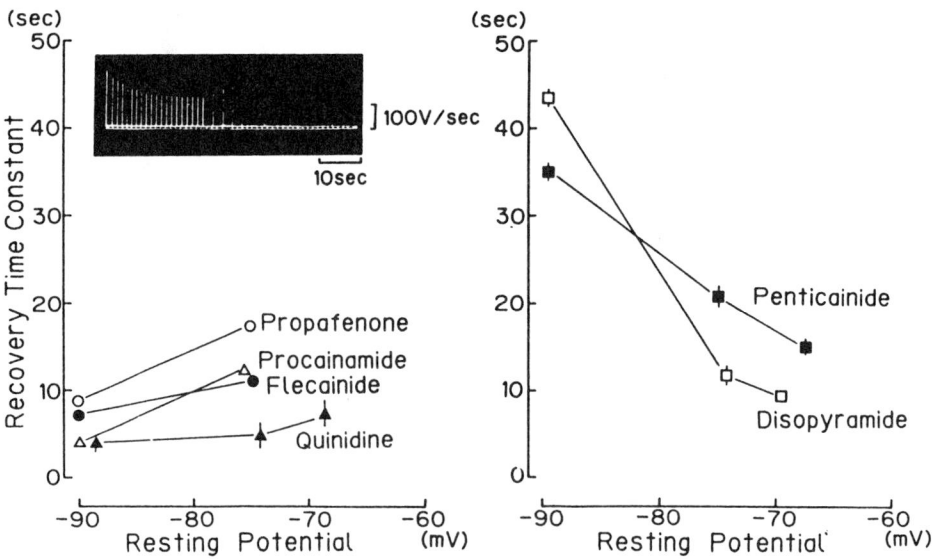

Figure 6. Effect of resting potential on recovery time constant. Minimal changes in the recovery time constant are observed in the drugs listed in the left graph, but the recovery time constants are lengthened markedly in disopyramide and penticainide as the resting potential is hyperpolarized.

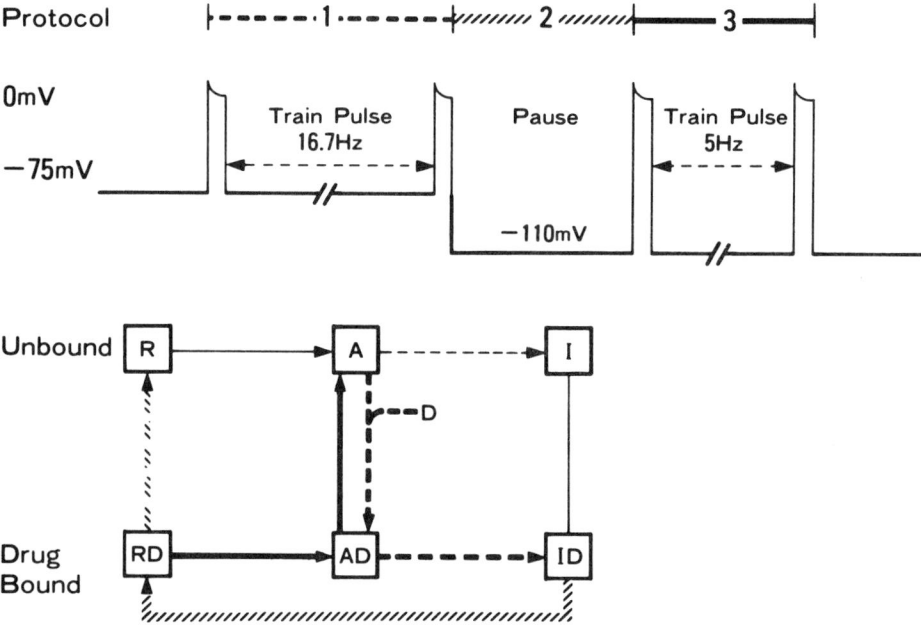

Figure 7. Stimulation protocol of testing the unbinding of disopyramide from activated state channel. Upper panel shows stimulation protocols. Lower panel depicts the drug-channel interaction suspected from the modulated receptor hypothesis. R, A, and I: resting, activated, and inactivated state of drug-free (unbound) channel, respectively. RD, AD, and ID represent the three states of drug-bound channel. See text for details.

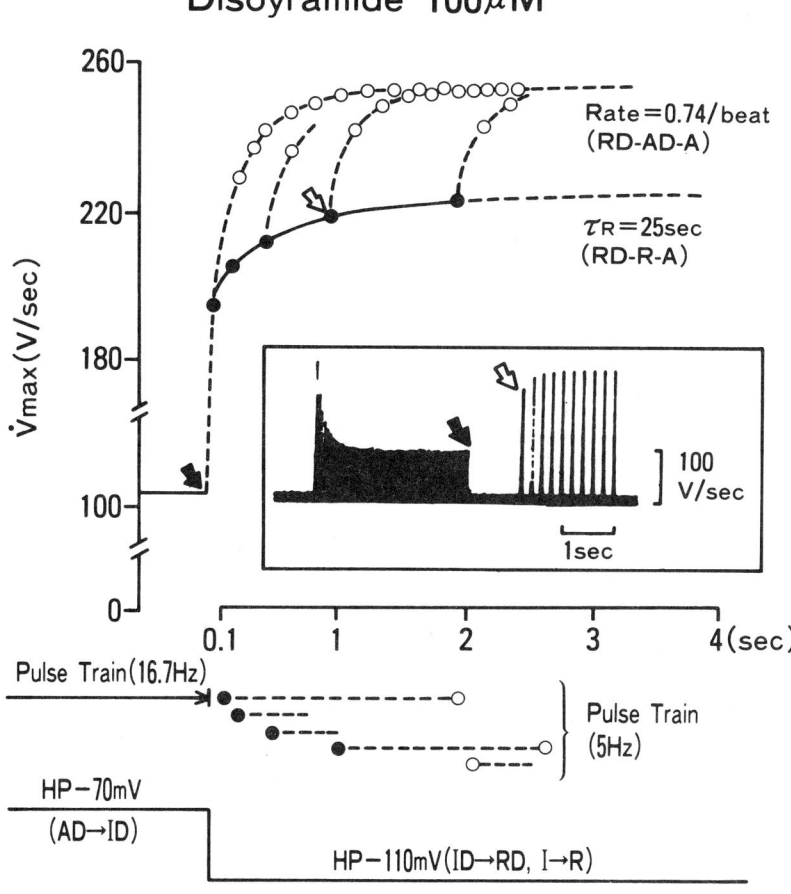

Figure 8. $\dot{V}_{max}$ recovery through the drug unbinding from the activated state channel. The difference of $\dot{V}_{max}$ indicated by a solid and open arrow in the inset indicates a sudden increase of the drug-free channel through the mechanisms of ID-RD-AD-A as illustrated in the lower panel of Figure 7. See text for details.

amide. The Class Ic drugs tested in this study had the affinity for binding preferentially to the activated state channel than to the inactivated channel and that they unbound mostly from the resting state channel with intermediate to slow rates.

It is concluded that the Class I drugs that are conventionally subclassified into Class Ia, Ib, and Ic do not have common profiles of the interaction with sodium channel, and that clinical studies should therefore be planned to determine whether or not the Class I drugs subclassified on the basis of the drug-channel interaction might also exhibit common pro-

files with respect to their clinical efficacy and arrhythmogenicity.

Reliability of V_{max} as an Indicator for Available Sodium Channel

It has been widely accepted that the maximum upstroke velocity ($\dot{V}_{max}$) of cardiac muscle is a conventional and good indicator for the sodium channel availability.[19,20] However, it has been also claimed that $\dot{V}_{max}$ is a qualitative, but not a quantitative indicator as com-

Table 2
Profiles of Binding and Unbinding Kinetics
for Class I Drugs

Drug	Binding and unbinding kinetics		
	Bind	Unbind	Recovery
Class Ib			
Lidocaine	I ≫ A	R	fast
Mexiletine	I ≫ A	R	fast
Tocainide	I ≫ A	R	fast
Aprinedine	I ≫ A	R	slow
Class Ia			
Quinidine	I < A	R > A	slow
Disopyramide	I < A	R ≪ A	slow
Class Ic			
Propafenone	I < A	R > A	slow
Flecainide			slow–very
	I < A	R > A	slow

pared with the peak sodium current (I_{Na} peak) measured by voltage-clamp techniques.[21,22] In fact, I_{Na} peak has proven to be a quantitative (within 1% of error) indicator for the sodium channel availability when the voltage-clamp experiment is done in a low sodium external medium at low temperature (below 26°C). However, it is not known whether such linearity is applicable to I_{Na} peak measured under physiological conditions at 37°C, because any voltage-clamp technique developed at the present is not enough to follow the very rapid excitatory sodium current under physiological conditions. The arguments for the nonlinear relationship between $\dot{V}_{max}$ and I_{Na} peak under the physiological condition depends only on speculations that are extrapolated from such limited voltage-clamp data.

In accordance with current knowledge[23,24] of the cardiac sodium current model that can reproduce both the I_{Na} clamp currents using a multichannel recording technique at 37°C and the upstroke of action potentials recorded from a guinea pig myocyte, the relationship between $\dot{V}_{max}$ and I_{Na} peak current becomes more linear as the rate constant for the activation gate is increased with the elevation of temperature. The linearity is

then assured within 10% of error as long as the action potential is elicited under physiological conditions and latency of the excitation is kept constant by changing the stimulation current.

References

1. Vaughan Williams EM: Classification of anti-arrhythmic drugs. In: E Sandoe, E Flensted-Jensen, KH Olesen (eds): *Symposium on Cardiac Arrhythmias*. Astra: Sodertalje, 1970, p. 449.
2. Singh BN, Hauswirth D: Comparative mechanisms of action of antiarrhythmic drugs. *Am Heart J* 87:367, 1974.
3. Harrison DC, Winkle RA, Sami M, Mason JW: Encainide: A new and potent antiarrhythmic agent. In: DC Harrison (ed): *Cardiac Arrhythmias: A Decade of Progress*. Boston, MA: Hall Medical, 1981, p. 315.
4. Estes NAM, Garan H, McGovern B, Ruskin JN: Class I antiarrhythmic agents: classification, electrophysiologic considerations, and clinical effects. In: HJ Reriser, LN Horowitz (eds): *Mechanisms and Treatment of Cardiac Arrhythmias: Relevance of Basic Studies to Clinical Management*. Baltimore, MD: Urban and Schwarzenberg, 1985, p. 183.
5. Honjo H, Watanabe T, Kamiya K, et al: Effects of propafenone on electrical and mechanical activities of single ventricular myocytes isolated from guinea-pig hearts. *Br J Pharmacol* 97:731, 1989.
6. Carmeliet E, Saikawa T: Shortening of the action potential and reduction of pacemaker activity by lidocaine, quinidine and procainamide in sheep cardiac Purkinje fibers. An effect on Na or K currents? *Circ Res* 50:257, 1982.
7. Hume JR: Properties of myocardial K^+ channels and their pharmacologic modulation. In: LM Hondeghem (ed): *Molecular and Cellular Mechanisms of Antiarrhythmic Agents*. Mount Kisco, NY: Futura Publishing Company, Inc., 1989, p. 113.
8. Hille B: Local anesthetics: hydrophilic and hydrophobic pathways for the drug receptor reaction. *J Gen Physiol* 69:497, 1977.
9. Hondeghem LM, Katzung BK: Time and voltage dependent interaction of antiarrhythmic drugs with cardiac sodium channels. *Biochem Biophys Acta* 472:373, 1977.
10. Toyama J: Classification of Class I drugs on the basis of the modulated receptor concept. In: J Toyama, LM Hondeghem (eds): *Current Topics in Antiarrhythmic Agents. Mode of Action and Clinical Usage*. Tokyo: Excerpta Medica, 1989, p. 175.

11. Kodama I, Toyama J, Yamada K: Open and inactivated sodium channel block by Class I antiarrhythmic drugs. *Jpn Heart J* 27(Suppl):83, 1986.

12. Kodama I, Honjo H, Kamiya K, Toyama J: Two types of sodium channel block by Class I antiarrhythmic drugs studied by using $\dot{V}_{max}$ of action potential in single ventricular myocytes. *J Mol Cell Cardiol* 22:1, 1990.

13. Courtney KR: Structure-activity relations for frequency-dependent sodium channel block in nerve by local anesthetics. *J Pharmacol Exp Ther* 213:114, 1980.

14. Campbell TJ: Importance of physio-chemical properties in determining the kinetics of the effects of Class I antiarrhythmic drugs on maximum rate of depolarization in guinea-pig ventricle. *Br J Pharmacol* 80:33, 1983.

15. Toyama J, Kamiya K, Kodama I, Yamada K: Frequency- and voltage-dependent effects of aprindine on the upstroke velocity ($\dot{V}_{max}$) of action potential in guinea pig ventricular muscles. *J Cardiovasc Pharmacol* 9:165, 1987.

16. Hiraoka M, Sunami A, Fan Z: Reassessment of the kinetics of the $\dot{V}_{max}$ block of action potentials by Class I antiarrhythmic agents in guinea pig papillary muscles. In: J Toyama, LM Hondeghem (eds): *Current Topics in Antiarrhythmic Agents. Mode of Action and Clinical Usage.* Tokyo: Excerpta Medica, 1989, p. 73.

17. Carmeliet E: Activation block and trapping of penticainide, a disopyramide analogue, in the Na^+ channel of rabbit cardiac Purkinje fibers. *Circ Res* 63:50, 1988.

18. Anno T, Hondeghem LM: Interactions of flecainide with guinea pig cardiac sodium channels. Importance of activation unblocking to the voltage dependence of recovery. *Circ Res* 66: 789, 1990.

19. Grant AO, Starmer CF, Straus HD: Antiarrhythmic drug action. Blockade of the inward sodium current. *Circ Res* 55:427, 1984.

20. Hondeghem LM: Validity of $\dot{V}_{max}$ as a measure of the sodium current in cardiac and nervous tissues. *Biophys J* 23:147, 1978.

21. Bean BP, Cohen CJ, Tsien RW: Block of cardiac sodium channels by tetrodotoxin and lidocaine: sodium current and $\dot{V}_{max}$ experiments. In: A Paes de Carvalho, BF Hoffman, M Lieberman (eds): *Normal and Abnormal Conduction in the Heart: Biophysics, Physiology, Pharmacology, and Ultrastructure*. Mount Kisco, NY: Futura Publishing Company, Inc., 1982, p. 189.

22. Fozzard HA, Hank DA, Sheets MF: The relationship between $\dot{V}_{max}$ and I_{Na} in cardiac Purkinje cells and their interpretation from single Na^+ channel analysis. In: LM Hondeghem (ed): *Molecular and Cellular Mechanisms of Antiarrhythmic Agents*. Mount Kisco, NY: Futura Publishing Company, Inc., 1989, p. 1.

23. Murray KT, Anno T, Benett PB, Hondeghem LM: Voltage clamp of the cardiac sodium current at 37°C in physiologic solutions. *Biophys J* 57:607, 1990.

24. Anno T, Murray KT, Taniguchi A, et al: Excitatory sodium currents of guinea pig ventricular myocytes under physiological conditions: mathematical perspectives of relationship between $\dot{V}_{max}$ and I_{Na}. (in press).

Chapter 17

β-Adrenoceptor Blockers as Antiarrhythmic Agents

Aurelio Duran
Robert J. Myerburg

β-Adrenoceptor blocking agents are among the most important therapeutic agents available in clinical cardiology, and are useful as antianginal, antihypertensive, and antiarrhythmic agents. The latter role of this class of drugs is especially important in the post-Cardiac Arrhythmia Suppression Trial (CAST) era,[1] because of serious new questions about the risk versus benefit status of membrane active antiarrhythmic therapy.[2] This comes at a time of an increasing fund of knowledge pertaining to neurohumoral influences on cardiac electrophysiology and the milieu promoting arrhythmogenesis. In addition to direct antiarrhythmic activity, a number of studies have demonstrated or suggested a beneficial effect of the β-adrenoceptor drugs in decreasing cardiac death in postmyocardial infarction patient populations (BHAT,[3] APSI,[4] MIAMI,[5] ISIS,[6] and TIMOLOL[7] studies). The reduction in mortality with these agents in this particular patient population is in the 30% range, although it is not clear if this is due to the antiarrhythmic, antisympathetic, or antiischemic effects of β-blockade, or to a combination. This significant beneficial response and the low incidence of toxicity, compared to other classes of antiarrhythmic drugs, makes a review of the role of these agents for treating arrhythmias relevant. The goal of this chapter is to review the pertinent electrophysiological principles and clinical data on the use of β-adrenoceptor drugs as antiarrhythmic agents.

Cardiac Electrophysiological Effects

β-Adrenoceptor blockers act principally as antagonists to the electrophysiological responses to the β-agonist effect of catecholamines. An additional electrophysiological effect of unclear clinical relevance noted with β-antagonists (especially propranolol) is the membrane active effect. This is only noted in some preparations with concentrations of drug beyond the usual therapeutic range,[8,9] and is manifest by a decrease in the rate of rise of phase 0 of the transmembrane action potential. These agents also inhibit the increase in the slope of phase 4 depolarization elicited by β-adrenergic stimulation. Also, although β-blockers themselves cause little ef-

From BN Singh, HJJ Wellens, M Hiraoka, (eds): *Electropharmacological Control of Cardiac Arrhythmias.* Mount Kisco, NY, Futura Publishing Company Inc., © 1994.

fect on resting transmembrane potentials or action potential amplitude, they antagonize the positive chronotropic response to catecholamine administration on the sinoatrial node and sites of ectopic pacemaker activity. Slowing of conduction and prolongation of refractory periods are the manifestations of β-blockade in atrioventricular nodal tissue. In Purkinje fibers, the increase in action potential amplitude, caused by sympathomimetic amines is antagonized by β-blockers.[10,11] These observations are the basis for presumed mechanisms of action on arrhythmias due to automaticity, triggered activity, and reentry.

The role of autonomic activity in cardiac arrhythmias and its modification by β-adrenoceptor blocking agents must be viewed from both systemic and regional perspectives. Cardiac and noncardiac conditions influence the balance between sympathetic and parasympathetic activity at a systemic level, thereby influencing the pattern of cardiac stimulation during autonomic fluctuations. Such changes are expressed by levels of circulating catecholamines, reflex modulations measured as heart rate variability and baroreceptor sensitivity,[12–16] and efferent and afferent nerve traffic between the heart and the central nervous system.[17–19] In addition, regional myocardial abnormalities are associated with regional changes in autonomic receptor/effector complexes, causing dispersion of cardiac electrophysiological responses to various levels of autonomic stimulation.[20] Both experimental data[21,22] and limited clinical data[23] on the effects of myocardial infarction on regional responses to adrenergic stimulation support this concept. Accordingly, the interaction between autonomic activity, its blockade, and cardiac electrophysiology is quite complex, but may have far reaching clinical and pathophysiological implications.

Supraventricular Arrhythmias

Sinus Tachycardia

Although not an inherently pathological rhythm, sinus tachycardia will occasionally re-

quire therapy with β-blockade, as in thyrotoxicosis, coronary insufficiency, or some persistent forms of sinus tachycardia. It is of note that in acute myocardial infarction, sinus tachycardia may reflect not only anxiety and a secondary high catecholamine state, but also significant myocardial damage. In such instances, the agents should be administered with close clinical observation due to their negative inotropic effects.

Ectopic Automatic Atrial Tachycardia

When present in adults, this category of arrhythmia may be paroxysmal or persistent, but is usually not chronic. The limited data available suggest that β-blocker therapy will lead to an increase in cycle length of the arrhythmia and impede atrioventricular conduction, but usually will not suppress or terminate the rhythm.[24] β-Blocker administration may be effective for the multifocal variety of ectopic atrial tachycardia, but therapy may be problematic because of the common association with chronic obstructive pulmonary disease.[25,26] Nonetheless, metoprolol has been used successfully to treat patients with this rhythm, even in the presence of pulmonary disease.[27]

Atrioventricular Nodal Reentrant Tachycardia

Atrioventricular nodal reentrant tachycardia accounts for approximately 60% of paroxysmal supraventricular tachycardias in adults and is a reentrant tachycardia created by disparity in refractoriness of dual atrioventricular nodal pathways. β-Blockers can be of value not only as a chronic prophylaxis against this tachyarrhythmia, but also short-term therapy to terminate acute paroxysms of the arrhythmia. Adrenergic activity enhances the likelihood of initiating atrioventricular nodal reentry. A high catecholamine state allows shorter coupling intervals of atrial premature beats by decreasing atrial refractory periods and enhancing antegrade slow and retrograde fast tract conduction in the common form of atrioventricular nodal reentry (slow/fast).[28] In the common form of this rhythm, β-blockers may break the tachycardia by either slow (antegrade) or fast (retrograde) pathway block. In the uncommon form (fast/slow), this rhythm appears to be terminated by slow pathway (retrograde) block.[29]

Atrial Flutter

As in ectopic atrial tachycardia, atrial flutter cycle length may increase and atrioventricular block increase in the presence of β-blockers. These agents may occasionally cause conversion to sinus rhythm in atrial flutter of short duration, but their usefulness is usually limited to ventricular rate control by the effect on atrioventricular conduction frequency.

Supraventricular Tachycardias Using Accessory Pathways (Wolff-Parkinson-White Syndrome)

Although the direct effect of β-adrenoceptor blockers on accessory pathway conduction is minimal,[30] these drugs can be of value in patients with Wolff-Parkinson-White syndrome because of atrioventricular nodal effects during reciprocating tachycardia. Nonetheless, use of β-blockers as lone agents in Wolff-Parkinson-White syndrome and atrial fibrillation is not recommended. Antegrade conduction via an accessory pathway can increase in the presence of impaired atrioventricular nodal conduction because of a consequent decrease in retrograde concealed conduction.[31]

Atrial Fibrillation

β-Adrenoceptor blockade can be of great value in the management of ventricular rate in atrial fibrillation, both as a lone agent or in combination with calcium blockers and/or digitalis. It is particularly useful in the setting of renal dysfunction, where digitalis elimination can be decreased and variable. In hypertrophic cardiomyopathy, where the use of digitalis is avoided, β-blockers may have some benefit for the primary abnormality, and may be particularly useful for concomitant atrial fibrillation. Although β-adrenoceptor blockade may convert atrial fibrillation into sinus rhythm in some instances, the major effect is modulation of conduction at the level of the atrioventricular node for control of ventricular rate response.

Premature Ventricular Contractions, Salvos, and Nonsustained Ventricular Tachycardia

In the presence of underlying structural heart disease, premature ventricular contractions usually indicate increased risk for sudden cardiac death, but numerous studies, the most significant of which is CAST,[1] have failed to demonstrate that suppression of premature ventricular contractions or nonsustained ventricular tachycardia will lead to a decrease in mortality. Nonetheless, these studies do not refute the concept that suppression of these arrhythmias (especially repetitive forms) may be beneficial, but rather point out that therapy with conventional antiarrhythmics is potentially dangerous. Potential benefits may be neutralized, in part or totally, by competing proarrhythmic risk. Therefore, in the patient with symptomatic premature ventricular contractions or nonsustained ventricular tachycardia, an efficacious antiarrhythmic with low potential for proarrhythmia and side effects would be valuable. β-Blockers fit this description and have been shown to be effective for premature ventricular contractions and nonsustained ventricular tachycardia suppression when used at appropriate dosages. In a placebo-controlled study, Woosley et al.[32] showed that chronic high-frequency ventricular arrhythmias, both premature ventricular contractions and nonsustained ventricular tachycardia could be effectively suppressed by propranolol in 75% of patients (response being defined as ≥ 70% suppression) when dosage regimens were individualized. Repetitive form suppression can be achieved even when premature ventricular contraction frequency was not suppressed significantly. The dosages that lead to desired results ranged from 160–960 mg/day of propranolol. This variability is probably due to a wide range in plasma propranolol levels in response to a given dosage, and possibly to variation in biological responses. Of the 32 patients studied, the only side effects were bronchospasm in a heavy smoker and five subjects who developed fatigue. It is this high degree of efficacy and low toxicity that makes β-blockers potentially attractive to use in the setting of premature ventricular contractions and nonsustained ventricular tachycardia in patients with and without structural heart disease. Whether premature ventricular contractions and/or repetitive form suppression contributed to the beneficial outcome in BHAT and other β-blocker trials in postmyocardial infarction patients remains conjectural (see Chapters 31 and 48). These studies were not designed to test the suppression hypothesis, and the fact that arrhythmias were suppressed does not lead to a conclusion regarding causation.

Exercise- and Catecholamine-Mediated Premature Ventricular Contractions and Ventricular Tachyarrhythmias

In animal models in clinical settings and in the electrophysiology laboratory, it has been noted that the circulating catecholamine state can have a direct effect on arrhythmia prevalence, inducibility, and cardioversion defibrillation thresholds.[33] The arrhythmias that fit in this category represent a variety of mechanisms. Exercise-induced premature ventricular contractions and nonsustained ventricular tachycardia may occur in patients with and without structural heart disease. In

such individuals, the arrhythmia may be troublesome, but only infrequently leads to sustained, life-threatening rhythms. They commonly respond to β-blockade.

Repetitive Monomorphic Ventricular Tachycardia

Repetitive monomorphic ventricular tachycardia typically occurs in young females without structural heart disease, is usually benign,[34,35] and requires no therapy. In those cases associated with structural disease, the benign nature is less clear.[36,37] When symptomatic, these patients complain of palpitations, and rare occasions syncope. Automaticity has been suggested as the mechanism for this arrhythmia.[36,38,39] In the symptomatic group, whether or not associated with structural heart disease, therapy with β-blockers can be valuable.

Sustained Monomorphic Ventricular Tachycardia

Sustained monomorphic ventricular tachycardia occurs most commonly in the setting of chronic coronary disease, and not commonly due to acute ischemia. It also occurs in nonischemic or hypertrophic cardiomyopathies and will occasionally present without structural heart disease.[40,41] Although the majority of patients with monomorphic ventricular tachycardia associated with underlying structural heart disease will have clinical ventricular tachycardia induced during electrophysiological testing, some patients will require administration of intravenous sympathetic amines in the electrophysiology laboratory for arrhythmia induction.[41–43] These observations, and at least one study focusing on the primary role of β-blockers in sustained ventricular tachycardia,[44] form a basis for considering the use of β-blockers in the management of this arrhythmia in selected patients. In the small series available,[45–47] the use of β-adrenergic blockers in patients with catecholamine-sensitive ventricular tachycardia seems promising, especially where enhanced automaticity is felt to be the underlying mechanism of the arrhythmia. At our institution, 17 patients with clinical ventricular tachycardia or ventricular fibrillation who were not inducible during baseline electrophysiological study, were inducible during repeat study during isoproterenol infusion. Upon repeat study during isoproterenol infusion and after β-blockade with propranolol intravenously, 14 of the 17 (85%) were inducible and 11 of these 14 patients were noninducible after electrophysiological study during oral propranolol therapy and isoproterenol infusion.[47] All of these patients remained event free during a mean follow-up period of 15 months.

β-Adrenergic blocking agents are generally viewed as having a limited primary role for the treatment of sustained ventricular tachycardia not mediated by catecholamines. However, there is increasing evidence for a specific role for this category of drugs in a number of forms of this arrhythmia (see Chapters 31 and 48). The probability of efficacy is a function of both the underlying etiology and specific electrophysiological mechanisms. β-Blocker responsive ventricular tachycardias may occur in virtually all clinical settings, ranging from electrophysiological disturbances in normal hearts to those with advanced myopathy and/or myocardial ischemia. The mechanisms underlying ventricular tachycardia that may be sensitive to β-adrenoceptor blockade include reentry, enhanced automaticity, and triggered activity, and usually can be discerned from one another clinically and in the electrophystology laboratory.

Ventricular tachycardia due to reentry caused by inhomogeneous refractoriness and unidirectional block[48,49] is usually inducible by programmed electrical stimulation and can be terminated by pacing. The reentrant rhythm can be susceptible to resetting with administration of extrastimuli and entrainment with incremental pacing.[50] The rationale for use of β-adrenergic antagonists in this setting is the modification of dispersion of refractoriness that is enhanced by high adrenergic tone[51] and regional differences in adrenergic receptors.[18,21,52,53]

Ventricular tachycardia also may be due to enhanced normal or abnormal automaticity. Cells with enhanced normal automaticity are fully polarized and have enhanced phase 4 depolarization that may be partially or completely inhibited by β-blockers.[54,55] Abnormal automaticity occurs in cells that have decreased maximum diastolic potentials, findings that have been demonstrated in myocardium obtained at the time of arrhythmia surgery in patients with ventricular tachycardia.[54,56] By enhancement of slow inward current, catecholamines are thought to contribute to automaticity and induction of ventricular rhythms.[57,78] By antagonizing this effect, β-blockers may suppress such sites of ectopic activity. This rhythm is not inducible by programmed extrastimuli, and occurs spontaneously with administration of catecholamines. It is typically not terminable by pacing, able to be reset with extrastimuli, or entrainable in the electrophysiology laboratory.

Triggered activity is defined as automatic activity that is "triggered" by preceding sets of stimuli. "Afterdepolarizations", which are current oscillations across membranes before full repolarization (early afterdepolarizations [EADs]) or at the onset of phase 4 (delayed afterdepolarizations [DADs]), are the triggering events. This form of ventricular tachycardia can be initiated and terminated by extrastimuli and incremental pacing. Therefore, it can be difficult to differentiate from ventricular tachycardia due to reentry. Ventricular tachycardia due to triggered activity would not be expected to be reset by extrastimuli.[56,59] Adrenergic stimulation may contribute to activation of a Ca^{2+} modulated Na^+ channel or of the slow inward Ca^{2+} channel. This phenomenon can be inhibited by β-receptor antagonists by diminution or inhibition of afterdepolarizations.[60]

In our laboratory, the usual protocol for assessment of patients with ventricular tachycardia induced during electrophysiological testing only during isoproterenol infusion includes evaluation of arrhythmia suppression with β-blockade. The patient receives intravenous propranolol for a total dosage of approximately 0.2 mg/kg. The electrophysiological study is then repeated while still receiving isoproterenol infusion. If the rhythm is suppressed, oral β-blockers are instituted and titrated to β-blockade as dictated by sinus rate, blood pressure, and/or symptoms. The electrophysiological study is then repeated while on an oral regimen.

Nonetheless, among patients with hemodynamically stable sustained monomorphic ventricular tachycardias that are not catecholamine-mediated, β-blockade has only limited efficacy for preventing inducibility.[61,64]

Polymorphic Ventricular Tachycardia and Ventricular Flutter

When unassociated with electrolyte abnormalities or proarrhythmia, the inducibility of rapid nonsustained or sustained polymorphic ventricular tachycardia, and some very rapid monomorphic ventricular tachycardias (cycle length ≤ 240 msec, ventricular flutter) should suggest the possibility of transient ischemia with underlying coronary artery disease.[65] If clinically appropriate, administration of anti-ischemic agents including β-blockade, and evaluation of coronary anatomy is in order. As with all arrhythmias, QRS complex analysis should include evaluation of multiple leads as polymorphic ventricular tachycardia can appear monomorphic when seen in only one vectorial projection. It appears that patients with rapid and/or hemodynamically unstable ventricular tachycardia/flutter/fibrillation (cycle length ≤ 240 msec) are more likely to respond to β-blockade than those with slower monomorphic ventricular tachycardia.[44] In this series, 29% of those coronary artery disease patients with unstable ventricular arrhythmias became noninducible after propranolol administration.

Long QT Interval Syndromes

These syndromes can either be congenital, iatrogenic (ie, induced by type 1A agents, phenothiazines, or tricyclics), or associated with metabolic abnormalities. The first of these congenital disorders to be described is the autosomal recessive Jervell-Lange-Neilson syndrome and is associated with deafness.[66] The second, the Romano-Ward syndrome, is an autosomal dominant disorder.[68] A large body of data suggest that the arrhythmias seen in patients with the congenital form of the disorder can be attributed to abnormalities in autonomic tone.[68,69] Adrenergic hyperactivity originating from the left stellate ganglion is considered to be a key factor in the mechanism of these arrhythmias. These young patients have a high risk of mortality—approximately 25% 3 years after their first syncopal event.[70] With β-adrenoceptor blocker therapy, the mortality rate in this group is reduced to 6%[70] (see Chapter 14). These patients will present with palpitations, stress-induced syncope/near-syncope, and a corrected QT interval of > 440 msec. Torsades de pointes terminating in lethal ventricular fibrillation is the cause of death in these patients. β-Blockade is not, however, indicated in pharmacologically-induced torsades de pointes.

Ventricular Fibrillation

Experimental studies have shown both adrenergically-mediated decreases in fibrillation thresholds[71] and prophylaxis against sudden cardiac death[23] with β-blockers in post-myocardial infarction patients with subsequent episodes of ventricular fibrillation and ventricular tachycardia.

Although the sensitivity and specificity of ventricular fibrillation induced in the electrophysiology laboratory is not as high as with monomorphic ventricular tachycardia, there are cardiac arrest survivors who clearly have reproducible ventricular flutter or fibrillation, which is induced by two or less extrastimuli.

Unfortunately, there is no large body of data available specifically addressing the potential efficacy of prophylaxis with β-blockers against sudden cardiac death in these patients, but observations in small groups[44] suggest the possibility that such therapy may be efficacious in carefully selected subgroups.[44,47] In this era where implantable cardioverter defibrillator backup is available, the use of such therapy could be safely evaluated.

Adverse Side Effects, Dosages, and Pharmacological Properties

All β-adrenergic blockers can be associated with a number of detrimental side effects. These include: (1) worsening of congestive heart failure due to negative ionotropic effect;

(2) precipitation or worsening of bronchospasm; (3) sinus node dysfunction; (4) atrioventricular nodal blockade; (5) blockade of sympathetically-mediated warning symptoms of hypoglycemia; (6) lethargy and mental blunting; (7) impotence; (8) depression; and (9) hypotension. In a given patient, the potential for and the consequence of these side effects, must be evaluated in conjunction with cardioselectivity, drug half-life, and underlying medical illness in order to choose a specific β-blocking agent. The doses and elimination kinetics of a number of β-adrenoceptor blockers are listed in Table 1.

Conclusions

β-Blockers can, by a variety of mechanisms ranging from direct effect on the cardiac conduction system to alterations in autonomic

Table 1

	Usual starting dose	Relative B_1 selectivity	B_1 potency ratio (propranolol = 1.0)	Plasma half-life	Predominant elimination mode	Lipid solubility
Acebutolol Hydrochloride	200 mg bid	+	0.3	3–4 hours	K	+ +
Atenolol	25–50 mg qd	+ +	1.0	6–9 hours	K	+
Esmolol Hydrochloride	load: 500 μg/kg/min IV: then 50 μg/kg/min × 4 minutes	+ +	0.01	10 minutes	H	+
Metoprolol Tartrate	50 mg bid	+ +	1.0	3–4 hours	H	+
Labetolol Hydrochloride	100 mg bid	0	0.3	3–4 hours	H	+
Nadolol	40 mg qd	0	1.0	14–24 hours	K	+
Oxprenolol Hydrochloride	—	0	0.5–1.0	2–3 hours	H	+ +
Pindolol	5 mg bid	0	6.0	3–4 hours	K	+ +
Propranolol Hydrochloride	10–40 mg q6h	0	1.0	3–4 hours	H	+ + +
Sotalol Hydrochloride	80 mg bid	0	0.3	8–10 hours	K	+
Timolol Malate	10 mg bid	0	6.0	4.5 hours	K	+

Adapted from: Frishman WH: *Clinical Pharmacology of the Beta-Adrenoreceptor Blocking Drugs.* 2nd edition, 1984, Norwalk, Appleton-Century-Crofts, Inc., p. 22; and Frishman WH: The beta blocking drugs. *Int J Cardiol* 2:172, 1982.

tone, alter the milieu that would allow arrhythmias to be initiated and sustained. Their use in supraventricular arrhythmias has been very successful for decades. Because of preliminary data suggesting efficacy, theoretical considerations, and their low toxicity profile, there exists significant potential for their use in certain malignant ventricular rhythms as well. Further studies specifically evaluating long-term follow-up in different rhythms and cardiac substrate need to be undertaken, particularly in the more rapid and unstable ventricular tachyarrhythmias.

References

1. The Cardiac Arrhythmia Suppression Trial (CAST) Investigators: Preliminary report: effects of encainide and flecainide on mortality in a randomized trial of arrhythmia suppression after myocardial infarction. *N Engl J Med* 321: 406, 1989.
2. Akhtar M, Breithardt GM, Coumel P, et al: CAST and beyond: implications of the Cardiac Arrhythmia Suppression Trial. *Circulation* 81: 1123, 1990.
3. β-Blocker Heart Attack Trial Research Group: A randomized trial of propranolol in patients with acute myocardial infarction. *JAMA* 247: 1707, 1982.
4. Boissel JP, Leizorovicz A, Picolet H, et al: Secondary prevention after high risk acute myocardial infarction with low dose acebutolol. *Am J Cardiol* 66:251, 1990.
5. Olsson G, Rehnquist N, Sjogren A, et al: Long-term treatment with metoprolol after myocardial infarction: effect on 3-year mortality and morbidity. *J Am Coll Cardiol* 5:1428, 1985.
6. ISIS-1 Collaborative Group: Randomized trial of intravenous atenolol among 16,027 cases of suspected acute myocardial infarction: ISIS-1. *Lancet* 2:57, 1986.
7. Norwegian Multicenter Study Group: Timolol-induced reduction in mortality and reinfarction in patients surviving acute myocardial infarction. *N Engl J Med* 304:801, 1981.
8. Lucchesi ER, Whitsitt LS, Brown NL: Propranolol in experimentally induced cardiac arrhythmias. *Can J Physiol Pharmacol* 44:543, 1966.
9. Morales-Aquilera A, Vaughn-Williams EM: The effects on cardiac muscle of β-receptor antagonists in relation to their activity as local anesthetics. *Br J Pharmacol* 24:332, 1965.
10. Rosen MR, Hordof AJ, Ilvento JP, Hoffman BF: Effects of adrenergic amines on electrophysiologic properties in automaticity of neonatal and adult canine Purkinje fibers.
11. Frishman WH: Beta-adrenergic blockers. *Med Clin North Am* 72:37, 1988.
12. Kleiger RE, Miller JP, Bigger JT, et al: Heart rate variability: a variable predicting mortality following acute myocardial infarction. *Am J Cardiol* 59:256, 1987.
13. Lombardi F, Sandrone G, Perpruner S, et al: Heart rate variability as an index of sympathovagal interaction after acute myocardial infarction. *Am J Cardiol* 60:1239, 1987.
14. Schwartz PJ, Vanoli E, Stramba-Badiale M, et al: Autonomic mechanisms and sudden death: new insights from analysis of baroreceptor reflexes in conscious dogs with and without myocardial infarction. *Circulation* 78:969, 1988.
15. Schwartz PJ, Billman GE, Stone HL: Autonomic mechanisms in ventricular fibrillation induced by myocardial ischemia during exercise in dogs with healed myocardial infarction: an experimental model for sudden cardiac death. *Circulation* 69:790, 1984.
16. Billman GE, Schwartz PJ, Stone HL: Baroreflex control of heart rate: a predictor of sudden death. *Circulation* 66:874, 1982.
17. Kolman B, Verrier RL, Lown B: The effect of vagus nerve stimulation upon vulnerability of the canine ventricle: role of sympathetic-parasympathetic interaction. *Circulation* 52:578, 1975.
18. Zipes DP, Barber MJ, Takahashi N, et al: Recent observations in autonomic innervation of the heart. In: DP Zipes, J Jalife (eds): *Cardiac Electrophysiology and Arrhythmias*. Orlando, FL: Grune and Stratton, 1985, p. 181.
19. Schwartz PJ, Stramba-Badiale M: Parasympathetic nervous system and cardiac arrhythmias. In: HE Kulbertus, G Frank (eds): *Neurocardiology*. Mount Kisco, NY: Futura Publishing Company, Inc., 1988, p. 179.
20. Watson RM, Schwartz JL, Maron JM, et al: Inducible polymorphic ventricular tachycardia and ventricular fibrillation in a subgroup of patients with hypertrophic cardiomyopathy at high risk for sudden death. *J Am Coll Cardiol* 10:761, 1987.
21. Kuo CS, Mura Kata K, Reddy CP, et al: Characteristics and possible mechanisms of ventricular arrhythmia dependent on the dispersion of action potential durations. *Circulation* 67:1356, 1983.
22. Kimura S, Bassett AL, Cameron JS, et al: Cellular electrophysiological changes during ischemia in isolated, coronary perfused cat ventricle with a healed myocardial infarction. *Circulation* 78:401, 1988.
23. Schwartz PJ, Motolese M, Pollavini G, et al: Sur-

gical and pharmacological antiadrenergic intervention in the prevention of sudden cardiac death after a first myocardial infarction. *Circulation* 72(III):358, 1985.

24. Gillette PC, Garson A: Electrophysiologic and pharmacologic characteristics of automatic atrial tachycardia. *Circulation* 56:571, 1977.

25. Wang K, Goldfarb B, et al: Multifocal atrial tachycardia. *Arch Intern Med* 137:161, 1977.

26. Shine KI, Kastor JA, Yinchah PM: Multifocal atrial tachycardia: clinical and electrocardiographic features in 32 patients. *N Engl J Med* 279:344, 1968.

27. Arsina EL, Solar M, et al: Metoprolol in the treatment of multifocal atrial tachycardia. *Crit Care Med* 15:591, 1987.

28. Huycke EC, Lai WT, Nguygn NX, et al: Role of intravenous isoproterenol in the electrophysiologic induction of atrial ventricular nodal reentrant tachycardia in patients with dual atrial ventricular nodal pathways. *Am J Cardiol* 64:1131, 1989.

29. Sung RJ, Elzner B, McAllister RG: Intravenous verapamil for termination of reentrant supraventricular tachycardias. *Am J Med* 93:682, 1980.

30. Denes P, et al: Effects of propranolol on anomalous pathway refractoriness and circus movement tachycardias in patients with pre-excitation. *Am J Cardiol* 41:1061, 1978.

31. Krikler BM, Spurrell RAJ: Verapamil in the treatment of paroxysmal supraventricular tachycardia. *Postgrad Med* 50:447, 1974.

32. Woosley RL, Kornhauser D, Smith R, et al: Suppression of chronic ventricular arrhythmias with propranolol. *Circulation* 60:819, 1979.

33. Ruffy MF, Schechtman K, Monje E: Beta-adrenergic modulation of direct defibrillation energy in anesthetized dog heart. *Am J Physiol* 248:H-674, 1985.

34. Gallavardin L: Extrasystolie ventriculaire a paroxysmes tachycardiques prolonges. *Arch Mal Coeur* 15:298, 1922.

35. Parkinson J, Popp C: Repetitive paroxysmal tachycardia. *Br Heart J* 9:241, 1947.

36. Buxton AE, Marchlinski FE, Doherty JU, et al: Repetitive monomorphic ventricular tachycardia: clinical and electrophysiologic characteristics in patients with and patients without organic heart disease. *Am J Cardiol* 54:997, 1984.

37. Kienzle MG, Martins JB, Constantin L, et al: Autonomic influence in repetitive monomorphic ventricular tachycardia. *Circulation* 74:II-127, 1986.

38. Constantin L, Leonard MT, Martins JB: Autonomic control of ventricular tachycardia: direct effects of beta-adrenergic blockade in 24-hour old canine myocardial infarction. *J Am Coll Cardiol* 9:336, 1987.

39. Palileo EV, Ashley WW, Swiryn S, et al: Exercise provocable right ventricular outflow tract tachycardia. *Am Heart J* 104:185, 1982.

40. Palileo EV, Ashley WW, Swiryn S: Exercise provocable right ventricular outflow tract tachycardia. *Am Heart J* 104:185, 1982.

41. Coumel P, et al: Role of the sympathetic nervous system in the non-ischemic ventricular arrhythmias. *Br Heart J* 47:137, 1982.

42. Friedman RA, Swerdlow CD, Echt DS, et al: Cilitation of ventricular tachyarrhythmia induction by isoproterenol. *Am J Cardiol* 54:765, 1984.

43. Reddy CP, Gettes LS: Use of isoproterenol as an aid to electric induction of chronic recurrent ventricular tachycardia. *Am J Cardiol* 44:705, 1979.

44. Huikuri H, Cox M, Interian A, et al: Efficacy of intravenous propranolol for suppression of inducibility of ventricular tachyarrhythmias with different electrophysiologic characteristics in coronary artery disease. *Am J Cardiol* 64:1305, 1989.

45. Olshansky B, Martins JB: Usefulness of isoproterenol facilitation of ventricular tachycardia induction during extrastimulus testing in predicting effective chronic therapy with beta-adrenergic blockade. *Am J Cardiol* 59:573, 1987.

46. DeCarlo L, Susser F, Winston S: The role of beta-blockade therapy for ventricular tachycardia induction with isoproterenol: a prospective analysis. *Am Heart J* 6:1347, 1990.

47. Interian A, Fernandez P, Robinson E, et al: Long-term effect of propranolol in ventricular tachycardia/fibrillation patients with isoproterenol dependent inducibility. *Circulation* 82(Suppl III):O 435, 1990.

48. Mines GR: On circulating excitations in heart muscle and their possible relation to tachycardia and fibrillation. *Trans R Soc Can* 8:43, 1914.

49. Mines GR: On dynamic equilibrium in the heart. *J Physiol (Lond)* 46:349, 1913.

50. Almendral JM, Stomato MJ, Rosenthal ME, et al: Re-setting response patterns during sustained ventricular tachycardia: relationship to the excitable gap. *Circulation* 74:722, 1986.

51. Frishman WH: *Clinical Pharmacology of Beta-Adrenoreceptor Blocking Drugs.* 2nd edition. Norwalk, CT: Appleton-Century-Crofts, Inc., 1984.

52. Giotti A, Ledda F, Mannaioni PF: Effects of noradrenalin and isoprenalin, in combination with alpha- and beta-receptor sustances on the action potential of cardiac Purkinje fibers. *J Physiol* 229:99, 1973.

53. Gaide MS, Myerburg RJ, Cameron JS, Bassett AL: Effects of sympathetic stimulation on ventricular refractory periods in cats with acute coronary ligation. *Experientia* 40:694, 1984.

54. Singer DH, Baumgarten CM, Ten-Eick RE: Cellular electrophysiology of ventricular and other dysrhythmias in diseased and ischemic heart. *Prog Cardiovasc Dis* 24:97, 1981.

55. Singh BN, Jewitt DE: β-Adrenoreceptor blocking drugs in cardiac arrhythmias. In: G Avery (ed): *Cardiovascular Drugs*. Volume 2. Baltimore, MD: University Park Press, 1977, p. 141.

56. Gilmore RF Jr, Hegger JJ, Prystowsky EM, Zipes DP: Cellular electrophysiological abnormalities of diseased human ventricular myocardium. *Am J Cardiol* 51:137, 1983.

57. Epstein SE, Braunwald E: Beta-adrenergic receptor drugs. *N Engl J Med* 275:1106, 1966.

58. Zipes DP, Besch HR Jr, Watanabe AM: Role of slow current in cardiac electrophysiology. *Circulation* 51:761, 1975.

59. Zipes DP: Genesis of cardiac arrhythmias: electrophysiologic considerations. In: E Braunwald (ed): *Heart Disease: A Textbook of Cardiovascular Medicine*. Philadelphia, PA: WB Saunders, 1988, p. 597.

60. Wit AL, Cranefield PF, Gadsby DC: Electrogenic sodium extrusion can stop triggered activity in the canine coronary sinus. *Circ Res* 29:1029, 1981.

61. Wellens HJJ, Bar FWHM, Lie KI, et al: Effects of procainamide, propranolol and verapamil on mechanisms of tachycardia in patients with chronic recurrent ventricular tachycardia. *Am J Cardiol* 40:579, 1977.

62. Duff HJ, Mitchell B, Wyse G: Antiarrhythmic efficacy of propranolol: comparison of low and high serum concentrations. *J Am Coll Cardiol* 8:959, 1986.

63. Brodsky MA, Allen BJ, Bessen M, et al: Beta-blocker therapy in patients with ventricular tachyarrhythmias in the setting of left ventricular dysfunction. *Am Heart J* 115:799, 1988.

64. Buxton AE, Waxman HL, Marchlinski FE, et al: Electropharmacology of non-sustained ventricular tachycardia. Effects of Class I antiarrhythmic agents, verapamil and propranolol. *Am J Cardiol* 53:738, 1984.

65. Tchen P, Atassi K, Jazayen M, et al: Etiology of polymorphic ventricular tachycardia in absence of prolonged QT. *J Am Coll Cardiol* 13:2, 1989.

66. Jervell A, Lange-Nielsen F: Congenital deaf mutism: functional heart disease with prolongation of the Q-T interval and sudden death. *Am Heart J* 54:59, 1957.

67. Romano C, Gemme G, Pongiglione R: Aritne cardiache rare en eta pediatrica. *Clin Pediatr* 45:656, 1963.

68. Jackman WM, Friday KJ, Anderson JL, et al: The long Q-T syndromes: a critical review, new political observations and a unified hypothesis. *Prog Cardiovasc Dis* 2:115, 1988.

69. Schwartz PJ: The idiopathic long Q-T syndrome: progress and questions. *Am Heart J* 2:399, 1985.

70. Schwartz PJ, Locati E: The idiopathic long Q-T syndrome: pathogenic mechanisms and therapy. *Eur Heart J* 6:103, 1985.

71. Lown B, Verrier R: Neurologic activity and ventricular fibrillation. *N Engl J Med* 294:1165, 1976.

Chapter 18

Molecular Mechanisms of Potassium Channel Block by Antiarrhythmic Drugs

Thomas J. Colatsky
Walter Spinelli
Christopher H. Follmer

The importance of potassium channel block in antiarrhythmic drug action has become more widely appreciated in recent years. Voltage-clamp studies have shown that even agents that exert their primary effects on sodium and calcium channels can suppress one or more of the various potassium currents underlying repolarization in the heart, and this ancillary activity may help to define the particular electrophysiological profile observed for each agent. In most cases, the presence of K^+ channel block is realized as a prolongation of the cardiac action potential, and it has been proposed that differences in the effects of Class I agents on repolarization and refractoriness can be used as a basis for their subclassification.[1] However, recent evidence suggests that significant K^+ channel block may be present when there are no overt changes in repolarization time course. For example, the Class IC agents flecainide and encainide block the delayed rectifier potassium current I_K in cat ventricular myocytes,[2,3] despite the fact that they appear to produce only small and variable effects on repolarization and refractoriness in animal studies and during clinical therapy.[4-6]

The findings of the Cardiac Arrhythmia Suppression Trial (CAST) have led to a renewed interest in selective block of myocardial K^+ channels as an antiarrhythmic mechanism. The synthesis and evaluation of new compounds targeting specific K^+ channels has yielded a chemically diverse family of investigational agents that selectively prolong repolarization without slowing cardiac conduction (see Chapters 31, 34, and 35). This chapter reviews the general properties of the K^+ channel blockers, and the molecular mechanisms by which they act.

Specificity of K^+ Channel Block

Table 1 summarizes the data currently available for the K^+ channel specificity of

From BN Singh, HJJ Wellens, M Hiraoka, (eds): *Electropharmacological Control of Cardiac Arrhythmias*. Mount Kisco, NY, Futura Publishing Company Inc., © 1994.

Table 1
Specificity of Antiarrhythmic Drugs for
Cardiac Potassium Channels

Class	Agent	I_{to}	$I_{K(dr)}$	I_{KI}
IA	Quinidine	Yes	Yes	Yes
	Disopyramide	Yes	Yes	Yes
IB	Lidocaine	No	No	No
IC	Flecainide	?	Yes	No
	Encainide	No	Yes	No
	Recainam	No	No	No
III	Clofilium	Yes	Yes	Yes
	Sotalol	Yes	Yes	Yes
	Amiodarone	No	Yes	?
	Dofetilide	No	Yes	No
	E-4031	No	Yes	No
	Tedisamil	Yes	Yes	No
	RP-58855	No	No	Yes

The presence or absence of block for each is assessed relative to therapeutically relevant concentrations.[19] I_{to}: transient outward current; $I_{K(dr)}$: delayed rectifier current; I_{KI}: inward rectifier current.

agents in the various Vaughan-Williams antiarrhythmic drug classes. With the exception of the Class I agents lidocaine and recainam, and the newer Class III agents such as E-4031 and dofetilide (UK-68,798), most antiarrhythmic drugs currently in clinical use block multiple K^+ channels at therapeutic or near-therapeutic concentrations. The Class I agents lidocaine and recainam act principally by blocking the excitatory sodium current, and show only weak actions at cardiac K^+ channels,[3,7] while the newer Class III agents appear to be highly selective for the rapidly activating component of delayed rectification (I_{Kr}),[8] with negligible effects on other inward and outward currents. The ubiquity of potassium channel block within all the antiarrhythmic classes suggests a possible reclassification scheme that uses the relative amounts of sodium and potassium channel block as the primary determinants of potential clinical activity.[9] As opposed to representing distinct classes of drugs, these Class I and Class III agents would be viewed under this scheme as representing a continuum between those compounds having little if any effect on potassium channels (eg, lidocaine) to those with little if any effect on sodium currents (eg, dofetilide). The Class IC and IA agents fall between these extremes.

Mechanisms of K^+ Channel Block

The interactions between Class I antiarrhythmics and the delayed rectifier K^+ channel have formed a useful paradigm for assessing general modes of drug-K^+ channel interaction in the heart. In particular, quinidine has been extensively examined in a variety of preparations, and except for studies in guinea pig ventricular myocytes,[10] appears to show the type of voltage dependence noted previously for block of neuronal delayed rectifier channels by tetraethylammonium and its related quaternary analogs[11] in that: (1) block appears to require channel opening; (2) the level and rate of block is increased at more positive membrane potentials; and (3) repolarization leads to the release of a drug from its binding site, leading to changes in the time course of the deactivation tail currents. An interaction of quinidine with open cardiac delayed rectifier channels has been observed in rabbit nodal cells[12] and in mouse fibroblasts expressing the human cardiac delayed rectifier channel (HK2).[13] Under conditions in which K^+ currents can be studied unambiguously, quinidine block is characterized by the type of voltage-dependence typically associated with the sodium channel blocking activity of Class I antiarrhythmics, rather than the reverse use dependence that has been postulated to govern K^+ channel block by Class III agents.[14]

We have recently observed a similar link to channel activation for block of the delayed rectifier current by the Class I agents flecainide and encainide, and by the Class III agents amiodarone and WAY-123,398. In these experiments, membrane currents were recorded using the single suction pipette voltage-clamp technique in freshly dissociated cat ventricular myocytes. In the preparations, the tail currents representing deactivation of the delayed rectifier current $I_{K(dr)}$ appeared to be completely suppressed by the Class III agent E-4031, suggesting that unlike guinea pig, only a single I_{Kr}-like component of delayed rectification is present.[2] Activation curves were constructed in the usual manner by plotting the peak tail current amplitude against test potential. Figure 1 illustrates a typical result obtained with the Class IC agent flecainide. At a concentration of 1.1 μM, flecainide suppressed the tail currents measured upon repolarization (compare Figures 1A and 1B). When activation curves are constructed by plotting

peak tail currents against the associated test potential (Figure 1C), it can be seen that flecainide is a more effective blocker of $I_{K(dr)}$ at positive potentials, and that only negligible changes in tail current amplitude occur at more negative potentials.

The difference in the degree of block observed at positive and negative potentials suggests that flecainide is blocking the delayed rectifier channel in a voltage-dependent manner. If data from these experiments are replotted as fractional block, they can be seen to track the activation curve very closely, suggest-

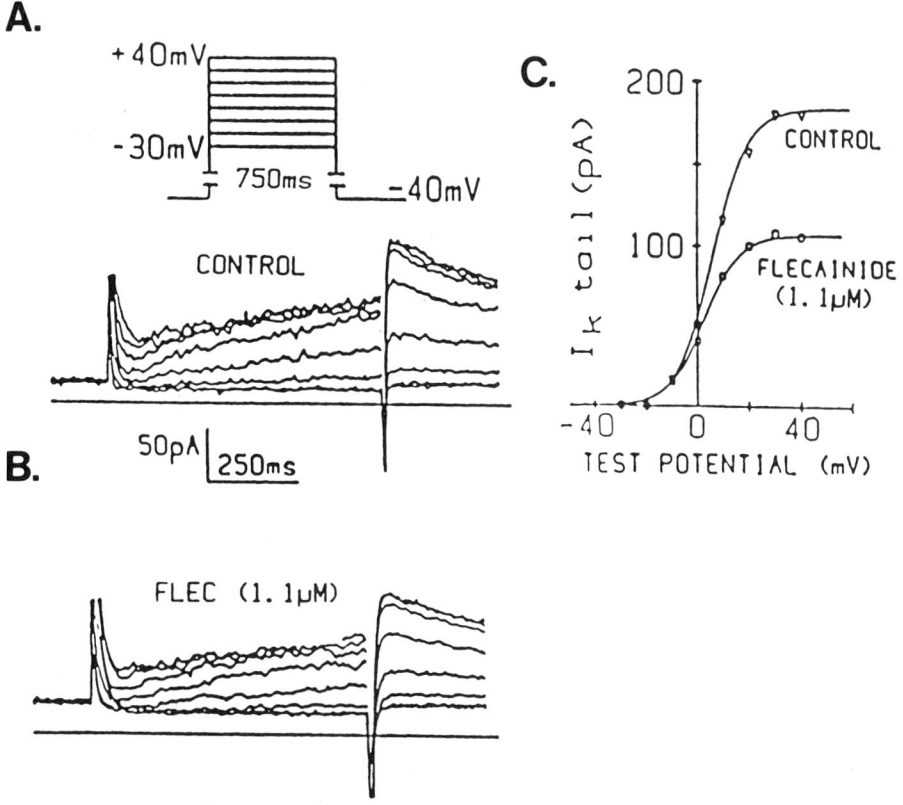

Figure 1. Effects of flecainide on the time-dependent outward current, I_K, in cat ventricular myocytes. A: Recordings of I_K elicited using 750-msec voltage-clamp steps from -40 mV to selected test potentials between -30 and $+40$mV. B: Flecainide (1.1 μM) decreased the outward current during the step and following repolarization by about 25%. Same preparation as in panel A. C: Activation curves determined by plotting peak tail current amplitude against test potential for an experiment similar to that shown in panels A and B. The solid line passing through the data points represents a simple Boltzmann distribution with a slope factor (k) of 6.7 mV and voltage mid-point ($V_{1/2}$) of $+6.4$ mV. Exposure to flecainide (1.1 μM) decreased the maximal tail current amplitude by 41%, shifted $V_{1/2}$ to $+2.7$ mV and increased k to 6.5 mV.

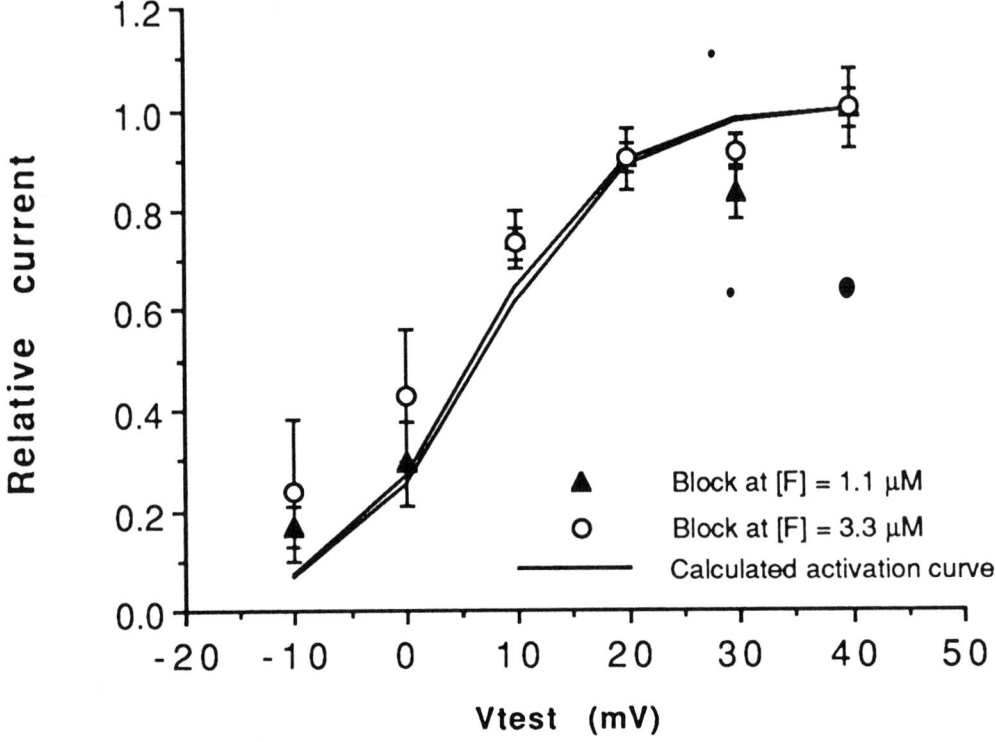

Figure 2. Relative tail current amplitude in the presence of flecainide at 1.1 μM (n = 6) and 3.3 μM (n = 7) is plotted for each test potential as a fraction of the tail current amplitude measured in the absence of drugs. The solid lines are the best-fit Boltzmann distributions for the data at each concentration of flecainide.

ing a link between block and channel activation. This is demonstrated in Figure 2, which summarizes data collected from a series of similar experiments performed using two different concentrations of flecainide (1.1 and 3.3 μM). The activation curves represented by the solid lines are calculated based on fits of the data obtained in the absence of drug for each set of experiments. While the agreement between the data and the activation curves is not exact, ie, there is a small (3–5 mV) negative shift at the higher concentration of flecainide, the amount of block tracks the activation curve fairly well, suggesting that block of I_K is somehow linked to channel activation. A similar relationship can also be obtained for the Class III agent WAY-123,398 (Figure 3), as well as for amiodarone (data not shown) and the Class IC

agent encainide,[3] and appears to be a fairly general property of blockers of the cardiac delayed rectifier current.

Interactions of the K^+ channel blockers with open channels are also reflected by the changes observed in the time course of the tail currents following repolarization (Figure 4). In the presence of drugs, delayed rectifier tail currents exhibit a distinct rising phase associated with a delayed time to peak and a slower rate of decay at later times. These changes in time course are similar to those reported for block of $I_{K(dr)}$ by quaternary ammonium ions in nerve,[11] and would be expected if drug blocked open channels released drugs upon repolarization and became available to conduct outward current transiently before deactivating. Crossover and

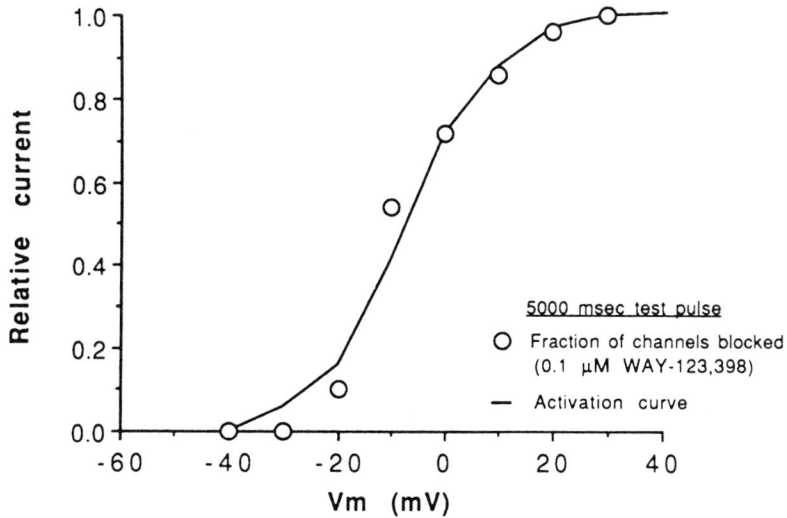

Figure 3. Data for the class III agent WAY-123,398 plotted in the same manner used for flecainide in Figure 2. The concentration (0.1 μM) represents the IC_{50} for block of $I_{K(dr)}$ in cat ventricular myocytes. In these experiments, test pulses were 5 seconds in duration. The solid line represents the fit to the Boltzmann distribution calculated prior to drug exposure.

blunting of tail currents have also been reported to occur with quinidine block of rabbit and human delayed rectifier channels.[12,13]

Reverse Use Dependence and K⁺ Channel Block

The drug channel interaction found for the agents studied above, ie, increasing block with depolarization and removal of block upon repolarization, resembles the conventional type of use and voltage dependence associated with the sodium channel blocking activity of the local anesthetics and the Class I antiarrhythmic agents. That this may be a general mode of drug channel interaction for agents acting on the delayed rectifier channel is suggested by more recent data using the Class III agents dofetilide and WAY-123,398.[15,16] However, it is well known that the ability of the Class III agents to prolong cardiac action potential is diminished at fast heart rates and accentuated by slow heart rates.[17,18] This is opposite to the use-dependent behavior of Class I agents, which show

enhanced pharmacological activity (ie, conduction slowing) at fast heart rates and reduced efficacy at slow heart rates.

Given that the mode of drug-K⁺ channel interaction appears to be conventional and not the reverse of that seen with the sodium channel blockers, the mechanism underlying the reverse use-dependence of the K⁺ channel blockers on action potential duration remains unclear. It is worth keeping in mind that Class III agents can still produce significant (15% to 30%) increases in action potential duration during premature stimulation at short cycle lengths, which may contribute to their greater overall efficacy in models of programmed electrical stimulation compared to fast channel blockers. It is likely that the blunting of the expected increase in action potential duration seen during rapid stimulation will involve changes in the importance of other current components to repolarization under these conditions (eg, calcium current inactivation, activation of pump currents).

Based on the observation that unblocking appears to occur principally via open channels, one might postulate that use-dependent

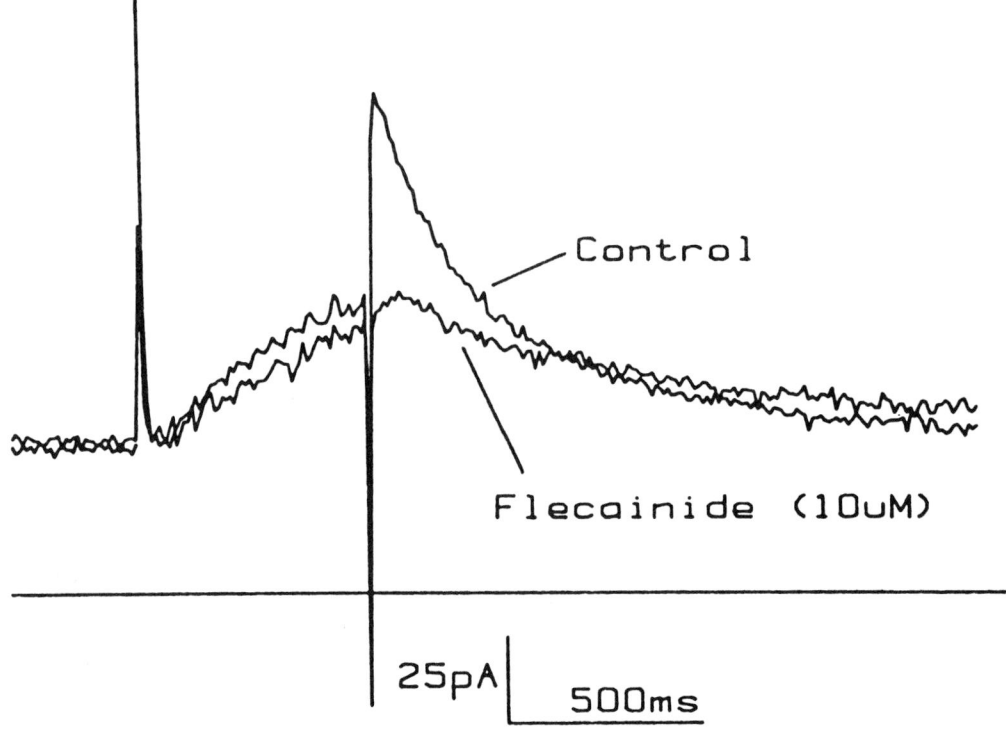

Figure 4. Tail currents elicited upon repolarization to −40 mV following 600-msec voltage-clamp steps to +50 mV are altered by flecainide (10 μM), reflecting unblocking from open channels. The bathing solution contained 0.2 mM CdCl₂ to speed the decay of the tail current (see Follmer et al.[20]).

effects will not be present at holding potentials where deactivation is sufficiently fast to "trap" drugs within the channel, ie, at negative potentials, but may occur at more depolarized levels where the channel closes slowly relative to drug binding. In preliminary studies, we have been unable to modulate the degree of $I_{K(dr)}$ block by altering the rate of pulsing when physiological holding potentials are used.[16] Using the Class III agent WAY-123,398, trains of depolarizations from −100 mV at cycle lengths of 300 to 2,500 msec failed to alter the amount of block observed after the first pulse. These results are consistent with the idea that block occurs rapidly (ie, during the first pulse) and does not reverse with repolarization to potentials at which the channels deactivate very rapidly. While we have not yet explored this behavior at more depolar-

ized holding potentials, use-dependent changes in I_K tail currents have been noted under these conditions for the Class III agent dofetilide.[15] Further studies are clearly needed to resolve this important question.

Conclusions

The diversity of the K^+ channels present in the heart and the variation in their regional distribution make them a rich source of targets for drug action. Only agents selective for the rapidly activating component of delayed rectification are generally available today; however, it is likely that new compounds with clear specificity for other K^+ channel subtypes will become available in the near future. This class of compounds will not only be very useful as probes of K$^+$ channel function in the heart, but should command considerable attention as an important new approach to the control of cardiac arrhythmias.

References

1. Harrison DC: Antiarrhythmic drug classification: new science and practical applications. *Am J Cardiol* 56:185, 1985.
2. Follmer CH, Colatsky TJ: Block of the delayed rectifier potassium current I$_K$ by flecainide and E-4031 in cat ventricular myocytes. *Circulation* 82:289, 1990.
3. Follmer CH, Cullinan CA, Colatsky TJ: Differential block of cardiac delayed rectifier current by class Ic antiarrhythmics: evidence for open channel block and unblock. *Cardiovasc Res* (in press).
4. Hellestrand KJ, Bexton RS, Nathan AW, et al: Acute electrophysiological effects of flecainide acetate on cardiac conduction and refractoriness in man. *Br Heart J* 48:140, 1982.
5. Somberg JC, Tepper D: Flecainide: a new antiarrhythmic agent. *Am Heart J* 112:808, 1986.
6. Davy J-M, Dorian P, Kantelip J-P, et al: Qualitative and quantitative comparison of the cardiac effects of encainide and its three major metabolites in the dog. *J Pharmacol Exp Ther* 237(3): 907, 1986.
7. Colatsky TJ: Mechanisms of action of lidocaine and quinidine on action potential duration in rabbit cardiac Purkinje fibers: an effect on steady-state sodium currents? *Circ Res* 50:17, 1982.
8. Sanguinetti MC, Jurkiewicz NK: Two components of cardiac delayed rectifier K$^+$ current. Differential sensitivity to block by class III antiarrhythmic agents. *J Gen Physiol* 96:195, 1990.
9. Colatsky TJ, Follmer CH: Potassium channels as targets for antiarrhythmic drug action. *Drug Dev Res* 19:129, 1989.
10. Balser JR, Bennett RB, Hondeghem LM, Roden DM: Suppression of time-dependent outward current in guinea pig ventricular myocytes. Actions of quinidine and amiodarone. *Circ Res* 69:519, 1991.
11. Armstrong CM: Interaction of tetraethylanmmonium ion derivatives with the potassium channels of giant axons. *J Gen Physiol* 58:413, 1971.
12. Furukawa T, Tsujimura Y, Kitamura K, et al: Time- and voltage-dependent block of the delayed K$^+$ current by quinidine in rabbit sinoatrial and atrioventricular nodes. *J Pharmacol Exp Ther* 251(2):756, 1989.
13. Snyders DJ, Knoth KM, Roberds SL, et al: Time-, voltage- and state-dependent block by quinidine of a cloned human cardiac potassium channel. *Mol Pharmacol* 41:322, 1992.
14. Hondeghem LM, Snyders DJ: Class III antiarrhythmic agents have a lot of potential but a long way to go. Reduced effectiveness and dangers of reverse use-dependence. *Circulation* 81:686, 1990.
15. Carmeliet E: Effect of UK-68,798 on delayed rectifier K$^+$ currents in cardiac myocytes. *Circulation* 84:II-176, 1991.
16. Spinelli W, Moubarak O, Colatsky TJ: Mechanism of delayed rectifier block by WAY-123,398, a new class III agent, in cat ventricular myocytes. *Circulation* 84:II-176, 1991.
17. Strauss HC, Bigger JT, Hoffman BF: Electrophysiological and beta-receptor blocking effects of MJ 1999 on dog and rabbit cardiac tissue. *Circ Res* 24:661, 1970.
18. Steinberg MI, Sullivan ME, Wiest SA, et al: Cellular electrophysiology of clofilium, a new antifibrillatory agent, in normal and ischemic canine Purkinje fibers. *J Cardiovasc Pharmacol* 3:881, 1981.
19. Colatsky TJ, Follmer CH, Starmer CF: Channel specificity in antiarrhythmic drug action: mechanism of potassium channel block and its role in suppressing and aggravating cardiac arrhythmias. *Circulation* 82:2235, 1990.
20. Follmer CH, Lodge NJ, Cullinan CA, Colatsky TJ: Modulation of the delayed rectifier I$_K$ by cadmium in cat ventricular myocytes. *Am J Physiol* 262:C75, 1992.

Chapter 19

Calcium Channel Blockers

Robert F. Gilmour, Jr.
Dante R. Chialvo
Jose Jalife

The potential roles of the calcium current I_{Ca} in impulse initiation and propagation in cardiac tissues have been studied extensively in recent years. Although our understanding of I_{Ca} remains incomplete, it seems clear that I_{Ca} contributes importantly to the generation of spontaneous impulses in the sinus node[1-4] and in depolarized myocardium and Purkinje fibers[5-8] and to the initiation of triggered activity.[9-13] Moreover, I_{Ca} mediates the upstrokes of normal sinus node and atrioventricular (AV) node action potentials[3,14] and slow response action potentials in depolarized myocardium and Purkinje fibers.[15-20]

The documented or suspected involvement of I_{Ca} in the generation of spontaneous or triggered impulses and in the propagation of action potentials in normal and injured cardiac cells suggests that inhibitors of I_{Ca} may exert a wide spectrum of antiarrhythmic effects. These include suppression of normal automaticity, abnormal automaticity, and triggered activity resulting from either early or delayed afterdepolarizations, and modulation of slow conduction, as it occurs normally in regions such as the AV node, or abnormally,

in acutely or chronically injured ventricular myocardium. The experimental observations that support each of these projected antiarrhythmic effects of calcium channel blockers will be considered individually. In addition, a potentially novel effect of calcium channel blockers on irregular electrical activity, as assessed using nonlinear dynamical systems theory, will also be discussed.

Suppression of Normal Automaticity

Although controversy exists regarding the ionic basis for diastolic depolarization in the sinus node,[2,4,21] experimental and clinical observations indicate clearly that the sinus node discharge rate is reduced by calcium channel blockers.[22-24] The negative chronotropic effects of drugs such as verapamil, nifedipine, and diltiazem probably reflect inhibition of L-type calcium current, although verapamil may also have a small inhibitory effect on T-type calcium current.[25] It has been proposed that crossover of the activation and

Supported by grants HL-40800 (RFG) and HL-39707 (RFG, DRC, JJ) from the National Institutes of Health, Bethesda, Maryland.
From BN Singh, HJJ Wellens, M Hiraoka, (eds): *Electropharmacological Control of Cardiac Arrhythmias*. Mount Kisco, NY, Futura Publishing Company Inc., © 1994.

inactivation curves for L-type calcium current may produce a significant window current at voltages within the pacemaker range.[2] In contrast, T-type calcium current exhibits little window current, but is activated significantly at membrane potentials that correspond to the latter half of diastolic depolarization.[1,2] Accordingly, inhibition of L-type calcium current would be expected to reduce inward current and, therefore the rate of diastolic depolarization throughout phase 4, whereas inhibition of T-type calcium current would affect primarily the latter half of phase 4.[1,2]

In intact animals or humans, reduction of the sinus node discharge rate by calcium channel blockers is offset to varying degrees by reflex activation of the sympathetic nervous system, secondary to peripheral vasodilation and reduction of arterial blood pressure.[22,23] Because the dihydropyridine derivatives such as nifedipine reduce blood pressure to a greater extent than verapamil or diltiazem, heart rate may actually increase after administration.[22,23]

Suppression of Abnormal Automaticity

Sustained depolarization has been shown to induce automaticity in cardiac tissues that are not normally automatic and to accelerate automaticity in tissues that normally exhibit relatively slow spontaneous discharge rates (eg, Purkinje fibers).[5-8] Although studied most extensively under experimental conditions where healthy tissue is depolarized using current injection, depolarization-induced automaticity is thought to occur under certain pathological conditions associated with the development of cardiac arrhythmias.[15,19]

In normal tissue depolarized by current injection, automaticity arising from membrane potentials less negative than -60 mV is suppressed by calcium channel blockers, whereas automaticity arising from more negative membrane potentials is not.[5-8] Similarly,

spontaneous activity in depolarized ventricular myocardium surviving myocardial infarction is abolished by calcium channel blockers.[15,19,26,27] The suppressant effects of calcium channel blockers on depolarization-induced automaticity probably reflect inhibition of the upstroke of spontaneous action potentials, rather than attenuation of phase 4 depolarization, although ionic mechanisms for the latter remain to be defined clearly.[8,28]

Suppression of Triggered Activity

Calcium channel blockers have been shown to suppress triggered activity arising from either early[12,13,29] or delayed[9,11,13,30] afterdepolarizations. Delayed afterdepolarizations reflect activation of the transient inward current following cyclic release of calcium from the sarcoplasmic reticulum.[31,32] The later phenomenon is more likely to occur under conditions of high $[Ca^{2+}]_i$. Suppression of delayed afterdepolarizations by calcium channel blockers probably reflects inhibition of calcium influx via I_{Ca} and a resultant decrease in $[Ca^{2+}]_i$, particularly under conditions that would otherwise promote calcium overload, such as exposure to toxic concentrations of cardiac glycosides.[9,11,30]

The ionic mechanisms for early afterdepolarizations have not been characterized completely, but reactivation of I_{Ca} during the plateau phase of prolonged action potentials appears to contribute to early afterdepolarizations and/or triggered responses under certain experimental conditions. In this regard, early afterdepolarizations induced by inhibition of I_K (using low $[K^+]_o$ and quinidine[29] or cesium[13]), promotion of I_{Ca} (using Bay K 8644[12,13]), or inhibition of I_{to} and I_K (using 4-aminopyridine [Figure 1]) are inhibited by calcium channel blockers. Moreover, it seems likely that the inhibitory effects of Mg^{2+} on early afterdepolarizations[29,33,34] can be attributed, at least in part, to reduction of I_{Ca}.[35] The suppressant effects of Mg^{2+} on early afterde-

Control   Verapamil

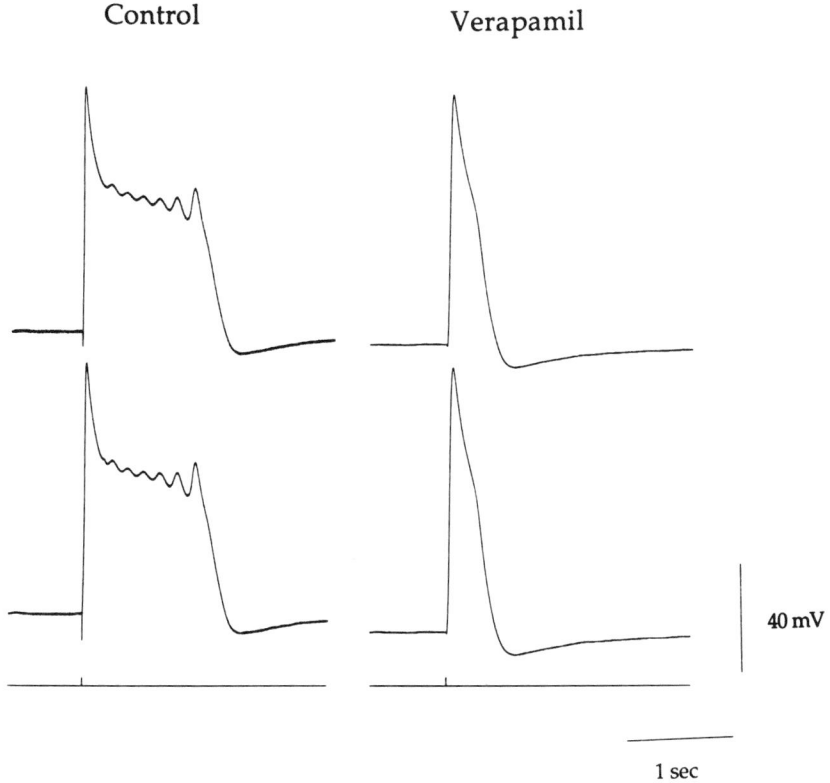

40 mV

1 sec

Figure 1. Effects of verapamil (1 μM) on early afterdepolarizations and triggered activity induced in a canine Purkinje fiber by superfusion with Tyrode's solution containing 10 mM 4-aminopyridine and 2.7 mM KCl. Recordings were obtained from two cells on opposite ends of the Purkinje fiber during pacing at a cycle length of 5,000 msec before (left panel) and after (right panel) 15 minutes of superfusion with verapamil.

polarizations produced in vitro may explain the ability of Mg^{2+} to prevent or terminate torsades de pointes-type arrhythmias observed experimentally[36] and clinically.[37]

Modulation of Normal Slow Conduction

Conduction through portions of the AV node occurs via action potentials that exhibit slowly rising upstrokes mediated by I_{Ca} (ie, slow response action potentials).[3,14] Accordingly, AV conduction times are prolonged by calcium channel blockers,[22–24] although, as discussed, this negative dromotropic effect may be offset to varying degrees by reflex changes in autonomic tone secondary to peripheral vasodilation. Accentuation of slow conduction by calcium channel blockers is useful for reduction of the ventricular rate during atrial fibrillation[26,38,39] and for the interruption of AV nodal reentry or AV reentry in association with an accessory pathway.[38–41] In both types of reentry, slow anterograde conduction through the AV node provides one limb of the reentry circuit, while more rapid retrograde conduction via the AV node or an accessory pathway provides the other. Interruption of reentry by calcium channel blockers most often is associated with block of slow anterograde conduction,[39–41] as would be expected from a selective suppression of slow response action potentials.

Modulation of Abnormal Slow Conduction

Sustained depolarization of atrial and ventricular myocardium and Purkinje fibers secondary to myocardial ischemia or other forms of injury inactivates fast sodium channels and, under the appropriate conditions, may thereby facilitate the induction of slow response action potentials.[15] Because slow response action potentials conduct slowly and are prone to block, they may mediate the unidirectional conduction block and slow conduction required for the initiation and maintenance of reentry within the atria or ventricles. Accordingly, suppression of slow response action potentials would be expected to correlate with an antiarrhythmic effect. In this regard, numerous experimental studies have shown that slow responses produced in models of simulated or actual myocardial ischemia are suppressed by calcium channel blockers,[15-20] yet clinical studies indicate that the antiarrhythmic effects of calcium channel blockers against ventricular tachyarrhythmias are limited.[42-44] However, agents that combine calcium channel blockade with blockade of sodium channels may be more effective antiarrhythmic agents, as suggested by studies of bepridil[26] and perhexilene.[45]

Although calcium channel blockers have not been found to be very effective for terminating existing arrhythmias associated with myocardial ischemia or infarction, pretreatment with calcium channel blockers may prevent the subsequent development of ventricular arrhythmias during acute myocardial ischemia.[46-52] This effect appears to be mediated by a reduction in the extent of ischemia-induced conduction delay. By inhibiting calcium influx via I_{Ca}, and thereby reducing intracellular calcium accumulation during ischemia, calcium channel blocking agents conceivably might attenuate ischemia-induced conduction delay by several mechanisms, including reductions of membrane depolarization,[47] action potential alternans,[53] and cyclic release of calcium from the sarcoplasmic reticulum.[54]

The observation that calcium channel blocking agents reduce conduction delay and the incidence of ventricular arrhythmias during acute myocardial ischemia suggests that these agents may be useful for the prevention of sudden death associated with an acute ischemic event. The results of clinical trials to test this hypothesis have been mixed, however, as discussed in more detail in Chapter 29 of this volume.

Modulation of Nonlinear Dynamical Behavior

One approach to the study of an apparently complex problem such as the mechanisms for cardiac arrhythmias is to assume that the system under study is multidimensional and that detailed information regarding the characteristics of each component of the system and the potential interactions between the components will be required to adequately explain the overall behavior of the system. A different approach is to assume that the behavior of a system is dominated by only a few components, with the proviso that at least one of the components be capable of exhibiting highly nonlinear behavior. An example of the potential usefulness of the latter approach is given by May,[55] who demonstrated that complex population dynamics could be explained entirely by the nonlinear response to alteration of a single variable. Specifically, he demonstrated that as resources for population growth were increased, the population at first rather predictably increased at an exponential rate. However, as resources were increased past a certain threshold, the population began to oscillate between two values. Moreover, further increases in resources caused the population to oscillate between, 4, then 8, then 16 values. At some still higher level of resources the population no longer exhibited periodic changes. Rather, very complex aperiodic changes in the population occurred.

The periodic changes in population with increasing allocation of resources is an example of a cascade of period doubling bifurca-

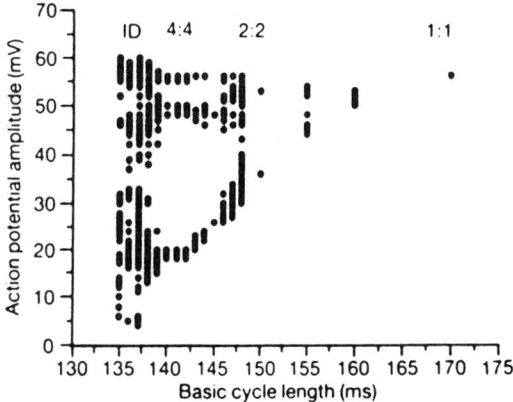

Figure 2. Period doubling bifurcations and chaos in canine ventricular muscle. Steady-state beat-to-beat changes in action potential amplitude are shown at different pacing cycle lengths. As the pacing cycle length was shortened, 1:1 locking was replaced first by 2:2 locking, then by 4:4 locking, and finally by irregular dynamics (chaos). (Reproduced with permission from Rreference 56.)

tions, where 1 begets 2 and 2 begets 4, etc. The culmination of this period doubling cascade is an aperiodic regime of deterministic chaos. Although the aperiodic activity (chaos) is extremely complex, it is predicted (ie, determined) by a simple nonlinear expression, the logistic equation (where next year's population x_{n+1} is a function of this year's population, x_n, and the resource allocation, r, according to $x_{n+1} = rx_n(1-x_n)$).

Recently, the relevance of period doubling bifurcations and low-dimensional chaos to the electrical behavior of cardiac tissue has been investigated using in vitro preparations of cardiac Purkinje fibers and ventricular muscle.[56–58] The results of these studies indicate that period doubling and chaos can be induced in regularly driven preparations by changing the stimulation rate (Figure 2), and that such activity can be predicted from a simple analytical model.[56] The basic elements of the model are illustrated in Figure 3.

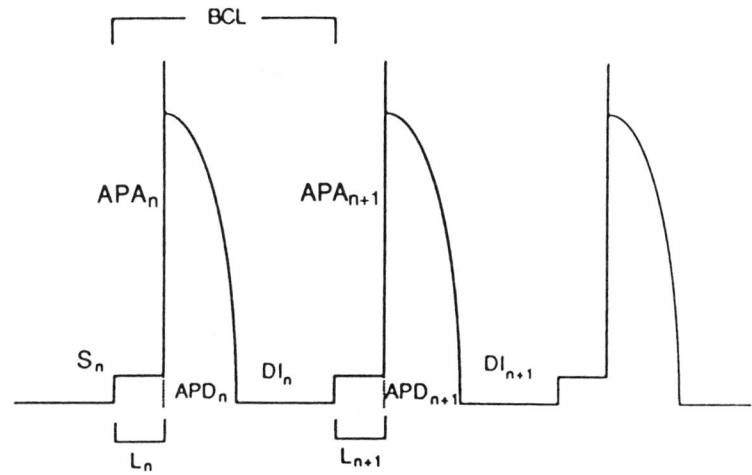

$$DI_n = BCL - L_n - APD_n$$

1) $L_{n+1} = F(DI_n)$ 3) $Th_{n+1} = Z(DI_n)$
2) $APD_{n+1} = G(DI_n)$ 4) $APA_{n+1} = Q(DI_n)$

Figure 3. Diagram illustrating components of the analytical model, where the diastolic interval (DI) equals the basic cycle length of pacing (BCL) minus latency to activation (L) and action potential duration (APD). L, APD, the excitability threshold (Th), and action potential amplitude (APA) are functions (F, G, Z, and Q, respectively) of the preceding DI.

From the analytical model it can be shown that chaotic behavior arises from the nonlinear dependence of the activated state of the cardiac cell on the preceding diastolic interval. The activated state is equivalent to the sum of the latency between delivery of the stimulus and the upstroke of the action potential (L) and the duration of the action potential (APD). At any given pacing cycle length (BCL), the diastolic interval (DI) can be calculated from the equation BCL = DI + L + APD; ie, the interval between stimuli encompasses the activated and the rest states. The relationships between APD or L and DI are determined using single premature stimuli delivered at the end of a train of stimuli. The relationship between DI and other relevant electrophysiological parameters, such as the current threshold for excitation or action potential amplitude, also can be determined using this protocol.

Examples of the dependence of latency and action potential duration on the preceding diastolic interval are shown in Figure 4. Summing these two functions produces a function with a region of steep negative slope at diastolic intervals of − 60 to − 125 msec and a region of ascending slope at shorter diastolic intervals. As illustrated in Figure 5, the steep slope and ascending region are necessary conditions for the development of chaotic activation. During rapid stimulation, increasingly larger oscillations of latency plus APD (and correspondingly of action potential amplitude) occur along the steeply sloped region of the function, until the trajectory leaves the steeply sloped region and encounters the ascending region of the function, where it is reflected back to the steeply sloped region. At this point the sequence repeats itself, although no two sequences are exactly the same. In the absence of an ascending limb, action potential

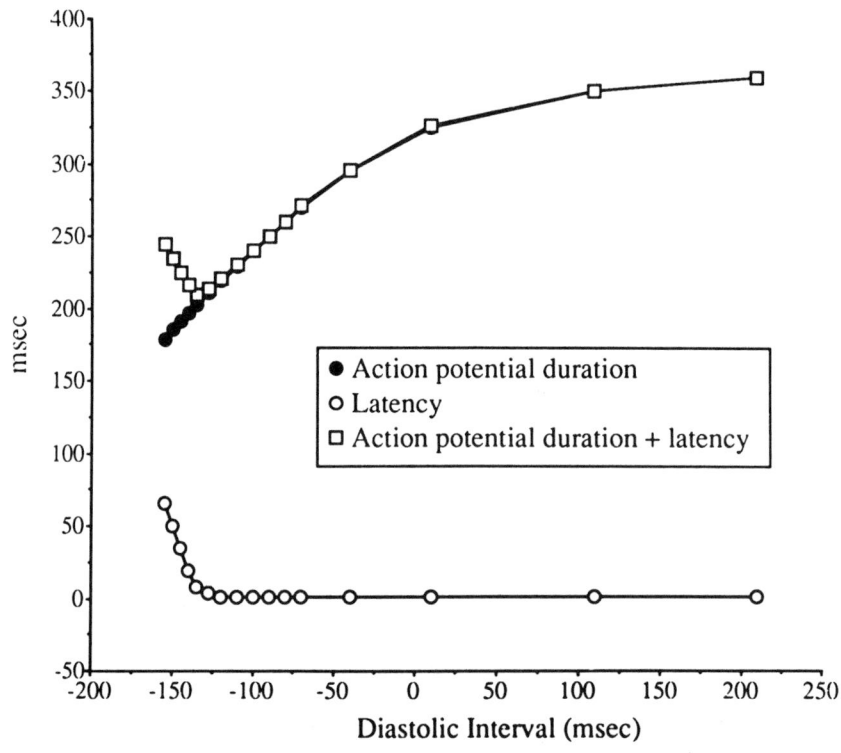

Figure 4. Relationship between diastolic interval and action potential duration (APD), latency, and the sum of APD and latency in a sheep cardiac Purkinje fiber (see inset).

A

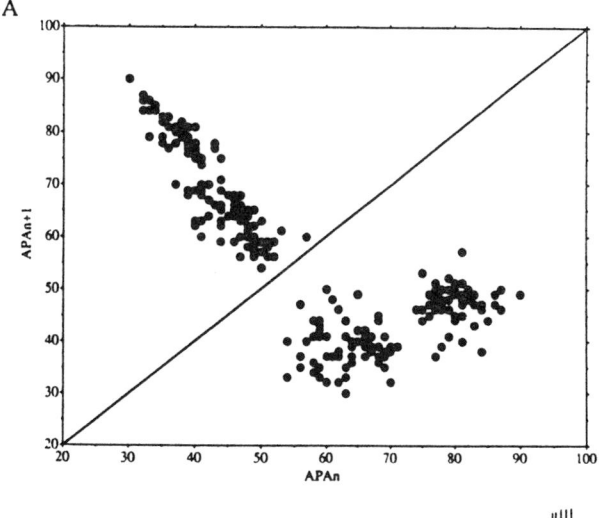

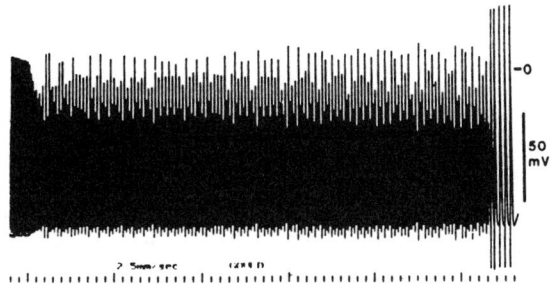

B

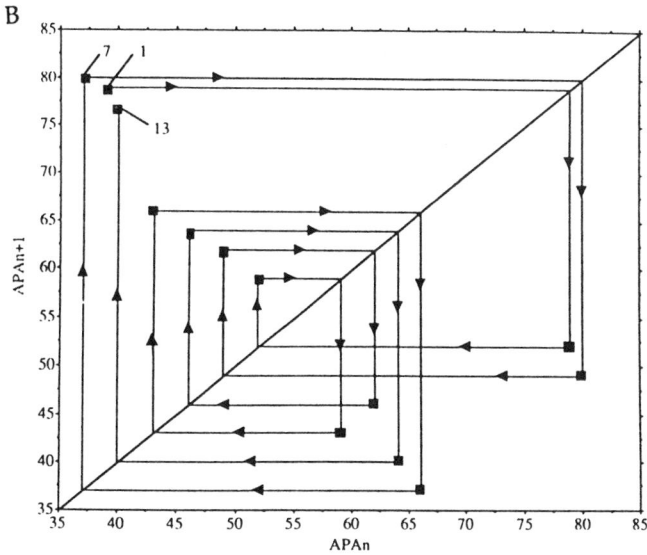

Figure 5. Low-dimensional chaos in a sheep cardiac Purkinje fiber. A: The upper panel is a one-dimensional return map for the series of transmembrane recordings shown in the lower panel. These recording were obtained by pacing the Purkinje fiber at cycle lengths of 185, 180 and 175 msec to produce 2:2 locking (left), chaos (middle), and 2:2 locking (right), respectively. For the return map, APA_{n+1} is plotted versus each preceding APA_n. APA_n and APA_{n+1} were linearly related (slope = 1.441, r^2 = 0.891) for $APA_n < 75$ mV. Note that the return map is the mirror image of the action potential duration (APD) plus latency function shown in Figure 4. B: Return map of a portion of the irregular dynamics shown in A. Arrows indicate the sequence of the map, starting at 1 and ending at 13 (upper left). (Reproduced with permission from reference 56.)

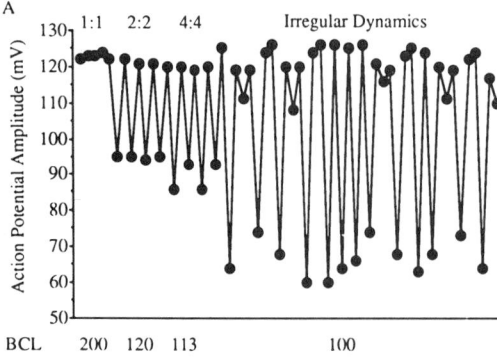

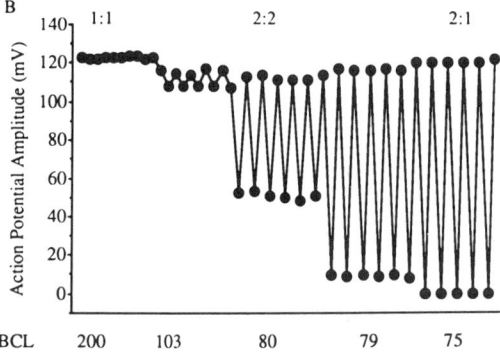

Figure 6. Effects of verapamil on period doubling bifurcations and chaos in a canine cardiac Purkinje fiber. A: Selected sections of the time series of steady-state action potential amplitude, illustrating the progression from 1:1 locking to 2:2, and 4:4 locking and to irregular dynamics as the pacing cycle length (BCL) was reduced from 200 to 120, 113 and 100 msec, respectively, during control. B: Loss of rate related higher order period doubling bifurcations and chaos following superfusion with verapamil (1 μM) for 30 minutes.

amplitudes labeled 1 and 7 in Figure 4 would be followed by conduction block. Accordingly, shortening the pacing cycle length in the absence of an ascending region causes 1:1 locking to be replaced by a single period doubling bifurcation (to 2:2) and then by 2:1 block, without intervening higher order period doubling bifurcations or chaos (Figure 2).

The results of the analytical and experimental models indicate that interventions that

decrease the slope of the relationship between APD and diastolic interval or prevent activation at short diastolic intervals (thereby eliminating the ascending limb of the function shown in Figure 4) will suppress period doubling bifurcations and chaos. Because calcium channel blockers are known to reduce the slope of APD restitution,[59] we investigated whether drugs such as verapamil might prevent the development of chaotic activation in isolated Purkinje fibers. As expected, verapamil did suppress chaotic activation, as shown in Figure 6. However, preliminary data suggest that this effect was related primarily to failure of activation at the shortest diastolic intervals, rather than to reduction of the slope of APD restitution.

Although previous experimental[46-52] and clinical[60] studies have linked the antiarrhythmic effects of verapamil during acute myocardial ischemia to a secondary effect of the drug, ie, a reduction of the electrophysiological consequences of ischemia, our observations suggest that verapamil may exert a direct antiarrhythmic effect under certain circumstances. Clearly, more studies are needed to determine whether suppression of chaotic activity by verapamil in vitro relates to clinically relevant arrhythmias.

References

1. Doerr Th, Denger R, Trautwein W: Calcium currents in single SA nodal cells of the rabbit heart studied with action potential clamp. *Pflügers Arch* 413:599, 1989.
2. Irisawa H, Hagiwara N: Ionic current in sinoatrial node cells. *J Cardiovasc Electrophysiol* 2: 531, 1991.
3. Irisawa H, Giles WR: Sinus and atrioventricular node cells: cellular electrophysiology. In: DP Zipes, J Jalife (eds): *Cardiac Electrophysiology: From Cell to Bedside.* Philadelphia, PA: WB Saunders, Co., 1990, p. 95.
4. Noble D: Ionic mechanisms in normal cardiac activity. In: DP Zipes, J Jalife (eds): *Cardiac Electrophysiology: From Cell to Bedside.* Philadelphia, PA: WB Saunders, Co., 1990, p. 163.
5. Elharrar V, Zipes DP: Voltage modulation of automaticity in cardiac Purkinje fibers. In: DP Zipes, JC Bailey, V Elharrar (eds): *The Slow In-*

ward Current and Cardiac Arrhythmias. The Hague: Martinus Nijhoff, 1980, p. 357.

6. Grant AO, Katzung BG: The effects of quinidine and verapamil on electrically induced automaticity in the ventricular myocardium of guinea pigs. *J Pharmacol Exp Ther* 196:407, 1976.

7. Imanishi S: Calcium-sensitive discharges in canine Purkinje fibers. *Jpn J Physiol* 21:443, 1971.

8. Imanishi S, Surawicz B: Automatic activity in depolarized guinea pig ventricular myocardium: characteristics and mechanisms. *Circ Res* 39:751, 1976.

9. Cranefield PF: Action potentials, afterpotentials and arrhythmias. *Circ Res* 41:415, 1977.

10. El-Sherif N, Craelius W, Boutjdir M, et al: Early afterdepolarizations and arrhythmogenesis. *J Cardiovasc Electrophysiol* 1:145, 1990.

11. Ferrier GR: Digitalis arrhythmias: role of oscillatory afterpotentials. *Prog Cardiovasc Dis* 19: 459, 1977.

12. January CT, Riddle JM: Early afterdepolarizations: mechanism of induction and block. A role for L-type Ca^{2+} current. *Circ Res* 64:977, 1989.

13. Marban E, Robinson SW, Weir WG: Mechanism of arrhythmogenic delayed and early afterdepolarizations in ferret muscle. *J Clin Invest* 78: 1185, 1986.

14. Zipes DP, Mendez C: Action of manganese ions and tetrodotoxin on atrioventricular nodal transmembrane potentials in isolated rabbit hearts. *Circ Res* 39:76, 1973.

15. Cranefield PF: *The Conduction of the Cardiac Impulse: The Slow Response and Cardiac Arrhythmias.* Mt. Kisco, NY: Futura Publishing Company, Inc., 1975.

16. Cranefield PF, Aronson RS, Wit AL: Effect of verapamil on the normal action potential and on a calcium-dependent slow response of canine cardiac Purkinje fibers. *Circ Res* 34:204, 1974.

17. Gilmour RF Jr, Zipes DP: Electrophysiological response of vascularized hamster cardiac transplants to ischemia. *Circ Res* 50:599, 1982.

18. Gilmour RF Jr, Heger JJ, Prystowsky EN, et al: Cellular electrophysiological abnormalities of diseased human ventricular myocardium. *Am J Cardiol* 51(1):137, 1983.

19. Singer DH, Baumgarten CM, Ten Eick RE: Cellular electrophysiology of ventricular and other dysrhythmias: studies on diseased and ischemic heart. *Prog Cardiovasc Dis* 24:97, 1981.

20. Spear JF, Horowitz LN, Hodess AB, et al: Cellular electrophysiology of human myocardial infarction. I. Abnormalities of cellular activation. *Circulation* 59:247, 1979.

21. DiFrancesco D: Current i_f and the neuronal modulation of heart rate. In: DP Zipes, J Jalife (eds): *Cardiac Electrophysiology: From Cell to Bedside.* Philadelphia, PA: WB Saunders, Co., 1990, p. 28.

22. Kawai C, Konishi T, Matsuyama E, et al: Comparative effects of three calcium antagonists, diltiazem, verapamil and nifedipine, on the sinoatrial and atrioventricular nodes. *Circulation* 63:1035, 1981.

23. Millard RW, Lathrop DA, Grupp G, et al: Differential cardiovascular effects of calcium channel blocking agents: possible mechanisms. *Am J Cardiol* 49:499, 1982.

24. Zipes DP, Fischer JC: Effects of agents which inhibit the slow channel on sinus node automaticity and atrioventricular conduction in the dog. *Circ Res* 34:184, 1974.

25. Bean BP: Classes of calcium channels in vertebrate cells. *Ann Rev Physiol* 51:367, 1989.

26. Prystowsky EN, Gilmour RF Jr: Role of slow channel blockers in the treatment of arrhythmias: basic considerations and clinical applications. In: JB Kostis, EA DeFelice (eds): *The Pharmacological Treatment of Cardiovascular Diseases.* New York, NY: Medical Examination Publishing Company, 1986, p. 213.

27. Spear JF, Horowitz LN, Moore EN: The slow response in human ventricle. In: DP Zipes, JC Bailey, V Elharrar (eds): *The Slow Inward Current and Cardiac Arrhythmias.* The Hague: Martinus Nijhoff, 1980, p. 309.

28. Katzung BG, Morgenstern JA: Effects of extracellular potassium on ventricular automaticity and evidence for a pacemaker current in mammalian ventricular myocardium. *Circ Res* 40: 105, 1977.

29. Nattel S, Quantz MA: Pharmacological response of quinidine induced early afterdepolarisations in canine cardiac Purkinje fibres: insights into underlying ionic mechanisms. *Cardiovasc Res* 22:808, 1988.

30. Hiraoka M, Okamoto Y, Sano T: Oscillatory afterpotentials in dog ventricular muscle fibers. *Circ Res* 48:510, 1981.

31. Kass RS, Lederer WJ, Tsien RW, et al: Role of calcium ions in transient inward current and aftercontractions induced by strophanthidin in cardiac Purkinje fibers. *J Physiol (Lond)* 281: 187, 1978.

32. Kass RS, Tsien RW, Weingart R: Ionic basis of transient inward current induced by strophanthidin in cardiac Purkinje fibers. *J Physiol (Lond)* 281:209, 1978.

33. Davidenko JM, Cohen L, Goodrow R, et al: Quinidine-induced action potential prolongation, early afterdepolarizations, and triggered activity in canine Purkinje fibers. *Circulation* 79:674, 1989.

34. Kaseda S, Gilmour RF Jr, Zipes DP: Depressant effect of magnesium on early afterdepolariza-

tions and triggered activity induced by cesium, quinidine, and 4-aminopyridine in canine cardiac Purkinje fibers. *Am Heart J* 118:458, 1989.

35. Lansman JB, Hess P, Tsien RW: Blockade of currents through single calcium channels by Cd^{2+}, Mg^{2+} and Ca^{2+}. Voltage and concentration dependence of Ca^{2+} entry into the pore. *J Gen Physiol* 88:321, 1986.

36. Bailie DS, Inoue H, Kaseda S, et al: Magnesium suppression of early afterdepolarizations and ventricular tachyarrhythmias induced by cesium in dogs. *Circulation* 77:1395, 1988.

37. Tzivoni D, Keren A, Cohen AM, et al: Magnesium therapy for torsades de pointes. *Am J Cardiol* 53:528, 1984.

38. Gilmour RF Jr, Zipes DP: The slow inward current and cardiac arrhythmias. *Am J Cardiol* 55:89B, 1985.

39. Rinkenberger RL, Zipes DP, Troup RJ, et al: Clinical and electrophysiologic effects of intravenous and oral verapamil in patients with supraventricular tachyarrhythmias. *Circulation* 62:996, 1980.

40. Sung RJ, Huycke EC, Keung EC, et al: Atrioventricular node reentry: evidence of reentry and functional properties of fast and slow pathways. In: DP Zipes, J Jalife (eds): *Cardiac Electrophysiology: From Cell to Bedside*. Philadelphia, PA: WB Saunders, Co., 1990, p. 513.

41. Wellens HJJ, Tan SL, Bar FWH, et al: Effect of verapamil studied by programmed electrical stimulation of the heart in patients with paroxysmal reentrant supraventricular tachycardia. *Br Heart J* 39:1058, 1977.

42. Buxton AE, Waxman HL, Marchlinski FE, et al: Electropharmacology of nonsustained ventricular tachycardia: effects of class I antiarrhythmic agents, verapamil and propranolol. *Am J Cardiol* 53:738, 1984.

43. Mason JW, Swerdlow CD, Mitchell B: Efficacy of verapamil in chronic, recurrent ventricular tachycardia. *Am J Cardiol* 51:1614, 1983.

44. Wellens HJJ, Bar FWHM, Lie KI, et al: Effect of procainamide, propranolol and verapamil on mechanisms of tachycardia in patients with chronic recurrent ventricular tachycardia. *Am J Cardiol* 40:579, 1977.

45. Vaughan Williams EM: *Antiarrhythmic Action and Puzzle of Perhexilene*. London: Academic Press, 1980.

46. Brooks WW, Verrier RL, Lown B: Protective effect of verapamil on vulnerability to ventricular fibrillation during myocardial ischaemia and reperfusion. *Cardiovasc Res* 14:295, 1980.

47. Clusin WT, Buchbinder M, Ellis AK, et al: Reduction of ischemic depolarization by the calcium channel blocker diltiazem. Correlation with improvement of ventricular conduction and

48. Elharrar V, Gaum WE, Zipes DP: Effect of drugs on conduction delay and incidence of ventricular arrhythmias induced by acute coronary occlusion in dogs. *Am J Cardiol* 39:544, 1977.

49. Gilmour RF Jr, Zipes DP: Effects of nitrendipine on ischemia-induced electrical changes in canine ventricle. In: A Scriabine, S Vanov, K Deck (eds): *Nitrendipine*. Baltimore, MD: Urban and Schwarzenberg, 1984, p. 209.

50. Kaumann JA, Aramendia P: Prevention of ventricular fibrillation induced by coronary artery ligation. *J Pharmacol Exp Ther* 164:326, 1977.

51. Nakaya H, Hattori Y, Sakuma I, et al: Effects of calcium antagonists on coronary circulation and conduction delay induced by myocardial ischemia in dogs: a comparative study with other coronary vasodilators. *Eur J Pharmacol* 73:272, 1981.

52. Peter T, Fujimoto T, Hamamoto H, et al: Electrophysiological effects of diltiazem in canine myocardium with special reference to conduction delay during ischemia. *Am J Cardiol* 49:602, 1982.

53. Lee HC, Mohabir R, Smith N, et al: Effect of ischemia on calcium-dependent fluorescence transients in rabbit hearts containing Indo 1. Correlation with monophasic action potentials and contraction. *Circulation* 78:1047, 1988.

54. Thandroyen FT, McCarthy J, Burton K, et al: Ryanodine and caffeine prevent ventricular arrhythmias during acute myocardial ischemia and reperfusion in rat heart. *Circ Res* 62:306, 1988.

55. May RM: Biological populations with non-overlapping generations: stable points, stable cycles and chaos. *Science* 186:645, 1974.

56. Chialvo DR, Gilmour RF Jr, Jalife J: Low dimensional chaos in cardiac tissue. *Nature* 343:653, 1990.

57. Chialvo DR, Jalife J: Nonlinear dynamics of cardiac excitation and impulse propagation. *Nature* 330:749, 1987.

58. Chialvo DR, Michaels DC, Jalife J: Supernormal excitability as a mechanism of chaotic dynamics of activation in cardiac Purkinje fibers. *Circ Res* 66:525, 1990.

59. Colatsky TJ, Hogan PM: Effects of external calcium, calcium channel blocking agents, and stimulation frequency on cycle length-dependent changes in canine cardiac action potential duration. *Circ Res* 46:543, 1980.

60. Vaage-Nilsen M, Rasmussen V, Fischer Hansen J, et al: Effect of verapamil on ischemia and ventricular arrhythmias after an acute myocardial infarction: prognostic implications. *J Cardiovasc Pharmacol* 18(Suppl 6):S26, 1991.

Chapter 20

Pharmacological Control of Experimental Atrial Arrhythmias: *Significance of Prolonging Excitation Wavelength*

Gregory K. Feld

The pharmacological control of reentrant atrial and ventricular arrhythmias has rapidly evolved over the past decade with the introduction of a variety of antiarrhythmic drugs that have markedly differing electrophysiological actions. Early antiarrhythmic drug development focused primarily on compounds that depress myocardial conduction velocity by blocking sodium channels, defined as Class I drugs. However, numerous clinical studies have shown that the Class I antiarrhythmic drugs have only limited efficacy, particularly in the treatment of atrial fibrillation and flutter.[1] In addition, they may produce serious side effects, organ toxicity, and life-threatening proarrhythmic effects. Further complicating matters is the fact that the electrophysiological effects of the Class I drugs are not pure in that they may produce a variety of effects other than sodium channel blockade, including inhibition of potassium and calcium channels and effects on the autonomic nervous system.

As a result of recent clinical trials showing increased mortality associated with the use of Class I antiarrhythmic drugs in a variety of arrhythmias,[2-4] research has shifted toward the development of new Class III antiarrhythmic drugs that selectively prolong repolarization. Partly as the basis for this shift in emphasis to the Class III antiarrhythmic drugs is the concept of control of arrhythmias by prolongation of wavelength, defined as the mathematical product of the refractory period and the conduction velocity in a reentrant circuit.[5,6] The wavelength of a reentrant tachycardia is by definition increased by prolongation of the refractory period and decreased by depression of conduction velocity.[5,6]

Theoretically, in anatomically determined reentrant arrhythmias with a fixed pathlength, Class III drugs that selectively prolong repolarization and wavelength might be expected to terminate and suppress tachycardia with minimal or no effects on conduction velocity or tachycardia rate, by eliminating the excitable gap in the reentrant circuit.[5,6] In contrast, functionally determined reentrant ar-

From BN Singh, HJJ Wellens, M Hiraoka, (eds): *Electropharmacological Control of Cardiac Arrhythmias*. Mount Kisco, NY, Futura Publishing Company Inc., © 1994.

rhythmias with a potentially variable path-length and no excitable gap, might be slowed, but not necessarily terminated by selective prolongation of repolarization.[5,6]

It can be further postulated that Class I antiarrhythmic drugs that slow conduction velocity and tachycardia rate might not terminate either form of reentrant arrhythmia if their net effect is to shorten wavelength and increase excitable gap. Alternatively, relatively pure Class I antiarrhythmic drugs (eg, Class Ic drugs that primarily depress conduction velocity) might terminate reentry if they cause complete conduction block in a critical zone of the reentry circuit, whereas Class I antiarrhythmic drugs with mixed effects (eg, Class Ia drugs that produce varying degrees of depression of conduction velocity and prolongation of refractoriness) might terminate reentry by narrowing or eliminating the excitable gap in the reentrant circuit, if their net effect is to prolong wavelength.

Despite these seemingly logical expectations, it has not been possible to accurately predict the mechanisms of action, nor the relative efficacy of the numerous antiarrhythmic drugs currently available. This is probably because of the highly variable electrophysiological effects of the antiarrhythmic drugs in vitro and in vivo, and the variability of the mechanisms of the arrhythmias they are used to treat. Thus, each drug must be independently studied in the treatment of specific arrhythmias to precisely assess their mechanisms of action, efficacy, and risk. However, since it is difficult and costly to study a large number of drugs in various arrhythmias in large numbers of patients, it may be useful to study experimental arrhythmia models to delineate the mechanisms of action, efficacy, and safety of new antiarrhythmic drugs prior to their use in humans.

Studies in a variety of experimental arrhythmia models have shown that arrhythmias due to reentry can be terminated and suppressed by the newer Class III antiarrhythmic drugs that primarily or selectively prolong myocardial refractoriness.[7-12] This chapter reviews the mechanisms of action and relative efficacy of the Class III antiarrhythmic drugs in the conversion and suppression of reentrant atrial arrhythmias in several experimental canine models, and compares and contrasts their effects to the Class I antiarrhythmic drugs.

Summary of Previously Published Studies

Mechanism of Atrial Reentrant Arrhythmias in Experimental Animal Models

Early experimental studies in rabbit and canine atrium demonstrated that sustained reentry could be produced in the presence of either a purely functional or an anatomical obstacle to conduction.[5,13-19] In arrhythmias resulting from reentry around an arc of purely functional conduction block (ie, so-called leading circle reentry) it has been shown that there may be no excitable gap or only a partially excitable gap, whereas in reentry around an anatomically-derived arc of block an excitable gap is expected.[5] These characteristics were demonstrated in early in vitro rabbit and in vivo canine experimental models of atrial reentry.[13-19] However, the relevance of the arrhythmias produced in these experimental models to clinical arrhythmias such as atrial flutter or fibrillation is uncertain.

In order to produce atrial reentrant arrhythmias that might have more clinical relevance, several new canine models of atrial reentry have been developed, including the sterile pericarditis, right atrial enlargement, right atrial Y-incision, and right atrial crush-injury models of atrial flutter.[20-29] Although in each of these models initiation of reentry may depend on an interplay between functionally and anatomically determined obstacles, sustained tachycardia in the sterile pericarditis and right atrial enlargement models is due to reentry around a functionally determined arc of block.[22-28] In contrast, reentry in the right atrial crush-injury and Y-incision models occurs around anatomical obstacles,[20,21,29] although only the right atrial crush-injury model has a fully excitable gap.[20,21] It is the anatomical obstacle models, particularly the right atrial crush-injury model, that may be most similar to human type 1 atrial flutter, which has been characterized as an anatomically determined macroreentry circuit, with an area of relatively slow conduction in the isthmus of tissue between the inferior vena cava and the tricuspid valve annulus, with a fully excitable gap, and from which double potentials can be recorded at the center of the reentry circuit.[20,21,30–34]

Electrophysiological Effects of Antiarrhythmic Drugs in Experimental Models of Atrial Reentrant Arrhythmias

Numerous studies on the effects of antiarrhythmic drugs in experimental models of atrial flutter have been published. Despite the variable efficacy in termination and suppression of atrial flutter in these different models, the electrophysiological effects of the various antiarrhythmic drugs are consistent and for the most part predictable from their known in vitro electrophysiological effects. Comparing similar intravenous doses (milligrams per kilogram) from published studies, the Class III drugs d-sotalol and N-acetylprocainamide (NAPA) prolonged atrial effective (ERP) and functional (FRP) refractory periods by 16% to 32%, while the Class I drugs disopyramide,

flecainide, recainam, procainamide, propafenone, and quinidine prolonged ERP and FRP by 20% to 67%.[7–12] In these same studies, the atrial flutter cycle length was prolonged 8% to 16% by the Class III drugs, and 31% to 78% by the Class I drugs.[7–12] Drug-induced changes in conduction velocity were similar to those of atrial flutter cycle length. Representative data from two studies in our crush-injury atrial flutter model comparing Class Ia, Ib, Ic, and III drugs are summarized in Table 1.[21,22]

On further comparison of these studies several points deserve additional comment.[7–12] At least in the studies by Hoffman et al.[9,11] it appears that the effects of the Class I drugs on ERP and FRP were on average somewhat greater than those of the Class III drugs. One possible explanation for this difference, compared to the comparable effects of the Class I and III drugs on atrial ERP and FRP in other published studies[7,8,10] is that Hoffman et al.[9,11] used relatively high doses of procainamide, flecainide, and propafenone infused as a bolus, followed by a constant maintenance infusion, which produced plasma concentrations that were higher than those considered therapeutic in humans. This may have caused an inordinate prolongation of ERP and FRP. In other reported studies maximal observed prolongation of ERP and FRP by the Class Ia, Ic, and III drugs was similar.[7,8,10]

Interestingly, in contrast to what has been observed in ventricular myocardium, the Class Ic drugs flecainide, propafenone, and re-

Table 1
Electrophysiological Effects of Intravenous Quinidine, Lidocaine, Recainam, d-Sotalol, and
N-Acetylprocainamide in the Canine Crush-Injury Model of Atrial Flutter

	CONT/QUIN (n = 15)	CONT/LIDO (n = 10)	CONT/REC (n = 10)	CONT/dSOT (n = 15)	CONT/NAPA (n = 15)
AERP	111 ± 25/155 ± 38*	112 ± 23/114 ± 21	120 ± 10/154 ± 24*	125 ± 17/166 ± 20*	127 ± 14/161 ± 15*
AFRP	148 ± 24/187 ± 53*	163 ± 22/153 ± 25#	143 ± 9/171 ± 26*	146 ± 13/189 ± 18*	148 ± 12/181 ± 16*
A-Ct	51 ± 11/60 ± 12*	NA/NA	53 ± 9/89 ± 12*	53 ± 8/57 ± 9#	44 ± 7/46 ± 8
AFcl	131 ± 26/171 ± 38*	145 ± 18/164 ± 28#	138 ± 10/215 ± 14*	140 ± 11/151 ± 15*	151 ± 21/170 ± 23*

A-Ct: right to left atrial conduction time during right atrial pacing at 150 msec cycle length; AERP: right atrial effective refractory period; AFRP: right atrial functional refractory period; AFcl: atrial flutter cycle length; CONT: control before drug; dSOT: d-sotalol; LIDO: = lidocaine; n: number of animals studied in each group; NA: not available; NAPA: N-acetylprocainamide; QUIN: quinidine; REC: recainam. All values are in milliseconds and presented as the mean ± 1 SD for all animals studied. # = $p < 0.05$; * = $p < 0.01$.

cainam produced significant increases (20% to 43%) in the atrial ERP and FRP.[8,9] Recent in vitro studies in canine and human atrial tissue have shown that the Class Ic drug flecainide may block the delayed rectifier potassium channel, thus prolonging atrial action potential duration and ERP in a use-dependent manner.[35] This effect is consistent with the observations described in the experimental canine atrial flutter models.[8,9]

The effects of the Class Ia and Ic antiarrhythmic drugs on atrial flutter cycle length also differed significantly, as would be predicted. For example, the Class Ic drugs flecainide, propafenone, and recainam prolonged atrial flutter cycle length by 56% to 78%, and the Class Ia drugs disopyramide, procainamide, and quinidine by 31% to 61%.[7–11] In these studies, prolongation of tachycardia cycle length appears to be more closely correlated to drug-induced changes in atrial conduction velocity, rather than refractory period.[7–11] However, since d-sotalol has no effect on sodium channel conductance it is likely that prolongation of refractory period may contribute to some extent to tachycardia slowing, possibly by reducing upstroke velocity of the action potential by impingement of atrial beats on the relative refractory period of each previous beat.

These observations on the electrophysiological effects of various Class I and III antiarrhythmic drugs should help one predict their efficacy and possible mechanisms of termination and suppression of specific experimental atrial tachycardia models. However, the results of these studies have shown that such predictions cannot always be made accurately.

Mechanisms of Action and Relative Efficacy of Various Antiarrhythmic Drugs in Experimental Atrial Reentrant Arrhythmias

The results of previously published studies on the effects of the Class I and III drugs in canine experimental models of atrial flutter have led to varying conclusions regarding the mechanism of arrhythmia termination and suppression.

Hoffman et al.[9,11] observed that termination of reentry in their Y-incision atrial flutter model by the Class I drugs correlated most closely with the degree of depression of conduction velocity and tachycardia cycle length. In contrast, termination by the Class III drug d-sotalol was associated with prolongation of refractoriness.[9] They also observed that d-sotalol and disopyramide decreased excitable gap, while flecainide increased excitable gap.[9,11] These findings are consistent with what one would predict from their known electrophysiological effects, drugs that selectively prolong ERP (ie, Class III) would increase wavelength and narrow excitable gap, drugs that predominately depress conduction velocity (ie, Class Ic) would increase excitable gap, and those that prolong ERP and depress conduction velocity (ie, Class Ia) would have varying effect depending on their relative effect on ERP and conduction velocity. However, in their model, both the Class I and III drugs, with the exception of the Class Ib drug lidocaine, were similarly highly effective in terminating atrial tachycardia.[9,11]

In no case was excitable gap eliminated by an antiarrhythmic drug and Hoffman et al.[9,11] concluded that narrowing or elimination of the excitable gap in the reentry circuit did not appear to be crucial to arrhythmia termination. However, in their discussion Hoffman et al.[9,11] conceded that excitable gap was not measured at the moment of termination of atrial tachycardia, but following reinduction of atrial flutter after drug infusion. Furthermore, local changes in conduction velocity and refractoriness in the reentrant circuit were not measured. Thus, a significant role of alteration in refractoriness and excitable gap could not be ruled out, even in the case of the Class I antiarrhythmic drugs.

Hoffman et al.[9,11] did make two additional, very important observations, which may in fact suggest a significant role of prolongation of refractoriness in termination of atrial reentry in their model. First, Class I drugs produced significant slowing and tachycardia cycle length oscillation, with termination due to abrupt conduction block usually occurring during a short cycle length. Second, termination of tachycardia by Class III drugs (eg, d-sotalol) was often preceded by a single premature activation and then subsequent conduction block. They postulated that this could be due to reflection in the reentry circuit or failure of lateral boundaries of the reentry circuit with interruption following an eccentric premature activation of the circuit.

In our own model of experimental canine atrial flutter[7,8] we observed a close correlation between termination and suppression of reentry with prolongation of refractoriness, but not depression of conduction velocity. This was the case for the Class Ia (quinidine), Class Ic (recainam), and Class III (NAPA and d-sotalol) drugs. Lidocaine, a Class Ib drug, mildly depressed conduction velocity but was ineffective in terminating or suppressing atrial flutter.[7,8] Furthermore, the efficacy of each drug was correlated with the degree to which it prolonged the ERP and FRP or the ratio of prolongation of the ERP and FRP to conduction velocity. As a result, the Class III drugs were more effective than the Class Ia drugs, which were in turn more effective than the Class Ic drugs, while the Class Ib drug lidocaine was least effective.[7,8] Thus, we concluded that prolongation of refractoriness and not conduction velocity, possibly by narrowing or eliminating the excitable gap, was critical to arrhythmia termination and suppression. Observations similar to those of our own were made by Okumura and co-worker[10] with NAPA and quinidine in the sterile pericarditis model of atrial flutter.

The differences in degree of efficacy of the various antiarrhythmic drugs used in these studies may relate in part to the different models used and the different methods of drug administration and dosages. For example, Hoffman et al.[9,11] used a bolus injection and achieved higher than usual therapeutic levels in their study compared to ours[7,8] or that of Okumura and co-worker.[10] Nonetheless, based on these studies it appears that several mechanisms may exist by which antiar-rhythmic drugs terminate experimental atrial reentrant arrhythmias.

New Experimental Results

With the advent of computerized mapping it is now possible to study the termination of reentrant arrhythmias by antiarrhythmic drugs in a more detailed manner than previously possible. Therefore, we studied the effects of the Class III antiarrhythmic drug d-sotalol on the termination of reentry in our canine crush-injury model of atrial flutter. We chose d-sotalol because it was reliably effective in terminating reentry in this model. The remainder of this chapter describes the results of this study.

Experimental Method

As in our previous experiments[20,21] we induced sustained atrial flutter by rapid atrial pacing or programmed stimulation after producing a crush-injury in the right atrial free wall, parallel to and about 1.5 cm above the tricuspid annulus, extending 1.5 to 2 cm from the base of the atrial appendage toward the intercaval zone (Figure 1). A 64-channel mapping system (Bard Electrophysiology, Inc., Haverhill, MA, USA) was used with a 56-electrode custom-shaped plaque covering the entire posterior right atrial epicardial surface or a higher density rectangular plaque covering just the crush-injury and the area of the reentry circuit (Figure 1).

Activation maps were obtained during sustained atrial flutter and at the moment of termination of atrial flutter during intravenous infusion of d-sotalol, 2 mg/kg over 10 minutes. Conduction time during atrial flutter (ie, a measure of conduction velocity) above and below the length of the crush-injury was determined from these activation maps, before and during infusion of d-sotalol. Atrial ERPs and FRPs were determined during sinus rhythm at bipolar plunge electrodes placed above and below the crush-injury, using decremental premature stimuli scanning diastole (S_1S_2 10-

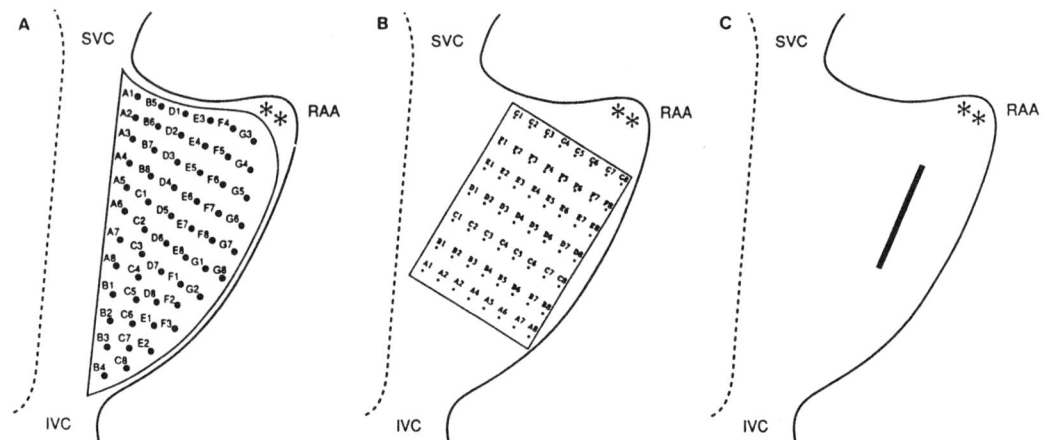

Figure 1. Schematic diagrams of the posterior right atrial surface showing positions of molded 56-electrode plaque (A), high-density rectangular plaque (B), and approximate location of crush-injury (C). IVC: inferior vena cava; RAA: right atrial appendage; SVC: superior vena cava.

msec intervals) following an 8-beat drive (S_1S_1 200 msec), before and after d-sotalol infusion. Atrial flutter cycle length was noted just prior to infusion of d-sotalol and just prior to termination of atrial flutter.

Results

Sustained atrial flutter was reproducibly induced in seven of nine dogs studied (Figure 2). The mean atrial flutter cycle length during control was 139 ± 16 msec (range 125–175), and increased by 15% to 161 ± 24 msec (range 134–210) during the d-sotalol infusion ($p < 0.01$). D-sotalol increased conduction time during atrial flutter by 8% from 34 ± 9 to 41 ± 7 msec above ($p < 0.05$) and by 7.5% from 47 ± 8 to 63 ± 13 msec below ($p < 0.05$) the crush-injury. Conduction time tended to be longer below than above the crush-injury, both before and after d-sotalol infusion, but this difference did not reach statistical significance. Atrial ERP was similar above (123 ± 12 msec) and below (134 ± 11 msec) the crush-injury at control. D-sotalol increased ERP by 29% and 35% to 160 ± 18 and 181 ± 27 msec above and below the

crush-injury ($p < 0.01$), respectively. Although there was an apparent trend for d-sotalol to increase ERP to a greater extent below the crush-injury than above (ie, 35% versus 29%), this trend was not statistically significant in this small group of animals. A similar effect of d-sotalol on FRP was observed.

In these experiments d-sotalol terminated sustained atrial flutter in each of the seven dogs studied. Termination occurred following the development of conduction block between the crush-injury and the tricuspid annulus in each dog. Conduction block occurred abruptly without significant cycle length alteration in 1 dog, following premature eccentric activation of the reentrant circuit with subsequent development of conduction block in 3 doys, and following premature eccentric activation of the reentrant circuit causing a transient fibrillatory activation pattern and then conduction block in 3 dogs. An example of each pattern of termination is shown in Figures 3–5.

These patterns of termination suggest several different mechanisms produced by d-sotalol, not dissimilar from those proposed by Hoffman et al.[9,11] The first mechanism, abrupt termination with minimal or no cycle length

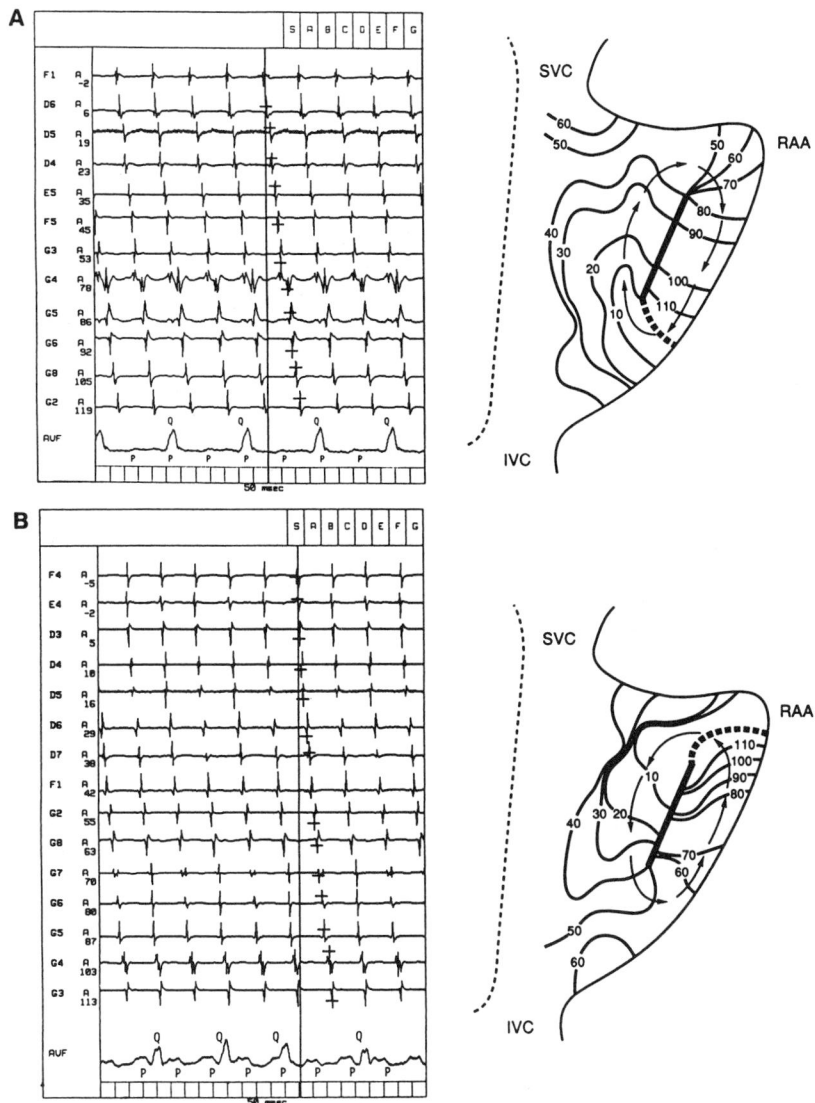

Figure 2. Epicardial electrograms from around the reentrant circuit (left panels) and activation patterns (right panels) during two episodes of sustained atrial flutter in one dog. Note counterclockwise (A) and clockwise (B) rotation of reentry, producing flat to inverted or upright P waves in electrocardiogram lead aVF, respectively. Activation time lines represent 10-msec intervals. Heavy solid line represents location of crush-injury. Heavy dashed line represents 0 activation time referenced to the atrial flutter P wave onset in surface electrocardiogram lead aVF. P: P wave or atrial flutter wave; Q: QRS; IVC: inferior vena cava; RAA: right atrial appendage; SVC: superior vena cava.

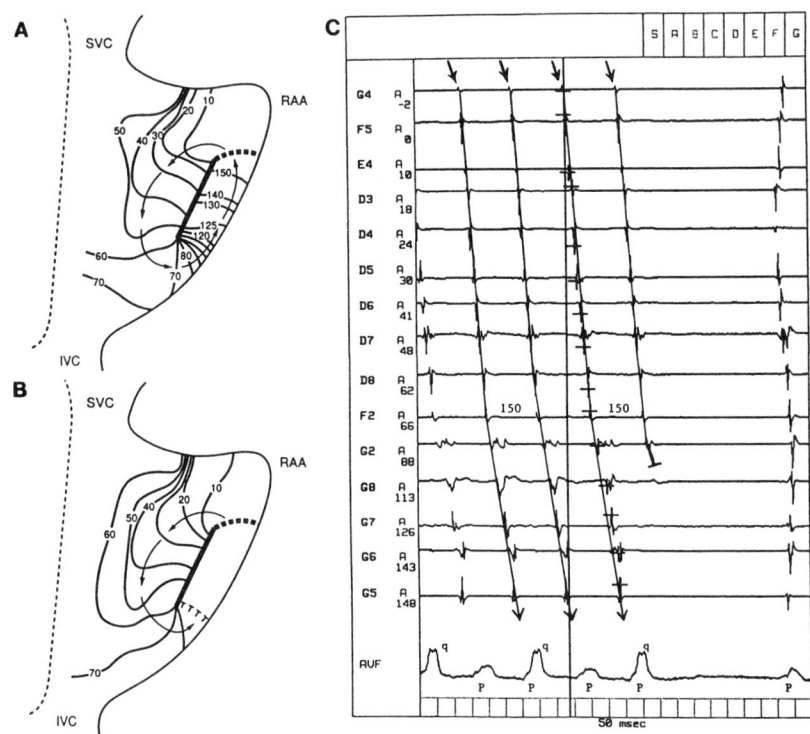

Figure 3. Activation patterns and epicardial electrograms during an episode of clockwise rotating atrial flutter that abruptly terminated during infusion of d-sotalol. Although there was slight slowing of atrial flutter rate prior to termination compared to control (130 msec), there was no cycle oscillation (150 msec) prior to termination. During the next-to-last beat of atrial flutter (A) bunching of isochrones is noted below the posterior end of the crush-injury, indicating localized conduction slowing. During the last beat of atrial flutter (B) abrupt block occurs in this same area between electrodes G2 and G8 (C). P: P wave or atrial flutter wave; Q: QRS; IVC: inferior vena cava; RAA: right atrial appendage; SVC: superior vena cava.

oscillation, is most likely due to prolongation of refractoriness with local elimination of excitable gap causing failure of impulse propagation. The second and third patterns of termination appear to be variations of the same mechanism, and likely represent failure of lateral boundaries of the reentrant circuit as originally described by Hoffman et al.[9,11] Failure of lateral boundaries allows an eccentric wave front to prematurely activate the reentrant circuit, leading to abrupt block below the crush-injury in the second pattern of termination, or repeated premature eccentric activation resulting in the third pattern of termination manifesting as a transient fibrillatory activation leading to conduction block. In both the second and third patterns of termination, prolongation of refractoriness is still the most likely mechanism for eventual failure of impulse propagation, even though failure of lateral boundaries initiates the process.

Although we have not yet performed similar mapping studies in this model of atrial flutter to assess the mechanisms of termination by Class I antiarrhythmic drugs, we did assess the potential proarrhythmic effects of the investigational Class Ic drug recainam, in the two animals in this study in which sustained atrial flutter was not inducible in the control state. Activation maps were obtained and refractory periods determined, in an identical manner to that described in the *Methods* section, before and after intravenous infusion of recainam, 10 mg/kg over 10 minutes followed by a constant maintenance infusion of 10 mg/kg per hour. Our hypothesis was that the pathlength around the crush-injury was not long enough in these two dogs to maintain an excitable gap that would allow sustained reentry, given the baseline conduction velocity, refractoriness, and wavelength of the right atrium. We postulated that slowing of conduction velocity would decrease the wavelength enough, such that it would be less than the anatomical pathlength around the crush-injury and produce an adequate excitable gap to allow reentry. In both of these animals, sustained atrial flutter at a relatively slow rate was easily induced with programmed stimulation after recainam infusion. The mechanism of atrial flutter was typical for this model, with counterclockwise reentry around the crush-injury, initiated by transient unidirectional block below the crush-injury during pacing (Figure 6). Thus, in addition to the lesser efficacy in terminating atrial flutter in this model compared to the Class Ia and III drugs,[7,8] the Class Ic drug recainam also has proarrhythmic

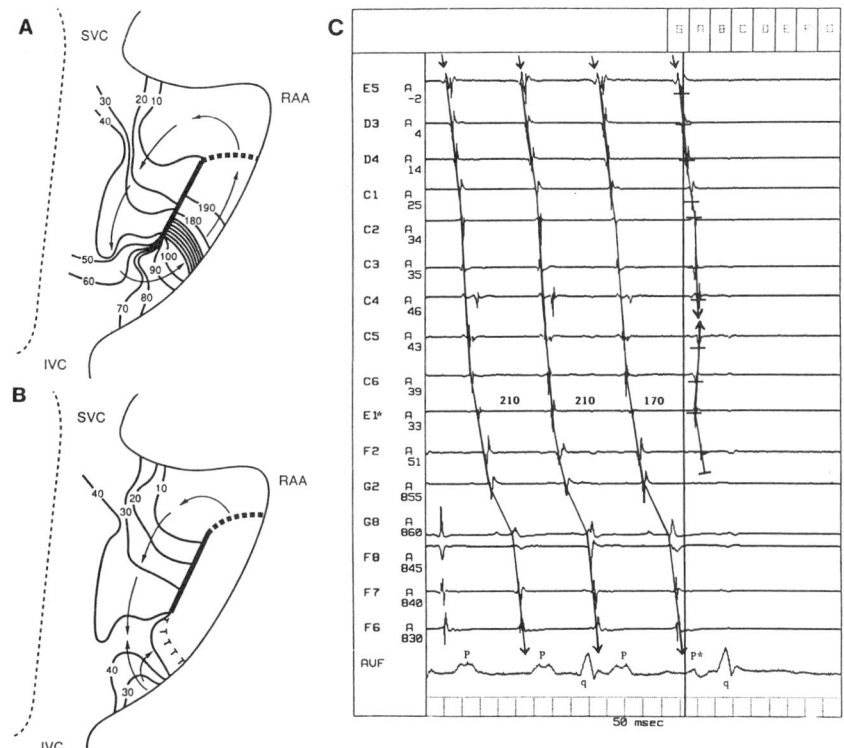

Figure 4. Activation patterns and epicardial electrograms during an episode of clockwise rotating atrial flutter that terminated abruptly following a single eccentric premature activation of the reentry circuit. During the next-to-last beat of atrial flutter (A) bunching of isochrones is noted inferior to the posterior end of the crush-injury, indicating localized conduction slowing. During the last beat of atrial flutter (B), a premature activation in the reentry circuit (cycle length 170 msec) is noted below the posterior end of the crush-injury (electrode E1), which conducts antidromically into the reentry circuit above the crush-injury, and orthodromically below the crush-injury. The premature orthodromic wave front then blocks beneath the posterior end of the crush-injury between electrodes G2 and G8 (C), terminating atrial flutter. P: P wave or atrial flutter wave; Q: QRS; IVC: inferior vena cava; RAA: right atrial appendage; SVC: superior vena cava.

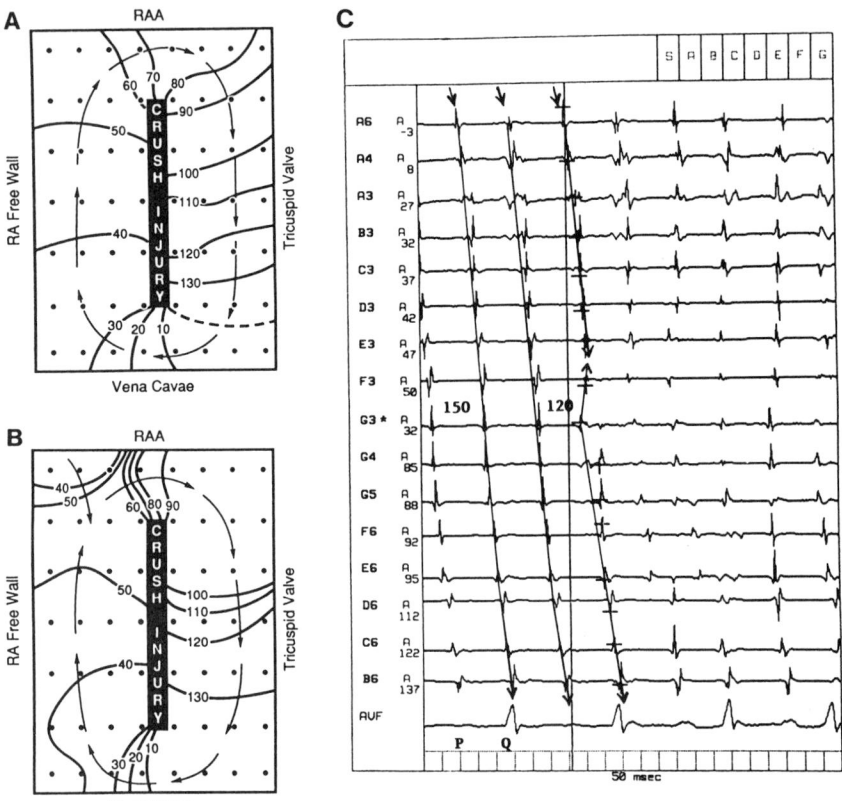

Figure 5. Activation patterns and epicardial electrograms during an episode of counterclockwise atrial flutter that terminated after transient fibrillatory activity induced by a single eccentric premature activation of the reentry circuit. Activation pattern (A) using high-density rectangular plaque during the next-to-last beat of atrial flutter. During the last beat of atrial flutter (B), a premature activation in the reentry circuit (cycle length 120 msec) is noted above the anterior end of the crush-injury (electrode G3), which conducts antidromically into the reentry circuit above the crush-injury, and orthodromically below the crush-injury. The first premature eccentric wave front sets up pattern of repeated eccentric wave fronts (C), producing an atrial fibrillation or type 2 atrial flutter pattern, which subsequently terminates with block below the anterior end of the crush-injury between electrodes E6 and D6 (not shown). P: P wave or atrial flutter wave; Q: QRS; IVC: inferior vena cava; RAA: right atrial appendage; SVC: superior vena cava.

potential, likely due to its potent depressant effects on conduction velocity. The potential for atrial proarrhythmia has also been observed in patients.[36]

Summary

The extensive investigation of the effects of antiarrhythmic drugs in the termination and suppression of atrial arrhythmias using experimental animal models has greatly enhanced our understanding of their effects. However, these studies have often raised as many questions as they have answered. Recent technological advances (eg, computerized mapping) have provided further insights into the mechanisms of action of antiarrhythmic drugs in experimental atrial reentrant arrhythmias.

A   **B**

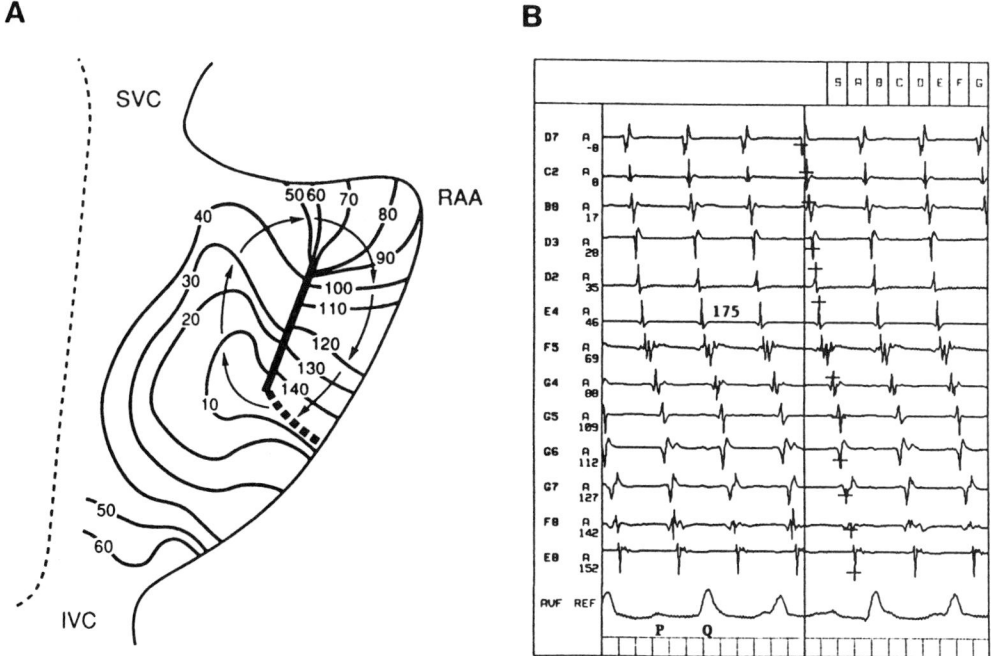

Figure 6. Activation patterns (A) and epicardial electrograms (B) during an episode of sustained atrial flutter induced by programmed stimulation after intravenous infusion of the Class Ic drug recainam. Sustained atrial flutter could not be induced in this dog during control. Atrial flutter cycle length is 175 msec due to pronounced effects of recainam on conduction velocity. P: P wave or atrial flutter wave; Q: QRS; IVC: inferior vena cava; RAA: right atrial appendage; SVC: superior vena cava.

Studies in the most clinically relevant models of atrial reentry, suggest that in therapeutically relevant concentrations the Class III drugs may be more effective than the Class Ia or Ic drugs in termination and suppression of atrial tachycardia. Furthermore, these studies suggest that prolongation of refractoriness is critically important to their antiarrhythmic effect. In contrast, depression of conduction velocity may be of lesser importance and may in fact be responsible for some forms of proarrhythmia.

Thus, the use of clinically relevant arrhythmia models to evaluate new antiarrhythmic drugs prior to human testing remains a valid and appropriate method to screen and guide the development of safer and more effective compounds for the treatment of atrial arrhythmias.

References

1. Feld GK: Atrial fibrillation, is there a safe and highly effective pharmacological treatment? *Circulation* 82:2248, 1990.
2. Ruskin J: The cardiac arrhythmia suppression trial (CAST). *N Engl J Med* 321:386, 1989.
3. Coplen SE, Antmann EM, Berlin JA, et al: Efficacy and safety of quinidine therapy for maintenance of sinus rhythm after cardioversion: a meta-analysis of randomized control trials. *Circulation* 82:1106, 1990.
4. Hine LK, Laird N, Hewitt P, et al: Meta-analysis of empirical long-term antiarrhythmic therapy after myocardial infarction. *JAMA* 262:3037, 1989.
5. Allessie MA, Lammers WJEP, Rensma PL, Bonke FIM: Flutter and fibrillation in experimental models: what has been learned that can be applied to humans? In: P Brugada, HJJ Wellens (eds): *Cardiac Arrhythmias: Where To Go From Here?* Mount Kisco, NY: Futura Publishing Company, Inc., 1987, p. 67.

6. Rensma PL, Allessie MA, Lammers WJE, et al: Length of excitation wave and susceptibility to reentrant atrial arrhythmias in normal conscious dogs. *Circ Res* 62:395, 1988.

7. Feld GK, Venkatesh N, Singh BN: Pharmacologic conversion and suppression of experimental canine atrial flutter: differing effects of d-sotalol, quinidine, and lidocaine and significance of changes in refractoriness and conduction. *Circulation* 74:197, 1986.

8. Feld GK, Venkatesh N, Singh BN: Effects of N-acetylprocainamide and recainam in the pharmacologic conversion and suppression of experimental canine atrial flutter: significance of changes in refractoriness and conduction. *J Cardiovasc Pharmacol* 11:573, 1988.

9. Spinelli W, Hoffman BF: Mechanisms of termination of reentrant atrial arrhythmias by class I and class III antiarrhythmic agents. *Circ Res* 65:1565, 1989.

10. Okumura K, Waldo AL: Effects of N-acetylprocainamide on experimental atrial flutter and atrial electrophysiologic properties in conscious dogs with sterile pericarditis: comparison with the effects of quinidine. *J Am Coll Cardiol* 9:1332, 1987.

11. Wu KM, Hoffman BF: Effect of procainamide and N-acetylprocainamide on atrial flutter: studies in vivo and in vitro. *Circulation* 76:1397, 1987.

12. Boyden PA: Effects of pharmacologic agents on induced atrial flutter in dogs with right atrial enlargement. *J Cardiovasc Pharmacol* 8:170, 1986.

13. Allessie MA, Bonke FIM, Schopman FJG: Circus movement in rabbit atrial muscle as a mechanism of tachycardia. *Circ Res* 33:54, 1973.

14. Allessie MA, Bonke FIM, Schopman FJG: Circus movement in rabbit atrial muscle as a mechanism of tachycardia. II. The role of nonuniform recovery of excitability in the occurrence of unidirectional block, as studied with multiple microelectrodes. *Circ Res* 39:168, 1976.

15. Allessie MA, Bonke FIM, Schopman FJG: Circus movement in rabbit atrial muscle as a mechanism of tachycardia. III. The "Leading Circle" concept: a new model of circus movement in cardiac tissue without the involvement of an anatomical obstacle. *Circ Res* 41:9, 1977.

16. Boineau JP, Schuessler RB, Mooney CB, et al: Natural and evoked atrial flutter due to circus movement in dogs. *Am J Cardiol* 45:1167, 1980.

17. Rosenbleuth A, Garcia Ramos J: Studies on flutter and fibrillation. *Am Heart J* 33:677, 1947.

18. Ioue H, Matsuo H, Takayanagi K, et al: Clinical and experimental studies of the effects of atrial extrastimulation and rapid pacing on atrial flutter cycle. *Am J Cardiol* 48:623, 1981.

19. Rytand DA: The circus movement (entrapped circuit wave) hypothesis and atrial flutter. *Ann Intern Med* 65:125, 1966.

20. Feld GK, Shahandeh-Rad F: Activation patterns in experimental canine atrial flutter produced by right atrial crush injury. *J Am Coll Cardiol* 20:441, 1992.

21. Feld GK, Shahandeh-Rad F: Mechanism of double potentials recorded during sustained atrial flutter in the canine right atrial crush-injury model. *Circulation* 86:628, 1992.

22. Page PL, Plumb VJ, Okumura K, et al: A new animal model of atrial flutter. *J Am Coll Cardiol* 8:872, 1986.

23. Shimizu A, Nazaki A, Rudy Y, et al: Multiplexing studies of effects of rapid atrial pacing on the area of slow conduction during atrial flutter in canine pericarditis model. *Circulation* 83:983, 1991.

24. Okumura K, Plumb VJ, Page PL, et al: Atrial activation sequence during atrial flutter in the canine pericarditis model and its effects on the polarity of the flutter wave in the electrocardiogram. *J Am Coll Cardiol* 17:509, 1991.

25. Shimizu A, Nozaki A, Rudy Y, et al: Onset of induced atrial flutter in the canine pericarditis model. *J Am Coll Cardiol* 17:1223, 1991.

26. Schols W, Gough WB, Restive M, et al: Circus movement atrial flutter in the canine sterile pericarditis model: activation patterns during initiation, termination and sustained re-entry in vivo. *Circ Res* 67:35, 1990.

27. Boyden PA: Effects of pharmacologic agents on induced atrial flutter in dogs with right atrial enlargement. *J Cardiovasc Pharmacol* 8:170, 1986.

28. Schols W, Gough W, Yang H, et al: Circus movement atrial flutter in the right atrial enlargement model: correlation of activation and refractory maps (abstract). *PACE* 14:II-627, 1991.

29. Frame LH, Page RL, Hoffman BG: Atrial re-entry around an anatomical barrier with a partially excitable gap: a canine model of atrial flutter. *Circ Res* 58:495, 1986.

30. Waldo AL, Wells JL, Plumb VJ, et al: Studies of atrial flutter following open heart surgery. *Ann Rev Med* 30:259, 1979.

31. Klein GJ, Guiraudon GM, Sharma AD, et al: Demonstration of macroreentry and feasibility of operative therapy in the common type of atrial flutter. *Am J Cardiol* 57:587, 1986.

32. Disertori M, Inama G, Vergara G, et al: Evidence of a reentry circuit in the common type of atrial flutter in man. *Circulation* 67:434, 1983.

33. Olshansky B, Okumura K, Hess PG, et al: Demonstration of an area of slow conduction in human atrial flutter. *J Am Coll Cardiol* 16:1639, 1990.

34. Olshansky B, Okumura K, Henthorn RW, et al: Characterization of double potentials in human atrial flutter: studies during transient entrainment. *J Am Coll Cardiol* 15:833, 1990.

35. Wang Z, Pelletier C, Talajic M, Nattel S: Effects of flecainide and quinidine on human atrial ac-tion potentials. Role of rate-dependence and comparison with guinea pig, rabbit, and dog tissues. *Circulation* 82:274, 1990.

36. Feld GK, Chen PS, Nicod P, et al: Possible atrial proarrhythmic effects of encainide and flecai-nide. *Am J Cardiol* 66:378, 1990.

Chapter 21

Mechanisms of Action of Class III Versus Class I Antiarrhythmic Agents on Ventricular Tachycardia in the Infarcted Heart

Peter B. Corr
Jianyi Wu

In patients with previous myocardial infarction, malignant ventricular arrhythmias are the major cause of sudden cardiac death. The electrophysiological mechanisms responsible for the development of these malignant arrhythmias have been evaluated extensively in experimental animals and humans.[1-3] Using three-dimensional mapping in vivo, we and others have shown that the primary mechanism underlying the maintenance of ventricular tachycardia in the days to weeks after infarction was intramural reentry.[4-6] More recently, we used three-dimensional mapping of the human heart in patients undergoing surgical correction for incessant ventricular tachycardia and showed that intramural reentry was the predominant underlying mechanism.[7] However, in the human heart, focal mechanisms without evidence of macroreentry also contribute to the maintenance of ventricular tachycardia.[7] Therefore, both reentrant and possibly nonreentrant or focal mechanisms contribute to the development of malignant arrhythmias in the infarcted human heart.

Based on findings from the Cardiac Arrhythmia Suppression Trial (CAST), it is clear that merely decreasing the incidence of premature ventricular complexes is not synonymous with decreasing the incidence of lethal arrhythmias leading to sudden cardiac death.[8] Indeed, the results of CAST clearly demonstrate that Class Ic agents encainide or flecainide, which slow conduction velocity markedly due to inhibition of the rapid inward Na^+ current (I_{Na}), actually increase the incidence of sudden cardiac death in patients with a previous myocardial infarction. Although the precise reasons for the detrimental effects of these agents are unknown, the negative ino-

Research from the authors' laboratory was supported in part by the National Institutes of Health grants HL-17646, SCOR in Ischemic Heart Disease, and HL-28995. Support was also through a postdoctoral fellowship grant (Dr. Wu) from the American Heart Association Missouri Affiliate.
From BN Singh, HJJ Wellens, M Hiraoka, (eds): *Electropharmacological Control of Cardiac Arrhythmias*. Mount Kisco, NY, Futura Publishing Company Inc., © 1994.

tropic effect and heterogeneous reduction in conduction velocity appear to be the most important factors.[9,10] At first glance, the results of CAST would suggest that Class Ic agents induced a simple proarrhythmic response in patients with a previous myocardial infarction. However, the fact that the increased death rate in patients treated with encainide or flecainide was constant over the first year[8] suggests an additional trigger was the lethal event in the presence but not in the absence of the drug.[11] Based on recent analysis of the CAST data, it appears that the fatal trigger may have been an acute ischemic event in the presence of a previous myocardial infarction.[12] This conclusion is supported by the fact that patients who were given placebos exhibited more angina and nonfatal myocardial infarctions, whereas the patients treated in CAST exhibited a marked increase in arrhythmic deaths, suggesting that the treated patients had a fatal myocardial infarction.[12] This is also supported by the fact that patients with non-Q wave infarcts were nine times more likely to die while being given encainide or flecainide compared to a placebo. As pointed out by Roden,[11] blockade of Na^+ channels with agents with very slow off-time dissociation kinetics such as flecainide and encainide has been shown to facilitate the development of ventricular fibrillation in the presence of acute ischemia in experimental animals. This arrhythmogenic effect may be due to the fact that Na^+ channel blocking agents would bind more readily to depolarized cells, enhancing the degree of regional conduction delay and thereby facilitating the development of reentrant arrhythmias.[11] Thus, in hindsight, the results of CAST are not particularly surprising, but their implications are that newer, more specific agents will be required to decrease the incidence of sudden cardiac death in patients with coronary artery disease.

The interruption or prevention of a reentrant circuit involves increasing the reentrant wavelength (λ), where $\lambda(M) =$ conduction velocity (M/sec) · refractory period (sec). Therefore, increasing either the refractory period or the conduction velocity or both, if of a sufficient magnitude, would theoretically interrupt any reentrant circuit. Although agents are available that can increase the refractory period, there are no consistent approaches to enhance or increase conduction velocity. The approach then has been to depress conduction velocity selectively in the hope of maintaining conduction in normal regions and extinguishing conduction in abnormal regions, and thereby preventing the maintenance of the reentrant circuit. Therefore, the question is not strictly whether to delay conduction or to prolong refractoriness but must take into account the following key questions:

1. What is the specificity of the response of the agent on conduction velocity versus the refractory period? In other words, can we do one without the other?

2. Is the effect of the agent on conduction velocity or the refractory period heterogenous? In other words, assuming we have a specific effect on the refractory period, is it going to be uniform across a defined region of the atria or ventricle?

3. Is the effect of a given agent different on normal versus abnormal tissue?

4. If the agent inhibits a specific channel, what is the time constant of drug binding and unbinding from the channel?

It is our contention that the failure of antiarrhythmic agents to affect sudden arrhythmic death relates to the answers to these questions. Both clinical and experimental evidence indicates that a nonuniformity between regional conduction velocity and refractory periods is a critical link in the development of reentrant arrhythmias, particularly in the presence of a previous myocardial infarction. This chapter reviews our recent findings related to the specificity of action of Class I versus Class III antiarrhythmic agents not only in normal tissue and cells, but also in diseased hearts in vitro and in vivo.

Can Class III Agents Result in a Selective Increase in Refractoriness?

By definition of a Class III effect, the answer to the above question should be yes.

However, the currently available Class III agents, amiodarone, bretylium, and racemic sotalol possess other distinct properties that deviate from a pure Class III effect that could either enhance or attenuate their antiarrhythmic efficacy.[13,14] For example, amiodarone has been shown to slow conduction velocity that is particularly prominent at faster heart rates or in depolarized tissue,[15,16] as might occur in the presence of ischemia. The effect of amiodarone to slow conduction velocity appears to be due not only to a depression of I_{Na} but also increasing the passive resistance to current flow,[17] possibly by decreasing gap junctional conductance. In addition, all three agents influence adrenergic neural function either at the presynaptic or postsynaptic level. Amiodarone will noncompetitively inhibit both α- and β-adrenergic receptors that can often preclude its use in certain patients.[18] Sotalol is a potent β-adrenergic blocking agent[19,20] that could contribute to its antiarrhythmic efficacy, but is also known to decrease ventricular function, particularly in patients with low ejection fractions who are at the highest risk for sudden cardiac death. Finally, bretylium can only be used intravenously and produces an initial sympathomimetic effect due to release of catecholamines from sympathetic neurons and subsequently an antiadrenergic effect due to inhibition of catecholamine release from sympathetic neurons in response to neurostimulation.[21] Thus, there is obviously the need for more specific Class III antiarrhythmic agents to test the hypothesis as to whether a specific increase in the refractory period of the atria or ventricle can lead to inhibition of arrhythmias, not only in experimental animals, but in humans.

Dofetilide, previously referred to as UK-68,798, is a new Class III antiarrhythmic agent currently undergoing clinical evaluation. We recently evaluated the ability of dofetilide to inhibit tachyarrhythmias induced by programmed electrical stimulation in dogs with a previous myocardial infarction.[22] Using three-dimensional mapping in vivo, the studies also were performed to assess the mechanisms underlying the genesis of ventricular tachycardia and ventricular fibrillation and to assess whether dofetilide produced an antiarrhythmic effect in the absence of an alteration in conduction velocity in infarct or peri-infarct regions. Although dofetilide did not alter PQ interval or QRS duration, the agent produced a significant increase in the QT (218–256 msec) and QTc (350–400 msec). The data pertaining to the effective refractory period in response to dofetilide are shown in Figure 1. Dofetilide produced a significant increase in the ventricular effective refractory period at a basic cycle length of either 300 or 250 msec with an analogous and similar increase as measured with the S_2 or S_3 stimulus. These results indicate that in the presence of a rapid change in rate or at very short coupling intervals (S_3) the Class III effect of dofetilide appears to be maintained. Thus, negative use dependence, which has been suggested as a major limitation of some Class III agents,[23] may not be prominent with dofetilide.

The results of the antiarrhythmic effect of dofetilide is shown in Figure 2. In animals with 5- to 8-day-old myocardial infarcts (n = 13), 3 animals (23%) developed ventricular fibrillation, 7 animals (54%) developed sustained ventricular tachycardia with a mean cycle length of 171 msec, and 3 animals (23%) were noninducible. Animals in which sustained ventricular tachycardia was induced prior to drug (dofetilide, 30 μg/kg) prevented the induction of sustained ventricular tachycardia in 6 of 7 animals (86%, $p < 0.05$). In the remaining animal, the cycle length of the ventricular tachycardia was increased from 166 to 220 msec. Dofetilide failed to prevent the induction of ventricular fibrillation in all 4 animals in which fibrillation was induced. None of the noninducible animals were affected by dofetilide. Thus, it appears that dofetilide will effectively prevent the induction of sustained ventricular tachycardia in dogs with a previous myocardial infarction, but fails to prevent the electrical induction of ventricular fibrillation.

The results using three-dimensional mapping in the presence and absence of dofetilide indicate that the agent did not affect conduction velocity in normal, peri-infarct, or infarct regions in the same hearts in which there was a marked increase in the ventricular effective refractory period (Figure 3). Thus, this agent appears to produce a specific increase in refractoriness without altering conduction velocity even in abnormal tissue. In this particular study,[22] the induction of ventricular fibrillation by programmed electrical stimulation occurred secondary to a rapid nonreentrant or focal mechanism in hearts in which the infarct size was substantially smaller than in the hearts of animals who exhibited sustained ventricular tachycardia. The failure of dofetilide to inhibit the induced ventricular fibrillation was secondary to the fact that the drug did not affect this focal or nonreentrant mechanism.[22] Other investigators also have demonstrated that the induction of ventricular fibrillation by programmed electrical stimulation is more likely to occur in animals with small infarcts, whereas sustained monomorphic ventricular tachycardia occurs in the presence of larger transmural infarcts.[24,25]

The induction of ventricular tachycardia in response to premature electrical stimuli occurs secondary to further slowing in conduction velocity as the premature impulse impinges on the relative refractory period. This leads to the development of the reentrant circuit, either confined to the epicardium overlying the infarct or involving the epicardium and endocardium leading to intramural reentry.[4,5] It is interesting to note that the prevention of ventricular tachycardia by dofetilide was due to the marked prolongation of the effective refractory period in the peri-infarct region in the absence of any change in conduction delay.[22] The drug-induced prolongation of the effective refractory period did not permit the slowly propagating wave front of excitation in the peri-infarct region (epicardial border zone) to reactivate the proximal region. Thus, it appears that dofetilide, and possibly other Class III antiarrhythmic agents, can produce a much more specific response and thereby effectively interrupt reentrant tachycardias without concomitant decreases in conduction velocity.

It is well known that ventricular fibrilla-

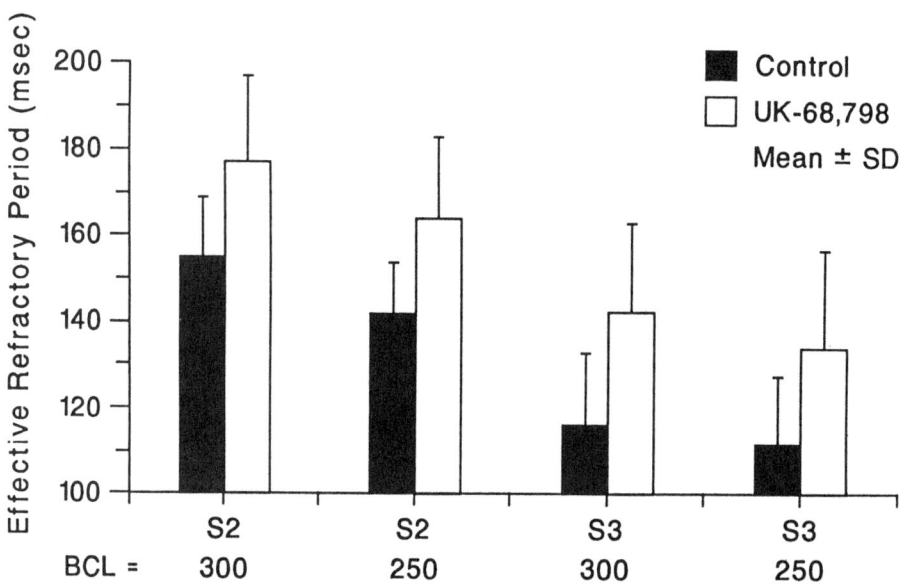

Figure 1. Influence of UK-68,798 (dofetilide) on the ventricular ERP during programmed electrical stimulation from the right ventricle for the first (S_2) and the second (S_3) premature stimulus at the basic cycle length (BCL) of either 300 msec or 250 msec. N = 16 for S_2; N = 6 for S_3. (Reproduced with permission from Reference 22.)

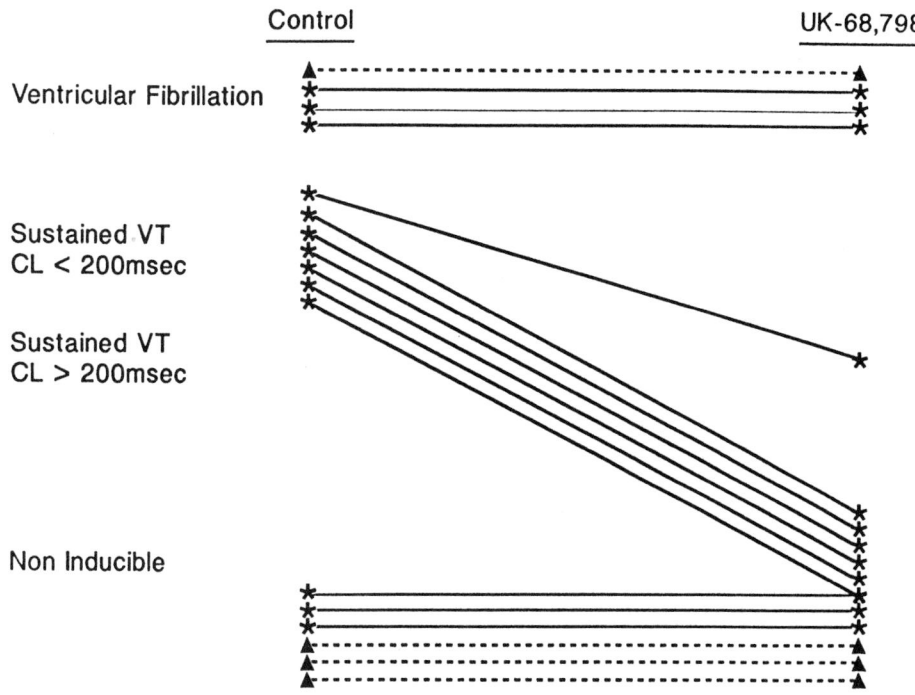

Figure 2. Influence of UK-68,798 (dofetilide) on arrhythmias induced by programmed electrical stimulation in individual dogs with a 5- to 8-day-old myocardial infarction (*—*) or with a 1- to 3-month-old myocardial infarction (▲---▲). CL: cycle length of the VT. (Reproduced with permission from Reference 22.)

tion can be induced by programmed electrical stimulation even in normal hearts,[26,27] suggesting the nonspecificity of the response and indicating that simply because a drug does not prevent induction of ventricular fibrillation by electrical stimuli, it cannot be inferred that the drug would be ineffective in preventing spontaneous induced ventricular fibrillation, for example in the ischemic heart. Indeed, dofetilide has been shown, albeit at very high doses (900 μg/kg, intravenously), to inhibit the induction of ventricular fibrillation in response to acute ischemia in animals with a previous myocardial infarction.[28]

Influence of Class I Versus Class III Antiarrhythmic Agents on Microscopic Propagation

As summarized, one specific Class III antiarrhythmic agent, dofetilide, appeared to

increase the refractory period specifically without altering conduction velocity. However, it is possible that an agent such as dofetilide could alter microscopic conduction that would not be detected by three-dimensional mapping in vivo despite simultaneously recording from 240 sites. These limitations were overcome by increasing the resolution of mapping to assess directly the effects of selective Class III agents compared to Class I antiarrhythmic agents.[29] We used a high-density recording grid that has been described in detail previously.[30] This grid electrode permits simultaneous recording from 224 electrode sites with an interelectrode distance of 350 μm.[30] Studies were performed using a structurally similar derivative of dofetilide, UK-66,914 or d-sotalol as the Class III antiarrhythmic agent, compared to the Class I agent procainamide. The concentration of each agent used was that which increased the effective

A Areas with Rapid Conduction Velocity

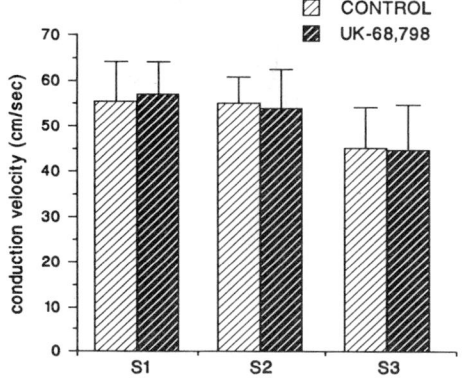

B Areas with Slow Conduction Velocity

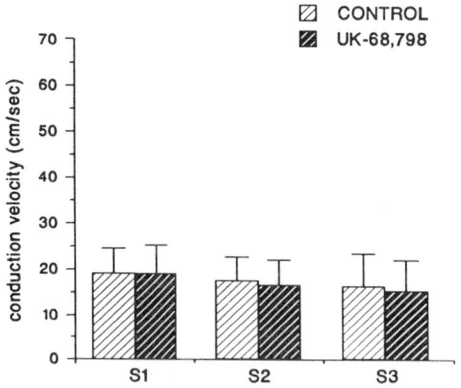

Figure 3. Comparison of the effects of UK-68,798 (dofetilide) on the conduction velocities in regions with normal or rapid conduction (A) or slow conduction (B). Values are expressed as mean ± SD during stimulation at a basic cycle length of 250 msec (S_1) or with premature stimulation (S_2 and S_3). (Reproduced with permission from Reference 22.)

refractory period in vitro in isolated endocardial tissue by 40 msec and for UK-66,914 was 6×10^{-7}M, for sotalol was 1.6×10^{-4}M and for procainamide was 5.5×10^{-4}M. Detailed mapping studies were then performed in subendocardial regions of the dog left ventricle adjacent to infarcts induced 14 to 21 days previously.[29] The isochronal activation maps obtained using this grid recording at a basic cycle length of stimulation of 500 msec in the control state and after treatment with UK-66,914 are shown in Figure 4. Although areas of conduction block and conduction slowing are apparent in the control state prior to UK-66,914, the Class III agent did not alter microscopic conduction velocity nor the extent of conduction block indicated by the darkened regions despite a 40-msec increase in the effective refractory period. Similarly, d-sotalol (1.6×10^{-4}M) failed to alter conduction velocity in normal or peri-infarct regions despite using concentrations achieved clinically.[31] In contrast, the response to procainamide was quite different (Figure 5). In the control state prior to procainamide, activation proceeded rapidly across the grid in a direction perpendicular to fiber orientation with only one area of inexcitability in the lower left-hand corner as indicated by the blackened region. After procainamide, at a concentration sufficient to increase the effective refractory period by 40 msec, there was a marked increase in the extent of conduction delay and block with regions of very slow conduction (1.7 cm/sec). Likewise, regions that were inexcitable prior to the drug demonstrated slowed propagation after treatment. The summarized data of the effect of UK-66,914 and procainamide on conduction velocity are shown in Figure 6. These findings demonstrate that UK-66,914 did not alter conduction velocity in normal or peri-infarct regions at a cycle length of 500 msec or in the presence of a premature stimulus (ie, 350 msec), despite a marked 40-msec increase in the effective refractory period. In contrast, procainamide produced a marked decrease in conduction velocity in regions exhibiting either a normal or very slow conduction velocity and could markedly enhance the extent of conduction block. This extensive conduction delay and block in the presence of procainamide occurred at concentrations achieved clinically.[32,33] The fact that conduction velocity was decreased by a greater percentage in regions exhibiting more rapid conduction velocity prior to the drug agrees with findings by others that this agent decreases conduction velocity to a greater extent in the

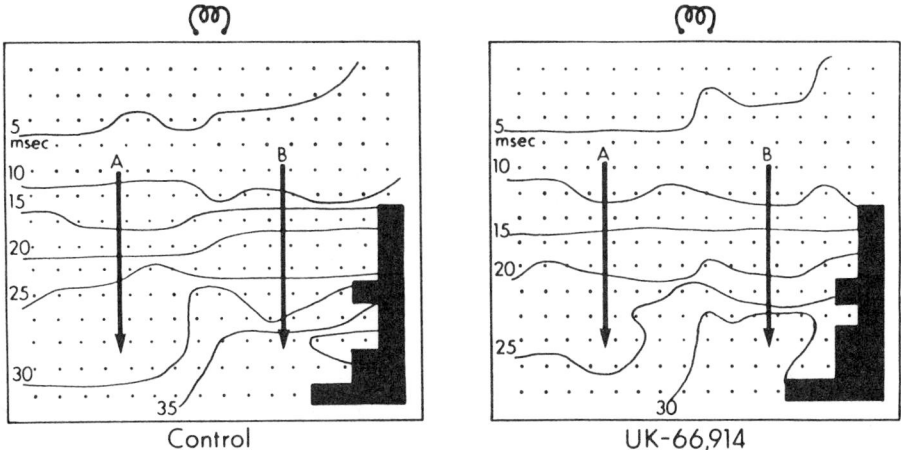

Figure 4. Isochronic activation sequence of the fourth S_1 (BCL = 500 msec) from the endocardial infarct border zone obtained from dogs with a 2-week-old myocardial infarction before and after treatment with UK-66,914 (6×10^{-7}M). The stimulation site is indicated by the symbol (♈). Each individual recording site is indicated by a dot. Areas of block are indicated by regions shaded black or thickened black lines. The direction of activation is indicated by the arrows. (Reproduced with permission from Reference 29.)

direction longitudinal to fiber orientation.[34] Finally, the fact that procainamide could elicit an increase in excitability in peri-infarct regions that were inexcitable prior to the drug further attests to the nonspecific and potential proarrhythmic effects of such a Class I agent.

This finding is in agreement with the suggestion by Colatsky and colleagues[35] that Class I antiarrhythmic agents that prolong refractoriness by delaying the recovery of Na^+ channels "carry some intrinsic potential for arrhythmia aggregation because they can introduce non-

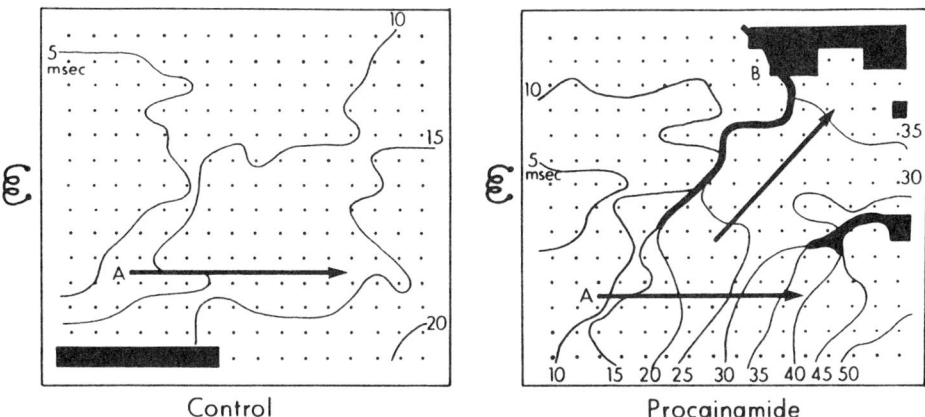

Figure 5. Isochronic activation maps of the fourth S_1 (BCL = 500 msec) before and after treatment with procainamide (5.5×10^{-4}M). Arrows indicate the direction of activation. B is the new site of functional conduction block. The stimulation site is indicated by the symbol (♈). Each individual recording site is indicated by a dot. Areas of block are indicated by regions shaded black or thickened black lines. The direction of activation is indicated by the arrows. (Reproduced with permission from Reference 29.)

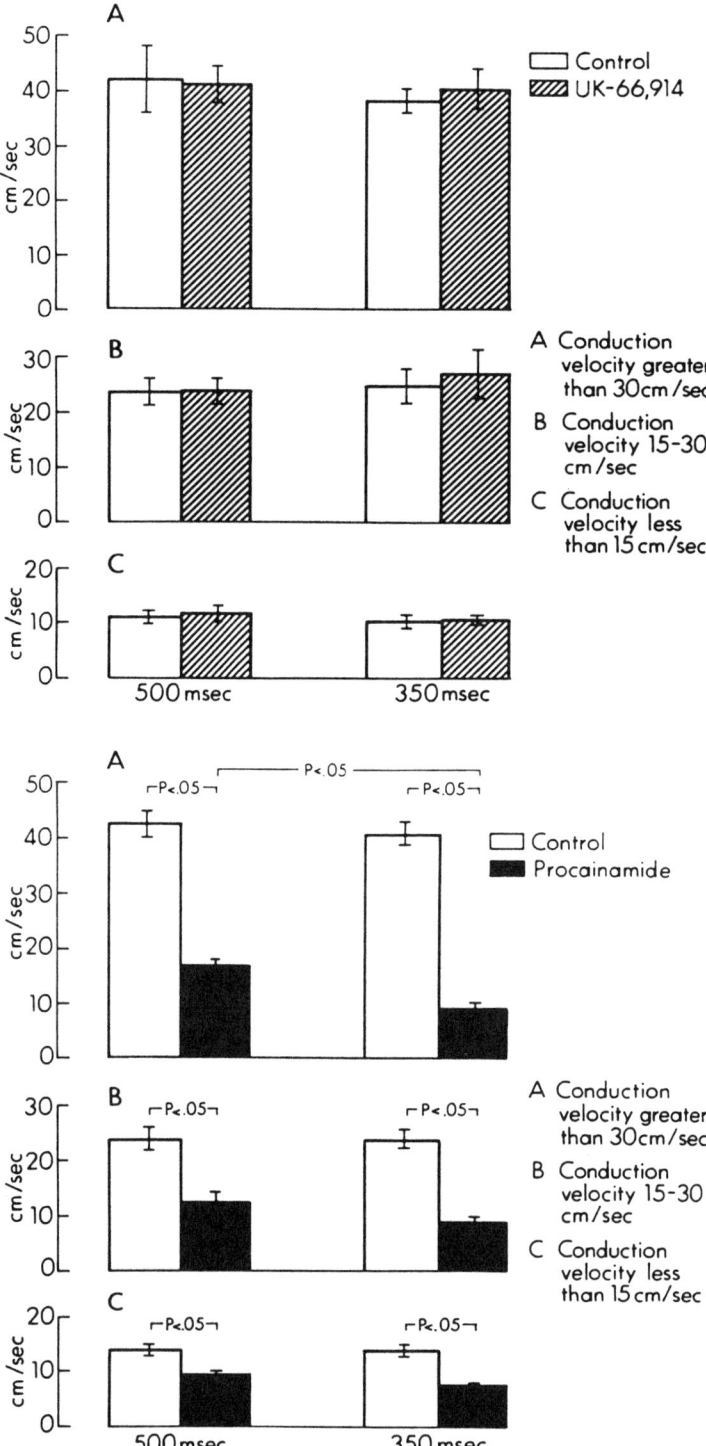

Figure 6. Mean apparent conduction velocity ($\pm$ SEM) for S_1 (BCL = 500 msec) and S_2 (CL = 350 msec) before and after treatment with UK-66,914 (left) and procainamide (right) for three levels of conduction velocity. A: conduction velocity > 30 cm/sec; B: conduction velocity = 15–30 cm/sec; C: conduction velocity < 15 cm/sec. (Reproduced with permission from Reference 29.)

uniformities" and increase the "window" over which slowed conduction and block can occur. It appears that the enhanced specificity of the newer Class III antiarrhythmic agents actually does lead to improved clinical efficacy against sustained ventricular tachycardia when compared to Class I agents such as procainamide.[36,37] This potential increased efficacy of Class III agents may occur with or without a concomitant increase in proarrhythmic potential. Obviously, if the more specific Class III agents are given to patients who already have prolonged QT intervals (ie, QTc > 440 msec) and/or hypokalemia, then the occurrence of drug-induced arrhythmias, including torsades de pointes ventricular tachycardia, will be increased. As new more specific ionic channel blocking agents are developed, it is likely that the specificity will be even greater, that the consistency of response at different heart rates will be achieved, and that the efficacy for prevention of life-threatening arrhythmias will improve. Even combination therapies such as an agent that blocks the delayed rectifier (I_K) and a β-adrenergic blocking agent to prevent sympathetic mediated attenuation of the block of I_K as shown recently[38] may be one approach. The specific blockade of the cyclic AMP-induced Cl^- current to prevent the rapid shortening of repolarization, for example during ischemia, may be another approach.[39] This I_{Cl} may mediate the extremely short cycle lengths[39] that we recently have shown occurs just prior to the transition from ventricular tachycardia to ventricular fibrillation in response to ischemia in vivo.[40]

Are There Real Differences Between the Newer Class III Antiarrhythmic Agents?

As summarized, the data would suggest that new Class III agents such as sotalol or dofetilide have fairly similar degrees of selectivity. However, because of the diversity of K^+ channels and multiple mechanisms controlling cardiac repolarization, it is likely that

these could have markedly different effects under varying conditions. There are at least six different ionic currents involved in cardiac repolarization including[41-46]: (1) the noninactivating sodium window current occurring during the plateau phase of the action potential; (2) the electrogenic Na^+/Ca^{2+} exchange current; (3) the decay of the L-type calcium current; (4) the activation of I_K; (5) the outward component of I_{K1}; and (6) the activation of the transient outward current (I_{to}). The problem relates to the fact that the net contribution of each current to repolarization and therefore the effect of blocking or attenuating a specific current will vary depending on species, as well as the area or region of myocardium evaluated.[35,42,43,46] Most data would suggest that the major current responsible for repolarization would be the delayed rectifier I_K and that the outward component of I_{K1} would contribute modestly to repolarization, but its major influence would be maintenance of the resting membrane potential. Because I_{K1} is the major background current, it is responsible for the passive input resistance. Previous results with d-sotalol are controversial and indicate that in addition to blocking I_K, this agent either does not alter or decrease I_{K1}.[13,47-49] Therefore, we recently evaluated the effects of dofetilide and d-sotalol on I_K and I_{K1} in guinea pig ventricular myocytes using whole-cell voltage-clamp procedures ($[K^+]_o$ = 5.4 mM; $[K^+]_i$ = 150 mM. I_K was activated positive to -30 mV ($V_{1/2}$ activation = 17.2 ± 0.53 mV, n = 8) and the tail current density for I_K at -40 mV was 4.0 ± 0.5 pA/pF. Dofetilide inhibited the I_{K-tail} current in a dose-dependent manner (maximal inhibition = 48% and IC_{50} = 1.92 μM). Dofetilide (10 μM) decreased the I_{K-tail} current by 42.9 ± 2.8%, but d-sotalol at the same concentration (10 μM) was far less potent and decreased the I_{K-tail} by only 17.6 ± 3.7%. Dofetilide (10 μM) significantly delayed the time of activation of I_K from 24.4 ± 0.8 to 32.1 ± 1.5 msec ($p < 0.05$) and increased the time constants of the tail current inactivation at -40 mV based on a 2 exponential fit, from τ_1 of 131.5 to 177.5 msec and τ_2 of 378.3 to 841.2 msec ($p < 0.05$), but had no effect on the voltage dependence of steady-state activation or the time constants of activation. The decrease in the I_K tail current by dofetilide was more effective ($p < 0.01$) at 250-msec depolarization steps ($53.9 \pm 1.1\%$; n = 6) than that at 2,000 msec ($43.7 \pm 2.3\%$; n = 6) indicating a potential reverse use dependence. In contrast, an equipotent dose of d-sotalol (100 μM) decreased I_K by $34.8 \pm 4.0\%$ and $36.8 \pm 5.7\%$ at voltage-clamp pulse durations of either 250 msec and 2,000 msec (n = 5), respectively, indicating a lack of use dependence. Interestingly, d-sotalol had no effects on the kinetics of activation or inactivation of I_K. d-Sotalol (100 μm) reduced the steady-state current of I_{K1} at -130 mV by $46.0 \pm 8.4\%$ with an increase in membrane resistance (R_{in}) of $62.1 \pm 12.8\%$. In contrast, an equipotent concentration of dofetilide (10 μM) produced only a small change in I_{K1} ($14.8 \pm 6.1\%$) with no change in R_{in}. Therefore, despite the close structural similarities between dofetilide and d-sotalol, dofetilide appears to be more specific than d-sotalol for blockade of I_K versus I_{K1}. Thus, dofetilide may be expected to possess a potent and specific Class III antiarrhythmic action because of its selective inhibition of I_K. In contrast, the proarrhythmic effect of d-sotalol may be enhanced by the increase of R_i leading to a larger voltage change in response to a given inward current, such as the transient inward current (I_{ti}). However, the increase in R_{in} might also be antiarrhythmic by increasing the length or space constant of the tissue permitting more effective transfer of current from cell to cell and facilitating conduction.[35] Therefore, despite differences in these two agents and in other new or old Class III antiarrhythmics, it is uncertain whether these or other differences could improve the antiarrhythmic efficacy and, at the same time, decrease the proarrhythmic potential.

Conclusion

The new Class III antiarrhythmic agents currently under development are likely to provide improved efficacy for the prevention and treatment of malignant ventricular arrhythmias, including sudden cardiac death. Since these agents appear to possess extensive differences relative to selectivity and specificity, it will be imperative that mechanistic comparative studies are performed with different agents, not only in isolated cells and tissue, but in diseased hearts of experimental animals, and ultimately in humans. It is clear that reentrant circuits underlie arrhythmogenesis in most forms of atrial arrhythmias in humans including paroxysmal atrial tachycardias due to atrioventricular node reentry or accessory bypass tracts and atrial fibrillation, all of which should be highly amenable to treatment with the new Class III antiarrhythmic agents. In contrast, malignant ventricular arrhythmias associated with early myocardial ischemia or more chronic arrhythmias in the presence of a previous myocardial infarction appear to be due not only to reentry, but also nonreentrant or focal mechanisms. The effectiveness of the newer Class III agents in this patient population with ischemic heart disease will require very careful evaluation, particularly since these nonreentrant or focal mechanisms are likely to be unresponsive to an agent that only increases the ventricular refractory period. The future is likely to involve combination therapy directed towards reentrant as well as nonreentrant mechanisms, including triggered rhythms. This combination approach might also decrease or abolish the potential proarrhythmic effects of some of the newer Class III agents, particularly those associated with early or delayed afterdepolarizations leading to triggered rhythms.

References

1. Janse MJ, Wit AL: Electrophysiological mechanisms of ventricular arrhythmias resulting from myocardial ischemia and infarction. *Physiol Rev* 69:1049, 1989.
2. Pogwizd SM, Corr PB: Electrophysiologic and biochemical mechanisms underlying malignant ventricular arrhythmias during early myocardial ischemia. In: G Heusch (ed): *Pathophys-*

iology and Rational Pharmacotherapy of Myocardial Ischemia. Darmstadt: Steinkopff, 1990, p. 137.

3. Gettes LS, Cascio WE: Effect of acute ischemia on cardiac electrophysiology. In: HA Fozzard, RB Jennings, E Haber, et al. (eds): *The Heart and Cardiovascular System: Scientific Foundations.* New York, NY: Raven Press, 1991, p. 2021.

4. Kramer JB, Saffitz JE, Witkowski FX, et al: Intramural reentry as a mechanism of ventricular tachycardia during evolving canine myocardial infarction. *Circ Res* 56:736, 1985.

5. Garan H, Fallon JT, Rosenthal S, et al: Endocardial, intramural, and epicardial activation patterns during sustained monomorphic ventricular tachycardia in late canine myocardial infarction. *Circ Res* 60:879, 1987.

6. Gough WB, Mehra R, Restivo M, et al: Reentrant ventricular arrhythmias in the late myocardial infarction period in the dog. *Circ Res* 57:432, 1985.

7. Pogwizd SM, Hoyt RH, Saffitz JE, et al: Reentrant and focal mechanisms underlie sustained ventricular tachycardia in humans. *Circulation* 82(Suppl III):III-587, 1990.

8. CAST Investigators: Preliminary report: effect of encainide and flecainide on mortality in a randomized trial of arrhythmia suppression after myocardial infarction. *N Engl J Med* 321:406, 1989.

9. Rosen MR, Wit AL: Arrhythmogenic actions of antiarrhythmic drugs. *Am J Cardiol* 59:10E, 1987.

10. Gottlieb SS: The use of antiarrhythmic agents in heart failure: implications of CAST. *Am Heart J* 118:1074, 1989.

11. Roden DM: CAST: implications for the use of antiarrhythmic agents in the setting of ischemic heart disease. *Coronary Artery Dis* 2:723, 1991.

12. Echt DS, Liebson PR, Mitchell B, et al: Mortality and morbidity in patients receiving encainide, flecainide, or placebo: the Cardiac Arrhythmia Suppression Trial. *N Engl J Med* 324:781, 1991.

13. Carmeliet E: Electrophysiologic and voltage clamp analysis of the effects of sotalol on isolated cardiac muscle and Purkinje fibers. *J Pharmacol Exp Ther* 232:817, 1985.

14. Cobbe SM: Modification of class III antiarrhythmic activity in abnormal myocardium (editorial). *Cardiovasc Res* 22:847, 1988.

15. Mason JW, Hondeghem LM, Katzung BG: Block of inactivated sodium channels of depolarization-induced automaticity in guinea pig papillary muscle by amiodarone. *Circ Res* 55:277, 1984.

16. Anderson KP, Walker R, Dustman T, et al: Rate-related electrophysiologic effects of long-term administration of amiodarone on canine ventricular myocardium in vivo. *Circulation* 79:948, 1989.

17. Levine J, Moore N, Kadish AH, et al: Mechanisms of depressed conduction from long term amiodarone therapy in canine myocardium. *Circulation* 78:684, 1988.

18. Bexton RS, Camm AJ: Drugs with a class III antiarrhythmic action. *Pharmacol Ther* 17:315, 1982.

19. Nattel S, Feder-Elituv R, Matthews C, et al: Concentration dependence of class III and beta-adrenergic blocking effects of sotalol in anesthetized dogs. *J Am Coll Cardiol* 13:1190, 1989.

20. Lish PM, Shelanski MV, LaBudde JA, et al: Inhibition of cardiac chronotropic action of isoproterenol by sotalol (MJ 1999) in rat, dog and man. *Curr Ther Res* 9:311, 1967.

21. Boura ALA, Green AF: The actions of bretylium: adrenergic neurone blocking and other effects. *Br J Pharmacol* 14:536, 1959.

22. Zuanetti G, Corr PB: Antiarrhythmic efficacy of a new class III agent, UK-68,798, during chronic myocardial infarction: evaluation using three-dimensional mapping. *J Pharmacol Exp Ther* 256:325, 1991.

23. Hondeghem LM, Snyders DJ: Class III antiarrhythmic agents have a lot of potential but a long way to go: reduced effectiveness and dangers of reverse use dependence. *Circulation* 81:686, 1990.

24. Steinberg JS, Bigger JT, Damm CJ: Predictors of ventricular tachycardia after experimental myocardial infarction: use of signal averaged ECG and infarct size. *Circulation* 80(Suppl II):II-36, 1989.

25. Denniss RA, Richards DA, Waywood JA, et al: Electrophysiological and anatomic differences between canine hearts with inducible ventricular tachycardia and fibrillation associated with chronic myocardial infarction. *Circ Res* 64:155, 1989.

26. Echt DS, Griffin JC, Ford AJ, et al: Nature of inducible ventricular tachyarrhythmias in a canine chronic myocardial infarction model. *Am J Cardiol* 52:1127, 1983.

27. Hamer AW, Karagueuzian HS, Sugi K, et al: Factors related to the induction of ventricular fibrillation in the normal canine heart by programmed electrical stimulation. *J Am Coll Cardiol* 3:751, 1984.

28. Black SC, Chi L, Mu D-X, et al: The antifibrillatory actions of UK-68,798, a class III antiarrhythmic agent. *J Pharmacol Exp Ther* 258:416, 1991.

29. Onufer JR, Dalrymple HW, Corr PB: Selective class III antiarrhythmic properties of a novel agent, UK-66,914, during chronic myocardial infarction. *J Cardiovasc Electrophysiol* 2:117, 1991.

30. Cohen ML, Hoyt RH, Saffitz JE, et al: A high density in-vitro extracellular electrode array: description and implementation. *Am J Physiol* 257(Heart Circ Physiol 26):H681, 1989.

31. Nademanee K, Feld G, Hendrickson J, et al: Electrophysiologic and antiarrhythmic effects of sotalol in patients with life-threatening ventricular tachyarrhythmias. *Circulation* 72:555, 1985.

32. Koch-Weser J, Klein SW: Procainamide dosage schedules, plasma concentrations, and clinical effects. *JAMA* 215:1454, 1971.

33. Bigger JT, Hoffman BF: Antiarrhythmic drugs. In: AG Gilman, TW Rall, AS Nies, et al. (eds): *Goodman and Gilman's The Pharmacological Basis of Therapeutics*. New York, NY: Pergamon Press, 1990, p. 840.

34. Kadish AH, Spear JF, Levine JE, et al: The effects of procainamide on conduction in anisotropic canine ventricular myocardium. *Circulation* 74:616, 1986.

35. Colatsky TJ, Follmer CH, Starmer CF: Channel specificity in antiarrhythmic drug action: mechanism of potassium channel block and its role in suppressing and aggravating cardiac arrhythmias. *Circulation* 82:2235, 1990.

36. Lidell C, Rehnquist N, Sjorgen A, et al: Comparative efficacy of oral sotalol and procainamide in patients with chronic ventricular arrhythmias: a multicenter study. *Am Heart J* 109:970, 1985.

37. Jordaens LJ, Colardyn F, Clement DL: A comparison of sotalol and procainamide in symptomatic ventricular tachycardia. *Cardiovasc Drugs Ther* 3:155, 1989.

38. Sanguinetti MC, Jurkiewicz NK, Scott A, et al: Isoproterenol antagonizes prolongation of refractory period by the class III antiarrhythmic agent E-4031 in guinea pig myocytes. *Circ Res* 68:77, 1991.

39. Hume JR, Harvey RD: Chloride conductance pathways in heart. *Am J Physiol* 261(Cell Physiol 30):C399, 1991.

40. Pogwizd SM, Corr PB: Mechanisms underlying the development of ventricular fibrillation during early myocardial ischemia. *Circ Res* 66:672, 1990.

41. Singh BM, Courtney KR: The classification of antiarrhythmic mechanisms of drug action: experimental and clinical considerations. In: DP Zipes, J Jalife (eds): *Cardiac Electrophysiology: From Cell to Bedside*. Philadelphia, PA: WB Saunders, 1990, p. 882.

42. Noble D: The surprising heart: a review of recent progress in cardiac electrophysiology. *J Physiol* 353:1, 1984.

43. Trube G: Potassium currents in isolated adult cardiac myocytes. In: HM Piper, G Isenberg (eds): *Isolated Adult Cardiomyocytes*. Boca Raton, FL: CRC Press, 1989, p. 75.

44. Pennefather P, Cohen IS: Molecular mechanisms of cardiac K$^+$-channel regulation. In: DP Zipes, J Jalife (eds): *Cardiac Electrophysiology: From Cell to Bedside*. Philadelphia, PA: WB Saunders, 1990, p. 17.

45. Tseng G-N, Robinson RB, Hoffman BF: Passive properties and membrane currents of canine ventricular myocytes. *J Gen Physiol* 90:671, 1987.

46. Doerr T, Denger R, Doerr A, et al: Ionic currents contributing to the action potential in single ventricular myocytes of the guinea pig studied with action potential clamp. *Pflügers Arch* 416:230, 1990.

47. Komeichi K, Tohse N, Nakaya H, et al: Effects of N-acetylprocainamide and sotalol on ion currents in isolated guinea-pig ventricular myocytes. *Eur J Pharmacol* 187:313, 1990.

48. Varro A, Nanasi PP, Lathrop DA: Effect of sotalol on transmembrane ionic currents responsible for repolarization in cardiac ventricular myocytes from rabbit and guinea pig. *Life Sci* 49:PL-7, 1991.

49. Berger F, Borchard U, Hafner D: Effects of (+)- and (±)-sotalol on repolarizing outward current and pacemaker current in sheep cardiac Purkinje fibres. *Naunyn-Schmiedeberg's Arch Pharmacol* 340:696, 1989.

Chapter 22

The Efficacy of Antiarrhythmic Drugs as Antifibrillatory Agents

Andrew C.G. Uprichard
Benedict R. Lucchesi

Sudden cardiac death is recognized as a major cause of mortality in the industrialized world. In medical terms, sudden death generally denotes death that is nonviolent, unexpected, witnessed, and instantaneous or occurs within a few minutes of an abrupt change in the previous clinical state.[1] Although there has been a decrease in the number of sudden cardiac deaths over the past 20 years, the number of fatalities in the United States, exceeds 300,000 per year. Of significance is the fact that as many as 60% of the fatal events occur in individuals without any prior history of heart disease.[2] Accounting for 50% of all cardiovascular deaths,[3] the problem of sudden death is compounded by the recent realization that not only has pharmacological management done little to improve the situation, but may in fact have contributed to the onset of the fatal events in susceptible individuals.[4] The dimensions of the problem have made sudden cardiac death one of the United States' most pressing unresolved clinical and public health concerns.

Sudden cardiac death may be considered to involve an interaction between structural derangements of the heart, transient functional disturbances, and the specific electrophysiological events responsible for the fatal arrhythmia.[3] Coronary atherosclerosis and its associated influences on the heart constitutes the major pathological finding in the vast majority of persons who succumb to sudden cardiac death. Patients who have experienced a major cardiovascular event are at high risk of sudden cardiac death during the first 6–18 months after the index event, suggesting a time dependence of risk and indicating the need for appropriate therapy in the early period.[5]

The Clinical Scenario

The role of drug intervention in the prevention of sudden death is based on the premise of there being treatable factors that might be identified in those at risk. One factor, recognized for many years, is the finding of chronic ventricular ectopy in patients after

Published investigations cited from this laboratory were supported by the National Institutes of Health, Heart, Lung and Blood Institute, Grant HL-05806-32.

From BN Singh, HJJ Wellens, M Hiraoka, (eds): *Electropharmacological Control of Cardiac Arrhythmias.* Mount Kisco, NY, Futura Publishing Company Inc., © 1994.

myocardial infarction.[6-11] The assumption was made that premature ventricular complexes (PVCs) appearing in the vulnerable phase of myocardial repolarization were responsible for the initiation of malignant arrhythmias in these individuals. Therefore, it seemed entirely appropriate that an agent capable of suppressing PVCs would be effective in preventing sudden death. Indeed, early studies with lidocaine, an effective agent in suppressing ectopy,[12] suggested that its use might be associated with a decreased incidence of ventricular fibrillation.[13] After this, however, there appeared a number of reports using several agents that failed to substantiate this claim, and when reviewed in early meta-analyses, appeared to suggest an adverse trend.[14,15] Nevertheless, the analyses were not without criticism for dissimilarities in study designs and populations, so it was not until the advent of the Cardiac Arrhythmia Suppression Trial (CAST) that the prescribing public was given a clear picture of the issue. CAST was designed specifically to address the question of whether PVC suppression was an appropriate surrogate for mortality in the postmyocardial infarction population. Encainide, flecainide, and moricizine were identified in the Cardiac Arrhythmia Pilot Study (CAPS)[16] as PVC killers and were considered to be the agents of choice for CAST. Despite ironic concern over the ethics of a placebo arm, it was included in the major multicenter study that used an elegant dose titration in a double-blind manner. Preliminary (CAST I) and final (CAST II) results from this study provided the definitive answer that the use of all three agents was associated with significant increases in arrhythmic deaths.[17,18] Furthermore, the adverse trends were apparent in all identified subgroups and, in view of the diverging curves, were felt to be ongoing throughout the trial.

An alternative clinical model for the testing of antiarrhythmic drugs is the unmasking of malignant reentrant arrhythmias by electrophysiological testing. An appropriately timed stimulus, delivered via an indwelling cardiac catheter, can induce ventricular tachyarrhythmias in patients at risk of life-threatening disturbances in cardiac rhythm.[19] Furthermore, the same arrhythmias may be prevented by the use of individualized drug therapy.[20,21] The induction of sustained ventricular arrhythmia is considered an objective endpoint by which to evaluate candidates for antiarrhythmic drug therapy. The rate at which inducible ventricular arrhythmias are suppressed during serial antiarrhythmic drug testing in survivors of sudden cardiac death ranges from 20% to 50%.[20,23,24] However, even when ventricular fibrillation is induced by programmed electrical stimulation in the electrophysiology laboratory, one cannot be sure that the substrate of the arrhythmia thus generated is identical to that pertaining at the time of sudden death, or that pharmacological prevention of stimulus-induced ventricular fibrillation reflects protection against sudden death. The question remains, therefore, of whether it is the fact that a patient's arrhythmia can be suppressed that is important, or if it is due to the associated drug therapy. In other words, is suppressibility per se associated with a good prognosis? To answer this would require a placebo controlled trial in which patients with suppressible arrhythmias were compared with patients whose arrhythmias could not be prevented, but before embarking on this we must first be assured that electrophysiological testing is an appropriate surrogate for mortality. The only study to date that addresses this question is the National Institutes of Health sponsored Electrophysiology Study Versus Electrocardiographic Monitoring (ESVEM) trial.[24] ESVEM uses mortality in determining the relative usefulness of electrophysiological testing and Holter monitoring in assessing several antiarrhythmics, including quinidine, procainamide, mexiletine, propafenone, sotalol and pirmenol, a Class Ia agent no longer being developed. An imipramine limb was removed shortly after the trial was initiated. Until this trial reports in 1993, electrophysiological testing cannot be recommended for routine use.

To summarize the clinical situation, while certain drugs (eg, lidocaine, bretylium, and amiodarone) do have the indication for the prevention of recurrent ventricular fibrillation, no pharmacological intervention has yet been shown to decrease the incidence of sudden cardiac death. Furthermore, there appears to be no relevant surrogate endpoint for the evaluation of potential new therapies. It is imperative, therefore, to devise appropriate animal models for early preclinical testing, based on an understanding of the pathophysiological milieu pertaining at the time of sudden death.

The Substrate and the Insult

Postmortem studies indicate that in the majority of cases, ventricular fibrillation is a primary event and not related to acute myocardial infarction.[25,26] Sudden cardiac death is known to occur most commonly in patients with previous myocardial ischemic injury secondary to advanced coronary artery atherosclerosis.[27–29] Furthermore, the finding in many cases of intracoronary thrombus without acute infarction suggests that ischemia, per se, may be acting as the trigger for the genesis of ventricular fibrillation in a vulnerable, electrically unstable ventricular myocardium. The electrophysiological properties of ischemic myocardium, such as increased excitability, shortening of the ventricular refractory period, slowing of conduction velocity, and increased inhomogeneity in recovery may provide the milieu for the emergence of reentrant rhythms in a heart critically deranged by previous infarction. The concept of ischemia in a region remote from the infarct related artery acting as the trigger for fatal ventricular arrhythmias was addressed by Schuster and Bulkley.[30] In a study of two groups of patients with early postinfarction angina, they found that patients with remote ischemia constituted a group of hemodynamically stable patients who faced an unexpectedly high mortality compared with those patients whose angina arose from the peri-infarcted region. Schwartz and co-workers[31,32] reproduced this phenom-

enon experimentally when they demonstrated a high incidence of ventricular fibrillation in a chronic model of myocardial infarction where additional ischemia was initiated using a hydraulic coronary artery occluder. Also using a canine model, Kabell and co-workers[33] demonstrated a diminution in infarct collateral blood flow with distant ischemia. Since this was preceded by delayed epicardial activity within the area of preexisting infarction, it suggested that ischemia might be influencing the substrate of an infarcted area of myocardium to render it more suitable for the emergence of lethal arrhythmias.

Coronary vasospasm has been considered to be a triggering mechanism for sudden death, especially since patients with atypical angina have demonstrated serious ventricular arrhythmias during episodes of spasm.[34] Although the majority of survivors of cardiac arrest give no previous or subsequent history of atypical angina, in one study sudden death was observed in 17% of 114 patients with coronary vasospasm followed for a mean of 24 months.[35]

Another mechanism to be considered in the genesis of lethal arrhythmias is the role of the autonomic nervous system. Alterations in autonomic tone are well recognized in acute myocardial ischemia and may be inherently arrhythmogenic by nature of the increase in myocardial oxygen consumption and alterations in refractoriness. Inhomogenous adrenergic stimulation has been shown to precipitate arrhythmias in a number of animal models,[36] while others have demonstrated a possible role of the sympathetic nervous system when acute ischemia is produced in the setting of previous myocardial infarction.[31,32,37] Specifically, sympathetic hyperactivity favors the onset of life-threatening cardiac arrhythmias, whereas vagal activation exerts a protective and antifibrillatory effect.[37] Direct neural recording of vagal activity to the heart confirmed that vigorous reflex vagal activation during acute myocardial ischemia is associated with protection from ventricular fibrillation.[38] Other factors contributing to the precipitating trigger in sudden death include

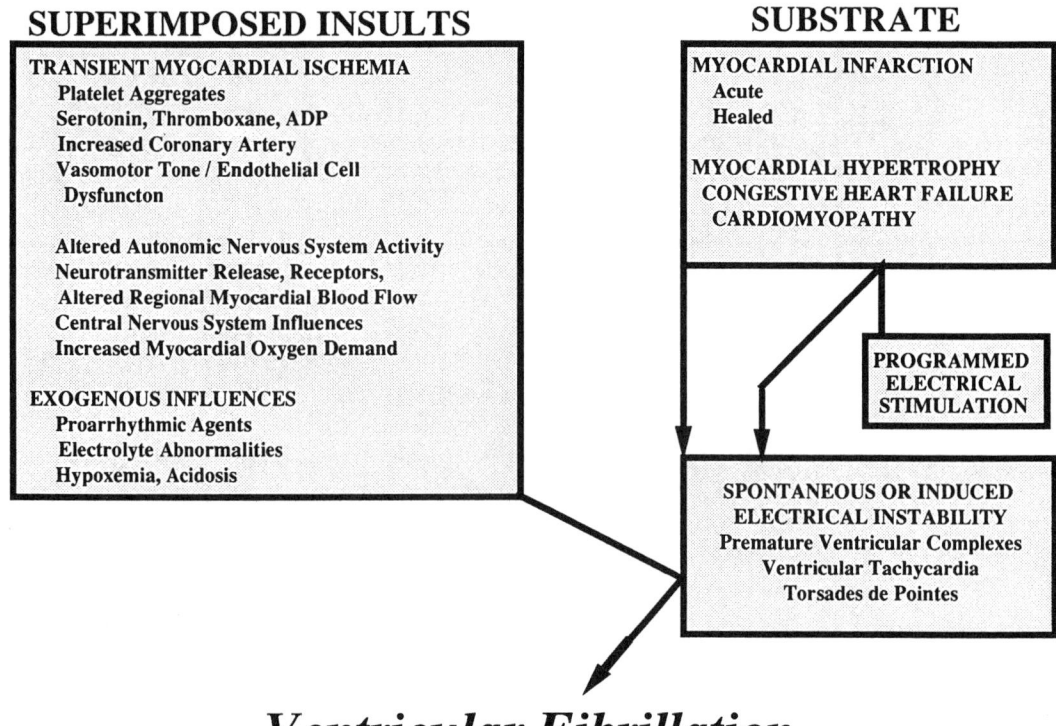

Figure 1. Diagram illustrating the potential "insults" capable of contributing to the emergence of fatal ventricular arrhythmias in a heart critically deranged from previous myocardial infarction. The use of programmed electrical stimulation in the postinfarction period is capable of unmasking the electrical instability that is ultimately responsible for the terminal arrhythmia.

those biochemical alterations (hypokalemia, hypomagnesemia, etc.) that are known to precipitate fatal arrhythmias in individuals at risk. Thus, a variety of factors may predispose the individual at risk to the development of lethal ventricular arrhythmias (Figure 1). Ischemia must be differentiated from infarction. There is a period of healing after myocardial infarction in which the necrotic mass of tissue is converted to a dense, fibrous scar. The healed phase of myocardial infarction is characterized by a chronic alteration in myocardial structure, that in itself, is electrically stable. However, the structural abnormality is capable of influencing electrophysiological parameters when other events are superimposed upon the heart. In contrast, ischemia is a transient event due to an absolute or relative reduction in regional myocardial blood flow.

The influence of ischemia on a structurally normal heart has a more favorable outcome compared to an ischemic event superimposed upon a heart previously subjected to myocardial infarction. There is compelling evidence to indicate that in contrast to a normal heart, regional myocardial ischemia superimposed upon the previously damaged heart is more likely to precipitate malignant and potentially lethal ventricular arrhythmia.[39–41]

Preclinical Models for Antifibrillatory Drug Efficacy

Until recently, whole animal models for the evaluation of antiarrhythmic activity have relied upon arrhythmogenesis by cardiotoxic agents, electrical stimuli, or arrhythmias associated with coronary artery occlusion, with or without reperfusion.[42] More complicated maneuvers include arrhythmias induced by catecholamines[43] or electrical stimuli[44,45] in the subacute phase of myocardial infarction. It is apparent, however, that while each of these techniques is capable of generating reliable and reproducible arrhythmias, they fail to provide an opportunity to examine the electrophysiological environment at the time of ventricular fibrillation, or to study pharmacological interventions aimed at preventing sudden death. Table 1 presents a summary of some of the more commonly used experimental models. The preclinical development of antiarrhythmic agents should emphasize the importance of designing animal models to address ventricular fibrillation, as it may repre-

sent one of the primary rhythm disturbance associated with sudden cardiac death. In light of the CAST results,[17] animal models that evaluate a drug's capacity to reduce the number of innocent ventricular premature depolarizations may be of limited value in new drug development. The ideal drug may be one that is effective against sustained ventricular tachycardia and ventricular fibrillation that occur spontaneously in the presence of previous myocardial injury. There may be a clear distinction between antiarrhythmic efficacy and antifibrillatory potential. It may not follow that the latter is simply an extension of the former.

The ventricular fibrillation threshold (VFT) has been considered to be a reflection of the electrical stability of the whole heart, and therefore a measure of its resistance to fibrillate.[46] Although used for some time as an indicator of antifibrillatory effectiveness, the model has come under criticism for an inability to correlate alterations in fibrillation thresholds with direct electrophysiological actions.[47] Despite procedural modifications such as determinations of VFT under normal and ischemic conditions,[48] it appears that, particularly where trains of current are used, there is a release of local stores of epinephrine. The total release of catecholamines would influence the outcome by lowering the fibrillation threshold.[49] If this is the case, the elevation of fibrillation thresholds seen with the β-adrenoceptor antagonists[50,51] may relate more to antagonism of the effects of stimulus-induced epinephrine release than to any direct antifibrillatory phenomenon.

Table 1
Experimental Methods for Evaluation of Antiarrhythmic Agents

A. Chemically-Induced Arrhythmias
   1. Aconitine
   2. Hydrocarbon-catecholamine
   3. Barium chloride
   4. Digitalis glycosides
   5. Potassium channel openers
B. Electrically-Induced Arrhythmias
   1. Ventricular fibrillation/defibrillation threshold
   2. Repetitive ventricular response
   3. Programmed electrical stimulation
C. Neurally-Induced Arrhythmias
   1. Application of stimuli to the lateral ventricle of the brain
   2. Electrical stimulation of the autonomic nervous system
   3. Emotional- or exercise-induced stress
D. Ischemia-Induced Arrhythmias
   1. Acute interruption of regional coronary artery blood flow (Harris one or two stage)
   2. Acute interruption of regional coronary artery blood flow followed by reperfusion
   3. Acute regional ischemia superimposed on a previously infarcted myocardium

---

The Conscious Canine Model of Ventricular Tachycardia and Sudden Cardiac Death

Our laboratory has described and made extensive use of a conscious canine model that was susceptible to the initiation of stimulus-induced ventricular arrhythmias in the subacute phase of anterior myocardial infarc-

Table 2
Characteristics of the Chronic Canine Model of Sudden Death

Features	Inducible	Noninducible
Anterior infarct size (% left ventricular mass)	24.7 ± 1.7	5.3 ± 1.1*
Time to ischemia (min)	196 ± 39	225 ± 30
Sudden ventricular fibrillation (< 1 hour)	11/15	2/15
Delayed ventricular fibrillation (< 24 hours)	3/15	0/15
Thrombus mass (mg)	7.2 ± 1.81	11.2 ± 2.3
Posterolateral infarct mass	19.0 ± 1.0 (n = 3)	16.7 ± 2.3 (n = 13)

* $p < 0.001$.
Summarized from Reference 53.

tion.[40,42] Of particular interest in this model was the finding that an additional ischemic insult (initiated by a 150 μA anodal current to the left circumflex coronary artery [LCA]) served as a reliable model for the spontaneous onset of ventricular fibrillation. The same study[40] also demonstrated that previous myocardial damage was a prerequisite for the observed high mortality, since dogs without anterior infarctions exhibited a low risk of ventricular fibrillation. A subsequent study[52] evaluated the model further by looking at the relationship between inducible ventricular tachycardia and the subsequent development of ventricular fibrillation. Results suggested that inducible arrhythmias (either sustained or nonsustained) were predictive of spontaneous ventricular fibrillation during posterolateral ischemia. The mass of previously injured myocardium was a critical determinant of both, since animals with inducible arrhythmias (24-hour mortality, 93%) had much larger infarct sizes (24.7 ± 1.7% of left ventricular mass) than the animals that were noninducible at baseline testing (24-hour mortality, 15%; infarct size 5.3 ± 1.1% of left ventricular mass) (Table 2). The use of this model enabled the evaluation of antiarrhythmic activity against arrhythmias thought to share the same reentrant basis as ischemic arrhythmias in humans.[44,53] In addition, the model permits one to discriminate between antiarrhythmic activity as determined with programmed electrical stimulation versus antifibrillatory activity in the postinfarcted heart subjected to an ischemic event in a region remote from the infarct related artery.

Methods

Mongrel dogs of either sex were anesthetized by the intravenous administration of sodium pentobarbital, intubated, and ventilated with room air. Using aseptic techniques, the left jugular vein is isolated and cannulated for subsequent drug administration. A left thoracotomy is performed, and the heart exposed and suspended in a pericardial cradle. The left anterior descending coronary artery (LAD) was dissected free at the tip of the left atrial appendage and the LCX isolated approximately 1 cm from its origin. Anterior wall infarction is achieved by a 2-hour occlusion of the LAD followed by reperfusion in the presence of a critical stenosis. An epicardial bipolar electrode was sutured to the left atrial appendage for subsequent atrial pacing. A bipolar plunge electrode was sutured onto the surface of the heart in the region of the right ventricular outflow tract (RVOT) for the subsequent introduction of extrastimuli during programmed electrical stimulation. In addition, two bipolar plunge electrodes were sutured to the left ventricular wall; one in the distribution of the LAD distal to the site of occlusion (infarct zone [IZ]) and the second in the distribution of the LCX (normal zone [NZ]). Finally, a 30-gauge electrode was inserted into the lumen of the LCX and secured by suturing to the heart wall. Figure 2 is a schematic representation of the instrumented canine heart as used in the model of sudden cardiac death.

Programmed electrical stimulation and electrophysiological testing was performed in the conscious, unsedated animal, 3 to 5 days after surgical preparation. After determination of the RVOT excitation threshold and refractory period, programmed stimulation continues with the introduction of double (S_2, S_3) and triple (S_2, S_3, S_4) extrastimuli (4-msec duration at twice RVOT excitation threshold) during sinus rhythm. Previous studies indicated that these stimulation methods will not induce arrhythmias in sham-operated animals.[40] Electrophysiological parameters from normal and infarcted myocardium were determined from the construction of strength-interval curves using data obtained from the NZ and IZ electrodes, respectively. Dogs with sustained or nonsustained ventricular tachycardia were randomly allocated to drug or vehicle groups, and electrophysiological testing and programmed stimulation are repeated in full after drug equilibration.

Upon completion of the post-treatment stimulation protocol, a direct anodal current of 150 μA was applied to the intimal surface of the LCX using a 9-V nickel-cadmium battery and variable resistor. Application of an anodal current to the intimal surface of the vessel results in injury and exposure of the underlying

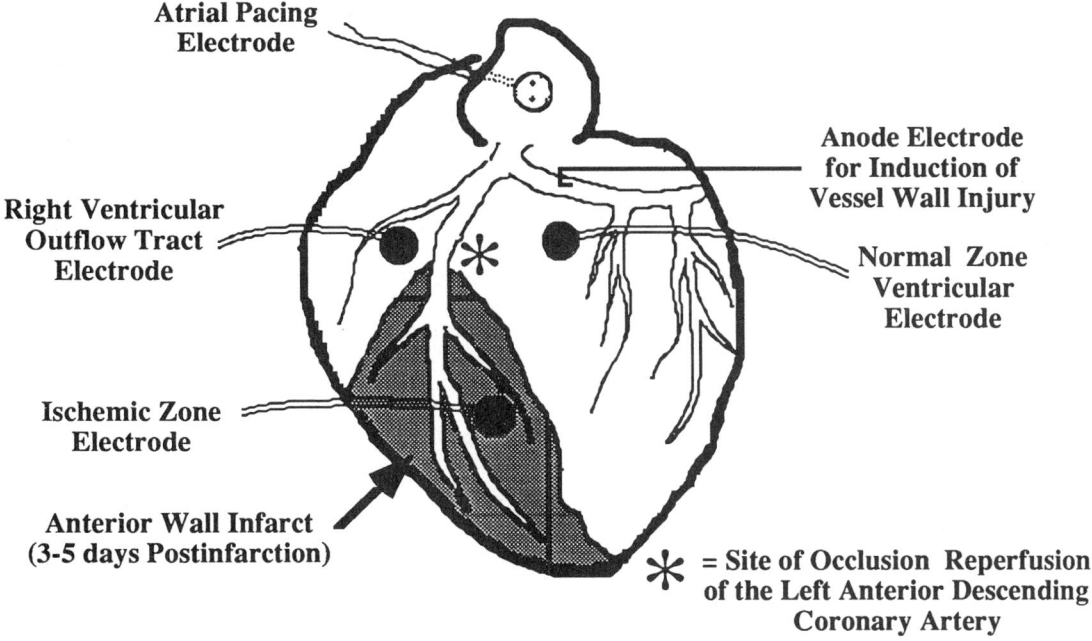

Figure 2. The conscious canine model of sudden death (surgical preparation). Anterior myocardial infarction is produced by a 2-hour occlusion of the left anterior descending coronary artery with subsequent reperfusion in the presence of a critical stenosis. An atrial bipolar epicardial electrode is illustrated, as well as bipolar plunge electrodes in normal myocardium (normal zone [NZ]), infarcted tissue (infarct zone [IZ]), and the right ventricular outflow tract (RVOT). The latter is subsequently used for the introduction of extrastimuli during programmed electrical stimulation, 3 to 5 days after surgery. A silver wire electrode is illustrated within the lumen of the left circumflex coronary artery (LCX). Ultimate introduction of a 150 μA anodal current results in acute posterolateral ischemia and a high incidence of ventricular fibrillation in the sudden death protocol.

collagen matrix. Platelet aggregates form on the denuded surface of the coronary artery accompanied by cyclic variations in blood flow and a high incidence of acute ventricular fibrillation within 1 hour from the onset of ischemia as determined by depression and/or elevation in the ST segment of the electrocardiogram.

Lead II of the electrocardiogram was recorded at preset intervals (30 seconds, every 15 minutes) by a programmable cardiocassette recorder. After 24 hours of continuous application of the anodal current or the development of ventricular fibrillation, the heart was excised and any thrombus in the LCX is removed and weighed. The heart was sectioned transversely and incubated in a 0.4% solution of triphenyltetrazolium chloride (TTC) for 15 minutes. Anterior and posterolateral areas of infarction are identified by their inability to reduce TTC enzymatically to a brick-red formazan precipitate. Infarct masses in the myocardial regions were quantified by computer assisted planimetry and expressed as a percentage of total left ventricular mass. Playback of the cardiocassette provides information regarding the time of onset of ischemia (as assessed by the appearance of ventricular ectopy and/or ST segment changes), the time from ischemia to death, and the percent change in heart rate before death.

Review of Results

When last reviewed, a total of 201 inducible, vehicle treated dogs had been studied in this laboratory; of these, 188 (94%) died within 24 hours of posterolateral ischemia in the sudden death protocol.[54] An interesting observation in many of the animals that die is the finding of variable periods of sustained monomorphic ventricular tachycardia before the onset of ventricular fibrillation; in this respect the model can be seen to resemble closely the clinical situation where ambulatory monitoring has identified sustained ventricular arrhythmias as the most common terminal mechanism in sudden death.[55–57] Phar-

macological protection in this model is apparent when animals survive the arrhythmias associated with the onset of acute posterolateral ischemia and ultimately develop second infarcts in the distribution of the LCX. The results of various pharmacological interventions in the conscious canine model of sudden death are summarized in Table 3.

What is immediately obvious from Table 3 is the apparent dichotomy of action of many

Table 3
Drug Efficacy in the Conscious Canine Model of Myocardial Infarction and Sudden Death

Agent	VT suppression (programmed stimulation)	24-Hour survival
Vehicle	−	6%*
Class I		
Quinidine	+	9%
Flecainide	−	14%
Class II		
Nadolol	−	56–63%
Dilevalol	−	20–60%
Sotalol	+	63%
Celiprolol	−	30%
Class III		
d-Sotalol	+	65%
Bretylium	+	60%
Amiodarone	−	40–80%
Clofilium	+	30%
CK 3579[1]	−	70%
Sematilide	+	60%
E-4031	−	60%
UK 68,798	−	42%
Class IV		
Diltiazem	−	10%
Bepridil	+	30–40%
Other		
Alinidine	−	60%
Meobentine	−	0%
Bethanidine	−	0%
Prazosin	−	50%
CGS 12970[2]	−	30%
R 68070[3]	−	30%

* = cumulative; [1] Class III with β$_1$-adrenoceptor antagonist properties; [2] Thromboxane synthetase (TS) inhibitor; [3] Combined TS inhibitor/receptor antagonist. Adapted from Reference 62.

antiarrhythmic agents when tested against the arrhythmias of programmed electrical stimulation and in their effects against ischemic ventricular fibrillation. In fact, it could be concluded that there is little, if any value in predicting antifibrillatory efficacy from a drug's effect on stimulus-induced ventricular tachycardia. It can be seen that clinically relevant plasma concentrations of the Class Ia agent quinidine were capable of preventing the induction of stimulus-induced arrhythmias, but were ineffective in preventing ventricular fibrillation.[58] Conversely, if we ignore for the present the confounding issues with sotalol, β-adrenergic receptor blockade appears to be offering some degree of protection in the sudden death model without influencing stimulus-induced VT,[59–62] a phenomenon shared by the specific bradycardic agent alinidine.[63] Studies with two calcium channel antagonists show bepridil to be antiarrhythmic without affecting mortality,[64] while diltiazem did not demonstrate any beneficial trends.[65] Studies with other agents not covered by the Vaughan-Williams classification offer little additional insight into the antiarrhythmic/antifibrillatory relationship.[66–70] Even in the group with the greatest overall effect in the sudden death model, only half of the Class III agents tested demonstrated a correlation with antiarrhythmic activity. Thus, it would seem reasonable to conclude that there is little prognostic value from suppression of ventricular tachycardia in this model, other than the ancillary electrophysiological data obtained at the time of testing, which frequently provide an insight into potential antifibrillatory mechanisms.

Clinical Significance of the Conscious Canine Model of Sudden Death

A striking observation from Table 3 is the apparent lack of activity of the Class I agents in preventing sudden death in the model. In light of what we have learned from CAST, the study with flecainide was particularly interesting in that 3 of 7 animals, noninducible at

baseline and therefore at low risk from posterolateral ischemia, failed to survive the sudden death protocol.[71] Thus, potential profibrillatory activity with flecainide had been suggested on the basis of preclinical studies several years before CAST. The Class Ic agents are characterized by their ability to slow conduction velocity with only minimal effects on the duration of the refractory period of the ventricular myocardium. Flecainide in particular is of interest in that it increases the ventricular effective refractory period and to a lesser extent, the action potential duration. Conversely, in Purkinje fibers, action potential duration is decreased as flecainide concentration increases.[72] In contrast to the actions of other antiarrhythmic agents that are sodium channel inhibitors, flecainide, like encainide, exerts a differential effect on repolarization in ventricular muscle and Purkinje fibers, an effect that is likely to aggravate heterogeneity of excitability and refractoriness on the heart and may worsen ventricular tachyarrhythmias under certain experimental and/or clinical situations.[72] Depending on the length of the reentrant circuit, slowing of conduction velocity without a coincident lengthening of the refractory period may result in multiple reentrant circuits.[73] Quinidine, as well as procainamide, two Class Ia antiarrhythmic agents, produce a prolongation of refractoriness and a rate-dependent depression of conduction velocity. The precise role of these electrophysiological effects in mediating an antiarrhythmic action is not clear. Studies with procainamide indicate that lesser slowing of conduction velocity and greater prolongation of refractoriness tend to abolish reentry within the reentrant circuit.[74] Drugs that prolong refractoriness appear more likely to be effective against tachycardia caused by reentry than are drugs that produce a slowing of conduction velocity as their major electrophysiological effect.[75]

The canine model of sudden cardiac death successfully identified the proarrhythmic action of flecainide. The antiarrhythmic and antifibrillatory effects of flecainide acetate during the early postinfarction period were evaluated in the conscious canine model of sudden cardiac death. Ventricular tachycardia remained inducible early after infarction in 8 of 9 dogs receiving an intravenous loading dose of flecainide (2.0 mg/kg body weight) and 7 of 8 dogs receiving saline vehicle. In both the drug and vehicle groups, there was no significant change in the ventricular refractory period or in the cycle length of the induced ventricular tachycardia. With a maintenance intravenous infusion of flecainide, 1.0 mg/kg per hour for 4 hours, the subsequent development of acute posterolateral ischemia resulted in ventricular fibrillation and sudden death in 7 of 8 flecainide treated and 8 of 8 vehicle treated dogs. Seven additional postinfarction dogs with noninducible tachycardia during pretreatment programmed stimulation, and therefore considered to be at low risk for developing ischemic ventricular fibrillation,[52] were given flecainide in an intravenous loading and maintenance dosing regimen. The subsequent occurrence of posterolateral ischemia resulted in the development of ventricular fibrillation in 3 of these 7 dogs. These findings suggest that flecainide acetate may not possess pharmacological properties useful in managing ventricular tachycardia or in preventing ischemic ventricular fibrillation in the presence of recent myocardial damage.[71,76]

The only pharmacological intervention shown to have a beneficial effect on sudden death is β-adrenergic receptor antagonism, where a number of studies in the postmyocardial infarction period have confirmed significant protection.[77–81] In this context there also appears to be a good correlation with the conscious canine model of sudden death, since protection has been demonstrated with a number of agents.[60–62,82] The antiarrhythmic and antifibrillatory potential of β-adrenoceptor antagonism, however, remains unclear; in particular, there is uncertainty over whether the drugs act by a direct antifibrillatory effect or via a primary anti-ischemic influence. This point is pursued in the following section.

Although no individual study with a Class III agent has yet demonstrated significant anti-

fibrillatory activity, suggestions of a beneficial trend are apparent in a recent meta-analysis.[83] The authors conducted an overview of randomized controlled trials of Class I and II antiarrhythmic agents and updated earlier overviews on Class II and IV antiarrhythmic drugs. A total of 137 trials involving 96,000 patients made up the study population. It was concluded that mortality increased significantly with Class I antiarrhythmic agents, reduced with Class II and III, and not significantly altered with Class IV drugs. The data suggest that amiodarone and β-adrenoceptor blocking agents are the only drugs likely to reduce mortality, while other agents may be ineffective or may actually increase the likelihood of a fatal arrhythmia. With the exception of the ESVEM trial mentioned earlier,[24] most of the major ongoing studies use amiodarone, with European and Canadian postmyocardial infarction trials and two placebo-controlled trials in heart failure: the VA CHF trial of antiarrhythmic therapy and the group study of heart failure survival in Argentina (GESICA).

Drug Protection in the Conscious Canine Model of Sudden Death: Direct or Indirect?

Except where ancillary electrophysiological properties are part of a particular agent's pharmacological profile, the β-adrenergic receptor antagonists as a group, appear to be devoid of a direct effect on the heart. Despite this, several studies have reported significant antiarrhythmic effects with these drugs, both in clinical[84] and experimental studies.[85,86] Our laboratory has examined several β-adrenoceptor blocking agents for potential antiarrhythmic and antifibrillatory activity in the canine model of sudden cardiac death. Nadolol, a noncardioselective agent, was studied in the sudden death protocol after pretreatment with 1 (n = 9) and 8 (n = 13) mg/kg, respectively. Respective survival figures were 56% and 63% ($p < 0.01$ versus placebo).[82] D-nadolol, an optical isomer devoid of β-adrenoceptor blocking properties, was ineffective. An interesting feature in this study was the observation that the majority of nadolol treated dogs that died, did so not from ventricular fibrillation, but as the result of complete heart block, severe bradycardia, and/or pump failure. This phenomenon was also observed in subsequent studies with dilevalol, the R,R-enantiomer of labetalol, where 75% of deaths were consequent upon severe bradyarrhythmias.[60,61] The administration of methylscopolamine to postinfarction animals pretreated with dilevalol, however, significantly reduced mortality (40% versus 100% vehicle treated, *p* < 0.05), suggesting that dilevalol, like nadolol, was capable of preventing ischemic ventricular fibrillation in this model, but that death was due to the unopposed effects of parasympathetic influences plus the inability of the sinoatrial node to manifest a positive chronotropic action due to the presence of β-adrenoceptor inhibition.

In a series of experiments with celiprolol, a Class II drug with intrinsic stimulant properties, it was significant that the drug was without effect in preventing sudden cardiac death.[62] In particular, ventricular fibrillation was responsible for each of the 7 deaths in the drug treated group. Although the model is not designed specifically to address the question of intrinsic cardiostimulant phenomena, it was noted that resting heart rates did not change after celiprolol administration and it is possible that this feature of the drug attenuated any protection during acute posterolateral ischemia. It has been demonstrated, for example, that the propensity of sympathetic stimulation to induce arrhythmias in the late myocardial infarction period may relate primarily to heart rate.[87] Previous studies have shown antagonism of the antiarrhythmic protection afforded by propranolol by overdrive atrial pacing.[88] In a recent review of several large prospective double-blind trials with β-adrenoceptor antagonists, Kjekshus[59] demonstrated an almost linear relationship between the reduction in resting heart rate and mortality and noted that drugs with intrinsic sympathomimetic activity produced small reduc-

tions in heart rate and lesser effects on mortality.[89] Although it is unclear whether celiprolol's stimulant properties are due entirely to partial agonism,[90] intrinsic sympathomimetic activity is cited as a possible reason why the drug failed to exert a beneficial influence upon ventricular arrhythmias in a group of patients with acute myocardial infarction.[91]

In an attempt to clarify the role of heart rate in the genesis of sudden death, we evaluated the antifibrillatory effects of alinidine, the N-allyl derivative of clonidine. Alinidine is one of a number of agents, the main pharmacological action of which appears to be a reduction in heart rate from a direct action on the sinus node.[92,93] Although capable of attenuating the chronotropic response to isoproterenol, these drugs do not operate by antagonism of β-adrenoceptors.[92,94] Similarly, there is evidence that the specific bradycardic action involves α-adrenergic or muscarinic receptors, or calcium channels.[92,94,95] However, studies in isolated tissues have shown a nonvoltage-dependent decrease in the slope of the slow diastolic depolarization, indicating that the drugs' effects may be mediated by restriction of current through anion selective channels.[95] In the canine model of sudden cardiac death, alinidine (1 mg/kg) produced a significant (*p* < 0.01) decrease in resting heart rate and prevented ventricular fibrillation in 6 of 10 animals studied (*p* < 0.05 versus concurrent placebo group). In a third group of dogs where constant atrial pacing maintained heart rates at predrug values throughout the sudden death protocol, mortality was 100% despite pretreatment with alinidine.[63] No changes were observed on parameters of ventricular refractoriness or conduction velocity.

Bradycardic agents, like the β-adrenoceptor antagonists, are capable of increasing perfusion pressure distal to a coronary artery stenosis,[96] an effect that for the bradycardic agents at least, appears to be attenuated by atrial pacing to control (predrug) heart rate values.[97] Thus, during posterolateral ischemia, drugs with a negative chronotropic action may contribute to an enhanced collateral flow in the ischemic bed secondary to slowing of heart rate, prolongation of diastole, and presumed reduction in myocardial oxygen consumption.

An additional property of the β-adrenoceptor antagonists is their ability to attenuate the potentially deleterious influence of enhanced adrenergic stimulation. In this respect, it is interesting to consider results in the sudden death model with the α_1-adrenoceptor antagonist prazosin. Despite an inability to alter electrocardiographic intervals, ventricular refractoriness, or the induction of ventricular tachycardia by programmed stimulation, pretreatment with 500 μg/kg of drug resulted in a 50% survival rate in the sudden death protocol ($p < 0.05$ versus placebo).[68] This may be of particular significance in view of the recent suggestion that α-adrenergic responsiveness may be enhanced under conditions of myocardial ischemia,[98,99] and that this is correlated with an increase in α-adrenoceptor concentration.[100] Although the relative contributions of α- and β-adrenergic influences in the genesis of ventricular fibrillation remain unclear, it has been suggested that α-mediated prolongation of action potential duration in ischemic areas may combine with β-mediated shortening of action potential duration in nonischemic areas to increase disparity in refractory periods and produce the arrhythmogenic milieu suitable for the emergence of fatal reentrant pathways.[101] Antagonism of either adrenergic pathway (by the respective adrenergic antagonist) could therefore be seen as an indirect reduction in the electrophysiological derangements leading to ventricular fibrillation, and explain the protection afforded by both the β-adrenoceptor antagonists and prazosin in the animal model of sudden cardiac death.

In identifying a common direct electrophysiological characteristic for antifibrillatory efficacy in the experimental model of sudden cardiac death, it becomes apparent that the greatest overall protection has been seen with agents that have as part of their pharmacological profile prolongation of the action potential duration (Class II activity). Studies with bretylium,[102] amiodarone,[103] sotalol,[104,105] and a number of experimental agents[106–108] have demonstrated significant protection in placebo controlled studies. The effects of clofilium, an alternative Class III drug, were less clear[109] and may relate to a failure to provide an appropriate dosing regimen.

Bretylium was introduced into clinical cardiology in the early 1980s and is currently one of the few drugs marketed as an antifibrillatory agent. Its electrophysiological properties include direct effects upon cardiac action potential duration and indirect effects mediated via its actions on the autonomic nervous system. Early studies with the drug demonstrated suppression of stimulus-induced ventricular tachycardia[110,111] and elevation in VFTs.[112] In the sudden cardiac death model, bretylium (10 mg/kg intravenous every 6 hours) resulted in significant prolongation of ventricular refractoriness and the survival of 6 of the 10 animals studied ($p < 0.05$ versus placebo). The exact antifibrillatory mechanism of the drug, however, remains obscure; while bretylium has been shown to exert similar electrophysiological effects in the denervated heart,[113] the significance of its autonomic effects upon the development of ventricular fibrillation are unknown. Furthermore, studies with bethanidine[66] and meobine[67] failed to prevent ventricular fibrillation and sudden death in the same model, despite similar structural and electrophysiological characteristics.

Amiodarone was originally introduced as an antianginal agent, but was subsequently found to have electrophysiological features attributable to each of the four classes of antiarrhythmic action.[114–116] In addition, the drug reduces the inotropic and chronotropic responses of other agents and has vasodilatory effects on the coronary and systemic vasculature.[117] Its outstanding property, however, is prolongation of the cardiac action potential, prompting its identification as a potential antifibrillatory agent. Despite the observation that alterations in action potential duration and ventricular refractoriness are apparent only with chronic dosing, studies in our laboratory have demonstrated significant antifibrillatory protection after long- and short-term oral therapy. Although no differences were observed in plasma or myocardial concentrations of amiodarone between the two dosing regimens, the greater survival in those animals treated for 10 days (80% versus 60% treated acutely) suggests that long-term therapy may have additional, as yet unidentified actions contributing to greater efficacy. It is known that the electrophysiological effects of amiodarone resemble closely those of hypothyroidism[118,119]; that this is not due to the iodine moiety of the drug has been shown in experiments where the administration of iodine has had no effect on cardiac action potentials.[120] However, the concomitant administration of amiodarone and thyroid hormone has prevented the repolarization changes seen with amiodarone alone, and thyroidectomy can protect postinfarction animals from ischemic ventricular fibrillation in the sudden death protocol.[121]

The effects of sotalol and its dextrorotatory enantiomer, d-sotalol, have been of particular importance in correlating the antifibrillatory potential of pharmacological agents with their known electrophysiological characteristics. Racemic sotalol is a noncardioselective β-adrenoceptor antagonist that produces a dose-dependent prolongation of action potential duration without associated Class I (membrane stabilizing) properties. The dextrorotatory optical isomer of sotalol, d-sotalol, however, while retaining the same cardiac electrophysiological profile, does not share to the same extent the parent compound's β-adrenoceptor blocking properties. The use of d-sotalol allows an assessment of the relative antifibrillatory action of the drug's direct electrophysiological effects divorced from the confounding influence of β-adrenoceptor antagonism. Initial studies with racemic sotalol demonstrated a 65% survival in animals treated with the drug and entered into the sudden death protocol.[104] The protective effect was associated with significant prolongation of the QT interval (an electrocardiographic parameter of action potential duration) and bridging diastolic electrical activity

of the lead II electrocardiogram, a phenomenon invariably followed by ventricular fibrillation in vehicle treated animals. In a subsequent study with the d-isomer, Lynch and co-workers[105] demonstrated similar electrophysiological and antifibrillatory effects, only without the attenuation of the ischemic increase in heart rate seen with the parent compound. This suggests that the observed antifibrillatory effect of d-sotalol was not related to antagonism of the β adrenoceptor, but stemmed directly from prolongation of action potential duration and the increase in the ventricular refractory period.

More recent studies from this laboratory have reinforced the positive trend seen with agents sharing the ability to prolong ventricular refractoriness. Thus, the experimental agents CK-3579 and sematilide,[106] E-4031,[107] and UK-68,798[108] have all produced protection in placebo controlled studies in the canine model of sudden cardiac death. Figure 3 is an example of drug protection in an animal treated with CK-3579.

Class III: One Activity, But Many Mechanisms

The Vaughan Williams classification was the first serious effort to classify antiarrhythmic agents based on what was known regarding common electrophysiological characteristics of the available drugs in the early 1970s.[122] It is widely recognized, however, that the classification is not without major inadequacies, not least of which being that the system is essentially a hybrid: Class I and IV represent agents that impair ion channels; Class II agents inhibit receptors; and Class III agents change an electrophysiological variable (the action potential duration).[123] Although actual mechanisms contributing to Class III effects were not known 20 years ago, the common feature now appears to be interruption of normal potassium efflux by antagonism of one or more of the potassium channels.[124] With the increased understanding of the role of various potassium channels in health and disease, an explo-

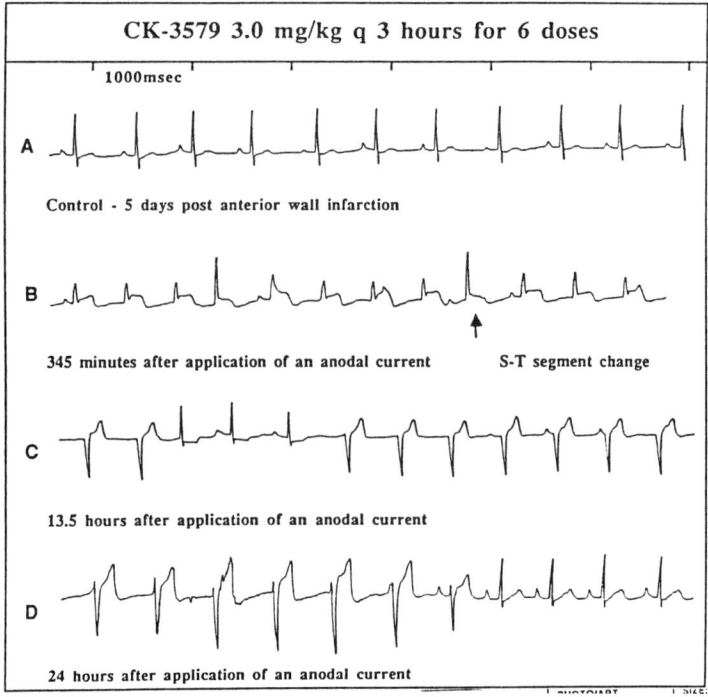

Figure 3. Drug protection in the conscious canine model of sudden death. Sinus tachycardia and ST segment elevation are apparent 345 minutes after application of a 150 µA anodal left circumflex artery (LCX) current in an animal responsive to baseline programmed electrical stimulation. The animal survived the ischemic insult and subsequently developed a posterolateral infarction as manifest by a Harris arrhythmia, evident at 13.5 hours and established at 24 hours. Example of a CK-3579 treated animal.

sion of publications on the subject and an ever-increasing number of newly discovered channels in various organ systems has occurred.[125] Figure 4 represents the number of citations in *Biological Abstracts* for the word channel adjacent to potassium (or K) compared with sodium (or Na) for the years 1970–1990. The increasing interest in potassium channels over the past decade appears exaggerated by the waning publications on sodium channels.

At the present time it is not known which of these several types of potassium channels is responsible for the action of the Class III antiarrhythmic agents, but evidence suggests the major effect of these drugs may be directed against the delayed rectifier channel, I_K.[126] Blockade of the I_K channel appears to cause the most pronounced prolongation of

repolarization in vitro, with the in vivo correlate of global increases in parameters of refractoriness. Blockage of the I_K, however, like any ubiquitous physiological channel, will have effects shared by all cardiac myocytes, normal and abnormal, ischemic and nonischemic. Bearing in mind the basic tenet of arrhythmia generation being a difference in electrophysiological characteristics between normal and abnormal myocardium, it can be seen that global increases in any parameter may be antiarrhythmic in one situation while proarrhythmic in another, if inhomogenous prolongation of refractoriness is associated with the emergence of reentrant pathways. Unlike the use dependence of Class I agents, Class III drugs appear in many cases to have a reverse use dependence with excessive prolongation of action potential duration at slow heart rates. This has been implicated as a possible cause of the reported long QT syndromes (with the associated risks of torsades de pointes and ventricular fibrillation) with these drugs.[126]

With the discovery of ATP-dependent potassium (K_{ATP}) channels regulating insulin release in the pancreatic islet β cells,[127] and their subsequent determination in the heart,[128] came the realization of a cardiac channel active only in pathological (hypoxic or ischemic) circumstances, where it could potentially play a crucial role in the genesis of fatal reentrant arrhythmias. Furthermore the functional or active K_{ATP} channels would become manifest only in myocardial cells in which intracellular ATP was decreased. The concept was supported by the finding that glyburide, a sulfonylurea that (like all members of its class) exerted an antidiabetic effect by promoting the closure of pancreatic K_{ATP} channels, could also reverse the electrophysiological consequences of ischemia in isolated myocardial cells.[129] At about the same time,

independent research demonstrated that glyburide was effective in preventing the development of ventricular fibrillation in isolated heart preparations under conditions of low intracellular ATP, whether the result of ischemia[130,131] or hypoxia.[132] More recently, this laboratory has confirmed a similar antifibrillatory effect in the rabbit isolated heart made hypoxic in the presence of pinacidil. Pinacidil is an antihypertensive agent that promotes intracellular potassium efflux and significantly reduces action potential duration via an agonist effect on K_{ATP} channels.[133] In the normoxic heart under atrial pacing, pinacidil is without discernible effects on cardiac rhythm, despite the fact that a significant decrease in ventricular effective refractory period occurs, presumably due to opening of the K_{ATP} channel. However, in the presence of pinacidil, but not in its absence, ventricular fibrillation occurs in over 90% of hearts made hypoxic for 12 minutes or occurs shortly after the heart is reoxygenated.[134] The induction of ventricular fibrillation in the presence of

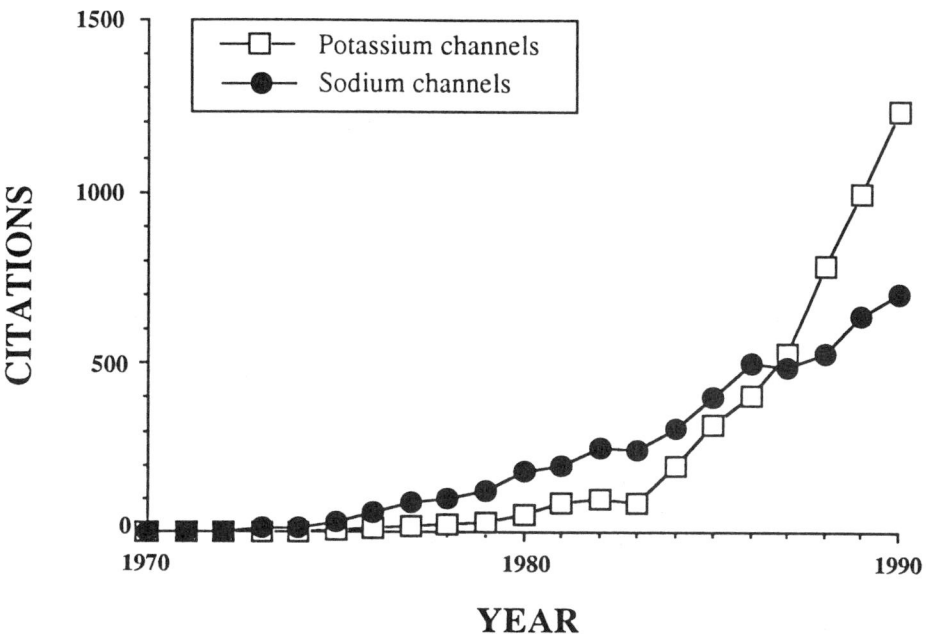

Figure 4. The number of citations in *Biological Abstracts* for the word *channel* adjacent to the terms *K* or *potassium*, *NA*, or *sodium*, for the period 1970–1990. (Modified with permission from Reference 137.)

pinacidil is dependent upon a decrease in myocardial cell ATP content, thereby suggesting that the myocardial K_{ATP} channel shows increased responsiveness to the agonist effects of pinacidil when it is disinhibited as a result of decreased cellular ATP. Glyburide, known for its ability to inhibit the K_{ATP} channel, prevents the pinacidil-induced decrease in the effective refractory period and significantly reduces the incidence of ventricular fibrillation in the hypoxic/reoxygenated perfused heart.[134] The profibrillatory action of pinacidil is unmasked by myocardial hypoxia or ischemia, either of which will decrease myocardial cell ATP content. It is anticipated that a lowering of myocardial ATP will favor opening of the K_{ATP} channel, especially in the presence of the agonist, pinacidil. The two events, lowering of cellular ATP and further opening of the K_{ATP} channel by the pinacidil, would favor the rapid outward movement of potassium and a marked decrease in the ventricular refractory period. Therefore, pharmacological interventions directed at blocking the K_{ATP} channel, thereby preventing a decrease in the ventricular refractory period, may provide a useful approach to the prevention of ventricular fibrillation, without necessarily possessing antifibrillatory activity as manifest by the reduction or prevention in premature ventricular depolarizations. Based on these observations, it is suggested that inhibition of K_{ATP} channel, by preventing potassium efflux, will antagonize reductions in the action potential duration and will prevent the shortening of refractoriness in ischemic and ATP depleted myocardial cells. By so doing, disparity in refractory periods can be avoided, and with it the risk of emergent ventricular reentrant arrhythmias.

Using a cohort of small infarct, noninducible dogs similar to those described above in the flecainide study, we evaluated the profibrillatory action of pinacidil in the sudden cardiac death model. Compared with a 24-hour mortality in the placebo group of 20% (incidence of ischemic ventricular fibrillation 6.7%), mortality in the pinacidil group was 87% (ischemic fibrillation 60%), a difference

statistically significant at the $p < 0.01$ level. Changes in arterial blood pressure did not reach statistical significance, indicating that the profibrillatory effect could not be explained on the basis of hypotension.[135] These studies lend further support for the pivotal role of the K_{ATP} channel in the genesis of fatal cardiac arrhythmias. In the search for the K_{ATP} channel antagonist to be developed as the first potential antifibrillatory agent, the hypoglycemic properties of the sulfonylureas made their evaluation particularly difficult in the intact animal. However, a number of unrelated compounds claim to have K_{ATP} blocking activity as part of their pharmacological profile. One in particular, 5-hydroxy decanoic acid purports to be a pure K_{ATP} channel antagonist and appears to attenuate ischemic ventricular fibrillation in preliminary studies with the chronic canine model of sudden death (unpublished results).

Conclusions

The lack of an effective and safe drug for the prevention of lethal arrhythmias and sudden cardiac death has served to stimulate renewed interest in the area of drug development and the introduction of several new candidate agents that share a common ability to prolong ventricular refractoriness. Equally important is the recognition that most antiarrhythmic agents have been evaluated with in vitro or in vivo models that have little relevance to the clinical situation of sudden cardiac death. As the recent CAST report[17,18] has emphasizd, the final analysis of a drug's ultimate utility will depend on appropriate clinical testing in patients who are at risk of developing sudden and unexpected life-threatening arrhythmias and/or ventricular fibrillation. We can no longer afford to use the more expedient and less dependable approach to evaluating new agents for their ability to reduce the frequency and/or complexity of ventricular depolarizations or their ability to modify the patient's response to programmed electrical stimulation. Despite the formidable task involved in the clinical assessment of an effective therapy for the prevention of ventricular fibrillation, the challenge could be made more readily attainable by preclinical assessment of a candidate drug, based upon studies conducted in relevant animal models using meaningful electrophysiological endpoints that occur spontaneously. To this end, we have used an animal model of sudden coronary death in which ventricular fibrillation develops within 1 hour from the onset of an ischemic event in a myocardial substrate that has been identified, through the use of programmed electrical stimulation, to be capable of supporting an arrhythmic mechanism. The conscious, postinfarcted, canine model has been used by us to confirm antifibrillatory activity in a number of marketed agents, propose antifibrillatory potential in several agents at exploratory stages of development and warn of profibrillatory dangers in others. Perhaps the last words should be those of Craig Pratt, MD, Chairman of the Cardiovascular and Renal Drugs Advisory Board of the US Food and Drug Administration, who writes: "Although a number of animal models of sudden death exist, it seems desirable to use the model with previous MI (healed scar) and new induction of ischemia, which may most closely emulate the situation seen in the CAST".[136] The significance of the animal model as a potential solution to a major public health problem becomes particularly important, especially at a time when there is increasing pressure to abandon the physiological approach to basic research by activists who oppose the use of animals in biomedical research.

Acknowledgments: The principal investigator (BRL) expresses sincere gratitude to the National Institutes of Health, Heart, Lung and Blood Institute for the uninterrupted support of our studies on the analysis of antiarrhythmic agents. Much of the work by the principal investigator's laboratory would not have been possible without the cooperation of colleagues in the pharmaceutical industry who provided the many drugs studied over the past 32 years. Lastly, the principal investigator acknowledges the dedication of the many pre- and postdoctoral fellows and faculty colleagues who partici-pated in our research program. The authors thank Ms. Laura Sell for editorial assistance in the preparation of this manuscript.

References

1. Roberts WC: Sudden cardiac death: definitions and causes. *Am J Cardiol* 57:1410, 1986.
2. Kannel WB, McGee DL, Schatzkin A: An epidemiological perspective of sudden death: 26 year follow up in the Framingham Study. *Drugs* 28:1, 1984.
3. Myerburg RJ, Kessler KM, Castellanos A: Sudden cardiac death. Structure, function, and time-dependence of risk. *Circulation* 85:I-2, 1992.
4. Buxton AE: Antiarrhythmic drugs: good for premature ventricular contractions but bad for patients? *Ann Interm Med* 116:420, 1992.
5. Moss AJ, DeCamilla J, David H: Factors associated with cardiac death in the post-hospital phase of myocardial infarction. In: HE Kulbertus, HJJ Wellens (eds): *Sudden Death*. The Hague: Martinus Nihoff Publishing, 1980, p. 237.
6. The Coronary Drug Project Research Group: Prognostic importance of premature beats following myocardial infarction. *JAMA* 223:116, 1973.
7. Moss AJ, Davis HT, DeCamilla J, Bayer LW: Ventricular ectopic beats and their relation to sudden and nonsudden cardiac death after myocardial infarction. *Circulation* 60:998, 1979.
8. Hinkle LE: The immediate antecedents of sudden death. *Acta Med Scand* 651:207, 1981.
9. The Multicentcr Postinfarction Research Group: Risk stratification and survival after myocardial infarction. *N Engl J Med* 309:331, 1983.
10. Mukharji J, Rude RE, Poole WK, et al: Risk factors for sudden death after myocardial infarction: two-year follow-up. *Am J Cardiol* 54:31, 1984.
11. Bigger JT, Fleiss JL, Kleiger R, et al: The relationships among ventricular arrhythmias, left ventricular dysfunction, and mortality in the 2 years after myocardial infarction. *Circulation* 69:250, 1984.
12. Gianelly R, von der Groeben JO, Spivack AP, Harrison DC: Effect of lidocaine on ventricular arrhythmias in patients with coronary heart disease. *N Engl J Med* 277:1215, 1967.
13. Lie KI, Wellens HJ, van Capelle FJ, Durrer D: Lidocaine in the prevention of primary ventricular fibrillation. *N Engl J Med* 291:1324, 1974.
14. Furberg CD: Effects of antiarrhythmic drugs

on mortality after myocardial infarction. *Am J Cardiol* 52:32C, 1983.

15. May GS, Furberg CD, Eberlein KA, Geraci BJ: Secondary prevention after myocardial infarction: a review of short-term acute phase trials. *Prog Cardiovasc Dis* 25:335, 1983.

16. The CAPS Investigators: The Cardiac Arrhythmia Pilot Study. *Am J Cardiol* 57:91, 1986.

17. CAST Investigators: Preliminary report: effect of encainide and flecainide on mortality in a randomized trial of arrhythmia suppression after myocardial infarction. *N Engl J Med* 321:406, 1989.

18. CAST II Investigators: Effect of the antiarrhythmic agent moricizine on survival after myocardial infarction. *N Engl J Med* 327:227, 1992.

19. Wellens HJ, Schuilenburg RM, Durrer D: Electrical stimulation of the heart in patients with ventricular tachycardia. *Circulation* 46:216, 1972.

20. Roy D, Waxman HL, Kienzle MG, et al: Clinical characteristics and long-term follow-up in 119 survivors of cardiac arrest: relation to inducibility at electrophysiologic testing. *Am J Cardiol* 52:969, 1983.

21. Ruskin JN: Role of invasive electrophysiological testing in the evaluation and treatment of patients at high risk for sudden cardiac death. *Circulation* 85:I-152, 1992.

22. Skale BT, Miles WM, Heger JJ, et al: Survivors of cardiac arrest: prevention of recurrence by drug therapy as predicted by electrophysiologic testing or ECG monitoring. *Am J Cardiol* 57:113, 1986.

23. Cupples LA, Gagnon DR, Kannel WB: Long- and short-term risk of sudden cardiac death: population at risk. *Circulation* 85:I-11, 1992.

24. The ESVEM Investigators: The ESVEM trial: electrophysiologic study versus electrocardiographic monitoring for selection of antiarrhythmic therapy of ventricular tachyarrhythmias. *Circulation* 79:1354, 1989.

25. Kuller L, Cooper M, Perper J: Epidemiology of sudden death. *Arch Intern Med* 129:714, 1972.

26. Baum RS, Alvares H, Cobb LA: Survival after resuscitation from out-of-hospital ventricular fibrillation. *Circulation* 50:1231, 1974.

27. Weaver WD, Lorch GS, Alvarez HA, Cobb LA: Angiographic findings and prognostic indicators in patients resuscitated from sudden cardiac death. *Circulation* 54:895, 1976.

28. Reichenbach DD, Moss NS, Meyer E: Pathology of the heart in sudden cardiac death. *Am J Cardiol* 39:865, 1977.

29. Goldstein S, Landis R, Leighton R, et al: Characteristics of the resuscitated out-of-hospital cardiac arrest victim with coronary heart disease. *Circulation* 64:977, 1981.

30. Schuster EH, Bulkley BH: Ischemia at a distant site after myocardial infarction: a cause of early postinfarction angina. *Circulation* 62:509, 1980.

31. Schwartz PJ, Stone HL: Left stellectomy in the prevention of ventricular fibrillation caused by acute myocardial ischemia in conscious dogs with anterior myocardial infarction. *Circulation* 62:1256, 1980.

32. Schwartz PJ, Billman GE, Stone HL: Autonomic mechanism in ventricular fibrillation induced by myocardial ischemia during exercise in dogs with healed myocardial infarction. An experimental preparation for sudden death. *Circulation* 69:790, 1984.

33. Kabell G, Brachmann J, Scherlag BJ, et al: Mechanisms of ventricular arrhythmias in multivessel coronary disease: the effects of collateral zone ischemia. *Am Heart J* 108:447, 1984.

34. Previtali M, Klersy C, Salerno JA, et al: Ventricular tachyarrhythmias in Prinzmetal's variant angina: clinical significance and relation to the degree and time course of ST segment elevation. *Am J Cardiol* 52:19, 1983.

35. Miller DD, Waters DD, Szlachcic J, Theroux P: Clinical characteristics associated with sudden death in patients with variant angina. *Circulation* 66:588, 1982.

36. Malliani A, Schwartz PJ, Zanchetti A: Neural mechanisms in life-threatening arrhythmias. *Am Heart J* 100:705, 1980.

37. Schwartz PJ, La Rovere MT, Vanoli E: Autonomic nervous system and sudden cardiac death. Experimental basis and clinical observations for post-myocardial infarction risk stratification. *Circulation* 85:I-77, 1992.

38. Schwartz PJ, Pagani M, Lombardi F, et al: A cardiocardiac sympatho-vagal reflex in the cat. *Circ Res* 32:215, 1973.

39. Myerburg RJ, Epstein K, Gaide MS, et al: Electrophysiological consequences of experimental acute ischemia superimposed upon healed myocardial infarction in cats. *Am J Cardiol* 49:323, 1982.

40. Patterson E, Holland K, Eller BT, Lucchesi BR: Ventricular fibrillation resulting from ischemia at a site remote from previous myocardial infarction. A conscious canine model of sudden coronary death. *Am J Cardiol* 50:1412, 1982.

41. Garan H, McComb JM, Ruskin JN: Spontaneous and electrically induced ventricular arrhythmia during acute ischemia superimposed on 2 week old canine myocardial infarction. *J Am Coll Cardiol* 11:603, 1988.

42. Lucchesi BR, Lynch JJ: Preclinical assessment of antiarrhythmic drugs. *Fed Proc* 45:2197, 1986.

43. Maling HM, Moran NC: Ventricular arrhythmias induced by sympathomimetic amines in unanesthetized dogs following coronary artery occlusion. *Circ Res* 5:409, 1957.
44. El-Sherif N, Scherlag BJ, Lazzara R, Hope RR: Re-entrant ventricular arrhythmias in the late myocardial infarction period. 1. Conduction characteristics in the infarction zone. *Circulation* 55:686, 1977.
45. Karagueuzian HS, Fenoglio JJ, Weiss MB, Wit AL: Protracted ventricular tachycardia induced by premature stimulation of the canine heart after coronary artery occlusion and reperfusion. *Circ Res* 44:833, 1979.
46. Moore EN, Spear JF: Ventricular fibrillation threshold. Its physiological and pharmacological importance. *Arch Intern Med* 135:446, 1975.
47. Euler DE, Scanlon PJ: Comparative effects of antiarrhythmic drugs on the ventricular fibrillation threshold. *J Cardiovasc Pharmacol* 11:291, 1988.
48. Axelrod PJ, Verrier RL, Lown B: Vulnerability to ventricular fibrillation during acute coronary artery occlusion and release. *Am J Cardiol* 36:776, 1975.
49. Euler DE: Norepinephrine release by ventricular stimulation: effect on fibrillation thresholds. *Am J Physiol* 238:H406, 1980.
50. Anderson JL, Rodier HE, Green LS: Comparative effects of beta-adrenergic blocking drugs on experimental ventricular fibrillation thresholds. *Am J Cardiol* 51:1196, 1983.
51. Patterson E, Lucchesi BR: Antifibrillatory properties of the beta-adrenergic receptor antagonists nadolol, sotalol, atenolol and propranolol, in the anesthetized dog. *Pharmacology* 28:121, 1984.
52. Wilber DJ, Lynch JJ, Montgomery DG, Lucchesi BR: Postinfarction sudden death: significance of inducible ventricular tachycardia and infarct size in a conscious canine model. *Am Heart J* 109:8, 1985.
53. Josephson ME, Horowitz LN, Farshidi A, Kastor JA: Recurrent sustained ventricular tachycardia. 1. Mechanisms. *Circulation* 57:431, 1978.
54. Uprichard ACG, Lucchesi BR: Antifibrillatory drugs. In: KH Dangman, DS Miura (eds): *Basic and Clinical Electrophysiology and Pharmacology of the Heart*. New York, NY: Marcel Dekker, 1991, p. 723.
55. Panidis JP, Morganroth J: Sudden death in hospitalized patients: cardiac rhythm disturbances detected by ambulatory echocardiographic monitoring. *J Am Coll Cardiol* 2:798, 1983.
56. Kempf FC, Josephson ME: Cardiac arrest recorded on ambulatory electrocardiograms. *Am J Cardiol* 53:1577, 1984.
57. Milner PG, Platia EV, Reid PR, Griffith LSC: Ambulatory electrocardiographic recordings at the time of fatal cardiac arrest. *Am J Cardiol* 56:588, 1985.
58. Patterson E, Lucchesi BR: Quinidine gluconate in chronic myocardial ischemic injury—differential effects in response to programmed stimulation and acute myocardial ischemia in the dog. *Circulation* 68:III-155, 1983.
59. Kjekshus J: Comments—beta blockers: heart rate reduction—a mechanism of benefit. *Eur Heart J* 6:29, 1985.
60. Lynch JJ, Nelson SD, MacEwen SA, et al: Antifibrillatory efficacy of concomitant beta adrenergic receptor blockade with dilevalol, the R,R-isomer of labetalol, and muscarinic receptor blockade with methylscopolamine. *J Pharmacol Exp Ther* 241:741, 1987.
61. Lynch JJ, Lucchesi BR: How are animal models best for the study of antiarrhythmic drugs? In: DJ Hearse, AS Manning, MJ Janse (eds): *Life-Threatening Arrhythmias and Infarction*. New York, NY: Raven Press, 1987, p. 169.
62. Uprichard ACG, Lynch JJ, Kitzen JM: Celiprolol, a β1–selective adrenoceptor antagonist with intrinsic stimulant properties, does not protect against ventricular tachycardia or ventricular fibrillation in a conscious canine model of myocardial infarction and sudden death. *J Pharmacol Exp Ther* 251:571, 1989.
63. Uprichard ACG, Chi L, Lynch JJ, et al: Alinidine protects against ischemic ventricular fibrillation in a conscious canine model: probable anti-ischemic mode of action. *J Cardiovasc Pharmacol* 14:475, 1989.
64. Lynch JJ, Montgomery DG, Ventura A, Lucchesi BR: Antiarrhythmic and electrophysiologic effects of bepridil in chronically infarcted conscious dogs. *J Pharmacol Exp Ther* 234:72, 1985.
65. Patterson E, Eller BT, Lucchesi BR: Effects of diltiazem upon experimental ventricular dysrhythmias. *J Pharmacol Exp Ther* 225:224, 1983.
66. Patterson E, Amalfitano DJ, Lucchesi BR: Development of ventricular tachyarrhythmias in the conscious canine during the recovery phase of experimental ischemic injury: effect of bethanidine administration. *J Cardiovasc Pharmacol* 6:470, 1984.
67. Zimmerman JM, Patterson E, Pitt B, Lucchesi BR: Antidysrhythmic actions of meobentine. *Am Heart J* 107:1117, 1984.
68. Wilber DJ, Lynch JJ, Montgomery DG, Lucchesi BR: Alpha-adrenergic influences in canine ischemic sudden death: effects of α_1-adreno-

ceptor blockade with prazosin. *J Cardiovasc Pharmacol* 10:96, 1987.

69. Kitzen JM, Lynch JJ, Uprichard ACG, et al: Failure of thromboxane synthetase inhibition to protect the postinfarcted heart against the induction of ventricular tachycardia and ventricular fibrillation in a conscious canine model of sudden coronary death. *Pharmacology* 37: 171, 1988.

70. Kitzen JM, Chi L, Uprichard ACG, Lucchesi BR: Effects of combined thromboxane synthetase inhibition/thromboxane receptor antagonism in two models of sudden death in the canine: limited role for thromboxane. *J Cardiovasc Pharmacol* 16:68, 1990.

71. Kou WH, Nelson SD, Lynch JJ, et al: Effect of flecainide acetate on prevention of electrical induction of ventricular tachycardia and occurrence of ischemic ventricular fibrillation during the early postmyocardial periods: evaluation in a conscious canine model of sudden death. *J Am Coll Cardiol* 9:359, 1987.

72. Ikeda N, Singh BN, Davis LD, Hauswirth O: Effects of flecainide on the electrophysiologic properties of isolated canine and rabbit myocardial fibers. *J Am Coll Cardiol* 5:303, 1985.

73. Brugada J, Boersma L, Kirchhof C, et al: Double wave re-entry as a mechanism of acceleration of ventricular tachycardia. *Circulation* 81: 1633, 1990.

74. Furukawa T, Rozanski JJ, Moroe K, et al: Efficacy of procainamide on ventricular tachycardia: relation to prolongation of refractoriness and slowing of conduction. *Am Heart J* 118: 702, 1989.

75. Sasyniuk BI, McQuillan J: Mechanisms by which antiarrhythmic drugs influence induction of reentrant responses in subendocardial Purkinje network of 1-day-old infarcted canine ventricle. In: DP Zipes, J Jalife (eds): *Cardiac Electrophysiology and Arrhythmias*. Orlando, FL: Grune & Stratton, 1983, p. 389.

76. Lynch JJ, DiCarlo LA, Montgomery DG, Lucchesi BR: Effects of flecainide acetate on ventricular tachyarrhythmia and fibrillation in dogs with recent myocardial infarction. *Pharmacology* 35:181, 1987.

77. Multicentre International Study: Improvement in prognosis of myocardial infarction by long-term β-adrenoceptor blockade using practolol. *Br Med J* 3:735, 1975.

78. Norwegian Multicenter Study Group: Timolol-induced reduction in mortality and reinfarction in patients surviving acute myocardial infarction. *N Engl J Med* 304:801, 1981.

79. Beta-Blocker Heart Attack Trial Research Group: A randomized trial of propanolol in patients with acute myocardial infarction. *JAMA* 247:1707, 1982.

80. Yusuf S, Peto R, Lewis J, et al: Beta blockade during and after myocardial infarction: an overview of the randomized trials. *Prog Cardiovasc Dis* 27:335, 1985.

81. The MIAMI Trial Research Group: Metoprolol in acute myocardial infarction (MIAMI): a randomised placebo-controlled international trial. *Eur Heart J* 6:199, 1985.

82. Patterson E, Lucchesi BR: Antifibrillatory actions of d,l-nadolol in a conscious canine model of sudden coronary death. *J Cardiovasc Pharmacol* 5:737, 1983.

83. Teo K, Yusuf S, Furberg C: Effect of prophylactic antiarrhythmic drug therapy on post-myocardial infarction mortality. *JAMA* (in press).

84. Rossi PR, Yusuf S, Ramsdale D, et al: Reduction of ventricular arrhythmias by early intravenous atenolol in suspected acute myocardial infarction. *Br Med J* 286:506, 1983.

85. Echt DS, Griffin JC, Ford AJ, et al: Nature of inducible ventricular arrhythmias in a canine chronic myocardial infarction model. *Am J Cardiol* 52:1127, 1983.

86. Gang ES, Bigger JT, Uhl EW: Effects of timolol and propranolol on inducible sustained ventricular tachyarrhythmias in dogs with subacute myocardial infarction. *Am J Cardiol* 53: 275, 1984.

87. El-Sherif N: Re-entrant ventricular arrhythmias in the late myocardial infarction period 6. Effects of the autonomic system. *Circulation* 58:103, 1978.

88. Hope RR, Williams DO, El-Sherif N, et al: The efficacy of antiarrhythmic agents during acute myocardial ischemia and the role of heart rate. *Circulation* 50:507, 1974.

89. Kjekshus J: Comments—beta blockers: heart rate reduction—a mechanism of benefit. *Eur Heart J* 6:29, 1985.

90. Wolf PS, Smith RD, Khandwala A, et al: Celiprolol—pharmacological profile of an unconventional beta-blocker. *Br J Clin Pract* 39:5, 1985.

91. Payrhuber K, Kratzer H, Kuhn P: Celiprolol in acute myocardial infarct. *Wien Klin Wochensch* 98:171, 1986.

92. Kobinger W, Lillie C, Pichler L: N-allyl-derivative of clonidine, a substance with specific bradycardic action at a cardiac site. *Naunyn-Schmiedeberg's Arch Pharmacol* 306:255, 1979.

93. Kobinger W, Lillie C, Pichler L: Cardiovascular actions of N-allyl-clonidine (ST 567), a substance with specific bradycardic action. *Eur J Pharmacol* 58:141, 1979.

94. Lillie C, Kobinger W: Actions of alinidine and AQ-A 39 on rate and contractility of guinea pig atria during β-adrenoceptor stimulation. *J Cardiovasc Pharmacol* 5:1048, 1983.

95. Millar JS, Vaughan Williams EM: Pacemaker selectivity: influence on rabbit atria of ionic environment and of alinidine, a possible anion antagonist. *Cardiovasc Res* 15:335, 1981.

96. Gross GJ, Lamping KG, Warltier DC, Hardman HF: Effects of three bradycardic drugs on regional myocardial blood flow and function in areas distal to a total or partial coronary occlusion in dogs. *Circulation* 69:391, 1984.

97. Gross GJ, Daemmgen JW: Effect of the new specific bradycardic agent AQ-A39 (falipamil) on coronary collateral blood flow in dogs. *J Cardiovasc Pharmacol* 10:123, 1987.

98. Juhasz-Nagy A, Aviado DM: Increased role of alpha-adrenoceptors in ischemic myocardial zones. *Physiologist* 19:245, 1976.

99. Sheridan DJ, Penkoske PA, Sobel BE, Corr PB: Alpha adrenergic contributions to dysrhythmia cardiac muscle. *Br J Pharmacol* 39:657, 1970.

100. Corr PB, Shayman JA, Kramer JB, Kipnis RJ: Increased alpha-adrenergic receptors in ischemic cat mycoardium. *J Clin Invest* 67:1232, 1981.

101. Vaughan Williams EM: Cardiac electrophysiological effects of selective adrenoceptor stimulation and their possible roles in arrhythmias. *J Cardiovasc Pharmacol* 7:S61, 1985.

102. Holland K, Patterson E, Lucchesi BR: Prevention of ventricular fibrillation by bretylium in a conscious canine model of sudden coronary death. *Am Heart J* 105:711, 1983.

103. Patterson E, Eller BT, Abrams GD, et al: Ventricular fibrillation in a conscious canine preparation of sudden coronary death—prevention by short- and long-term amiodarone administration. *Circulation* 68:857, 1983.

104. Patterson E, Lynch JJ, Lucchesi BR: Antiarrhythmic and antifibrillatory actions of the beta adrenergic receptor antagonist, dl-sotalol. *J Pharmacol Exp Ther* 230:519, 1984.

105. Lynch JJ, Coskey LA, Montgomery DG, Lucchesi BR: Prevention of ventricular fibrillation by dextrorotatory sotalol in a conscious canine model of sudden coronary death. *Am Heart J* 109:949, 1985.

106. Chi L, Mu D-X, Driscoll EM, Lucchesi BR: Antiarrhythmic and electrophysiologic actions of CK-3579 and sematilide in a conscious canine model of sudden coronary death. *J Cardiovasc Pharmacol* 16:312, 1990.

107. Chi L, Mu D-X, Lucchesi BR: Electrophysiology and antiarrhythmic actions of E-4031 in the experimental animal model of sudden coronary death. *J Cardiovasc Pharmacol* 17:285, 1991.

108. Black SC, Chi L, Mu D-X, Lucchesi BR: The antifibrillatory actions of UK-68,798, a class III

antiarrhythmic agent. *J Pharmacol Exp Ther* 258:416, 1991.

109. Kopia GA, Eller BT, Patterson E, et al: Antiarrhythmic and electrophysiologic actions of clofilium in experimental canine models. *Eur J Pharmacol* 116:49, 1985.

110. Patterson E, Gibson JK, Lucchesi BR: Postmyocardial infarction reentrant ventricular arrhythmias in conscious dogs: suppression by bretylium tosylate. *J Pharmacol Exp Ther* 216:453, 1981.

111. Patterson E, Gibson JK, Lucchesi BR: Prevention of chronic canine ventricular arrhythmias with bretylium tosylate. *Circulation* 64:1045, 1981.

112. Anderson JL, Patterson E, Conlon M, et al: Kinetics of antifibrillatory effects of bretylium: correlation with myocardial drug concentrations. *Am J Cardiol* 46:583, 1980.

113. Namm DH, Wang CM, El-Sayad S, et al: Effects of bretylium on rat cardiac muscle: the electrophysiological effect and its uptake and binding in normal and immunosympathectomized rat hearts. *J Pharmacol Exp Ther* 193:194, 1975.

114. Bexton RS, Camm AJ: Drugs with a class III antiarrhythmic action. 1. Amiodarone. *Pharmacol Ther* 17:315, 1982.

115. Gloor HO, Urthaler F, James TN: Acute effects of amiodarone upon the canine sinus node and atrioventricular junctional region. *J Clin Invest* 71:1457, 1983.

116. Mason JW, Hondeghem LM, Katzung BG: Block of inactivated sodium channels and of depolarization-induced automaticity in guinea pig papillary muscle by amiodarone. *Circ Res* 55:277, 1984.

117. Charlier R: Cardiac actions in the dog of a new antagonist of adrenergic excitation which does not produce competitive blockade of adrenoceptors. *Br J Pharmacol* 39:668, 1970.

118. Freedberg AS, Papp JG, Vaughan Williams EM: The effect of altered thyroid state on atrial intracellular potentials. *J Physiol* 207:357, 1970.

119. Johnson PN, Freedberg AS, Marshall JM: Action of thyroid hormone on the transmembrane potentials from sinoatrial node cells and atrial muscle cells in isolated atria of rabbits. *Cardiology* 58:273, 1973.

120. Singh BN, Vaughan Williams EM: The effects of amiodarone, a new anti-anginal drug, on cardiac muscle. *Br J Pharmacol* 39:657, 1970.

121. Venkatesh N, Lynch JJ, Uprichard ACG, et al: Hypothyroidism renders protection against lethal ventricular arrhythmias in a conscious canine model of sudden death. *J Cardiovasc Pharmacol* 18:703, 1991.

122. Vaughan Williams EM: Classification of anti-

dysrhythmic drugs. *Pharmacol Ther* 1:115, 1975.

123. Task Force of the Working Group on Arrhythmias of the European Society of Cardiology: The Sicilian gambit: a new approach to the classification of antiarrhythmic drugs based on their actions on arrhythmogenic mechanisms. *Circulation* 84:1831, 1991.

124. Colatsky TJ, Follmer CH: K$^+$ channel blockers and activators in cardiac arrhythmias. *Cardiovasc Drug Rev* 7:199, 1989.

125. Cook NS: The pharmacology of potassium channels and their therapeutic potential. *Trends Pharmacol Sci* 9:21, 1988.

126. Colatsky TJ, Follmer CH, Starmer CF: Channel specificity in antiarrhythmic drug action: mechanism of potassium channel block and its role in suppressing and aggravating cardiac arrhythmias. *Circulation* 82:2235, 1990.

127. Cook DL, Hales CN: Intracellular ATP directly blocks K$^+$ channels in pancreatic B-cells. *Nature* 311:271, 1984.

128. Noma A: ATP-regulated K$^+$ channels in cardiac muscle. *Nature* 305:147, 1983.

129. Fosset M, De Weille JR, Green RD, et al: Antidiabetic sulfonylureas control action potential properties in heart cells via high affinity receptors that are linked to ATP-dependent K channels. *J Biol Chem* 263:7933, 1988.

130. Kantor PF, Coetzee WA, Dennis SC, Opie LH: Effects of glibenclamide on ischemic arrhythmias. *Circulation* 76:IV-17, 1987.

131. Wolloben CD, Sanguinetti MC, Siegl PKS: Influence of ATP-sensitive potassium channel modulators on ischemia-induced fibrillation in isolated rat hearts. *J Mol Cell Cardiol* 21:783, 1989.

132. Siegl PKS, Scott AL, Sanguinetti MC: Inhibition of anoxia- and BRL 3495-induced shortening of cardiac refractory period by the sulfonylurea, glyburide, in isolated ferret papillary muscle (abstract). *J Mol Cell Cardiol* 20(Suppl III):S32, 1988.

133. Smallwood JK, Steinberg MI: Cardiac electrophysiological effects of pinacidil and related pyridylcyanoguanidines: relationship to antihypertensive activity. *J Cardiovasc Pharmacol* 12:102, 1988.

134. Chi L, Black S, Kuo PI, et al: Actions of pinacidil at a reduced potassium concentration: a direct cardiac effect possibly involving the ATP-dependent potassium channel. *J Cardiovasc Pharmacol* 21:179, 1993.

135. Chi L, Uprichard ACG, Lucchesi BR: Profibrillatory actions of pinacidil in a conscious canine model of sudden coronary death. *J Cardiovasc Pharmacol* 15:452, 1990.

136. Pratt CM: FDA guidelines for antiarrhythmic drug development. *Choices in Cardiology* 5:44, 1991.

137. Robertson DW, Steinberg MI: Potassium channel modulators: scientific applications and their therapeutic promise. *J Med Chem* 33:1529, 1990.

Chapter 23

Experimental Determinations of Antiarrhythmic and Proarrhythmic Drug Action in Reentrant Ventricular Tachycardia

Bruce C. Hill
Rachel A.J. Summers
Kenneth R. Courtney

In the quest to design and optimize antiarrhythmic drugs, what are appropriate experimental tests of antiarrhythmic drug action? The experimentalist has an ever-increasing spectrum of techniques to use in attempting to characterize various actions of drugs, but it is far from clear which tests are pertinent toward the drugs' clinical behavior. Commonly used tests start at the cardiac cellular membrane level and move up in examining effects on successively more complex systems: patch clamp measurements of isolated ionic currents, microelectrode determinations of drug effects on action potentials, mapping studies that detect drug action on activation sequences, and susceptibility of canine infarcts to arrhythmias. Studies on the cellular level have provided classifications such as that of Singh and Vaughan Williams.[1-3] This classification groups drugs into four classes relating to their effects on action potential characteristics (and their underlying ionic currents) and β-adrenergic response. What does such a classification tell us about how a drug will affect specific types of arrhythmias? We have developed tests that help to answer this question in a specific case: Class I versus Class III drug action in ventricular tachycardia (VT) caused by reentry.

Reentry is understood to cause VT in human infarcts[4] and in an experimental model of chronic canine infarct,[5] and antiarrhythmic efficacy has been demonstrated in both settings by a drug's ability to prevent induction of VT by programmed stimulation. Using an in vitro model of VT, we have developed three tests to determine other drug actions on VT in addition to effects on inducibility by programmed stimulation. These are illustrated schematically in Figure 1. One of these assays measures the frequency of stimulation required to produce VT. A continuous

From BN Singh, HJJ Wellens, M Hiraoka, (eds): *Electropharmacological Control of Cardiac Arrhythmias*. Mount Kisco, NY, Futura Publishing Company Inc., © 1994.

NEW MEASURES OF ANTIARRHYTHMIC AND PROARRHYTHMIC DRUG ACTION

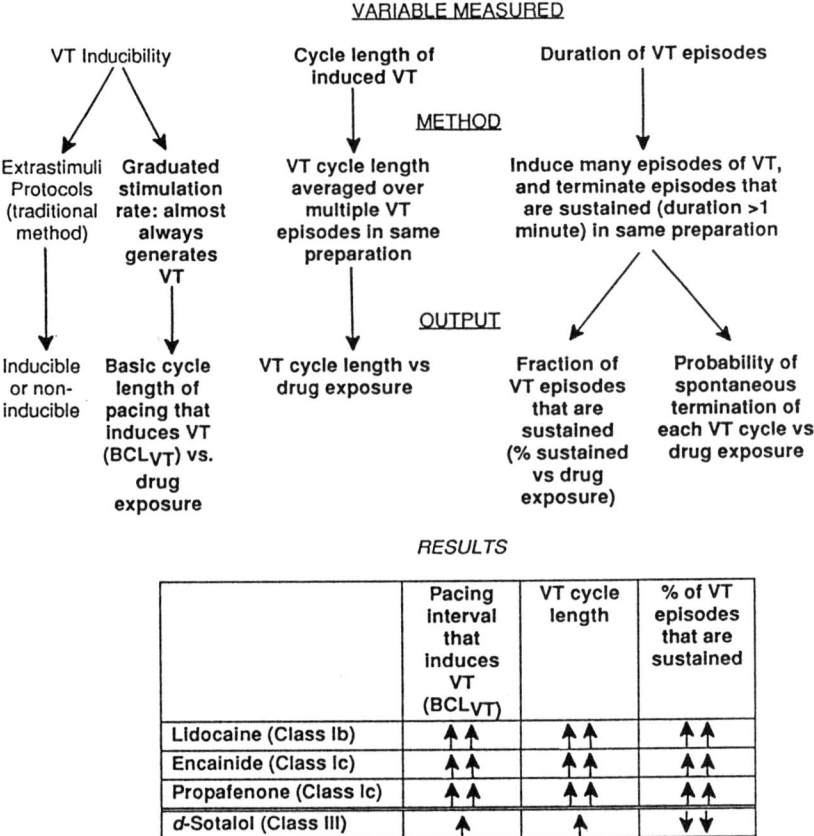

Figure 1. Overview of experimental measures of antiarrhythmic and proarrhythmic drug action in reentrant ventricular tachycardia (VT). Bold lettering indicates techniques and results of our new assays.

train of stimulation with slowly increasing frequency is applied to the heart. This aggressive stimulation protocol almost always succeeds in generating VT, with or without the drug being present. This test differs from the common technique of determining if premature stimulation in the presence of the drug succeeds or fails to induce VT. We consider a drug effect to be antiarrhythmic if it requires that a faster stimulation rate be applied before VT is generated, and proarrhythmic if slower stimulation rates will start VT. Another variable that we measure is the rate of the VT that results from our induction procedure. Since

a slow VT may be tolerated much better than a fast one, a drug's effect of substantially slowing the VT rate is antiarrhythmic. The third variable we measure is perhaps the most important: the duration of the episodes of the induced VT. Our protocols allow induction of multiple episodes of VT, and we have found that there are profound differences in the likelihood of spontaneous termination of a VT episode in the presence of different drugs. An arrhythmic episode that only lasts a few beats will certainly not cause the hemodynamic compromise of a sustained VT, and it may be less likely to lead to ventricular fibrillation.

Thus, enhancement of the probability of spontaneous termination may be a potent antiarrhythmic effect, whereas reducing this probability is an undesirable proarrhythmic drug action. We present our results by counting the number of episodes that are sustained (lasting longer than 1 minute) and the number that are nonsustained (terminating spontaneously in less than 1 minute). Drug effects are then displayed as the dose-dependent ratio of the number of sustained episodes to the total number of episodes. We also present an alternative index to describe drug effects on termination: the probability of termination with each cycle of the VT.

The Model: Reentry in the Left Ventricular Subepicardium of Isolated Rabbit Heart

Most experimental studies of drug action on VTs arising from reentry have been performed using the chronic canine infarcted heart in vivo.[5] Our studies use a preparation in which reentry causes VT, but it is neither canine, chronic, infarcted, nor in vivo. It consists of an isolated Langendorff perfused rabbit heart that has been treated with a cryogenic procedure to produce a substrate for reentry (Figure 2). The technique has previously been described in detail.[6,7] Briefly, the procedure is to circulate liquid nitrogen for 6 minutes through a cannula inserted through the mitral valve into the left ventricle with the heart immersed in a 30°C bath of Tyrode's solution. The epicardial surface is exposed to the warm, oxygenated Tyrode's solution in the bath and thus kept alive while the endocardial and midwall tissue is killed by freezing. After thawing, the heart is returned to perfusion for a 30-minute equilibration period before any electrophysiological measurements are made. The perfusate is normal Tyrode's solution to which bovine serum albumin is added to enhance electrophysiological stability.[8] Internal left

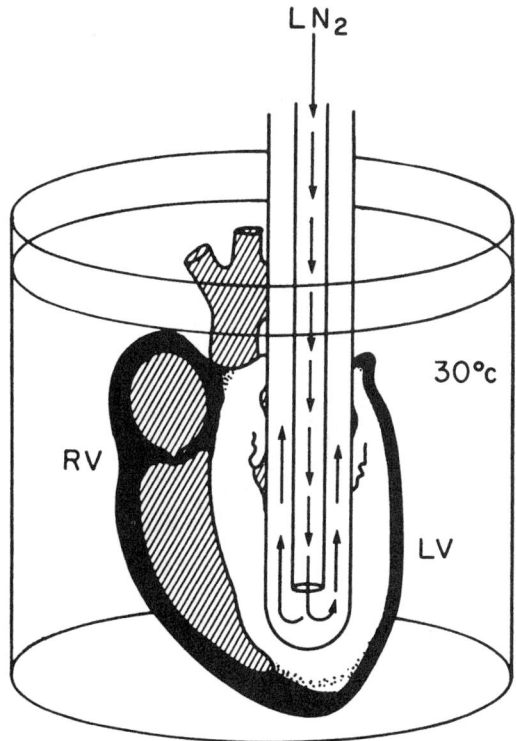

Figure 2. Cryogenic freezing technique used with rabbit heart to create thin left ventricular (LV) subepicardial conduction layer that supports reentrant ventricular tachycardia (VT). Liquid nitrogen (LN₂) is circulated through a freezing tube for 6 minutes, freezing LV endocardium and mid-wall (indicated as white areas). Left ventricular subepicardium and right ventricular (RV) free wall are protected from freezing by contact with warm stirred Tyrode's solution. (Reproduced with permission from Reference 7.)

ventricular (LV) temperature is maintained at 38.5 ± 0.5°C.

This freezing procedure kills the LV endocardial and mid-wall tissue while sparing the outer 1 mm of subepicardium and epicardium (Figure 3). The cells in this surviving thin layer have normal action potential upstroke velocity and duration[6] and are able to support reentrant activation around a functional barrier[6,9–11] or around an epicardial lesion produced by touching a cryoprobe to the surface.[12–14]

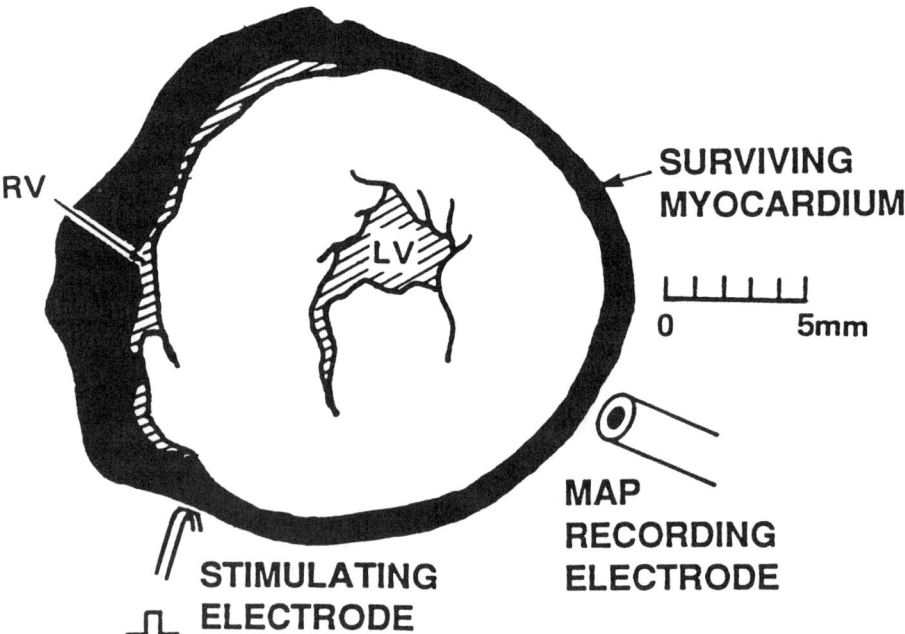

Figure 3. Tracing of cross section of Langendorff perfused rabbit heart after cryogenic procedure shown in Figure 2. Heart was stained with tetrazolium dye[7] that renders surviving right ventricle (RV) and thin rim of subepicardial left ventricle (LV) dark; killed tissue is white. This section was taken mid-way between base and apex; placement of stimulating and monophasic action potential (MAP) recording electrode is shown. (Reproduced with permission from Reference 15.)

Electrophysiological Methods

Electrical stimulation to the epicardium was applied through bipolar electrodes located on the LV anterior surface adjacent to the interventricular groove, as illustrated in Figure 3. Activation was recorded from a monophasic action potential (MAP) electrode on the LV lateral free wall. Effective and functional refractory periods (ERP, FRP) were determined by increasing the coupling interval of a premature stimulus (twice diastolic threshold, constant current mode) following 20 regularly paced beats until capture was seen as the recording electrode. Conduction time (CT) was measured as the delay between delivery of a stimulus and activation at the recording electrode, located 10–15 mm away. Other details of the stimulation and recording were as previously described.[7,15]

Experimental Protocols

The protocols measured electrophysiological variables (ERP, FRP, CT) and VT characteristics (pacing cycle length that induced VT, VT cycle interval, and proportion of VT episodes with durations greater than 1 minute) under control conditions and during exposure to increasing concentrations of antiarrhythmic drugs. Three of the drugs were Class I: lidocaine (Sigma Chemical Co., St. Louis, MO), encainide (Mead-Johnson Pharmaceutical Co., Evansville, IN), and propafenone (Knoll Pharmaceuticals, Whippany, NJ). One Class III drug, d-sotalol (Bristol Myers, New York, NY), was also tested. Each preparation was exposed to three levels of a particular drug at relative concentrations of approximately 1, 2, and 4. The intermediate level for each drug was chosen in preliminary experiments so as to increase ERP by 20% to 30%

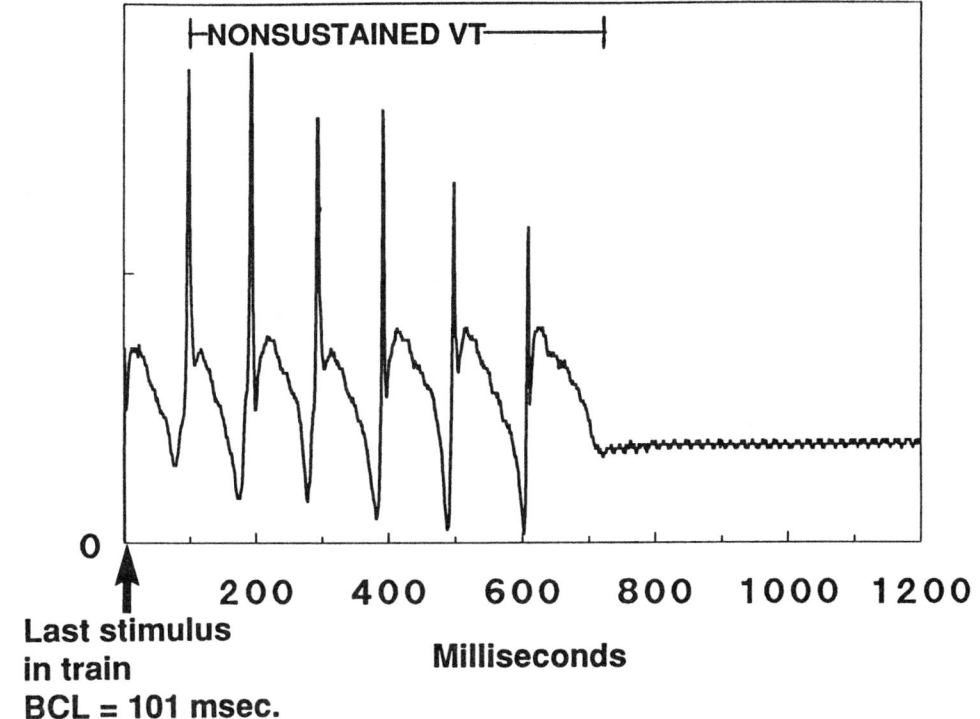

├─NONSUSTAINED VT───────┤

0

Last stimulus in train

Milliseconds

A **BCL = 101 msec.**

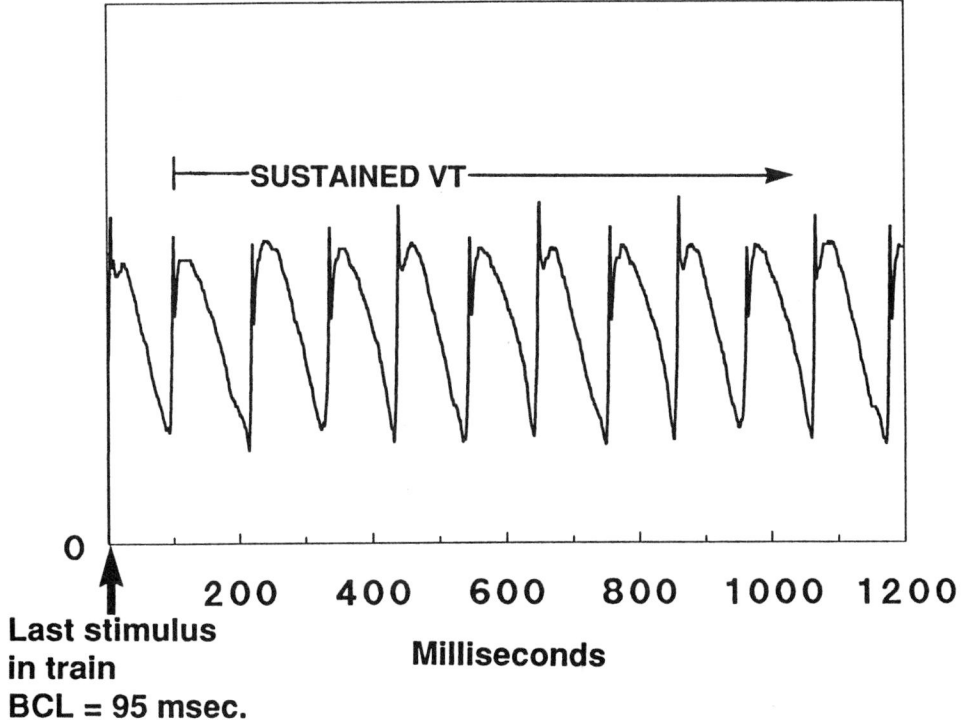

├─SUSTAINED VT───────────→

0

Last stimulus in train

Milliseconds

B **BCL = 95 msec.**

Figure 4. A: Fast pacing (basic cycle length = 101 msec) resulted in a nonsustained ventricular tachycardia (VT) consisting of six extra nondriven beats. **B:** Another episode of VT in the same preparation did not spontaneously terminate. After 1 minute, such episodes were terminated by pouring cool Tyrode's solution over the left ventricular (LV) surface and then rewarming. (Reproduced with permission from Reference 15.)

at a moderately fast drive rate (200-msec basic cycle length [BCL] of pacing).

Effective and functional refractory periods and CT were measured under control conditions by pacing at BCLs of 300, 200, 180, 160, and 150 msec. Measurements were then continued as the BCL was reduced in 10-msec increments (ie, 140, 130, 120 msec, etc.) until either a VT was produced or we could not achieve 1 : 1 following of the response to the stimulus.

We then initiated VTs with pacing at fast BCLs using a stimulator having a continuously variable rate. We determined the onset of VT by observing the recording electrode's signal on an oscilloscope as the BCL was gradually reduced. The oscilloscope trigger was synchronized to the delivery of the stimulus. When the pacing rate was slow, the recorded activity was synchronous with this stimulus. When the BCL was reduced to a critical value, the response lost its synchronization with the stimulus, thereby signaling the onset of a VT episode. Stimulation was halted at this time, and we continued to record the response from the MAP electrode. Since both the stimulus train and the responses were continuously recorded during this process, we could reconstruct the onset of each VT episode and determine the pacing BCL that generated it (eg, BCL = 101 msec in Figure 4A). This value of BCL is defined as BCL_{VT}.

Each episode of VT either terminated spontaneously (classified as nonsustained; eg, Figure 4A) or, if it persisted for 1 minute (classified as sustained; eg, Figure 4B), was terminated by pouring cool Tyrode's solution over the left ventricle. After such cooling, Tyrode's solution at 40°C was then poured over the ventricle to rewarm it quickly. The stimulation procedure for generating another VT was then repeated, and in this manner we generated as many episodes of VT as possible in 30 minutes (typically 25–40 episodes).

We then repeated these procedures under conditions of drug exposure. Each preparation was exposed to increasing concentrations of either lidocaine (free base form, 7.5, 15, and 30 μM), encainide (1, 2, and 4 μM), propafenone HCl (0.1, 0.3, and 0.6 μM) or d-sotalol (25, 50, and 100 μM). Each drug was applied to five preparations. After each increase in drug concentration, we waited 15 minutes before repeating the 30-minute period of stimulating VT episodes.

We also carried out two control experiments to determine if time-dependent changes occurred in the VT characteristics. Each preparation was subjected to four runs of the VT induction protocols without being exposed to drugs. We changed Tyrode's solution between runs and used the same waiting times as in the drug studies. Thus, these control preparations were measured at intervals similar to those of the drug exposed preparations.

Data Analysis

We used 1/CT as an indication of the average conduction velocity (CV) across the epicardial surface and for each preparation normalized the control values at the slow pacing rate (BCL = 300 msec) to 100%. The values of CV following drug exposure and fast pacing are, therefore, presented relative to these normalized control values. In the same way, the values of ERP and FRP during fast pacing and/ or drug exposure are presented as means of each preparation's relative value of that variable compared to its control value at the slow pacing rate.

BCL_{VT} was measured as the average of the last four stimulus cycle lengths before the stimulus was turned off. Tachycardia cycle lengths were measured as the mean interval between the first 10 consecutive beats of the VT episode. If the episode lasted for fewer than 10 beats, the mean was taken from the total number of extra beats.

Results

We have reported that action potential duration in control hearts of this preparation remain relatively constant for at least 3 hours.[7]

We also found in control hearts no time-dependent variations in VT induction characteristics, cycle time, and spontaneous termination that would account for the effects seen during drug exposure.[15]

Spontaneous Ventricular Tachycardia Termination: Class I Drugs Have the Opposite Effect from d–Sotalol

The most striking of our findings is that the Class I drugs increased the incidence of episodes of sustained VT, while the Class III drug d-sotalol decreased it (Figure 5). Our aggressive VT initiation procedure resulted in multiple episodes of VT under all control conditions and in most drug exposed conditions. The only drug that prevented VT induction was d-sotalol at high concentrations in two preparations (Figure 5D).

The fraction of episodes of VT that were sustained increased in a dose-dependent manner for every preparation exposed to Class I drugs. This increase was statistically significant in 4 of 5 propafenone preparations, 3 of 5 encainide preparations, and 3 of 5 lidocaine preparations ($p < 0.025$, Cochran's test of linear trend of proportions[16]). The fraction of sustained episodes decreased in a dose-dependent manner for all preparations exposed to d-sotalol, with the decrease being significant in 3 of the 5 preparations ($p < 0.002$).

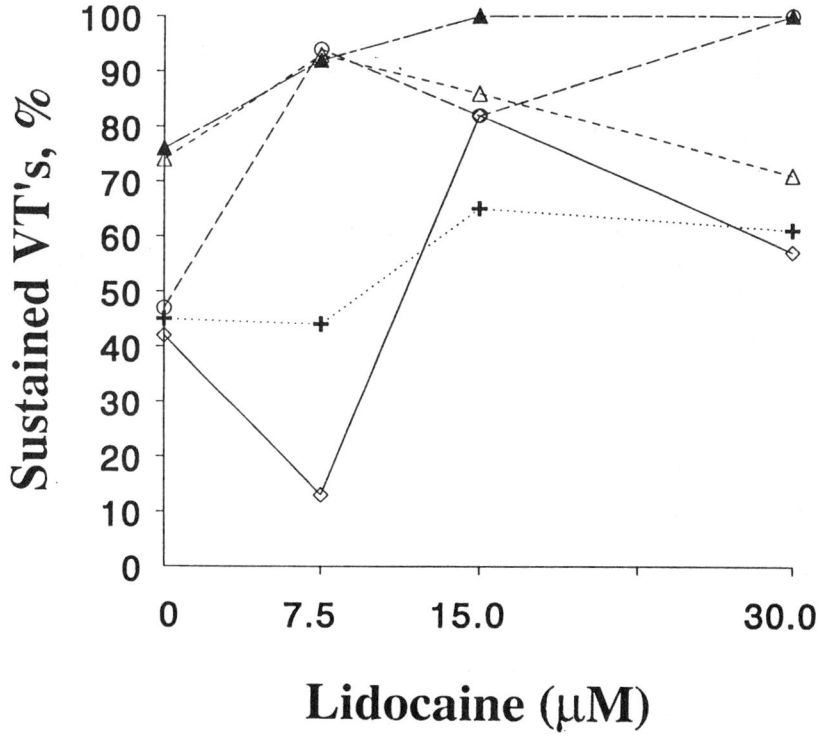

Figure 5. Fraction of ventricular tachycardia (VT) episodes that were sustained (duration > 1 minute) as a function of exposure to lidocaine (a), encainide (b), propafenone (c), and d-sotalol (d). Two of the preparations exposed to d-sotalol (#311 and #710) could not be stimulated to produce VT at the higher drug concentrations. The fraction of sustained episodes increased in a concentration-dependent manner with exposure to the three Class I drugs (a, b, and c) while decreasing with exposure to d-sotalol. (Modified with permission from Reference 15.)

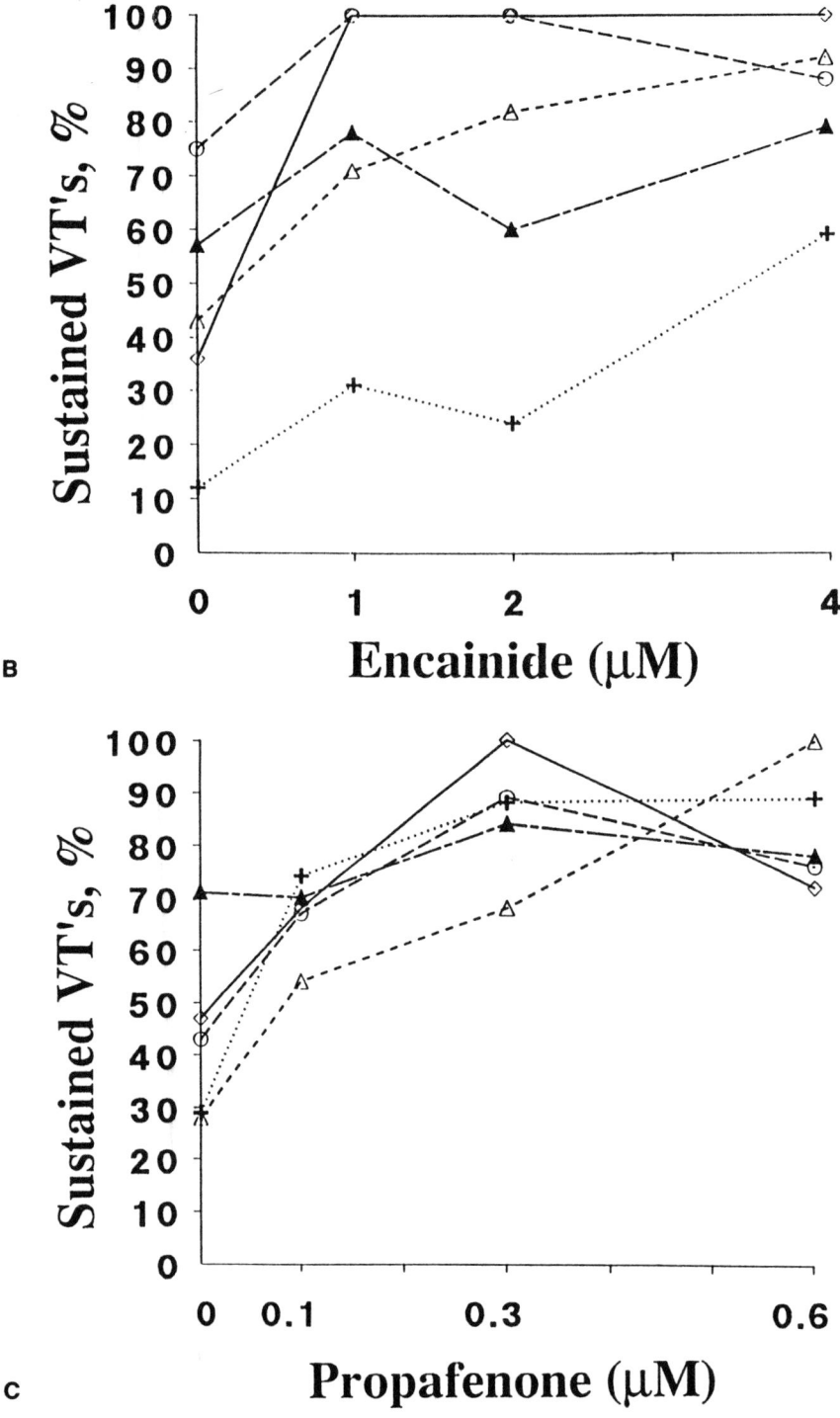

B

C

Figure 5. *(continued)*

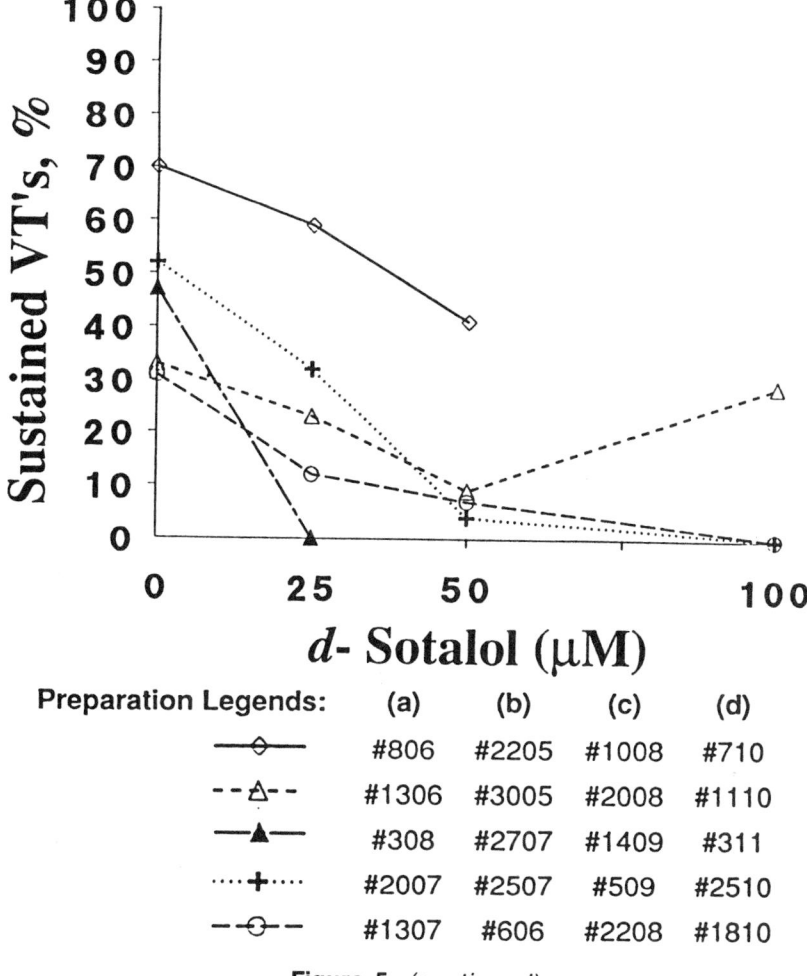

Figure 5. *(continued)*

Basic Cycle Length for Ventricular Tachycardia Induction: All Drugs Increased It

The mean BCL of pacing that induced VT (BCL$_{VT}$) was prolonged by the Class I drugs and d-sotalol (Figure 6); ie, VT was induced at slower pacing rates. All preparations showed a perfect correlation of increasing BCL$_{VT}$ with increasing drug concentration (r_S = 1.0, Spearman's rank correlation coefficient). The perfect correlation for 5 of 5 preparations exposed to each drug is highly significant ($p <$ 0.0001).

Exposure to the high doses of the Class I drugs prolonged BCL$_{VT}$ relatively more than exposure to d-sotalol. The average increase in BCL$_{VT}$ was 198% for lidocaine, 184% for encainide, and 203% for propafenone, compared to 158% for d-sotalol.

Ventricular Tachycardia Cycle Interval: All Drugs Slowed Ventricular Tachycardia

The VT cycle interval increased with increasing dosage for each drug; ie, the VT rate was slowed. Figure 7 shows that all drugs had an increasing VT cycle interval that was correlated with increasing concentration (r_S = 1.0 for all encainide, propafenone, and d-sotalol

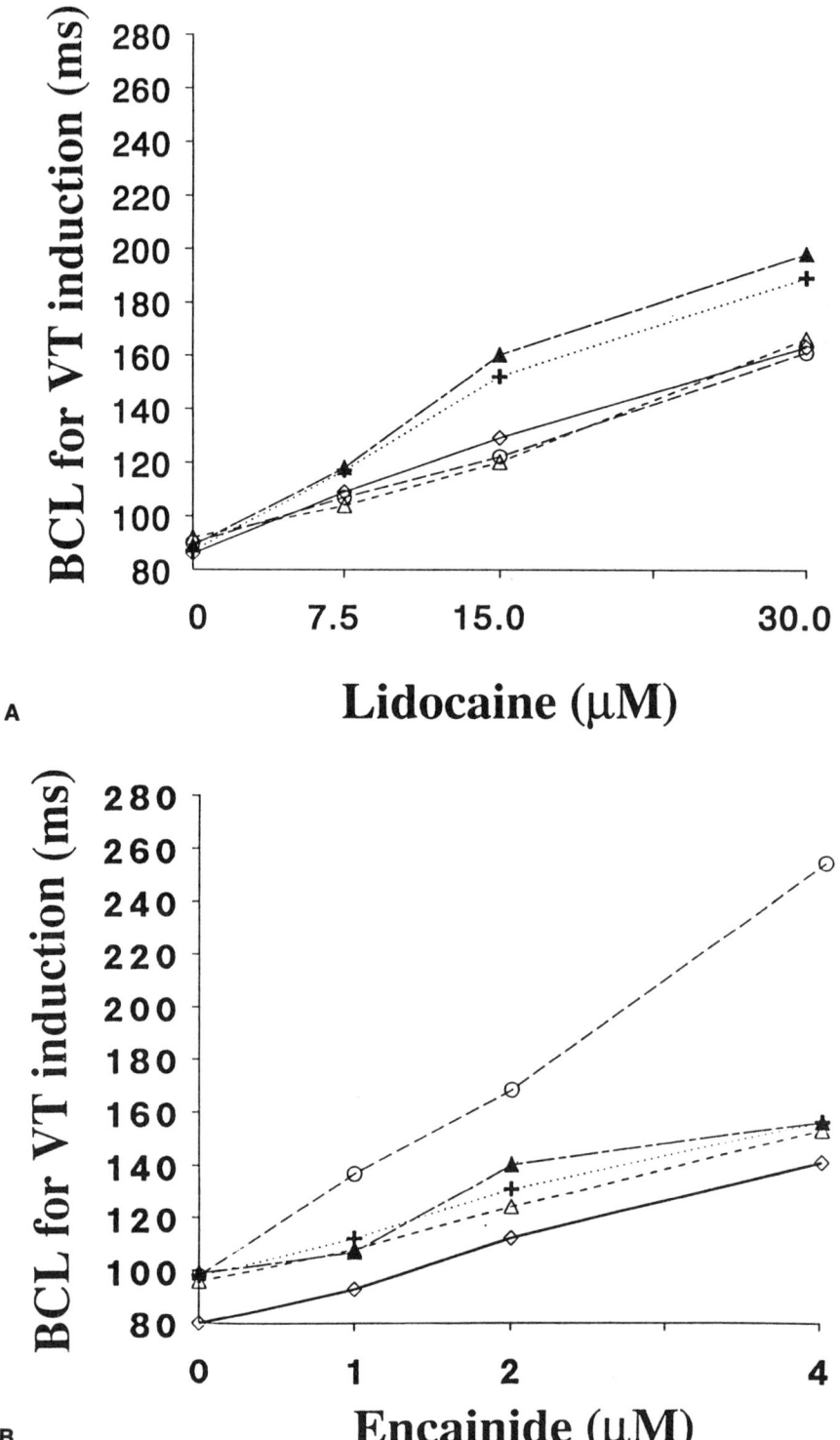

A

Lidocaine (μM)

B

Encainide (μM)

Figure 6. Basic cycle length of pacing at which ventricular tachycardia (VT) was induced (BCL$_{VT}$) as a function of exposure to lidocaine (a), encainide (b), propafenone (c), and d-sotalol (d). Preparation legends are the same as in Figure 5. All drugs produced a concentration-dependent increase in BCL$_{VT}$; increase was smallest for d-sotalol. (Modified with permission from Reference 15.)

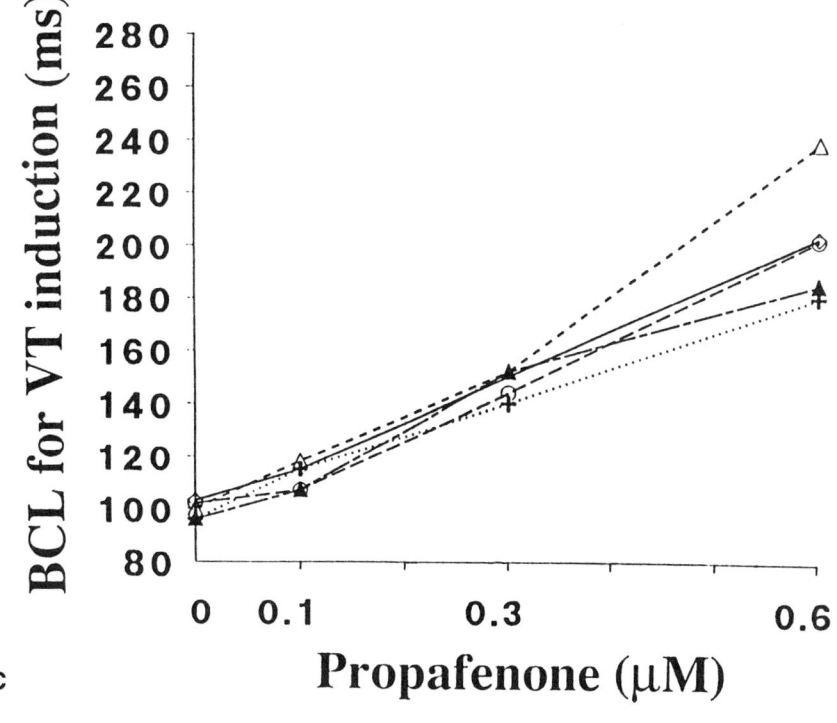

C

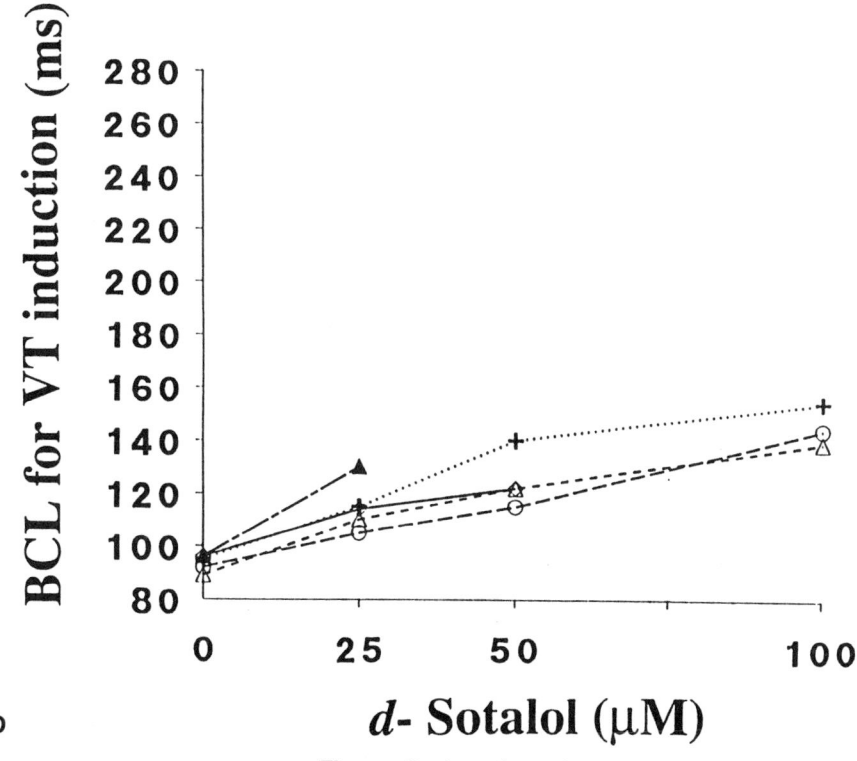

D

Figure 6. *(continued)*

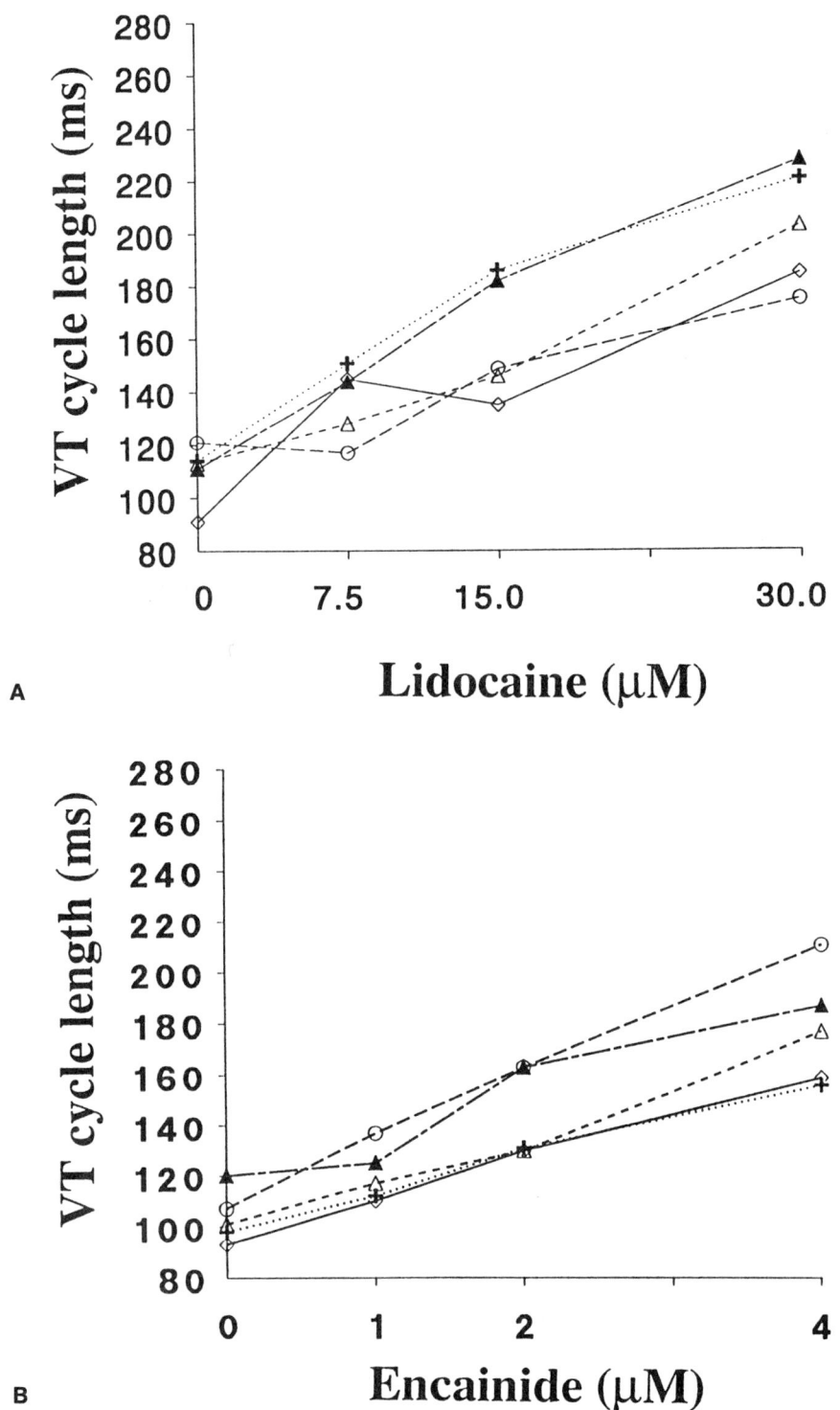

Figure 7. Cycle length of ventricular tachycardia (VT) as a function of exposure to lidocaine (a), encainide (b), propafenone (c), and d-sotalol (d). All drugs produced dose-dependent slowing; d-sotalol had the smallest effect. Preparation legends are the same as in Figure 5. (Modified with permission from Reference 15.)

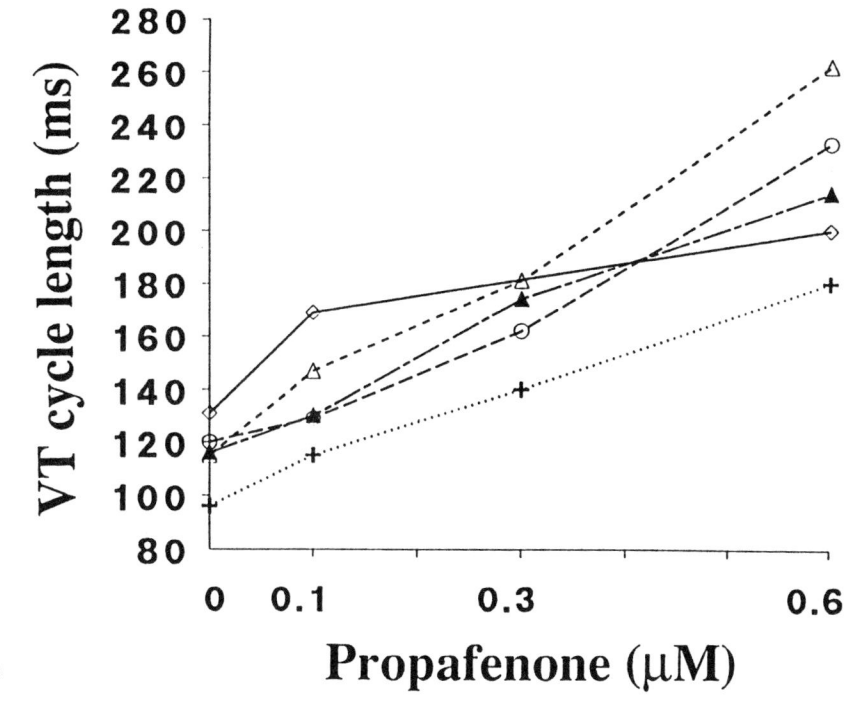

C

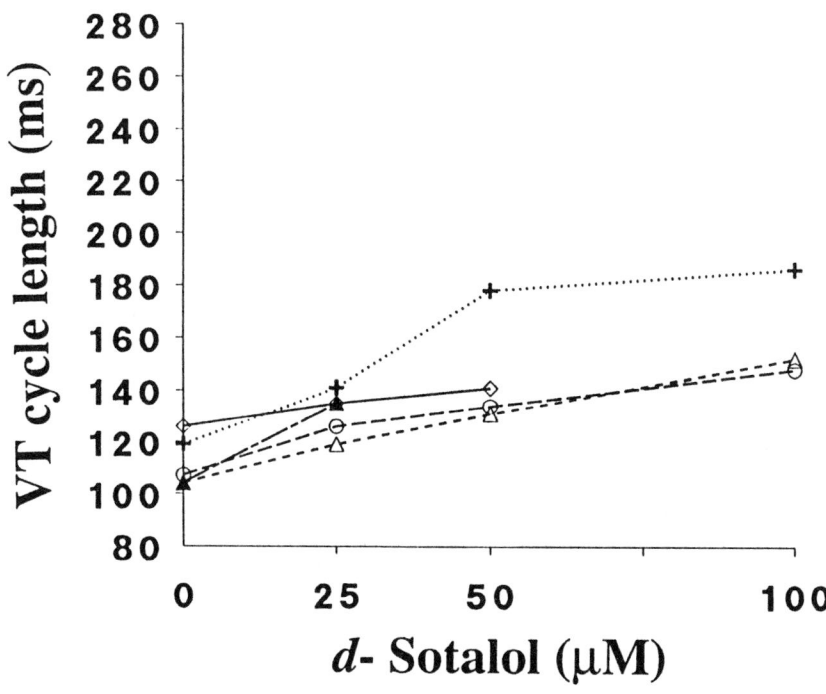

D

Figure 7. *(continued)*

preparation, $r_S > 0$ for all lidocaine preparations). These correlations across 5 of 5 preparations exposed to each drug are significant ($p < 0.04$ for lidocaine, $p < 0.001$ for all others).

The Class I drugs at high concentrations prolonged the VT intervals relatively more than d-sotalol did: 185% for lidocaine, 172% for encainide, and 190% for propafenone, compared to 147% for d-sotalol.

Drugs Effects on Refractory Period and Conduction Velocity

The effects of all four drugs are shown in Table 1. The results obtained at three different pacing intervals are presented; not every preparation could be measured during drug exposure at faster intervals (200 and 160 msec) because episodes of VT were generated (eg, Figure 6) or 1:1 following the response to the stimulus was lost. Under drug-free conditions there was no change in CV as BCL was decreased to 160 msec. However, all Class I drugs caused a frequency- and dose-dependent slowing, while d-sotalol produced only minimal velocity reduction at high exposures and fast rates. All drugs prolonged refractory periods at each drive rate as compared to the control values at that rate, and this prolongation was greater at the higher drug concentrations.

Discussion

What do these results tell us about desirable and undesirable actions of drugs on arrhythmias? We believe that the tests we have described are most relevant to VT arising in the presence of myocardial scarring caused by a chronic infarct (a condition existing in many survivors of myocardial infarction who are at elevated risk for sudden cardiac death). We have described new measures of pro- and antiarrhythmic action within an experimental model of this condition in the belief that broad classifications of drug action, such as that of Singh and Vaughan Williams,[1-3] are best interpreted within the context of an ar-

rhythmia whose cause is known. For instance, our finding that d-sotalol causes VTs to terminate quickly is likely correlated with its Class III action of action potential prolongation, whereas the velocity depression resulting from the sodium channel block of Class I agents likely causes their proarrhythmic effect of reducing spontaneous termination. The same Class III action that results in antiarrhythmic action against ventricular reentry, however, produced proarrhythmic early afterdepolarizations in the presence of lowered potassium.[17,18] Conversely, the depression of sodium current that depresses CV and is probably proarrhythmic for sustained reentry may prevent such abnormal automaticity.[19] Ultimately, we may be able to develop a drug that optimizes antiarrhythmic action against all forms of VT. A helpful approach to that task is using assays such as ours to test effectiveness against arrhythmias arising from well-known causes.

In the context of reentry, our results indicate two substantial drawbacks that seem to be associated with drugs that delay conduction by sodium channel block: arrhythmias are generated at slower pacing rates, and, more importantly, any particular episode of VT is more likely to be sustained rather than spontaneously terminating. The Class III action of d-sotalol also seems to allow VTs to start at slower pacing rates, but not as slow as the Class I drugs for a given degree of prolongation of refractoriness. Unlike the Class I drugs, d-sotalol increased the likelihood that an arrhythmia would spontaneously terminate.

The propensity for reentrant VT to start at slower rates during exposure to the Class I drugs may be caused by shortening of the wavelength (WL) of refractoriness associated with these drugs.[20] This wavelength is the spatial extent of refractory tissue lying behind the excitation front of a traveling cardiac impulse and is the product of the FRP and the CV: WL = FRP × CV.[21] This wavelength must be smaller than the length of the reentrant circuit for a reentrant impulse to not collide with its own tail of refractoriness.

The effect of fast pacing under drug-free

Table 1
Electrophysiological Effects of Lidocaine, Encainide, Propafenone, and d-Sotalol

	n	Conduction velocity	FRP	ERP
		Absolute values at slow drive rate (BCL = 300 msec)		
Control	19	(relative values only)	153 ± 3 msec	136 ± 4 msec
		Relative values at slow drive rate (BCL = 300 msec)		
Control	19	100%	100%	100%
Lidocaine				
7.5 μM	5	106 ± 6%	117 ± 3%	119 ± 3%
30 μM	5	98 ± 9%	159 ± 5%	161 ± 3%
Encainide				
1 μM	4	92 ± 4%	107 ± 1%	110 ± 4%
4 μM	4	62 ± 1%	127 ± 5%	134 ± 5%
Propafenone				
0.1 μM	5	97 ± 2%	109 ± 3%	114 ± 5%
0.6 μM	5	65 ± 6%	128 ± 6%	132 ± 10%
d-Sotalol				
25 μM	5	102 ± 3%	117 ± 5%	121 ± 2%
100 μM	5	93 ± 4%	137 ± 3%	140 ± 5%
		Relative values at intermediate drive rate (BCL = 200 msec)		
Control	19	98 ± 1%	86 ± 1%	87 ± 1%
Lidocaine				
7.5 μM	5	94 ± 6%	100 ± 2%	102 ± 3%
30 μM	4	65 ± 10%	134 ± 5%	137 ± 4%
Encainide				
1 μM	4	89 ± 3%	94 ± 1%	96 ± 2%
4 μM	3	57 ± 1%	108 ± 1%	113 ± 4%
Propafenone				
0.1 μM	5	91 ± 2%	92 ± 2%	96 ± 4%
0.6 μM	3	47 ± 6%	115 ± 10%	111 ± 20%
d-Sotalol				
25 μM	5	99 ± 2%	96 ± 1%	98 ± 2%
100 μM	3	92 ± 4%	113 ± 4%	117 ± 4%
		Relative values at fast drive rate (BCL = 160 msec)		
Control	19	98 ± 1%	77 ± 1%	79 ± 1%
Lidocaine				
7.5 μM	5	86 ± 5%	90 ± 2%	89 ± 3%
30 μM	2	60 ± 8%	100 ± 4%	110 ± 4%
Encainide				
1 μM	4	86 ± 3%	84 ± 2%	84 ± 3%
4 μM	3	53 ± 2%	99 ± 3%	93 ± 4%
Propafenone				
0.1 μM	5	86 ± 2%	85 ± 3%	87 ± 3%
0.6 μM		No preparations could be stimulated at this fast drive rate.		
d-Sotalol				
25 μM	5	96 ± 3%	84 ± 2%	84 ± 3%
100 μM	2	91 ± 4%	96 ± 1%	99 ± 1%

All values given ± SEM. BCL: basic cycle length; FRP: functional refractory period; ERP: effective refractory period.

conditions is to shrink the wavelength. At fast rates the refractory period is reduced. This is primarily due to shortening of the action potential duration. At very fast rates, close to the maximum stimulation rate of the tissue, there is also a modest reduction in CV. These two factors combine to cause a rate-dependent decrease in wavelength, as seen in Figure 8. For these figures, relative values of wavelength were calculated from the measurements of FRP and CV, with all values normalized to 100% at a pacing BCL = 300 msec. On the same graphs histograms are plotted showing the distribution of BCLs that started VT episodes (BCL_{VT}). Under control conditions, VTs were generated in the range of BCL_{VT} = 80–110 msec. At these rates, the wavelength was 50% to 60% of its value at BCL = 300 msec. During exposure to Class I drugs, the wavelength was reduced to this

range at slower pacing rates (BCL > 140 msec in these examples), and VTs were generated at these slower rates.

The Class I drug effects on wavelength result from two opposing actions: the drugs increase the FRP while decreasing the CV. If these effects were equal, they would cancel each other in the equation WL = FRP × CV, and the wavelength would not be affected by the drugs. However, the relative effects of the drugs are frequency dependent, as can be seen for lidocaine (Figure 8A). At BCL = 300 msec, lidocaine prolongs refractoriness relatively more than it reduces CV. The net effect is to increase the wavelength over its control value at this rate. At faster rates (BCL < 200 msec) this relationship reverses: lidocaine's depression of CV is more pronounced than its enhancement of refractoriness, and wavelength is reduced relative to the control wave-

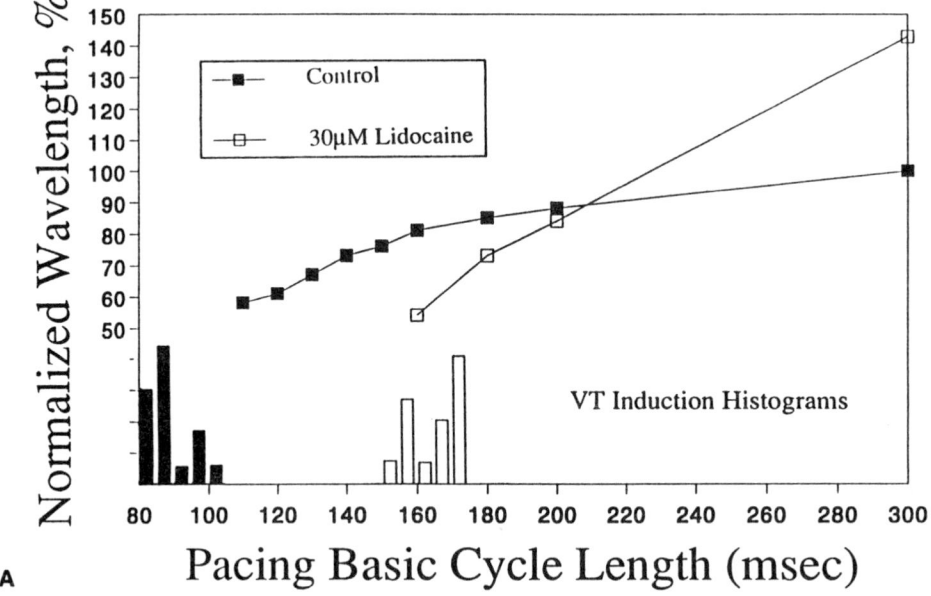

A

Figure 8. Frequency-dependent changes in the wavelength of refractoriness plotted with histograms showing distribution of basic cycle lengths (BCLs) that induced ventricular tachycardia (VT). Lidocaine (a) prolonged the wavelength at the slow (300 msec) pacing interval, but shortened it at intervals less than 200 msec. Encainide (b) and propafenone (c) shortened wavelengths at all pacing intervals used. The wavelength at which VTs are induced appears to be similar in the control and drug exposed condition. The effect of all three Class I drugs was to shift both the wavelength curve and the VT induction histograms to the right. As a result, VTs were induced at slower pacing intervals during exposure to these drugs. A: preparation #806; B: preparation #2707; C: preparation #509.

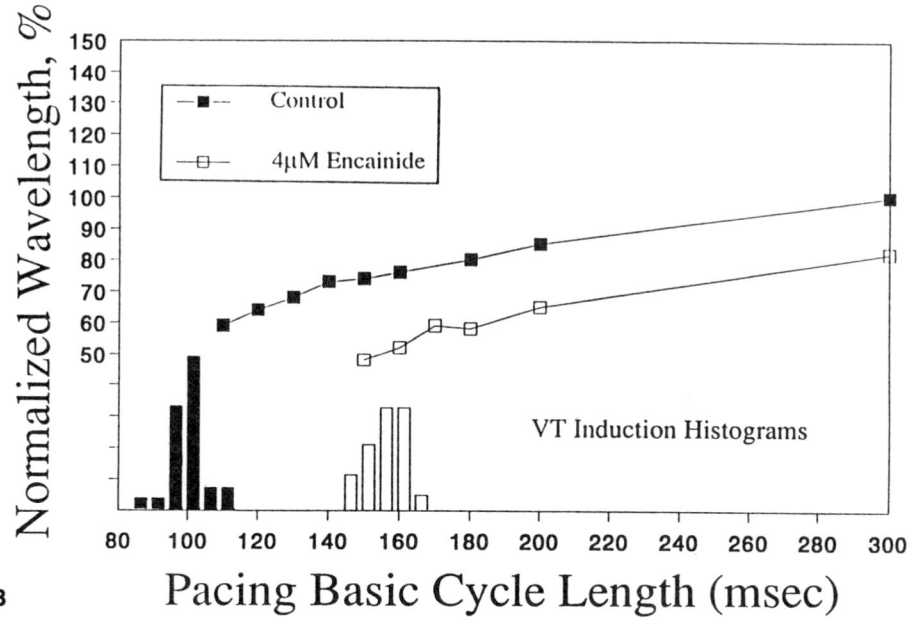

B

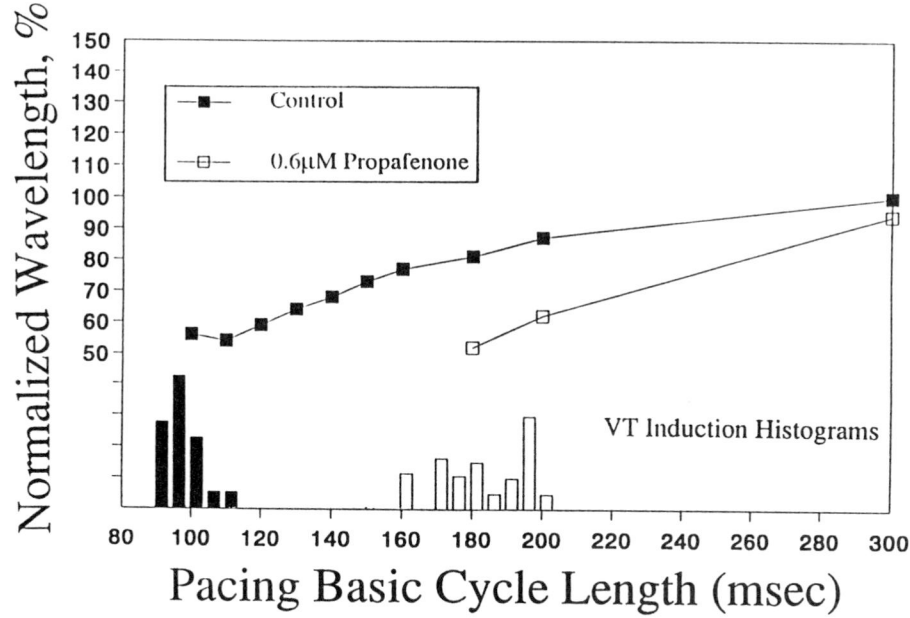

C

Figure 8. *(continued)*

length. The crossover point at 200 msec occurs close to the time constant for lidocaine unbinding from sodium channels[22]; at pacing intervals faster than this, the partial block of sodium channels is increased, and substantial velocity reduction occurs. Encainide and propafenone both have much slower time constants for drug unbinding (> 10 seconds[22]) and thus slow CV even at BCL = 300 msec (Table 1). Consequently, wavelength is reduced relative to controls at all pacing rates tested.

The net result, for all three Class I drugs tested, is that the curve of wavelength versus pacing BCL is shifted to the right: wavelength reduction occurs at slower pacing rates during drug exposure. If this shift is sufficiently large, the wavelength may get reduced to its critical size for supporting reentry at heart rates that are at the high end of the normal physiological range. It is likely that such an effect underlies the occurrence of exercise-induced VT seen in patients being treated with flecainide, another Class I drug with slow time constant for unbinding from sodium channels.[22] In the case of these drugs, the relative value of prolonging refractoriness versus depressing conduction is easily assessed as regards VT initiation: when velocity is reduced more than refractoriness is prolonged, proarrhythmic tendencies appear.

The effect of d-sotalol on wavelength is not as easy to assess. Even at relatively fast rates (BCL = 160), there was no significant depression of velocity, even at 100 μM concentration (Table 1). The FRP, however, was prolonged relative to controls at that rate, and thus the wavelength was increased. As we attempted to measure CV (by measuring CT) at rates very close to those that initiated VT, we observed alternans in action potential duration and CT that prevented assessing relative changes in CV. Thus we do not have wavelength data at the pacing rates that induced VT. It appears that wavelength reductions by d-sotalol, if they occur, may only appear over a narrow range of pacing rates very close to those that induce VT.

Drug Effects on the Stability of Ventricular Tachycardia

One of the advantages of this preparation is that multiple episodes of VT can be induced and tested for their tendency to spontaneously terminate. Since VT does not lead to either ventricular fibrillation or hemodynamic compromise in this model, it is possible to allow

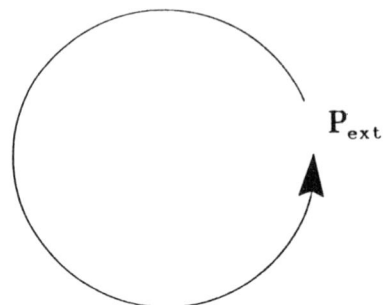

$$\mathbf{Prob(n)} = (\mathbf{P_{ext}})(1 - \mathbf{P_{ext}})^{n-1}$$

Figure 9. Derivation of geometric distribution for spontaneous termination of reentry. For each pass an impulse makes around a reentrant circuit, a fixed probability of extinction, P_{ext}, can be assigned. After $(n - 1)$ cycles, the probability that it has not extinguished is $(1 - P_{ext})^{n-1}$. Therefore, the probability that the reentry will terminate on the *n*th pass is given by $P_{ext}(1 - P_{ext})^{n-1}$

the episodes to persist long enough to classify an arrhythmia as "sustained" (our criterion was duration greater than 1 minute) and to determine the fraction of episodes that met this criterion. Moreover, drug concentrations can be precisely maintained in the perfusate so that concentration-dependent trends in VT stability can be seen.

We saw that all three Class I drugs increased the propensity toward sustained VT (ie, increased VT stability), while the single Class III drug tested decreased it. Increases in VT stability during exposure to another Class Ic drug, flecainide, have recently been observed in this model[11] and in a canine atrial tricuspid ring model of reentry.[23] The measure of stability that we present, the fraction of episodes lasting longer than 1 minute, was chosen to be analogous to classification of clinical arrhythmias as sustained or nonsustained. The choice of 1-minute duration was arbitrary; a different duration would yield different numbers, although the dose-dependent trends would still appear. Is there a way to characterize more completely the distributions of durations of VT episodes? Such a characterization would be very helpful in making decisions as to the "danger" of short runs of VT in clinical settings.

A useful approach is to consider an impulse traveling around a reentrant circuit. There is a fixed probability of extinction, P_{ext}, associated with each pass around the circuit (Figure 9). The probability that the reentry will extinguish on the nth cycle is therefore given by

$$Prob(n) = P_{ext}(1 - P_{ext})^{n-1} \qquad (1)$$

This is a geometric distribution that has been used by statisticians to analyze failure rates. Can the single parameter of this distribution, P_{ext}, provide a reasonable quantification of our observations? Figure 10 shows that it can work quite well. This scheme for quantifying short

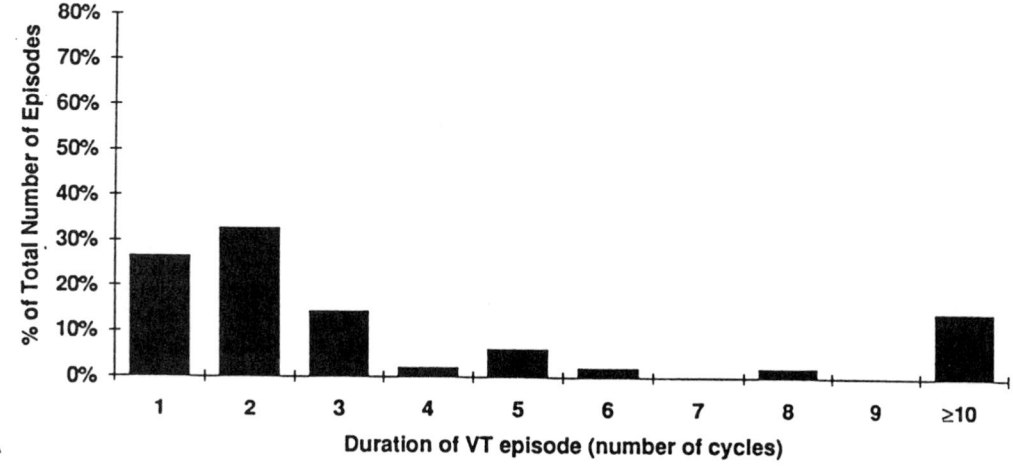

A

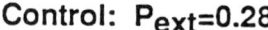

Control: $P_{ext}=0.28$

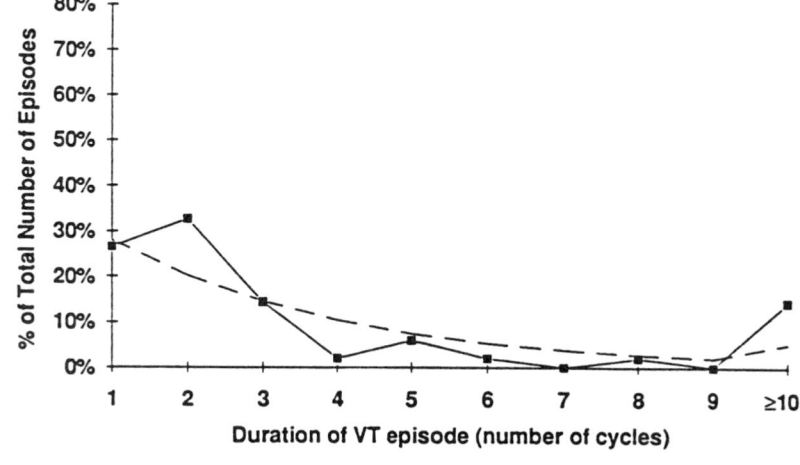

B

Figure 10. Data from drug-free preparation showing distribution of ventricular tachycardia (VT) episodes as a function of the number of cycles in the episode before termination. A: Histograms of data; B: Same data plotted (solid line) along with least-squares fit of geometric distribution for spontaneous termination (dashed line), which yields $P_{ext} = 0.28$. Preparation #2507.

runs of VT can be used in several ways. If one clinician considers that runs of more than 30 activations are dangerous then a simple calculation can be made to estimate the likelihood that a run will last longer or shorter than this. Another observer who thinks shorter runs are dangerous can make an estimation of risk for those cases. All that is needed is to estimate the single parameter P_{ext}. This can be done by generating a frequency histogram of VT episodes as a function of number of cycles in the episode, as in Figure 10A. A least-squares fit of Equation 1 to the histogram data will generate P_{ext}. These P_{ext} estimates may also prove useful in grading the differences in the arrhythmogenic substrate in different patients.

How do antiarrhythmic drugs influence the extinction probability P_{ext}? In the case of encainide (Figure 11) we find that P_{ext} decreases with drug exposure, meaning that an

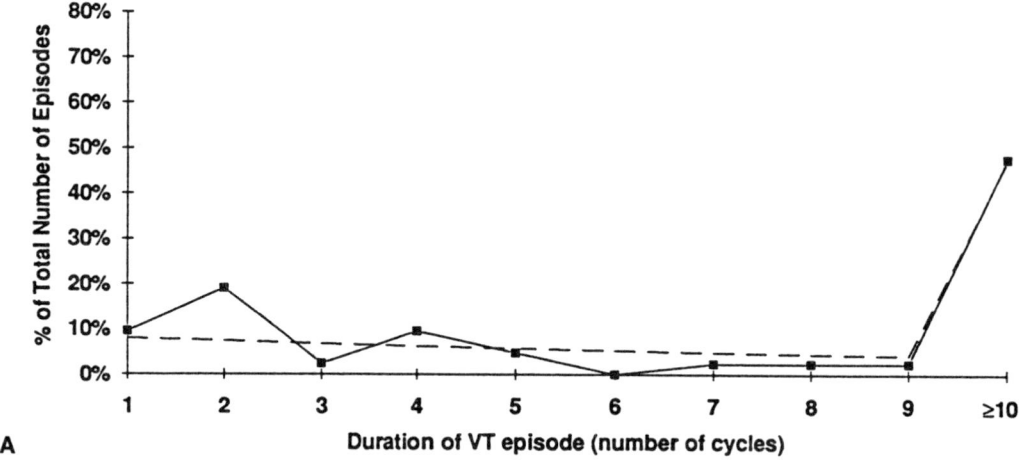

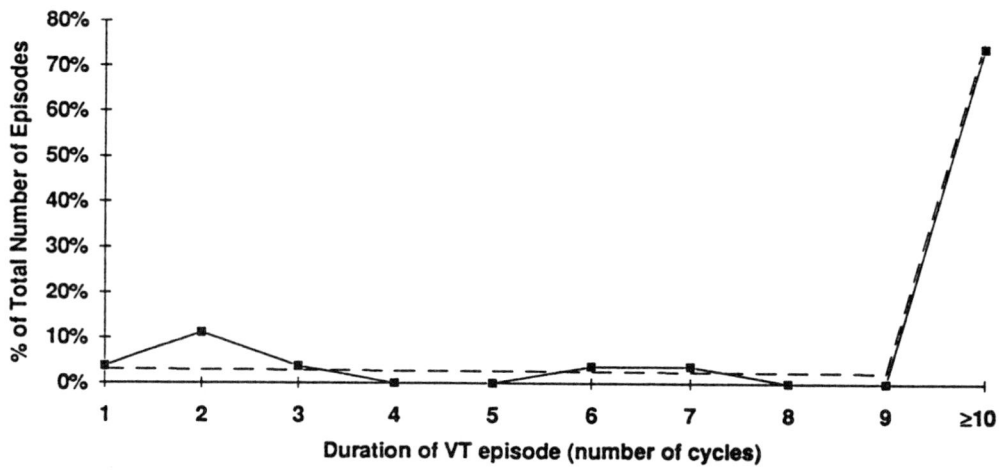

Figure 11. Effects of encainide on P_{ext}. As encainide concentration was increased, P_{ext} changed from 0.28 (control) → 0.08 (1 μM) → 0.15 (2 μM) → 0.03 (4 μM). Preparation #2507, as in Figure 10. Graphs show geometric distribution fit (dashed lines) and data (solid lines).

episode of VT is more likely to be sustained (ie, less likely to extinguish) with drug treatment.

Summary

We have described new assays of antiarrhythmic and proarrhythmic drug action on one particular form of arrhythmia: VT caused by reentry. We found that all drugs tested were antiarrhythmic in one test (they slowed VT rates) and proarrhythmic in another (allowing VTs to be generated at slower pacing rates). There was a difference between Class I drugs and d-sotalol in the third measure: the Class I drugs appear to decrease the likelihood of spontaneous termination of VT while d-sotalol increases this probability. As with all experimental models of clinical conditions, one must be aware of the differences between this in vitro model of VT and human VT. In the rabbit heart preparation, reentry occurs in a thin layer of ostensibly normal myocardial cells without the heterogeneous scarring often found in human infarcts. In this respect the arrhythmia resembles VT seen in the epicardial border zone of canine infarcts, when the thin surviving tissue lies over chronically infarcted muscle and reentry is around a functional (as opposed to anatomical) obstacle.[24] We would hope that these assays will add to the picture of how drugs affect VT and will help to understand better how their basic electrophysiological actions impact on their clinical profile. In attempting to establish rational bases for developing new therapeutic agents, it should prove helpful to have in vitro tests not only for reentry, but also for arrhythmias caused by afterdepolarizations and acute ischemia. At the very least, the picture of drug action that evolves can suggest which clinical conditions may be helped or harmed by the drug. At best, the tests would efficiently screen the many possible compounds currently being developed and help identify the strongest candidates having the fewest undesirable proarrhythmic actions.

References

1. Singh BN, Vaughan Williams EM: A third class of antiarrhythmic action. Effects on atrial and ventricular intracellular potentials and other pharmacological actions on cardiac muscle of MJ 1999 and AH 3474. *Br J Pharmacol* 39:675, 1970.
2. Vaughan Williams EM: A classification of antiarrhythmic actions reassessed after a decade of new drugs. *J Clin Pharmacol* 24:129, 1984.
3. Singh BN, Vaughan Williams EM: A fourth class of antiarrhythmic action? Effect of verapamil on ouabain toxicity, on atrial and ventricular intracellular potentials, and on other features of cardiac function. *Cardiovasc Res* 6:109, 1972.
4. Surawicz B: Ventricular arrhythmias: why is it so difficult to find a pharmacologic cure? *J Am Coll Cardiol* 14:1401, 1989.
5. Janse MJ, Wit AL: Electrophysiological mechanisms of ventricular arrhythmias resulting from myocardial ischemia and infarction. *Physiol Rev* 69:1049, 1989.
6. Schalij MJ: *Anisotropic Conduction and Ventricular Tachycardia.* Maastricht, The Netherlands: University of Limburg; 1988. Thesis.
7. Hill BC, Hunt AJ, Courtney KR: Reentrant tachycardia in a thin layer of ventricular subepicardium: effects of d-sotalol and lidocaine. *J Cardiovasc Pharmacol* 16:871, 1990.
8. Kates RE, Yee Y-G, Hill I: Effect of albumin on the electrophysiologic stability of isolated perfused rabbit hearts. *J Cardiovasc Pharmacol* 13:168, 1989.
9. Allessie MA, Schalij MJ, Kirchhof CJHJ, et al: Experimental electrophysiology and arrhythmogenicity. Anisotropy and ventricular tachycardia. *Eur Heart J* 10(Suppl E):2, 1989.
10. Allessie MA, Schalij MJ, Kirchhof CJ, et al: Electrophysiology of spiral waves in two dimensions: the role of anisotropy. *Ann N Y Acad Sci* 591:247, 1990.
11. Brugada J, Boersma L, Kirchhof C, et al: Proarrhythmic effects of flecainide. Experimental evidence for increased susceptibility to reentrant arrhythmias. *Circulation* 84:1808, 1991.
12. Brugada J, Boersma L, Kirchhof CJH, et al: Reentrant excitation around a fixed obstacle in uniform anisotropic ventricular myocardium. *Circulation* 84:1296, 1991.
13. Brugada J, Mont L, Boersma L, et al: Differential effects of heptanol, potassium, and tetrodotoxin in reentrant ventricular tachycardia around a fixed obstacle in anisotropic myocardium. *Circulation* 84:1307, 1991.
14. Brugada J, Brugada P, Boersma L, et al: On the mechanisms of ventricular tachycardia acceler-

ation during programmed electrical stimulation. *Circulation* 83:1621, 1991.

15. Hill BC, Summers RAJ, Courtney KR: d-Sotalol has opposite effects from encainide and propafenone on the proportion of episodes of ventricular tachycardia that are sustained in an experimental substrate for reentry. *J Cardiovasc Pharmacol* 19:493, 1992.

16. Cochran WG: Some methods for strengthening the common Chi-square test. *Biometrics* 10: 417, 1954.

17. El-Sherif N, Craelius W, Boutjdir M, et al: Early afterdepolarizations and arrhythmogenesis. *J Cardiovasc Electrophysiol* 1:145, 1990.

18. Sasyniuk BI, Valois M, Toy W: Recent advances in understanding the mechanisms of drug-induced torsades de pointes arrhythmias. *Am J Cardiol* 64:29J, 1989.

19. Lazzara R, Szabo B, Patterson E, et al: Mechanisms for proarrhythmia with antiarrhythmic drugs. In: DP Zipes, J Jalife (eds): *Cardiac Electrophysiology: From Cell to Bedside*. Philadelphia, PA: WB Saunders Co., 1990, p. 402.

20. Rensma PL, Allessie MA, Lammers WJEP, et al: Length of excitation wave and susceptibility to reentrant atrial arrhythmias in normal conscious dogs. *Circ Res* 62:395, 1988.

21. Wiener N, Rosenblueth A: The mathematical formulation of the problem of conduction of impulses in a network of connected excitable elements, specifically in cardiac muscle. *Arch Inst Cardiol Mex* 16:205, 1946.

22. Courtney KR: Progress and prospects of optimum antiarrhythmic drug design. *Cardiovasc Drugs Ther* 1:117, 1987.

23. Frame LH, Rhee EK, Fei H, et al: Proarrhythmic and antiarrhythmic effects of flecainide on nonsustained reentry around the canine atrial tricuspid ring in vitro. *PACE* 14:1728, 1991.

24. Dillon SM, Allessie MA, Ursell PC, et al: Influences of anisotropic tissue structure on reentrant circuits in the epicardial border zone of subacute canine infarcts. *Circ Res* 63:182, 1988.

Chapter 24

Proarrhythmic Consequences of Pharmacologically Prolonged Repolarization: *Experimental Considerations*

Nabil El-Sherif
Mohamed Boutjdir
William B. Gough
Mark Restivo

Several interventions, including a large number of pharmacological agents, can cause prolongation of cardiac repolarization. Drugs that prolong cardiac repolarization exhibit strong antiarrhythmic properties, so-called Class III action.[1] By lengthening cardiac refractoriness, these drugs can slow or terminate tachyarrhythmias. These drugs can also have an antifibrillatory effect[2] because they can limit the ability of cardiac tissue to be re-excited at a very fast and irregular rate, which is a hallmark of cardiac fibrillation. Conversely, prolongation of repolarization can have proarrhythmic effects. One possible mechanism is the development or accentuation of dispersion of repolarization between contiguous myocardial sites, long considered a substrate for reentrant arrhythmias.[3] Another mechanism that has been widely investigated in the last several years is early afterdepolarization-induced triggered arrhythmias.[4] Prolongation of repolarization can be the priming step for the development of early afterdepolarizations (EADs), which have been implicated in the genesis of the syndrome of long QTU and torsades de pointes. The latter, is a polymorphic ventricular tachyarrhythmia that can degenerate into ventricular fibrillation.[5] The following report briefly examines the experimental evidence of the proarrhythmic consequences of pharmacologically prolonged cardiac repolarization.

Supported in part by National Institutes of Health Grant HL 36680 and by the Veterans Administration Medical Center Research Funds.

From BN Singh, HJJ Wellens, M Hiraoka, (eds): *Electropharmacological Control of Cardiac Arrhythmias.* Mount Kisco, NY, Futura Publishing Company Inc., © 1994.

Early Afterdepolarization-Induced Triggered Activity

Three steps are required for the manifestation of EAD-induced triggered activity[4]: (1) Critical prolongation of the repolarization phase that requires a reduction of net outward current. This can result from an increase of one or more inward currents, a decrease of one or more outward currents or from both. A balance of net inward and outward currents, even momentarily, is followed by: (2) a net depolarizing current carrying the charge for the EAD; and (3) propagation of EADs, which are generated locally at one or more sites, to capture the entire heart resulting in an extrasystole. There is evidence that EAD-induced activity can be enhanced or suppressed by influencing one or more of these three steps.

Definition of Early Afterdepolarizations

An EAD has been defined as a depolarizing potential that begins prior to the completion of repolarization and causes an interruption or retardation of normal repolarization.[6,7] The depolarizing deflection that may arise from the delayed repolarization wave was not considered as part of the EAD. This definition was applied primarily to phase 3 delayed repolarization and depolarizing deflections with a take-off potential in the vicinity of -60 mV. Other investigators have also come to recognize the delay or hump in phase 3 repolarization as the EAD[8,9] with the membrane potential never moving in a positive direction during the hump in the absence of reexcitation (local or propagated response) or electrotonic interaction.[9] As will be discussed, the distinction between lengthening of the repolarization phase, which requires a net decrease of repolarizing (outward) current and the occurrence of a depolarizing wave, which requires a net inward current, is valid as these two events can have different ionic mechanisms and, under certain conditions, could be perturbed separately. The lengthening of the repolarization phase could be considered the priming step for the possible occurrence of a second depolarizing potential before completion of repolarization. The depolarizing potential may spread locally by conduction or electrotonic transmission (subthreshold) or result in a regenerative response that activates the entire heart resulting in an extrasystole. However, it seems more appropriate to reserve the term EAD to the depolarizing deflection (whether or not it can result in a regenerative action potential) rather than to the priming event of prolonged repolarization. This is particularly true in case of phase 2 EADs where a prolonged and sometimes flattened plateau provides no real hint as to whether or not an EAD will arise.

Electrotonic interactions between neighboring regions with disparate repolarization phases can give rise to deflections simulating EADs in multicellular preparations and in recordings from the intact heart. However, EADs have been shown to represent a genuine oscillation of membrane voltage in isolated single myocytes[10,11] (Figure 1) and in short segments of Purkinje fibers.[12,13]

Early afterdepolarizations could arise at the end of a prolonged phase 2 from a take-off potential around -30 mV (Figures 2B and 3) or from a hump in phase 3 at a take-off potential of approximately -60 mV (Figures 2C and 4). A series of phase 2 EADs tend to arise from progressively more negative transmembrane potential until final repolarization terminates the series (Figure 3). This behavior of phase 2 EADs is most evident in isolated Purkinje preparations or when Purkinje fibers are uncoupled from muscle fibers.[14] Both phase 2 and phase 3 EADs could be observed simultaneously in Purkinje fibers under a variety of interventions, including exposure to quinidine,[15,16] cesium,[17] barium,[18] and hypoxia plus epinephrine.[19] Triggered activity from phase 3 EADs manifest at rates considerably slower than those associated with phase 2 EADs.[15,16] Quinidine-induced phase 2, but not phase 3 EADs, could be abolished by increased extracellular magnesium $(Mg^{2+})_o$.[15]

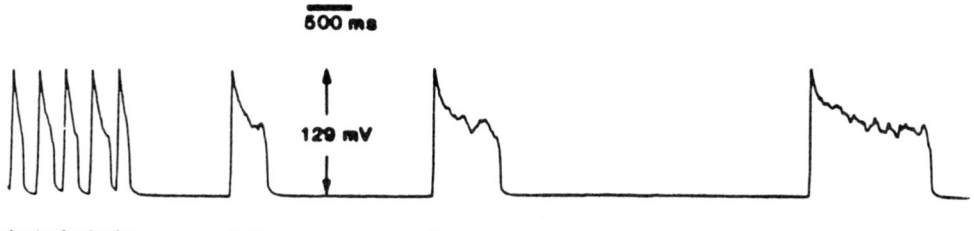

Figure 1. Current clamp recordings of action potential from a neonatal rat myocyte elicited with 100-pa pulses, 2-msec duration, obtained after exposure to anthopleurin-A (100 nM). Action potentials at a cycle length of 350 msec (left) were significantly prolonged and showed 2:1 alternation of action potential duration. At a slower driving frequency marked prolongation of action potential duration occurred and early afterdepolarizations developed during the prolonged plateau phase in the form of irregular depolarizations of up to 10 mV in amplitude. (Reproduced with permission from Reference 4.)

Ionic Mechanisms of Prolonged Repolarization

Under normal physiological conditions inward currents during phase 2 could be carried by sodium through a sodium window current[20] or a slowly inactivating sodium current,[21] by calcium through the calcium channel and a calcium window current,[22,23] and by the electrogenic Na/Ca exchange.[24] Outward currents include a number of potassium currents, of which the inward rectifier I_{K1} and the delayed rectifier I_K, are the two most commonly involved (ie, depressed) when Class III pharmacological agents result in prolonged repolarization. Other outward currents are generated by the transient outward current (I_{to}) and by the Na-K pump (I_p). The importance of the I_{to} varies with cardiac tissue and species.[25] The role of nonspecific cation channels that may appear in response to increased intracellular calcium $[Ca^{2+}]_i$ is not clear.[26] Although the magnitude and kinetics of some of the above currents have been described, the interaction between these currents in a quantitative way during the repolarization phase is not well understood. It is also important to note that during phase 2 repolarization membrane conductance is low, so that only small changes in net inward or outward currents can result in significant changes in membrane potential. The currents involved in the

transition to phase 3 and the rapid change in membrane potential during this phase include, the time- and voltage-dependent decay of I_{Ca}, the I_p, the time-dependent increase of I_K, and the progressive increase of conductance of I_{K1}. The role of the Na/Ca exchange current is less clear.

The ionic mechanisms of pharmacologically-induced prolonged repolarization and EAD formation are complex. Several pharmacological agents act by affecting more than one ionic current either in a synergistic or opposing directions. More important, the synergistic effects of other interventions are frequently required for critical lengthening of repolarization and the generation of EADs. A slow driving rate as well as a low extracellular $[K^+]_o$ usually play a significant synergistic effect. The slow driving rate probably acts by reducing the I_p.[27] Low $[K^+]_o$ will decrease potassium conductance, which in turn will affect a number of currents including I_K, I_{K1}, I_p, and I_f.[28]

The majority of pharmacological agents that prolong repolarization could be grouped as acting predominantly through one of four different mechanisms: (1) A delay of one or both potassium currents, I_K and I_{K1}, as in the case of quinidine,[29–31] N-acetyl procainamide,[32] cesium,[33] sotalol,[34] bretylium,[2] clofilium,[35] and other new Class III antiarrhythmic agents.[36,37] This action could possibly be specifically antagonized by drugs that activate the

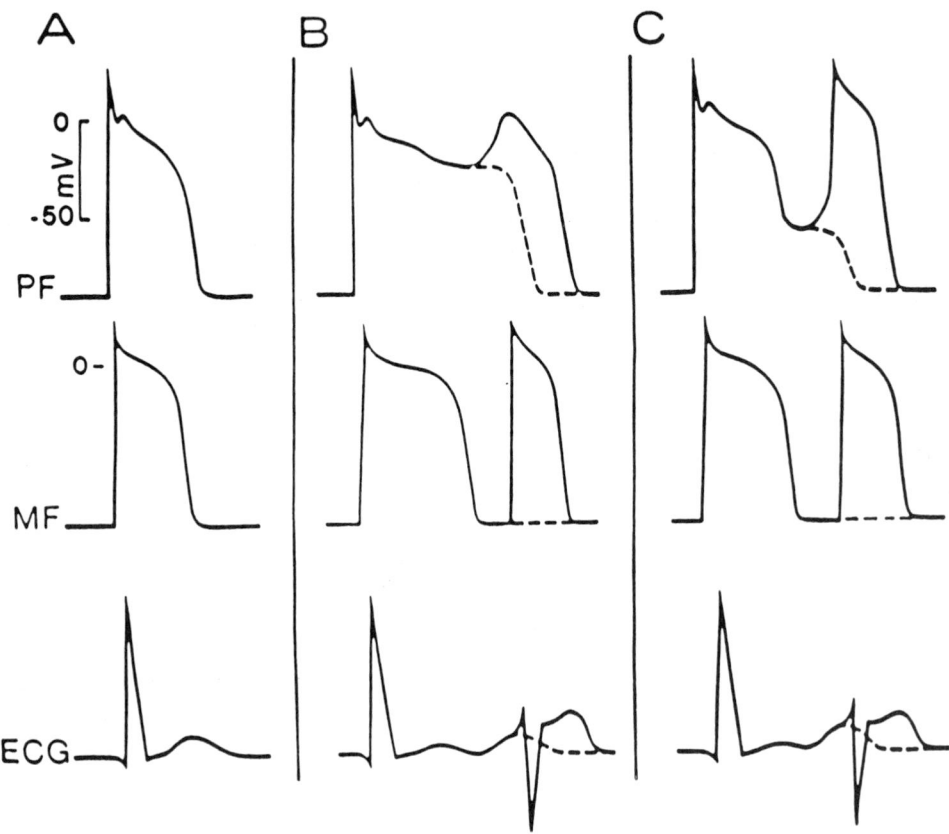

Figure 2. Diagrammatic representation of transmembrane action potentials from a Purkinje fiber (PF) and an adjacent muscle fiber (MF) and the surface electrocardiogram (ECG) to illustrate the changes associated with the development of prolonged repolarization, early after-depolarization (EAD), and EAD-triggered action potential. A: Control recording; B: Phase 2 EAD. Note that the first step is marked prolongation and flattening of the plateau of the PF (dotted section). Prolongation of repolarization of the MF is relatively less pronounced. The EAD is a depolarizing potential that arises from the prolonged plateau at an approximate take-off potential of −25 to −30 mV. The EAD may or may not succeed in conducting to the adjacent MF. The mechanism of conduction of phase 2 EAD is not clear. The surface ECG shows the development of a prominent U wave (dotted section) that corresponds in time with the terminal part of the PF prolonged plateau and/or with the EAD arising from the plateau. Successful conduction of EAD generated in Purkinje network to overlying myocardium is essential for the occurrence of a ventricular premature complex in the ECG. The latter may seem to arise from the prominent U wave; and C: Phase 3 EAD. Note that the first step is an interruption and retardation of the fast phase 3 repolarization (dotted section). The EAD is a depolarizing potential that arises from the hump on phase 3 at an approximate take-off potential of −60 mV. The EAD may or may not result in a triggered action potential that conducts to adjacent MF. The changes in surface ECG is similar to those described for phase 2 EAD. (Reproduced with permission from Reference 4.)

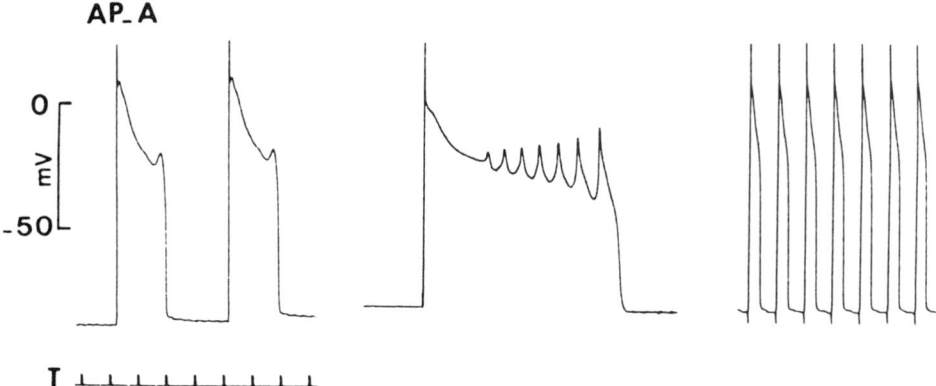

Figure 3. Action potential recordings from a Purkinje fiber in a canine endocardial preparation exposed to anthopleurin-A (AP-A, 50 μg/L) showing phase 2 early afterdepolarization (EAD). A: The preparation was stimulated at a cycle length of 4 seconds. AP-A significantly prolonged the action potential duration and an EAD developed from late phase 2; B: When the preparation was stimulated at a cycle length of 8 seconds a series of EADs developed arising from progressively more negative transmembrane potential until final repolarization terminated the series; and C: When the preparation was stimulated at a cycle length of 1 second the action potential duration shortened and EADs were suppressed. Time marker (T) represents 1-second intervals. (Reproduced with permission from Reference 4.)

potassium channel such as pinacidil and cromakalin[38]; (2) Suppression of I_{to}, as in the case of 4-aminopyridine (4-AP), which was shown to prolong repolarization and induce EADs preferentially in canine subepicardial M cells, which are reported to have prominent I_{to}[39]; (3) An increase of I_{Ca}, as in the case of Bay K 8644. This action could be reversed by calcium channel blockers[13]; and (4) A delay of I_{Na} inactivation as in the case of aconitine,[40] veratridine,[41,42] batrachotoxin,[43] a diphenyl-methylpiperazine-indole derivative (DPI),[44] and the sea anemone toxins anthopleurin-A and ATX-II.[10,45-47] This action could be antagonized by drugs that block I_{Na} and/or the slowly inactivating sodium current such as tetrodotoxin and lidocaine.[48] Since these drugs can shorten prolonged repolarization they can also suppress EADs induced by the first two mechanisms.[13]

Quinidine, the most common agent involved in the acquired long QTU syndrome and torsades de pointes, prolongs repolarization by a voltage-dependent block of I_K and at higher concentrations of I_{K1}.[29-31] Quinidine also blocks other currents like I_{Na} sodium window current, I_f, and I_{to}.[49-52] Block of these currents can shorten repolarization and reduce the chance for the development of EADs. However, quinidine block of I_{Na} is use and concentration dependent[53] while block of I_K is reverse use dependent.[30] Thus, in the presence of a slow driving rate and an optimal concentration of quinidine, more inhibition of I_K and simultaneously less or no block of I_{Na} can result in sufficient prolongation of repolarization and provide the priming step for the development of EADs. Similar to quinidine, the chance that other drugs that block both inward and outward currents, ie, lidoflazine and bepridil, will produce EADs depends on block of the predominating outward current.[16]

Cesium prolongs repolarization probably by decreasing I_{K1} and I_{K1}.[33] Block of I_K and possibly of I_{K1} is also the mechanism of prolonged repolarization by sotalol, d-sotalol,[34] bretylium,[2] and clofilium.[35] Interestingly enough, d-sotalol, bretylium, and clofilium prolong repolarization and produce EADs preferentially in ischemic Purkinje fibers obtained from 1-day-old canine infarcts com-

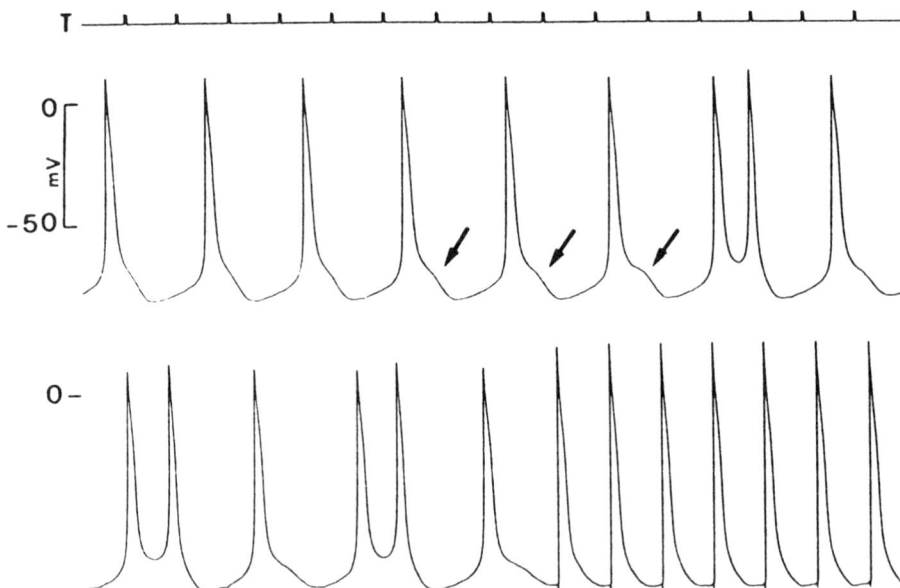

Figure 4. Action potential recordings from a Purkinje fiber in a canine endocardial preparation exposed to low [K]o illustrating phase 3 early afterdepolarizations (EAD). The recordings in top and bottom panels are continuous. The upper panel shows spontaneous automaticity at a cycle length of 1900 msec. Note the marked delay of late phase 3 repolarization that became more pronounced in successive beats (marked by arrows). Eventually, a premature action potential arose from the hump on phase 3. Early afterdepolarization-induced action potential occurred in alternate beats giving rise to a trigeminal rhythm (first half of lower panel). When the preparation was paced at a cycle length of 1 second (the second half of the lower panel) the EAD was markedly suppressed. Time marker (T) represents 1-second intervals. (Reproduced with permission from Reference 4.)

pared to normal fibers (Figure 5).[54] The mechanism of this differential sensitivity is not clear, but may be related to differences in binding of the drugs or some abnormalities of ionic currents in the ischemic fibers.

Bay K 8644 prolongs repolarizations and produces EADs by a voltage- and use-dependent increase of I_{Ca}, primarily by increasing mean open times of L-type calcium channels.[13] Drugs that delay I_{Na} inactivation prolong repolarization through an enhanced sodium window current[20] or a slowly inactivating sodium current.[21] Recent single channel studies have raised uncertainty regarding the existence of a sodium window current by identifying sodium channels whose kinetic behavior could underlie the macroscopic sodium window current. These studies described sodium channels that have slow inacti-

vation kinetics and tend to burst open repetitively during sustained depolarization.[47,55–59] Bursting behavior of normal cardiac sodium channels is rare. It has been estimated as once in 2,000–5,000 depolarizations per channel by Patlak and Ortiz,[56] as once in 2,700 depolarizations per channel by Kiyosue and Arita,[59] and once in 2,305 depolarizations per channel by El-Sherif et al.[47] (Figure 6). ATX-II has been shown to increase the fraction of sodium channels with late kinetics and greatly enhance their bursting behavior (Figure 7).[47]

The Depolarizing Current for Early Afterdepolarizations

The depolarizing charge for EADs could be through the calcium channel, the sodium channel, or the electrogenic Na/Ca exchange. There is strong evidence that EADs induced by the calcium channel agonist Bay K 8644 result from the time- and voltage-dependent reopening of L-type calcium channels within their window voltage range during the action potential plateau (Figure 8) and that this recovery of inward current shifts the balance of membrane currents toward depolarization.[13,23] When depolarization is initiated, additional L-type calcium channels could then be recruited to open from a closed state(s), thereby augmenting the depolarizing calcium current. Other investigators have suggested that the depolarizing current for quinidine-induced EADs is also a voltage-dependent cal-

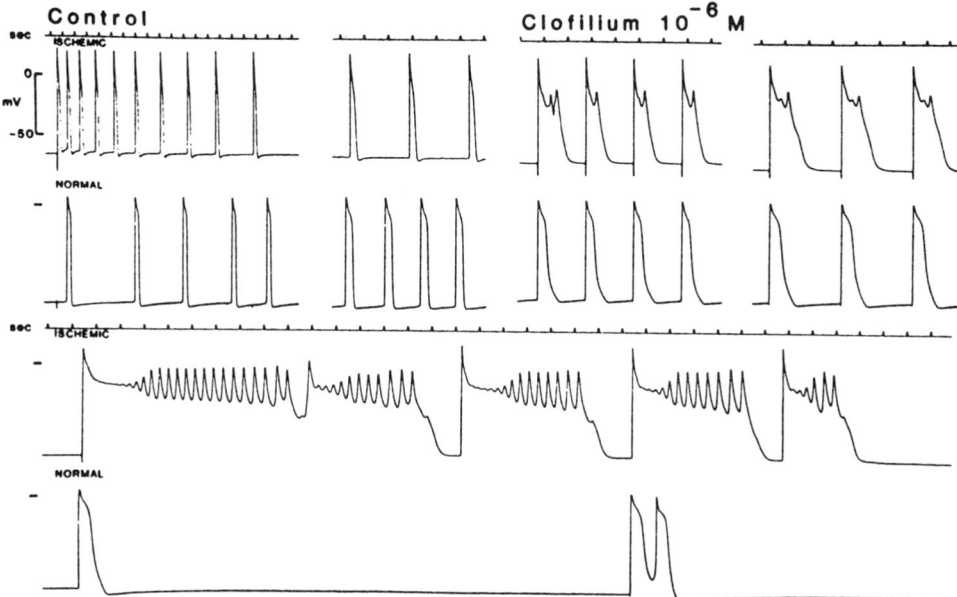

Figure 5. Transmembrane action potentials recorded from normal canine Purkinje fiber and ischemic subendocardial Purkinje fiber 1 day after infarction, demonstrating triggered activity from early afterdepolarizations (EADs) in the ischemic fiber when perfused with clofilium. Under control condition in Tyrode's solution both fibers showed diastolic depolarization. In the ischemic preparation, triggered activity from delayed afterdepolarizations was observed. One stimulus evoked an action potential that was followed by a delayed afterdepolarization, which in turn initiated spontaneous action potential formation. The triggered activity started with a cycle length of 900 msec that gradually increased to a cycle length of approximately 3 seconds. After further superfusion, only a slow pacemaker activity persisted at a cycle length of 2.5 seconds. After introducing clofilium into the perfusate at 10^{-6}M and pacing at a cycle length of 2 seconds EADs occurred during the plateau of the action potential of the ischemic Purkinje at a coupling interval of 500 msec. The normal action potential was only prolonged in phases 2 and 3, and showed no early or delayed afterpotentials. At a driven cycle length of 3 seconds, repolarization of the ischemic cell was more prolonged and was accompanied by EADs. When the preparation was permitted to remain quiescent for periods longer than 30 seconds (bottom tracing) EADs developed in the ischemic fiber at a low membrane potential (in the range of -15 to -35 mV) and continued with a cycle length of 300 to 500 msec extending the duration of the action potential to beyond 10 seconds. Generally, the membrane potential of the nadir of the EADs became progressively greater during the plateau until repolarization was completed or reexcitation occurred. The normal Purkinje fiber showed slowing of late phase 3 repolarization consistent with EAD at high membrane potential that gave rise to a single triggered action potential. (Reproduced with permission from Reference 70.)

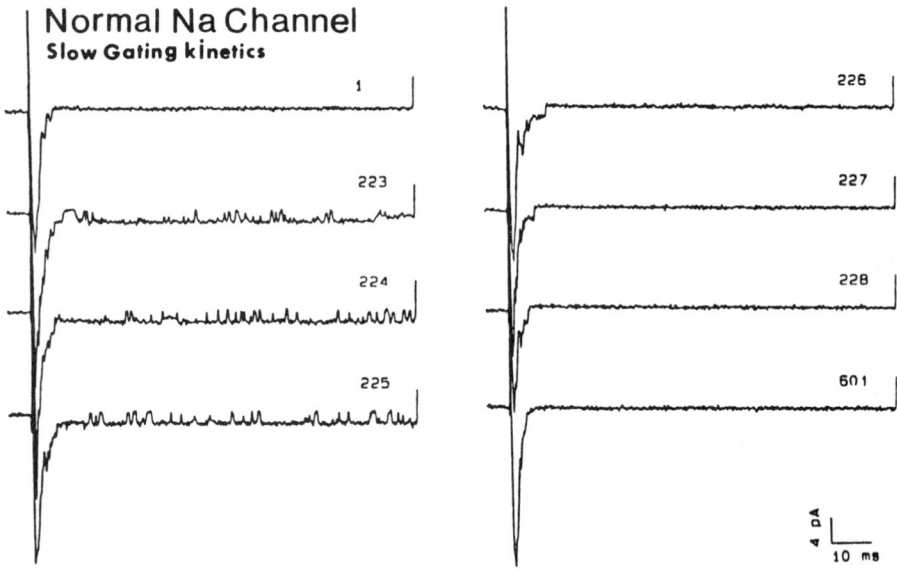

Figure 6. Bursting behavior of normal sodium channels in a macropatch from a rabbit cardiac myocyte estimated to have 16 channels. The pipette filling solution contained (in millimoles) NaCl 280, CaCl$_2$ 1, MgCl$_2$ 1, tetramethylammonium 10, and HEPES 10. The bath solution contained (mM) potassium aspartate 150, MgCl$_2$ 2, HEPES 10. Examples from a total of 601 sweeps recorded for a potential step to -20 mV from a holding potential of -120 mV. Five sweeps showed prolonged bursting activity grouped as three successive sweeps (223–225) and as two successive sweeps (not shown). Although it is impossible to be certain that the long-lived bursting represented the activity of a single channel, the rarity of the event makes it very likely. If it is assumed that all 16 channels in the patch had an equal chance of such bursting behavior, then the probability of occurrence for each channel can be estimated approximately as the observed frequency divided by the number of channels (ie, 5/601 ÷ 16 = 1/1,923). (Reproduced with permission from Reference 47.)

cium current.[14] The calcium channel blockers nifedipine and verapamil were shown to eliminate the EAD without altering the plateau prolongation.[14] This observation provides indirect but persuasive evidence that ionic current underlying the priming step of plateau prolongation and the depolarizing current for the EADs in the case of quinidine are distinct and could be manipulated separately. Similarly, calcium channel blockers were shown to block cesium-induced EADs in vitro[60] and torsades de pointes arrhythmias in vivo.[61] Magnesium was also shown to block EADs induced by both quinidine[15] and cesium[62] while having less significant effect on the prolonged repolarization phase. These observations are consistent with the efficacy of magnesium in

abolishing torsades de pointes in patients with quinidine-induced long QTU, but with slight or no change in the QTU interval.[63] Magnesium probably acts by a membrane stabilizing effect[15] and/or by a calcium channel blocking effect.[64]

Some investigators have suggested that the Na/Ca exchange current may provide the depolarizing charge for the EADs.[65] However, other investigators have shown that chelation of $[Ca^{2+}]_i$ by BAPTA as well as inhibition of oscillatory calcium release from the sarcoplasmic reticulum by ryanodine failed to suppress cesium-induced EADs.[60]

There is little evidence that the calcium channel and/or the Na/Ca exchange current provide the depolarizing charge for EADs induced by drugs that delay sodium inactivation. Both inorganic (cobalt) and organic (verapamil) calcium channel blockers, as well as inhibitors of oscillatory calcium release from the sarcoplasmic reticulum (ryanodine and 10 mM caffeine) failed to abolish EADs induced by the sea anemone toxin ATX-II.[48]

A unified concept for the charge carrier of EADs may not be warranted. Early afterdepolarizations could be viewed as being caused by an imbalance between multiple voltage- and time-dependent inward and outward currents whose magnitudes, voltage, and time de-

pendence vary between cell type, species, and physiological state. Total membrane currents are small at plateau voltages, therefore, small changes in outward and inward currents could cause potentials to depolarizing or repolarizing directions. In this regard, it has been suggested that time- and voltage-dependent changes in the background current, mainly produced by I_K and I_{K1}, might be involved in the genesis of repetitive EADs, in association with recovery from inactivation of L-type calcium current,[42] or a persistent sodium inward current.[47]

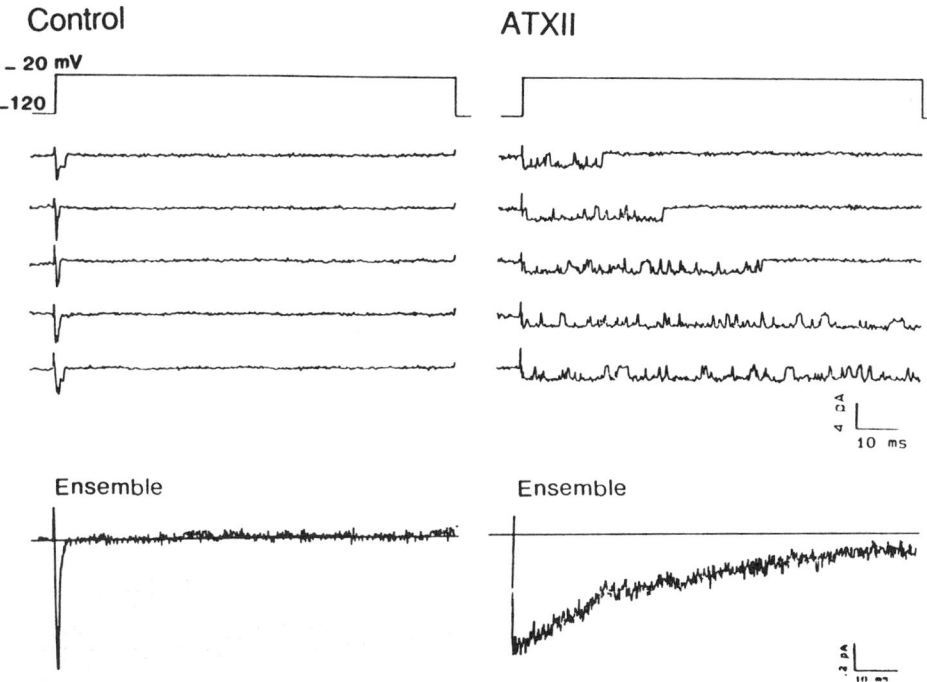

Figure 7. Sequential recordings of single sodium channel current responses during depolarizing steps from −120 to −20 mV from two rabbit cardiac myocytes. Left panel: Recordings under control conditions from a patch estimated to have three channels. Right panel: Recordings from a patch estimated to have a single channel exposed to 1,000 nM sea anemone toxin ATX-II. Solutions were as described in Figure 6. The upward spike in each sweep marks the time at which voltage was changed. At −20 mV, control sodium channels opened briefly, on average only once, very soon after the potential step. By contrast, the sodium channel exposed to ATX-II showed long-lasting bursts consisting of repetitive long openings interrupted by brief closures. Some of the bursts lasted for the entire duration of the potential step. The ensemble currents from both patches are shown on the bottom. The control ensemble current shows fast relaxation. Conversely, the ensemble current of the sodium channel exposed to ATX-II shows markedly slowed relaxation with the current failing to relax completely by the end of the 95-msec step. (Reproduced with permission from Reference 47.)

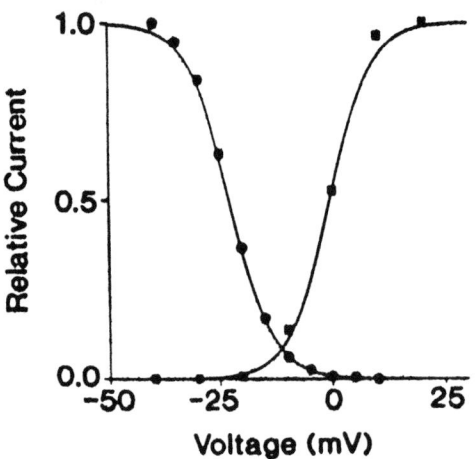

Figure 8. L-type calcium channel current activation and inactivation relations in single cardiac Purkinje cells. The figure shows Boltzmann fits through normalized peak currents for steady-state inactivation (circles) and activation (squares). The window voltage range is predicted by the overlap of the curves between about −30 and −0 mV. (Reproduced with permission from Reference 23.)

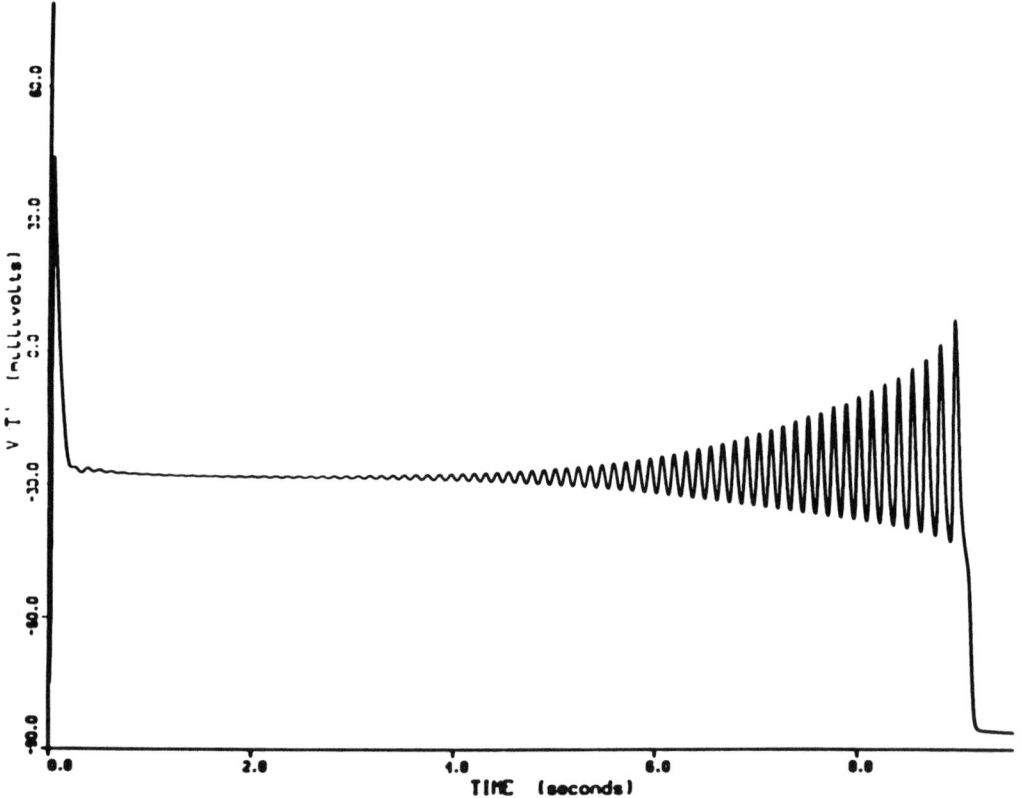

Figure 9. Computer simulation of a cardiac Purkinje cell action potential in which sodium inactivation rate was decreased by tenfold resulting in multiple oscillations during the course of the markedly prolonged plateau phase. See text for details.

Computer Modeling of Early Afterdepolarizations

In the experimental setting, trying to focus on specific ionic currents believed responsible for EAD generation may be compromised because there may be some doubt about the completeness of blockade of a specific ion channel or chelation of an ionic species. Therefore, we investigated the genesis of EADs in a computer model of electrical activity. One of the benefits of a computer model in studying EAD formation is that there is no doubt about blockade or chelation.

The model used was based on 14 ionic currents (including voltage-gated and pump currents) for Purkinje fibers using modified DiFrancesco-Noble equations of a Hodgkin-Huxley formalism. The simulations were performed on either a Digital Equipment Corporation VAX or a Convex computer at the Engineering Computing Center at Rutgers University, Piscataway, New Jersey.

Based on our experimental observations with the sea anemone toxins model for EADs,[11,47,48,66] we simulated delayed sodium inactivation in the computer model in an attempt to elucidate the mechanism of EAD formation.[67] Equations for sodium inactivation (variable h in the Hodgkin-Huxley equations) are shown. Delayed sodium inactivation was simulated by reducing the rate that inactivation gates go from open to closed state (β_h). Inspection of inactivation variables indicate that a reduction in β_h, a voltage-dependent variable, increases the time constant for inactivation (τ_h) and the availability ($h\infty$) in a voltage-dependent manner. The change in $h\infty$ results in a rightward shift of the inactivation curve and increases the overlap in inactivation and activation curves. Though the inactivation parameters ($h\infty$-$j\infty$) included a baseline slow inactivation component, the generation of EADs was accomplished without any further change in the time course of inactivation.

$$open \underset{\beta}{\overset{\alpha}{\rightleftharpoons}} closed$$

$$\tau_h = \frac{1}{\alpha_h + \beta_h}$$

$$h_\infty = \frac{\alpha_h}{\alpha_h + \beta_h}$$

Figure 9 shows a simulated action potential in which β_h was decreased tenfold. For the control simulation (not shown) the action potential duration was 400 msec. The action potential shown has a duration of more than 9 seconds and exhibits multiple depolarizations (EADs) during the course of the plateau phase. Note that the amplitude of the oscillations increase with time until a strong outward current eventually terminated the oscillations and brought the action potential to resting potential. We have been able to demonstrate oscillations of this type (not shown) even when all equations for calcium currents were eliminated from the simulation.

Another way of visualizing the imbalance of currents and their time course during EAD formation is the use of phase plane trajectories. A phase plane trajectory is a plot of membrane potential (V) versus the first temporal derivative of potential (dV/dt) at each instant of time. The relation for membrane current is $I_{total} = -C \, dV/dt$; where I_{total} is the total membrane current, C is the membrane capacitance, and V is the membrane potential. Therefore, membrane current is directly proportional to dV/dt. Figure 10 shows the phase plane trajectory for the same action potential shown in Figure 9. In the experimental setting, this technique can be useful for analyzing EAD formation.

Propagation of Early Afterdepolarization-Induced Activity

With few exceptions[60,68] EADs were shown to be readily induced in Purkinje fibers rather than in myocardial fibers in vitro. In

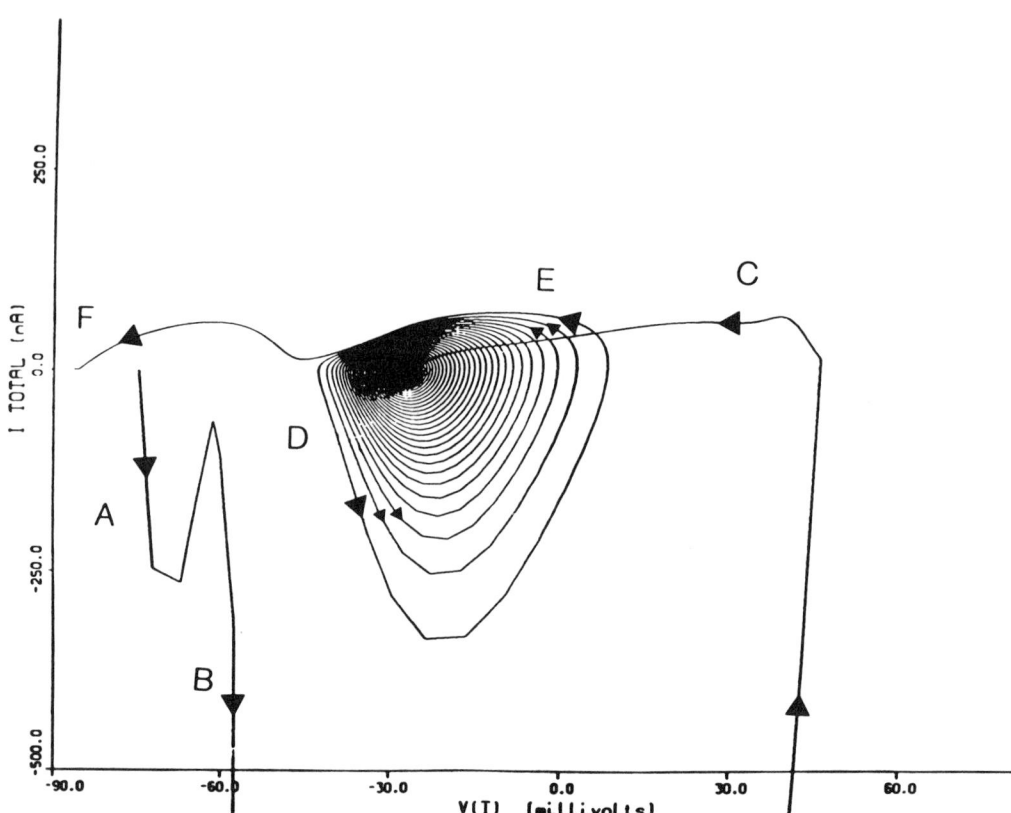

Figure 10. Phase plane trajectory for the simulated action potential shown in Figure 9. The abscissa is a membrane potential; the ordinate is scaled by the membrane capacitance of a Purkinje cell to reflect total membrane current. Following standard motion, inward currents are represented by negative values. In the example shown here a 250 nA stimulus was applied to elicit an action potential (A). The downward deflection of the fast inward current begins at a threshold value around −60 mV. Because the magnitude of the fast inward current is much greater than the EAD currents, the trajectory during upstroke is not shown in its entirety. During phase 2 (B), the total current is near 0. Because of the fine balance of inward and outward currents small oscillation in membrane potential ensued. Early afterdepolarization can be visualized in the phase plane by the concentric semicircular trajectories centered around a point at approximately −30 mV. The trajectory of the oscillations began in the core and moved outward until the outward current was of sufficient magnitude to repolarize the cell (F). Inward current movements are indicated by (D) in the figure; the take-off potential for each depolarization is the point where the trajectory crosses the 0 current axis in the downward direction (D). Net outward movement, repolarizations, are indicated by (E). Note that in this instance the maximum outward currents during each oscillation was much less than the maximum inward current developed during that oscillation.

the intact heart, EADs generated at one or more sites in the Purkinje network must propagate to ventricular myocardium and activate the entire heart to induce an extrasystole. Several investigators have studied the propagation of EADs. Mendez and Delmar[19] investigated the propagation of EADs induced in ca-

nine false tendons to an attached papillary muscle separated by a latex partition. Early afterdepolarizations that arose at relatively positive take-off potential failed to propagate, while EADs with take-off potential of about −55 mV excited the papillary muscle. Similar observations were reported by Kupersmith and Hoff (1985) when Purkinje fibers were placed in a double chamber divided by rubber partition and EADs generated in one segment were observed to propagate to the normal segment. El-Sherif et al.[65] studied the propagation of EADs in a Purkinje muscle preparation exposed to anthopleurin-A. The drug resulted in marked lengthening of plateau and development of EADs preferentially in Purkinje fibers compared to adjacent muscle fibers. Conduction of EADs from Purkinje to muscle fibers was relatively slow (up to 100 msec). Similar observations could be seen in Purkinje muscle preparations exposed to ATX-II (Figure 11). It was suggested that the conduction delay occurred predominantly at the Purkinje

muscle junction. However, electrotonic interactions because of marked disparity of repolarization between Purkinje and adjacent muscle fibers may also play a significant role. In fact, the mechanism of propagation of phase 2 EADs is not entirely clear and some form of electrotonic transmission or reflection[69] that could be repetitive in nature, cannot be excluded.

An interesting aspect of EAD propagation was shown in a study by Gough and et al.[70] in endocardial strips from 1-day-old canine infarcts exposed to clofilium. The preparations had adjacent normal and ischemic tissue. Clofilium preferentially induced action potential prolongation and EADs in ischemic Purkinje

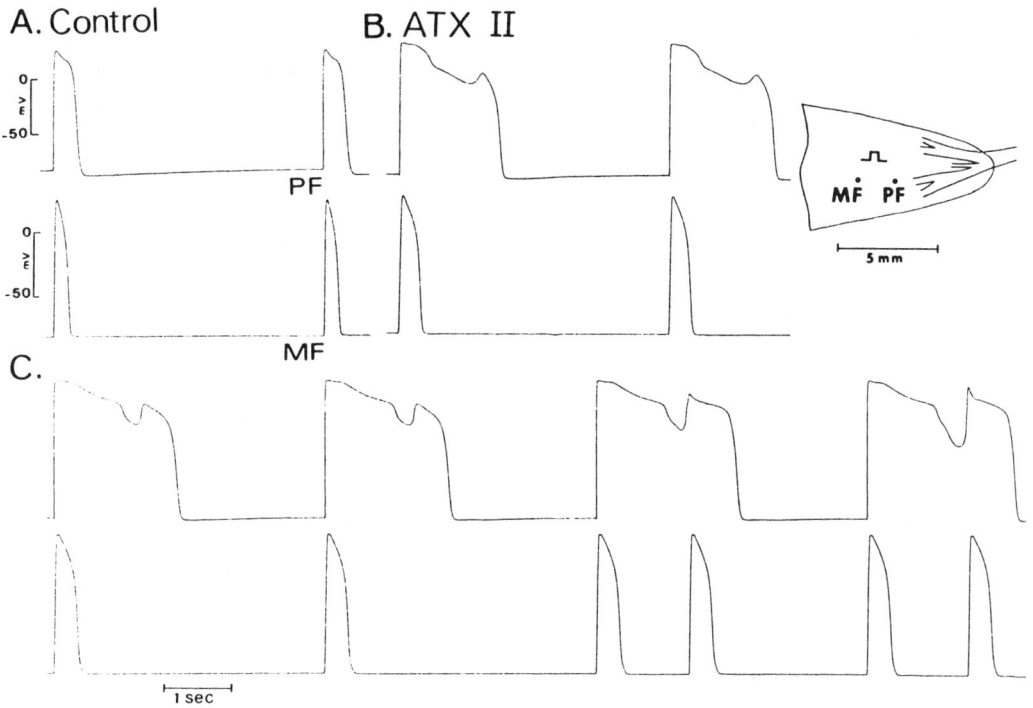

Figure 11. Simultaneous recordings of action potentials from a Purkinje fiber (PF) and muscle fiber (MF) in canine papillary muscle preparation. Sketch of the preparation and the site of recordings is shown on the right. The preparation was paced at a constant cycle length of 4 seconds. Panel A is control recordings. Recording in B and C were obtained after exposure of the preparation to ATX-II (2 × 10⁻⁷ M) for 20 and 22 minutes, respectively. ATX-II resulted in prolongation of action potential duration of both PF and MF, but the changes were more marked in PF. In B, only PF developed an EAD. In C, the EAD triggered an action potential that conducted to MF with a conduction delay of 70 to 80 msec (measured from the onset of EAD to the onset of MF action potential) giving rise to a bigeminal rhythm.

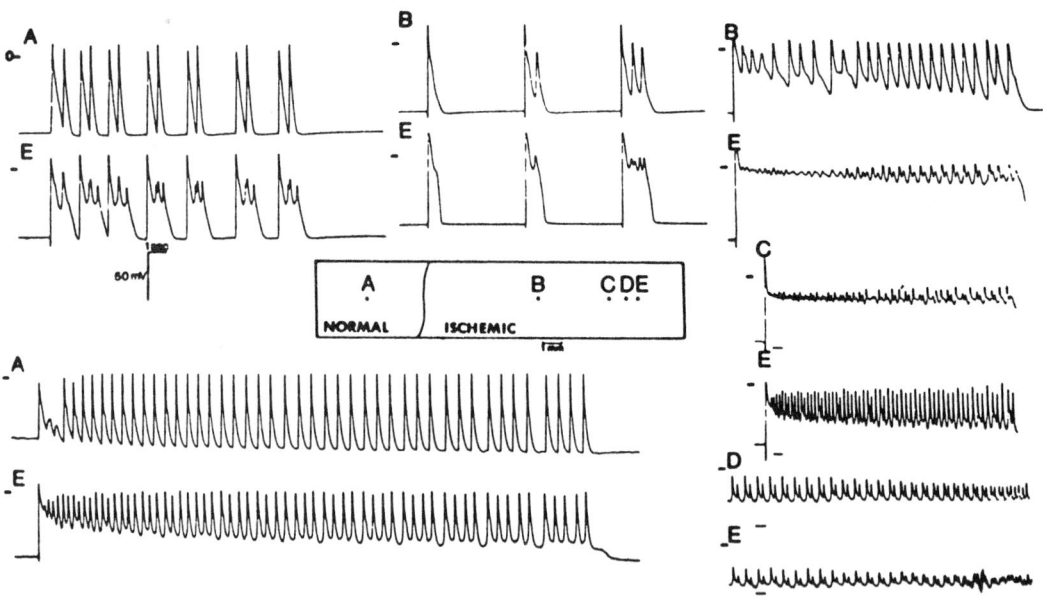

Figure 12. In vitro recordings from a canine endocardial preparation 1 day postinfarction. Transmembrane potentials were recorded from a normal site in the basal papillary muscle (site A) and the adjacent ischemic sites (sites B to E) during superfusion of 10^{-6} M clofilium and illustrate the ability of clofilium-induced early afterdepolarizations (EADs) in ischemic endocardium to trigger activity in adjacent normal tissue. Simultaneous records from site A (normal) and site E (ischemic) show that not all EADs induced triggered activity in the ischemic region produced 1:1 activity in the normal area. A single stimulus to the ischemic area produced a rapid succession of action potential, with up to three EADs (500-msec cycle length) in each. No more than one of these EADs was accompanied by activity in normal tissue. The resultant rhythm in the normal tissue was a bigeminal rhythm that became quiescent when the ischemic area became quiescent. After a pause of longer than 1 minute, a single stimulus to the ischemic area produced an action potential 30-msec long at site E (lower left). Activity at site A resembled aborted premature action potentials for two beats and then a sustained burst of activity (600-msec cycle length). The relation of EAD-induced triggered activity (cycle lengths as short as 250 msec) at site E to activity at site A soon resembled varying degrees of Wenkebach conduction, terminating finally when conduction was 5:4. The transmission of EADs from one area of the ischemic region to other areas within the ischemic region was not homogeneous. To determine the distance over which there was synchrony of activity in the ischemic area, activity separated by 1.5 mm (sites C and E) and 0.5 mm (sites D and E) were studied. The closest resemblance to synchrony was observed between sites D and E (lower right). This record included only plateau activity, and not the entire action potential. The horizontal bar to the left of each recording is 0 mV. Note the compressed time scale in pairs C and E and D and E. The horizontal bar beneath each record represents 1 second. (Reproduced with permission from Reference 70.)

fibers. An arrhythmia equivalent to torsades de pointes developed in ischemic tissue. However, conduction block from ischemic to normal tissue prevented the expression of that arrhythmia in the normal tissue (Figure 12). This correlated with the in vivo expression of clofilium-induced arrhythmia in the form of

bursts of ventricular rhythms at a rate considerably slower than the rate of EAD-induced activity in ischemic tissue in vitro.

Because EADs are generated preferentially in Purkinje network and have to propagate to overlying myocardium to be expressed as an arrhythmia in the intact heart, it is entirely possible that this expression could be enhanced or suppressed by interventions that act predominantly on EAD transmission. Under certain circumstances catecholamines may enhance the expression of EADs as an arrhythmia both by augmenting the calcium current providing the depolarizing charge for the EADs and by facilitating its propagation in the intact heart.[14,16] Low concentration of catecholamines may favor EAD-induced activity while high concentration may have the opposite effect if marked acceleration of heart rate occurs.[14,16] Using monophasic action potential (MAP) recordings in vivo some investigators have shown that β-adrenergic blockade can prevent the expression of cesium-induced EADs as sustained arrhythmia without eliminating the EADs.[71] This suggests a significant role of circulating catecholamines in facilitating EAD transmission in the intact heart.

In Vivo Models of Pharmacologically-Induced Long QTU and Torsades de Pointes

Several experimental models of pharmacologically-induced torsades de pointes have been described. Some of these studies failed to recognize the possibility that different electrophysiological mechanisms may account for polymorphic ventricular tachyarrhythmias induced under different circumstances. In two experimental models of quinidine-induced torsades de pointes, the arrhythmia was initiated by premature stimuli in the presence of a toxic dose of quinidine.[72,73] In one of the studies, acute ischemia was also superimposed on quinidine toxicity. Both studies analyzed epicardial activation patterns during induced polymorphic ventricular tachyarrhythmias that resembled torsades de pointes and showed that each change in QRS morphology was associated with a change in the site of the earliest epicardial breakthrough.

The relevance of these experimental studies to clinical examples of quinidine-induced torsades de pointes can be questioned

on two accounts. First, the polymorphic ventricular tachyarrhythmia was induced by premature stimulation in both studies. This is quite different from the mode of initiation of the acquired form of torsades de pointes, which is characteristically bradycardia dependent. Second, both studies used toxic concentrations of quinidine. Clinical examples of quinidine-induced torsades de pointes are commonly associated with low or normal levels of quinidine concentration.[74] This observation is substantiated by several in vitro studies in which canine Purkinje fibers were shown to develop prolonged repolarization and EADs in the presence of hypokalemia, bradycardia, and a low quinidine concentration.[14,15,75] An example of a polymorphic ventricular tachyarrhythmia resembling torsades de pointes that could be induced by premature stimulation in circumstances other than those associated with acquired torsades de pointes was demonstrated by El-Sherif et al.[76] In this study, polymorphic ventricular tachyarrhythmia resembling torsades de pointes was induced in the canine postinfarction heart and was shown to be due to the presence of more than one asynchronous reentrant circuit.

Two in vivo experimental models in the dog have produced tachycardia-dependent QTU prolongation and polymorphic ventricular tachyarrhythmias that may resemble the clinical form of acquired long QTU and torsades de pointes. The two drugs used were cesium[77,78] and the sea anemone polypeptides anthopleurin-A[65] and ATX-II.[79] Despite the in vivo similarity between the two models, these drugs are known to induce prolonged repolarization and EADs through markedly different ionic mechanisms. In both in vivo models MAP recordings by a contact electrode technique demonstrated EAD-like deflections more prominent in endocardial than in epicardial recordings.[65,78] In the anthopleurin-A and ATX-II models the EAD-like deflection in endocardial MAP recordings corresponded to a prominent U wave in surface electrocardiographic leads.[65,79] Ventricular premature depolarizations could arise from the U or TU complex and initiate polymorphic ventricular

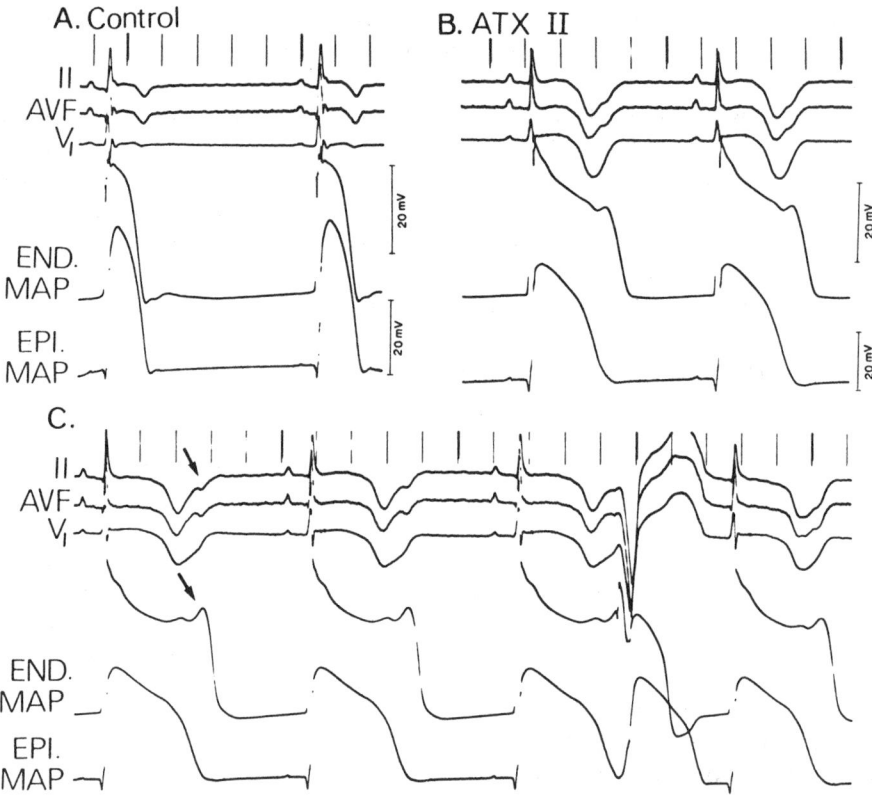

Figure 13. Simultaneous recordings of endocardial (End) monophasic action potential (MAP), epicardial (EPI) MAP, and surface ECG from a dog before and after administration of ATX-II (25 μg/kg). A: Control recording at a cycle length of 1,240 msec. Recordings in B and C were obtained 10 and 12 minutes, respectively, after administration of ATX-II. The drug resulted in marked prolongation of phase 2 of the endocardial MAP and the development of an EAD at the end of phase 2. The epicardial MAP was also prolonged, but its duration was 40–100 msec shorter than the endocardial MAP and it failed to show EAD. The QTU interval was also prolonged and showed the development of a distinct second deflection suggestive of a U wave. This deflection was synchronous with the EAD in the endocardial MAP. In C, a premature ventricular depolarization arose from the peak of the EAD.

tachyarrhythmia that terminated spontaneously or degenerated into ventricular fibrillation (Figures 13 and 14). The development of TU alternans coincided with the occurrence of 2:1 alternation of EADs in endocardial MAP.[65] These observations suggested that the prominent U wave in the long QTU syndrome may represent EADs generated in the Purkinje network. However, the nature of endocardial MAP recording in the in vivo heart is not well defined. The MAP recording may reflect activity generated in Purkinje fibers and in subendocardial muscle fibers. Mere differences in

repolarization between Purkinje and adjacent muscle can produce MAP deflections very much similar to phase 3 EADs in normal endocardial preparations.[80]

Role of Early Afterdepolarizations and Dispersion of Repolarization in Torsades de Pointes

There is strong evidence that the initiating beat of pharmacologically-induced torsades de pointes represents an action potential triggered by an EAD arising from the Purkinje network. It could also be postulated that the first beat of torsades de pointes is the result of marked dispersion of repolarization between contiguous sites, resulting in reactivation of the site with shorter action potential by currents flowing during prolonged repolarization (a form of reflection).[69] This mechanism, however, requires a region with sharp transition between cells with different repolarization characteristics because electrotonic effects favor more gradual transition between contiguous zones. Conversely, the electrophysiological mechanism(s) of subsequent beats in torsades de pointes is less certain. These beats could result from a succession of triggered action potentials arising from EADs,

from electrotonic reflection, or from circus movement reentry due to dispersion of repolarization or from a combination of more than one mechanism.

In normal hearts, the dispersion of MAP durations at different endocardial sites ranges from 21 to 64 msec[81,82] while in patients with long QTU and torsades de pointes the dispersion between right ventricular endocardial sites[81] or between right and left ventricular sites[83] (Figure 15) could be in excess of 200 msec. The reasons for this marked dispersion of repolarization in different regions of the heart are not clear. Circus movement reentry will require that the first or subsequent triggered action potential encounter myocardial regions that have not fully repolarized. Although the first ectopic beat of torsades de

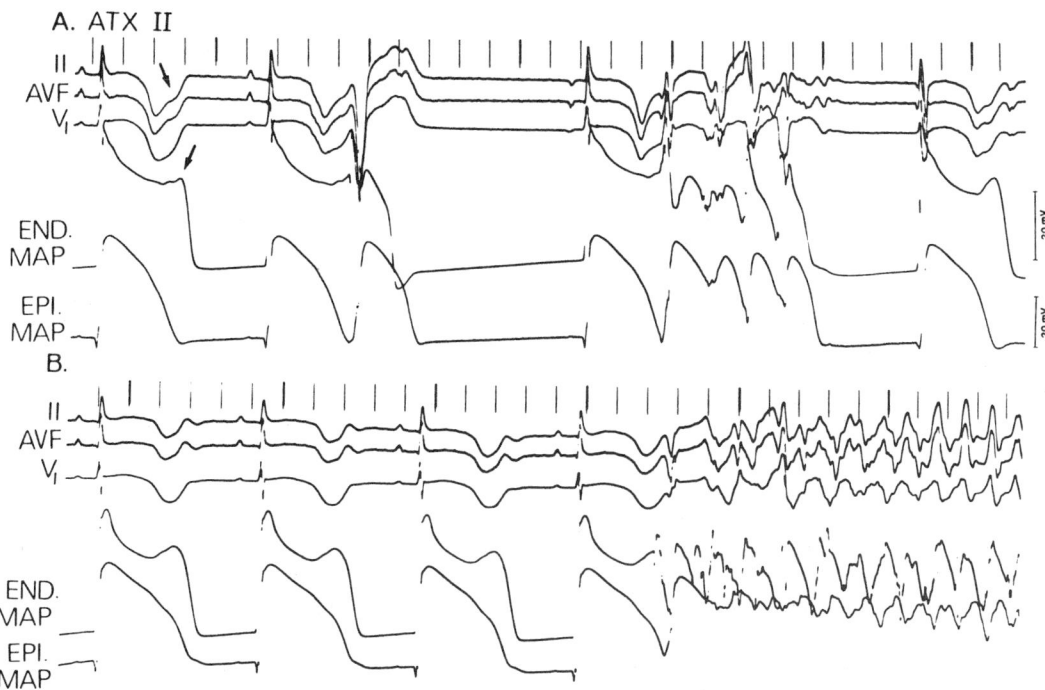

Figure 14. Simultaneous recording of endocardial (END) monophasic action potential (MAP), epicardial (EPI) MAP, and surface ECG from the same experiment shown in Figure 13. The recordings were obtained 14 and 16 minutes, respectively, following the administration of ATX-II (25 μg/kg). A shows a 4-beat run of polymorphic ventricular tachycardia, while B shows a polymorphic ventricular tachycardia that degenerated into ventricular fibrillation. The first premature ventricular depolarization in both tachyarrhythmias arose from the peak of an EAD in the endocardial MAP.

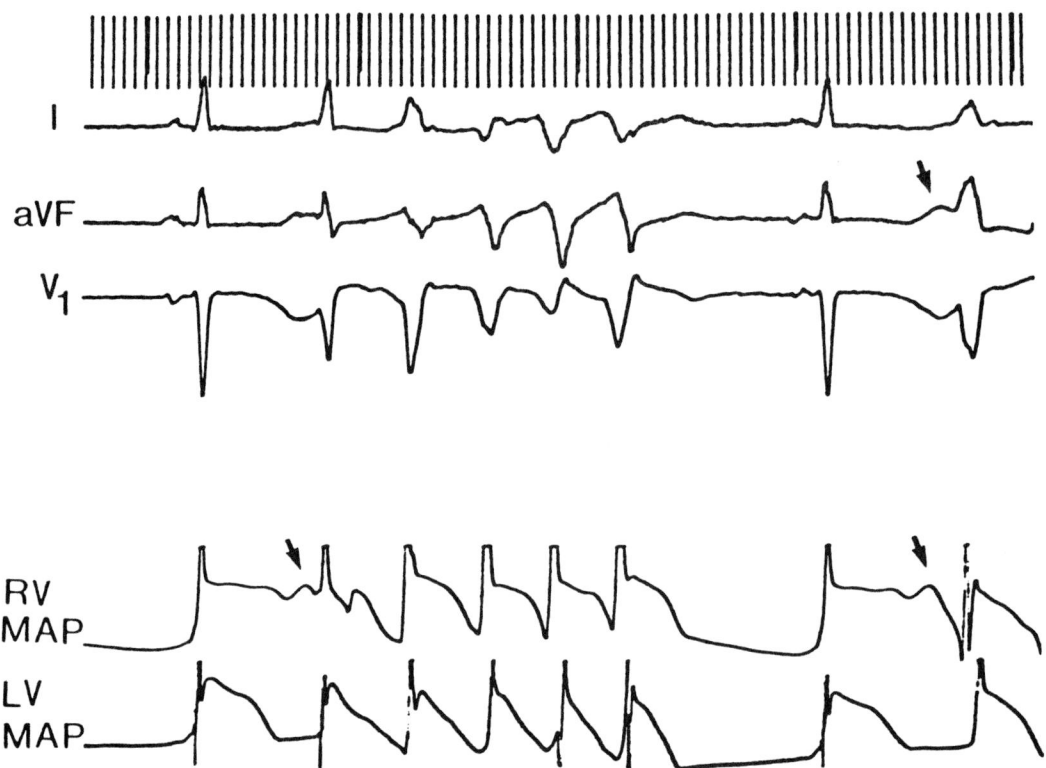

Figure 15. Simultaneous recording of monophasic action potential (MAP) from apical sites in the right ventricle (RV) and left ventricle (LV) in a patient with acquired long QTU and torsades de pointes who was receiving procainamide. The MAP from the RV site was markedly prolonged (640 msec) and showed a deflection at the end of the plateau consistent with early afterdepolarization (EAD) that corresponded to a prominent late deflection in the long QTU segment (both marked by arrows). Conversely, the MAP recording from the LV site had a much shorter duration (380 msec) and failed to show an EAD. The dispersion of repolarization between RV and LV sites was 260 msec. The torsades de pointes tachycardia was initiated by a premature depolarization that seemed to arise from the peak or on the descending limb of the EAD in the RV MAP. The premature action potential occurred 200 msec after the end of repolarization of the LV MAP. (Reproduced with permission from Reference 4.)

pointes represents an R-on-TU phenomenon, it usually arises from the terminal part of a markedly prolonged action potential, has relatively long coupling intervals to the preceding action potential, and probably would encounter mostly fully repolarized myocardial sites. Therefore, it may be less likely to result in circus movement reentry. Most experimental models of circus movement reentry have shown that for successful reentry to occur a critically timed premature beat should originate from the region with shorter refractoriness.[84–86]

Furthermore, the first ectopic action potential is always associated with a much shorter action potential duration compared to the preceding sinus beat (Figure 15). However, the decrease in action potential duration in response to the first or subsequent short cycles need not be the same at all myocardial zones. It is possible that an abnormal adjustment of action potential duration to shortening of the cardiac cycle length plays an important role in the mechanism of torsades de pointes.[87] Thus, the critical degree of dispersion of repolarization that may underlie possible circus movement reentry in torsades de pointes may not be the one associated with the first sinus beat, even though it is usually the largest. Rather, it may be the persistent dispersion of repolarization at subsequent short cycles that could create the electrophysiological prerequisite for circus movement reentry. A definite role of dispersion of repolarization and circus movement reentry in pharmacologically-induced torsades de pointes must await detailed tridimensional activation maps in appropriate experimental models.

References

1. Vaughn Williams EM: Delayed ventricular repolarization as an antiarrhythmic principle. *Eur Heart J* 6:145, 1985.
2. Bacaner MB, Clay JR, Shrier A, Brachu RM: Potassium channel blockade: a mechanism for suppressing ventricular fibrillation. *Proc Natl Acad Sci USA* 83:2223, 1985.
3. Han J, Moe GK: Nonuniform recovery of excitability in ventricular muscle. *Circ Res* 14:44, 1964.
4. El-Sherif N, Craelius W, Boutjdir M, Gough WB: Early afterdepolarizations and arrhythmogenesis. *J Cardiovasc Electrophysiol* 1:145, 1990.
5. Dessertenne F: La tachycardie ventriculaire a deux foyers opposes variables. *Arch Mal Coeur* 59:263, 1966.
6. Cranefield PF: Action potentials, afterpotentials, and arrhythmias. *Circ Res* 41:415, 1977.
7. Cranefield PF, Aronson RS: *Cardiac Arrhythmias: The Role of Triggered Activity and Other Mechanisms.* Mount Kisco, NY: Futura Publishing Company, Inc., 1988.
8. Trautwein W: Mechanisms of tachyarrhythmias and extrasystoles. In: E Sandoe, E Flenested-Jensen, KH Olesen (eds): *Symposium on Cardiac Arrhythmias.* Sodertalje, Sweden: AB Astra, 1970, p. 53.
9. Coraboeuf E, Deroubaix E, Coulombe A: Acidosis-induced abnormal repolarization and repetitive activity in isolated dog Purkinje fibers. *J Physiol (Paris)* 76:97, 1980.
10. Isenberg G, Ravens U: The effects of anemonia sulcata toxin (ATX II) on membrane currents of isolated mammalian myocytes. *J Physiol* 357:127, 1984.
11. Craelius W, Chen VKH, El-Sherif N: Sodium current modifications by anthopleurin-A and their role in early afterdepolarizations (abstract). *J Am Coll Cardiol* 11(2):253A, 1988.
12. January CT, Riddle JM, Salata JJ: A model for early afterdepolarizations: induction with the Ca^{2+} channel agonist Bay K 8644. *Circ Res* 62:563, 1988.
13. January CT, Riddle JM: Early afterdepolarizations: mechanism of induction and block. A role for L-type Ca^{2+} current. *Circ Res* 64:977, 1989.
14. Nattel S, Quantz MA: Pharmacological response of quinidine induced early afterdepolarizations in canine Purkinje fibers: insights into underlying ionic mechanisms. *Cardiovasc Res* 22:808, 1988.
15. Davidenko JM, Cohen L, Goodrow R, Antzelevitch C: Quinidine-induced action potential prolongation, early afterdepolarizations, and triggered activity in canine Purkinje fibers. Effects of stimulation rate, potassium, and magnesium. *Circulation* 79:674, 1989.
16. Sasyniuk BI, Valois M, Toy W: Recent advances in understanding the mechanisms of drug-induced Torsade de Pointes. *Am J Cardiol* 64(20):29J, 1989.
17. Damiano BP, Rosen MR: Effects of pacing on triggered activity induced by early afterdepolarizations. *Circulation* 69:1013, 1984.
18. Takanaka C, Singh BN: Barium-induced non-driven action potentials as a model of triggered potentials from early afterdepolarizations: significance of slow channel activity and differing effects of quinidine and amiodarone. *J Am Coll Cardiol* 15:213, 1990.
19. Mendez C, Delmar M: Triggered activity: its possible role in cardiac arrhythmias. In: D Zipes, J Jalife (eds): *Cardiac Electrophysiology and Arrhythmias.* Orlando, FL: Grune & Stratton, 1985, p. 311.
20. Attwell D, Cohen I, Eisner D, et al: The steady state TTX sensitive ("window") sodium current in cardiac Purkinje fibers. *Pflügers Arch* 379:137, 1979.
21. Gintant GA, Datyner NB, Cohen IS: Slow inactivation of a tetrodotoxin-sensitive current in canine cardiac Purkinje fibers. *Biophys J* 45:509, 1984.
22. Cohen NM, Lederer WJ: Calcium current in isolated neonatal rat ventricular myocytes. *J Physiol* 391:169, 1987.
23. Hirano Y, Moscucci A, January CT: Direct measurement of L-type Ca^{2+} window current in heart cells. *Circ Res* 70:445, 1992.
24. Earm YE, Noble D: A model of the single atrial cell: relation between calcium current and calcium release. *Proc R Soc* 240:83, 1990.
25. Gintant GA, Cohen IS, Datyner NB, Kline RP: Time-dependent outward currents in the heart. In: HA Fozzard, E Haber, RB Jennings, et al. (eds): *The Heart and Cardiovascular System.* New York, NY: Raven Press, 1991, p. 1121.

26. Kass RS, Tsien RW: Fluctuations in membrane current driven by intracellular calcium in cardiac Purkinje fibers. *Biophys J* 38:259, 1982.

27. Gadsby DC, Cranefield PF: Two levels of resting potential in cardiac Purkinje fibers. *J Gen Physiol* 70:725, 1977.

28. Noble D: Ionic bases of rhythmic activity in the heart. In: DP Zipes, J Jalife (eds): *Cardiac Electrophysiology and Arrhythmias*. Orlando, FL: Grune & Stratton, 1985, p. 3.

29. Hiraoka M, Sawada K, Kawano S: Effects of quinidine on plateau currents of guinea-pig ventricular myocytes. *J Mol Cell Cardiol* 18:1097, 1986.

30. Roden DM, Bennett PB, Synders DJ, et al: Quinidine delays I_K activation in guinea pig myocytes. *Circ Res* 62:1055, 1988.

31. Salata JJ, Wasserstrom JA: Effects of quinidine on action potentials and ionic currents in isolated canine ventricular myocytes. *Circ Res* 62:324, 1988.

32. Komeichi K, Tohse N, Nakaya H, et al: Effects of N-acetylprocainamide and sotalol on ion currents in isolated guinea-pig ventricular myocytes. *Eur J Pharmacol* 187:313, 1990.

33. Isenberg G: Cardiac Purkinje fibers: cesium as a tool to block inward rectifying potassium currents. *Pflügers Arch* 365:99, 1976.

34. Carmeliet E: Electrophysiologic and voltage clamp analysis of the effects of sotalol on isolated cardiac muscle and Purkinje fibers. *J Pharmacol Exp Ther* 323:817, 1985.

35. Arena JP, Kass RS: Block of heart potassium channels by clofilium and its tertiary analog: relationship between drug structure and type of channel block. *J Pharmacol Exp Ther* 34:60, 1988.

36. Gwilt M, Arrowsmith JE, Blackburn KJ, et al: UK-68,798: a novel, potent and highly selective Class III antiarrhythmic agent which blocks potassium channels in cardiac cells. *J Pharmacol Exp Ther* 256(1):318, 1991.

37. Sanguinetti MC, Jurkiewicz NK: Two components of cardiac delayed rectifier K^+ current. Differential sensitivity to block by Class III antiarrhythmic agents. *J Gen Physiol* 96:195, 1990.

38. Fish FA, Prakash C, Roden DM: Suppression of repolarization-related arrhythmias in vitro and in vivo by low-dose potassium channel activators. *Circulation* 82:1362, 1990.

39. Antzelevitch C, Sicouri S, Litovsky, et al: Heterogeneity within the ventricular wall. Electrophysiology and pharmacology of epicardial, endocardial, and M cells. *Circ Res* 69:1427, 1991.

40. Nilius B, Boldt W, Benndorf K: Properties of aconitine-modified sodium channels in single cells of mouse ventricular myocardium. *Gen Physiol Biophys* 5:473, 1986.

41. Barnes S, Hille B: Veratridine modifies open sodium channels. *J Gen Physiol* 91:421, 1988.

42. Hiraoka M, Sunami A, Fan Z, Sawanobori T: Multiple ionic mechanisms of early afterdepolarizations in isolated ventricular myocytes from guinea-pig hearts. *Ann NY Acad Sci* 64:33, 1992.

41. Huang L-Y M, Moran N, Ehrenstein G: Batrachotoxin modifies the gating kinetics of sodium channels in internally perfused neuroblastoma cells. *Proc Natl Acad Sci USA* 79:2082, 1982.

44. Kohlhardt M, Froke U, Herzig JW: Modification of single cardiac Na^+ channels by DPI 201–106. *J Membrane Biol* 89:163, 1986.

45. Hashimoto K, Ochi R, Inu J, Miura Y: The ionic mechanism of prolongation of action potential duration of cardiac ventricular muscle by anthopleurin-A and its relationship to the inotropic effect. *J Pharmacol Exp Ther* 215:479, 1980.

46. Schreibmayer W, Kazerani H, Tritthart HA: A mechanistic interpretation of the action of toxin II from anemonia sulcata on the cardiac sodium channel. *Biochim Biophys Acta* 901:273, 1987.

47. El-Sherif N, Fozzard HA, Hanck DA: Dose-dependent modulation of the cardiac sodium channel by sea anemone toxin ATXII. *Circ Res* 70:285, 1992.

48. Boutjdir M, El-Sherif N: Pharmacological evaluation of early afterdepolarizations induced by sea anemone toxin (ATXII) in dog heart. *Cardiovasc Res* 25:815, 1991.

49. Colatsky TJ: Mechanisms of action of lidocaine and quinidine on action potential duration in rabbit cardiac Purkinje fibers. *Circ Res* 50:17, 1982.

50. Lee KS, Hime JR, Geles W, Brown AM: Sodium current depression by lidocaine and quinidine in isolated ventricular cells. *Nature* 291:325, 1981.

51. Carmeliet E, Saikawa T: Shortening of the action potential and reduction of pacemaker activity by lidocaine, quinidine, and procainamide in sheep cardiac Purkinje fibers. *Circ Res* 50:257, 1982.

52. Imaizumi Y, Giles WR: Quinidine-induced inhibition of transient outward current in cardiac muscle. *Am J Physiol* 253:H704, 1987.

53. Hondeghem LM, Katzung BG: Antiarrhythmic agents: the modulated receptor mechanism of action of sodium and calcium channel blocking drugs. *Ann Rev Pharmacol Toxicol* 24:387, 1984.

54. Gough WB, El-Sherif N: The differential response of normal and ischaemic Purkinje fibres to clofilium, d-sotalol and bretylium. *Cardiovas Res* 23:554, 1989.

55. Kunze DL, Lacerda AE, Wilson DL, Brown AM: Cardiac Na currents and the inactivating, reopening and waiting properties of single cardiac Na channels. *J Gen Physiol* 86:697, 1985.

56. Patlak JB, Ortiz M: Slow currents through single sodium channels of the adult rat heart. *J Gen Physiol* 86:89, 1985.

57. Grant AO, Starmer CF: Mechanisms of closure of cardiac sodium channels in rabbit ventricular myocytes: single-channel analysis. *Circ Res* 80:897, 1987.

58. Fozzard HA, Hanck DA, Makielski JA, et al: Sodium channels in cardiac Purkinje cells. *Experientia* 43:1162, 1987.

59. Kiyosue T, Arita M: Late sodium current and its contribution to action potential configuration in guinea pig ventricular myocytes. *Circ Res* 64:389, 1989.

60. Marban E, Robinson SW, Wier WG: Mechanism of arrhythmogenic delayed and early afterdepolarizations in ferret muscle. *J Clin Invest* 78:1185, 1986.

61. Aliot E, Szabo B, Sweidan R, Lazzara R: Prevention of torsades de pointes with calcium channel blockade in an animal model (abstract). *J Am Coll Cardiol* 5:492, 1985.

62. Bailie DS, Inoue H, Kaseda S, et al: Magnesium suppression of early afterdepolarizations and ventricular tachyarrhyhtmias induced by cesium in dogs. *Circulation* 77:1395, 1988.

63. Tzivoni D, Keren A, Cohen AM, et al: Magnesium therapy for torsade de pointes. *Am J Cardiol* 53:528, 1984.

64. Lansman JB, Hess P, Tsien RW: Blockade of currents through single calcium channels by Cd^{2+}, Mg^{2+}, and Ca^{2+}. Voltage and concentration dependence of Ca^{2+} entry into the pore. *J Gen Physiol* 88:321, 1986.

65. Szabo B, Sweidan R, Patterson E, et al: Increased intracellular Ca^{2+} may be important also for early afterdepolarizations (abstract). *J Am Coll Cardiol* 9:210A, 1987.

66. El-Sherif N, Zeiler RH, Craelius W, et al: QTU prolongation and polymorphic ventricular tachyarrhythmias due to bradycardia-dependent early afterdepolarizations. *Circ Res* 63:286, 1988.

67. Restivo M, Kowtha V, Boutjdir M, et al: Mechanism of early afterdepolarization formation by delayed sodium inactivation. (abstract). *J Mol Cell Cardiol* 27(Suppl I):5, 1990.

68. Sicouri S, Antzelevitch C: Quinidine-induced early afterdepolarizations (EAD) develop slowly in canine ventricular muscle (abstract). *FASEB J* 15:A1277, 1988.

69. Antzelevitch C, Jalife J, Moe GK: Characteristics of reflection as a mechanism of reentrant arrhythmias and its relationship to parasystole. *Circulation* 61:182, 1980.

70. Gough WB, Hu D, El-Sherif N: Effects of clofilium in ischemic subendocardial Purkinje fibers one day post-infarction. *J Am Coll Cardiol* 11:431, 1988.

71. Hanich RF, Levine JH, Spear JF, Moore EN: Automatic modulation of ventricular arrhythmias in cesium chloride-induced long QT syndrome. *Circulation* 77:1149, 1988.

72. Inoue H, Murakawa Y, Toda I, et al: Epicardial activation pattern of torsade de pointes in canine hearts with quinidine-induced long QTU interval but without myocardial infarction. *Am Heart J* 111:1080, 1986.

73. Bardy GH, Ungerleider RM, Smith WM, Ideker RE: A mechanism of torsade de pointes in a canine model. *Circulation* 67:52, 1983.

74. Jackman WM, Clark M, Friday KJ, et al: Ventricular tachyarrhythmias in the long QT syndrome. *Med Clin North Am* 68:1079, 1984.

75. Roden DM, Hoffman BF: Action potential prolongation and induction of abnormal automaticity by low quinidine concentrations in canine Purkinje fibers. Relationship to potassium and cycle length. *Circ Res* 56:857, 1985.

76. El-Sherif N, Mehra R, Gough WB, Zeiler RH: Ventricular activation patterns of spontaneous and induced ventricular rhythms in canine one day old myocardial infarction. Evidence for focal and reentrant mechanism. *Circ Res* 51:152, 1982.

77. Brachmann J, Scherlag BJ, Rosenshtraukh LV, Lazzara R: Bradycardia-dependent triggered activity: relevance to drug-induced multiform ventricular tachycardia. *Circulation* 68:846, 1983.

78. Levine JH, Spear JF, Guarnieri T, et al: Cesium chloride-induced long QT syndrome: demonstration of afterdepolarizations and triggered activity in vivo. *Circulation* 72:1092, 1985.

79. El-Sherif N, Boutjdir M, Henkin R: Role of Purkinje and muscle fibers in a new model of Torsade de Pointes due to early afterdepolarizations (abstract). *Circulation* 78(4)II:158, 1983.

80. Gough WB, Henkin R: The early afterdepolarization as recorded by the monophasic action potential technique: fact or artifact (abstract). *Circulation* 80:II-130, 1989.

81. Bonati V, Roli A, Botti G: Recording of monophasic action potentials of the right ventricle in long QT syndromes complicated by severe ventricular arrhythmias. *Eur Heart J* 4:168, 1983.

82. Franz MR, Bargheer K, Raffenbeul W, et al: Monophasic action potential mapping in human subjects with normal electrocardiograms: direct evidence of the genesis of the T wave. *Circulation* 75:379, 1987.

83. Habbab MA, El-Sherif N: Drug-induced Torsade de Pointes. Role of early afterdepolarizations and dispersion of repolarization. *Am J Med* 89:241, 1990.

84. Allessie A, Bonke FIM, Schopman JG: Circus movement in rabbit atrial muscle as a mechanism of tachycardia. II. The role of nonuniform recovery of excitability in the occurrence of unidirectional blocks, as studied with multiple microelectrodes. *Circ Res* 39:168, 1976.

85. Gough WB, Mehra R, Restivo M, et al: Reentrant ventricular arrhythmia in the late myocardial infarction period in the dog. 13. Correlation of activation and refractory maps. *Circ Res* 57:432, 1985.

86. Kuo CS, Munakata K, Reddy CP, Surawicz B: Characteristics and possible mechanism of ventricular arrhythmias dependent on the dispersion of action potential durations. *Circulation* 67:1356, 1983.

87. Attwell D, Lee JA: A cellular basis for the primary long QT syndromes. *Lancet* I:1136, 1988.

PART IV

Clinical Considerations and Therapeutic Implications

Chapter 25

Programmed Electrical Stimulation Versus Electrocardiographic Monitoring Guided Therapy for Ventricular Tachyarrhythmias

Wolfram Grimm
Mark E. Josephson

The therapy of patients with ventricular tachyarrhythmias should prevent sudden cardiac death and recurrence of potentially lethal arrhythmias as sustained ventricular tachycardias (VT) and/or decrease symptoms. Importantly, clinical presentation of the arrhythmia (ie, well-tolerated VT versus cardiac arrest) as well as the type and severity of the underlying heart disease may reflect differences in the anatomical and electrophysiological substrate and are of the utmost importance for therapy and prognosis of patients with tachyarrhythmias. Therefore, it is mandatory that these arrhythmias are not grouped together in terms of diagnostic evaluation, effects of pharmacological therapy, and clinical outcome.

Since empiric therapy, with the exception of β-blocker therapy in patients after myocardial infarction, clearly failed to reduce sudden death from ventricular arrhythmias, electrocardiographic (Holter) monitoring and programmed ventricular stimulation (PES) are the two clinical techniques most commonly used to guide antiarrhythmic drug therapy[1-4] in patients with ventricular tachyarrhythmias. Newer techniques like the signal-averaged ECG or heart rate variability measurements may be useful in identifying patients at risk for potentially lethal arrhythmias, in addition to clinical parameters such as low ventricular ejection fraction despite their modest positive predictive value. However, to date, these techniques cannot be used to guide antiarrhythmic therapy.[5-12] Of note, positive signal-averaged ECGs in patients with recurrent VT remain positive in almost all patients after successful long-term drug therapy, catheter ablation, or device therapy. Although the disappearance of late potentials in patients undergoing subendocardial resection for recurrent VT may indicate the removal of the substrate of the arrhythmia, a positive postop-

Supported in part by grants HL28093 and HL07346 from the National Heart, Lung, and Blood Institute, Bethesda, Maryland. Dr. Grimm is supported by a grant from the German Science Foundation, University of Marburg, Germany. From BN Singh, HJJ Wellens, M Hiraoka, (eds): *Electropharmacological Control of Cardiac Arrhythmias*. Mount Kisco, NY, Futura Publishing Company Inc., © 1994.

erative signal-averaged ECG by no means predicts failure of the procedure.

This chapter discusses the preference of programmed ventricular stimulation over Holter monitoring to guide pharmacological therapy in patients with potentially lethal ventricular tachyarrhythmias. Importantly, only about 30% to 50% of these patients have induction of ventricular tachyarrhythmias suppressed with available antiarrhythmic drugs.[13,14] In patients considered for nonpharmacological forms of therapy including surgical or catheter ablation of VT or implantable cardioverter defibrillator therapy with or without antitachycardia pacing capabilities, electrophysiological testing is mandatory, and Holter monitoring alone cannot be used to guide therapy.

The role of programmed ventricular stimulation and Holter monitoring in guiding therapy in patients with known ventricular tachyarrhythmias, which will be discussed, must be differentiated from the role of both techniques to identify patients at high risk for sudden cardiac death who never had malignant ventricular tachyarrhythmias. In the latter patients, both Holter monitoring and programmed stimulation are limited by a low positive predictive accuracy when used independently from other variables such as positive signal-averaged ECG and impaired left ventricular function as discussed elsewhere.[15]

Programmed Ventricular Stimulation

The gold standard for programmed ventricular stimulation guided therapy is noninducibility of sustained VT or ventricular fibrillation (VF) that has been reproducibly initiated in the absence of drugs. This is based on two assumptions: (1) the induced arrhythmia is identical to the patient's spontaneous arrhythmia; and (2) the laboratory response to drugs predicts the clinical response during long-term therapy. Some investigators have suggested that the relative ease of VT or VF

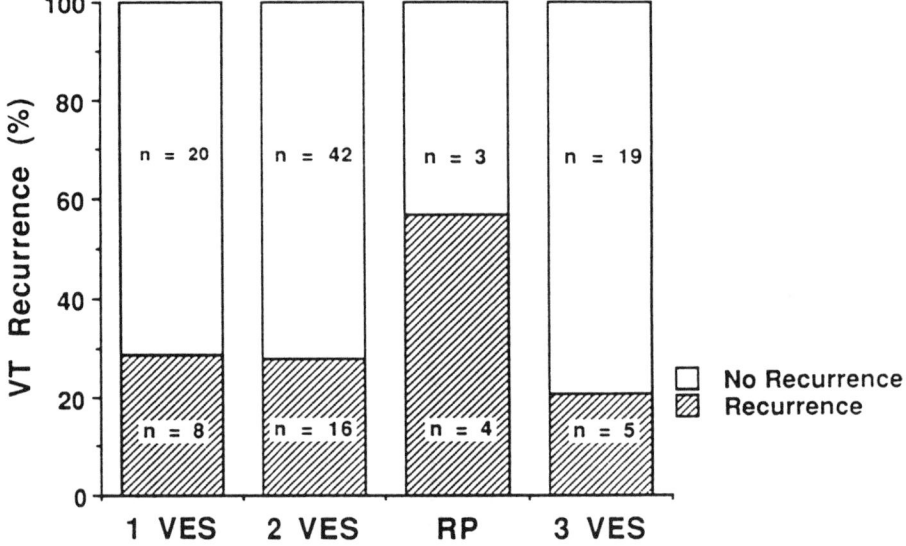

Figure 1. Relationship of mode of initiation of ventricular tachycardia (VT) to outcome. The mode of VT initiation is shown on the horizontal axis. Of note, there is no difference in recurrence rate (dotted bars) and freedom from recurrence (white bars) based on the mode of induction. Only seven patients had VT induced by rapid pacing (RP). VES: ventricular extrastimuli. (Adapted with permission from Reference 17.)

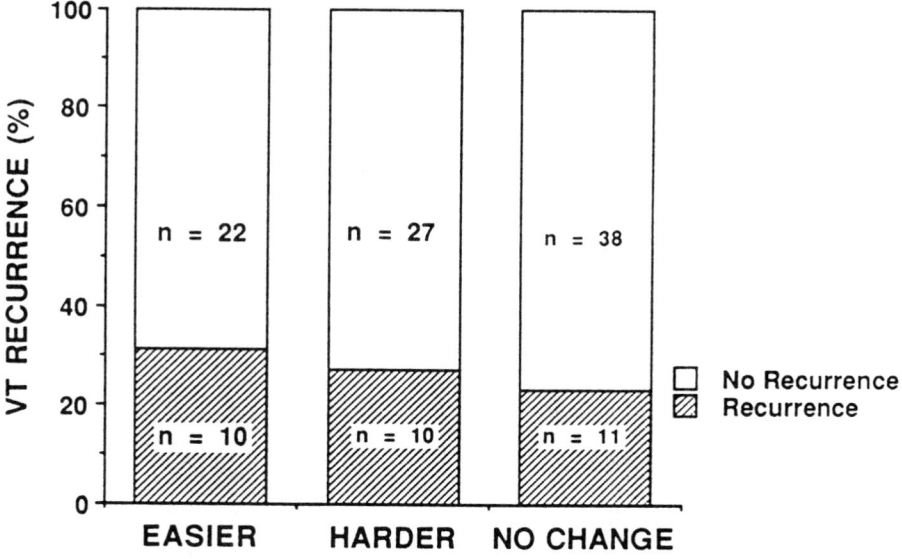

Figure 2. The relationship of relative ease of initiation of ventricular tachycardia (VT) to recurrence rate. The effect of antiarrhythmic agents on the relative ease of induction (ie, the number of extrastimuli used) is shown on the horizontal axis. Of note, the relative ease of induction had no influence on recurrence rate (dotted bars) and freedom of recurrence (white bars). (Adapted with permission from Reference 17.)

initiation might be useful.[16] We have found neither the absolute number of extrastimuli (Figure 1) nor the relative ease of induction (Figure 2) to be a useful predictor of outcome.[17] Swerdlow and colleagues[18] suggested that the induction of 15 beats or less was predictive of a good outcome. As it is uncommon for an arrhythmia to last more than 15 or 20 complexes without being sustained, 15 complexes represent the statistical likelihood of an arrhythmia to be nonsustained rather than a magical number.

The sensitivity and specificity of ventricular stimulation critically depends on the mode of stimulation (Figure 3): the more vigorous the programmed stimulation, the higher the sensitivity of inducing VT, but the lower the specificity. The use of different stimulation protocols in different laboratories complicates the comparison of reported results. The most important intrinsic factors of the stimulation protocol that affect sensitivity are: (1) the number of extrastimuli delivered; (2) the number of stimulation sites; (3) the drive cycle

lengths; and (4) the current strengths applied.[19–24] In our laboratory, we recommend the use of up to three extrastimuli at twice diastolic threshold current delivered during at least two drive cycle lengths from at least two right ventricular sites.[15] In addition, we use rapid ventricular pacing, decreasing the cycle length to 250 msec or to the cycle length at which loss of 1:1 capture occurs, and pacing from left ventricular sites in patients with uniform sustained VT, in whom the stimulation protocol described above failed to induce the arrhythmia, although the additional yield of inducing uniform VT with rapid pacing or left ventricular stimulation is small (2%–5%).[15]

Using this protocol, 95% of patients presenting with sustained uniform VT in the setting of coronary artery disease had uniform VT reproducibly initiated in our laboratory (Figure 4). In patients with cardiac arrest, however, sustained uniform VT was induced in slightly more than 50% of patients. In addition, about 30% of patients had polymorphic VT or VF induced by PES (Figure 4). The in-

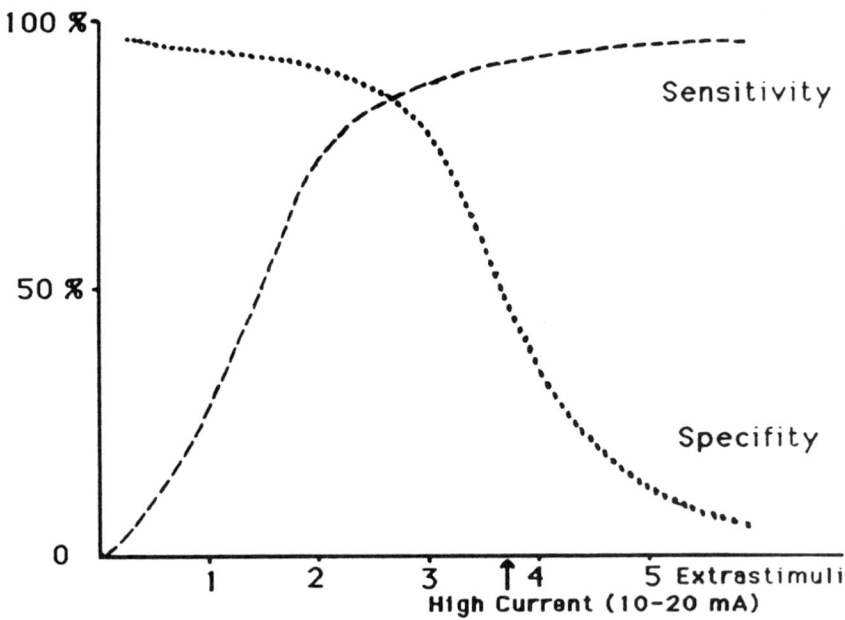

Figure 3. Relationship between sensitivity and specificity of induced arrhythmias by programmed stimulation. An increasingly aggressive stimulation protocol is shown on the horizontal axis, from a single extrastimulus to five extrastimuli. See text for discussion. (Reproduced with permission from Reference 72.)

duction of polymorphic VT in patients presenting with uniform VT most likely represents a nonspecific response to PES without clinical significance. Reproducibly-induced polymorphic VT or VF in patients with chronic ischemic heart disease who survived a cardiac arrest, however, may be more significant, since half of cardiac arrests may be initiated by polymorphic VT or VF.

In our experience, patients with chronic ischemic heart disease presenting with tolerated, sustained uniform VT have a very low incidence of recurrent VT (9%) during 2-year follow-up, if the tachycardia had been noninducible by PES guided drug therapy (Figure 5). The results of programmed stimulation guided therapy with Class I drugs from laboratories using similar stimulation protocols as described above are summarized in Table 1. Inducibility of sustained VT or VF ranged from 43% of patients presenting with cardiac arrest in the study of Poole and colleagues[25] to 95% of patients presenting with uniform VT in the

series reported by Horowitz et al.[26] Importantly, the negative predictive accuracy of programmed ventricular stimulation with Class I antiarrhythmic agents defined as freedom of arrhythmia recurrence or sudden cardiac death, if an antiarrhythmic agent is found which renders the arrhythmia noninducible, is very good (80% to 90%, Table 1). The positive predictive accuracy of programmed stimulation defined as the ability to predict recurrence of the arrhythmia or sudden cardiac death, if no antiarrhythmic drug is found to render the arrhythmia noninducible, is only about 30% to 50% in most studies. This moderate positive predictive accuracy may in part, be due to the short mean follow-up of 1 to 2 years in most reported series, and the unknown natural history of the clinical arrhythmias. Although the number of patients with VT or VF recurrence increases with follow-up duration, as demonstrated for example by the actuarial incidence of appropriate shocks in patients with implantable cardioverter defi-

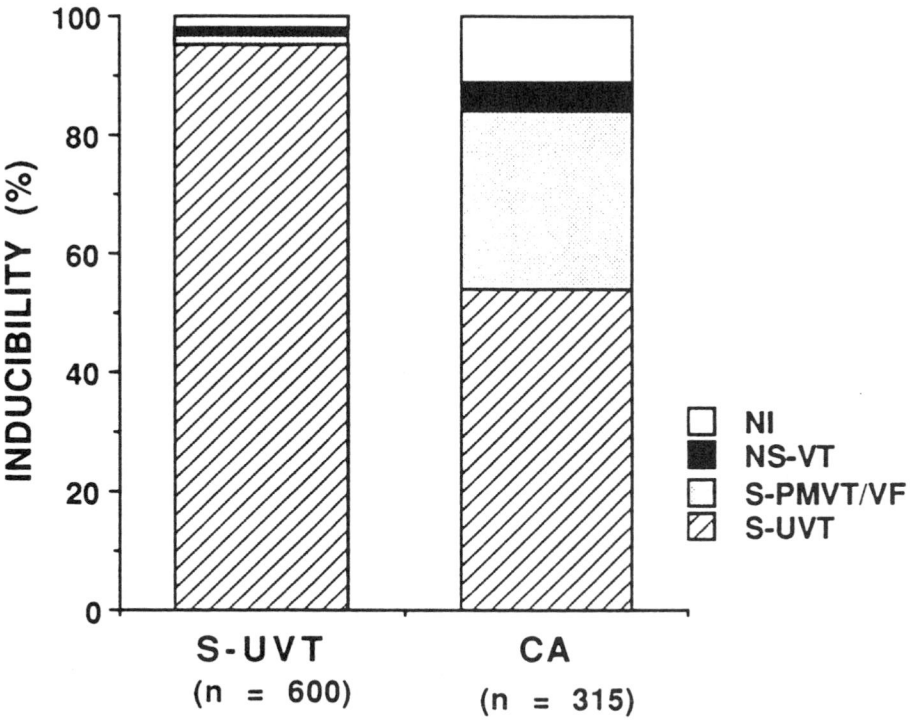

Figure 4. Inducibility of ventricular tachycardia (VT) in patients presenting with uniform VT and cardiac arrest in coronary disease. The bar diagrams show the incidence of inducible arrhythmias in patients presenting with sustained uniform ventricular tachycardia (S-UVT) on the left and cardiac arrest (CA) on the right. In patients presenting with VT, 95% have sustained uniform VT induced. In patients presenting with cardiac arrest, sustained uniform VT and polymorphic VT or fibrillation (S-PMVT/VF) are the most commonly initiated arrhythmias. Non-sustained VT (NS-VT) is less commonly induced. No inducible arrhythmia (NI) is observed in about 15%. (Adapted from with permission Reference 15.)

brillator,[27,28] a significant number of patients with documented VT or VF remain free of arrhythmia recurrence despite persistent tachycardia inducibility during PES. However, we believe that any method to guide therapy of these malignant arrhythmias overpredicting failure is less hazardous than underpredicting success, since the latter error may mean death of the patient. For the case of hemodynamically well tolerated uniform VT, recurrences are usually well tolerated, and survival may not be significantly influenced by recurrence as predicted by persistent inducibility.[29] In survivors of cardiac arrest, however, recurrence is more likely to be fatal. Of note, the results of PES guided drug therapy in patients with aborted sudden cardiac deaths are diver-

gent in the two largest reported series.[25,30] Wilber and colleagues[30] found a 1-year incidence of cardiac arrest recurrence of 12% of 91 patients, in whom inducible arrhythmias had been suppressed, and in 33% of 36 patients, in whom inducible arrhythmias persisted. Importantly, the 1-year incidence of recurrent cardiac arrest in patients with noninducible VT on drugs was only 1% to 2% in the subgroup with an ejection fraction > 30%. In contrast to Wilber et al.[30] and other investigators,[31,32] Poole and colleagues[25] did not find that noninducibility by PES guided therapy with Class I drugs predicted a better prognosis than persistent inducibility of baseline-induced tachyarrhythmias. The underlying cardiac disease was chronic ischemic heart dis-

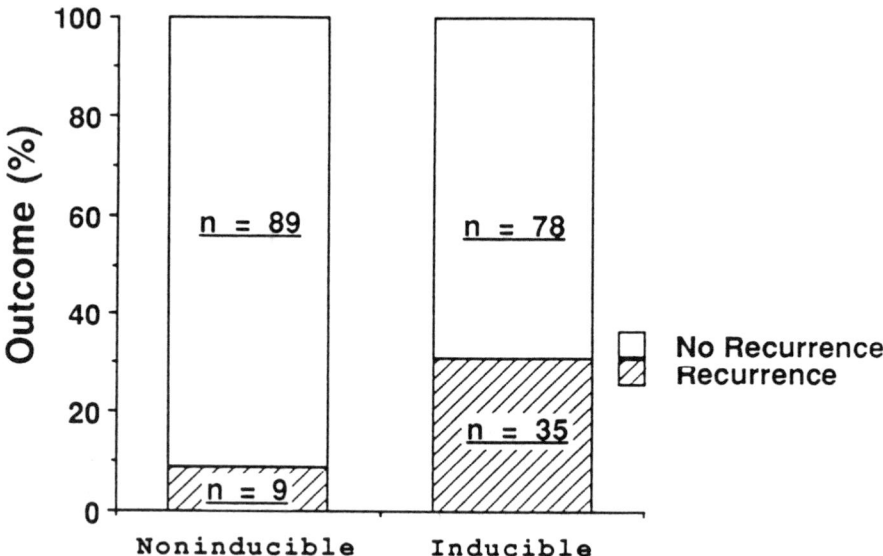

Figure 5. Incidence of recurrent ventricular tachycardia (VT) during 2-year follow-up on Class I drugs in patients presenting with hemodynamically tolerated, sustained, uniform VT. The bars show the incidence of recurrent VT relative to persistent inducibility (left) and suppression of VT induction (right) during electrophysiological testing. Positive predictive value was 31% and negative value was 91%. (Adapted with permission from Reference 15.)

Table 1
Programmed Ventricular Stimulation in Patients with Sustained Ventricular Tachyarrhythmias

	Number of pts.	Cardiac arrest	Inducibility of VT/VF	Mean FU (months)	# of Pts followed	Drug tested	PES predictive value positive	negative
Horrowitz (1982)[26]	111	0%	95%	18	111	Class I	91%	93%
Swerdlow (1983)[38]	239	38%	86%	15	105	Class I*	34%	89%
Roy (1983)[31]	119	100%	61%	17	42	Class I*	22%	83%
Skale (1986)[32]	62	100%	74%	22	41	Class I†*	37%	100%
Kim (1986)[39]	52	8%	Prerequisite	18	52	Class I	30%	60%
Wilber (1988)[30]	166	100%	52%	21	127	Class I†*	33%	88%
Poole (1990)[25]	241	100%	43%	30	92	Class I*	NA§	NA§
Josephson (1992)[15]	211	0%	95%	24	211	Class I	31%	91%

* Some patients who did not have inducibility of VT or VF suppressed by Class I drugs were followed on amiodarone.
† Some patients had induction of VT suppressed on amiodarone.
§ In this study, survival was not improved by noninducibility during PES guided drug therapy.
Pts: patients; FU: follow-up; PES: programmed ventricular stimulation; NA: not available; VT: ventricular tachyarrhythmias; VF: ventricular fibrillation.

ease in approximately 70% of patients in both series,[25,30] and therefore, cannot explain the divergent results in both studies.

While sustained uniform VT may also occur in patients with hypertrophic or dilated cardiomyopathy, cardiac arrest due to polymorphic VT and/or VF is 10 times as common as hemodynamically tolerated VT. In the setting of idiopathic cardiomyopathy, conflicting data still exist as to the predictive value of antiarrhythmic therapy that proved effective in preventing VT inducibility.[14,33–36] Moreover, most patients with cardiomyopathy do not respond to antiarrhythmic therapy as indexed by noninducibility of sustained VT during PES. Therefore, the implantable cardioverter defibrillator is usually the therapy of choice in patients with idiopathic cardiomyopathy and hemodynamically poorly tolerated, sustained ventricular tachyarrhythmias.

In contrast to Holter monitoring, electrophysiological testing is useful in predicting the effect of antiarrhythmic drugs on tachycardia cycle length.[15] A recent analysis by Waller et al.[29] of 258 patients with inducible sustained VT baseline showed a similar reduction in sudden cardiac death mortality in the group of patients in whom VT became noninducible during serial drug testing as compared to the group of patients in whom tachycardia remained inducible, but the VT cycle length increased more than 100 msec and the tachycardia was well tolerated. Increase in cycle length of induced VT after drug administration, however, did not prevent arrhythmia recurrence. Notably, only 13% of patients in the study from Waller at al.[29] presented with a cardiac arrest. In contrast to these findings, a recent study by Sousa and colleagues[37] of 31 patients with aborted sudden death revealed a 2-year actuarial incidence of sudden death of 31% in the 11 patients in whom antiarrhythmic drugs suppressed VT induction or resulted in hemodynamically stable induced VT. In the majority of these 11 patients, however, therapy included amiodarone. For amiodarone, the value of programmed stimulation is not yet established.

Electrocardiographic (Holter) Monitoring

The Holter monitoring approach assumes that ventricular ectopic activity is a marker for sustained arrhythmias and that abolition or significant reduction of this ambient ectopy will prevent recurrences of sustained ventricular arrhythmias (VPC hypothesis). In the Cardiac Arrhythmia Suppression Trial (CAST), however, Holter guided treatment with encainide and flecainide lead to a 3.6-fold increase in arrhythmic deaths compared to the placebo group in patients after myocardial infarction.[40] Of note, this deleterious effect occurred despite over 80% suppression of VPCs and over 90% suppression of nonsustained VT. Although high-risk patients with sustained VT or VF had been excluded from the CAST study or died during the titration phase resulting in low mortality in the placebo group, and although it is not clear whether the CAST findings can be extrapolated to other antiarrhythmic agents,[40–42] two conclusions regarding Holter guided therapy can be drawn: (1) abolition of ventricular ectopy does not confirm freedom from VT or VF (death of the VPC hypothesis); and (2) Holter monitoring cannot predict deleterious proarrhythmic effects of drugs. These conclusions are confirmed by previous observations that 30% to 50% of VT or VF recurrences in the absence of acute ischemia are not triggered by VPCs,[17] and up to 50% of patients with VT or VF have no or insufficient ventricular ectopy to be used to assess antiarrhythmic ectopy.[43] Furthermore, the high hourly and daily variability of arrhythmia frequency and complexity does not only reduce the applicability of Holter monitoring to approximately 50% of patients with sustained tachyarrhythmias, but also makes the definition of a therapeutic end point difficult. If, for example, abolition of all nonsustained VT is considered a therapeutic end point, at least five episodes of nonsustained VT must be recorded in the baseline state.[44] Since only a few patients would be eligible for Holter guided therapy using absence of nonsustained VT as therapeutic end point, most studies like CAST[40] or the Electrophysiological Study Versus Electrocardiographic Monitoring (ESVEM) trial[45] use 90% reduction in mean VT count, and 70% to 80% reduction in VPCs as criteria for drug efficacy. In a prospective study by Pratt and colleagues,[46] 25% of 80 patients with documented VT, cardiac arrest, or syncope of cardiac origin showed less than 10 ventricular premature depolarizations per hour on Holter, and the majority of patients did not have runs of nonsustained VT during a mean of 22 hours of Holter monitoring. In this study, 65% of patients had sustained VT induced by PES. Of note, VT inducibility did not correlate with frequency or complexity of ventricular ectopy during Holter monitoring.

Programmed Ventricular Stimulation Versus Holter Monitoring

To date, only one prospective randomized study by Mitchell and colleagues[47] compared Holter guided therapy to electrophysiological testing in a small patient population (Table 1). In this study, electrophysiological testing appeared to predict drug efficacy more accurately than did Holter monitoring, similar to the findings of Chua and co-workers,[48] Platia and colleagues[49] and Skale et al.[32] (Table 2). Very small patient numbers and limitations of the study protocols in the former studies formed the rationale for the ESVEM study.[45,50] At the time of this writing 486 patients with more than 10 VPCs per hour and inducible VT or VF in the baseline state have been randomized to Holter monitoring or PES guided drug therapy, but the predictive values of both methods have not been published. Of note, although the baseline electrophysiological study in the ESVEM trial consists of up to three extrastimuli at two right ventricular sites and two basic drive cycle lengths, a third extrastimulus or second right ventricular site during serial drug testing is only used in patients in whom a third extrastimulus or second pacing site was required for tachycardia induction in the baseline study. We believe that complete protocols with triple extrastimuli are necessary in order to assure that a predicted success is a success. Since many of the drugs tested in the ESVEM study slow conduction not only in the reentry circuit itself, but also in the tissue between the right ventricular pacing site and the reentry circuit, which is almost always located in the left ventricle in patients with coronary artery disease, a third extrastimulus or second ventricular pacing site might sometimes be necessary to overcome slowing of conduction in the intervening tissue after drug administration. Therefore, the omission of completing the whole stimulation protocol on each drug regimen in order to confirm

---

Table 2
Programmed Stimulation Versus Holter Monitoring in Patients with Sustained Ventricular Tachyarrhythmias

	Number of pts.	Mean FU (months)	PES predictive value		Holter predictive value	
			positive	negative	positive	negative
Chua (1983)[48]	95	15	55%	94%	17%	73%
Platia (1984)[49]	44	18	88%	94%	70%	50%
Skale (1986)[32]	62	22	40%	100%	NA	56%
Mitchell (1987)[47]	57	26	NA*	NA*	NA*	NA*
ESVEM (1991)[45]	486	36	NP	NP	NP	NP

* 18% arrhythmia recurrence in PES guided group and 45% arrhythmia recurrence in Holter monitoring-guided group.
PES: progr. stimulation; Pts: patients; NA: not available; NP: not yet published; FU: follow-up.

noninducibility of VT most likely results in a lower negative predictive value for arrhythmia recurrence in the electrophysiological study limb than could be expected from the results of previous studies (Table 1). Moreover, patients presenting with tolerated VT, and patients with hemodynamically unstable VT and VF have been grouped together. The end points should be different; ie, for VT it should be recurrent VT and/or sudden cardiac death, while for VF it should be sudden cardiac death. Since the incidence of sudden cardiac death will be low in patients presenting with tolerated VT, the ESVEM trial will probably show that there is no difference in sudden cardiac death rate between Holter and PES guided therapy. For recurrence of VT, PES prediction should be better.

The hypothesis that drugs often render tachycardias noninducible by slowing conduction in the intervening tissue between stimulus site and reentry circuit rather than in the circuit itself is supported by a recent study from our laboratory.[51] In more than half of the patients in whom no tachycardia was inducible on drugs, a tachycardia could be initiated when the current was increased to 10 mA. The clinical significance of this finding remains to be determined by long-term follow-up of these patients. Jazayeri and colleagues[52] showed that isoproterenol administration allowed reinitiation of VT in 10 of 17 patients rendered noninducible with Class I drugs. The patients, in whom isoproterenol lead to reinitiation of VT during PES, had a higher incidence of spontaneous VT recurrence during follow-up.

Whereas more patients with sustained ventricular tachyarrhythmias qualify for programmed stimulation guided therapy than for Holter guided therapy as discussed above, more patients are assessed to be effectively treated with Class I agents by Holter monitoring than by programmed stimulation. Of note, the results of both techniques were discordant in more than 50% of patients in the study by Kim and colleagues.[53] In the majority of discordant cases the drug was assessed to be effective by Holter criteria but ineffective by PES

criteria. Unfortunately, the predictive accuracy of each method could not be evaluated due to the lack of clinical follow-up.

Amiodarone

Since only 30% to 50% of patients with ventricular tachyarrhythmias respond to antiarrhythmic therapy with type I drugs based on serial electrophysiological testing (ie, noninducibility of sustained VT), amiodarone is often used after type I agents have failed despite its considerable side effects. The usefulness of programmed stimulation guided therapy with amiodarone is still controversial.[54-71] Noninducibility on amiodarone correlates with an excellent clinical response with a negative predictive value of 80% to 100%. However, the incidence of noninducibility on amiodarone is low (10%–20%), and the majority of patients who remain inducible do well: only about 40% of the patients in whom VT or VF remains inducible have a recurrence.[72] A study by Gottlieb et al.[73] suggests that in patients who presented with cardiac arrest, 25% of recurrences during amiodarone therapy will still be cardiac arrest, regardless of how slow the induced arrhythmia has been during electrophysiological testing, or even if the arrhythmia was rendered noninducible by amiodarone.

Similar to type I agents, Holter criteria more frequently predict efficacy of amiodarone than does programmed stimulation. A recent review of several reported series[72] revealed that efficacy of amiodarone by Holter criteria appeared to have a similarly good negative predictive value as programmed stimulation. The positive predictive value for Holter monitoring appeared to be even greater than that for programmed stimulation. Most of these studies, however, had been nonrandomized, retrospective, or included only a very small patient population. The results from ongoing prospective clinical trials like the Conventional Versus Amiodarone Drug Evaluation Study (CASCADE), Canadian Amiodarone Myocardial Infarction Arrhythmia Trial

(CAMIAT), the European Myocardial Infarction Arrhythmia Trial (EMIAT), and the second clinical trial conducted by Veterans Administration investigators in the United States will contribute to clarify the potential benefit of amiodarone.[74-76]

Sotalol

Sotalol is a noncardioselective β-blocking agent with potent Class III antiarrhythmic effects.[77-79] Similar to the use of intravenous procainamide for prediction of inducibility with oral procainamide[80] or other Class I agents[81] during electrophysiological testing in patients with uniform VT, the response to intravenous sotalol during programmed stimulation appears to predict the response to oral sotalol.[82] In contrast to β blockers without Class III effects, sotalol has been found to suppress frequent ventricular ectopy very effectively during Holter monitoring[83-87]; significant, dose-dependent suppression of VPCs with sotalol, defined as more than 75% arrhythmia reduction, was found in 56% to 83% of patients with frequent ventricular ectopy,[83,86] and appears to compare favorably with standard Class I agents.[86]

In contrast to the controversy regarding the effect of amiodarone on VT/VF inducibility and the subsequent clinical outcome, the available data on sotalol are more consistent (Table 3). Notable, all studies published after 1986 and listed in Table 3 had been performed using a stimulation protocol with up to three ventricular extrastimuli for assessment of sotalol efficacy. Importantly, the negative predictive value of sotalol by PES defined as lack of clinical arrhythmia recurrence or sudden cardiac death, if sustained VT or VF was not inducible on the drug, appears to be excellent and ranges from 80% to 100% (Table 3). In addition, sotalol appears to be slightly more effective at preventing VT and/or VF induction than Class I agents. However, the ability of programmed stimulation to predict arrhythmia recurrence on sotalol (positive predictive accuracy) varies from 0% to 100%. This variability may be due in part to the small number of patients followed on sotalol despite persistent inducibility of sustained VT as well as differences in stimulation protocol, definition of therapeutic end points, patient selection, and duration of clinical follow-up.

In an uncontrolled multicenter study reported by Kehoe et al.,[95] the incidence of ar-

Table 3
Sotalol in Patients with Sustained Ventricular Tachyarrhythmias Refractory to Other Antiarrhythmic Drugs

	Number of pts.	Noninducibility with oral Sotalol	Follow-up on Sotalol		PES predictive accuracy		PES/ Holter correlation
			(months)	# of pts	Recurrence	No recurrence	
Senges (1984)[88]	18†	69%* (iv)	16	9	NA	91%	No
Nademanee (1985)[89]	33	45%* (iv)	9	25	60%	73%	Yes
Steinbeck (1986)[90]	34	32%*	13	22	100%	94%	No
Gonzales (1988)[91]	45	20%	20	18	27%	100%	NA
Singh (1988)[92]	14	58%	19	14	NA	NA	No
Ruder (1989)[93]	39	20%	12	24	44%	83%	No
Kuchar (1989)[94]	42	24%	8	14	0%	78%	NA
Kehoe (1990)[95]	236*	31%	12	151§	14%	87%	NA
Kus (1992)[96]	22	45%	23	6	NA	100%	NA

* Only 2 ventricular extrastimuli used. All other studies used up to 3 extrastimuli at 2 sites and 2 drive cycle lengths.
† Eight patients had no previous drug trials.
§ Only 106 of 236 patients underwent PES baseline, and only 68 of these 106 patients were discharged on sotalol.
PES: programmed ventricular stimulation; Pts: patients; iv: intravenously; NA: not available.

rhythmia recurrence on sotalol during a short follow-up of 12 months appeared to be independent from persistent inducibility during PES and independent from VPC suppression during Holter monitoring. Since only 9 of 68 patients assessed by PES in this study had clinical arrhythmia recurrences, the lack of a difference in outcome of drug responders and nonresponders by PES most likely reflects a type II statistical error. Furthermore, patients presenting with VT and VF, and patients with coronary and noncoronary artery disease have been grouped together in this study. Analogous to Class I drugs, sotalol more frequently resulted in a significant suppression of VPCs (more than 75% reduction) during Holter monitoring than in suppression of inducibility of VT (more than 9 beats): 51% of patients responded to Holter criteria, and only 31% of patients had no VT induced during PES, respectively. All patients in this study, however, had failed at least three previously administered antiarrhythmic drugs. If sotalol had been tried as a first-line agent, the relative efficacy might have been different.

It is of note, that only one study listed in Table 3 by Nademanee and colleagues[89,97] found a positive correlation between the effect of sotalol on VT inducibility by PES and the effect of sotalol on VPC suppression during Holter monitoring. In all other studies, either no correlation between Holter and EPS result was found,[88,90,92,93] or the correlation had not been evaluated.[91,94–96]

Proarrhythmic Drug Effects

Four examples of ventricular proarrhythmia are generally accepted[15,98]: fascicular (bidirectional) VT in digitalis toxicity; torsades de pointes (eg, Class Ia and III drugs); the development of incessant, but tolerated VT (eg, Class Ia and Ic drugs); and the development of a sine wave-like ventricular arrhythmia, which may be difficult to cardiovert (Class Ic drugs). These arrhythmias cannot be predicted by programmed ventricular stimu-

lation or Holter monitoring. As the natural history of malignant arrhythmias remains unknown in the individual patient, the definition of proarrhythmia, except the examples mentioned, is a problem. Holter monitoring clearly failed to predict lethal proarrhythmic effects of encainide and flecainide the CAST study, although the drugs suppressed VPCs very effectively. Conversely, we also believe that electrophysiological testing cannot be used to predict proarrhythmic drug effects in patients with spontaneous VT or VF. Proposed definitions for proarrhythmic drug effects during electrophysiological testing include: (1) VT induction only on drug; (2) induction of new VT morphologies; (3) induction of faster and/or more poorly tolerated VT; and (4) VT easier to induce; (5) VT more difficult to terminate. The effects of drugs on tachycardia termination do not reflect their efficacy on tachycardia initiation and have nothing to do with proarrhythmia. This is confirmed by a recent study from our laboratory.[99] Tachycardia termination by infusion of procainamide did not prevent reinduction of sustained VT in 54% of patients immediately after termination. As discussed, we have never found the relative ease of tachycardia induction or the absolute number of extrastimuli useful in predicting arrhythmia recurrence (Figures 1 and 2). Therefore, easier VT induction after administration of a drug cannot be defined as proarrhythmia. Finally, the clinical significance of new and/or faster VT morphologies after drug administration or inducible VT on drug only by no means proves a proarrhythmic drug effect. When completion of the whole stimulation protocol is performed, many patients already have multiple VT morphologies induced at baseline (Figure 6). New VT morphologies after drug administration despite completion of the stimulation protocol baseline can be induced in up to 50% of patients after incremental dosing of procainamide in our experience.[100] Presuming reentry as the mechanism of uniform VT, new VT morphologies could possibly be: (1) changes in the properties of the reentry circuit of the baseline VT; (2) unmasking of a previously

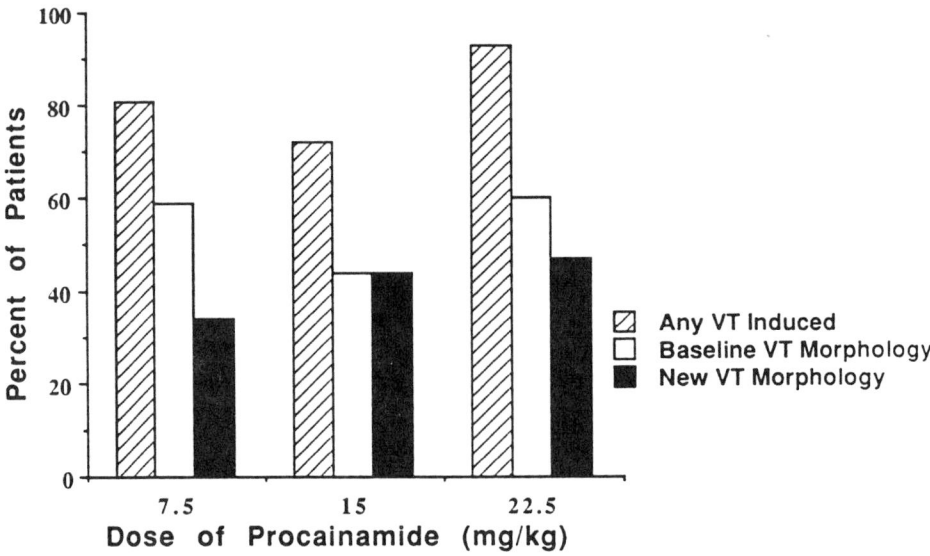

Figure 6. Effect of incremental dosing of procainamide on inducibility of ventricular tachycardia (VT) in patients with inducible, sustained, uniform VT in the baseline, drug-free state. Completion of the stimulation protocol was attempted in all studies. Of 32 patients, 10 (29%) had two VT morphologies induced at baseline. Approximately one half of patients had "new" VT morphologies (black bars) induced after incremental intravenous loading doses of a total of 7.5, 15, and 22.5 mg/kg of procainamide. About 20% to 30% of patients had new and baseline VT morphologies induced at each particular dose of procainamide. (Adapted with permission from Reference 100.)

hidden reentry circuit; or (3) creation of a new circuit. The clinical significance of these new VT morphologies, however, remains to be determined.

Evaluation of Drug Effects on the Arrhythmia Substrate

To date, the precise mechanism of action of antiarrhythmic agents in ventricular arrhythmias in vivo remains unknown.[15,101] As a consequence, antiarrhythmic therapy is empirically chosen whether its efficacy is assessed by Holter monitoring or programmed stimulation. However, only electrophysiological testing allows to study the effects of drugs on the arrhythmia substrate in vivo.[101] If the substrate can be rendered incapable of supporting sustained reentry, then no arrhythmia will result, regardless of the trigger or other

factors involved. Drug effects on VT in humans can be analyzed by electrophysiological studies, eg, using resetting and entrainment. Three possible effects of antiarrhythmic drugs on the reentry circuit are shown in Figure 7: (1) primary prolongation of refractoriness; (2) primary slowing of conduction; and (3) primary lengthening of the circuit barriers. Preliminary data from our laboratory[102] suggest that eg, procainamide increases VT cycle length by decreasing conduction velocity in fully recovered tissue or by changing the pathway of the impulse, rather than by prolongation of refractoriness within the reentry circuit. Class I antiarrhythmic agents, however, have very limited efficacy in suppressing VT induction as discussed above. Moreover, in a retrospective evaluation of randomized anitarrhythmic drug trials (without PES testing), Class I agents almost uniformly demonstrated an adverse effect on mortality, whereas sympathetic antagonists (Class II) were almost invariably benefi-

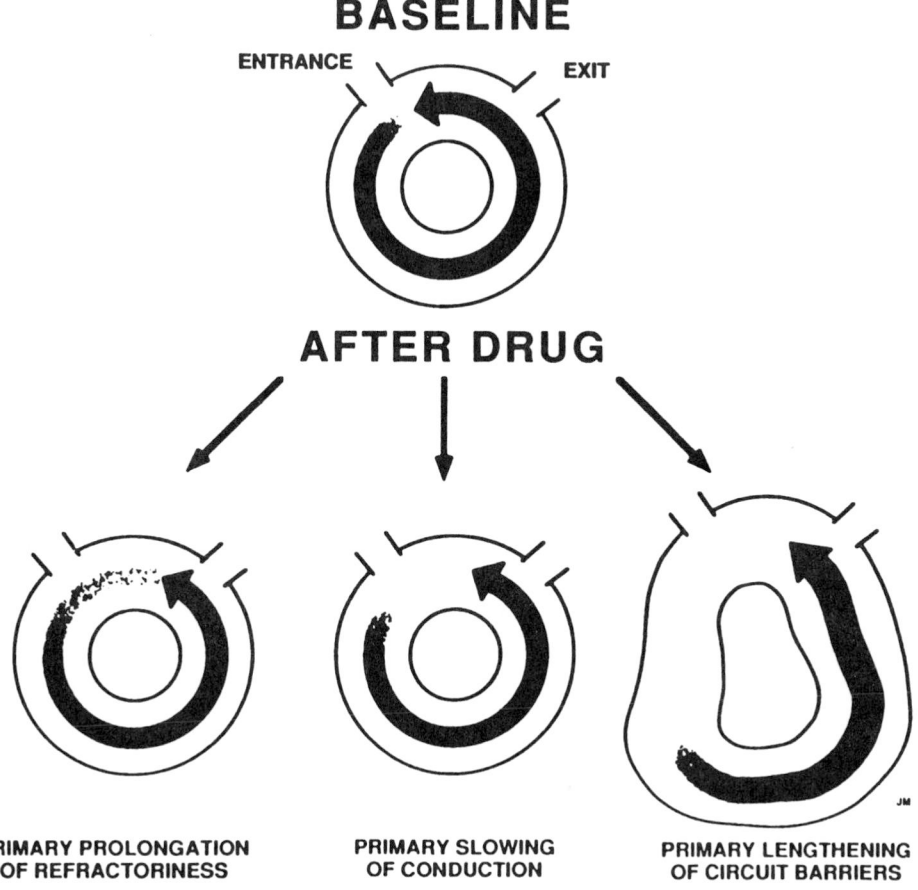

BASELINE

ENTRANCE   EXIT

AFTER DRUG

PRIMARY PROLONGATION
OF REFRACTORINESS

PRIMARY SLOWING
OF CONDUCTION

PRIMARY LENGTHENING
OF CIRCUIT BARRIERS

Figure 7. Possible mechanisms of drug effects on a reentrant circuit with separate, fixed entrance and exit sites. The black portion of the arrow represents fully refractory tissue while the dotted portion represents partially refractroy tissue. (Adapted with permission from Reference 15.)

cial.[103] Class III antiarrhythmic drugs like sotalol appear to be slightly more effective at preventing VT and/or VF induction than Class I agents by prolonging the effective refractory period by lengthening cardiac repolarization. Moreover, sotalol and amiodarone both exert sympathetic antagonism. These β-adrenergic blocking properties of amiodarone have been recently demonstrated to make its electrophysiological effects more resistant to reversal by catecholamines as compared to Class I agents.[104] The use of amiodarone, however, is limited by its side effects and the unpredictability of its efficacy by PES or Holter, especially in patients with cardiac arrest as dis-

cussed. Sotalol, however, also does not represent the ideal antifibrillatory agent because of up to a 5% incidence of torsades de pointes tachycardias.[95] The reverse use-dependent effects of sotalol may contribute to this proarrhythmic effect.[105,106] However, the reason for the very low incidence of torsades de pointes related to amiodarone despite marked QT interval prolongation is unclear[104,107]; it may be due in part to amiodarone's calcium antagonistic effects suppressing the development of early afterdepolarizations, which were thought to be responsible for torsades de pointes.[108]

Experimental electrophysiological data

showed that d-sotalol can terminate reentry by two mechanisms[109]: (1) by increasing ventricular refractoriness in reentry circuits with short excitable gaps; and (2) by fixed block at vulnerable sites within the circuit. Whether lengthening of action potential duration and concomitant prolongation of refractoriness in reentry circuits with short excitable gaps also is the mechanism of sotalol and newer pure Class III agents[110] can only be evaluated by electrophysiological testing, not by Holter monitoring.

Summary

Although most of the data discussed are derived from retrospective uncontrolled studies with relative small numbers of patients, the bulk of the evidence suggests that programmed stimulation is preferable to Holter monitoring in guiding therapy in patients with sustained ventricular tachyarrhythmias. Programmed stimulation is not only useful in guiding pharmacological therapy, but since it is the most successful and reproducible method of replicating the clinical arrhythmias, it is absolutely mandatory for the development of nonpharmacological therapy including pacing, defibrillation, catheter ablation, or surgically directed ablation of arrhythmias. The excellent negative predictive value of programmed ventricular stimulation with classical antiarrhythmic agents appears to be true also for newer agents like sotalol. However, the use of PES still remains controversial with amiodarone.

The limitations of PES guided drug therapy include: (1) the inability to repeatedly induce the clinical arrhythmia, particularly in patients with cardiac arrest; (2) the limited specificity of induced polymorphic arrhythmias; (3) the unknown specificity of induced, but never before observed uniform VT; (4) the limited positive predictive value (which is less hazardous than falsely predicting a good outcome); 5) the influence of patient population both in terms of disease state and arrhythmia presentation on PES predictive accuracy;

(6) the inability to predict proarrhythmic drug effects; (7) the lack of a generally accepted stimulation protocol and therapeutic end points; and (8) the lack of knowledge of the natural history of the arrhythmia.

The use of Holter monitoring to guide pharmacological therapy is limited by: (1) the absence of significant arrhythmias during the monitoring period in up to 50% of patients with sustained tachyarrhythmias; (2) the significant hourly and daily variability of ventricular ectopy; (3) failure to predict proarrhythmic drug effects; (4) abolition of arrhythmias on Holter does not confirm freedom from VT or VF; and (5) persistence of arrhythmias does not preclude a good outcome (also see Chapter 47).

Finally, pharmacological therapy, whether guided by Holter monitoring or programmed stimulation, is limited by the lack of uniformly successful drugs, their potential for arrhythmogenesis, narrow toxic to therapeutic ratios, the lack of steady-state conditions, and, last but not least, a limited patient compliance. Only electrophysiological testing allows to study drug effects on the arrhythmia substrate in vivo with possible therapeutic and prognostic consequences in the future. Whether the use of Holter monitoring in combination with programmed stimulation is useful in patients whose tachycardias remain inducible requires further investigation.[111]

References

1. Mason JW, Winkle RA: Electrode-catheter arrhythmia induction in the selection and assessment of arrhythmic drug therapy for recurrent ventricular tachycardia. *Circulation* 58:971, 1978.
2. Horwitz LN, Josephson ME, Farshidi A, et al: Recurrent sustained ventricular tachycardia. 3. Role of the electrophysiological study in selection of antiarrhythmic regimens. *Circulation* 58:986, 1978.
3. Ruskin JN, DiMarco JP, Garan H: Out-of-hospital cardiac arrest: electrophysiologic observations and selection of long-term antiarrhythmic therapy. *N Engl J Med* 303:607, 1980.
4. Josephson ME, Horowitz LN: Electrophysiologic approach to therapy of recurrent sus-

tained ventricular tachycardia. *Am J Cardiol* 43:631, 1979.

5. Bigger JT, Fleiss JL, Steinman RC, et al: Frequency domain measures of heart period variability and mortality after myocardial infarction. *Circulation* 85:164, 1992.

6. Jarrett JR, Flowers NC: Signal-averaged electrocardiography: history, techniques, and clinical applications. *Clin Cardiol* 14:984, 1991.

7. Nalos PC, Pappas JM, Nyitray W, et al: Prospective community evaluation of the signal-averaged electrocardiogram in predicting malignant ventricular arrhythmias: beneficial outcome with electrophysiology guided therapy. *Clin Cardiol* 14:963, 1991.

8. Steinberg JS, Regan A, Sciacca RR, et al: Predicting arrhythmic events after acute myocardial infarction using the signal-averaged electrocardiogram. *Am J Cardiol* 69:13, 1992.

9. Simson MB, Kindwall E, Buxton AE, et al: Signal averaging of the ECG in the management of patients with ventricular tachycardia: prediction of antiarrhythmic drug efficacy. In: P Brugada, HJJ Wellens (eds): *Cardiac Arrhythmias: Where To Go From Here?* Mount Kisco, NY: Futura Publishing Company, Inc., 1987, p. 299.

10. Simson MB: The role of the signal averaged electrocardiography in identifying patients at high risk for lethal ventricular tachyarrhythmias. *PACE* 14:944, 1991.

11. Farrell TG, Bashir Y, Cripps T, et al: Risk stratification for arrhythmic events in postinfarction patients based on heart rate variability, ambulatory electrocardiographic variables and the signal-averaged electrocardiogram. *J Am Coll Cardiol* 18:687, 1991.

12. Buxton AE, Simson MB, Falcone RA, et al: Results of signal-averaged electrocardiography and electrophysiologic study in patients with nonsustained ventricular tachycardia after healing of acute myocardial infarction. *Am J Cardiol* 60:80, 1987.

13. Rae AP, Greenspan AM, Spielman SR, et al: Antiarrhythmic drug efficacy for ventricular tachyarrhythmias associated with coronary artery disease as assessed by electrophysiologic studies. *Am J Cardiol* 55:1494, 1985.

14. Rae AP, Spielman SR, Kutalek SP, et al: Electrophysiologic assessment of antiarrhythmic drug efficacy for ventricular tachyarrhythmias associated with dilated cardiomyopathy. *Am J Cardiol* 59:291, 1987.

15. Josephson ME: *Clinical Cardiac Electrophysiology: Techniques and Interpretation.* 2nd Edition. Malvern: Lea and Febiger, (in press).

16. Poser R, Lombardi F, Podrid PJ, et al: Aggravation of arrhythmia induced with antiarrhythmic drugs during electrophysiologic testing. *Am Heart J* 110:9, 1985.

17. Josephson ME: Use of electrophysiological testing to select antiarrhythmic drug therapy for ventricular arrhythmias. In: MR Rosen, MJ Janse, AL Wit (eds): *Cardiac Electrophysiology: A Textbook.* Mount Kisco, NY: Futura Publishing Company, Inc., 1990, p. 1137.

18. Swerdlow CD, Winkle RA, Mason JW: Prognostic significance of the number of induced ventricular complexes during assessment of therapy for ventricular tachyarrhythmias. *Circulation* 68:400, 1983.

19. Mann DE, Luck JC, Griffin JC, et al: Induction of clinical ventricular tachycardia using programmed stimulation: value of third and fourth extrastimuli. *Am J Cardiol* 52:501, 1983.

20. Brugada P, Green M, Abdollah H, et al: Significance of ventricular arrhythmias initiated by programmed ventricular stimulation: the importance of the type of ventricular arrhythmia induced and the number of premature stimuli required. *Circulation* 69:87, 1984.

21. Herre JM, Mann DE, Luck JC, et al: Effect of increased current, multiple pacing sites and number of extrastimuli on induction of ventricular tachycardia. *Am J Cardiol* 57:102, 1986.

22. Morady F, DiCarlo LA Jr, Liem LB, et al: Effects of high stimulation current of the induction of ventricular tachycardia. *Am J Cardiol* 56:73, 1985.

23. Brugada P, Abdollah H, Heddle B, et al: Results of a ventricular stimulation protocol using a maximum of 4 premature stimuli in patients with documented or suspected ventricular arrhythmias. *Am J Cardiol* 52:1214, 1983.

24. Richards DA, Cody DV, Denniss AR, et al: Ventricular electrical instability: a predictor of death after myocardial infarction. *Am J Cardiol* 51:75, 1983.

25. Poole JE, Mathisen TL, Kudenchuk PJ, et al: Long-term outcome in patients who survive out of hospital ventricular fibrillation undergo electrophysiologic studies: evaluation by electrophysiologic subgroups. *J Am Coll Cardiol* 16:657, 1990.

26. Horowitz LN, Spielman SR, Grennspan AM, et al: Role of programmed stimulation in assessing vulnerability to ventricular arrhythmias. *Am Heart J* 103:604, 1982.

27. Fogoros RN, Elson JJ, Bonnet CA: Actuarial incidence and pattern of occurrence of shocks following implantation of the automatic implantable cardioverter defibrillator. *PACE* 12:1465, 1989.

28. Gross JN, Song SL, Buckingham T, et al: Influence of clinical characteristics and shock oc-

currence on ICD patient outcome: a multicenter report. *PACE* 14:1881, 1991.

29. Waller TJ, Kay HR, Spielman SR, et al: Reduction in sudden death and total mortality by antiarrhythmic therapy evaluated by electrophysiologic drug testing: criteria of efficacy in patients with sustained ventricular tachyarrhythmia. *J Am Coll Cardiol* 10:83, 1987.

30. Wilber BJ, Garan H, Finkelstein D, et al: Out-of-hospital cardiac arrest: use of electrophysiologic testing in the prediction of long-term outcome. *N Engl J Med* 318:19, 1988.

31. Roy D, Waxman HL, Kienzle MG, et al: Clinical characteristics and long-term follow-up in 119 survivors of cardiac arrest: relation to inducibility at electrophysiologic testing. *Am J Cardiol* 52:969, 1983.

32. Skale BT, Miles WM, Heger JJ, et al: Survivors of cardiac arrest: prevention of recurrence by drug therapy as predicted by electrophysiologic testing or electrocardiographic monitoring. *Am J Cardiol* 57:113, 1986.

33. Poll DS, Marchlinski FE, Buxton AE, et al: Usefulness of programmed stimulation in idiopathic dilated cardiomyopathy. *Am J Cardiol* 58:992, 1986.

34. Milner PG, DiMarco JP, Lerman BB: Electrophysiological evaluation of sustained ventricular tachyarrhythmias in idiopathic dilated cardiomyopathy. *PACE* 11:562, 1988.

35. Fananapazir L, Epstein SE: Hemodynamic and electrophysiologic evaluation of patients with hypertrophic cardiomyopathy surviving cardiac arrest. *Am J Cardiol* 67:280, 1991.

36. Naccarelli GV, Prystowsky EN, Jackman WM, et al: Role of electrophysiologic testing in managing patients who have ventricular tachycardia unrelated to coronary artery disease. *Am J Cardiol* 50:165, 1982.

37. Sousa J, Rosenheck S, Calkins H, et al: Results of electrophysiologic testing and long-term prognosis in patients with coronary artery disease and aborted sudden death. *Am Heart J* 122:1001, 1991.

38. Swerdlow CD, Winkle RA, Maso JW: Determinants of survival in patients with ventricular tachyarrhythmias. *N Engl J Med* 308:1436, 1983.

39. Kim SG, Seiden SW, Felder SD, et al: Is programmed stimulation of value in predicting the long-term success of antiarrhythmic therapy for ventricular tachycardias? *N Engl J Med* 315:356, 1986.

40. The Cardiac Arrhythmia Suppression Trial (CAST) Investigators: Preliminary report: effect of encainide and flecainide on mortality in a randomized trial of arrhythmia suppression after myocardial infarction. *N Engl J Med* 321:406, 1989.

41. Pratt CM, Moye LA: The Cardiac Arrhythmia Suppression Trial: background, interim results and implications. *Am J Cardiol* 65:20B, 1990.

42. Luederitz B: The Cardiac Arrhythmia Suppression Trial (CAST). In: B Luederitz, S Saksena (eds): *Interventional Electrophysiology.* Mount Kisco, NY: Futura Publishing Company, Inc., 1991, p. 95.

43. Josephson ME: Treatment of ventricular arrhythmias after myocardial infarction. *Circulation* 74:653, 1986.

44. Pratt CM, Slymen DJ, Wierman AM, et al: Analysis of the spontaneous variability of ventricular arrhythmias: consecutive ambulatory electrocardiographic recordings of ventricular tachycardia. *Am J Cardiol* 56:67, 1985.

45. The ESVEM Investigators: The ESVEM Trial: electrophysiologic study versus electrocardiographic monitoring for selection of antiarrhythmic therapy of ventricular tachyarrhythmias. *Circulation* 79:1354, 1989.

46. Pratt CM, Thornton BC, Magro SA, et al: Spontaneous arrhythmia detected on ambulatory electrocardiographic recording lacks precision in predicting inducibility of ventricular tachycardia during electrophysiologic study. *J Am Coll Cardiol* 10:97, 1987.

47. Mitchell LB, Duff HJ, Manyari DE, et al: A randomized clinical trial of the noninvasive and invasive approaches to drug therapy of ventricular tachycardia. *N Engl J Med* 317:1681, 1987.

48. Chua W, Roth H, Summers C, et al: Programmed stimulation versus ambulatory monitoring for therapy of malignant arrhythmias (abstract). *Circulation* 67:III-55, 1983.

49. Platia EV, Reid PR: Comparison of programmed electrical stimulation and ambulatory electrocardiographic (Holter) monitoring in the management of ventricular tachycardia and ventricular fibrillation. *J Am Coll Cardiol* 4:493, 1984.

50. Mason JW and the ESVEM Investigators: Unsustained VT as a predictor of spontaneous sustained VT in the ESVEM study (abstract). *Circulation* 84:II-348, 1991.

51. Hook BG, Buxton AE, Marchlinski FE, et al: Reversal of antiarrhythmic drug-induced suppression of sustained ventricular tachycardia by increased pacing current strength during programmed stimulation. *Circulation* 82: III-82, 1990.

52. Jazayeri MR, VanWyhe G, Avitall B, et al: Isoproterenol reversal of antiarrhythmic effects in patients with inducible sustained ventricular tachyarrhythmias. *J Am Coll Cardiol* 14: 705, 1989.

53. Kim SG, Seiden SW, Matos JA, et al: Discordance between ambulatory monitoring and programmed stimulation in assessing efficacy of class Ia antiarrhythmic agents in patients with ventricular tachycardia. *J Am Coll Cardiol* 6:539, 1985.

54. Kim SG, Felder SD, Figura I, et al: Value of Holter monitoring in predicting long-term efficacy and inefficacy of amiodarone used alone and in combination with class Ia antiarrhythmic agents in patients with ventricular tachycardia. *J Am Coll Cardiol* 9:169, 1987.

55. Nademanee K, Hendrickson J, Kannan R, et al: Antiarrhythmic efficacy and electrophysiologic actions of amiodarone in patients with life-threatening ventricular arrhythmias: potent suppression of spontaneously occurring tachyarrhythmias versus inconsistent abolition of induced ventricular tachycardia. *Am Heart J* 103:950, 1982.

56. Morady F, Scheinman MM, Hess DS: Amiodarone in the management of patients with ventricular tachycardia and ventricular fibrillation. *PACE* 6:609, 1983.

57. Naccarelli GV, Fineberg NS, Zipes DP, et al: Amiodarone: risk factors for recurrence of symptomatic ventricular tachycardia identified at electrophysiologic study. *J Am Coll Cardiol* 6:814, 1985.

58. Veltri EP, Reid PR, Platia EV, et al: Amiodarone in the treatment of life-threatening ventricular tachycardia: role of Holter monitoring in predicting long-term clinical efficacy. *J Am Coll Cardiol* 6:806, 1985.

59. DiCarlo LA Jr, Morady F, Sauve MJ, et al: Cardiac arrest and sudden death in patients treated with amiodarone for sustained ventricular tachycardia or ventricular fibrillation: risk stratification based on clinical variables. *Am J Cardiol* 55:372, 1985.

60. Veltri EP, Griffith LSC, Platia EV, et al: The use of ambulatory monitoring in the prognostic evaluation of patients with sustained ventricular tachycardia treated with amiodarone. *Circulation* 74:1054, 1986.

61. Stamato NJ, Marchlinski FE: Role of Holter monitoring in the management of patients with ventricular tachycardia treated with amiodarone. *Clin Prog Electrophysiol Pacing* 4: 395, 1986.

62. Marchlinski FE, Buxton AE, Flores BT, et al: Value of Holter monitoring in identifying risk for sustained ventricular arrhythmia recurrence on amiodarone. *Am J Cardiol* 55:709, 1985.

63. Sokoloff NM, Spielman SR, Greenspan AM, et al: Utility of ambulatory electrocardiographic monitoring for predicting recurrence of sustained ventricular tachyarrhythmias in patients receiving amiodarone. *J Am Coll Cardiol* 7:938, 1986.

64. Toivonen L, Kadish A, Morady F: A prospective comparison of class IA, B, and C antiarrhythmic agents in combination with amiodarone in patients with inducible, sustained ventricular tachycardia. *Circulation* 84:101, 1991.

65. Kadish AH, Buxton AE, Waxman HL, et al: Usefulness of electrophysiologic study to determine the clinical tolerance of arrhythmia recurrences during amiodarone therapy. *J Am Coll Cardiol* 10:90, 1987.

66. Greenspon AJ, Volosin KJ, Greenberg RM, et al: Amiodarone therapy: role of early and late electrophysiologic studies. *J Am Coll Cardiol* 11:117, 1988.

67. Morady F, Sauve MJ, Malone P, et al: Long-term efficacy and toxicity of high-dose amiodarone therapy for ventricular tachycardia or ventricular fibrillation. *Am J Cardiol* 52:975, 1983.

68. Veltri EP, Reid PR, Platia EV, et al: Results of late programmed electrical stimulation and long-term electrophysiologic effects of amiodarone therapy in patients with refractory ventricular tachycardia. *Am J Cardiol* 55:375, 1985.

69. Horowitz LN, Greenspan AM, Spielman SR, et al: Usefulness of electrophysiologic testing in evaluation of amiodarone therapy for sustained ventricular tachyarrhythmias associated with coronary heart disease. *Am J Cardiol* 55:367, 1985.

70. Kadish AH, Buxton AE, Waxman HL, et al: Usefulness of electrophysiologic study to determine the clinical tolerance of arrhythmia recurrences during amiodarone therapy. *J Am Cardiol* 10:90, 1987.

71. Herre JM, Sauve MJ, Malone P, et al: Long-term results of amiodarone therapy in patients with recurrent sustained ventricular tachycardia or ventricular fibrillation. *J Am Coll Cardiol* 13: 442, 1989.

72. Gottlieb C, Josephson ME: The preference of programmed stimulation-guided therapy for sustained ventricular arrhythmias. In: P Brugada, HJJ Wellens (eds): *Cardiac Arrhythmias: Where To Go From Here?* Mount Kisco, NY: Futura Publishing Company, Inc., 1987, p. 421.

73. Gottlieb CD, Berger MD, Miller JM, et al: What is an acceptable risk for cardiac arrest patients treated with amiodarone? *Circulation* 78:II-500, 1988.

74. Cairns JA, Connolly SJ, Gent M, et al: Post-myocardial infarction mortality in patients with ventricular premature depolarizations: Canadian Amiodarone Myocardial Infarction Arrhythmia Trial (CAMIAT) Pilot Study. *Circulation* 84:550, 1991.

75. The CASCADE Investigators: Cardiac arrest in Seattle: conventional versus amiodarone drug evaluation (The CASCADE Study). *Am J Cardiol* 67:578, 1991.

76. Furberg CD, Yusuf S: Antiarrhythmics and VPD suppression. *Circulation* 84:928, 1991.

77. Levy S, Collet F: Clinical pharmacology of new pharmacologic agents: sotalol, flecainide, and moricizine. In: B Luederitz, S Saksena (eds): *Interventional Electrophysiology*. Mount Kisco, NY: Futura Publishing Company, Inc., 1991, p. 115.

78. Antonaccio MJ, Gomoll A: Pharmacology, pharmacodynamics and pharmacokinetics of sotalol. *Am J Cardiol* 65:12A, 1990.

79. Singh BN: Expanding clinical role of unique class III antiarrhythmic effects of sotalol. *Am J Cardiol* 65:84A, 1990.

80. Marchlinski FE, Buxton AE, Vassallo JA, et al: Comparative electrophysiologic effects of intravenous and oral procainamide in patients with sustained ventricular arrhythmias. *J Am Coll Cardiol* 4:1247–54, 1984.

81. Waxman HL, Buxton AE, Sadowski LM, et al: The response to procainamide predicts the response to other medications. *J Am Coll Cardiol* 6:298, 1985.

82. Kopelman HA, Woosley RL, Lee JT, et al: Electrophysiologic effects of intravenous and oral sotalol for sustained ventricular tachycardia secondary to coronary artery disease. *Am J Cardiol* 61:1006, 1988.

83. Deedwania PC: Suppressant effects of conventional β blockers and sotalol on complex and repetitive ventricular premature complexes. *Am J Cardiol* 65:43A, 1990.

84. Anderson JL, Askins JC, Gilbert EM, et al: Multicenter trial of sotalol for suppression of frequent, complex ventricular arrhythmias: a double-blind, randomized, placebo-controlled evaluation of two doses. *J Am Coll Cardiol* 8:752, 1986.

85. Anastasiou-Nana MI, Gilbert EM, Miller RH, et al: Usefulness of d,l sotalol for suppression of chronic ventricular arrhythmias. *Am J Cardiol* 67:511, 1991.

86. Anderson JL: Effectiveness of sotalol for therapy of complex ventricular arrhythmias and comparisons with placebo and class I antiarrhythmic drugs. *Am J Cardiol* 65:37A, 1990.

87. Singh SN, Cohen A, Chen J, et al: Sotalol for refractory sustained ventricular tachycardia and nonfatal cardiac arrest. *Am J Cardiol* 62:399, 1988.

88. Senges J, Langfelder W, Jauernig R, et al: Electrophysiologic testing in assessment of therapy with sotalol for sustained ventricular tachycardia. *Circulation* 69:577, 1984.

89. Nademanee K, Feld G, Hendrickson J, et al: Electrophysiologic and antiarrhythmic effects of sotalol in patients with life-threatening ventricular tachyarrhythmias. *Circulation* 72:555, 1985.

90. Steinbeck G, Bach P, Haberl R: Electrophysiologic and antiarrhythmic efficacy of oral sotalol for sustained ventricular tachyarrhythmias: evaluation by programmed stimulation and ambulatory electrocardiogram. *J Am Coll Cardiol* 8:949, 1986.

91. Gonzales R, Scheinman MM, Herre JM, et al: Usefulness of sotalol for drug-refractory malignant ventricular arrhythmias. *J Am Coll Cardiol* 12:1568, 1988.

92. Singh SN, Cohen A, Chen Y, et al: Sotalol for refractory ventricular tachycardia and nonfatal cardiac arrest. *Am J Cardiol* 62:399, 1988.

93. Ruder MA, X T, Lebsack C, et al: Clinical experience with sotalol in patients with drug-refractory ventricular arrhythmias. *J Am Coll Cardiol* 13:145, 1989.

94. Kuchar DL, Garan H, Venditti FJ, et al: Usefulness of sotalol in suppressing ventricular tachycardia or ventricular fibrillation in patients with healed myocardial infarcts. *Am J Cardiol* 64:33, 1989.

95. Kehoe RF, Zheutlin TA, Dunnington CS, et al: Safety and efficacy of sotalol in patients with drug-refractory ventricular tachyarrhythmias. *Am J Cardiol* 65:58A, 1990.

96. Kus T, Campa MA, Nadeau R, et al: Efficacy and electrophysiologic effects of oral sotalol in patients with sustained ventricular tachycardia caused by coronary artery disease. *Am Heart J* 123:82, 1992.

97. Nademanee K, Singh BN: Effects of sotalol on ventricular tachycardia and fibrillation produced by programmed electrical stimulation: comparison with other antiarrhythmic agents. *Am J Cardiol* 65:53A, 1990.

98. Bigger JT, Sahar DI: Clinical types of proarrhythmic response to antiarrhythmic drugs. *Am J Cardiol* 59:2E, 1987.

99. Callans DJ, Marchlinski FE: Dissociation of termination and prevention of inducibility of sustained ventricular tachycardia with infusion of procainamide: evidence for distinct mechanisms. *J Am Coll Cardiol* 19:111, 1992.

100. Grimm W, Cho G, Marchlinski FE: Effects of incremental doses of procainamide on patients with sustained uniform ventricular tachycardia (abstract). *PACE* (in press).

101. Hook BG, Josephson ME: Effect of drugs on arrhythmia substrate in vivo. In: *Current Topics in Cardiology*. New York, NY: Elsevier Science Publishing Company, Inc., 1991, p. 297.

102. Stamato NJ, Frame LH, Rosenthal ME, et al:

Procainamide induced slowing of ventricular tachycardia with insights from analysis of resetting response patterns. *Am J Cardiol* 63: 1455, 1989.

103. Pitt B: The role of β-adrenergic blocking agents in preventing sudden cardiac death. *Circulation* 85(Suppl I):I107, 1992.

104. Calcins H, Sousa J, El-Atassi R, et al: Reversal of antiarrhythmic drug effects by epinephrine: quinidine versus amiodarone. *J Am Coll Cardiol* 19:347, 1992.

105. Schmitt C, Brachmann J, Karch M, et al: Reverse use-dependent effects of sotalol demonstrated by recording monophasic action potentials of the right ventricle. *Am J Cardiol* 68: 1183, 1991.

106. Hondeghem LM, Snyders DJ: Class III antiarrhythmic agents have a lot of potential but a long way to go. *Circulation* 81:686, 1990.

107. Lazara R: Amiodarone and torsades de pointes. *Ann Intern Med* 111:549, 1989.

108. Takanaka C, Singh BN: Barium-induced non-driven action potentials as a model of triggered automaticity and early afterdepolarisations: differing effects of amiodarone and quinidine and significance of slow-channel activity. *J Am Coll Cardiol* 15:213, 1990.

109. Frame LH, Hailing F: D-sotalol terminates reentry by two mechanisms with different dependence on the duration of the excitable gap. *Circulation* 84:II-507, 1991.

110. Sedgwick ML, Rasmussen HS, Cobbe SM: Clinical and electrophysiologic effects of intravenous dofetilide (UK-68,798), a new class III antiarrhythmic drug, in patients with angina pectoris. *Am J Cardiol* 69:513, 1992.

111. Kim SG: The management of patients with life-threatening ventricular tachyarrhythmias: programmed stimulation or Holter monitoring (either or both)? *Circulation* 76:1, 1987.

Chapter 26

Significance of the Cardiac Arrhythmia Suppression Trial (CAST) in the Survivors of Acute Myocardia Infarction

Raymond L. Woosley

The Cardiac Arrhythmia Suppression Trial (CAST)[1] has not only had a profound impact on the practice of cardiology but has also greatly influenced the attitudes of physicians in cardiology and many other disciplines. The trial brought into sharp focus the importance of placebo controls in judging the effects of therapy and the potential pitfalls of using surrogate end points for mortality and survival in clinical disorders.

Although cardiologists were initially reluctant to accept the findings of CAST,[2] similar results obtained in other studies[3–5] have convinced all but the most unyielding skeptics. There have been a number of practical consequences that have stemmed from the results of CAST. For example, the findings of CAST have led to changes in the Food and Drug Administration (FDA) approved labeling of antiarrhythmic drugs, the practice of cardiology in general and in the area of arrhythmias, and in the development of new drugs. We expand on these issues in this chapter and discuss other perhaps broader implications of the results of CAST when considered in relation to the more recently released data from CAST II.

Antiarrhythmic Drug Labeling

Prior to the results of CAST, the FDA approved indications for antiarrhythmic drugs consisting of a list of electrocardiographic descriptors for a wide variety of supraventricular and ventricular arrhythmias with less consideration of the clinical setting for the arrhythmias. After a complete review of the results of CAST, the FDA required that the manufacturers and sponsors of most currently available antiarrhythmic drugs restrict indications for these drugs to the treatment of ventricular arrhythmias that in the judgment of the physician are life-threatening. The manufacturers' labeling for these drugs recommends that they not be used in patients with less severe ventricular arrhythmias, "even if the patients

From BN Singh, HJJ Wellens, M Hiraoka, (eds): *Electropharmacological Control of Cardiac Arrhythmias.* Mount Kisco, NY, Futura Publishing Company Inc., © 1994.

are symptomatic." An exception is flecainide, which has FDA approval for the treatment of supraventricular tachycardia in patients with structurally normal hearts.[6] Clearly, in this subset of patients the risk of proarrhythmic reactions is low and the risk benefit ratio justifies their use. The FDA is currently reviewing labeling of the older drugs such as quinidine. It is likely that the provisions of drug labeling for therapeutic use of antiarrhythmic compounds may fall within the scope of such a change if the meta-analytic data presented elsewhere in this volume (see Chapter 26) holds up to the continuing scrutiny of drug effects relative to end points such as mortality.

Patterns of Antiarrhythmic Drug Use Following CAST

After the conclusion of CAST, many patients previously taking encainide and flecainide were switched to therapy with mexiletine and other drugs that were perceived as being safer.[4] It was widely felt that had conventional drugs such as quinidine and mexiletine been used in CAST, the outcome might have been different. However, as the results of other studies, including CAST II, became available, physicians realized that other antiarrhythmic drugs may cause similar harm, although the degree of harm may be less for the drugs with lower potency.[2] The number of new prescriptions for antiarrhythmic drugs fell steadily for several months after CAST was interrupted, but eventually stabilized at a low level.[2] Encainide sales decreased so much that the manufacturer voluntarily removed the drug from the United States market. This decrease in sales, which is likely to continue, has the potential to adversely affect the development of new drugs—at least those that act by slowing conduction—for the prevention of sudden death. The important issue is whether all Class I agents might increase mortality or at the very least whether they have a measurable potential to prolong survival by suppressing ventric-

ular arrhythmias. In this regard, CAST II data are of much significance.

It is noteworthy that, as with CAST (best labeled CAST I), the Data Safety Board monitoring CAST II also terminated the trial before its completion because of excess mortality in treatment limb.[7] The first 14-day period of treatment with moricizine in postinfarct patients with high-density premature ventricular contractions (PVCs) and with left ventricular ejection fractions less than 40% was associated with excess mortality (17 of 665 patients died or had cardiac arrests) as compared with no treatment or placebo (3 of 660 patients died or had cardiac arrests). At the completion of the long-term phase, there were 49 deaths or cardiac arrests due to arrhythmias in patients allocated to moricizine and 42 in patients assigned to placebo. The difference did not reach statistical significance but it is difficult not to interpret this trend as being deleterious in light of the frankly adverse effects of the drug on survival during the first 14 days of the trial.

An additional but major change in the practice of cardiology has been the increased use of implantable cardioverter defibrillator devices. This has surely fueled concern about the increased mortality seen with antiarrhythmic drugs in CAST. It also is influenced by the recent increased availability of the devices. Nevertheless, antiarrhythmic drugs remain essential for the effective treatment of those patients who have very frequent recurrences of serious arrhythmias or those for whom a device is not technically feasible or in whom devices alone are insufficient treatment for controlling arrhythmias.

Impact on Research and New Drug Development

Shortly after the results of CAST were made public several drugs with electrophysiological actions similar to those of encainide and flecainide were withdrawn from clinical testing. Development of 3-methoxy-O-desmethyl encainide, the second major metabolite of encainide, was halted within months of CAST's interruption. Other agents that have been withdrawn include ACC-9358, quinacainol, pirmenol, indecainide, recainam, and cibenzoline. This may have been unfortunate because several of the drugs had distinct pharmacological advantages over encainide or flecainide in certain clinical settings. For example, ACC-9358 appeared to be a rapidly acting sodium channel blocker with a pharmacokinetic profile that indicated it could be safely given as a rapid intravenous injection.[8] The negative inotropic actions of flecainide[9] and the active metabolites of encainide[10] make acute intravenous therapy with these agents difficult if not impossible.

CAST created a general concern about the effects of antiarrhythmic drugs on mortality. This concern will have a major effect on future drug development. Because encainide, flecainide, and probably other antiarrhythmic drugs increase mortality,[3–5] the effects of an investigational drug on mortality must be considered during development. That does not necessarily mean that every drug sponsor must conduct a CAST-like study to gain approval for marketing. However, drug sponsors will most likely be required to demonstrate that any negative effect on mortality is no greater than that for drugs previously approved for treatment of life-threatening arrhythmias. As was the case with flecainide, it is likely that drug sponsors will also be required to show that drugs for treatment of less severe arrhythmias are relatively safe in that population before they can be approved. If sponsors want their drugs to be recommended for suppression of prognostically significant arrhythmias, such as PVCs, they are likely to be required to demonstrate that it reduces mortality in a trial similar to CAST. However, the exact form that the antiarrhythmic drug approval might take, remains unclear. Undoubtedly, it will be shaped in light of the ongoing developments.

Significance of CAST

The significance of CAST is that it has reinforced several axioms that had been over-

looked in our desire to reduce the mortality due to sudden cardiac death. Physicians had been encouraged by the results of clinical trials evaluating other risk factors, such as hypertension and hyperlipidemia, to conclude that suppression of a risk factor equaled a clinical benefit. Several surveys of physician practice habits prior to CAST showed that cardiologists routinely prescribed antiarrhythmic drugs for patients with PVCs after myocardial infarction.[2,11,12] The basis for this practice stemmed from the management of patients with acute myocardial infarction in which the theoretical value of the Lown grading system for ventricular arrhythmias had been accepted.[13] Now, however, the overwhelming conclusion is that the surrogate end point, PVCs, is an invalid end point for potential reduction in mortality in both the setting of acute myocardial infarction[14] and in the convalescent phase as examined in CAST. This has raised new concerns and deliberation about the use of surrogate end points in developing drugs and in treating illnesses in general.

CAST called attention to another old axiom that may warrant reinforcing. Many physicians feel compelled to do everything possible to help their patients and felt that suppressing their potentially lethal ventricular arrhythmias was essential because the drugs were available and had that potential.[15,16] Now we know that, in this case, doing everything for the patient carried with it harm.

It is current practice by many cardiologists to risk-stratify patients with asymptomatic nonsustained ventricular tachycardia and reduced ventricular function. They obtain a signal-averaged electrocardiogram and conduct an electrophysiological study including programmed ventricular stimulation. This exposes these patients to additional medical expense and the risks and stress inherent in the electrophysiological procedure. More importantly, it often leads to the prescription of antiarrhythmic drug therapy guided by the results of programmed ventricular stimulation in spite of the total absence of evidence that these drugs will provide any clinical benefit or improved mortality. Some physicians go so far as to implant an automatic defibrillator in asymptomatic patients for whom effective drug therapy cannot be found. This practice is clearly unsupported by any clinical data that clearly identify the natural history of these patients without confounding factors such as empirical antiarrhythmic drug therapy.

Prior to CAST, physicians generally believed that the antiarrhythmic drugs were likely to be effective at preventing sudden death. Actually, many felt that it would be unethical to perform a placebo controlled trial in these patients who were presumed to be at high risk for developing sudden death or serious arrhythmias (personal observation). Because of the realization that the drugs may cause harm, even in high-risk populations, it is now possible (if not imperative) to conduct placebo-controlled trials of antiarrhythmic drugs in patients with severe left ventricular dysfunction and nonsustained ventricular tachycardia such as the Multicenter Unsustained Ventricular Tachycardia Trial (MUST trial) and the amiodarone trials that are currently being conducted[17] or those that have already provided preliminary data of interest.[18]

New Proarrhythmias

The increase in deaths in the CAST patients treated with encainide and flecainide was a previously unrecognized form of harm. The time course of the occurrence of deaths in CAST (Figure 1) is constant and indicates that the harm is unlike the arrhythmia worsening that occurs early after initiating antiarrhythmic therapy. The time course has led several authors to hypothesize that the deaths may be due to an adverse interaction with randomly occurring ischemic events.[19,20] This hypothesis is supported by several lines of indirect evidence. As shown in Table 1, there were fewer cases of nonfatal myocardial infarction and new or worsened angina in the CAST treatment arm randomized to encainide or flecainide.[20] One possible interpretation is that the drugs converted nonfatal infarction

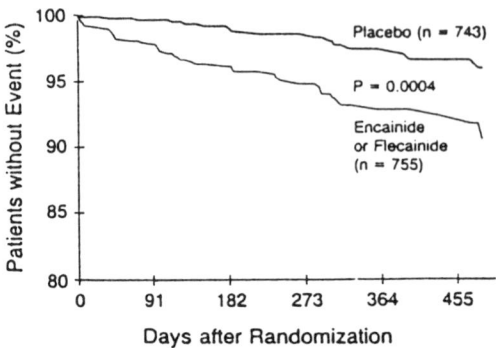

Figure 1. Actuarial probabilities of freedom from death or cardiac arrest due to arrhythmia in 1,498 patients receiving encainide or flecainide or corresponding placebo. The number of patients at risk of an event is shown along the bottom of the figure. (Reproduced with permission from Reference 1.)

and anginal events to fatal events. This is also supported by the results with antiarrhythmic drugs in animal models of ischemic heart disease. As shown in Figure 2, Nattel et al.[21] reported that pretreatment with aprindine caused an increased incidence of ventricular tachycardia or fibrillation in dogs during coronary occlusion. Similar results were obtained with lidocaine in an ischemic pig model.[22] Dawson et al.[23] found that the major active metabolite of encainide, O-desmethyl encainide (ODE), reduced the threshold for electrical fibrillation in dogs with prior myocardial infarction. Kou et al.[24] found that flecainide was either ineffective or increased serious arrhythmias in their model of ischemia in the setting of prior infarction. There seems to be

Table 1
Nonfatal Infarction and New Angina in CAST

Outcome	Placebo	Active drug
Death and cardiac arrest	26	63
Nonfatal infarction	33	19
New/increasing angina	88	65
Total	148	147

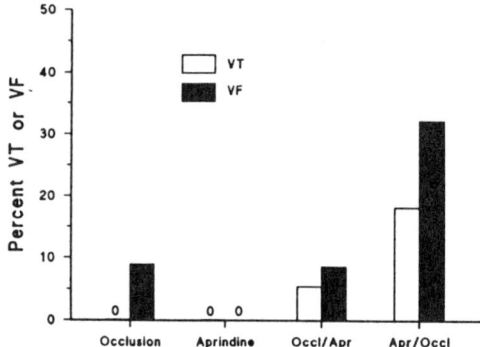

Figure 2. Influence of aprindine on the prevalence of ventricular tachycardia or ventricular fibrillation in dogs after coronary occlusion. The figure demonstrates the incidence of ventricular tachycardia or ventricular fibrillation in four groups of dogs. From left to right, the groups are (1) coronary occlusion alone; (2) aprindine alone without occlusion; (3) coronary occlusion followed by aprindine administration, and (4) aprindine treatment prior to coronary occlusion. (Adapted from with permission Reference 19.)

a remarkable consistency of results when sodium channel blockers are evaluated in models that incorporate acute ischemia.

New Concerns

One of the remarkable findings of CAST was the very low mortality in patients who responded to antiarrhythmic drugs.[25,26] There is no clear understanding of this phenomenon but it raises serious questions about other uncontrolled trials with these and perhaps many other drugs. For ethical reasons, it has been impossible to conduct a controlled trial in patients with sustained ventricular tachycardia. Several studies have evaluated antiarrhythmic drugs using programmed ventricular stimulation. All have found that those patients for whom an effective drug regimen can be found, ie, one that prevents induction of VT, have a much better outcome that those who remain inducible on all tested drug regimens.[27-29] It is certainly possible that, as in CAST, response to therapy identifies a popula-

tion at lower risk of recurrence or sudden death. This is supported by the observation that the left ventricular ejection fraction (the most powerful predictor of outcome) was much higher in patients whose inducible ventricular arrhythmias were suppressed by antiarrhythmic drugs compared to those who were not suppressed (42% ± 17% versus 30% ± 15%).[30] This indicates that the patients who respond and receive chronic antiarrhythmic drug therapy may simply be a population selected to have a better outcome for reasons totally unrelated to the drugs.[26] This possibility supports the need for a randomized comparison of the effects of antiarrhythmic drugs on mortality in patients with severe life-threatening ventricular arrhythmias.

Lessons for the Future

CAST demonstrated that drugs that have been developed because of their ability to block normal sodium channels increase mortality in patients with ischemic heart disease. It also emphasized the critical importance of appropriate and concurrent controls as well as clinically relevant end points (especially cardia and total mortality) in the conduct of clinical trials to prolong survival. The inadequacy of surrogate end points also clearly emerged from CAST I and CAST II. As other experience accumulates, it is becoming clear that most, if not all, of the newly developed potassium channel blocking drugs have a significant incidence of torsades de pointes.[31] Therefore, it may be unwise to develop drugs directed against normal sodium or potassium channels, ie, normal physiological processes. On the contrary, it would seem more reasonable that efforts should be directed to the determination of the mechanistic link between ischemia (see Chapter 10) and other forms of substrate derangements (see Chapter 47) and ventricular fibrillation. With this information it might be possible to develop specific agents to prevent arrhythmias before they become manifest in normal myocardial tissue and thereby lead to sudden death.

References

1. CAST Investigators: Preliminary report: effect of encainide and flecainide on mortality in a randomized trial of arrhythmia suppression after myocardial infarction. *N Engl J Med* 321: 406, 1989.

2. Reiffel JA, Cook JR: Physician attitudes toward the use of Type IC antiarrhythmics after the Cardiac Arrhythmia Suppression Trial (CAST). *Am J Cardiol* 66:1262, 1990.

3. Impact Research Group: International mexiletine and placebo antiarrhythmic coronary trial: I. report on arrhythmia and other findings. *J Am Coll Cardiol* 4:1148, 1984.

4. Morganroth J, Goin JE: Quinidine-related mortality in the short-to-medium-term treatment of ventricular arrhythmias. *Circulation* 84:1977, 1991.

5. Hine LK, Laird NM, Hewitt P, et al: Meta-analysis of empirical long-term antiarrhythmic therapy after myocardial infarction. *JAMA* 262:3037, 1989.

6. Pritchett EL, Wilkinson WE: Mortality in patients treated with flecainide and encainide for supraventricular arrhythmias. *Am J Cardiol* 67:976, 1991.

7. The Cardiac Arrhythmia Suppression Trial II Investigators: Effect of the anti-arrhythmic agent moricizine on survival after myocardial infarction. *N Engl J Med* 327:227, 1992.

8. Pavlou HN, Funck-Brentano C, Lineberry MD, et al: Prospective pharmacokinetically based development of effective infusion regimens for ACC-9358, a new antiarrhythmic drug. *Clin Pharmacol Ther* 49:314, 1991.

9. Franciosa JA, Wilen M, Weeks CE, et al: Pharmacokinetics and hemodynamic effects of flecainide in patients with chronic low output heart failure (abstract). *J Am Coll Cardiol* 1:699, 1983.

10. Barbey JT, Thompson KA, Echt DS, et al: Antiarrhythmic activity, electrocardiographic effects and pharmacokinetics of the encainide metabolites O-desmethyl encainide and 3-methoxy-O-desmethyl encainide in man. *Circulation* 77: 380, 1988.

11. Vlay SC: How the university cardiologist treats ventricular premature beats: a nationwide survey of 65 University Medical Centers. *Am Heart J* 110:904, 1985.

12. Morganroth J, Bigger JT Jr, Anderson JL: Treatment of ventricular arrhythmias by United States cardiologists: a survey before the Cardiac Arrhythmia Suppression Trial results were available. *Am J Cardiol* 65:40, 1990.

13. Lown B, Wolf M: Approaches to sudden death from coronary heart disease. *Circulation* 44: 130, 1971.

14. MacMahon S, Collins R, Peto R, et al: Effects of prophylactic lidocaine in suspected acute myocardial infarction. *JAMA* 260:1910, 1988.

15. Morganroth J: Premature ventricular complexes. *JAMA* 252:673, 1984.

16. Bigger JT Jr: Antiarrhythmic treatment. An overview. *Am J Cardiol* 53(Suppl):8B, 1984.

17. Cairns JA, Connolly SJ, Gent M, et al: Post-myocardial infarction mortality in patients with ventricular premature depolarizations. *Circulation* 84:550, 1991.

18. Ceremuzynski L, Kleczar E, Krzeminiska-Pakula M, et al: Effect of amiodarone on mortality after myocardial infarction: a double-blind, placebo-controlled, pilot study. *J Am Coll Cardiol* 20: 1056, 1992.

19. Woosley RL: Antiarrhythmic drugs. *Ann Rev Pharmacol Toxicol* 31:427, 1991.

20. Echt DS, Liebson PR, Mitchell LB, et al: Mortality and morbidity in patients receiving encainide, flecainide, or placebo: The Cardiac Arrhythmia Suppression Trial. *N Engl J Med* 324:781, 1991.

21. Nattel S, Pedersen DH, Zipes DP: Alterations in regional myocardial distribution and arrhythmogenic effects of aprindine produced by coronary artery occlusion in the dog. *Cardiovasc Res* 15:80, 1981.

22. Carson DL, Cardinal R, Savard P, et al: Relationship between an arrhythmogenic action of lidocaine and its effects on excitation patterns in acutely ischemic porcine myocardium. *J Cardiovasc Pharmacol* 8:126, 1986.

23. Dawson AK, Roden DM, Duff HJ, et al: Differential effects of O-desmethyl encainide on induced and spontaneous arrhythmias in the conscious dog. *Am J Cardiol* 54:654, 1984.

24. Kou H, Nelson SD, Lynch JJ, et al: Effect of flecainide acetate on prevention of electrical induction of ventricular tachycardia and occurrence of ischemic ventricular fibrillation during the early postmyocardial infarction period: evaluation in a conscious canine model of sudden death. *J Am Coll Cardiol* 9:359, 1987.

25. Hallstrom AP, Greene HL, Huther ML: The healthy responder phenomenon in non-randomized clinical trials. *Statistics Med* 10:1621, 1991.

26. Wyse DG, Hallstrom A, McBride R, et al: Events in the cardiac arrhythmia suppression trial (CAST): mortality in patients surviving open label titration but not randomized to double-blind therapy. *J Am Coll Cardiol* 18:20, 1991.

27. Ruskin JN, DiMarco JP, Garan H: Out-of-hospital cardiac arrest: electrophysiologic observations and selection of long-term antiarrhythmic therapy. *N Engl J Med* 303:607, 1980.

28. Mason JW, Winkle RA: Electrode-catheter arrhythmia induction in the selection and assess-

ment of antiarrhythmic drug therapy for recurrent ventricular tachycardia. *Circulation* 58: 971, 1978.

29. Shannon JA, Hammill SC, Gersh BJ: Predictive value of early electrophysiologic testing in determining long-term outcome with amiodarone treatment in patients with sustained ventricular tachycardia. *Mayo Clin Proc* 66:1114, 1991.

30. Wilber DJ, Garan H, Finkelstein D, et al: Out-of-hospital cardiac arrest: use of electrophysiologic testing in the prediction of long-term outcome. *N Engl J Med* 318:19, 1988.

31. Hondeghem LM, Snyders DJ: Class III antiarrhythmic agents have a lot of potential but a long way to go. Reduced effectiveness and dangers of reverse use dependence. *Circulation* 81:686, 1990.

Chapter 27

Critical Analysis of Various Approaches to the Prevention of Sudden Death

Koon K. Teo
Salim Yusuf

It is believed that a substantial proportion of people with underlying cardiovascular disease die from sudden cardiac death. In the United States alone it has been estimated that about 500,000 sudden cardiac deaths occur annually. The true extent of this is not known since the exact proportion of cardiac deaths that is classified as being sudden varies depending on the population, the underlying disease, and the definition of sudden death. Epidemiologic studies such as the Framingham study have suggested that approximately two thirds of deaths classified as being sudden and of cardiac origin occurred in individuals who were not known previously to have heart disease.[1]

Several studies in patients with cardiac disease have reported a relationship between the presence or frequency of ventricular arrhythmia and subsequent mortality.[2] Some other studies have indicated that about 3 of 4 sudden deaths are due to ventricular tachycardia (VT) or ventricular fibrillation (VF).[3]

The traditional approach to preventing sudden death is based on the above informa-tion, with the following rationale: "because patients with frequent ventricular arrhythmia are at high risk of sudden death (presumably due to VT or VF in most cases), then suppression of these ambient ventricular arrhythmias should lead to a reduction in sudden death, which in turn should lead to a reduction in total death."

This approach has formed the basis for the prevention of sudden death by pharmacological means and has led to the widespread use of antiarrhythmic agents in patients presumed to be at high risk for sudden death. A large number of randomized clinical trials have been carried out over the last two decades based on this rationale. The data from these trials are reviewed below.

Results from Trials of Antiarrhythmic Agents

An overview of the results of the various randomized trials evaluating the effects of antiarrhythmic agents in patients with myocar-

From BN Singh, HJJ Wellens, M Hiraoka, (eds): *Electropharmacological Control of Cardiac Arrhythmias.* Mount Kisco, NY, Futura Publishing Company Inc., © 1994.

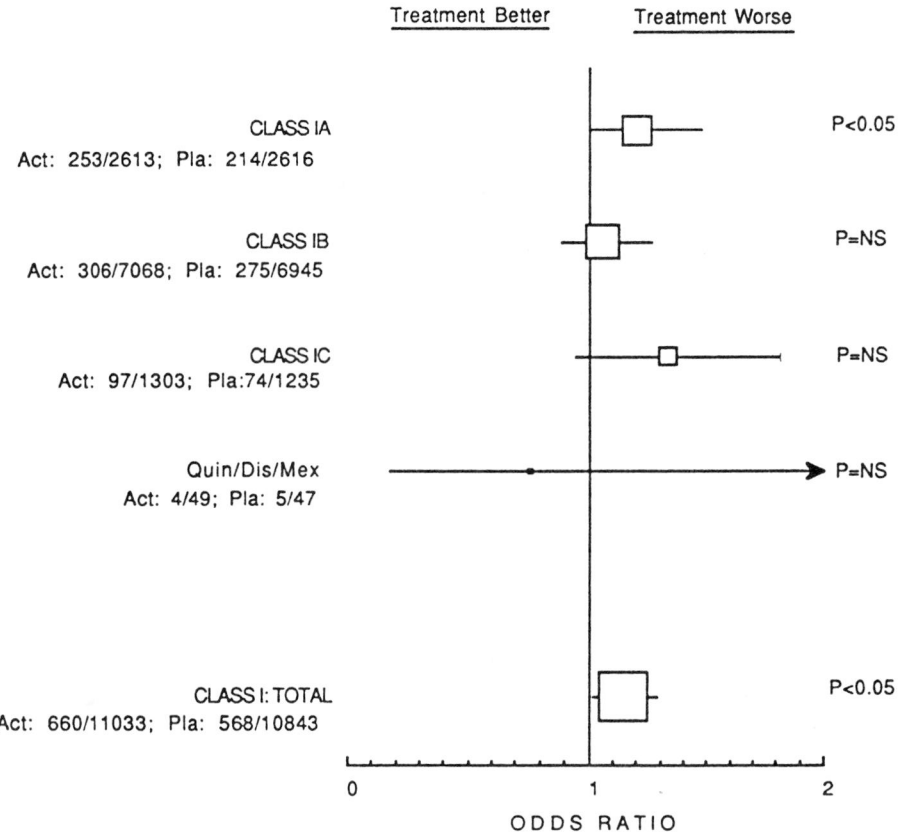

SUMMARY OF TRIALS OF CLASS 1 ANTIARRHYTHMIC AGENTS

Figure 1. Effects of Class I antiarrhythmic agents on mortality. Typical odds ratio by subclasses IA, IB, and IC (plus a small trial of three agents). Mortality data (number of deaths/number allocated treatment) are provided for active treatment (Act) and placebo or control (Pla). Areas of squares are proportional to the variance for each. Bars indicate 95% confidence intervals. Portions to left of vertical line (corresponding to odds ratio < 1) indicate reduced risk with treatment; portions to right of vertical line indicate increased risk with treatment. Note that overall Class I and subclass IA significantly increased the risk of death and subclasses IB and IC showed trends toward excess risk.

dial infarction has been conducted and the results summarized in Figures 1 and 2. Altogether 51 trials of Class I agents, 55 trials of Class II agents, 7 trials of Class III agents (amiodarone), and 24 trials of Class IV agents were included.[4,5]

There were 16 trials of Class IA agents (quinidine, procainamide, disopyramide, imipramine, and moricizine) involving 5,229 patients. There were 253 deaths among 2,613 patients allocated to active treatment com-

pared to 214 among 2,616 control patients. The excess in mortality among treated patients was statistically significant (odds ratio 1.21, 95% confidence interval [CI] 1.00 to 1.47, $p < 0.05$). Class IB agents (lidocaine, tocainide, phenytoin, and mexiletine) were evaluated in 32 trials with a total of 14,013 patients. Among these, 306 of the 7,068 patients allocated to active treatment died, compared to 275 of the 6,945 control patients (odds ratio 1.06, 95% CI 0.89 to 1.26, p = NS). Six trials evaluated

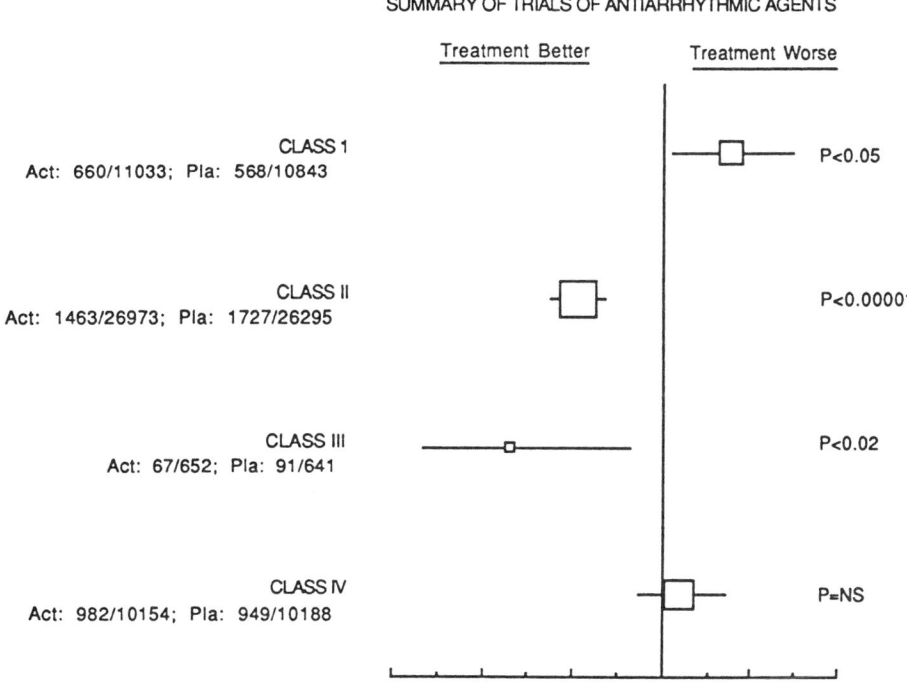

Figure 2. Effects of antiarrhythmic agents on mortality. Typical odds ratio by classes (I to IV) of agents. Explanatory notes are as in Figure 1. Note that Classes II and III significantly reduced risk, Class I significantly increased the risk of death, and Class IV showed a nonsignificant trend toward increased risk.

Class IC agents (aprindine, encainide and flecainide) in 2,538 patients. There were 97 deaths among 1,303 patients treated actively compared to 74 deaths among 1,235 controls (odds ratio 1.31, 95% CI 0.95 to 1.79, p = NS). Overall, there were 660 deaths among 11,033 patients allocated to active treatment with Class I agents and 566 deaths among 10,843 controls (odds ratio 1.15, 95% CI 1.02 to 1.29, $p < 0.05$) (Figure 1).

Separate examination of the data on individual Class I agents either showed harm or appeared unpromising. Individually and collectively, there is no evidence that Class I agents reduce the risk of death. Instead, Class I antiarrhythmic agents appear to significantly increase the risk of death in those patients given these agents prophylactically after myocardial infarction.

Among the various trials of Class I agents, the Cardiac Arrhythmia Suppression Trial (CAST)[6] deserves further elaboration. In this study, patients with frequent ventricular arrhythmias after myocardial infarction were identified by 24-hour Holter recordings. In each patient, one of three drugs (encainide, flecainide, or moricizine) was identified. Patients were then randomized to receive the active agent or placebo. The trial was stopped early when a statistically significant two- to threefold excess in total mortality and sudden arrhythmic death in patients treated with encainide or flecainide, as compared to those with placebo emerged. The second part of CAST (CAST-II) was continued with moricizine versus placebo. At the time the study with encainide and flecainide was terminated, there was a favorable trend toward a lower mortality among the small numbers of patients who received moricizine compared to placebo. It is disturbing, however, to note that when CAST-II was ultimately terminated, an excess in mortality was also found with moricizine, compared to placebo.[7]

In CAST, there was an increase in both nonarrhythmic deaths and sudden arrhythmic deaths. The substantial increase in presumed arrhythmic deaths and nonfatal cardiac arrests implies a proarrhythmic action of these drugs. The increase in nonarrhythmic cardiac mortality suggests that the drugs may also have other adverse consequences such as precipitation of heart failure. This excess in mortality and cardiac arrests was seen in all identified subgroups of patients (eg, those with normal and impaired left ventricular ejection fraction, frequent and relatively infrequent arrhythmia, presence or absence of previous myocardial infarction, presence or absence of other medications, etc.).

There are several implications from CAST for the assessment of antiarrhythmic therapy. First, only large studies are likely to have sufficient events to provide reliable information on benefit or harm. Previous smaller studies on encainide and flecainide were not able to do so conclusively. Similarly, there was a favorable trend with moricizine early in CAST that reversed with the inclusion of more patients. Indeed, databases on these agents suggested that they were safe. Second, although these drugs were associated with increased risk of death, they have been found to be quite effective in suppressing ventricular arrhythmias. Therefore, studies using suppression of arrhythmia as the primary end point can be misleading. This end point does not indicate whether sudden cardiac death can be successfully prevented. Third, although it may be reasonable to make limited extrapolation of the CAST results to other Class IC agents, or perhaps to all Class I agents, it may not be appropriate to generalize the CAST findings to all antiarrhythmic agents. Each one may need to be evaluated for its effects on clinical outcomes. Furthermore, the risk-benefit ratio of antiarrhythmic drugs may vary in different types of patients who have different underlying conditions and arrhythmic substrate. It may be necessary to evaluate these drugs in different populations.

Nevertheless, the disturbing adverse trends seen in the trials of Class I agents in patients after myocardial infarction appear consistent. It seems that none of the Class I agents tested thus far is likely to reduce mortality, and this observation must make us exceedingly cautious in considering the use of these agents in most patients.

Other overviews have reported similar results with other Class I agents.[8–11] Lidocaine has been shown to reduce the incidence of VF during acute myocardial infarction, but it has not been associated with a decrease in total mortality. MacMahon et al.[9] have shown that in the lidocaine trials there was a trend toward an increase in mortality, which appears to be due to an increase in asystole. A meta-analysis of long-term studies by Hine et al.[10] reported similar findings. Morganroth et al.[11] compared the effects of procainamide and quinidine to encainide or flecainide. In this analysis, mortality rates were higher in the former group compared to the latter group. These data suggest that the adverse effects observed with encainide, flecainide, and moricizine in CAST is likely to be seen with a number of other antiarrhythmic agents such as procainamide and quinidine.

By contrast, trials of Class II agents, β blockers, have shown conclusively that these agents reduce mortality during the acute phase of myocardial infarction and when treatment is initiated later and continued for 1 to 2 years following infarction. In 29 short-term trials of the use of β blockers in the early hours of infarction, there were 530 deaths in 14,535 patients randomized to active β blockade compared to 603 deaths in 14,435 control patients (odds ratio 0.87, 95% CI 0.77 to 0.98, $p < 0.02$). In the 26 long-term trials, 934 patients out of 12,438 patients allocated to active treatment died compared to 1,124 deaths among 11,860 control patients (odds ratio 0.77, 95% CI 0.70 to 0.84, $p < 0.0001$). Overall, there were 1,464 deaths in 26,973 patients randomized to active treatment and 1,727 deaths in 26,295 patients randomized to control (odds ratio 0.81, 95% CI 0.75 to 0.87, $p <$ 0.00001).[5] Additionally, there was a reduction in nonfatal cardiac arrest in the short-term trials ($p < 0.02$), and a reduction in sudden death in the long-term trials ($p < 0.001$).[12,13] These findings suggest that major arrhythmic events were being prevented by β blockade (Figure 2).

There are only limited data on amiodarone. Seven randomized trials of amiodarone on 1,293 patients have been carried out. Although only one trial reported a statistically significant reduction in mortality, 6 of the 7 trials reported trends toward a beneficial effect. Overall, 67 out of 652 patients who were allocated active treatment and 91 out of 641 control patients died. Although the reduction in death with amiodarone is statistically significant, the CIs are wide (odds ratio 0.66, 95% CI 0.47 to 0.93, $p < 0.02$) (Figure 2).[5] While these promising data are encouraging, more definitive answers are likely to become available when the several ongoing trials with amiodarone (Canadian Amiodarone Myocardial Infarction Trial, European Myocardial Infarction Trial, The Veterans Affairs and Argentine Trials in Heart Failure) are completed.

The results from the overview of trials lead us to an important conclusion: there is little relationship between the ability of drugs to suppress ventricular arrhythmia and their effects on survival. Although Class I agents effectively suppress arrhythmias, they either have a neutral or harmful effect on survival. Conversely, although β blockers have been shown to have limited effectiveness in suppressing ventricular arrhythmias, these agents have been proven conclusively to reduce mortality and prevent sudden death and VF. It is interesting to speculate that the benefits of amiodarone may relate less to its ability to suppress arrhythmias than to its antifibrillatory properties and its ability to produce β blockade and slow heart rate.

Heterogeneity of Sudden Death

It is becoming clearer that sudden death is heterogeneous and it is likely to be related, in varying degrees, to other factors such as ischemia, atherosclerosis, imbalances in neurohormonal and electrolyte status and other cardiac and noncardiac causes. This is illustrated by the summary in Table 1, which shows the autopsy findings from a study on patients who died suddenly.[14] Therefore, alternate approaches to the prevention of sudden death need to be considered. The remaining sections of this chapter will examine the heterogeneity of sudden death and consider alternate approaches to its prevention.

The failure of antiarrhythmic therapy in preventing sudden death may be because clinically recognized sudden death is a composite of some quite different processes. It is possible that some drugs may be beneficial on some of these processes and yet may be harmful on others. The net clinical effect then depends on the balance between potential benefit (eg, reduction in VF) and harm (eg, increased risk of asystole). There are, however, only limited data available on the exact initiating and terminal arrhythmic events. This is due to the practical difficulty of obtaining recordings of cardiac rhythm preceding and

Table 1
Autopsy Findings in Sudden Death
(<6 Hours of Symptoms) in the
Wandsworth Study

Causes	Males (n = 238)	Females (n = 84)
Ischemic heart disease	65.1%	40.5%
Other cardiac[1]	5.9%	11.9%
Extracardiac	26.5%	41.7%[2]
Uncertain	2.5%	5.9%

Adapted from Reference 14.
[1] autopsy findings of left ventricular hypertrophy, mitral valve prolapse, aortic stenosis, myocardial disease, anomalies of coronary arteries, right ventricular dysplasia, etc.
[2] chiefly due to pulmonary embolism, subarachnoid hemorrhage.

during episodes of sudden and nonsudden deaths. Limited data are available from the following sources: (1) recordings at the time of resuscitation of out-of-hospital cardiac arrests; (2) recordings during the early hours of myocardial infarction before patients were admitted to hospital; (3) recordings among patients admitted to hospital with acute myocardial infarction; and (4) recordings obtained by chance among patients who had a Holter monitor and were being evaluated or treated with antiarrhythmic therapy.

The results of these studies are summarized in Table 2. Most subjects studied in these reports were not random samples of patients suffering from the particular disease conditions. Instead, recordings were coincidentally obtained when the events occurred. Therefore, whether the studies are representative is questionable. The results may be confounded by the effects of concomitant therapy, the differences in disease processes, and the delay from the onset of the event to the beginning of recording. For example, in patients receiving a drug that is proarrhythmic, the proportion of deaths ascribed to VT or VF may be exaggerated. Conversely, drugs that increase the risk of asystole or heart block might alter the proportions of the various causes of death. Some studies have suggested that if recordings were obtained earlier during a cardiac arrest, VT or VF is more likely to be recorded, whereas with increasing delay, asystole is likely to be observed. This may explain the

considerable variation in the proportion of sudden deaths (25% to 75%) that were ascribed to ventricular tachyarrhythmia in various conditions. Moreover, in patients hospitalized after acute myocardial infarction,[15] or those with heart failure,[16] a significant proportion of sudden death may be due to asystole or electromechanical dissociation.

The proportion of sudden cardiac death compared to other cardiac deaths varies by the type of patient or the presence and severity of heart failure. The contribution of ventricular tachyarrhythmia to all cardiac deaths may be small, perhaps as low as 10% to 15% in some patients with severe left ventricular dysfunction, heart failure, or late after myocardial infarction. Deaths due to ventricular tachyarrhythmias could also be as high as 40% to 50% of cardiac deaths during further follow-up among those resuscitated from out-of-hospital cardiac arrest. As a result, even if 80% to 90% of deaths due to ventricular tachyarrhythmia are prevented by an ideal and highly effective therapy (which has no adverse effects and does not merely change the mode of death), the maximum theoretical benefit is likely to be only about a 30% to 40% reduction in cardiac mortality, unless the intervention has beneficial effects on other mechanisms of death. In practice, the expected benefit is likely to be less marked for a number of reasons. The heterogeneity of cardiac deaths classified as sudden[14] suggests that any particular intervention is unlikely to be effective in the

Table 2
Causes of Sudden Death in Various Conditions

Study	Condition	Causes of death		
		VT/VF	Asystole	E-M dissociation/ cardiac rupture
Schaffer & Cobb[3]	Out-of-hospital cardiac arrest	65–75	10–15	10–15
Schaffer & Cobb[3]	Prehospital acute MI	80	10	10
Volpi et al.[15]	In-hospital acute MI	15–20	10–15	65–69
Luu et al.[16]	Severe heart failure	20–30	60–70	5–10

Adapted from Yusuf S, Teo KK. *J Cardiovasc Electrophysiol* 1991; 2(suppl):S233.
E-M: electromechanical; MI: myocardial infarction.

majority of cases. Even in sudden deaths due to cardiac arrhythmias, the intervention may have been used in a population in which the contribution of tachyarrhythmic deaths to all cardiac deaths is lower. Further, the intervention may also be only partially effective in preventing tachyarrhythmic deaths. Some interventions may increase the risk of death due to other causes (eg, asystole), or it may change the mode of death such as patients destined to suffer death due to VF may die from heart failure. All these factors should lead us to expect a more modest effect (15% or 20%) on total mortality.

Alternative Approaches to Prevention of Sudden Death

Risk factors for sudden cardiac death among a general population are the same as those for the development of ischemic heart disease. Therefore, it is reasonable to assume that reduction of common risk factors such as cigarette smoking, elevated cholesterol levels, hypertension, or prevention of thrombosis may prevent sudden death. This assumption is supported by observational, pathological, and interventional studies that are all suggestive of the important role of ischemia in causing sudden death. Studies of the prognostic significance of ischemic changes during exercise testing indicate that patients with a positive exercise test are at greater risk of cardiac death but not of recurrent infarction.[17] Extensive atherosclerosis and platelet microthrombi have been demonstrated in the hearts of patients suffering sudden cardiac death in some pathological studies. Moreover, at least three randomized trials of antiplatelet agents have reported a significant reduction in nonfatal cardiac arrest or sudden death.[18–20] These data suggest a role for ischemia, due either to coronary narrowing or acute platelet microdeposits, in the pathogenesis of sudden death or presumed sudden death.

It is also important to consider modulation of the balance between the sympathetic and parasympathetic systems as a potential cause for sudden death. It is now possible to investigate autonomic control of the circulation by analysis of heart rate variability.[21] Reduced variability has been suggested to be due to sympathetic overstimulation or diminished parasympathetic tone. A decreased heart rate variability has been reported to be associated with increased mortality in patients with myocardial infarction[22] and in heart failure.[23]

Several of the interventions, eg, β blockade, physical exercise, cervical ganglionectomy, and amiodarone, that appear to reduce sudden death also reduce the heart rate. For example, an overview of the trials of physical rehabilitation following acute myocardial infarction demonstrates a significant reduction in sudden death but not reinfarction.[24] In animal experiments, increase in vagal tone and physical training have both been found to increase the fibrillation threshold during coronary occlusion.[25] Cervical ganglionectomy has been shown to be effective in reducing the risk of sudden death in a randomized trial following myocardial infarction.[26] This may be indicative of a reduction in sympathetic activity or an increase in parasympathetic activity.

Hypokalemia and hypomagnesemia have been shown to be associated with frequent ventricular arrhythmia.[27] Moreover, magnesium has been shown to be important for the maintenance of adequate intracellular levels of potassium and may be crucial in preventing ventricular arrhythmia.[28] Epidemiologic studies have also reported that in areas deficient in magnesium in the drinking water, cardiovascular mortality is increased.[29] The effect of magnesium in reducing the frequency of ventricular arrhythmia in the acute phase and also several weeks after myocardial infarction has been reported. In an overview of all randomized trials, the infusion of magnesium was associated with a significant reduction in mortality.[30] A recent trial (the Second Leicester Intravenous Magnesium Intervention Trial or LIMIT-2) on 2,300 acute myocardial infarction patients treated with magnesium sulfate infusion or saline also indicated a significant reduction in 28-day mortality (7.9% mortality rate in the active group versus 10.4% in the control group; $p < 0.04$).[31] Large prospective randomized trials are currently planned or underway to evaluate the effect of magnesium infusion in acute myocardial infusion and oral supplementation in heart failure.

Use of Implantable Cardiac Defibrillators to Prevent Sudden Death

As a result of the failure of conventional antiarrhythmic drugs (especially Class I agents) in preventing sudden death, many investigators and physicians have recently turned to nonpharmacological approaches such as surgery (endocardial resection, stellate ganglionectomy, etc.) or the implantation of devices that recognize VT or VF and deliver a shock. The greatest interest has been generated by work on the implantable cardiac defibrillator (ICD). Many workers in this field believe that the available data indicate that the ICD reduces the incidence of sudden death (and consequently overall mortality) markedly and that such data are so compelling[32] that formal evaluation in prospective studies may not be necessary.

It is of interest to examine the types of studies that have been conducted. They fall into six categories according to the relative reliability of their findings. The problems with each category are summarized in Table 3. It is clear that studies that belong to categories 5 and 6 are likely to be most reliable, those in categories 3 and 4 are of intermediate reliability, and those in categories 1 and 2 are the least reliable. However, the claims of benefit of the ICD are largely based on patient series (categories 1 and 2) that have major limitations in evaluating any therapy.[32,33] Therefore, even the direction of effect from these studies is unreliable. The case series by Newman et al.,[34] which compares the outcome among patients who received the ICD with those receiving amiodarone requires some elaboration. While the authors of this study attempt to overcome some of the problems by matching key

baseline prognostic characteristics, even this study is not free from potential biases. For example, there may have been differences in prognostic features that had not been used in matching, ancillary therapies that may have been different, and there may be differences in the time elapsed from the index event to entry into the series. There can be longer delays from the index cardiac arrest to receiving an ICD (due to delays in referrals, electrophysiological testing, etc.) so that a higher proportion of the early deaths may have occurred prior to receiving the ICD. Conversely, pharmacological treatment may have started earlier in patients receiving amiodarone and thus this group may include a proportion of the high-risk group that are excluded from the ICD arm. With such a design, no true intention to treat analysis can be carried out. In several of the studies that claimed a benefit from the ICD, including that by Newman et al.[34] there was a substantial "reduction" in nonarrhythmic deaths suggesting the possibility of bias in patient selection, ie, good risk patients were selected to receive the ICD, whereas poor risk patients were managed conservatively.

Proper evaluation of this question requires that patients should be randomized to receive the ICD or alternative therapy in trials. A preliminary report from a small randomized study indicates no benefit on total mortality.[35] However, larger studies of longer duration are needed to reliably address this question. Several such studies are planned or are underway.

Conclusions

It is clear that the traditional approach to suppressing ambient arrhythmias with antiarrhythmic agents as a means of preventing sudden death is unpromising. It is also evident that sudden death is a heterogeneous condition and is the manifestation of several different processes (ventricular tachyarrhythmia, asystole, electromechanical dissociation, and cardiac rupture). It is reasonable that a multifactorial approach be used to prevent sudden death.

Table 3

Overview of Studies Evaluating the Efficacy of the Implantable Cardiac Defibrillators on Survival: Different Approaches and Their Limitations

Type of study	Results	Limitations
1. Comparison of a series with ICD vs. a separate historical control series from the same or another center.	Claims for reduced sudden death. However, lower nonsudden death with ICD is apparent in some series, suggesting biases in patient selection.[32]	1. Marked differences in patient selection, concomitant therapy and CABG surgery. 2. Biases due to differences in time from cardiac arrest to entry into study (eg, may be longer in studies of ICD, so highest risk patients may have died before entry).
2. Comparison of actual with "projected" sudden death rates based on number of "appropriate" shocks.	Claims for reduced sudden death.[33]	1. Validity of ascertaining "appropriate" shocks dubious. 2. Large number of shocks may be inappropriate. 3. ? Reversible episodes of VT or fast AF may be shocked.
3. Comparison with historical matched controls within the same institution.	Reduced sudden death. But increase in deaths due to heart failure. Difference in mortality only apparent for about 2 years.[34]	1. No assurance that all prognostic features matched. 2. No assurance that all other treatments similar. 3. Biases due to differences in time from cardiac arrest to entry into study.
4. Concurrent matched controls.	No study	No guarantee that selection biases or referral biases can be avoided.
5. Concurrent randomized controls.	Preliminary results of an ongoing study[35] shows no benefit on total mortality, but apparent effect on sudden death.	Primary endpoint should be CV or total mortality to avoid classification bias. Need for study or at least 600 to 800 patients who survived cardiac arrest.
6. Concurrent randomized controls + use of devices that can record the rhythm at the time of ICD discharge.	No study	Would be ideal study if it has 600 to 800 survivors of cardiac arrest and uses CV or total mortality as the end points.

Adapted from Yusuf S, Teo KK: *J Cardiovasc Electrophysiol* 2(suppl):S233, 1991; and from Connally S, Yusuf S: *Am J Cardiol* 69:959, 1992.

ICD: implantable cardiac defibrillator; CABG: coronary artery bypass graft; VT: ventricular tachycardia; AF: atrial fibrillation; CV: cardiovascular.

The convincing reduction of sudden death by β blockers appears to be mediated only in part by its antiarrhythmic effects. Reduction of sudden death by β blockers may be due to a combination of its effects on heart rate, reduction in sympathetic tone, relief of ischemia, and prevention of cardiac rupture. There is some evidence that relief of ischemia by surgery, prevention of thrombi formation by antiplatelet agents, use of magnesium, use of amiodarone, and increasing parasympathetic tone by exercise may each prevent sudden death. For high-risk patients, the ICD may be a useful adjunct. However, before these interventions become part of the routine clinical approach to prevent sudden death, they should each be evaluated rigorously.

Acknowledgment: This chapter relies considerably on a previous publication by the authors on a similar topic (Yusuf S, Teo KK: Approaches to prevention of sudden death: need for fundamental reevaluation. *J Cardiovasc Electrophysiol* 2(Suppl): S233, 1991.).

References

1. Kannel WB, McGee DL, Schatzkin A: An epidemiologic perspective of sudden death: 26 year follow up in the Framingham Study. *Drugs* 28(Suppl 1):1, 1984.
2. Bigger JT Jr, Fleiss JL, Kleiger R, et al: The relationships among ventricular arrhythmias, left ventricular dysfunction, and mortality in the 2 years after myocardial infarction. *Circulation* 69:250, 1984.
3. Schaffer WA, Cobb LA: Recurrent ventricular fibrillation and modes of death in survivors of out-of-hospital ventricular fibrillation. *N Engl J Med* 293:259, 1975.
4. Teo KK, Yusuf S, Furberg CD: Effect of antiarrhythmic drug therapy on mortality following myocardial infarction (abstract). *Circulation* 82(Suppl III):197, 1990.
5. Teo KK, Yusuf S, Furberg C: Effects of prophylactic antiarrhythmic drug therapy in acute myocardial infarction. An overview of results from the randomized controlled trials. *JAMA* 270:158, 1993.
6. Cardiac Arrhythmia Suppression Trial (CAST) Investigators: Preliminary report: effect of encainide and flecainide on mortality in a randomized trial of arrhythmia suppression after myocardial infarction. *N Engl J Med* 321:406, 1989.
7. The CAST-II Investigators: Results partly presented at the 64th Scientific Sessions of the American Heart Association, November, 1991 (plus personal communications).
8. DeSilva RA, Hennekens CH, Lown B, Casscells W: Lignocaine prophylaxis in acute myocardial infarction: an evaluation of randomized trials. *Lancet* 2:855, 1981.
9. MacMahon S, Collins R, Peto R, et al: Effects of prophylactic lidocaine in suspected acute myocardial infarction. An overview of results from the randomized, controlled trials. *JAMA* 260:1910, 1988.
10. Hine LK, Laird NM, Hewitt P, Chalmers TC: Meta-analysis of emperical long-term antiarrhythmic therapy after myocardial infarction. *JAMA* 262:3037, 1989.
11. Morganroth J, Goin JE: Quinidine-related mortality in the short-to-medium term treatment of ventricular arrhythmias. A meta-analysis. *Circulation* 84:1977, 1991.
12. Yusuf S, Peto R, Lewis J, et al: Beta blockade during and after myocardial infarction: an overview of randomized trials. *Prog Cardiovasc Dis* 27:335, 1985.
13. ISIS-1 (First International Study of Infarct Survival) Collaborative Group: Mechanisms for the early mortality reduction produced by β-blockade started early in acute myocardial infarction. *Lancet* 1:921, 1988.
14. Thomas AC, Knapman PA, Krikler DM, Davies MJ: Community study of the causes of "natural" sudden death. *Br Med J* 297:1453, 1988.
15. Volpi A, Maggioni AP, Franzosi MG, et al: Ventricular fibrillation complicating myocardial infarction. *N Engl J Med* 318:382, 1988.
16. Luu M, Stevenson WG, Stevenson LW, et al: Diverse mechanism of unexpected cardiac arrest in advanced heart failure. *Circulation* 80:1675, 1989.
17. Yusuf S: Design of studies to critically evaluate if detection of asymptomatic ST-segment deviation (silent ischemia) is medical or public health importance. In: BN Singh (ed): *Silent Myocardial Ischemia and Angina. Prevalence, Prognostic and Therapeutic Significance.* New York, NY: Pergamon Press, 1988, p. 206.
18. Anturane Reinfarction Trial Research Group: Sulfinpyrazone in the prevention of sudden death after myocardial infarction. *N Engl J Med* 302:250, 1980.
19. Lewis HD Jr, Davis JW, Archibald DG, et al: Protective effects of aspirin against myocardial infarction and death in men with unstable angina: results of Veterans Administration Cooperative Study. *N Engl J Med* 309:396, 1983.

20. ISIS-2 (Second International Study of Infarct Survival) Collaborative Group: Randomized trial of intravenous streptokinase, oral aspirin, both or neither among 17,187 cases of suspected acute myocardial infarction. *Lancet* 2: 349, 1988.

21. Pagani M, Lombardi F, Guzetti S, et al: Power spectral analysis of heart rate and arterial pressure variabilities as a marker of sympatho-vagal interaction in man and conscious dog. *Circ Res* 59:178, 1986.

22. Kleiger RE, Miller P, Bigger JT, Moss AJ: Multicenter Post Infarction Research Group: decreased heart rate variability and its association with increased mortality after acute myocardial infarction. *Am J Cardiol* 59:256, 1987.

23. Takase B, Kurita A, Uehata A, et al: Prognostic importance of heart rate variability in patients with diabetes mellitus, congestive heart failure, and coronary artery disease (abstract). *Circulation* 80:III-354, 1990.

24. O'Connor GT, Buring J, Yusuf S, et al: Overview of randomized trials of physical rehabilitation following myocardial infarction. *Circulation* 80:234, 1989.

25. Posel D, Noakes T, Kantor P, et al: Exercise training after experimental myocardial infarction increases the ventricular fibrillation threshold before and after the onset of reinfarction in the isolated rat heart. *Circulation* 80: 138, 1989.

26. Schwartz PJ, Motolese M, Pollavini G, et al: Surgical and pharmacological antiadrenergic interventions in the prevention of sudden death after a first myocardial infarction (abstract). *Circulation* 72:III-355, 1985.

27. Dyckner T: Serum magnesium in acute myocardial infarction. Relation to arrhythmias. *Acta Med Scand* 207:59, 1980.

28. Wester PO, Dyckner T: Intracellular electrolytes in cardiac failure. *Acta Med Scand* 707(Suppl):33, 1986.

29. Anderson TW, Neri LC, Schreiber GB, et al: Ischemic heart disease, water hardness and myocardial magnesium. *Can Med Assoc J* 113:199, 1976.

30. Teo KK, Yusuf S, Collins R, et al: Effects of intravenous magnesium in suspected acute myocardial infarction: overview of randomized trials. *Br Med J* 303:1499, 1991.

31. Wood KL, Fletcher S, Roffe C, Haider Y: A randomized trial of intravenous magnesium sulphate in suspected acute myocardial infarction: results of the second Leicester Intravenous Magnesium Intervention Trial (LIMIT-2). *Lancet* 339:1553. 1992.

32. Winkle RA, Mead RH, Ruder MA, et al: Long term outcome with the automatic cardio-verter defibrillator. *J Am Coll Cardiol* 13:1353, 1989.

33. Tchou PJ, Kadri N, Anderson J, et al: Automatic implantable cardioverter defibrillators and survival of patients with left ventricular dysfunction and malignant ventricular arrhythmias. *Ann Intern Med* 109:529, 1988.

34. Newman D, Herre J, Sauve MJ, et al: The automatic implantable cardioverter defibrillator and patient survival: a case controlled study (abstract). *J Am Coll Cardiol* 13:65A, 1989.

35. Kuck KH, Siebels J, Schneider M, et al: Preliminary results of a randomized trial, AICD vs drugs (abstract). *Rev Eur Tech Biomed* 12:110, 1990.

Chapter 28

Impact of Calcium Channel Blockers on Mortality in Survivors of Acute Myocardial Infarction

Peter H. Held
Salim Yusuf

Calcium channel blockers relieve pain in stable angina pectoris. Their role in the treatment of acute myocardial infarction has, however, not been investigated until recently. This chapter presents the results of the clinical trials and discusses their implications. In order to avoid selection or systematic biases, the data from all randomized trials are presented, regardless of their results.

Calcium channel blockers have many properties that could potentially be beneficial during and after acute myocardial infarction. The proposed mechanisms of action vary somewhat among the different available agents, depending on their different ancillary properties. All calcium channel blockers are thought to cause coronary vasodilatation and thereby relieve ischemia. Calcium channel blockers have been shown effective in the treatment of vasospastic angina, but whether significant coronary vasodilatation in acute myocardial infarction by the use of these drugs can be achieved is not clear. Other potentially beneficial effects include reductions in afterload (and thus wall stress), a negative inotropic effect, and with some calcium channel blockers, reductions in heart rate. All these effects could be expected to reduce myocardial oxygen demand, which in turn reduces infarct size. Reduction in myocardial oxygen demand may also be beneficial during long-term secondary prevention. One further proposed beneficial effect during the acute phase of myocardial infarction is the reduction of cellular calcium overload occurring early after reperfusion.

There are a large number of different calcium blockers available. Although they share many of the abovementioned properties, there are important differences that might influence their clinical effects. The agents belonging to the dihydropyridine group (eg, nifedipine) may cause reflex tachycardia while the other two commonly used agents, diltiazem and verapamil, tend to reduce heart rate.

Calcium channel blockers have been extensively studied in animal experiments dur-

Supported by a grant from the Swedish Heart and Lung Foundation.

ing myocardial ischemia. Several of the agents have been shown to reduce the size of myocardial infarction when administered before or within a few minutes after coronary occlusion.[1] These promising experimental data have been the basis for a large number of clinical trials in patients with a suspected or recent myocardial infarction, studying at least five different agents. Such trials are necessary to assess the clinical role of these drugs in order to assess the balance between beneficial and adverse effects. Calcium channel blockers may cause various adverse effects such as hypotension, reflex tachycardia, heart failure, coronary steal, and atrioventricular block, which might outweigh any possible benefit in terms of mortality and major morbidity.

Available Trials

Twenty-three randomized controlled trials of calcium channel blockers in the early phase or following acute myocardial infarction have been reported.[2-24] Five different agents have been tested, but most of the experience has been obtained with nifedipine, verapamil, and diltiazem. Many of these trials were small, studying different aspects of myocardial ischemia while some were large interventional studies with mortality as the outcome of primary interest. However, even the larger trials have been too small to have high statistical power to detect the moderate-sized treatment effects (such as a 15% to 20% difference) that are generally plausible. For this reason and to avoid selection biases, the data will be discussed both for individual trials and with the data combined by appropriate statistical methods.[25] Details about design and results of individual trials have been published elsewhere.[26]

Patients included in the early interventional trials generally had a suspected myocardial infarction while patients included in the long-term trials had a confirmed prior infarction. Most trials excluded patients with low blood pressure, severe heart failure, or shock. In trials using verapamil or diltiazem, patients were often excluded if they had atrioventricular block. Recently, two additional trials[27,28] that studied the effect of calcium channel blockers on angiographic changes in the coronary vessels have been reported. Both included patients with coronary disease of varying severity and many had a previous myocardial infarction. The results of these trials will be discussed in the context of the postinfarction trials to examine the consistency of the results in secondary prevention.

Trial Results

Nifedipine

Nifedipine belongs to the dihydropyridine group and is the most extensively studied agent. Overall 9464 patients have been included in 13 trials.[2-14] The primary end point was infarct size or left ventricular function in most of the trials while three trials were primarily designed to study mortality.[9,13,14] There are no indications of benefit on any outcome (infarct development, death, or infarct size) regardless of the type of trial, duration of treatment, or type of patient studied. In 12 of the trials, treatment started early and most often within 6–12 hours of onset of pain. In two relatively large mortality trials[9,14] patients were entered up to 24 and 48 hours after start of symptoms, respectively. The majority of patients in these trials were, however, randomized early. In the SPRINT-II trial,[14] 75% of the patients were entered within 3 hours of the onset of pain. One mortality trial delayed treatment start until 7–21 days after the infarction.[13] The target dose varied in the different trials between 40 and 120 mg/day, divided in 3 to 6 doses. The duration of treatment varied in the small studies from 2 days to 2 two weeks and in the mortality trials from 1 to 6 months.

None of the nine trials studying infarct size reported any significant differences in mortality compared to the control patients. In two trials enzyme release was nonsignificantly lower in the treated group[5,8] while in the rest, including the 3 largest,[2,10,12] enzyme release was nonsignificantly higher in the nifedipine group. Three trials were designed specifically to study the effects on mortality.[9,13,14] The largest[9] randomized 4,491 patients with suspected myocardial infarction to nifedipine 40 mg/day or placebo. There was no difference in the number of patients developing a definite infarction. At the end of the 28-day treatment period, 150 patients died in the nifedipine group compared to 141 in the placebo group (not significant [NS]). In SPRINT I,[13] 2,276 patients were randomized to nifedipine 3 mg/day or placebo 1–3 weeks after the acute phase. This study was stopped by the study's Safety Committee due to lack of effect after an average of 10 months of follow-up. Sixty-five patients died in each group (NS). In the SPRINT II[14] trial, 1,358 patients at high risk (anterior or recurrent myocardial infarction, history of angina or hypertension, and patients with enzymatically large infarcts) were randomized as early as possible to nifedipine 60 mg/day or placebo. The study was also stopped by the Safety Committee due to a trend toward increased mortality in the nifedipine group during the early phase. At this time, 105 patients had died in the nifedipine

group compared to 90 patients in the placebo group (NS).

Additional mortality data are available from all of the smaller trials except one.[8] Table 1 presents the data for the larger trials and Figure 1 presents the combined estimate for the effect of nifedipine on mortality. The overall odds of death indicates that mortality was 13% higher in the nifedipine group than among placebo treated patients (NS). This trend toward more deaths in the nifedipine treated group is further supported by related data from trials of unstable angina and angiographic trials. These data will be discussed.

The available data on reinfarction in the above trials support the lack of benefit by nifedipine. In the six trials that chose to report the reinfarction rate, there were 124 of 3645 (3.4%) events in the nifedipine group compared to 111 of 3,680 (3.0%) in the placebo group (Figure 2).

Verapamil

Verapamil has been studied in four randomized, controlled trials on a total of about

Table 1
Mortality in Trials of Calcium Channel Blockers in Myocardial Infarction

Trial	Active	Control	Odds ratio	2p
Nifedipine				
Wilcox[9]	150/2240	141/2251	1.07	NS
SPRINT-I[13]	64/1130	65/1146	1.02	NS
SPRINT-II[14]	105/680	90/678	1.19	NS
9 small trials[2–7,10–12*]	46/560	34/581	1.14	NS
Subtotal	365/4731	330/4733	1.13	NS
Diltiazem				
MDPIT[22]	166/1232	167/1234	0.99	NS
3 small trials[19–21]	14/342	14/343	1.00	NS
Subtotal	180/1574	181/1577	0.99	NS
Verapamil				
DAVIT-I[17]	149/1729	145/1718	1.02	NS
DAVIT-II[18]	84/878	107/897	0.78	NS
2 small trials[15,16]	0/37	2/34	0.16	NS
Subtotal	233/2644	254/2649	0.91	NS
Lidoflazine				
Myocardial infarction study group[23]	178/904	167/888	1.06	NS
Total	956/9823	932/9847	1.03	NS

* Data missing from one small trial.[8]

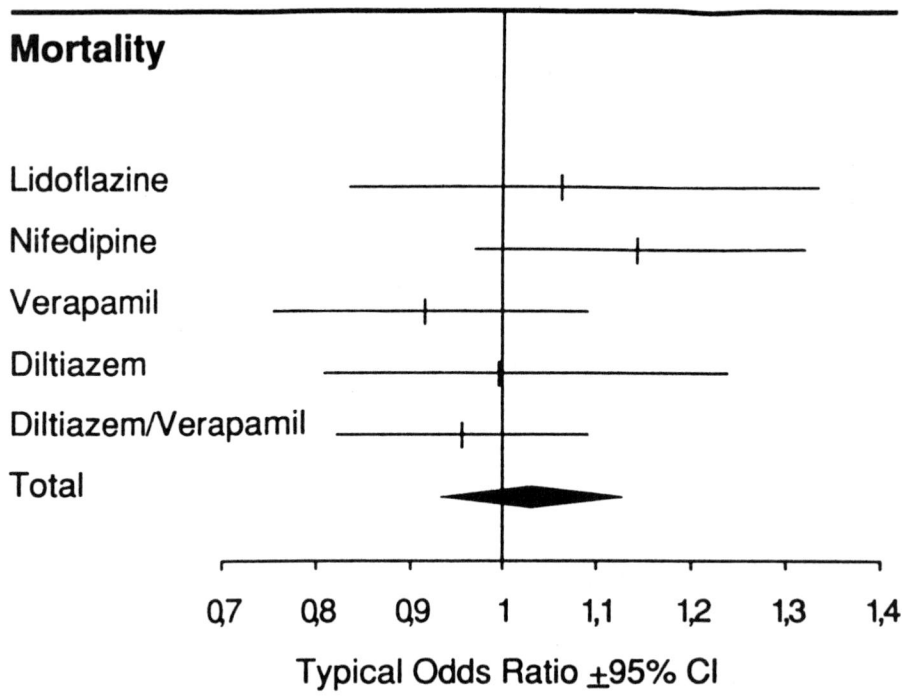

Figure 1. Typical odds of death by drug used are plotted. The bars indicate 95% confidence intervals. Portions to left of verticle line indicate reduced risk with treatment; portions to the right of vertical line indicate increased risk with treatment. The size of the bars corresponds to the number of events in each category of trial. No agent seems to reduce mortality.

5,300 patients.[15–18] The overall data on mortality appear more promising than the nifedipine results, although there is no statistically significant benefit in any single trial. One small short-term trial[15] studied the effect of intravenous verapamil (5–10 mg/h) on infarct size and reported a significant reduction in creatine kinase-MB release. In contrast, a substudy to a large mortality trial found a trend in the opposite direction with higher enzyme levels in the verapamil group.[17,29] Two relatively large mortality trials have been reported. In DAVIT I[17] 3,447 patients with a suspected myocardial infarction were randomized as early as possible to verapamil 0.1 mg/kg intravenously followed by 120 mg orally three times per day. Patients on β blockers or calcium channel blockers were excluded. Out of the 3,447 patients, 2,011 were found to not have an infarct and were withdrawn from treatment during the initial hospitalization.

The remaining 717 verapamil and 719 placebo patients were to be treated for 6 months. About 30% of these patients were withdrawn during the trial, mainly due to early side effects like atrioventricular or sinoatrial block, heart failure, or angina pectoris. An intention-to-treat analysis shows that after 6 months 149 of 1,729 patients in the verapamil group died compared to 145 of 1,718 patients in the placebo group (NS, Table 1). The data on reinfarctions were slightly more promising, with 50 events in the verapamil group as compared to 60 in the placebo treated group (p = NS).

Retrospective analyses of the mortality data in DAVIT I[17] seem to indicate that an early excess of mortality in the verapamil group was balanced by a later beneficial effect. This kind of analysis has to be very carefully interpreted and was the basis for a decision to design a new trial[18] to study the effect of initiating late treatment. In DAVIT II[18] the primary end point

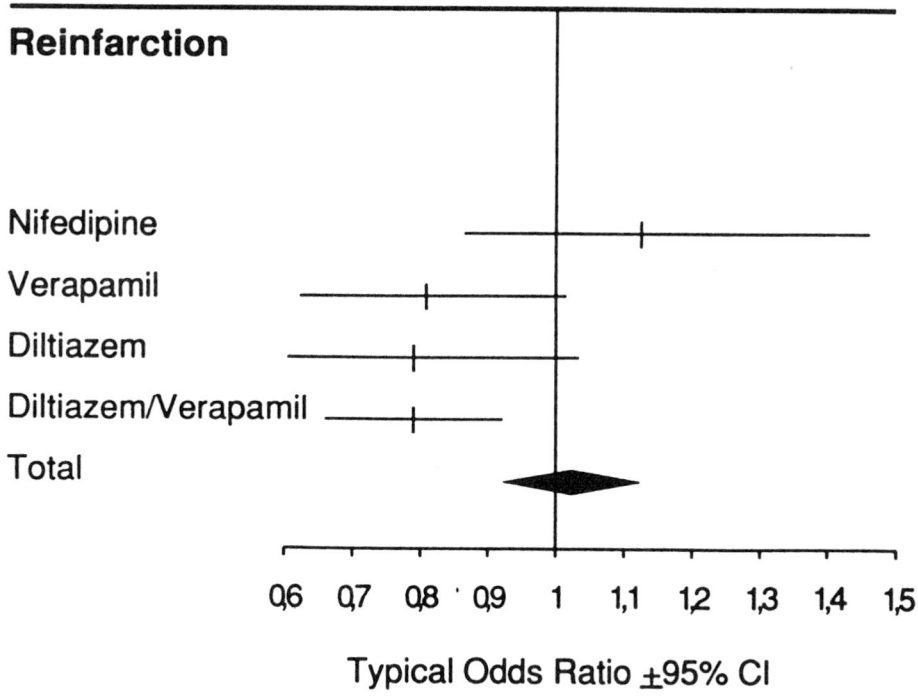

Figure 2. Typical odds of reinfarction by drug used. Bars as in Figure 1. Verapamil and diltiazem show a trend toward lower risk and the combined estimate is marginally statistically significant.

was mortality after 18 months of treatment and a secondary end point was death or reinfarction. Patients on β blockers were excluded. The trial aimed to recruit 2,100 patients, but finally randomized 878 to verapamil and 897 to placebo treatment. After an average of 16 months of treatment 95 patients had died in the verapamil group compared to 119 in the placebo group. This 21% reduction in the verapamil group is not statistically significant and should be viewed in the context of the earlier experience with verapamil. If all mortality data in the four verapamil trials are combined, a nonsignificant reduction in the odds of death of about 9% is achieved (Figure 1).

In DAVIT II a trend toward a lower number of reinfarctions in the verapamil treated group was observed, 84 of 878 (9.6%) versus 107 of 897 (11.9%). This is equivalent to a 22% decrease, but is not statistically significant. The secondary end point of the first major event (death or reinfarction) again shows about a

21% reduction which, however, does not quite reach conventional levels of significance.[30] If one views the totality of data on reinfarction in the four verapamil trials, there is a 20% reduction, which is not statistically significant (Figure 2). The results with verapamil should also be considered in light of the results obtained with other calcium channel blockers that lower heart rate such as diltiazem.

Diltiazem

Diltiazem has many similarities to verapamil in its mechanism of action. Both agents reduce heart rate. Four randomized trials in acute myocardial infarction on a total of about 3,100 patients are available.[19–22] Three of these studies were acute short-term trials, while one was designed as a mortality trial.[22] One trial that included only patients with non-

Q wave infarction evaluated the effects of dilti- azem on short-term reinfarction rate.[19] This trial randomized 576 patients within 24–72 hours of onset of symptoms to treatment with 90 mg every 6 hours of diltiazem or placebo. Of interest is that 65% of the patients received treatment with a β blocker at baseline. At the end of the 14-day treatment period, 11 of 287 diltiazem and 9 of 289 placebo treated patients had died. The number of reinfarctions were 15 of 287 in the diltiazem group and 27 of 289 among placebo treated patients. If a conven- tional two-sided statistical test is used, this promising difference in reinfarction rate is of borderline statistical significance ($p = 0.06$). No data on the severity of the reinfarctions or results on long-term follow-up are available. Two other small trials reported small and non- significant reductions in infarct size.[20–21] Only one large trial has been conducted with diltia- zem.[22] Patients under 75 years of age and with a documented myocardial infarction were eli- gible. Patients with atrioventricular block, se- vere heart failure, and bradycardia were ex- cluded. Patients were randomized to receive diltiazem 60 mg four times a day or placebo. Treatment continued for up to 52 months with a mean of 25 months. The trial was originally planned to study the effects of treatment on total mortality as the primary end point. When it became clear that 1-year mortality was lower than expected, the planned sample size of 2,000 was increased to 2,500 patients and the end point was changed to cardiac death or reinfarction. Approximately 54% of the pa- tients were concomitantly treated with a β blocker. At the end of the treatment period there was no difference in mortality; 166 deaths of 1,232 patients occurred in the diltia- zem group compared to 167 of 1,234 patients in the placebo group. Nonfatal reinfarctions seemed to be less common in the diltiazem group (99 versus 116, NS). In a subgroup anal- ysis, a trend toward more deaths and reinfarc- tions among patients with pulmonary conges- tion on x-ray was found, while a beneficial trend was observed among patients without congestion. These subgroup findings have to be interpreted very carefully.[31] The overall mortality and reinfarction rates in the diltia- zem trials are shown in Figures 1 and 2. Over- all there is no difference in mortality while there is a nonsignificant trend toward a lower number of reinfarctions. The results are very similar to that reported in the verapamil trials.

Lidoflazine

Although not generally available, lidoflaz- ine was the first calcium channel blocker to be studied in a randomized trial of acute myo- cardial infarction.[23] Its properties are slightly different from the other major agents. It has been shown to relieve angina. In the only available trial 1,792 patients were randomized to receive lidoflazine 60 mg three or four times a day or equivalent placebo. Treatment was started within 2 months of infarction and continued for up to 5 years. Mortality was the main end point and no benefit was found. There were 178 deaths among 904 patients treated with lidoflazine compared to 167 of 888 placebo treated patients. No data on the incidence of reinfarction are available.

Overall Mortality

As described, none of 23 randomized controlled trials were able to report any statis- tically significant change of mortality by treat- ment with a calcium channel blocker. The trials differ in their use of agent and in their starting time and duration of treatment. Figure 3 shows the overall results divided in groups according to the type of trial. The results seem to be worse if treatment is started early after infarction, but there are no statistically signifi- cant differences. The early data are, however, dominated by nifedipine trials. Figures 1 and 2 show the overall pooled mortality and rein- farction data from all trials divided by agent used and for all the trials of all agents together. There is no indication of benefit with respect to mortality with any single drug. There is in fact a worrisome trend toward more deaths among nifedipine treated patients than among controls.

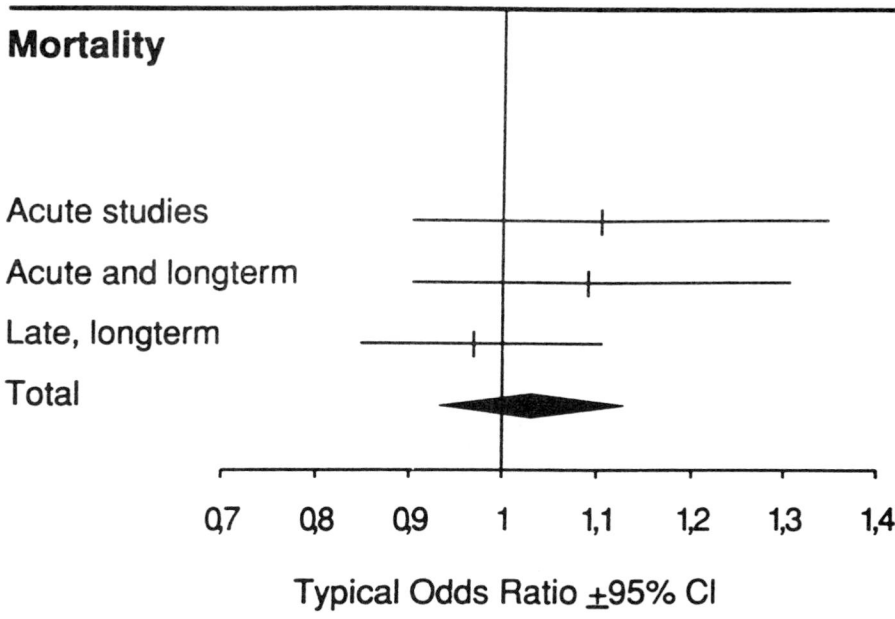

Figure 3. Typical odds of death by treatment start and duration of treatment. All agents analyzed together. About 6,500 patients were included in the early trials; 4,800 in acute studies were treatment continued for up to 6 months, and 8,400 in long-term trials. Bars as in Figure 1. No benefit can be found.

It appears that both diltiazem and verapamil reduce the risk of reinfarction by 20% (Figure 2). The combined data from both classes of agents is nominally significant ($p <$ 0.01). With nifedipine there appears to be a trend toward a higher number of reinfarctions among treated patients. These data need to be carefully interpreted. The three main agents do have different ancillary properties that may be of importance. In particular, verapamil and diltiazem decrease heart rate while nifedipine may increase heart rate. The degree of heart rate reduction has previously been proposed to be related to the degree of mortality reduction in the β blocker trials.[32] Based on retrospective findings in a previous overview[26] we postulated that heart rate reduction by calcium channel blockers might be beneficial and that agents that increase heart rate may be harmful. The DAVIT II trial[18] of verapamil (included above) have since been published and the results appear to support our hypothesis.[30] If the diltiazem and verapamil data are

combined (Figures 1 and 2) there is a 5% reduction in the odds of death (95% confidence interval of -18% to $+9\%$; NS) while reinfarctions are reduced by 21% (95% confidence interval from -33% to -6%; $p < 0.01$).

Possible Harmful Effects of Dihydropyridine Calcium Channel Blockers

The disappointing results reported with nifedipine in the infarction trials are supported by data from two recent angiographic trials of nifedipine and nicardipine.[27,28] These trials are often discussed in isolation rather than in the context of data from all trials of calcium channel blockers in ischemic heart disease. Lichtlen et al.[27] randomized 425 patients with stable angina to receive 80 mg per day of nifedipine or placebo for 3 years. Approximately one third had suffered a previous myocardial infarction and all had documented

Table 2
Mortality in Trials of the Dihydropyridine Calcium Blockers

	Active	Control	Odds ratio	95% Confidence intervals
Myocardial infarction				
Held[26] (overview)	365/4731	330/4733	1.13	0.97–1.32
Angiographic trials				
Waters[28]	2/192	3/191	0.66	0.06–1.90
Lichtlen[27]	12/214	2/211	4.40	1.50–12.60
Unstable angina				
Held[26] (overview)	12/477	7/462	1.78	0.71–4.49
Total	391/5614	342/5597	1.17	1.01–1.36*

* p < 0.05.
Nifedipine was used in all trials except for the one by Waters in which nicardipine was tested.

coronary disease. There was no difference in the primary end point of angiographic progression or regression. Fewer patients developed new lesions, but this difference was not statistically significant.[33] There were, however, 12 deaths in the nifedipine group compared with 2 deaths in the placebo group (*p* < 0.05) while similar numbers of patients were reported to develop a nonfatal reinfarction (Tables 2 and 3). Although the excess mortality in this trial may have been exaggerated by an imbalance in noncardiac deaths, there was also a considerable excess of cardiac deaths that appear to be consistent with the data from the trials of myocardial infarction. Waters et al.[28] randomized 383 patients with angina to treatment with the dihydropyridine nicardipine 90 mg per day for 2 years. There was no difference in the proportion of patients demonstrating progression or regression of existing lesions. In a subgroup of 217 patients with minimal disease fewer treated patients developed new lesions. There were 2 deaths and 14 patients who suffered a myocardial infarction in the treatment group compared to 3 deaths and 8 patients with infarction in the placebo group. The results of these two major angiographic trials are thus consistent with the previous data on nifedipine in acute myocardial infarction and reinforces the unfavorable trend toward more deaths and reinfarctions in the treated group.

Another area closely related to the trials of acute myocardial infarction is unstable angina pectoris. Three randomized trials of a total of approximately 1,000 patients studying the effects of nifedipine have been published.[26,34–36] Two of the trials used placebo as control while in one trial patients were randomized to nifedipine or standard treat-

Table 3
Reinfarction in Trials of the Dihydropyridine Calcium Channel Blockers

	Active	Control	Odds ratio	95% Confidence intervals
Myocardial infarction trials				
Held[26] (overview)	124/3,646	111/3,680	1.14	0.68–1.92
Angiographic trials				
Waters[28]	14/192	8/191	1.77	0.75–4.18
Lichtlen[27]	8/214	7/211	1.13	0.40–3.17
Total	146/4052	126/4082	1.19	0.93–1.52

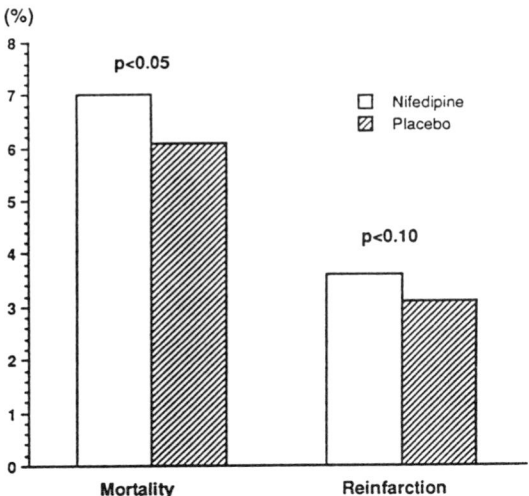

Figure 4. Percent mortality and infarction rates in the trials of dihydropyridine calcium blockers.

ment.[36] Overall, there were 12 deaths out of 477 in the nifedipine group compared to 7 deaths out of 462 in the placebo group. This difference is not statistically significant, but the trend toward more deaths in the nifedipine group reinforces the excess mortality observed in trials of myocardial infarction and coronary artery disease. It may therefore be prudent to analyze all the available data together. In Tables 2 and 3 meta-analyses of both mortality and reinfarction data have been performed. The overall results indicate a 17% increase in mortality ($p < 0.05$) and a 19% increase in the risk of reinfarction ($p = 0.10$). The adverse trends in both outcomes appears in trials of myocardial infarction, unstable angina, and stable coronary artery disease (Figure 4).

Subgroup Results

Differential effects in various subgroups of patients in clinical trials may often be observed. The interpretation of such subgroup findings, especially if they are not specified in advance, is difficult. Guidelines for the interpretation of subgroups effects have been pub-

lished.[31] Generally, in trials without clear overall differences, multiple subgroup analyses could produce misleading results by chance. In such trials, primary emphasis should be on the overall results. Exploratory subgroup analyses using interaction statistics may be appropriate for the generation of specific hypotheses to be tested in other trials. If consistent results appear in all independent trials (not just another selected trial), then there may be some credibility to such claims of preferential subgroup effects.

Two subgroups of patients have been particularly discussed in the context of the calcium channel blocker trials: patients with non-Q wave infarction and patients with depressed left ventricular function. In the following sections these claims are discussed.

Non-Q Wave Myocardial Infarction

A debate regarding the possibility of a beneficial effect, particularly among patients with a non-Q wave infarction, was initiated by the result in the previously described diltiazem trial by Gibson et al.[19] A promising trend of borderline statistical significance toward fewer reinfarctions (but not in mortality) in the treated group was found. Data on non-Q wave myocardial infarction are available from only three more trials. In the MDPIT trial[22] 634 patients with a non-Q wave myocardial infarction were randomized to diltiazem or placebo treatment. A trend toward a lower number of reinfarctions in the diltiazem group (25 of 296; 8.4%) compared to the placebo group (37 of 338; 10.9%) was noted, but was not statistically significant.[37] If the available data on diltiazem are combined a marginally significant reduction in the number of reinfarctions is achieved ($p < 0.05$). Similar data with a nonsignificant trend to a lower number of reinfarctions have recently been published from the DAVIT II trial.[38] However, care has to be taken in the interpretation because data are not available from a large number of trials. It is not known whether this is because such data were not collected or whether the data were not promising enough to be published. In the small nifedipine trial by Eisenberg et al.[6] no difference in reinfarction rate or mortality was found. Although the available diltiazem and verapamil data on reinfarction among patients with a non-Q wave infarction seem to be consistent with the overall trend toward fewer reinfarctions with heart rate reducing agents, it is unclear whether this is different from the effects among patients with Q wave myocardial infarction.

Patients With Left Ventricular Dysfunction

The calcium channel blockers all have varying degrees of negative inotropic effects. This has been a problem in the treatment of chronic heart failure where many patients experience worsening symptoms when treated by these drugs.[39,40] Patients with severe heart failure have not been included in the postin-farction trials. Patients with milder left ventricular dysfunction have, however, been studied and the results have been reported separately in some trials. The MDPIT trial[22] subdivided the patients according to the presence or absence of pulmonary congestion. Among the 490 patients with baseline pulmonary congestion there was a statistically significant increase in mortality in the diltiazem group, while there was a nonsignificant trend in the opposite direction among patients without pulmonary congestion. In a further analysis, diltiazem was found to increase the risk of developing heart failure and this risk was increased with lower left ventricular ejection fraction (Figure 5).[41] In the recent DAVIT II trial[18] an interaction between the presence of clinical heart failure and the treatment effect with verapamil was apparent. There was no difference in mortality or reinfarction among patients with heart failure, whereas a favorable trend was observed among patients with no heart failure. Although similar data are not

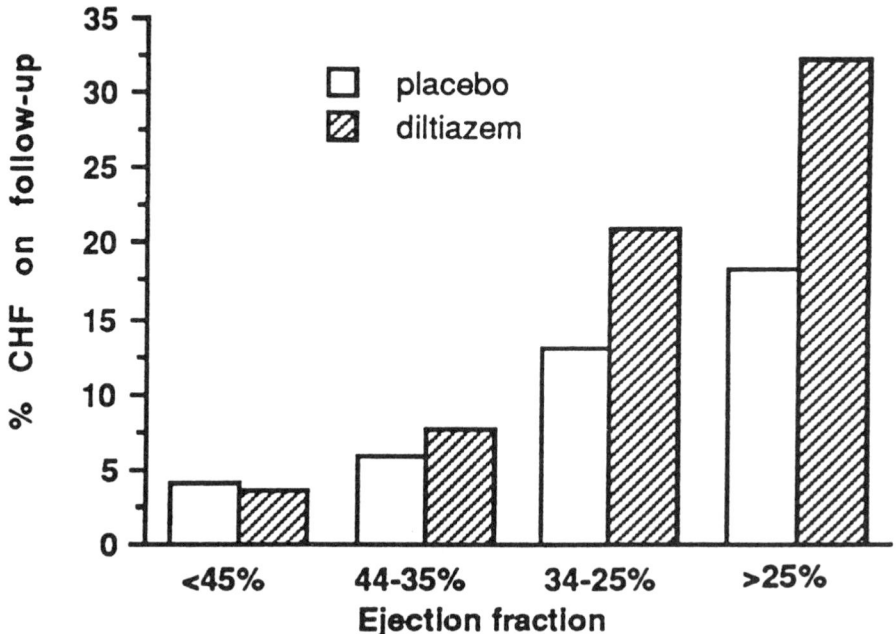

Figure 5. Percent of patients with new or worsened congestive heart failure in the MDPIT trial during study period, defined by baseline left ventricular ejection fraction. The proportion of patients developing heart failure is progressively larger as baseline ejection fraction is reduced. (Reproduced with permission from Reference 41.)

available from all trials it seems reasonable to recommend great caution when using a calcium channel blocker in patients with signs or symptoms of left ventricular dysfunction. In fact, two recent editorials have suggested that calcium channel blockers are contraindicated in heart failure.[40,42] This seems to contrast with the results obtained with β blockers. Although β blockers have a clearly negative inotropic effect, patients with mild to moderate heart failure appear to benefit the most.[43] It has been suggested that reflex activation of renin and other neurohormones by calcium channel blockers might be harmful in this situation whereas β blockers tend to reduce renin levels and blunt the impact of elevated catecholamines in congestive heart failure.[44]

Combination Therapy

The combination of a β blocker and a calcium channel blocker may increase the likelihood of side effects such as heart failure and atrioventricular block. Most trials allowed for the use of β blockers. In the nifedipine trials an average of about 20% of the patients in the placebo and the active treatment arms received β blockade. To test the possibility of an interaction, the large trial by Wilcox et al.[9] stratified randomization according to the use of β blockers on admission. However, no difference in mortality was observed. In total, 827 patients were on a β blocker and of these 38 of 406 (9.3%) in the nifedipine group compared to 38 of 421 (9.0%) in the placebo group died. In the diltiazem trials β blockers were allowed and frequently used. The verapamil mortality trials excluded patients receiving β blockers from participation. The possible problem of an interaction in side effects and efficacy was thus avoided but the interpretation and generalization of the results of the verapamil trials becomes more limited.

Calcium channel blockers could theoretically be beneficial in conjunction with thrombolytic treatment. After a period of ischemia and after thrombolysis a large amount of potentially deleterious calcium may accumulate in the myocardial calls. Early treatment with a calcium channel blocker in this situation has been tested in only one trial.[12] Seventy-four patients were randomized to nifedipine and 75 to placebo treatment in combination with thrombolytic and angioplastic revascularization. No benefit on reocclusion rate (15 of 74 nifedipine and 10 of 75 placebo treated patients), mortality (10 of 74 nifedipine and 6 of 75 placebo), or reinfarction rate (12 of 74 nifedipine and 8 of 75 placebo) was demonstrated.

Calcium Channel Blockers in Secondary Prevention

From a careful review of all the relevant data it is clear that the evidence favoring the calcium channel blockers in secondary prevention after an acute myocardial infarction is much weaker than for β blockers[25] or antiplatelet agents.[45] Even if one subdivides the data by the type of calcium blocker and focuses on the most promising (verapamil and diltiazem), the evidence of benefit on nonfatal reinfarction is only modest, and there is no indication of a reduction in mortality. In contrast, the dihydropyridine calcium blockers appear to increase the risk of death and reinfarction. In the choice of agents for secondary prevention it is therefore reasonable to recommend the use of β blockers and aspirin over any calcium channel blocker. In case of intolerance or contraindications to a β blocker a calcium channel blocker that slows heart rate might be considered as an alternative.

References

1. Kloner RA, Braunwald E: Effects of calcium antagonists on infarcting myocardium. *Am J Cardiol* 59:84B, 1987.
2. Sirnes PA, Overskeid K, Pedersen TR, et al: Evaluation of infarct size during the early use of nifedipine in patients with acute myocardial infarction. The Norwegian nifedipine multicenter trial. *Circulation* 70:638, 1984.
3. Muller JE, Morrison J, Stone PH, et al: Nifedi-

pine therapy for patients with threatened and acute myocardial infarction: a randomized, double-blind, placebo-controlled comparison. *Circulation* 69:740, 1984.

4. Gordon GD, Mabin TA, Isaacs S, et al: Hemodynamic effects of sublingual nifedipine in acute myocardial infarction. *Am J Cardiol* 53:1228, 1984.

5. Gottlieb SO, Becker L, Weiss JL, et al: Nifedipine in acute myocardial infarction: an assessment of left ventricular function, infarct size, and infarct expansion in a double-blind randomized trial. *Br Heart J* 59:411, 1988.

6. Eisenberg PR, Lee RG, Biello DR, et al: Chest pain after nontransmural infarction: the absence of remediable coronary vasospasm. *Am Heart J* 110:515, 1985.

7. Branagan JP, Walsh K, Kelly P, et al: Effect of early treatment with nifedipine in suspected acute myocardial infarction. *Eur Heart J* 7:859, 1986.

8. Loogna E, Sylven C, Groth T, Mogensen L: Complexity of enzyme release during acute myocardial infarction in a controlled study with early nifedipine treatment. *Eur Heart J* 6:114, 1985.

9. Wilcox RG, Hampton JR, Banks DC, et al: Trial of early nifedipine in acute myocardial infarction: the TRENT study. *Br Med J* 293:1204, 1986.

10. Walker L, Mackenzie A, Adgey J: Effect of nifedipine on enzymatically estimated infarct size in the early phase of acute myocardial infarction. *Br Heart J* 39:403, 1988.

11. Jaffe AS, Biello DR, Sobel BE, Geltman EM: Enhancement of metabolism of jeopardized myocardium by nifedipine. *Int J Cardiol* 15:77, 1987.

12. Erbel R, Pop T, Meinertz T, et al: Combination of calcium channel blocker and thrombolytic therapy in acute myocardial infarction. *Am Heart J* 115:529, 1988.

13. The Israeli SPRINT Study Group: Secondary prevention reinfarction Israeli nifedipine trial (SPRINT). A randomized intervention trial of nifedipine in patients with acute myocardial infarction. *Eur Heart J* 9:354, 1988.

14. SPRINT Study Group: the secondary prevention re-infarction Israeli nifedipine trial (SPRINT) II: design and methods, results. *Eur Heart J* 9(Suppl 1):350A, 1988.

15. Bussman WD, Ser W, Gruengrass M: Reduction of creatine kinase and creatine kinase—Mb indexes of infarct size by intravenous verapamil. *Am J Cardiol* 54:1224, 1984.

16. Crea F, Deanfield J, Crean P, et al: Effects of verapamil in preventing early postinfarction angina a reinfarction. *Am J Cardiol* 55:900, 1985.

17. Danish Study Group on Verapamil in Myocar-

dial Infarction: verapamil in acute myocardial infarction. *Eur Heart J* 5:516, 1984.

18. The Danish Study Group on Verapamil in Myocardial Infarction: Effect of verapamil on mortality and major events after acute myocardial infarction (The Danish Verapamil infarction trial II—DAVIT II). *Am J Cardiol* 66:779, 1990.

19. Gibson RS, Boden WE, Theroux P, et al: Diltiazem and reinfarction in patients with non-Q wave myocardial infarction. *N Engl J Med* 315:423, 1986.

20. Zannad F, Amor M, Karcher G, et al: Effect of diltiazem on infarct size estimated by enzyme release, serial thallium-201 single photon emission computed tomography and radionuclide angiography. *Am J Cardiol* 61:1172, 1988.

21. Machecourt J, Cassagnes J, Andre-Fouet X, et al: Proceedings of X World Congress of Cardiology, Washington, DC: American Heart Association, 1986.

22. Multicenter Diliazem Postinfarction Trial Research Group: The effect of diltiazem on mortality and reinfarction after myocardial infarction. *N Engl J Med* 319:385, 1988.

23. Myocardial Infarction Study Group: Secondary prevention of isehemic heart disease: a long term controlled lidoflazine study. *Acta Cardiol* 34(Suppl 24):7, 1979.

24. Eichler HG, Mabin TA, Commerford PJ, et al: Tiapamil, a new calcium antagonist: hemodynamic effects in patients with acute myocardial infarction. *Circulation* 71:779, 1985.

25. Yusuf S, Peto R, Lewis J, et al: Beta blockade during and after myocardial infarction: an overview of the randomized trials. *Prog Cardiovasc Dis* 17:335, 1985.

26. Held P, Yusuf S, Furberg C: Calcium channel blockers in acute myocardial infarction and unstable angina: an overview. *Br Med J* 299:1187, 1989.

27. Lichtlen PR, Hugenholtz PG, Rafflenbeul W, et al: Retardation of angiographic progression of coronary artery disease by nifedipine. Results of the International Nifedipine Trial on Antiatherosclerotic Therapy (INTACT). *Lancet* 335:1109, 1990.

28. Waters D, Lesperance J, Francetich M, et al: A controlled trial to assess the effect of a calcium channel blocker upon the progression of coronary artery atherosclerosis. *Circulation* 82:1940, 1990.

29. Thuesen L, Jorgensen JR, Kvistgaard HJ, et al: Effects of verapamil on enzyme release after early intravenous administration in acute myocardial infarction: double blind randomized trial. *Br Med J* 286:1107, 1983.

30. Yusuf S, Held P, Furberg C: Update of effects of calcium antagonists in myocardial infarction

or angina in light of the second Danish verapamil infarction trial (DAVIT-II) and other recent studies. *Am J Cardiol* 67:1295, 1991.

31. Yusuf S, Wittes J, Probstfield J, Tyroler HA: Analysis and interpretation of treatment effects in subgroups of patients in randomized clinical trials. *JAMA* 266:93, 1991.

32. Kjekshus JK: Importance of heart rate in determining β-blocker efficacy in acute and long-term myocardial infarction intervention trials. *Am J Cardiol* 57:43F, l986.

33. Yusuf S, Garg R: Randomized trials to assess the long-term effects of therapies on angiographic end points. *Chest* 99:1243, 1991.

34. Gerstenblith G, Ouyang P, Achuff SC, et al: Nifedipine in unstable angina. A double-blind, randomized trial. *N Engl J Med* 306:885, 1982.

35. Holland Interuniversity Nifedipine/Metoprolol Trial (HINT) Research Group: Early treatment of unstable angina in the coronary care unit: a randomized, double-blind, placebo controlled comparison of recurrent ischemia in patiens treated with nifedipine or metoprolol or both. *Br Heart J* 56:400, 1986.

36. Muller JE, Turi ZG, Pearle DL, et al: Nifedipine and conventional therapy for unstable angina pectoris: a randomized, double blind comparison. *Circulation* 69:728, 1984.

37. Boden W: Management of non-Q-wave myocardial infarction: role of diltiazem versus β-blocker therapy. *J Cardiovasc Pharmacol* 16: S55, 1990.

38. The Danish Study Group on Verapamil in Myocardial Infarction: Secondary prevention with verapamil after myocardial infarction. *Am J Cardiol* 66:331, 1990.

39. Elkayam U, Amin J, Mehra A, et al: A prospective, randomized, double-blind, crossover study to compare the efficacy and safety of chronic nifedipine therapy with that of isosorbide dinitrate and their combination in the treatment of chronic congestive heart failure. *Circulation* 82:1954, 1990.

40. Calcium antagonist caution (editorial). *Lancet* 337:885, 1991.

41. Goldstein RE, Boccuzzi SJ, Cruess D, et al: Diltiazem increases late-onset congestive heart failure in postinfarction patients with early reduction in ejection fraction. *Circulation* 83:52, 1991.

42. Packer M: Calcium channel blockers in congestive heart failure. The risk of "physiologically rational" therapy. *Circulation* 82:2254, 1990.

43. Chadda K, Goldstein S, Byington R, Curb JD: Effect of propranolol after acute myocardial infarction in patients with congestive heart failure. *Circulation* 73:503, 1986.

44. Packer M: Pathophysiological mechanisms underlying the adverse effects of calcium channel-blocking drugs in patients with chronic heart failure. *Circulation* 80:IV-59, 1989.

45. Anitplatelet Trialists' Collaboration: Secondary prevention of vascular disease by prolonged antiplatelet treatment. *Br Med J* 296:320, 1988.

Chapter 29

Antiarrhythmic Drug Therapy Based on Combination of Class III and Antiadrenergic Activity

Y. Bashir
A. John Camm

Although amiodarone and sotalol are widely regarded as prototype Class III antiarrhythmic drugs,[1,2] their impressive clinical efficacy may depend on the additive effects of lengthening of repolarization with subsidiary mechanisms such as inhibition of sympathetic drive. The concept of merging antiarrhythmic actions, either within a single agent or by use of drug combinations, in order to enhance pharmacological control of cardiac arrhythmias is entirely logical given the multifactorial pathogenesis of most clinically important rhythm disorders. In particular, ventricular tachyarrhythmias in patients with coronary artery disease arise from a complex interaction between the electrophysiological substrate (usually an area of delayed conduction in the infarct border zone) and modulating influences, including increased neurosympathetic activity, mechanical wall stress (via contraction excitation feedback), and myocardial ischemia.

Rationale for Combining Class III Drugs with β Blockers

Class III drugs exert their potent antiarrhythmic effects by uniformiy lengthening action potential duration and refractoriness and are less likely to cause hemodynamic depression or to promote proarrhythmic focal reentry than Class I drugs that act primarily by slowing conduction.[3] There are theoretical grounds for believing that the combination of Class III activity with the antiadrenergic and anti-ischemic properties of β blockers may be particularly effective as antiarrhythmic therapy:

(a) The role of the autonomic nervous system in arrhythmogenesis is increasingly recognized[4-6]: neurosympathetic activation contributes to the development of malignant ventricular arrhythmias during acute myocardial ischemia, in postinfarction survivors, and

From BN Singh, HJJ Wellens, M Hiraoka, (eds): *Electropharmacological Control of Cardiac Arrhythmias.* Mount Kisco, NY, Futura Publishing Company Inc., © 1994.

in patients with impaired left ventricular function. Although β blockers alone are relatively ineffective against reentrant ventricular arrhythmias,[7] they do elevate ventricular fibrillation threshold under both ischemic and non-ischemic conditions,[8] and they are still the only pharmacological agents that have been conclusively shown to prevent sudden arrhythmic death in clinical practice.[9]

(b) Both clinical and experimental studies have shown that sympathetic stimulation can reverse the electrophysiological effects of antiarrhythmic drugs.[10–12] There is increasing evidence that the delayed rectifier potassium current I_K in myocardial tissues is subject to β-adrenergic regulation,[13] and this seems to be the mechanism by which isoproterenol antagonizes action potential prolongation by Class III agents.[12] Thus, β blockers may preserve Class III activity during periods of increased sympathetic activity.

(c) An important limitation of Class III drugs is their reduced activity at rapid heart rates and short coupling intervals, so-called reverse use dependence.[14] β-Blockers will tend to maximize Class III antiarrhythmic efficacy by slowing the heart rate.

(d) During periods of acute myocardial ischemia, Class III drug effects are substantially reversed[15] (Figure 1), but β blockers may continue to provide cardioprotection: Kupersmith et al.[16] reported that propranolol abolished action potential shortening in ischemic myocardium although it had no effect on ventricular repolarization under control conditions.[16]

In contrast to Class I drugs, both β blockers and Class III agents seem to be effective in preventing sudden death after myocardial infarction.[17] In the Beta-Blocker Heart Attack Trial (BHAT), the beneficial effect of propran-

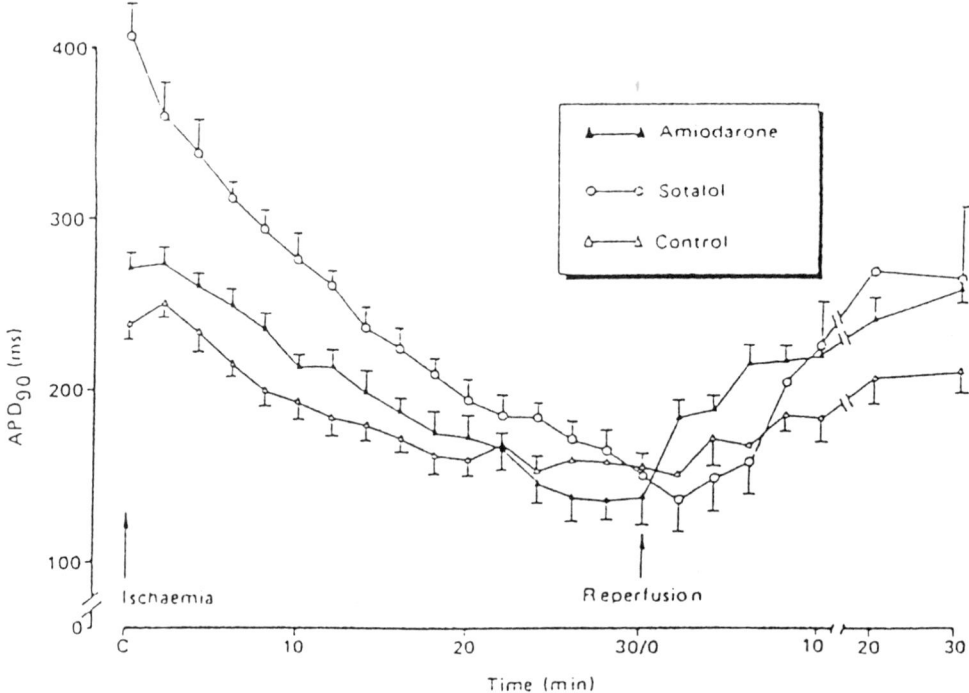

Figure 1. Effect of myocardial ischemia on action potential duration (APD_{90}) and Class III drug activity in arterially perfused rabbit interventricular septum. At baseline, amiodarone and sotalol prolonged APD_{90} compared to controls. In response to acute ischemia, APD_{90} shortened in all three groups and the Class III effects of both drugs were reversed. Following reperfusion, Class III action was reestablished. (Reproduced with permission from Reference 15.)

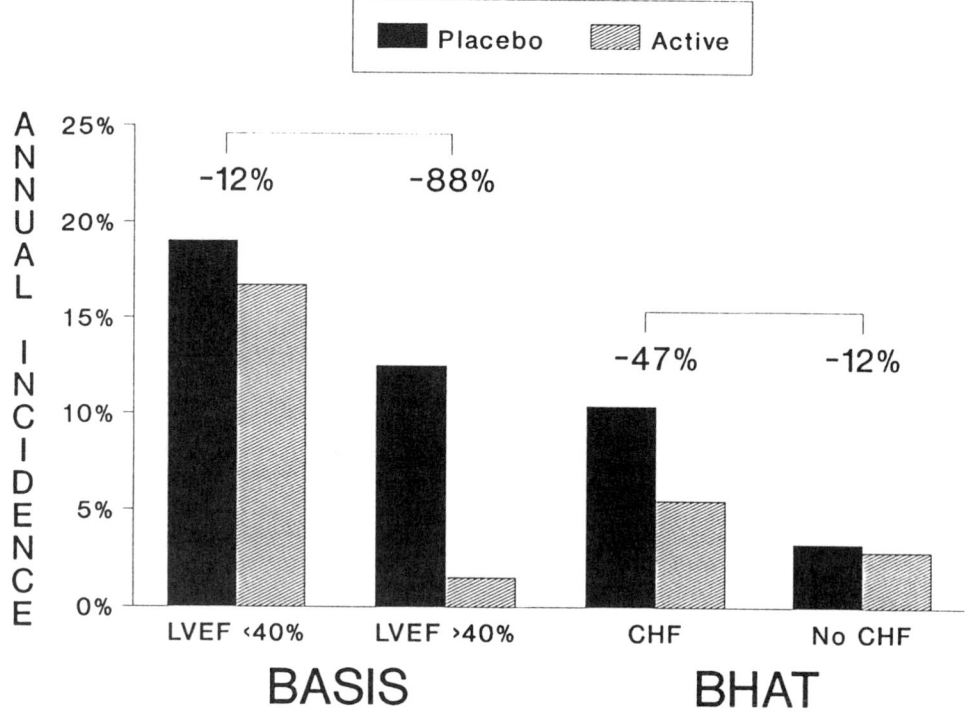

Figure 2. Complementary protective effects of Class III drugs and β blockers in postinfarction survivors grouped according to left ventricular (LV) function. In the Basel Antiarrhythmic Study of Infarct Survival (BASIS), amiodarone reduced the annual incidence of arrhythmic events (including sudden death) to a greater extent in patients with preserved LV function (LVEF > 40%) than in patients with impaired LV function (88% versus 12%). In contrast, in the Beta-Blocker Heart Attack Trial (BHAT), propranolol produced a greater reduction in sudden death rate among patients with prior congestive heart failure (CHF) than in those without a history of heart failure (No CHF) (47% versus 12%). (Adapted with permission from References 18 and 19.)

olol was largely due to a reduction in sudden deaths among patients with evidence of poor left ventricular function and/or heart failure at entry,[18] whereas in the Basel Antiarrhythmic Study of Infarct Survival (BASIS), amiodarone was more protective in patients with preserved left ventricular function (Figure 2).[19] Thus, combination therapy might yield a complementary improvement in efficacy, although as yet there have been no clinical studies addressing this possibility.

Disadvantages of Class III/ β Blocker Combinations

Antiarrhythmic drug combinations may exert cumulative negative inotropic effects, and there is always concern about further depressing myocardial contractility and precipitating hemodynamic deterioration in patients with impaired ventricular function. In fact, low-dose β blockade is surprisingly well tolerated and often produces clinical and hemodynamic improvement in patients with congestive heart failure due to either coronary artery disease or idiopathic dilated cardiomyopathy,[20–22] possibly by altering diastolic function and upregulating β receptors. Furthermore, Class III drugs augment myocardial contractility in vitro,[23] and used in combination might offset the negative inotropic influence of β blockers but preserve their favorable effects on diastolic relaxation/filling.

Another potential problem is that both Class III drugs and β blockers depress sinus node activity and atrioventricular conduction and may induce symptomatic bradycardias. Slowing of the heart rate also favors the development of early afterdepolarizations (EADs) and triggered activity, which is probably the underlying mechanism in drug-induced torsades de pointes, the most characteristic form of proarrhythmia with Class III agents.[24] Conversely, sympathetic blockade tends to reduce EAD amplitude[25] and this may offset the risk of bradycardia-dependent triggered activity.

Despite these theoretical risks, the use of Class III/β blocker combinations in clinical practice has been associated with a surprisingly low incidence of adverse hemodynamic, bradycardic, or proarrhythmic effects.

Antiarrhythmic Drugs with Both Class III and Antiadrenergic Properties

β Blockers (with the exception of sotalol) do not produce any consistent changes in electrophysiological parameters of ventricular myocardium acutely,[7] but Raine and Vaughan Williams[26] have reported that following long-term administration, in vitro action potential duration may be prolonged by as much as 25%. This raises the interesting possibility that the cardioprotective effects of all β blockers on electrical stability might be partly due to Class III activity. Clinical studies in humans using measurement of the surface QT interval or of right ventricular monophasic action potential duration constant rate pacing have confirmed

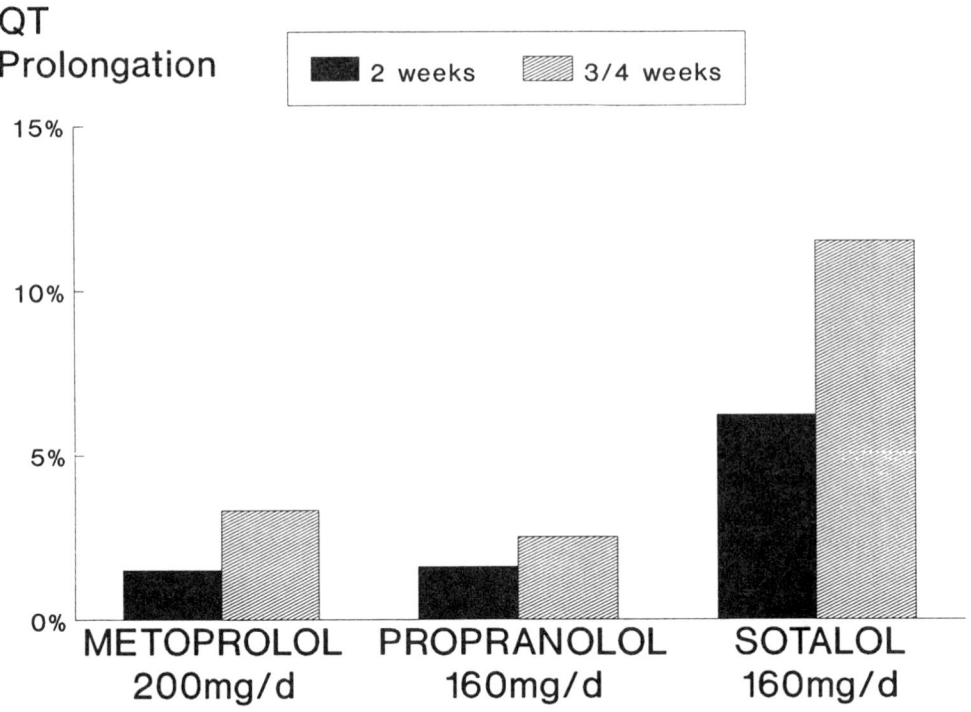

Figure 3. Comparative effects of sotalol and conventional β blockers on ventricular repolarization. The percent prolongation (compared to baseline) of the QT interval during constant rate ventricular pacing with metoprolol, propranolol, and sotalol after 2 and 3–4 weeks. Sotalol exhibited a much greater Class III effect (+11.5%) than metoprolol (+3.3%) and propranolol (+2.5%). (Adapted with permission from References 28 and 29.)

the onset of delayed repolarization during chronic β blockade,[27-29] but the observed changes were very slight (2%–4%). Direct comparisons against sotalol,[29,30] which typically prolong repolarization by more than 10%, also suggest that the Class III effects of conventional β blockers are trivial and unlikely to be of any clinical significance (Figure 3).

Although the sympatho-inhibitory properties of amiodarone were recognized some time ago,[31] it is only recently that Kadish et al.[32] have presented evidence for a clinically significant antiadrenergic effect: the peak heart rate response to isoprenaline stimulation was attenuated by approximately 20% within 2 days of starting oral amiodarone therapy, preceding the onset of delayed repolarization (Figure 4). Amiodarone is arguably the most potent antiarrhythmic agent currently

available for the treatment of recurrent ventricular tachyarrhythmias,[33] and may also reduce the incidence of sudden death in high-risk postinfarction survivors.[34,35] β Adrenergic antagonism probably contributes to this impressive antiarrhythmic profile, although other potentially important features include Class I activity and the absence of reverse use dependence.

Sotalol is the classic example of an antiarrhythmic agent combining Class II and III activities, being a nonselective β blocker that markedly prolongs action potential duration via effects on potassium conductance.[2] Comparative studies have shown that sotalol is more effective than the conventional β-blocking agents nadolol and propranolol in suppressing total and repetitive ventricular ectopic frequency (Figure 5).[36,37] Its antiarryth-

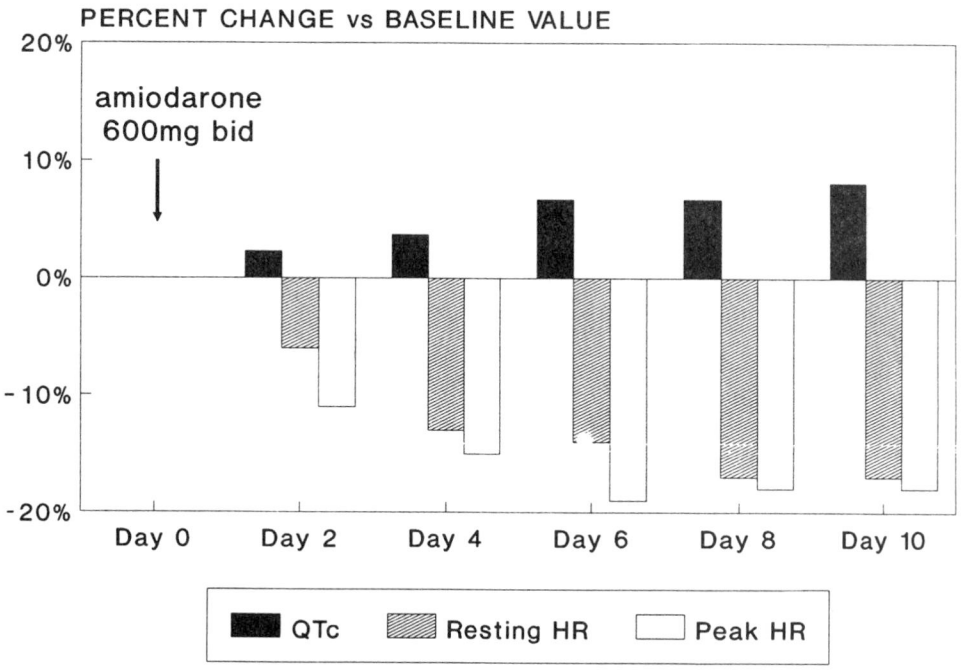

Figure 4. Time course of β adrenergic antagonism during treatment with oral amiodarone (600 mg, b.i.d.) in eight patients with recurrent ventricular tachycardia (VT). Amiodarone caused a progressive reduction in the resting heart rate and peak heart rate during isoproteronol infusion (maximum 50 ng/kg per minute), preceding the onset of QTc prolongation. (Adapted with permission from Reference 32.)

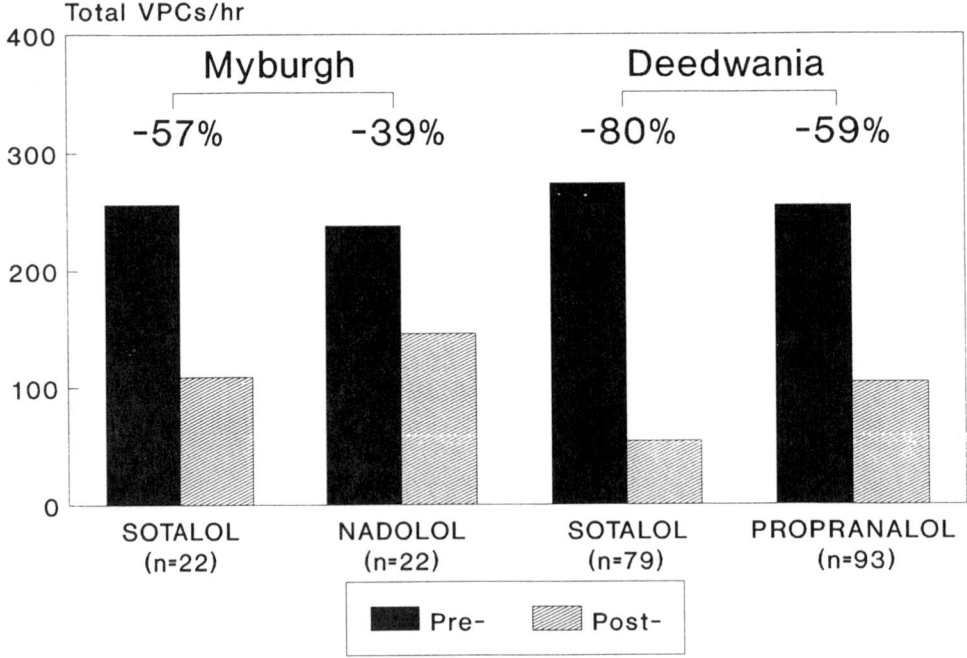

Figure 5. Comparative efficacy of sotalol and conventional β blockers in suppression of ventricular ectopic activity. In the crossover study of Myburgh et al.[36] sotalol suppressed VPC frequency by 57% compared to 39% with nadolol. In the parallel group study of Deedwania,[37] sotalol caused an 80% reduction compared to 59% with propranolol. (Adapted with permission from References 35 and 36.)

mic efficacy in the treatment of sustained ventricular tachyarrhythmias is broadly similar to amiodarone.[38] Because the β-blocking activity of sotalol is predominantly derived from the levo-isomer l-sotalol, whereas the dextro- and levo-isomers are equipotent in prolonging cardiac repolarization,[39] it is possible to separate the relative contributions of antiadrenergic and Class III activities to overall antiarrhythmic efficacy by comparing racemic dl-sotalol with d-sotalol. Kwan et al.[40] reported that dl-sotalol markedly increases the experimental ventricular fibrillation threshold in cats under both nonischemic and ischemic conditions compared to the equivalent dose of d-sotalol (Figure 6a). Although dl-sotalol also prolonged ventricular refractoriness to a greater extent than d-sotalol, these results suggest that the antifibrillatory properties of sotalol are more related to β blockade

than Class III activity. Similarly, in an isolated tissue model, dl-sotalol was significantly more effective than d-sotalol in preventing ventricular arrhythmias during acute ischemia[41]: action potential prolongation by both agents was lost but dl-sotalol prevented conduction slowing whereas d-sotalol increased transmural conduction time, thereby promoting reentry. In contrast, the isomers were equally effective in suppressing inducible ventricular tachycardia (VT) in a canine postinfarction model.[42] In a comparative clinical study, Brachmann et al.[43] found no significant difference between dl- and d-sotalol in suppressing inducibility of VT (11 of 28 versus 10 of 28 patients). Thus, the very limited available data suggests that β-blocking activity significantly contributes to the antifibrillatory action of sotalol but not to its antiarrhythmic activity against reentrant arrhythmias (Figure 6).

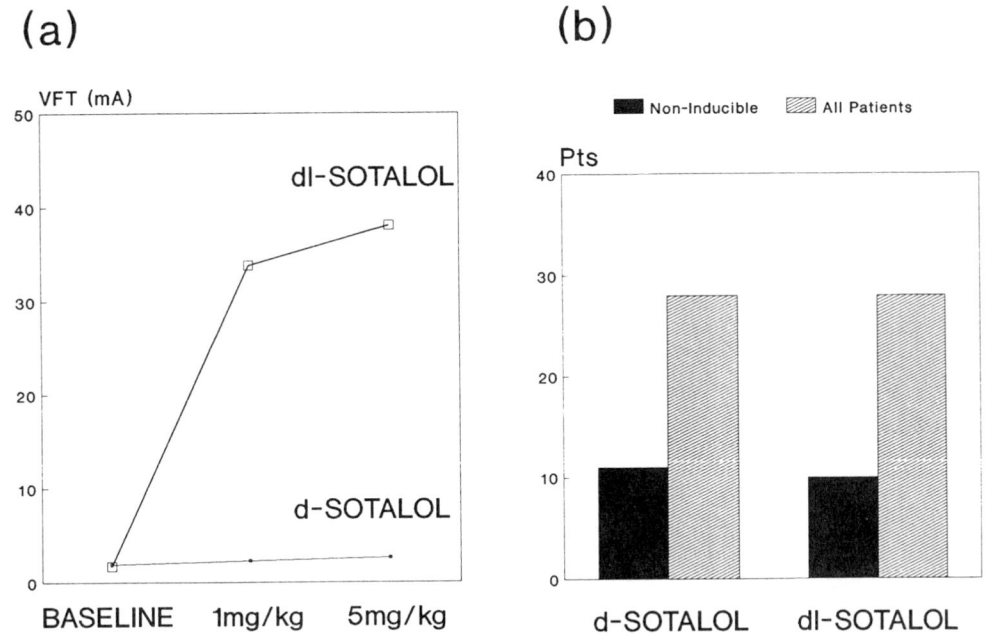

Figure 6. Comparative antifibrillatory and antiarrhythmic efficacy of dl-sotalol and d-sotalol. (a) Effect of d- and dl-sotalol (1 and 5 mg/kg) on ventricular fibrillation threshold (VFT) (mA) in cats. (b) Effect of d-sotalol (1.5–2.0 mg/kg) and dl-sotalol (1.5 mg/kg) on inducibility of sustained ventricular tachycardia (VT) in 28 patients. These results suggest that the antifibrillatory properties of sotalol may depend on β-blocking effect. (Adapted with permission from References 40 and 43.)

Combination of Amiodarone with β Blockade

The antiadrenergic activity of amiodarone alone is relatively weak, and addition of a β blocker may be required in some patients to achieve the optimum blend of Class II and Class III effects. Following Brodsky's report of excellent short and long-term results with low-dose β blockade/Class I combinations in patients with VT and impaired left ventricular function,[44] three recent studies have examined the benefits of adjuvant β blockade with amiodarone for controlling recurrent, drug-refractory ventricular tachyarrhythmias. Tonet et al.[45] retrospectively reported their experience in 20 patients with recurrent episodes of VT despite treatment with amiodarone and multiple other drug regimens. Severe left ventricular dysfunction was present in half of the subjects. Despite these adverse features, addition of low-dose β blockade resulted in short-term control of arrhythmias in all patients, with complete suppression of inducible VT in 4 of 15 who underwent electrophysiological testing. Adjuvant therapy was surprisingly well tolerated hemodynamically. All 20 patients were discharged on amiodarone/β blocker combinations and during a mean follow-up period of 14 months there were three deaths from congestive heart failure, but only one patient experienced a nonfatal recurrence of VT. We have prospectively studied a very similar study population of 20 patients with amiodarone resistant VT, multiple drug failures, and poor left ventricular function (mean ejection fraction 28%). Using an open randomized crossover design,[46] we compared inducibility of VT and exercise tolerance on amiodarone alone (i) and in combination with either metoprolol (ii) or xamoterol (iii). Xamoterol is a β blocker with intrinsic sympathomimetic activity that produces clinical and hemodynamic improvement in mild to moderate heart failure.[47] Our experience contrasted with Tonets' as regards hemodynamic tolerance: adjuvant metoprolol caused worsening heart failure or symptomatic hypotension in 25% of patients but xamoterol was excellently tolerated and signficantly improved exercise capacity compared to the other two regimens. The antiarrhythmic efficacy of the two β blockers was similar: sustained VT was inducible in all 20 patients on amiodarone alone and addition of xamoterol completely suppressed four cases and converted four others to nonsustained VT. Apart from slowing sinus cycle length, neither adjuvant altered ventricular conduction or refractoriness. Fifteen patients were discharged on amiodarone/β blocker combinations, and during a mean follow-up of 13 months there were three nonfatal VT recurrences, but no sudden deaths. Finally, a recent multicenter study of nadolol in VT included a subgroup of 24 patients with inducible VT despite treatment with amiodarone for longer than 6 months (mean LV ejection fraction 30%) in whom the immediate and long-term efficacy of adjuvant treatment with nadolol was assessed using a strict parallel study approach.[48] At acute drug testing, addition of nadolol suppressed inducible VT in 4 of 24 cases (17%) and all of these patients remained free of arrhythmias during follow-up. Ventricular tachycardia recurred in 7 of 20 patients who remained inducible at baseline. Out of the total study population of 60 patients, 7 experienced hemodynamic deterioration (5 withdrawals), although it is not clear how many of these patients were in the amiodarone subgroup. However, antibradycardia pacemakers were required in 6 of 24 patients receiving both amiodarone and nadolol, a relatively high proportion compared to the other two studies in which only 2 of 35 patients on long-term amio-

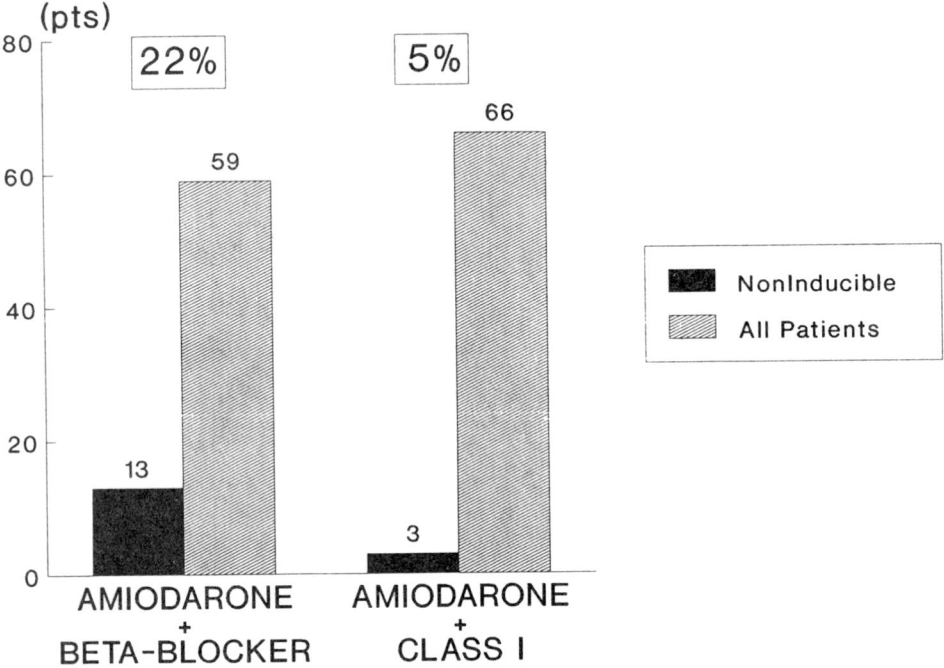

Figure 7. Pooled data from five studies showing the superior efficacy at acute electropharmacological testing of adjuvant β blockade in amiodarone resistant ventricular tachycardia (VT) (22% suppression of inducible VT) compared to combination therapy with a Class I agent (5% suppression). (Adapted with permission from References 45, 46, 48, 49, and 50.)

darone/β blocker combinations were paced.[45,46]

Thus, combination therapy with amiodarone and β blockade may be highly effective even in some difficult patients with drug refractory ventricular tachyarrhythmias, and seems to cause surprisingly few hemodynamic or proarrhythmic problems in spite of underlying poor left ventricular function. Pooling the data from the three studies,[45,46,48] adjuvant β blockade suppressed inducibility of VT in 13 of 59 cases (22%) with successful long-term arrhythmia control; these patients would otherwise have required nonpharmacological therapy with the attendant expenses and risks. Furthermore, there were some patients with frequent/incessant VT in whom adjuvant β blockade failed to suppress inducible VT, but nevertheless reduced the incidence of spontaneous episodes sufficiently, so that it was feasible to implant a defibrillator with antitachycardia pacing capabilities.

In contrast, addition of a Class I drug to amiodarone seldom results in complete suppression: in two recent papers,[49,50] inducibility of VT was only prevented acutely in 3 of 66 (5%) (Figure 7). Furthermore, there is very little data on the long-term efficacy and safety of amiodarone/Class I combination therapy in patients with reduced left ventricular function, and obviously this is of some concern in the aftermath of the Cardiac Arrhythmia Suppression Trial.

Conclusions

There are compelling theoretical reasons for believing that combining Class III and antiadrenergic activities will result in a complementary increase in antiarrhythmic and antifibrillatory potency, and indeed this might partly count for the efficacy of existing agents such as amiodarone and sotalol. Adjuvant low-dose β blockade in combination with amiodarone may be surprisingly effective and well tolerated in over 20% of cases of drug refractory ventricular tachyarrhythmias, even if underlying ventricular function is severely impaired.

References

1. Singh BN, Zipes DP: Basic concepts and clinical applications. *Am Heart J* 106:787, 1983.
2. Singh BN: Historical development of the concept of controlling cardiac arrhythmias by lengthening repolarization: particular reference to sotalol. *Am J Cardiol* 65:3A, 1990.
3. Singh BN: Controlling cardiac arrhythmias: to delay conduction or to prolong refractoriness? *Cardiovasc Drugs Therapy* 3:671, 1989.
4. Verrier RL, Hagestad EL: Role of the autonomic nervous system in sudden death. In: ME Josephson (ed): *Sudden Cardiac Death*. Philadelphia, PA: FA Davis Company, 1985, p. 41.
5. Schwartz PJ, Vanoli E, Stramba-Badiale, et al: Autonomic mechanisms and sudden death: new insights from the analysis of baroreceptor reflexes in conscious dogs with and without a myocardial infarction. *Circulation* 78:969, 1988.
6. Podrid PJ, Fuchs T, Candinas R: Role of the sympathetic nervous system in the genesis of ventricular arrhythmia. *Circulation* 82(Suppl I): 103, 1990.
7. Venditti FJ, Garan H, Ruskin JN: Electrophysiologic effects of β-blockers in ventricular arrhythmias. *Am J Cardiol* 60:3D, 1987.
8. Anderson JL, Rodier HE, Green LS: Comparative effects of β-adrenergic blocking drugs on experimental ventricular fibrillation thresholds. *Am J Cardiol* 51:1196, 1983.
9. Yusuf S, Peto R, Lewis J, et al: β-Blockade during and after myocardial infarction: an overview of the randomised trials. *Prog Cardiovasc Dis* 27: 335, 1985.
10. Morady F, Kou WH, Kadish AH, et al: Antagonism of quinidine's electrophysiologic effects by epinephrine in patients with ventricular tachycardia. *J Am Coll Cardiol* 12:388, 1988.
11. Jazayeri MR, Wyhe G, Avitall J, et al: Isoproterenol reversal of antiarrhythmic effects in patients with inducible sustained ventricular tachyarrhythmias. *J Am Coll Cardiol* 14:705, 1989.
12. Sanguinetti MC, Jurkiewicz NK, Scott A, Siegl PK: Isoproteronol antagonizes prolongation of refractory period by the class III antiarrhythmic agent E-4031 in guinea pig myocytes. Mechanism of action. *Circ Res* 68:77, 1991.
13. Duchatelle-Gourdon I, Hartzell HC, Lagrutta AA: Modulation of the delayed rectifier K current in frog cardiomyocytes by β-adrenergic agents and magnesium. *J Physiol (London)* 415: 251, 1989.
14. Hondeghem LM, Snyder DJ: Class III antiarrhythmic agents have a lot of potential but a long way to go. Reduced effectiveness and dan-

gers of reverse use-dependence. *Circulation* 81:686, 1990.

15. Cobbe SM: Modification of class III antiarrhythmic activity in abnormal myocardium. *Cardiovasc Res* 22:847, 1988.

16. Kupersmith J, Shiang H, Litwak RS, Herman MV: Electrophysiological and antiarrhythmic effects of propranolol in canine acute myocardial ischemia. *Circ Res* 38:302, 1976.

17. Teo K, Yusuf S, Furberg C: Effect of antiarrhythmic drug therapy on mortality following myocardial infarction. *Circulation* 82(Suppl III):III-197, 1990.

18. Chadda K, Goldstein S, Byington R, Cub JD: Effect of propranolol after acute myocardial infarction in patients with congestive heart failure. *Circulation* 73:503, 1986.

19. Pfisterer M, Burkart F, Kiowski W: Protective effect of amiodarone after myocardial infarction in patients with complex ventricular and preserved but not impaired LV function. *Circulation* 78(Suppl III):III-197, 1990.

20. Swedberg K, Hjalmarson A, Waagstein F, Wallentin I: Beneficial effects of long-term β-blockade in congestive cardiomyopathy. *Br Heart J* 44:117, 1990.

21. Charlap S, Lichstein E, Frishman WH: β-Adrenergic blocking drugs in the treatment of congestive heart failure. *Med Clin North Am* 73:373, 1989.

22. Fisher ML, Gottlieb SS, Hamilton B, et al: Beneficial effects of metoprolol in CHF associated with coronary artery disease: a randomised trial. *Circulation* 84(Suppl II):II-312, 1991.

23. Josephson MA, Singh BN: Haemodynamic effects of class III antiarrhythmic agents. In: BN Singh (ed): *Control of Cardiac Arrhythmias by Lenghthening Repolarization.* Mount Kisco, NY: Futura Publishing Company, Inc., 1988, p. 153.

24. Lazzara R, Szabo B, Patterson E, Scherlag BJ: Mechanisms for proarrhythmia with antiarrhythmic drugs. In: DP Zipes, J Jalife (eds): *Cardiac Electrophysiology From Cell to Bedside.* Philadelphia, PA: WB Saunders Company, 1990, p. 402.

25. Ben-David J, Zipes DP: Differential response to right and left ansae subclaviae stimulation of early afterdepolarizations and ventricular tachycardia induced by cesium in dogs. *Circulation* 78:1241, 1988.

26. Raine AEG, Vaughan Williams EM: Adaptation to prolonged β-blockade of rabbit atrial, Purkinje and ventricular potentials, and of papillary muscle contraction. *Circ Res* 48:804, 1981.

27. Edvardsson N, Olsson SB: Effects of acute and chronic β-receptor blockade on ventricular repolarisation in man. *Br Heart J* 45:628, 1981.

28. Edvardsson N, Olsson SB: Induction of delayed repolarization during chronic β-receptor blockade. *Eur Heart J* 6(Suppl D):163, 1985.

29. Creamer JE, Nathan AW, Shennan A, Camm AJ: Acute and chronic effects of sotalol on ventricular repolarization using constant rate pacing. *Am J Cardiol* 57:1092, 1988.

30. Way BP, Forfar JC, Cobbe SM: Comparison of the effects of chronic oral therapy with atenolol and sotalol on ventricular monophasic action potential duration and effective refractory period. *Am Heart J* 116:740, 1988.

31. Polster P, Broekhuysen J: The adrenergic antagonism of amiodarone. *Biochem Pharmacol* 39;668, 1970.

32. Kadish AH, Chen RF, Schmaltz S, Morady F: Magnitude and time course of β-adrenergic antagonism during oral amiodarone therapy. *J Am Coll Cardiol* 16:1240, 1990.

33. Herre JM, Sauve MJ, Malone P, et al: Long-term results of amiodarone therapy in patients with recurrent sustained VT or VF. *J Am Coll Cardiol* 13:442, 1989.

34. Burkart F, Pfisterer M, Kiowski W, et al: Effect of antiarrhythmic therapy on mortality in survivors of myocardial infarction with asymptomatic complex ventricular arrhythmias: Basel Antiarrhythmic Study of Infarct Survival. *J Am Coll Cardiol* 16:1711, 1990.

35. Ceremuzynski L, Kleczar E, Krezeminska-Pakula M, et al: Effect of amiodarone on mortality after myocardial infarction. *J Am Coll Cardiol* 20:1056, 1992.

36. Myburgh DP, Smith R, Diamond TH, et al: A comparison of the efficacy of sotalol and nadolol in the suppression of ventricular ectopic beats. *S Afr Med J* 63:263, 1983.

37. Deedwania PC: Suppressant effects of conventional β-blockers and sotalol on complex and repetitive ventricular premature complexes. *Am J Cardiol* 65:43, 1990.

38. Kehoe RF, Zheutlin TA, Dunnington CS, et al: Safety and efficacy of sotalol in patients with drug-refractory sustained ventricular tachyarrhythmias. *Am J Cardiol* 65:58A, 1990.

39. Kato R, Yabek S, Ikeda N, et al: Electrophysiologic effects of dextro- and levo-isomers of sotalol in isolated cardiac muscle and their in vivo pharmacokinetics. *J Am Coll Cardiol* 7:116, 1986.

40. Kwan YW, Solca AM, Gwilt M, et al: Comparative antifibrillatory effects of d- and dl-sotalol in normal and ischemic ventricular muscle of the cat. *J Cardiovasc Pharmacol* 15:233, 1990.

41. Pasnani JS, Ferrier GR: Pro- and antiarrhythmic effects of d- and dl-sotalol are mediated by actions on conduction in an isolated tissue model of ventricular tachycardia. *Circulation* 84(Suppl II):II-506, 1991.

42. Lynch JJ, Wilder DJ, Montgomery DG, et al: Anti-arrhythmic and antifibrillatory action of the l- and d-isomers of sotalol. *J Cardiovasc Pharmacol* 6:1132, 1984.

43. Brachmann J, Schmitt C, Waldecker B, et al: Comparative efficacy of the d-isomer and racemic sotalol in patients with sustained ventricular tachycardia. *Eur Heart J* 11(Suppl):401, 1990.

44. Brodsky MA, Allen BJ, Bessen M, et al: β-Blocker therapy in patients with ventricular tachyarrhythmias in the setting of left ventricular dysfunction. *Am Heart J* 115:799, 1988.

45. Tonet J, Frank G, Fontaine G, Grosgogeat Y: Efficacy and safety of low doses of β-blocker agents combined with amiodarone in refractory ventricular tachycardia. *PACE* 11:1984, 1988.

46. Bashir Y, Paul VE, Griffith MJ, et al: Adjuvant xamoterol or metoprolol for control of amiodarone-resistant ventricular tachycardia in patients with impaired left ventricular function. *Br Heart J* 66:107, 1991.

47. The German and Austrian Xamoterol Study Group: A double-blind placebo-controlled comparison of digoxin and xamoterol in chronic heart failure. *Lancet* i:489, 1988.

48. Leclercq J-F, Leenhardt A, Lemarec H, et al: Predictive value of electrophysiologic studies during treatment of ventricular tachycardia with the β-blocking agent nadolol. *J Am Coll Cardiol* 16:413, 1990.

49. Marchlinski FE, Buxton AE, Kindwall KE, et al: Comparison of individual and combined effects of procainamide and amiodarone in patients with sustained ventricular tachyarrhythmias. *Circulation* 78:583, 1988.

50. Toivonen L, Kadish A, Morady F: A prospective comparison of Class IA, B and C antiarrhythmic agents in combination with amiodarone in patients with inducible sustained ventricular tachycardia. *Circulation* 84:101, 1991.

PART V

Controlling Cardiac Arrhythmias by Prolonging Repolarization

Chapter 30

Control of Cardiac Arrhythmias by Prolonging Repolarization: *Historical Development of the Concept and Emerging Perspectives*

Bramah N. Singh

The approach to controlling cardiac arrhythmias by prolonging repolarization is not new, but only in the last decade or two has the concept become reality. The era of antiarrhythmic therapy was ushered in by the introduction into clinical therapeutics of quinidine, the archetype of antiarrhythmic compounds in 1918. The two major mechanisms for the genesis of arrhythmias—enhanced automaticity and reentry—had been proposed, but had not been completely verified experimentally. Subsequently, as techniques for studying the basic properties of myocardial fibers became available, much research followed to determine the fundamental mode of actions of the compound. However, Sir Thomas Lewis had recognized the significance of changes in the refractory period as a major determinant of the drug's beneficial effect in atrial fibrillation.[1] Microelectrode studies in isolated cardiac muscle[1] showed that quinidine produced not only slowing of myocardial conduction, but also caused a delay in cardiac repolarization. One might have expected an increase in myocardial refractoriness by either effect. Thus, both properties had the potential not only to abort, but also to prevent cardiac arrhythmias. As it turned out in retrospect, they both had the proclivity to aggravate or induce life-threatening disorders of rhythm. However, the latter possibility was not recognized until much later and indeed, only in recent years has it emerged as one of the crucial issues in contemporary cardiology.

For many years it has been appreciated that delaying the fast channel mediated conduction per se might slow the tachycardia cycle length and terminate the tachycardia by blocking conduction in the reentrant circuit. Electrophysiological studies over many decades also focused on the nature of cardiac arrhythmias. As the knowledge of fundamental mechanisms of cardiac dysrhythmias expanded from studies involving in vitro and in vivo experimental models, the actions of antiarrhythmic agents began to be correlated with their effects on the processes of normal and abnormal impulse generation and conduction

From BN Singh, HJJ Wellens, M Hiraoka, (eds): *Electropharmacological Control of Cardiac Arrhythmias.* Mount Kisco, NY, Futura Publishing Company Inc., © 1994.

and subsequently on triggered automaticity (see Chapter 6).

In the 1950s and 1960s, it was thought that blocking myocardial conduction was the main basis for the salutary action of quinidine.[2] Undoubtedly, such a belief at that time was bolstered by the newly reported link between prolonged repolarization and the propensity to spontaneous ventricular fibrillation and sudden death as described by Jervell and Lange-Nielsen in the congenital long QT interval syndrome.[3] This was promptly confirmed in other types of the so-called long QT interval syndromes. The occurrence of paroxysms of polymorphic ventricular tachycardia accompanied by syncope in the setting of drug-induced QT prolongation further supported the arrhythmogenic potential of prolonged ventricular repolarization.[4] In the case of quinidine, the so-called quinidine syncope was found to be due to paroxysmal ventricular tachycardia and fibrillation occurring in the context of prolonged cardiac repolarization. Thus, in the case of drugs that lengthen repolarization, it became widely accepted that they exerted proarrhythmic reactions in the form of a distinctive polymorphic ventricular tachycardia, designated torsades de pointes by Dessertenne in 1966.[5] The fact that in the case of delayed conduction, a prerequisite for the development of reentrant arrhythmias,[6] a proarrhythmic reaction due to drug-induced slowing of conduction may also induce reentrant ventricular tachycardia and fibrillation and carried a striking lethal potential was not appreciated until much later. This is scarcely surprising since, in sharp contrast to torsades de pointes, such arrhythmias were not remarkably different in rate or form from those occurring spontaneously in untreated patients. The effect of a drug such as quinidine, which may aggravate or even produce a new arrhythmia by delaying conduction could not be readily distinguished from the naturally occurring ventricular arrhythmias. Thus, the focus on the proarrhythmic effects of quinidine centered largely, if not exclusively, on its proclivity to induce torsades de pointes in association with prolonged repolarization.

Against this background, it might have been difficult if not impossible to conceive that lengthening of the action potential duration (APD) might be a potent antifibrillatory mechanism.

In the case of quinidine, electrophysiological considerations clearly suggest that the lengthening of repolarization must, however, contribute to the prolongation of refractoriness. This is likely to result in an antifibrillatory action[1] perhaps best exemplified in the case of atrial fibrillation. Whether an antifibrillatory effect of the compound is clinically meaningful in the case of ventricular arrhythmias has been difficult to confirm.

During the decades that followed the demonstration of the dual action of quinidine, the description of the congenital long QT interval syndrome, and the recognition of the occurrence of torsades de pointes, there have been various developments. Perhaps the most striking has been the development of β-adrenergic blocking drugs that neither slow conduction nor prolong refractoriness in the manner exhibited by quinidine and related compounds such as disopyramide or procainamide. Their electrophysiological properties stemmed from their propensity for reversing the deleterious actions of catecholamines. Of particular importance, however, was the synthesis and characterization of relatively pure molecules that exert one (eg, delay in conduction as exemplified by encainide and flecainide) or the other (eg, delay in repolarization as exemplified by sotalol) actions of quinidine. These compounds have provided the opportunity to critically evaluate the role of delaying conduction versus that of prolonging myocardial refractoriness in controlling arrhythmias. The controversy on the relative merits of delaying conduction versus prolonging repolarization as antiarrhythmic mechanisms continues. This is an exceedingly complex issue, not yet fully clarified. It may well be that it is the critical balance between changes in conduction versus those in refractoriness as modulated by autonomic transmitters that might determine the circumstances in which arrhythmias might be aborted or prevented and those in which the myocardial substrate might exhibit a particular form of a proarrhythmic reaction (see Chapters 8, 14, and 47). This chapter deals with the development of the concept that lengthening of the APD and refractoriness in the absence of concomitant change in conduction might be a preferable directional change in the substrate for the control of arrhythmias in general.

Origins of the Delineation of the Class III Concept

During the course of a systematic investigation of the properties of a number of β-receptor antagonists, Singh and Vaughan Williams[7] and Singh[8] found that the β-blocking drug sotalol (MJ 1999), besides having the propensity to block β-receptors competitively, lengthened the intracellularly measured action potentials in mammalian myocardial fibers (Figure 1). It also prolonged the QTc interval of the surface electrocardiogram in anesthetized guinea pigs. By inference, the drug prolonged the effective refractory period (ERP). Sotalol protected experimental animals from ventricular fibrillation due to cardiac glycoside intoxication.[7,8] Its overall effects could not, however, be explained on the basis of β blockade alone since numerous β blockers (alprenolol, pindolol, oxprenolol, propranolol, practolol, AH3474) studied under identical conditions in the same laboratory did not exhibit the phenomenon of concentration-dependent prolongation of the APD. The sole exception was INPEA, another β blocker that not only increased the APD in cardiac muscle but, unlike sotalol, it inhibited the maximal rate of depolarization.[9] Also, unlike sotalol, the drug had a nitro group as a parasubstituent in the aromatic ring of its chemical structure. Sotalol has a methanesulphonyl substitution in the same position of the aromatic ring. However, unlike quinidine or procainamide, sotalol produced no significant changes in depolarization over a wide range of concentrations. Thus, at that time, it was believed that sotalol exhibited electrophysiological proper-

ties that were unique.[7,8] It was postulated that the simple lengthening of the APD constituted a significant and discrete mechanism (the so-called Class III action) for the control of cardiac arrhythmias.[7,8]

It is noteworthy that previously Kaumann and Olsson[10] reported that in kitten papillary muscle sotalol augmented contractility coincident with the lengthening of the APD (Figure 2). These changes were associated with the development of aftercontractions that themselves were accompanied by what was subsequently termed early afterdepolarizations (EADs) (Chapter 6). However, in this study the significance of neither the proarrhythmic nor the antiarrhythmic correlates of prolonged cardiac repolarization was appreciated. It merits emphasis that sotalol is not a pure compound, but combines two discrete and unrelated actions—β blockade and the property of prolonging the cardiac action potential in most myocardial fibers. Since the original description of the compound from gross in vitro and in vivo experimental observations, the issue of its overall clinical efficacy has become complicated by the knowledge that β blockade per se exhibits a number of potent antiarrhythmic and antifibrillatory actions that have a bearing on its demonstrated potency for reducing sudden death in a number cardiac disorders (Chapters 14, 17, 27, 29, 47). Little was known about these actions when the electrophysiological effects of sotalol were first delineated in isolated cardiac preparations.[8] For these reasons, the initial focus was on the drug's propensity to prolong the APD as a distinct antiarrhythmic mechanism.

Are the Antifibrillatory Actions of Sotalol Accounted Solely by its β-Blocking Actions?

At the time the idea of controlling cardiac arrhythmias by simply lengthening APD was formally enunciated in the early 1970s,[7,8] there was little supportive clinical and experimental data to uphold the concept. Since then, two lines of experimental and clinical evi-

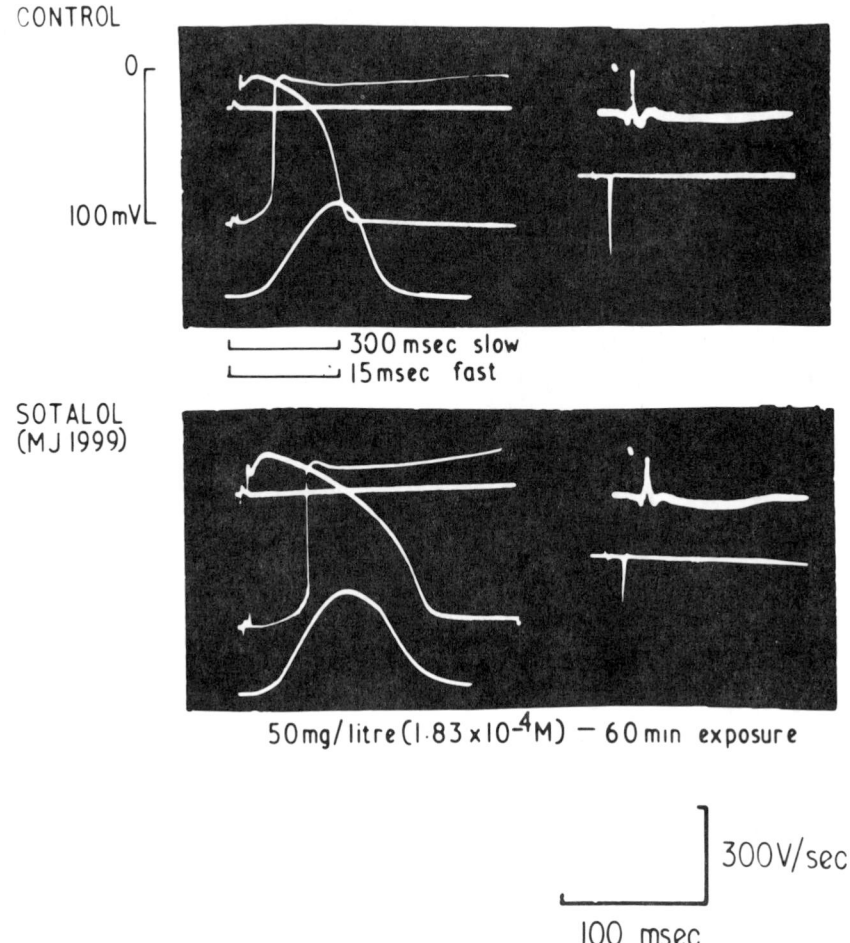

CONTROL

300 msec slow
15 msec fast

SOTALOL
(MJ 1999)

50 mg/litre (1·83 × 10⁻⁴ M) — 60 min exposure

300 V/sec

100 msec

Figure 1. The effects of varying concentrations of sotalol (MJ 1991) on intracellularly recorded action potentials from feline papillary muscle. The top trace on the left of each of the two panels indicates 0 potential; middle trace indicates transmembrane action potential at slow and fast sweep speeds; bottom trace indicates isometric tension. On the top right of each panel is the surface electrogram; the bottom trace depicts the rate of rise of depolarization of the action potential. The vertical and horizontal lines outside the panel show voltage and time calibrations. Note that sotalol lengthens the action potential duration (APD) without affecting depolarization. It also increases the amplitude of the isometric tension. This pattern of electrophysiological changes has been found in all cardiac tissues. (Reproduced with permission from Reference 7.)

dence have been of fundamental importance. The first is the emerging database that is consistent with the notion that isolated lengthening of the APD is indeed a mechanism to prevent ventricular and atrial fibrillation.[11–14] The second is the accumulated knowledge that β blockers are effective in a varying spectrum of patients with ventricular arrhythmias in which they prolong survival. The evidence for these lines of thought are briefly summarized.

Potential Role of Prolonging Cardiac Repolarization

In the 20 years since it was first suggested, lengthening of repolarization appears an

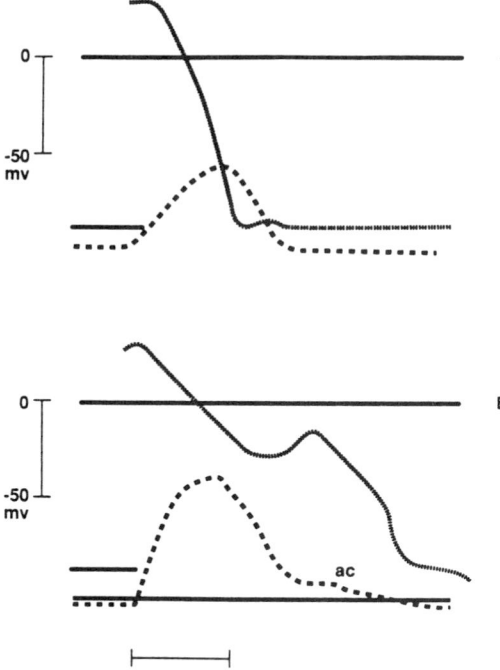

Figure 2. Effects of sotalol (MJ 1991) on feline papillary muscle action potential and isometric tension. A: The top trace shows 0 potential; middle trace shows transmembrane action potential; bottom trace shows isometric tension. B: The action potential from the fiber as in (A). Note that after sotalol, the action potential duration (APD) increased considerably. The plateau phase of the action potential exhibits voltage oscillations (early afterdepolarizations [EADs]), which are associated with aftercontractions (ac). Also noteworthy is the increase in the overall amplitude of contraction coincident with the lengthening of the APD. The figure represents three components of Class III action: (i) long APD and hence refractoriness as a basis for the drug's antifibrillatory action; (ii) augmented contractility; and (iii) the propensity to develop EADs (basis for torsades) when repolarization is markedly increased. (Modified with permission from Reference 10.)

effective approach for terminating as well as preventing the development of atrial and ventricular fibrillation, even in the absence of any change in conduction velocity.[1,13,15–17] The underlying electrophysiological principle is relatively simple. There are a number of clini-

cal correlates of such an antifibrillatory phenomenon. For example, atrial fibrillation is common in the case of hyperthyroidism, a state in which the atrial APD is markedly shortened. The very converse occurs in the case of hypothyroidism.[1,16,18] Many years ago, it was found that in patients with atrial fibrillation converted to sinus rhythm by electrical eonversion, relapses occurred more frequently in those whose atrial action potential (hence, ERP) was much shorter than in those whose APD was longer.[19] It was reasonable to presume that the longer action potential contributed to the electrical stability of the atrial tissue that reduced the probability of fibrillation.[1] It is also known that the marked shortening of the atrial APD effected by vagal stimulation predictably induced atrial fibrillation that was prevented by the administration of sotalol.[20] The issue has not been as clear in the case of ventricular arrhythmias. However, the electrophysiological principle is compelling[13] as is the expanding clinical data (see Chapters 33 and 47). The isolated increase in the ERP produces widening of the cycle length of sustained tachycardia and prevents it from deteriorating into fibrillation; the increase in the excitation wavelength of a reentrant circuit makes the arrhythmia difficult to sustain by precluding the establishment of a stable circuit. Although these considerations had not gone any steps beyond theoretical speculations, and as cited recently by Meinertz,[21] it was suggested 23 years ago that "antiarrhythmic drugs with Class III actions are of great interest clinically since they do not appear to depress excitability, conduction velocity, or myocardial contractility . . . These are clear indications for extensive clinical evaluation of Class III drugs in the management of cardiac arrhythmias in humans."[8]

Adrenergic Modulation of Sotalol's Class III Action—Is it Clinically Relevant?

The evidence that β blockers reduce sudden death in the survivors of acute infarction now is firm.[22,23] This class of drugs also reduces mortality in the congenital long QT interval syndrome.[24] Recent evidence indicates that they may also be effective in controlling symptomatic sustained monomorphic ventricular tachycardia.[25] In fact, they may be superior to Class I agents in prolonging survival in those with aborted sudden death.[26] In the animal ischemia model of sudden death, β blockers prevent the deterioration of ventricular tachycardia to ventricular fibrillation.[27] For example, it was found that the β blocker, nadolol,[28] given prior to programmed electrical stimulation, prevented the development of ventricular fibrillation in about 60% of dogs. However, the precise mechanism of the overall salutary effect of β blockers in these various settings is not clear. It appears multifactorial (Chapters 17, 27 and 47). It is likely due to the reversal of the arrhythmogenic consequences of sympathetic stimulation. An important issue is that their overall beneficial effect is correlated with the magnitude of the bradycardia they produce. By reducing heart rate β blockers may reduce dispersion of refractory period in the ischemic myocardium as has been reported during vagal stimulation.[29] The latter effect may be critical in its action as its beneficial effect in the survivors of acute infarction correlates well with decreases in heart rate.[30] Whatever the mechanisms that are finally established as mediating the salutary effects of β blockers on mortality in patients with ischemic heart disease, it is clear that antifibrillatory agents of the future cannot ignore the importance of incorporating an antiadrenergic action as an integral component of their overall molecular property.[7,14,15,31] This simple electrophysiological concept for controlling arrhythmias by lengthening repolarization is further exemplified more compellingly by the expanding database on the properties[32] and the clinical utility of amiodarone (see Chapter 34). While this agent has complex biological and pharmacodynamic profiles, its dominant electrophysiological action during chronic drug administration is a striking prolongation of myocardial repolarization with an accompanying lengthening

of the ERP. As in the case of sotalol, the changes in repolarization produced by amiodarone is antiadrenergically modulated resulting in marked sinus bradycardia by noncompetitive sympathetic inhibition or by as yet undefined mechanisms (see Chapter 34).

Amiodarone: The Development of a Unique Antifibrillatory and Antiarrhythmic Drug

It is of historical interest that amiodarone, verapamil, sotalol, and propranolol were all synthesized in about 1962 for the treatment of myocardial ischemia, the first two as coronary vasodilators, and the last two as those reducing myocardial oxygen consumption. It is complete serendipity that both amiodarone and sotalol have now become the major antiarrhythmic agents especially for the treatment of cardiac arrhythmias. They are prototypes of future antifibrillatory agents for mortality reduction in patients with life-threatening ventricular arrhythmias. It is noteworthy that the myocardial substrate for 70% to 80% of patients with such arrhythmias is ischemic heart disease. Thus, the anti-ischemic actions of both sotalol and amiodarone may be crucial to their overall utility as antifibrillatory actions in the setting of coronary artery disease.

The synthesis of amiodarone stemmed from attempts to create a potent coronary vasodilator from the khellin molecule in the 1950s at Labaz Research Center in Brussels, Belgium. The historical details of the development of precursors of amiodarone has been recounted by Broekhuysen.[33] The first compound that incorporated the benzofuran moiety of the khellin molecule was benzarone that was not iodinated. The compound that followed was more potent as a coronary vasodilator as a result of the addition of iodine atoms in the aromatic ring in the outer position. It was designated benziodarone, but the drug was abandoned during clinical investigation when it produced hepatoxicity with jaundice.

Amiodarone was developed next during a systematic search for substituted phenols.[33] In early clinical usage the drug was found to exert significant antianginal actions[34] in line with the objectives for its synthesis and development and despite the concern that during its metabolism in the body great deal of free iodine was liberated, the early therapeutic promise led to the drug's continued study as an antianginal agent. This was undoubtedly encouraged by the report by Charlier et al.[35] on its unusual pharmacological profile. In in vitro studies the drug antagonized α and β stimulation in a noncompetitive manner, it produced vasodilatation, but the most striking observation was the development of bradycardia and a reduction in oxygen consumption during chronic drug administration in dogs. Of particular interest was the observation on the temporal sequence of onset and offset times for heart rate changes. At a fixed dose, the peak heart rate reduction occurred at approximately 6 weeks; and even after 12 weeks of withdrawal of the drug, return to baseline values had not occurred. Thus, it became of interest to determine the electrophysiological effects of the drug in the experimental laboratory.

Professor Z.M. Bacq approached the University Laboratory of Pharmacology at Oxford (Dr. EM Vaughan Williams) for characterization of the electrophysiological properties of amiodarone. It became one of a series of cardioactive compounds (sotalol, alprenolol, inpea, mexiletine, lidocaine, diphenylhydantoin, verapamil, pindolol, AH3474) that were evaluated by a variety of techniques as a part of research for the fulfillment of the requirements of Doctor of Philosophy dissertation in the University at Oxford.[8] It promptly became obvious that the conventional superfusion studies could not be carried out because the drug could not be dissolved in water; contact with saline led to immediate precipitation.

In line with the approach indicated by the studies of Charlier et al.[35] in dogs, intraperitoneal amiodarone at varying intervals was given to rabbits and the atria and ventricles were removed and studied in vitro by the standard microelectrode techniques.

Amiodarone was found to increase the APD between 11% and 30% following 1–6 weeks of chronic administration; the spontaneous sinus frequency was reduced but the maximal rate of depolarization was reduced only about 10% at a driving frequency of 1 Hz in the ventricular myocardium.[8,31]

It was assumed that the major effect of the drug (Figure 3) was the prolongation of the APD with the inevitable increases in the absolute as well as the ERP—a Class III effect (Figure 2). The preliminary data was presented by Vaughan Williams at an International Meeting on Cardiac Arrhythmias in Elsinore in Denmark in 1970.[36] The data had been reported in full during the same year.[31] It was suggested that as in the case of sotalol,[7] the property exhibited by amiodarone during chronic treatment represented an example of Class III antiarrhythmic action although it was recognized that the drug was a complex molecule and had numerous subsidiary electrophysiological actions. Dr. Mauricio Rosenbaum (personal communication), present at the Elsinore symposium, was intrigued by the unique electropharmacological properties of amiodarone and its potential for an antiarrhythmic action when given orally. Dr. Rosenbaum decided to import the drug into Argentina (and subsequently arrange its manufacture) and test it clinically in ventricular and supraventricular arrhythmias. He reported his initial observations in 1984[37] and 1986.[38] These landmark reports in the *American Journal of Cardiology* drew relatively prompt attention in the United States; they initiated an era of intense clinical and experimental interest in the compound worldwide. It does not appear to have reached peak (see Chapters 34 and 39). The interest in the compound continues to grow.

Following the initial work at Oxford, the author's own early interest had been in the possibility that a major component of the drug's action, at least as far as the effect on repolarization was concerned, stemmed from the drug's inhibitory action of thyroid hormones with a measure of cardiospecificity.[16,31] The details behind such a hypothesis

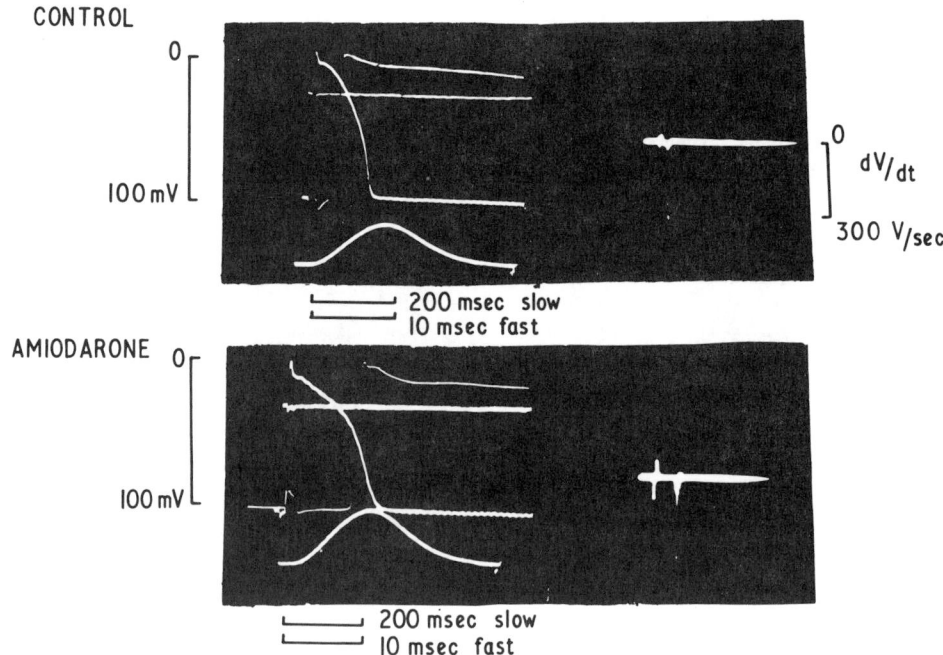

Figure 3. The effects of chronic amiodarone administration on the characteristics of transmembrane potentials in rabbit ventricular myocardium. The upper panel shows a typical recording from the ventricular muscle of a control rabbit, thc lower one from one treated with amiodarone 20 mg/kg intraperitoneally for 6 weeks. In each panel, the upper trace represents 0 potential; the middle trace, represents the transmembrane potential at slow and fast sweep speeds. In the right upper trace is shown the extracellular electrogram and in the lower trace, the differentiated signal of the rate of rise of phase 0 of the action potential. Note that the major effect of the drug was to increase the time course of repolarization (and by inference, the effective refractory period [ERP]) with a minimal effect on the upstroke velocity of phase 0. (Reproduced with permission from Reference 31.)

have been summarized elsewhere.[13,39] Therefore, it was important to exclude the possibility that amiodarone acted by producing generalized hypothyroidism. A series of patients with ischemic heart disease were given 600 mg/day of amiodarone for 6 weeks and their thyroid function tests were performed. There was a time-dependent decrease in heart rate accompanied by an increase in the QTc interval reaching a peak at about 6 weeks at which time the drug was stopped. Amiodarone increased the levels of T4, with a marginal decrease in T3, and no change in thyrotropin (TSH).[40] It was concluded that the drug acted by inhibiting the peripheral conversion of T4 to T3, an effect that was confirmed a year later by Burger et al.[41] Amiodarone thyroid interaction remains under investigation; it is now evident that while iodine released by the drug may induce altered thyroid state and the drug also inhibits peripheral conversion of thyroxine to triiodothyronine but neither of these properties accounts for the virtually identical electrophysiological effects of chronic amiodarone administration and that seen in chronic hypothyroidism. The possibility remains that the drug may exert at least part of its action by cardiospecifically inhibiting T_3 action.

Since these early observations, which are merely of historical interest, a great deal has been learned about the diversity of the drug's electrophysiological and pharmacodynamic actions (Chapters 34 and 47). Its efficacy in supraventricular and ventricular arrhythmias remains unrivalled as does its side effect profile.

To date, there are three types of antiarrhythmic agents—β blockers, sotalol, and amiodarone—which appear to offer the best scope for mortality reduction in patients with cardiac disease by preventing the occurrence of ventricular fibrillation. Their effects are in sharp contrast to those of Class I agents and calcium channel blockers in different subsets of patients with respect to mortality reduction. All three attenuate sympathetic excitation; sotalol and amiodarone share the common property of lengthening the APD and refractoriness, amiodarone having additional electrophysiological effects and exceedingly complex pharmacokinetic properties and membrane effects.[13,32] The clinical profiles of these agents, which have been studied for a few decades, may permit tentative conclusions regarding which components of their electrophysiological properties are linked to their clinical antifibrillatory and profibrillatory actions. The synthesis and characterization of the so-called pure Class III compounds are likely to provide insights into the precise significance of lengthening of the APD per se in preventing atrial and ventricular fibrillation.

What is the Rationale for Developing a Pure Class III Antifibrillatory Agent?

Given the premise that sodium channel blockers are unlikely to retain their previous preeminent role in the treatment of the majority of cardiac arrhythmias (Chapters 22, 23, 27, and 47), there is an increasing impetus to develop newer Class III compounds as substitutes or alternatives to the prototype agents sotalol and amiodarone. The limitations of these two agents are well defined. The major shortcomings of sotalol is its high degree of β-blocking activity and the incidence of torsades de pointes; the latter has been reported to be between 3% and 5% in the usual or the higher end of therapeutic doses.[15] Amiodarone has neither the β blocker side effects nor

does it produce a significant incidence of torsades de pointes. Conversely, the drug produces a wide range of side effects some of which (eg, pulmonary fibrosis and hepatoxicity) may be potentially lethal, especially at high doses. Therefore, the question of whether some or all of the limitations of sotalol and amiodarone might be overcome by creating compounds that exhibited profiles of a pure Class III agent, ie, one in which the electrophysiological effect was confined to the propensity for producing an isolated lengthening of the APD and the ERP arose. Inherent in this line of reasoning is the assumption that the major beneficial effects of sotalol and amiodarone stem from their most striking effect on myocardial repolarization. As an isolated entity, such a property has been designated as a pure Class III action. Compounds with such a property are essentially potassium channel blockers. The potential molecular basis of their actions is discussed in Chapter 18. But against the background of the demonstrated efficacy of β blockers, sotalol and amiodarone, one may well ask why there is now a need for a pure Class III agent?

A number of reasons may be cited. The creation of a pure compound may permit combination therapy with compounds of known pharmacological actions and predictable side effects. By the study of structure activity relationships, it might be possible to define the ionic current basis for the antiarrhythmic, as well as for the proarrhythmic correlates of prolonged cardiac repolarization.[13] The differing effects of pure class III agents may provide a diversity of electropharmacological probes to explore these important practical and theoretical issues.

The most important hallmark of a Class III antiarrhythmic agent is its antifibrillatory action in the atria and ventricles. It is equally characteristic of this class of antiarrhythmic agents that, given the appropriate clinical circumstances, they will produce a variable incidence of torsades de pointes as a reasonably specific proarrhythmic effect.[13] There are emerging data that prolonged cardiac repolarization is associated with an elevation of ventricular fibrillation threshold and a lowered defibrillation threshold. Lengthened repolarization has also been found to prevent the induction of ventricular tachycardia and fibrillation, but pure Class III agents do not appear to exert a major premature ventricular contraction suppressant effect.

Numerous such compounds have now been synthesized and are undergoing clinical and experimental evaluation. The early experimental and clinical data on some of these compounds are presented in Chapters 35 through 43. As will be noted, most are para-substituted benzamides (dofetilide, sematilide, ibutilide, E-4031) resembling sotalol, but without β-blocking actions; others are derivatives of Inpea (eg, almokalant) and some have more complex structures (eg, MS-551, ambasilide). These differences have a bearing on their precise electrophysiological profiles. In the case of the parasubstituted benzamides, the electrophysiological profile is reasonably predictable. In isolated tissues, these compounds produce concentration related increases in the APD and in the ERP. There is no effect on conduction velocity in atrial or ventricular muscle nor in Purkinje fibers. Similarly, a lack of slow channel blocking action or interactions with autonomic transmitters is associated with little or no change in the atrioventricular node under the action of these compounds. Thus, on the surface electrocardiogram these agents produce no effect on the AH, HV, or QRS intervals but they may slightly widen the RR intervals by virtue of their prolonging the APD in the sinus node fibers thereby delaying the onset of the next action potential. However, this is usually a modest effect; the net effect on heart rate is small.

A number of pure Class III agents have been studied in the Lucchesi model of sudden death in experimental animals. For example, Lynch et al.[42] recently reported that E-4031 prevented the development of ventricular fibrillation in 70% of dogs compared to 30% in the control series when 300 μg/kg of the compound was administered intravenously prior to programmed electrical stimulation. Similar data have been reported for the dex-troisomer of sotalol,[43] a compound with a weak β-blocking activity.[44] D-sotalol essentially functions as a pure Class III agent, although it has somewhat greater bradycardic action.

As the list of these so-called Class III agents and the data on their antifibrillatory and proarrhythmic actions increase, it is becoming clear that there is a variable spectrum for not only their antifibrillatory actions, but also for their proclivity to induce torsades de pointes for a given degree of prolongation of repolarization. Thus, it is clearly important to define the circumstances under which these agents as a class produce antifibrillatory or antiarrhythmic actions and under which they exert proarrhythmic actions relative to the fundamental electrophysiological correlates of these effects.[13,17] Therefore, the challenge is to define the basis for the observed differences in the antifibrillatory and proarrhythmic effects of the older and newer Class III compounds in terms of measurable electrophysiological parameters in vitro and in vivo experimental models.

Potential Problems With the Newer Class III Agents

The refractory period in the heart decreases as the stimulus frequency increases. An increase in the ERP in cardiac muscle is considered the critical determinant of an antifibrillatory action in cardiac muscle.[13] Thus, an ideal antifibrillatory agent is one that increases the ERP and the APD as the tachycardia cycle length is shortened. Such an agent should have no significant effect at physiological heart rates. As indicated by Hondeghem and Snyders,[45] that whereas sodium channel block is most pronounced at fast rates, the lengthening of the APD and hence the voltage-dependent ERP is most striking at slow rates in the case of Class IA agents (quinidine, procainamide, disopyramide), sotalol, and most newer Class III compounds. This phenomenon has been termed reversed use or rate dependence. However, it must be emphasized that, quantitatively, the frequency-dependent effect of all Class III agents is not identical. Ambasilide (see Chapter 42) is of particular interest in that it lengthens the APD in ventricular muscle as well as in Purkinje fibers, but it produces a greater shortening of the APD in Purkinje fibers than in ventricular muscle at higher (30 to 120 beats per minute) stimulation frequencies. However, the differential effect may be less striking at higher frequencies.

There are, however, two instances in which lengthening of the repolarization time and ERP, compared to baseline, increase or fail to decrease as the stimulus frequency is increased. The first is the case with the chronic administration with amiodarone. Anderson et al.[46] administered 30 mg of amiodarone to dogs over a 3-week period and measured its rate-dependent effects at the end of this period and compared the effects to the results in an untreated series of animals (control). There was a strong correlation between the test site ERP and the repolarization interval. The increases in the repolarization interval and the refractory periods resulting from amiodarone treatment did not vary with the cycle length over a wide range of stimulation frequencies (200 to 1,000 msec). This effect has now been verified in humans.[47] The second set of relevant observations are those of Wang et al.[48]; these results deal with the Class Ic drug flecainide that in ventricular tissue exerts a markedly depressant effect on conduction but with a minimal effect on the ERP[49] despite producing a powerful block of the delayed rectifier potassium current on isolated ventricular myocytes.[50] Wang et al.[48] showed that in the atrial transmembrane potentials recorded by the standard microelectrode technique, flecainide and quinidine both demonstrated use dependency in blocking the fast sodium channel function as indicated by $\dot{V}_{max}$ of the rising phase of the action potential. In contrast, flecainide markedly increased the APD (and the ERP) as the rate was increased, whereas quinidine exhibited the characteristic reversed use dependency previously reported in the ventricle. This appears to be an example of the Class III action con-

fined to the atrial myocardium at high stimulation frequencies; it provides an unusual electropharmacological probe to determine the ionic current profile of an ideal antiarrhythmic agent with a wider application. Such an effect is consistent with in vivo data in experimental animals in which increases in the refractory period were found to be more predictable determinants of conversion of atrial flutter than decreases in conduction velocity (see Chapter 20). Another potentially unfavorable feature of most of the Class III agents (with the possible exception of ambasilide and amiodarone during chronic drug administration) is their differential effects on ventricular muscle versus Purkinje fibers. Whereas these agents consistently produce increases in ventricular muscle in a concentration-dependent fashion, their effects in the Purkinje fibers are considerably greater for any given drug level (see Chapters 37 and 39). There is evidence that EADs readily develop in Purkinje fibers at a time when the membrane does not oscillate in contiguous ventricular myocardium.[51] Again, if such a phenomenon were applicable to the clinically occurring torsades de pointes, drugs that prolong the APD disproportionately more in the Purkinje fibers compared to ventricular muscle are likely to induce torsades de pointes more readily than those that do not. This issue will require detailed study in the case of individual Class III agents under development.

Conclusions

In recent years, there has been growing concern regarding the gravity of the proarrhythmic effects of Class I agents. Focus has therefore begun to shift to antifibrillatory compounds that act essentially by prolonging myocardial repolarization with little or no effects on conduction. Against this changing background, the role of adrenergic blockade needs to be critically evaluated. It is clear that the β blocker data in a variety of subset of patients emphasize the importance of β blockade as a major antiarrhythmic mechanism in its own right while being an integral component in more complex molecules as such sotalol and amiodarone. There is clinical and experimental evidence that such drugs exert a varying spectrum of antifibrillatory and proarrhythmic (characterized by torsades de pointes) actions for a given degree of prolongation of repolarization. These differences are not readily accountable in terms of specificity of their actions for single or multiple repolarizing myocardial ion currents. Third, there are differences between the so-called pure Class III agents such as sematilide, dofetilide, and E-4031 and more complex compounds such as sotalol and amiodarone that also exert antiadrenergic actions. It is unclear whether one should aim at the development of such antifibrillatory compounds with relatively simple molecules with clearly defined electrophysiological profiles in terms of actions on ion channels, currents, receptors, and pumps. Similarly, it remains uncertain whether it might be preferable to develop compounds with complex electropharmacological profiles that may better match with complex substrates to reverse or correct the arrhythmogenic milieu in different subsets of patients.

References

1. Singh BN, Nademanee K: Control of arrhythmias by selective lengthening of cardiac repolarization: theoretical considerations and clinical observations. *Am Heart J* 109:421, 1985.
2. Sekiya A, Vaughan Williams EM: A comparison of the antifibrillatory actions and effects on intracellular cardiac potentials of pronethalol, disopyramide and quinidine. *Br J Pharmacol* 21:473, 1963.
3. Jervell A, Lange-Nielsen F: Congenital deaf-mutism, functional heart disease with the prolongation of the QT interval and sudden death. *Am Heart J* 56:59, 1957.
4. Selzer A, Wray HW: Quinidine syncope and paroxysmal ventricular fibrillation occurring during treatment of chronic atrial arrhythmias. *Circulation* 30:17, 1964.
5. Dessertenne F: La tachycardie ventriculaire a deux foyers opposés variables. *Arch Mal Coeur* 59:253, 1966.
6. Wit AL, Cranefield PF: Re-entrant excitation as a cause of cardiac arrhythmias. *Am J Physiol* 235:H1, 1978.
7. Singh BN, Vaughan Williams EM: A third class of antiarrhythmic action. Effects on atrial and ventricular intracellular potentials, and other pharmacological actions on cardiac muscle, of MJ 1999 and AH 3474. *Br J Pharmacol* 39:675, 1978.
8. Singh BN: *Pharmacological Actions of Certain Drugs and Hormones: Focus on Studies of Antiarrhythmic Mechanisms*. Oxford, United Kingdom: Hertford College, University of Oxford; 1971. D. Phil. Thesis.
9. Singh BN, Vaughan Williams EM: Effects on cardiac muscle of the β-adrenoceptor blocking drugs INPEA and LB46 in relation to their local anesthetic action on nerve. *Br J Pharmacol* 43:10, 1971.
10. Kaumann AJ, Olson C: Temporal relationship between long-lasting aftercontractions and action potentials in cat papillary muscles. *Science* 163:293, 1968.
11. Singh BN (ed): *Control of Cardiac Arrhythmias by Lengthening Repolarization*. Mount Kisco, NY: Futura Publishing Company Inc., 1988.
12. Singh BN (ed): Control of cardiac arrhythmias with sotalol, a broad-spectrum antiarrhythmic with β-blocking effects and Class III activity. *Am J Cardiol* 765:1A, 1990.
13. Singh BN, Sarma JSM, Zhang ZH, Takanaka C: Controlling cardiac arrhythmias by lengthening repolarization: rationale from experimenal findings and clinical considerations. *Ann NY Acad Sci* 644:187, 1992.
14. Singh BN, Courtney K: On the classification of anti-arrhythmic mechanisms: experimental and clinical correlations. In: DP Zipes, J Jalife (eds): *Cardiac Electrophysiology: From the Cell to Bedside*. Philadelphia, PA: WB Saunder Company, 1990, p. 882.
15. Singh BN: Antiarrhythmic action of DL-sotalol in ventricular and supraventricular arrhythmias. *J Cardiovasc Pharmacol* 20(2):575, 1992.
16. Singh BN: Amiodarone: historical development and pharmacologic profile. *Am Heart J* 106:788, 1983.
17. Singh BN: When is QT prolongation anti-arrhythmic and when is it pro-arrhythmic? *Am J Cardiol* 63:867, 1988.
18. Freedberg AS, Papp JG, Vaughan Williams EM: The effects of altered thyroid state on atrial intracellular potentials. *J Physiol* 207:357, 1970.
19. Gavrilescu S, Luca C: Right atrium monophasic action potentials during atrial flutter and fibrillation in man. *Am Heart J* 90:199, 1975.
20. Bertrix L, Timour-Chah Q, Lang J, et al: Protec-

tion against ventricular and atrial fibrillation by sotalol. *Cardiovasc Res* 20:358, 1986.

21. Meinertz T: Clinical implications of new insights into mechanism of antiarrhythmic drug action. *J Cardiol Pharmacol* 20:S23, 1992.

22. Singh BN: Advantages of β-blockers versus antiarrhythmic drugs and calcium-channel antagonists in secondary prevention in survivors of myocardial infarction. *Am J Cardiol* 66:9, 1990.

23. Yusuf S, Teo KK: Approaches to prevention of sudden death: need for fundamental re-evaluation. *J Cardiovasc Electrophysiol* 2(3):S233, 1991.

24. Schwartz PJ: The idiopathic long QT syndrome: progress and questions. *Am Heart J* 109:399, 1985.

25. Steinbeck G, Andresen D, Bach P, et al: A comparison of electrophysiologically-guided antiarrhythmic drug therapy with β-blocker in patients with symptomatic, sustained ventricular tachyarrhythmias. *N Engl J Med* 327:987, 1992.

26. Hallstrom AP, Cobb LA, Yu BH, et al: An antiarrhythmic drug experience in 941 patients resuscitated from an initial cardiac arrest between 1970 and 1985. *Am J Cardiol* 68:1025, 1991.

27. Lynch JJ, Lucchesi BR: How are animal models best used for the study of antiarrhythmic drugs? In: DJ Hearse, AS Mouring, MJ Janse (eds): *Life-Threatening Arrhythmias During Ischemia and Infarction*. New York, NY: Raven Press, 1987, p. 169.

28. Patterson E, Lucchesi BR: Antifibrillatory actions of nadolol. *J Pharmacol Exp Ther* 223:144, 1982.

29. Kent KM, Smith ER, Redwood DR, Epstein SE: Electrical stability of acutely ischemic myocardium. Influences of heart rate and vagal stimulation. *Circulation* 67:291, 1973.

30. Kjekshus JK: Importance of heart rate in determining β-blocking efficacy in acute and longterm myocardial infarction trials. *Am J Cardiol* 57:43F, 1986.

31. Singh BN, Vaughan Williams EM: The effect of amiodarone, a new anti-anginal drug, on cardiac muscle. *Br J Pharmacol* 39:657, 1970.

32. Nattel S, Talajic M, Fermini B, Roy D: Amiodarone: pharmacology, clinical actions, and relationships between them. *J Cardiovasc Electrophysiol* 3:266, 1992.

33. Broekhuysen J: Pharmacology of amiodarone—history and prospects. In: DM Krikler, WJ McKenna, DA Chamberlain (eds): *Amiodarone and Arrhythmias*. Oxford: Pergamon Press, 1983, p. 5.

34. Vastesaeges M, Guillot P, Rasson G: Étude clinique d'une nouvelle medication anti-angoreuse. *Acta Cardiol (Brux)* 51:767, 1967.

35. Charlier R, Deltour E, Baudine A, Chaillet F: Pharmacology of amiodarone, and anti-anginal drug with a new biological profile. *Arzneimittel-Forschung* 18:1408, 1968.

36. Vaughan Williams EM: The classification of antiarrhythmic drugs. In: E Sandoe, K Flenestedt-Jensen, KH Olesen (eds): *Symposium on Cardiac Arrhythmias*. Sodertalje, Sweden: Astra, 1970.

37. Rosenbaum MB, Chiale PA, Ryba D, et al: Control of tachyarrhythmias with the Wolff-Parkinson-Syndrome by amiodarone hydrochloride. *Am J Cardiol* 34:215, 1974.

38. Rosenbaum MB, Chiale PA, Halpern MS, et al: Clinical efficacy of amiodarone as an anti-arrhythmic agent. *Am J Cardiol* 38:934, 1976.

39. Singh BN, Nademanee K: Amiodarone and thyroid function: clinical implications during antiarrhythmic therapy. *Am Heart J* 106(4):857, 1983.

40. Pritchard DA, Singh BN, Hurley PJ: Effects of amiodarone on thyroid function in patients with ischemic heart disease. *Br Heart J* 37:856, 1975.

41. Burger A, Dinichert C, Nicod P, et al: Effects of amiodarone on serum triiodothyronine, thyroxine and thyrotropin: a drug influencing peripheral metabolism of thyroid hormones. *J Clin Invest* 58:255, 1976.

42. Lynch JJ Jr, Heaney LA, Wallace AA, et al: Suppression of lethal ischemic ventricular arrhythmias by the Class III agent E4031 in a canine model of previous myocardial infarction. *J Cardiovasc Pharmacol* 15:764, 1990.

43. Lynch JJ, Coskey LA, Montgomery DG, Lucchesi DR: Prevention of ventricular fibrillation by dextro-rotatory sotalol in a conscious canine model of sudden coronary death. *Am Heart J* 109:949, 1985.

44. Kato R, Yabek S, Ikeda N, et al: Electrophysiologic effects of dextro and levo-isomers of sotalol in isolated cardiac muscle and their in vivo pharmacokinetics. *J Am Coll Cardiol* 7:116, 1986.

45. Hondeghem LM, Snyders DJ: Class III antiarrhythmic agents have a lot of potential but a long way to go: reduced effectiveness and dangers of reverse use dependence. *Circulation* 81:686, 1990.

46. Anderson KP, Walker R, Dustman T, et al: Rate-related electrophysiologic effects of long term administration of amiodarone on canine ventricular myocardium in vivo. *Circulation* 79:948, 1989.

47. Sager PT, Uppal P, Follmer C, et al: The frequency-dependent electrophysiologic effects of amiodarone in humans. *Circulation* 88:1063, 1993.

48. Wang Z, Pelletier LC, Talajic M, Nattel S: Effects of flecainide and quinidine on human atrial action potentials. *Circulation* 82:274, 1990.

49. Ikeda N, Singh BN, Davis LD, Hauswirth C: Effects of flecainide on the electrophysiologic properties of isolated canine and rabbit myocardial fibers. *J Am Coll Cardiol* 5:303, 1985.

50. Follmer CH, Colatsky TJ: Block of the delayed rectifier potassium current I_k by flecainide and E-4301 in cat ventricular myocytes. *Circulation* 82:289, 1990.

51. El-Sherif N, Craelius W, Boutjdir M, Gough WB: Early afterdepolarizations and arrhythmogenesis. *J Cardiovasc Electrophysiol* 1:145, 1990.

Chapter 31

Circadian Rhythmicity of Heart Rate and Myocardial Repolarization:
Implications for the Prevention of Ventricular Fibrillation

Jonnalagedda S.M. Sarma
Bramah N. Singh

In recent years there has been a great deal of interest in the phenomenon of the circadian rhythmicity of cardiovascular disease.[1] It is now known that sudden death, fatal and nonfatal myocardial infarction, and cerebral strokes exhibit a circadian rhythmicity of occurrence, the fewest cases being seen between the hours of midnight and 6 AM.[1,2] There is a steep increase on awakening with the peak at about 1 and 3 PM with a slow decline in frequency thereafter. The pattern is most distinctive in the manifestations of coronary artery disease especially that for silent and symptomatic myocardial ischemia.[3] That such a pattern is defined essentially by the effects of catecholamines is now well appreciated.[4] It is consistent with the observations that such major determinants of oxygen consumption such as heart rate and blood pressure also demonstrate virtually identical circadian periodicity.

From the standpoint of therapeutic impact on reducing arrhythmia mortality, it is of particular interest that in the BHAT[5] trial the pattern of sudden death followed the pattern of distribution similar to that in heart rate. The lowest rates were seen when the heart rates were slowest.[5] It is known that bradycardia has a protective effect against the development of sudden arrhythmic death.[6] Similarly, the ventricular refractory period is longer during slower heart rates and its dispersion in myocardial ischemia lower than during tachycardia.[7]

For these reasons, it became of interest to determine the circadian rhythmicity of ventricular repolarization as reflected in the QT interval in relation to the heart rate and their interaction especially with respect to the modulation by the activity of the two limbs of the autonomic nervous system. The impetus to study these phenomena was also derived from the growing interest in controlling cardiac arrhythmias by the homogeneous prolongation

Supported in part by grants from the Veterans Administration Research Service (Washington, DC) and the American Heart Association, the Greater Los Angeles Affiliate, California.
From BN Singh, HJJ Wellens, M Hiraoka, (eds): *Electropharmacological Control of Cardiac Arrhythmias.* Mount Kisco, NY, Futura Publishing Company Inc., © 1994.

of cardiac repolarization.[8] Our data reported here are derived from observations in: (1) patients with chronic stable angina treated with the long-acting β blocker nadolol[9]; (2) normal subjects and in those with hypothyroidism before and after hormone replacement[10]; and (3) those treated chronically with amiodarone.[11] These clinical situations were selected for study for specific reasons. The effect of β blockade was considered of obvious clinical importance as it is an intervention that without doubt curtails mortality in different subsets of patients at risk for sudden death (see Chapters 14, 17, 30, and 47). Nadolol is a specific β blocker with an elimination half-life exceeding 24 hours, but one that does not prolong cardiac depolarization. Hypothyroidism was chosen as a test clinical situation because it represents what appears to be a naturally occurring Class III mechanism characterized by a uniform lengthening of repolarization associated with bradycardia[12] and a reduced probability of cardiac arrhythmias (see Chapter 22). The actions of amiodarone are complex but closely resemble those demonstrated in hypothyroid cardiac muscle with an unusually potent antiarrhythmic and antifibrillatory efficacy in supraventricular and ventricular tachyarrhythmias (see Chapter 34). There is a component of its pharmacological action that overlaps with β blockade.

Methodological Considerations

The data reported here have been obtained from 24-hour Holter recordings at specified times in different subsets of patients or normal subjects. The focus has been on the circadian rhythmicity of myocardial repolarization relative to that of heart rate and that of fluctuations of autonomic tone as determined by power spectra.

Circadian Rhythmicity of Heart Rate and QTc Intervals

The data on the circadian variation of RR and rate normalized QT (QTc) intervals were

obtained using a programmable wave form analyzer and an IBM compatible computer.[10] The RR and QT intervals were measured at 5- to 10-minute intervals of real time and stored on the computer. The measured QT intervals were normalized for cardiac cycle length using an exponential formula validated earlier.[10,13] The heart rate (in beats per minute) was computed as the inverse of RR, expressed in minutes.

Power Spectral Analysis

The simultaneous power spectra of RR and QT intervals were obtained from each Holter recording at times corresponding to minimum and maximum mean heart rate values during the day. The minimum and maximum heart rates occurred around 3 AM and 1 PM, respectively (Figure 1A). Power spectra were calculated from 256 consecutive sinus beats by fast Fourier analysis. The measured values were interpolated to obtain evenly sampled RR and QT intervals. Baseline drift in the data was subtracted by a data smoothing algorithm. Since only the variability, but not the actual value is important for spectral estimations, the QT interval in this case was measured to the peak of T wave. It was verified that the T wave morphology did not change within the 256 consecutive beats. The time domain data was multiplied by Hanning window function to minimize spectral leakage. (See Marple[14] for a detailed mathematical treatment of digital spectral analysis.) The computer programs for power spectral analysis were developed in our laboratories using ASYST Scientific Software (Keithley Asyst, Taunton, MA).

The spectral bands within the frequency range 0.025–0.375 Hz were divided into seven equal intervals of 0.05 Hz width. The square root of the area under the spectrum within each frequency band was calculated as a measure of the frequency specific standard deviation (variability) of RR or QT interval, defined at the center of the frequency band.

The spectral coherence between RR and QT spectra in each case was obtained by a

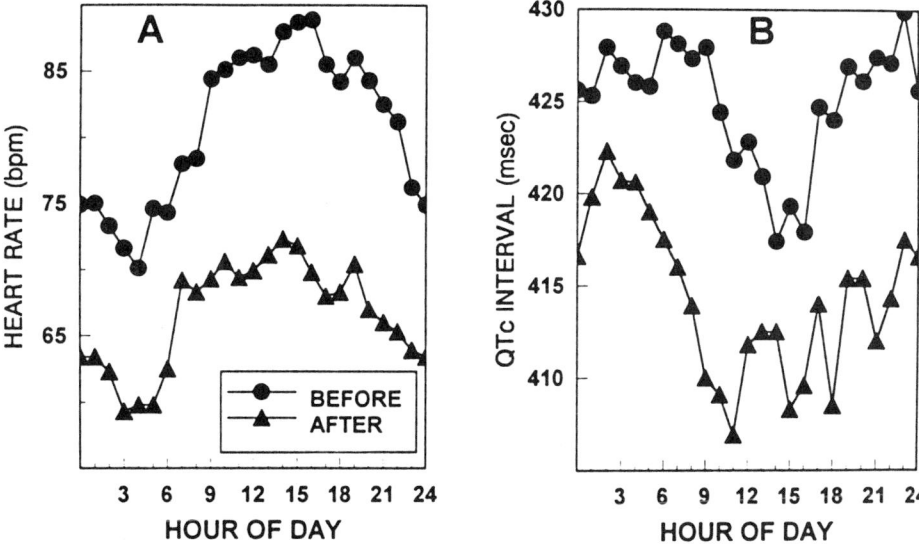

Figure 1. The mean circadian variation of heart rate (A) and QTc interval (B) in 12 subjects, before (circles) and after (triangles) 3 weeks of nadolol therapy.

bivariate spectral analysis program (BMDP Statistical Software, Los Angeles, CA, USA).

Statistical Analysis

Analysis of variance with repeated measures was used to compare the circadian variation and frequency specific variability curves obtained before and after nadolol treatment. When significant differences were obtained, paired or unpaired *t*-tests with appropriate corrections were used to identify which areas of the curves contribute to the overall differences. BMDP Software was used for statistical analysis.

Studies in β-Blocked Patients

Background

Of all the antiarrhythmic agents that have been studied in controlled clinical trials in survivors of acute infarction, β blockers remain the only class of agents that have been shown most definitively to reduce sudden death.[15,16] These agents also reduce sudden death in the congenital long QT syndrome[17] and in the survivors of aborted sudden death.[18] The primary mechanism of their beneficial actions in various subsets of patients is however unknown.

In recent years, the possibility has been raised whether compounds such as amiodarone, sotalol, and β blockers that have the potential to prevent ventricular fibrillation might act by influencing refractory period, either by prolonging it or by reducing its dispersion. Raine and Vaughan Williams[19] reported that β blockers, acebutalol and propranolol, induced a modest but significant increase in the action potential duration (APD) without an effect on myocardial depolarization. This effect was, of course, not as striking as it was for sotalol (see Chapter 30) whose structural characteristics differed from those of conventional β blockers. Raine and Vaughan Williams[19] interpreted their findings as being due to an adaptive phenomenon in response to prolonged β blockade; subsequently, it was suggested that the prolongation of the APD by β blockade might contribute to the observed beneficial effect in postinfarct survivors. The effect of β blockers on the APD in humans has been conflicting.[19] However, there have been no data on the circadian rhythmicity of QT or QTc interval (as an index of myocardial refractory period) in humans. The fact that β blockade in the BHAT trial[5] produced a salutary effect over the entire 24 hours suggested that it might be of interest to examine the effects of sympathetic inhibition on the QTc intervals relative to circadian rhythmicity.

We therefore studed the dynamic temporal variability of QT and RR simultaneously by studying RR and QT interval changes in both time and frequency domains from Holter recordings in a series of patients with chronic stable angina before and during steady-state treatment with nadolol. The control Holter recordings were obtained under drug-free (except nitroglycerine) conditions prior to the initiation of nadolol therapy. The patients were treated with incremental doses of nadolol (40, 80, 160 mg/day), increased at intervals of 1 week, for a total treatment period of 3 weeks. Second Holter recordings were obtained at the end of this period. The interrelationship between RR and QT spectra within different frequency bands was evaluated by spectral coherence, a measure of linear association between the two variables, similar to squared correlation.

Influence on Circadian Rhythmicity of RR and QTc Intervals

The mean data from 12 patients are shown in Figure 1 (A and B). Nadolol treatment significantly reduced the heart rate ($p < 0.01$) throughout the 24-hour period (Figure 1A) with an attenuation of the circadian variation due to the drug. The QTc interval showed a significant circadian variation both before and after nadolol treatment ($p < 0.01$), and shortened throughout the day after nadolol treatment (Figure 1B), with borderline significance ($p = 0.06$). The 24-hour mean QTc of the entire group was within the normal range before (425 ± 43 msec) and after (414 ± 32 msec).

Nadolol significantly increased the frequency-specific variability of the cardiac cycle length below the frequency of 0.25 Hz at 3 AM (Figure 2B) suggesting that the RR power spectrum under the present conditions is primarily determined by the vagal activity. Although there was a tendency for increased variability at 1 PM (Figure 2A), it was not statistically significant. In general, the variability of the QT interval was significantly lower ($p < 0.001$) than that of the RR interval (Figure 2). The QT variability plots were similar between day and night (Figure 2C and 2D). The frequency specific variability of the QT interval showed a tendency to increase below 0.25 Hz but did not attain statistical significance.

The frequency spectra of simultaneously measured RR and QT intervals were generally dissimilar in morphology except at the low frequency end (Figure 3). The RR spectral amplitudes were significantly higher than those of QT (Figure 3). The coherence between RR and QT spectra was consistently higher than 0.75 at low frequencies near 0.05 Hz, but variable at higher frequencies. The RR and QT intervals measured from 256 consecutive sinus beats under the conditions of Holter recording showed no apparent relationship to each other even when QT was plotted against a weighted average of preceding RR intervals.[9] This is in contrast to the measured values over a 24-hour period or during exercise when QT was related to RR through an exponential function.[10,13]

Conclusions

In our patient population, chronic β blockade shortened the QTc interval over the entire 24 hours although the change was of borderline significance. This is at variance with the in vitro data in rabbits reported by Raine and Vaughan Williams[19] as well as with the in vivo data reported by Vincent et al.[20] in chronically treated conscious dogs. The difference could not be accounted for by inadequate β blockade in humans as there was a marked attenuation at the circadan rhythmic-

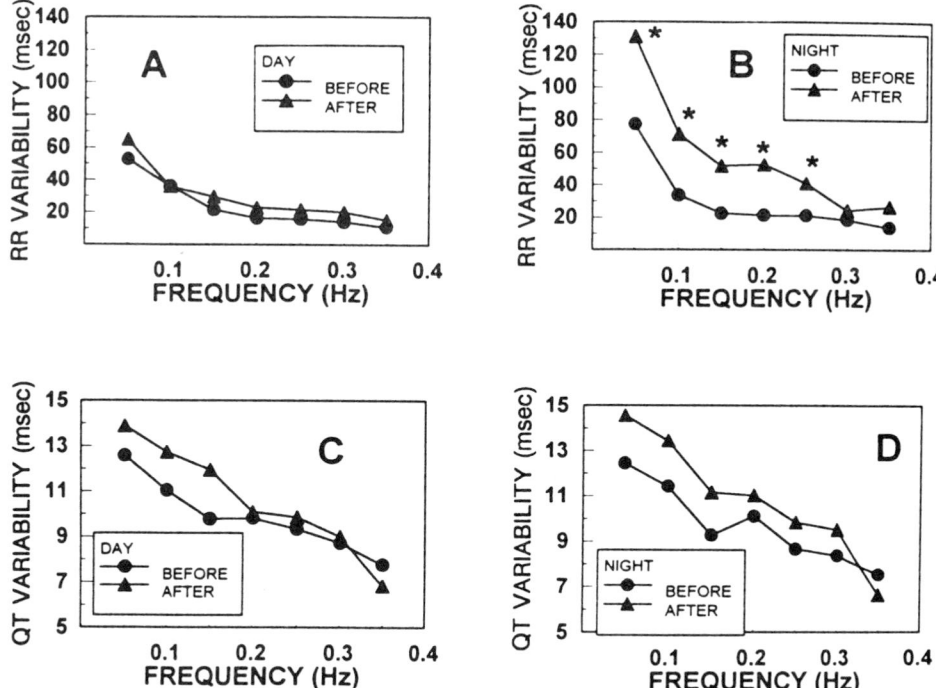

Figure 2. Frequency specific variability of RR interval during the day at about 1 PM (A) and at night at about 3 AM (B); and the variability of corresponding QT interval during the day (C) and at night (D) before (circles) and after (triangles) nadolol treatment. Asterisks indicate significant changes due to nadolol treatment ($p < 0.05$). The variability was measured as the square root of the area under the power spectral curve within a frequency band ($\pm$ 0.025 Hz) around the frequency specified for each data point above. The variability measured this way may be thought of as frequency specific standard deviation. The QT intervals were not normalized for RR (see text).

ity of heart rate characteristic of β blockade.[9] The shortening of the QT interval under the influence of nadolol is likely to be due to a decrease in the degree of dispersion of ventricular repolarization as suggested by a marked shortening in two patients in whom the baseline QTc was abnormally long.[9] The absence of an effect of nadolol on QT variability in the frequency range in which vagal activity predominates, indicates the insensitivity of ventricular repolarization to vagal action. Our data suggest that the relationship between RR and QT intervals depends on the frequency of variability and is not well defined at frequencies above 0.05 Hz.

The increased vagal activity at night by nadolol is likely due to the loss of sympathetic opposition to the circadian vagal dominance. Similar sympathovagal interactions have been described in the literature.[21,22] The lack of a significant increase of RR variability at the time of maximum circadian heart rate may be due to sympathetic dominance minimally opposed by parasympathetic tone. Thus, the time of the day may be an important determinant of the effects of autonomic interventions on the heart rate variability, even in the case of long-acting drugs like nadolol.

Studies in Hypothyroid Patients

As indicated elsewhere (see Chapters 30 and 34), thyroidectomy in experimental ani-

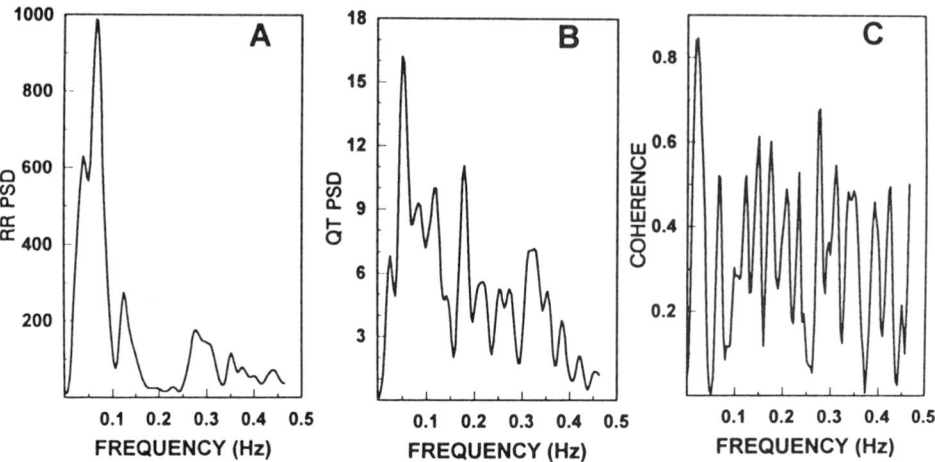

Figure 3. Typical RR (A) and QT (B) power spectra, and their coherence plot (C). Coherence is a measure of frequency specific linear association, similar to squared linear correlation coefficient, between two variables. Note the similarity of the two spectra only at low frequencies. PSD: power spectral density.

mals produces lengthening of the APD in atria and ventricles.[23,24] In this situation, there is reduction in β receptor density and a blunted effect of sympathetic stimulation.[25,26] Despite the significant prolongation of the QT or QTc interval of the surface electrocardiogram and the accompanying bradycardia, the incidence of torsades de pointes is extremely low except when associated with a marked degree of hypokalemia. Such a combination of electrophysiological parameters might be considered favorable for antifibrillatory actions.

We therefore determined the circadian rhythmicity of heart rate and the QTc interval in a series of hypothyroid patients (n = 10) before and after hormone replacement for a period of at least 12 weeks when the clinical and biochemical indexes of hypothyroidism had been normalized.[10] The mean data are summarized in Figure 4 in which data from an euthyroid control group are included. Before the introduction of replacement hormone therapy, the 24-hour heart rate compared to a matched control group was lower. In the latter there was distinct pattern of QTc distribution over the 24 hours, the longest intervals occurring between 12 midnight and 6 AM, with the subsequent tendency for a marked increase as the subjects woke up. The acrophase was between 1 PM and 2 PM. Thus, the circadian rhythmicity for the QTc was out of phase with that in heart rate that, as might be expected, was lowest between midnight and 6 AM. In the case of hypothyroid patients before they were given hormone therapy, the QTc intervals over the entire 24 hours were significantly longer but the circadian pattern was not altered. After hormone replacement therapy, the mean QTc intervals over the 24 hours were significantly shortened but they remained abnormally prolonged despite the normalization of the biochemical and clinical indexes of hypothyroidism. In contrast, with hormone replacement hypothyroid-induced bradycardia was not only corrected but compared to the normal euthyroid controls there appeared to be an overshoot (Figure 4).

The overall data permitted several conclusions. First, in hypothyroid patients, the QTc interval is longer than in normal euthyroid patients. Second, hormone replacement normalizes the hypothyroid-induced bradycardia after about 12 weeks of therapy but the effect on repolarization, while being reduced, remains considerably prolonged indicating a dichotomy between the mechanisms for the

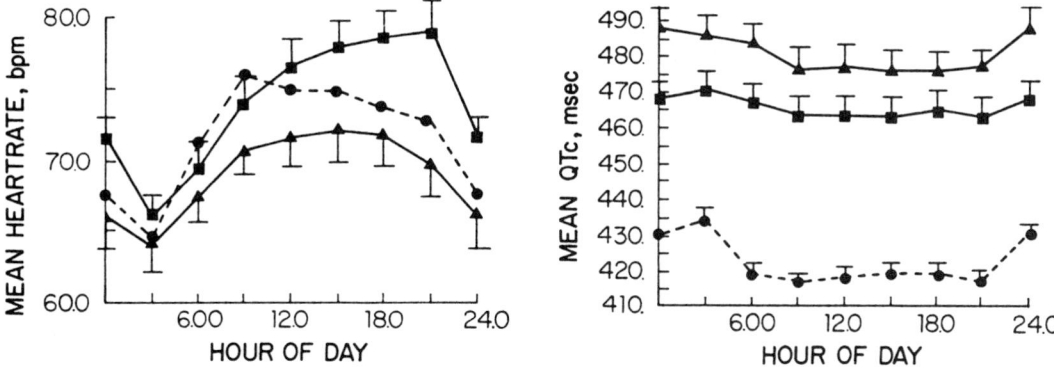

Figure 4. Circadian variation of heart rate and QTc interval in hypothyroid (triangles), euthyroid (squares), and control (circles) groups. Error bars (not plotted for control heart rates) represent standard error of the mean. Data for hypothyroids and euthyroids are from same patients before and after thyroid hormone replacement; data for control subjects are from six normal euthyroid volunteers in a similar age group.

control of heart rate and of the duration of ventricular repolarization. The prolonged QTc in the patients under replacement therapy with T4 alone may be due to an altered relative distribution of thyroid hormones (T3 and T4) in the ventricular myocardium.[27] Thus, these patients may enjoy partial protection from ventricular fibrillation under clinically euthyroid conditions.

Studies in Amiodarone Patients

Background

As indicated in Chapters 30, 34, and 47, the antiarrhythmic and antifibrillatory actions of amiodarone remains unparalleled. The complexity of its electropharmacological actions has been discussed in Chapter 34. The reasons behind the drug's unusual potency as an antiarrhythmic agent remains unclear. However, two features of its action are of particular importance. The first is its antiadrenergic actions that is almost of the same magnitude as that of β-blocking drugs at least with respect to the effects on heart rate during chronic drug administration. The second and

perhaps the most striking feature of its action is the marked lengthening of the APD.[28] This is reflected in the consistent increase in the QT and QTc intervals on the surface electrocardiogram.[29] It is generally assumed that both the drug's antiadrenergic and QT prolonging effects are central to its potency as an antifibrillatory agent. Therefore, it is clearly important to determine whether the drug provides a continuous protection against ventricular fibrillation by exerting these effects over 24 hours without peaks and troughs of therapeutic actions.

We therefore determined the effects of the commonly used regimens of amiodarone on the circadian rhythmicity of the QT interval determined by a computer assisted technique and corrected for heart rate changes with an exponential formula[10] from Holter recordings in patients undergoing therapy for ventricular arrhythmias.

Studies on the Circadian Rhythmicity of Heart Rate and QT Intervals

The study population consisted of three groups of male patients studied prior to and during short- and long-term treatment with amiodarone for ventricular arrhythmias. The three groups were as follows: group 1: 10 subjects (age 68.6 ± 4.1 years, range 61–75 years) awaiting amiodarone therapy; group 2: 11 subjects (age 68.7 ± 2.6 years, range 65–74 years) including all patients from group 1, who completed 3–6 months (4.6 ± 1.7) of amiodarone therapy; group 3: 13 separate subjects (age 65.8 ± 11.8 years, range 35–87 years) who had been on amiodarone therapy for 1–10 (4.7 ± 2.9) years. All patients had documented coronary artery disease or dilated cardiomyopathy and were considered for amiodarone therapy after one or more conventional antiarrhythmic agents failed to control their ventricular arrhythmias. Patients for chronic amiodarone therapy were chosen by virtue of their being on a stable dose of amiodarone for at least 3 months; all patients were chemically and clinically euthyroid at the time of the 24-hour Holter recordings. All patients studied were given loading doses followed by maintenance doses of amiodarone.

Heart Rate Changes

The effects of amiodarone on the pattern of circadian periodicity of heart rate after 3 to 6 months of treatment and following continuous maintenance therapy exceeding 12 months compared to the baseline pattern based on data from 24-hour ambulatory electrocardiogram recordings are shown in Figure 5. Heart rate was reduced over 24 hours of amiodarone therapy, which exerted a bradycardic response over the entire 24 hours

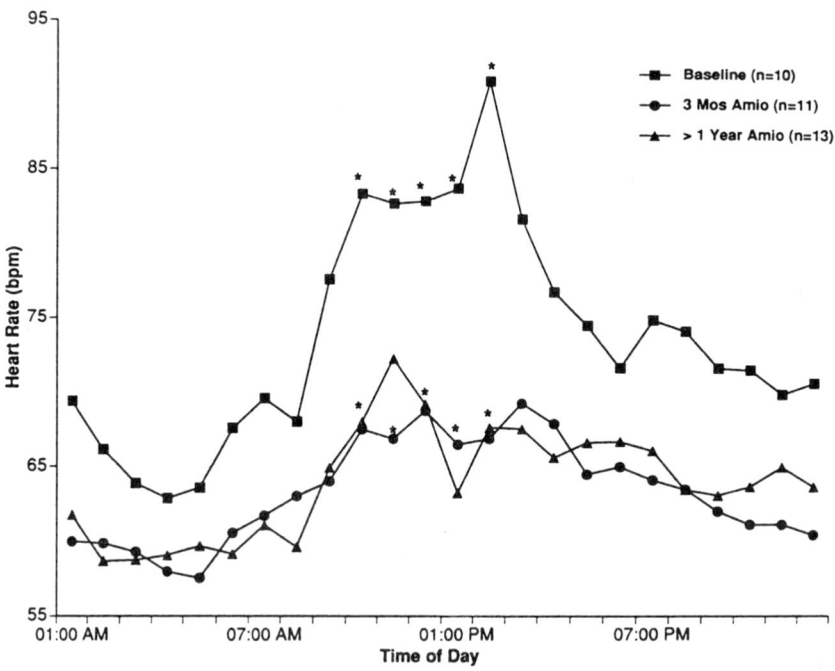

Figure 5. Effects of chronic amiodarone treatment on the circadian rhythmicity of heart rate in patients with cardiac arrhythmias. Amiodarone reduced the heart rate over the entire 24 hours, but the effect was most pronounced between 10 AM and 2 PM. The asterisks denote the hours at which pairwise comparisons revealed statistically significant differences between the two treated groups and the baseline. Note that the drug effect had reached steady state between 3 and 6 months of treatment and in both groups the circadian pattern was attenuated but not abolished (see text for details).

with an attenuation, but not an abolition of the normal circadian rhythmicity compared to the control group. The pattern resembled that after β blockade. The overall bradycardic effect appeared to reach a steady state between 3 and 6 months of therapy, there being no statistically significant difference in heart rate when compared to that after 12 months of maintenance therapy.

Changes in QT and QTc Circadian Rhythms Induced by Amiodarone

The mean data on the circadian rhythmicity of QT intervals as affected by chronic amiodarone therapy is shown in Figure 6; the corresponding pattern following the correction for heart rate (QTc) is presented in Figure 7. A significant increase in the QT interval over the 24 hours between the mean baseline values and the corresponding values for the

group of patients treated with amiodarone for 3 to 6 months ($p < 0.001$) and for the group treated for over a year ($p < 0.0001$). There was also a significant difference ($p < 0.001$) between the effects on the QT interval between the group treated for 3 to 6 months and that treated for over a year. This pattern of differences remained when the QT interval was corrected for heart rate changes. For the baseline group (n = 10), the mean ($\pm$ SD) QTc was 450 $\pm$ 55 msec. It was significantly ($p < 0.001$) longer (518 $\pm$ 43 msec) in the group (n = 11) treated for 3 to 6 months and also significantly ($p < 0.0002$) longer (581 $\pm$ 61 msec) in the group (n = 13) treated for over a year. There was also a significant difference between the two treatment groups ($p < 0.009$).

There was a prominent circadian pattern to the QT intervals under baseline conditions with the intervals during the sleeping hours (midnight and 6 AM) being markedly pro-

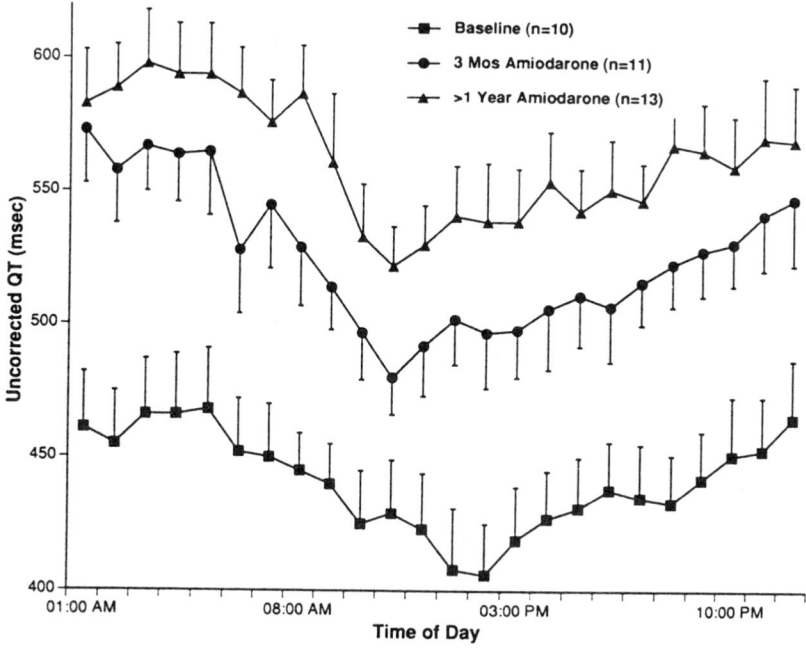

Figure 6. The circadian rhythmicity of uncorrected QT interval as influenced by chronic amiodarone treatment. The data are mean $\pm$ SEM. Note that the QT interval prolongation continued beyond 3–6 months, but the circadian rhythmicity was maintained as a reflection of heart rate variability (see Figure 5).

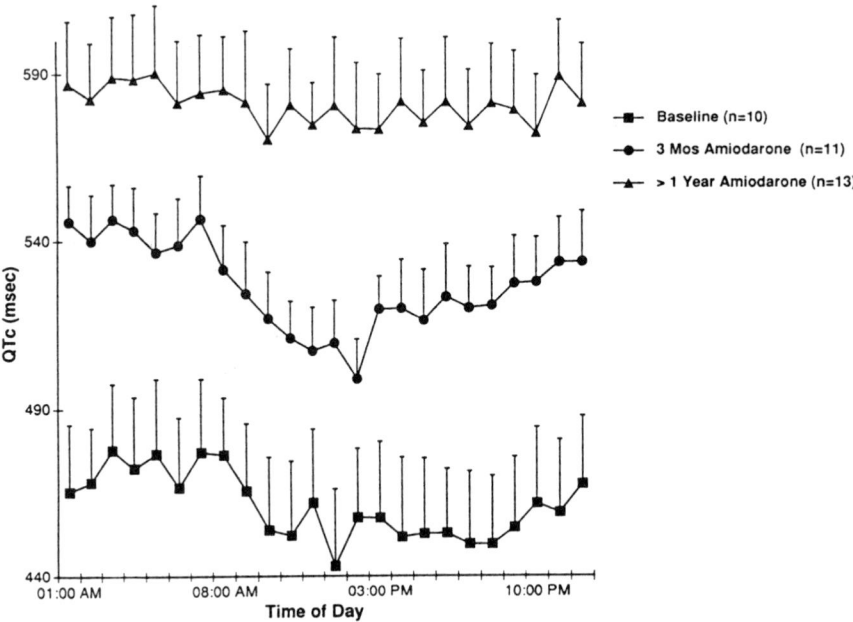

Figure 7. The circadian rhythmicity of corrected QT interval (QTc) as influenced by chronic amiodarone treatment. The data are mean ± SEM. When the QT was corrected for heart rate changes, the differences among the baseline and the treated groups were maintained, but the circadian rhythmicity of QTc after 3 to 6 months of treatment was attenuated and was abolished when drug administration exceeded 1 year.

longed compared to those during the waking hours. The overall periodicity of the QT interval was thus out of phase with that of the heart rate (see Figures 5 and 6). Our baseline data on QT intervals are consistent with the report of Cinca et al.,[30] who found a significant lengthening of the right ventricular effective refractory period between midnight and 7 AM in paced human subjects. These findings indicate that variations in the ventricular effective refractory period during the course of the 24 hours are due essentially to those in myocardial repolarization modulated by varying autonomic tone. Our data on β blockade suggests that the change is essentially due to the withdrawal of the sympathetic influence at night. Compared to the baseline, amiodarone prolonged the uncorrected QT length over the entire 24-hour interval in a parallel fashion at all heart rates. Although amiodarone significantly increased the QT interval in both treatment groups, it exerted little effect on the

overall pattern of the circadian rhythmicity of the uncorrected QT interval (Figure 6), which reflects direct dependence on the circadian rhythmicity of the heart rate.

Cosinor analyses on the QTc interval showed that 80% of the baseline patients exhibited a significant single cosine curve periodicity, whereas, only 66% of the patients treated for 3–6 months, and less than 50% of the chronically treated patients showed such periodicity. This analysis confirmed the gradual loss of circadian periodicity of QTc due to amiodarone treatment.

Conclusions

The data indicate a number of features of amiodarone action that have practical and theoretical implications. The reduction in heart rate over 24 hours conforming to the normal circadian rhythmicity albeit attenuated indicates a significant antiadrenergic potency for the drug in line with the animal data. The dissociation in the time course of changes in heart rate and QT intervals induced by amiodarone is consistent with differing sensitivities of these two parameters to fluctuations in sympathetic tone. Of particular importance is the observation that QT interval lengthening did not reach steady state for about a year despite the normal loading doses of the drug followed by adequate maintenance regimens. Finally, the reduced temporal variability of the QTc over 24 hours is consistent with a lessened heterogeneity of APDs as appeared to be the case with β blockade.

Implications for the Future Development of Antifibrillatory Compounds

The data on the effects of hypothyroidism, β blockade and chronic amiodarone treatment provide a number of insights for the development of newer antiarrhythmic drugs. In each case, there is blunting of the sympathetic nervous system activity that per se might constitute a significant antifibrillatory action (see Chapter 11). β Blockers and amiodarone have documented antifibrillatory actions with a potential to prolong survival in different subsets of patients, especially those with ischemic heart disease. Thyroid gland ablation has not been used as a therapeutic modality but a number of features of hypothyroidism closely overlap with those of chronic amiodarone administration. In both cases as well as with β blockade, there is likelihood of a marked anti-ischemic effect, a low propensity for proarrhythmic reactions despite significant bradycardia and, in the case of hypothyroidism and chronic amiodarone treatment, a marked degree of QT prolongation.

Pure Class III Agents

In the synthesis and characterization of the newer Class III agents (see Chapters 35–43), the focus has been on the isolated

prolongation of the APD. Our data have a bearing on the merit as well as the demerits of such an approach. Clearly, from the study of structure activity relationships it might be possible to minimize or delete some of the components of the pharmacological actions of the existing compounds such as sotalol and amiodarone and arrive at molecules that are devoid of adverse reactions. This is clearly so with the deletion of the β blocker effects as in the case of d-sotalol and the expanding plethora of agents that are parasubstituted methanesulphonyl benzamides derived from the sotalol molecule. The synthesis of such compounds is based on the assumption that adrenergic inhibition may not be critical for controlling cardiac arrhythmias. The bulk of the data from mortality studies with β blockers and amiodarone are contrary to this view. As indicated elsewhere (see Chapter 47), the critical determinant of the outcome of therapy with respect to mortality might depend on the nature of match or mismatch between the intervention and the vulnerable substrate. It is known that myocardial substrate is an exceedingly complex clinical entity subject to extrinsic and intrinsic modulating factors, both deleterious and beneficial, as a function of time and varying clinical course. It is therefore likely that the match of the drug with the substrate is more likely to succeed if the compound had an array of pharmacological properties counteracting a range of arrhythmogenic influences thereby stabilize the vulnerable myocardium.

Importance of β Blockade and Amiodarone

Our current data on the circadian rhythmicity of β blockade and especially that of amiodarone is of particular interest in this regard. Previously, we showed that amiodarone significantly reduced spatial dispersion in patients with cardiac arrhythmias, whereas this did not occur in the case of sotalol or the pure Class III agent sematilide.[31] We demonstrate that both β blockade and amiodarone also decrease the temporal dispersion of repolarization documented in 24-hour Holter recordings; β blockade appeared to induce such a change by shortening the abnormally long action potentials, whereas amiodarone may act by producing a differential effect resulting in a uniformly prolonged repolarization.

Currently, there are little data on the effects of the so-called Class III agents. However, it is known that these agents, at least those that block the delayed rectifier current (see Chapter 34), prolong the APD more in the Purkinje fibers than in the ventricular muscle. This is likely to augment rather than decrease spatial, and possibly temporal, dispersion of QT. Conversely, in the case of chronic amiodarone administration, Gallagher et al.[32] have shown that the effect of the drug in prolonging the APD in canine Purkinje fibers is much less than that reported for ventricular myocardium. Such an effect is likely to reduce the existing heterogeneity in myocardial refractoriness.

Our data raise the possibility that amiodarone might exert a differential effect on the myocardial action potentials of varying durations, prolonging to a greater extent those with a shorter repolarization time and the converse in the case of those fibers repolarizing more slowly. This will result in a reduced degree of spatial QT variability. If the spatial variability of repolarization is indeed reduced by amiodarone as suggested by the experimental data, there is likely to be a correspondingly less temporal variability in repolarization in vivo as the drug's antiadrenergic effects will tend to attenuate the beat-to-beat variations in the QT interval due to sympathetic excitation. It is noteworthy that our data did in fact demonstrate this phenomenon in patients who had attained the steady-state drug effect with respect to repolarization. This is also suggested by our data on hypothyroidism in which a similar pattern of the circadian rhythmicity of heart rate and the QTc interval was found.

The slow evolution of changes in repolarization as a function of time and the close similarity between the electrophysiological effects of chronic amiodarone action and those of the hypothyroid myocardium[33–35] has led to the hypothesis that the drug, an iodinated compound, might exert in part its action by selective inhibition of myocardial thyroid nuclear receptors (see Chapter 34).

Potential Significance of Long Therapeutic Half-Lives of Antiarrhythmic Agents

From Holter monitoring and in-hospital monitoring it has become increasingly clear that ventricular tachycardia deteriorating into ventricular fibrillation is the most common mode of arrhythmic deaths in patients with advanced structural heart disease. The process does not last for more than a few minutes. Thus, if an antiarrhythmic or antifibrillatory agent were to be effective, its electrophysiological actions mediating the salutary effect needs to be maintained continuously without troughs of subtherapeutic periods. In practice, this is rarely, if ever, possible with conventional antiarrhythmic compounds. Whether the newer Class III agents might differ in this regard for the present remains unclear.

The use of 24- or 48-hour Holter recordings permit the delineation of the continuous drug effects on heart rate and the QT intervals as an index of refractoriness. When combined with power spectral analysis for determining the nature of vagosympathetic modulation, 24- to 48-hour Holter analysis of RR and QT intervals becomes an important technique for the evaluation of antifibrillatory mechanisms in the development of newer compounds. This is suggested by our data on amiodarone.

Perhaps, the most significant findings in the case of amiodarone in this regard is slowing of heart rate and the lengthening of the QTc induced by amiodarone are slower in reaching steady state than previously thought; the former reached steady state by 3 to 6 months, the latter considerably later. Amiodarone attenuated the circadian rhythmicity of heart rate and QTc. In the case of QTc, the drug abolished the circadian periodicity at steady state while markedly reducing QTc variability over the 24 hours. These findings have significant clinical implications. In terms of its bradycardic action, amiodarone resembles β blockers, the effects of which in reducing sudden death in survivors of acute myocardial infarction correlate with heart rate reduction.[36,37] Preliminary data suggest that amiodarone might also be effective in this regard[38] and its bradycardic action that approaches that of β blockers might be contributory to its overall antifibrillatory propensity.[36] The fact that the steady-state effect of the drug on the QTc interval, an index of antifibrillatory action if homogeneously prolonged, is not reached for 6 months or longer is consistent with numerous reports that the largest numbers of sudden deaths on the drug occur in the first 3 to 6 months following the initiation of drug therapy with a very markedly reduced incidence thereafter.[39,40] Finally, our data suggest that the remarkable effectiveness of amiodarone in the control of malignant ventricular arrhythmias might in part stem from the sustained bradycardic effect in concert with the continuous sustained homogeneous lengthening of myocardial repolarization constituting a potent antifibrillatory mechanism.

Conclusions

In the development of newer antifibrillatory agents, essentially those that act primarily by prolonging the APD, there is a clear need to include a component of their action that blunts sympathetic excitation. Whether a simple combination of a pure Class III agent with β blockade might result in an effective and safe antifibrillatory agent remains unclear. It is unlikely to differ markedly from dl-sotalol. The findings with amiodarone indicate that in the search for the ideal antifibrillatory compound attention may need to focus on a complex molecule with a diversity of pharmacological properties, especially with prolonged therapeutic effects. Such an agent needs to have a sympathetically mediated bradycardic

effect with a potential for inducing sustained and continuous prolongation of the refractory period with an attenuation or abolition of the circadian periodicity of myocardial repolarization. As suggested elsewhere,[41] amiodarone is such a prototype.

References

1. Muller JE, Ludmer PL, Willich SN. Circadian variation in the frequency of sudden cardiac death. *Circulation* 75:131, 1987.
2. Marler J, Price T, Clark GL: Morning increase in onset of ischemic stroke. *Stroke* 1:795, 1989.
3. Rocco MB, Nabel EG, Selwyn AP: Circadian rhythms and coronary artery disease. *Am J Cardiol* 59:13C, 1987.
4. Townsend MM, Smith AJ: Factors influencing the urinary excretion of free catecholamines in man. *Clin Sci* 44:253, 1973.
5. Peters RW, Muller JE, Goldstein S, et al: Propranolol and the circadian variation in the frequency of sudden cardiac death: the BHAT experience (abstract). *Circulation* 76(Suppl 4): IV-364, 1987.
6. Castelli WP, Levy D, Wilson WPF, et al: Sudden death. The view from Framingham. In: J Kostis, M Sanders (eds): *The Prevention of Sudden Cardiac Death.* New York, NY: Wiley-Liss Publications, 1990, p. 1.
7. Kent KM, Smith ER, Redwood DR, Epstein SE: Electrical stability of acutely ischemic myocardium. Influence of heart rate and vagal stimulation. *Circulation* 67:291, 1973.
8. Singh BN (ed): *Control of Cardiac Arrhythmias by Lengthening Repolarization.* Mt, Kisco, NY: Futura Publishing Company, Inc., 1988.
9. Sarma JSM, Singh N, Shoenbaum MP, et al: Circadian and power spectral changes of RR and QT intervals during treatment with nadolol: evidence for differential autonomic modulation of heart rate and ventricular repolarization. (submitted).
10. Sarma JSM, Venkataraman K, Nicod P, et al: Circadian rhythmicity of rate-normalized QT interval in hypothyroidism and its significance for the development of class III antiarrhythmic agents. *Am J Cardiol* 66:959, 1990.
11. Antimisiaris M, Sarma JSM, Schoenbaum MP, et al: Effects of amiodarone on the circadian rhythmicity of ventricular repolarization as an index of myocardial refractoriness: significance for the control of sudden cardiac death. (submitted).
12. Singh BN, Sarma JSM, Zhang ZH, Takanaka C: Controlling cardiac arrhythmias by lengthen-

ing repolarization: rationale from experimental findings and clinical considerations. *Ann NY Acad Sci* 644:187, 1992.

13. Sarma JSM, Sarma RJ, Bilitch M, et al: An exponential formula for heart rate dependence of QT interval during exercise and cardiac pacing in humans. Re-evaluation of Bazett's formula. *Am J Cardiol* 54:103, 1984.

14. Marple SL: *Digital Spectral Analysis with Applications.* Englewood Cliffs, NJ: Prentice Hall, Inc., 1987.

15. Singh BN: Advantages of β blockers versus antiarrhythmic agents and calcium antagonists in secondary prevention after myocardial infarction. *Am J Cardiol* 66:9C, 1990.

16. Yusuf S, Teo KK: Approaches to prevention of sudden death. Need for fundamental reevaluation. *J Cardiovasc Electrophysiol* 2:S233, 1991.

17. Schwartz PJ: Idiopathic long QT syndrome: progress and questions. *Am Heart J* 109:399, 1985.

18. Hallstrom AP, Cobb LA, Yu BH, et al: An antiarrhythmic drug experience in 941 patients resuscitated from an initial cardiac arrest between 1970 and 1985. *Am J Cardiol* 68:1025, 1991.

19. Raine AEG, Vaughan Williams EM: Adaptation to prolonged β-blockade of rabbit atrial, Purkinje, and ventricular potentials, and papillary muscle contraction. Time-course of development of and recovery from adaptation. *Circ Res* 48:804, 1981.

20. Vincent A, Werquin S, Caron J, et al: Effects of acute and chronic administration of acebutolol on the right ventricular effective refractory period in conscious dogs. *J Cardiovasc Pharmacol* 21:7, 1993.

21. Morady F, Kou WH, Nelson SD, et al: Accentuated antagonism between β-adrenergic and vagal effects on ventricular refractoriness in humans. *Circulation* 77:289, 1988.

22. Martins JB, Zipes DP: Effects of sympathetic and vagal nerves on the recovery properties of the endocardium and epicardium of the canine left ventricle. *Circ Res* 46:100, 1980.

23. Sharp NA, Neal DS, Parsons RL: Influence of thyroid hormone levels on electrical and mechanical properties of rabbit papillary muscle. *J Mol Cell Cardiol* 17:119, 1985.

24. Freedberg AS, Papp JG, Vaughan Williams EM: The effect of altered thyroid state on atrial intracellular potentials. *J Physiol (Lond)* 207:357, 1970.

25. Nokin P, Clinet M, Schoenfeld P: Cardiac β-adrenoreceptor modulation by amiodarone. *Biochem Pharmacol* 32:2473, 1983.

26. Gagnoe JP, Bevos C, Clinet M, Nokin P: Amiodarone: biochemical aspects and hemodynamic effects. *Drugs* 29(Suppl 3):1, 1985.

27. Sarma JSM, Lev-Ran A, Pollard LM, et al: Circadian and power spectral changes in heart rate and QT interval during acute hypothyroidism (abstract). *PACE* 16:879, 1993.

28. Singh BN, Vaughan Williams EM: The effect of amiodarone, a new anti-anginal drug, on cardiac muscle. *Br J Pharmacol* 39:657, 1970.

29. Pritchard DA, Singh BN, Hurley PJ: Effects of amiodarone on thyroid function in patients with ischemic heart disease. *Br Heart J* 37:856, 1975.

30. Cinca J, Moya A, Figueras J, et al: Circadian variations in the electrical properties of the human heart assessed by sequential bedside electrophysiologic testing. *Am Heart J* 112:315, 1986.

31. Cui G, Sen L, Sager P, et al: Comparison of QT dispersion and RR interval induced by sematilide, amiodarone and sotalol (abstract). *Circulation* 86:I-393, 1992.

32. Gallagher JD, Bianchi J, Gessman LJ: A comparison of the electrophysiologic of acute and chronic amiodarone administration on canine Purkinje fibers. *J Cardiovasc Pharmacol* 13:723, 1989.

33. Singh BN: Electropharmacology of amiodarone. In: BN Singh, (ed): *Control of Arrhythmias by Lengthening of Repolarization.* Mt. Kisco, NY: Futura Publishing Company, Inc., 1988, p. 367.

34. Nademanee K, Hendrickson JA, Melmed S, et al: Pharmacokinetic significance of serum reverse T3 levels during amiodarone treatment: a potential method for monitoring chronic drug therapy. *Circulation* 66(1):202, 1982.

35. Singh BN, Venkatesh N, Nademanee K, et al: The historical development, cellular electrophysiology and clinical pharmacology of amiodarone. *Prog Cardiovasc Dis* 31:249, 1989.

36. Singh BN: Advantages of β-blockers versus antiarrhythmic drugs and calcium-channel antagonists in secondary prevention in survivors of myocardial infarction. *Am J Cardiol* 66:9, 1990.

37. Kjekshsus JK: Importance of heart rate in determining β-blocking efficacy in acute and long-term myocardial infarction trial. *Am J Cardiol* 57:43, 1986.

38. Burkhart F, Pfisterer M, Kiowski W, et al: Effect of antiarrhythmic therapy on mortality in survivors of myocardial infarction with asymptomatic complex ventricular arrhythmias: Basel Antiarrhythmic Study of Infarct Survival (BASIS). *J Am Coll Cardiol* 16:1711, 1990.

39. Herre JM, Sauve MJ, Malone P, Scheinman M:

Long-term results of amiodarone therapy in patients with recurrent sustained ventricular tachycardia or ventricular fibrillation. *J Am Coll Cardiol* 12:442, 1989.

40. Nademanee K, Stevenson W, Weiss JN, Singh BN: The role of amiodarone in the survivors of sudden arrhythmic deaths. In: BN Singh (ed): *Control of Cardiac Arrhythmias by Lengthening Repolarization.* Mt. Kisco, NY: Futura Publishing Company, Inc., 1988, p. 489.

41. Singh BN, Ahmed R, Sen L: Prolonging cardiac repolarization as an evolving anti-arrhythmic principle. In: D Escaude, NR Standen (eds): *K+ Channels in Cardiovascular Medicine: From Gene to Patient.* Heidelberg, Germany: Springer-Verlag Publishers, 1993, (in press).

Chapter 32

Plasma Concentration Response Relations for Class III Antiarrhythmic Drugs: *Are Pharmacokinetics Important?*

Dan M. Roden

The intensive study of the relationship between an administered dose of a drug, the resultant concentrations of drug and its metabolites in plasma, and the beneficial and undesirable effects of drug therapy has two important consequences. First, specific situations in which changes in drug dosing are required for effective therapy can be identified. A simple example is reduction in dose for a predominantly renally-excreted drug in patients with renal failure. In such a case, monitoring plasma concentrations to ensure that they remain within an appropriate therapeutic range is often a useful adjunct to patient management. Second, situations in which drug doses or the plasma concentrations they achieve do not correlate well with drug effect may be identified. In this case, further studies of the mechanisms underlying such lack of correlation may lead to fundamental insights into variables which control drug action in patients.

The central theme of clinical pharmacokinetics is the study of the relationships among dose, plasma concentration, and responses. Pharmacokinetic questions that are addressed during drug development include whether there is a dose or concentration below which no effect occurs, whether there is a dose or concentration above which toxicity is likely, and whether some or all of the effects observed during treatment (and in particular the adverse effects) can be related to plasma concentrations. Adverse or beneficial effects occurring at very low concentrations should raise the possibility of either an unidentified pharmacokinetic phenomenon (eg, toxicity residing in one isomer or an unidentified active metabolite) or unexplained sensitivity to drug action. Thus, the relationship between administered drug dose and resultant effect is often conceptualized as two separate processes: the relationship between administered dose and resultant drug concentrations in plasma and at effector sites (pharmacokinetics) and the relationship between drug concentrations and response (pharmacodynamics).

From BN Singh, HJJ Wellens, M Hiraoka, (eds): *Electropharmacological Control of Cardiac Arrhythmias.* Mount Kisco, NY, Futura Publishing Company Inc., © 1994.

Sources of Variability in Drug Action: Pharmacokinetics

Active Metabolites and Genetically Determined Drug Metabolism

The notion that variable drug disposition results in altered drug concentrations and hence response to drug therapy is central to pharmacokinetic studies. In addition to the example of disease states indicated above, interindividual variability in drug disposition can also result from genetic factors.[1] The clinical consequences of such genetically determined polymorphisms of drug metabolism depend on the relative activities of the parent drug and any metabolites whose formation is under genetic control, as well as the extent to which other pathways of drug disposition are available.[2,3] The simplest example is a drug whose metabolites are inactive and whose disposition is controlled by a single isozyme. In such a case, a defect in the isozyme would lead to an increase in parent drug concentrations with attendant increased drug effect, and perhaps toxicity. Alternatively, metabolites can be much more potent than the parent drug,[4,5] have different activities from the parent drug,[6] or interact with the parent drug.[7,8] In such cases, defective metabolism of the parent drug may well lead to decreased drug action.

The most widely studied polymorphism is that of debrisoquine 4-hydroxylase, P450IID6.[9,10] This enzyme is responsible for the biotransformation of a number of β blockers and antiarrhythmic agents, including metoprolol, bufuralol, encainide, propafenone, and flecainide. A further twist on this story is provided by the observation that quinidine is a potent inhibitor of P450IID6.[11-14] Thus, in patients in whom this enzyme is active (extensive metabolizers), the coadministration of even a subtherapeutic dose of quinidine may markedly perturb drug disposition and effect. Conversely, in patients in whom the isozyme is inactive (poor metabolizers), the coadministration of quinidine results in no change in drug disposition and effect. Thus, genetically determined drug metabolism can not only result in variable plasma concentrations of parent drug and metabolites, but also in genetically determined drug interactions. None of the compounds discussed in this volume (Figure 1) are specifically known to undergo such polymorphic metabolism. Ibutilide, almokalant, and amiodarone are known to have active metabolites, while NAPA, sotalol, sematilide, and dofetilide are thought not to have active metabolites.

Chirality

Another variable that can impact on drug disposition and resultant action is the presence of an atom (usually carbon), termed a chiral center, with four different substituent groups that can then exist in two mirror image conformations or stereoisomers.[2] Of the compounds addressed (Figure 1), sotalol, ibutilide, almokalant, and RP58826 have chiral centers, but are administered as racemates (50/50 mixtures of stereoisomers). Some pharmacological properties are strongly influenced by such optical activity. For example, for β blockers, one isomer is more potent than the other; as described elsewhere, l-sotalol is an order of magnitude more potent a β blocker than d-sotalol. Other β blockers such as metoprolol or propranolol have even higher eudismic ratios, often exceeding 100:1.

Action potential prolongation and/or potassium channel block may also be stereoselective. For example, only S-(+)-disopyramide prolongs action potentials in canine cardiac Purkinje fibers, while the R-(−)-isomer shortens them.[15] Similarly, quinine shortens cardiac action potentials in the same preparation, while they are prolonged by quinidine.[15] It is likely that these differences reflect differences in potassium channel block. As discussed elsewhere, the isomers of RP58826 are not equipotent as K$^+$ channel blockers, and the active isomer, RP62719, is undergoing clinical trials. Conversely, d- and l-sotalol are equally potent in prolonging action potentials and in blocking K$^+$ channels.[16,17] The K$^+$

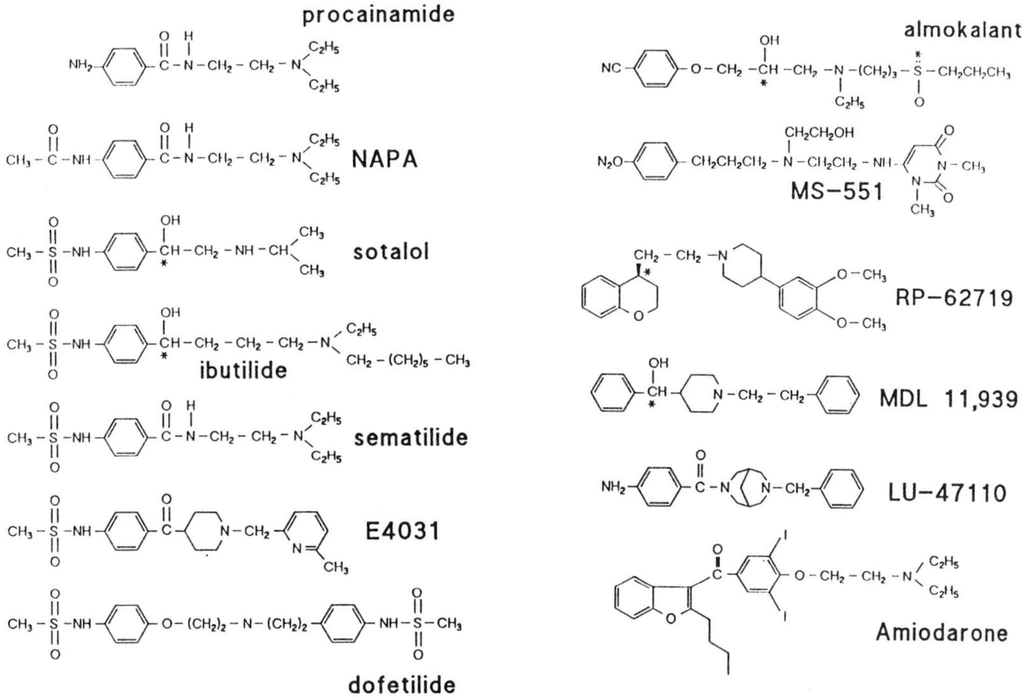

Figure 1. Structural formulas for Class III agents. Chiral centers are indicated by an asterisk (*).

channel blocking activity of the isomers of ibutilide and of almokalant have not yet been reported.

It is not a given that administration of a single enantiomer, rather than a racemate, will necessarily provide better treatment. Even if individual isomers have different pharmacokinetics, isomer specific treatment should not be entertained unless a difference in pharmacological actions between the isomers is identified. Certainly, if adverse effects are clearly identified with one isomer while beneficial effects are either nonstereoselective or reside in the other isomer, then isomer specific treatment may be justified. Such may be the case with sotalol, where the intolerance to β blockade that occurs in some patients might be overcome by use of the d-isomer. Isomer specific therapy is cumbersome, requiring either synthesis of a specific isomer or separation (resolution) of a racemate. In addition, at least in theory, administration of a pure isomer can lead to re-racemization in vivo.

Thus, the presence of multiple isomers or of active metabolites is not itself a contraindication to further drug development. Rather, the contribution of individual isomers and metabolites to pharmacological effect should be characterized. In addition, the possibility that metabolites might modulate the actions of parent drug (eg, by competing for access to a receptor site on an ion channel[7]) or that pharmacokinetic interactions between isomers or between parent drug and metabolites[18,19] that alter parent drug disposition can occur or should be entertained.

Pharmacokinetic Issues for Class III Agents

Initial pharmacokinetic studies of any new drug should include characterization of route(s) of metabolism and excretion, the presence and activity of metabolites, the possibility of enantiospecific therapy, and a consideration of the impact of disease or concomitant drug therapy on drug disposition. For Class III agents, a number of other questions are also important. For example, studies of drug interactions should not only include those that might alter drug disposition, but also those that might alter drug effect. These include not only cardioactive agents such as digitalis preparations or β blockers, but also drugs that target potassium channels. For example, we and others have shown that potassium channel activation can reverse the action potential prolonging effects of potassium channel block in vitro and in experimental models.[20,21] Thus, the notion that drugs that activate potassium channels might blunt the effects of potassium channel blockers should be investigated.

Sources of Variability in Drug Action: Pharmacodynamics

Response Variables

In studies of the relationship between plasma drug concentration and effect, explicit definitions of end points for evaluating drug action should be formulated prospectively. A surrogate variable, such as QT interval prolongation for Class III agents, is often used to gauge drug action in clinical trials. Such surrogates have a certain appeal because they are readily obtained; however, it is critical to recognize that changes in a surrogate variable are not equivalent to drug efficacy. Thus, changes in QRS duration or in ventricular ectopic frequency (surrogate variables) during encainide or flecainide therapy did not translate into reduction in mortality (drug efficacy) during CAST.[22] Just as failure of plasma concentration measurements to predict drug actions (surrogate or otherwise) can drive further research, a failure of surrogate variables to predict true drug efficacy should also prompt reevaluation of the assumptions underlying mechanisms of drug action. Methods to assess the QT interval, a primary response variable

for Class III antiarrhythmic agents, may require refinement. Data are now becoming available to suggest that dispersion of repolarization may be an important predictor for torsades de pointes[23,24]; methods to evaluate such dispersion should be further assessed. Methods to deal with U wave quantification and methods to appropriately rate correct (or not), and when to measure the QT interval in relation to dosing and (as discussed elsewhere) as a function of time during the day are other areas that are now receiving increasing attention. Another issue is a prospective definition of torsades de pointes. For example, it is not unusual to see ventricular tachycardia assume a polymorphic appearance, coincident with institution of a QT prolonging drug (Figure 2). It is certainly not clear that such a case should be classified as drug-induced torsades de pointes.

QT Response Variability

An important issue with respect to studies of the relationship between plasma concentration and effect for Class III agents is whether in fact changes in indexes of repolarization (the most readily available being the QT interval) actually predict drug efficacy. As early as 1970, Heissenbuttel and Bigger[25] reported that the extent of change in the QTc was very poorly correlated with plasma quinidine ($r = 0.28$). While it could be argued that this failure of correlation might reflect the presence of active metabolites of quinidine, further studies by our group do not support the concept that heterogeneous quinidine metabolism results in exaggerated QT responses in some patients.[26,27] Moreover, when we studied intravenous sematilide in patients with isolated ventricular ectopic depolarizations, a similar finding was noted[28]: although a fairly good correlation was identified between plasma concentration of sematilide and change in QTc, occasional patients had much greater changes in QTc at usual sematilide concentrations. Since sematilide does not undergo extensive metabolism and is excreted largely un-

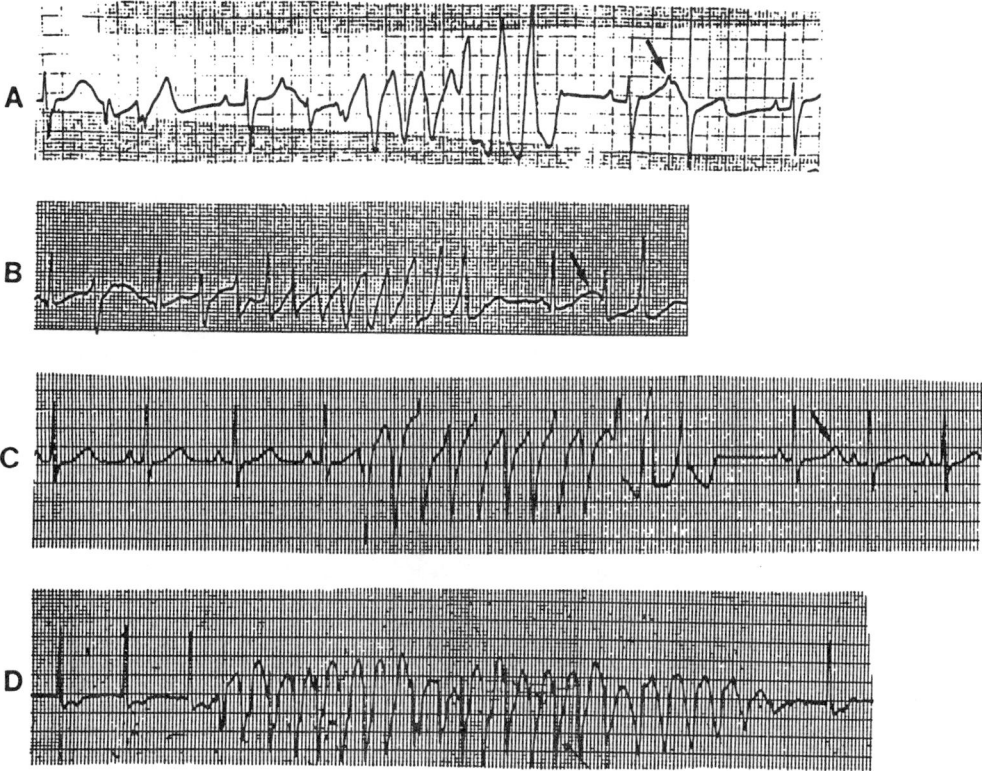

Figure 2. Four examples of polymorphic ventricular tachycardia. The first two, recorded during quinidine therapy, are accompanied by marked cycle length-dependent fluctuations of a long QT interval (arrows) and are examples of torsades de pointes. The last was recorded in a patient with acute myocardial ischemia receiving no antiarrhythmic agents. The QT interval is short and cycle length modulation is absent; this is not torsades de pointes. The third example illustrates the difficulty in strictly defining torsades de pointes. This is recorded during sotalol therapy from a patient with monomorphic nonsustained ventricular tachycardia at baseline. Note the tachycardia is now polymorphic and the posttachycardia QT is markedly prolonged.

changed by the kidneys, variable metabolism cannot be invoked to explain this variable response. Rather, a variable QT response to sematilide in this instance reflects interindividual variability in sensitivity to the QT prolonging effect of the drug, for reasons that have not yet been identified.

In a recent placebo controlled, dose ranging study of intravenous dofetilide in patients with inducible sustained ventricular tachyarrhythmias, we also found marked heterogeneity in the extent to which a given dose of drug prolonged the QT interval.[29] In that study, an increase in QT interval by more than 100 msec was only observed in two subjects. In one of the two, torsades de pointes developed, while in the second, the arrhythmia was rendered noninducible. In 3 of 18 other patients who received dofetilide in that trial, and in 1 of 6 who received placebo, tachycardias were also rendered uninducible, but with less than 25 msec increases in QT. The finding that arrhythmia suppression can occur in the absence of a substantial QT change during treatment with a Class III agent is compatible with previous reports using sotalol: in no studies of sotalol efficacy in patients with sustained ventricular tachycardia is a correlation between the extent of QT change and uninducibility reported.[30-35] Whether this reflects difficulties with the QT measurement or the possibility that Class III agents render at least some arrhythmias noninducible by acting at a local site without necessarily prolonging the QT interval will require further study.

Torsades de Pointes After Intravenous Infusion

In both the studies with sematilide and with dofetilide described above, one patient developed torsades de pointes shortly after an intravenous dose of drug. Similarly, as described elsewhere in this volume, torsades de pointes has occurred shortly after intravenous treatment with ibutilide and almokalant. Although these findings are compatible with a dose related adverse drug effect, they also raise the possibility that large intravenous boluses of Class III agents may be, for some as yet unidentified reason, particularly likely to produce torsades de pointes. For example, it is conceivable that rapid drug delivery results

in heterogenous drug delivery to the myocardium and therefore marked heterogeneity in the extent to which action potentials are prolonged; this in turn might increase the likelihood that an early afterdepolarization elicited at a site with a particularly long action potential could propagate to adjacent sites with shorter action potentials and hence produce torsades de pointes. Obviously, further studies in which drug delivery is much slower, including by the oral route, will be required to address such possibilities.

Pharmacodynamic Considerations for Drug Dosing

Drug treatment regimens that result in high peak trough ratios of plasma drug concentrations may carry at least the theoretical risk that in order to maintain trough plasma concentrations above a given minimum effective concentration, undesirable high peak concentrations may be required. As shown in Figure 3, variability in plasma concentration is less with an 8-hourly regimen than with a

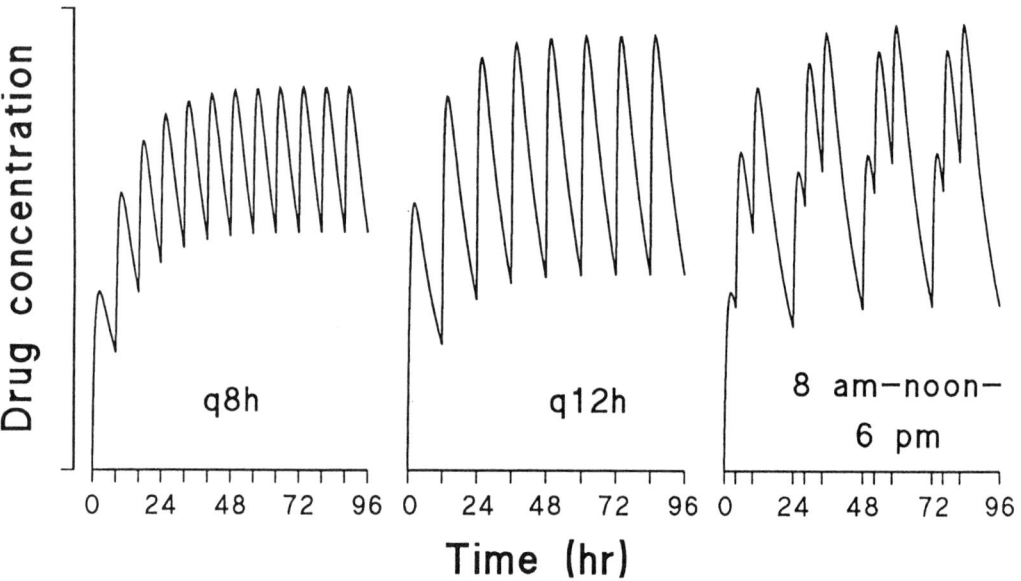

Figure 3. Simulations of plasma concentration time relationships for three different dosing regimens: every 8 hours, 12 hours, and three times a day with meals. Note that fluctuations are as great with a realistic three times a day regimen as with every 12 hours.

12-hourly one; however, it is important to note that a practical three times per day regimen (eg, with breakfast, lunch, and dinner) can produce as much, or more, variability in plasma concentrations as a theoretical 12-hourly one. Thus, the recognition that patients may not take their pills by the clock is an argument for simple dosing regimens (such as twice daily). Slow release formulations can also reduce this intradose variability in plasma concentration.

Summary

An intensive evaluation of the relationship between administered drug and resultant plasma concentrations and effect for Class III agents has, therefore, been important for two reasons. First, the determinants of drug disposition (renal function, drug metabolism, distribution, etc.) have been identified; appropriate and straightforward studies to characterize the impact of disease states, active metabolites, and stereoisomers can be proposed, and for many of the drugs discussed in this volume, have been performed or are underway. Second, the relationship between plasma drug concentration and resultant antiarrhythmic and electrocardiographic activities has suggested that an antiarrhythmic effect can be present with minimal QT prolongation. Thus, at least preliminary data suggests that guidelines that permit generous QT prolongation in the hopes of capturing further responders may result in an undesirable incidence of torsades de pointes.

References

1. Eichelbaum M: Defective oxidation of drugs: pharmacokinetic and therapeutic implications. *Clin Pharmacokinet* 7:1, 1982.
2. Turgeon J, Murray KT, Roden DM: Effects of drug metabolism, metabolites and stereoselectivity on antiarrhythmic drug action. *J Cardiovasc Electrophysiol* 1:238, 1990.
3. Drayer DE, Reidenberg MM: Clinical consequences of polymorphic acetylation of basic drugs. *Clin Pharmacol Ther* 22:251, 1977.
4. Roden DM, Duff HJ, Altenbern D, Woosley RL: Antiarrhythmic activity of the O-desmethyl metabolite of encainide. *J Pharmacol Exp Ther* 221:552, 1982.
5. Elharrar V, Zipes D: Effects of encainide and metabolites (MJ14030 and MJ9444) on canine cardiac Purkinje and ventricular fibers. *J Pharmacol Exp Ther* 220:440, 1982.
6. Roden DM, Reele SB, Higgins SB, et al: Antiarrhythmic efficacy, pharmacokinetics and safety of N-acetylprocainamide in man: comparison to procainamide. *Am J Cardiol* 46:463, 1980.
7. Bennett PB, Woosley RL, Hondeghem LM: Competitive interactions of lidocaine (L) and one of its metabolites, glycine xylidide (GX), with cardiac sodium channels. *Circulation* 78:692, 1988.
8. Funck-Brentano C, Light RT, Lineberry MD, et al: Pharmacokinetic and pharmacodynamic interaction of N-acetyl procainamide and procainamide in man. *J Cardiovasc Pharmacol* 14:364, 1989.
9. Idle JR, Mahgoub A, Lancaster R, Smith RL: Hypotensive response to debrisoquine and hydroxylation phenotype. *Life Sci* 22:979, 1978.
10. Eichelbaum M, Gross AS: The genetic polymorphism of debrisoquine/sparteine metabolism—clinical aspects. *Pharmacol Ther* 46:377, 1990.
11. Speirs CJ, Murray S, Boobis AR, et al: Quinidine and the identification of drugs whose elimination is impaired in subjects classified as poor metabolizers of debrisoquine. *Br J Clin Pharmacol* 22:739, 1986.
12. Funck-Brentano C, Kroemer HK, Woosley RL, Roden DM: Genetically-determined interaction between propafenone and low dose quinidine: role of active metabolites in modulating net drug effect. *Br J Clin Pharmacol* 27:435, 1989.
13. Otton SV, Inaba T, Kalow W: Competitive inhibition of sparteine oxidation in human liver by β-adrenoceptor antagonist and other cardiovascular drugs. *Life Sci* 34:73, 1984.
14. Turgeon JT, Pavlou H, Funck-Brentano C, Roden DM: Genetically-determined steady-state interaction between encainide and quinidine in patients with arrhythmias. *J Pharmacol Exp Ther* 255:642, 1990.
15. Mirro MJ, Watanabe AM, Bailey JC: Electrophysiological effects of the optical isomers of disopyramide and quinidine in the dog: dependence on stereochemistry. *Circ Res* 48:867, 1981.
16. Kato R, Ikeda N, Yabek SM, et al: Electrophysiologic effects of the levo- and dextrorotatory isomers of sotalol in isolated cardiac muscle and their in vivo pharmacokinetics. *J Am Coll Cardiol* 7:116, 1986.

17. Carmeliet E: Electrophysiologic and voltage clamp analysis of the effects of sotalol on isolated cardiac muscle and Purkinje fibers. *J Pharmacol Exp Ther* 232:817, 1985.

18. LeLorier J, Grenon D, Latour Y, et al: Pharmacokinetics of lidocaine after prolonged intravenous infusions in uncomplicated myocardial infarction. *Ann Intern Med* 87:700, 1977.

19. Suzuki T, Fujita S, Kawai R: Precursor-metabolite interaction in the metabolism of lidocaine. *J Pharmacol Sci* 73:136, 1984.

20. Fish F, Prakash C, Roden DM: Suppression of repolarization-related arrhythmias in vitro and in vivo by low dose potassium channel activators. *Circulation* 82:1362, 1990.

21. Spinelli W, Sorota S, Siegal M, Hoffman BF: Antiarrhythmic actions of the ATP-regulated K^+ current activated by pinacidil. *Circ Res* 68:1127, 1991.

22. Echt DS, Liebson PR, Mitchell LB, et al: Mortality and morbidity in patients receiving encainide, flecainide, or placebo. *N Engl J Med* 324:781, 1991.

23. Day CP, McComb JM, Campbell RWF: QT dispersion: an indication of arrhythmia risk in patients with long QT intervals. *Br Heart J* 63:342, 1990.

24. Hii J, Wyse DG, Gillis AM, et al: Dispersion of precordial QT intervals as a marker of torsades de pointes: disparate effects of class Ia drugs and amiodarone. *Circulation* 84:II-596, 1991.

25. Heissenbuttel RH, Bigger JT Jr: The effect of oral quinidine on intraventricular conduction in man: correlation of plasma quinidine with changes in QRS duration. *Am Heart J* 80:453, 1970.

26. Thompson KA, Blair IA, Woosley RL, Roden DM: Comparative electrophysiologic effects of quinidine, its major metabolites and dihydroquinidine in canine cardiac Purkinje fibers. *J Pharmacol Exp Ther* 241:84, 1987.

27. Thompson KA, Murray JJ, Blair IA, et al: Plasma concentrations of quinidine, major metabolites, and dihydroquinidine in patients with torsades de pointes. *Clin Pharmacol Ther* 43:636, 1988.

28. Wong W, Pavlou HN, Birgersdotter UM, et al: Pharmacology of the class III antiarrhythmic agent sematilide in patients with arrhythmias. *Am J Cardiol* 69:206, 1992.

29. Echt DS, Lee JT, Murray KT, et al: A randomized, double-blind, placebo-controlled dose-ranging study of intravenous UK-68,798 (dofetilide) in patients with inducible sustained ventricular tachyarrhythmias. *Circulation* 84:II-714, 1991.

30. Senges J, Lengfelder W, Jauernig R, et al: Electrophysiologic testing in assessment of therapy with sotalol for sustained ventricular tachycardia. *Circulation* 69:577, 1984.

31. Nademanee K, Feld G, Hendrickson J, et al: Electrophysiologic and antiarrhythmic effects of sotalol in patients with life-threatening ventricular tachyarrhythmias. *Circulation* 72:555, 1985.

32. Singh SN, Cohen A, Chen Y, et al: Sotalol for refractory sustained ventricular tachycardia and nonfatal cardiac arrest. *Am J Cardiol* 62:399, 1988.

33. Gonzalex R, Scheinman MM, Herre JM, et al: Usefulness of sotalol for drug-refractory malignant ventricular arrhythmias. *J Am Coll Cardiol* 12:1568, 1988.

34. Kuchar DL, Garan H, Venditti FJ, et al: Usefulness of sotalol in suppressing ventricular tachycardia or ventricular fibrillation in patients with healed myocardial infarcts. *Am J Cardiol* 64:33, 1989.

35. Ruder MA, Ellis T, Lebsack C, et al: Clinical experience with sotalol in patients with drug-refractory ventricular arrhythmias. *J Am Coll Cardiol* 13:145, 1989.

Chapter 33

Sotalol and d-Sotalol:
Electrophysiology, Pharmacology, and Role in Controlling Cardiac Arrhythmias

Michael J. Antonaccio
Bramah N. Singh

Sotalol (MJ 1999) (Figure 1) is 4'-(2-iso-propylamino-1-hydroxyethyl) methanesulfon-amide, which is a competitive antagonist at β-adrenergic receptor sites with no selectivity for β_1 or β_2 receptors. In addition, sotalol also increases the action potential duration (APD) and increases cardiac refractoriness, criteria that satisfy Class III antiarrhythmic activity (see Chapter 30). Sotalol is a mixture of d- and l-isomers, both of which have equal Class III activity but only the l-isomer retaining most of the β-adrenoceptor blocking activity. The focus of this chapter is on the electrophysio-logical and pharmacological properties of so-talol and its isomers relative to their effects on experimental and clinical cardiac arrhythmias.

β-Adrenoceptor Blockade

Sotalol is a competitive, nonselective β-adrenoceptor antagonist with little or no membrane stabilizing activity or intrinsic sym-pathomimetic activity, although it has positive inotropic activity as will be discussed.[1,2] The pA2 for dl-sotalol was very consistently found to be between 6.1 and 6.4, depending on the preparation used.[3-5]

The relative affinity (pKd) of d- and dl-sotalol for ^{125}I-pindolol in cat ventricular membranes was 5.0 ± 0.01 and 6.3 ± 0.03, yielding a ratio of 20 ± 1.0.[6] The blocking potency of d-sotalol (pKd) in this study was 5.4 ± 0.09.

Exposure of the isolated rabbit papillary muscle to 10^{-4} M sotalol attenuated the me-chanical contractile effects evoked by isopro-terenol.[7] The mean concentration of isopro-terenol producing 50% of the maximal in-crease in developed tension (ED50) in the absence of an antagonist was 2.5×10^{-8} M. In the presence of racemic sotalol, the value was 3.0×10^{-6} M; with d-sotalol, the ED50 value was 2.1×10^{-7} M. The potency ratios (given by the ratio [ED50 after drug]/[ED50 before drug]) were 122.7 and 8.5 for dl- and d-sotalol,

From BN Singh, HJJ Wellens, M Hiraoka, (eds): *Electropharmacological Control of Cardiac Arrhythmias*. Mount Kisco, NY, Futura Publishing Company Inc., © 1994.

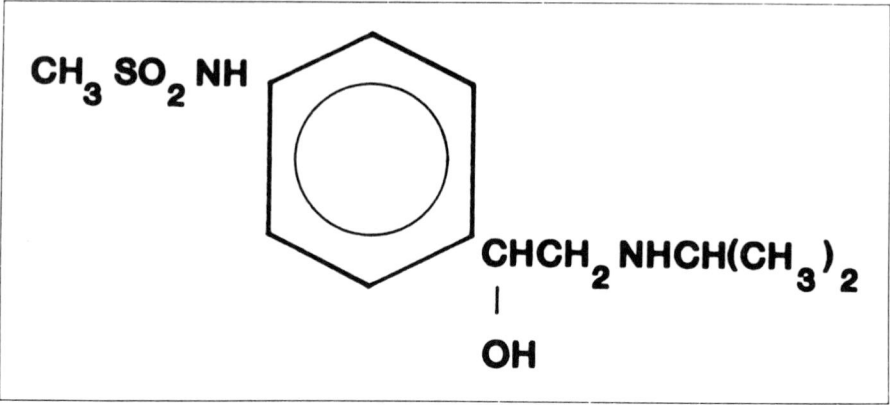

Figure 1. Chemical structure of sotalol.

respectively. Thus, the parent racemic drug displayed approximately 14 times the β-blocking potency of the d-isomer.

In a variety of isolated tissues, including the rat uterine horn rabbit and kitten right atria, rabbit and kitten papillary muscle, and perfused feline heart[3,7–12] sotalol was found to have little or no direct effect while producing rightward shifts of dose-response curves to β-adrenoceptor agonists.

In animals, sotalol also produced competitive blockade of both β_1 and β_2 adrenoceptors. In anesthetized dogs, the threshold blocking dose of sotalol against isoproterenol-induced tachycardia was 78 mg/kg administered intravenously, with maximal blockade occurring at 625 mg/kg intravenously.[10] In conscious rats, the oral dose producing 50% inhibition of isoproterenol-induced tachycardia was 6.3 and 15.5 mg/kg after 0.5 and 30 hours posttreatment.[11] In various preparations of anesthetized dogs, propranolol was found to be between 4 and 10 times as potent as sotalol.[11,13] The calculated pA2 values for racemic sotalol in anesthetized dogs was 6.6 for both heart rate and diastolic blood pressure changes induced by isoproterenol, whereas they were 5.4 and 5.5 for d-sotalol

Table 1
Characteristics of β-Adrenoceptor Antagonists

Drug	Potency (propranolol = 1)	Local anesthetic activity	IS A	Cardioselectivity
Sotalol	0.3	0	0	−
Nadolol	0.5	0	0	−
Timolol	5–10	0	0	−
Bunolol	50	0	0	−
Atenolol	1	0	0	+
Metoprolol	0.5–2	±	0	+
Propranolol	1	+ +	0	−
Labetalol	0.3	+	±	−
Acebutolol	0.3	+	+	+
Alprenolol	0.3–1	+	+ +	−
Oxprenolol	0.5–1	+	+ +	−
Pindolol	5–10	±	+ + +	−

and 6.8 and 7.1 for l-sotalol, respectively.[14] The large differences in the in vitro and in vivo potencies of sotalol compared with propranolol are undoubtedly related to the oral bioavailability of sotalol compared with the poor bioavailability of propranolol.

The relative characteristics of sotalol to other β-adrenoceptor antagonists with respect to potency, local anesthetic (membrane stabilizing) activity, intrinsic sympathomimetic activity and cardioselectivity are listed in Table 1.[15]

In Vitro Electrophysiological Actions

Effects on the Cardiac Action Potential

In 1970, Singh and Vaughan Williams[16] examined the effects of various β-adrenoceptor antagonists on several parameters of cardiac intracellular action potentials. They found that sotalol (then known as MJ 1999) greatly prolonged APD, whereas standard β adrenoreceptor antagonists including alprenolol had no effect on repolarization rates. Sotalol did not significantly affect the resting membrane potential or the maximum rate of depolarization, whereas other β adrenoreceptor antagonists including propranolol, practolol, and oxprenolol were found to have no effect on APD but significantly decreased the maximum rate of depolarization (Figure 2).[17] Strauss et al.[5] also found that sotalol increased APD as well as refractory period in both canine ventricular muscle and Purkinje fibers; however, the effects on Purkinje fibers were more sensitive and of a greater magnitude. In addition, these investigators showed that the effect of sotalol to increase APD was directly related to cycle length and that this effect was also much more dramatic in Purkinje fibers relative to ventricular muscle. Since these original reports, many other investigators have confirmed the ability of sotalol to in-

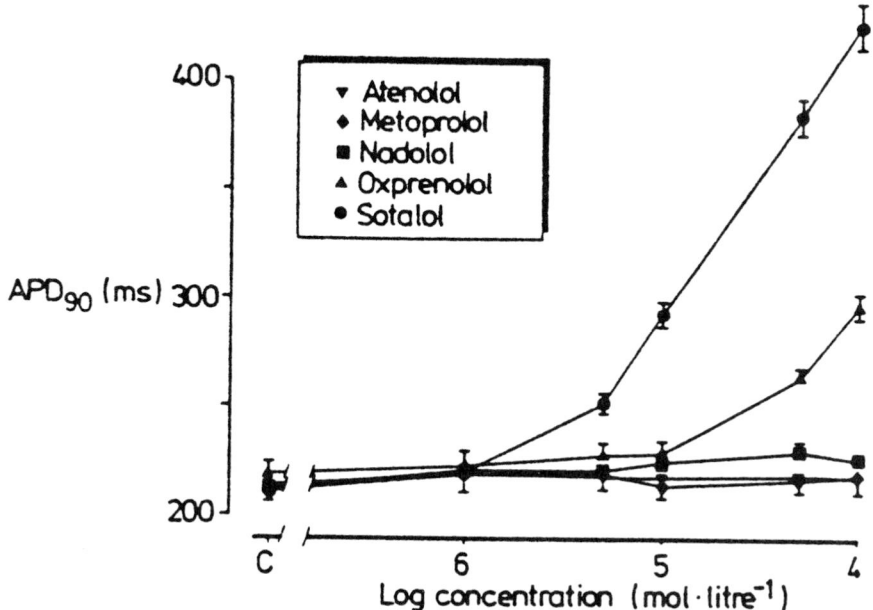

Figure 2. Effects of increasing concentrations of atenolol, metoprolol, nadolol, oxprenolol, and sotalol on action potential duration (APD) at 90% repolarization (APD$_{90}$). (Reproduced with permission from Reference 7.)

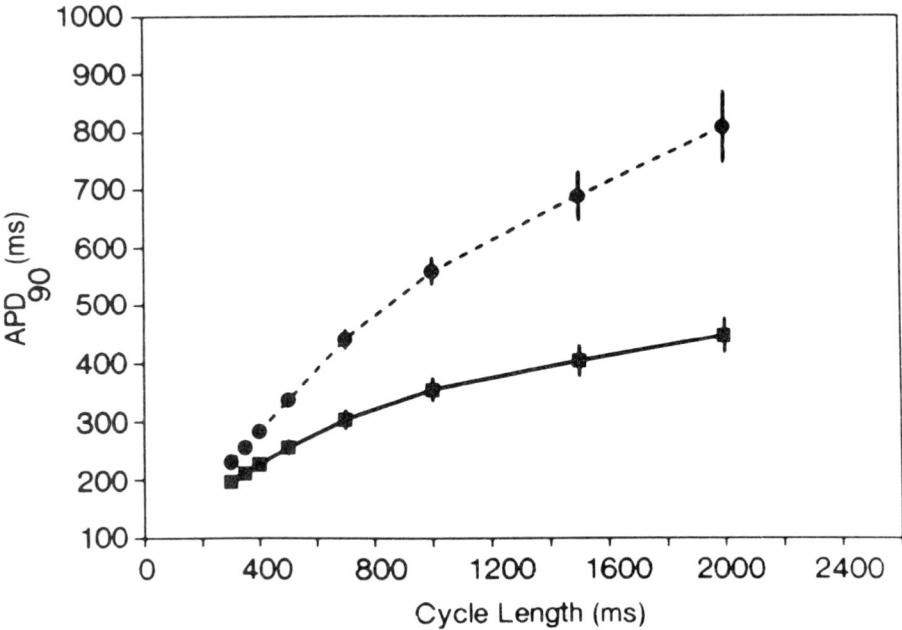

Figure 3. Rate-dependent effect of sotalol (30 mM) on dog Purkinje fiber action potential duration (APD) at 90% repolarization (APD_{90}). (Reproduced with permission from Reference 23.)

crease APD, its inverse correlation with heart rate (Figure 3), and lack of effect by sotalol on resting membrane potential and maximum rate of depolarization.[5–7,18–25] These effects have been shown to reside with equal potency and efficacy in the d-isomer of sotalol as well, and are not a consequence of β adrenoceptor antagonism since other β adrenoceptor antagonists do not have these properties nor is d-sotalol as effective a β antagonist as is sotalol.[1,2,7,17] The relative ability of d-, l- and dl-sotalol to increase APD with respect to decreasing the maximum rate of depolarization is shown in Figure 4. An exception to the APD prolongation caused by sotalol is the recent report that d-sotalol is not able to increase the APD of isolated papillary muscles or the effective refractory period (ERP) of perfused rat hearts.[26] This was attributed to the short resting APD and the lack of any discernible tail current in rat cardiac tissue. However, in another study using rats both d- and dl-sotalol were effective in reducing reperfusion-in-duced arrhythmias in both Sprague-Dawley and Wistar rats and also significantly increased APD and ERPs of septal myocardial cells in both strains.[27]

Effects on Myocardial Ion Channels

Both d- and dl-sotalol increase APD primarily by blocking the time-dependent outward delayed rectifier K^+ current (I_k). As demonstrated by Carmeliet[18] and shown in Figure 5, both d- and dl-sotalol decreased I_k in a concentration related manner, the IC50 being obtained at 10^{-5} M and total inhibition at 10^{-4} M, a concentration range consistent with the ability of sotalol to prolong APD. d- and dl-Sotalol did not change activation kinetics nor was the effect related to β adrenoceptor antagonism, but could be totally explained by a reduction in the number of conducting I_k channels, single channel conductance or the mean open time.

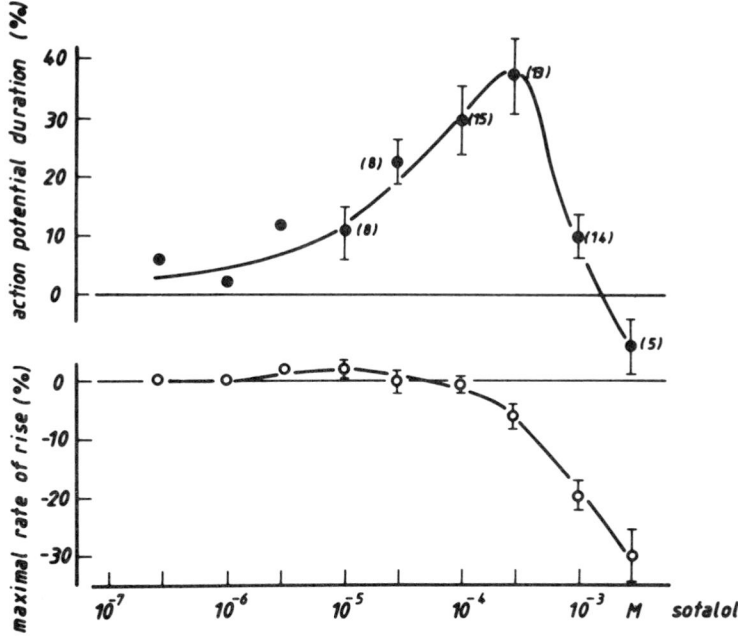

Figure 4. Percent change in action potential duration (APD) and maximal rate of rise of guinea pig papillary muscle preparations as a function of sotalol concentration. Values for dl-, d-, and l-sotalol were pooled since they were not different from each other. (Reproduced with permission from Reference 18.)

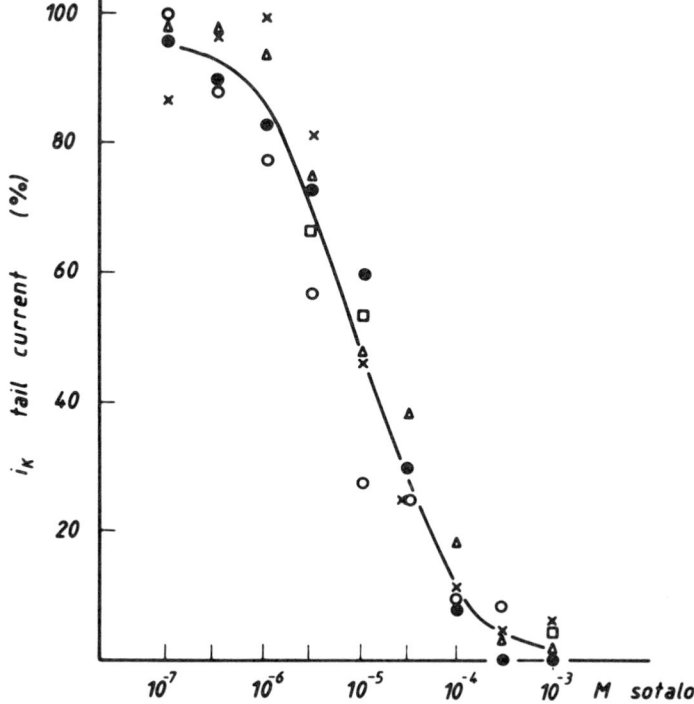

Figure 5. Dose-response relationship for the effect of dl-sotalol on the amplitude of the delayed rectifier current in rabbit Purkinje fibers. (Reproduced with permission from Reference 18.)

Recently, it has been shown that the delayed rectifier current results from the activation of two separate outward K^+ currents; namely, a very rapid current, I_{kr} and a slowly activating current I_{ks}.[28]

Class III antiarrhythmic agents, including d-sotalol, inactivate I_{kr} but not I_{ks}.[28] Both d- and dl-sotalol, especially at high concentrations, can also inhibit the background or inward rectifying K^+ current (I_{k1}) and thereby decrease resting potential by a few millivolts as shown by Carmeliet[18] and Courtney and Hill[29] although others have not seen this effect.[25] Similarly, Berger et al.[21] have found that d- and dl-sotalol decrease the transient outward K^+ current (I_{to}) in sheep Purkinje fibers, but this effect has been specifically excluded in rabbit myocardium.[25]

At concentrations below 0.5 mM, sotalol has little or no effect on the maximum rate of depolarization[5,16–18,21–25] and, as might be anticipated from such a lack of effect, no inhibitory action on the fast sodium channel (I_{Na}).[18,25] Similarly, sotalol has no appreciable effect on the slow, inward calcium channel.[18,25] The effects of sotalol on various ion currents that are responsible for its actions to increase APD are shown in Table 2.

After exposure to high concentrations of either d- or dl-sotalol, the APD becomes markedly prolonged and during the sustained plateau, the membrane potential begins to oscillate with an early afterdepolarization (EAD) associated with an aftercontraction.[16,17,30–34]

Like the APD prolongation activity of sotalol, the EADs and aftercontractions produced by the drug are probably related to excessive Ca^{2+} entering the myocyte through Ca^{2+} channels during the plateau phase of the APD since: (1) doubling the Ca^{2+} concentration increased aftercontractions induced by sotalol by over 300%[30]; and (2) agents that reduce Ca^{2+} influx either directly (such as the Ca^{2+} channel blocker verapamil[31] or indirectly (such as the K^+ ATP channel activator nicorandil[33]) are capable of blocking both the APD prolongation and EADs produced by d- and dl-sotalol. Class I agents that reduce APD such as mexiletine and lignocaine are also capable of reducing the APD prolongation and EADs produced by sotalol.[33–36]

Sotalol and Early Afterdepolarizations

The membrane oscillations during the plateau of the APD and the EADs induced by sotalol may have clinical relevance since they may be causally related to an unusual arrhythmia seen in approximately 4% of patients receiving sotalol; namely, torsades de pointes. This arrhythmia is often associated with marked bradycardia, prolonged QT, and hypokalemia (see Chapter 8) and appears to be initiated by triggered activity sometimes caused by high doses of sotalol.[37–39]

Table 2
Effects of Sotalol on Cardiac Ion Channels

K^+-Channels	Effect
I_K (time-dependent outward delayed rectifier)	
$\quad I_{KR}$ (rapidly activating component)	$++++$
$\quad I_{KS}$ (slowly activating component)	0
I_{KI} (inward rectifier)	$+$
I_{TO} (transient [inactivating] outward current)	$1\pm$
K^+_{ATP}	
	0
Na^+ channels	0 (except at > [mM])
Ca^{2+} channels	0

Sotalol Action During Electrolyte Perturbations and in Disease

An important and complicated aspect of sotalol's effect on APD prolongation is its interaction with elevated extracellular K^+ as well as its effects on K^+ leakage in ischemic cardiac tissue. Under conditions of mild hypoxia, the ability of sotalol to lengthen APD was preserved.[40] In contrast, under severe hypoxic conditions, the Class III effect of sotalol was lost within 5 minutes of exposure to hypoxia.[41] However, the extent of shortening of the baseline APD under these severe conditions is much greater than normal and since the ability of sotalol to prolong APD is directly related to resting APD,[42] these findings are not surprising and are probably not strictly related to hypoxia itself. The effect of sotalol in lengthening APD and ERP are preserved under conditions of elevated extracellular K^+, which caused partial depolarization.[19] Even under these conditions of partial depolarization, there was no evidence of a hidden Class I action for sotalol.[19]

The effects of ischemia on the action of sotalol were examined in the isolated, arterially perfused interventricular septum of the rabbit.[43] Prior to ischemia, sotalol increased APD by 52%; however, during 30 minutes, 0 flow ischemia, there was a gradual diminution of the sotalol APD prolongation. Interestingly, Hicks and Cobbe[44] reported that sotalol and its isomers markedly attenuated the increases in extracellular K^+ that occurred during severe myocardial ischemia (30 minutes of global 0 flow), even though the prolongation of APD was lost. In contrast, the β blocker atenolol was without effect on $[K^+]_o$.

These data with sotalol under various in vitro conditions are very difficult to interpret since preservation of the Class III effect of sotalol in tissues from infarcted areas has been demonstrated[45] and in vivo studies indicate that sotalol increases QTc and refractoriness within the infarcted area after coronary ligation. Finally, prolongation of APD in nonischemic myocardium will always occur after sotalol that may be sufficient to prevent arrhythmias (although potentially increasing dispersion of repolarization).[41]

In Vivo Electrophysiological Actions of Sotalol

Experimental Observations

Sotalol and d-sotalol prolong QT and QTc intervals without any significant effect on QRS or PR intervals.[14,17,46–50] These prolonging effects on QT intervals are also demonstrable when heart rates are maintained constant by pacing, unlike the shortening of QT that occurs after β adrenoceptor antagonism with metoprolol.[46,49] Both d- and dl-sotalol also concomitantly increased ventricular refractory periods both in normal and ischemic tissues.[46,49] In contrast, neither compound had any effect on ventricular activation time nor on excitation thresholds.[2,31] Also, neither d- nor dl-sotalol had any effect on atrial (PA interval), His-Purkinje (HV intervals) or ventricular (HS interval) conduction velocity, whereas both compounds significantly slowed atrioventricular (AV) nodal conduction.[14] Sinus cycle lengths were increased by both d- and dl-sotalol, presumably as a consequence of both β adrenoceptor blockade and QTc prolongation.

Substantially higher concentrations of sotalol are required for the Class III effects of sotalol than for its β-blocking effect. Nattel et al.[51] determined the relative β-blocking and Class III effects in dogs and showed that half-maximal β blockade occurred at a sotalol concentration of 0.8 ± 0.3 mg/mL whereas the concentrations required for half-maximal effects on atrial and ventricular refractoriness were 6.9 ± 1.2 mg/mL and 6.8 ± 2.8 mg/mL, respectively (Figure 6).

Effects in Humans

In a double-blind study, intravenous sotalol (0.3 or 0.6 mg/kg) increased right atrial

Sotalol Concentration - Response Relationships in Anesthetized Dogs

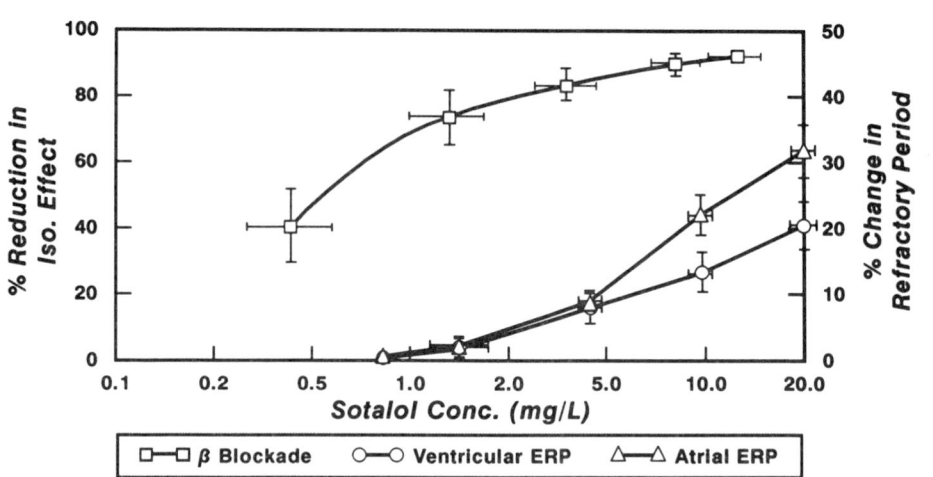

Figure 6. β Adrenergic blocking effects and Class III actions (ERP) of sotalol in anesthetized dogs. (Reproduced with permission from Reference 51.)

monophasic APD by 44 msec ($p < 0.01$), whereas propranolol (0.15 or 0.2 mg/kg) had no effect.[52] The QT interval, atrial and ventricular effective refractory period (VERP), and right ventricular monophasic action potential were also significantly prolonged by sotalol but not propranolol. A similar increase in atrial APD in human subjects has also been reported by Haywood and Taggart.[53] Sotalol (0.6 mg/kg intravenously) was also found to

Table 3
Electrophysiological Effects of Sotalol in Patients With Sustained Ventricular Tachycardia

	Baseline (n = 20)	I.V. Sotalol (n = 13)	Mean % change	Oral sotalol (n = 13)	Mean % change
SCL	825 ± 180	1031 ± 250[a]	39	1108 ± 293[a]	39
AH	120 ± 38	161 ± 37[a]	34	191 ± 50[a]	45
WCL	365 ± 78	442 ± 78[a]	29	451 ± 70[a]	26
AVNRRP	492 ± 69	543 ± 62	15	545 ± 56	11
QTc	397 ± 50	440 ± 40[b]	11	—	—
QT	344 ± 51	415 ± 34[a]	22	447 ± 66[a]	39
AERP	241 ± 39	313 ± 65[a]	33	295 ± 24[a]	34
RVERT	240 ± 18	282 ± 31[a]	23	287 ± 23[a]	20
HV	60 ± 18	61 ± 20[b]	2	—	—
RR	738 ± 163	955 ± 182[b]	29	—	—

SCL: sinus cycle length; AH: atrio-His interval; WCL: Wenckebach cycle length; AVNRRP: Atrioventricular node relative refractory period; HV: HIS-ventricular interval; RR: R-wave to R-wave interval; QT: QT interval; AERP: atrial effective refractory period; RVERP: right ventricular effective refractory period. Modified from Reference 57, with permission.
[a] Statistically significant compared with baseline values.
[b] Data from Kopelman et al.[56] (n = 33).

increase AV nodal conduction time, His-Purkinje conduction time, QT interval, and retrograde refractory period of specialized ventricular tissue.[54] In a double-blind crossover comparison of long-term (4 weeks) oral therapy with sotalol (160 mg b.i.d.) or metoprolol (100 mg b.i.d.) in postmyocardial infarction patients, QT interval was significantly prolonged by sotalol but not metoprolol, with no change in QRS interval despite equieffective β blockade.[55]

In patients with life-threatening sustained ventricular tachycardia (VT), sotalol administered either intravenously (100–160 mg) or orally (mean dose 612 ± 206 mg) caused significant increases in the sinus cycle length, Wenckebach cycle length, and RR, AH, QT, and QTc intervals but was without effect on the QRS or HV intervals.[56,57] Atrial and ventricular

refractory periods were also significantly prolonged by both intravenous and oral sotalol (Table 3).

In patients with frequent (more than 30 per hour) premature ventricular contractions (PVCs), orally administered sotalol (80–640 mg/day) caused dose related increases in the QT and QTc intervals (Figure 7), which were also correlated with sotalol plasma levels.[1] PR intervals were slightly increased whereas QRS intervals were unchanged (Figure 7). In a comparative trial in patients with similar arrhythmia profiles, both sotalol (640 mg/day) and propranolol (240 mg/day) caused a small but significant increase in the PR interval, but did not alter QRS duration. As noted, both drugs caused similar reductions in heart rate and also increased the QT intervals, but the effect of sotalol was much greater. When the

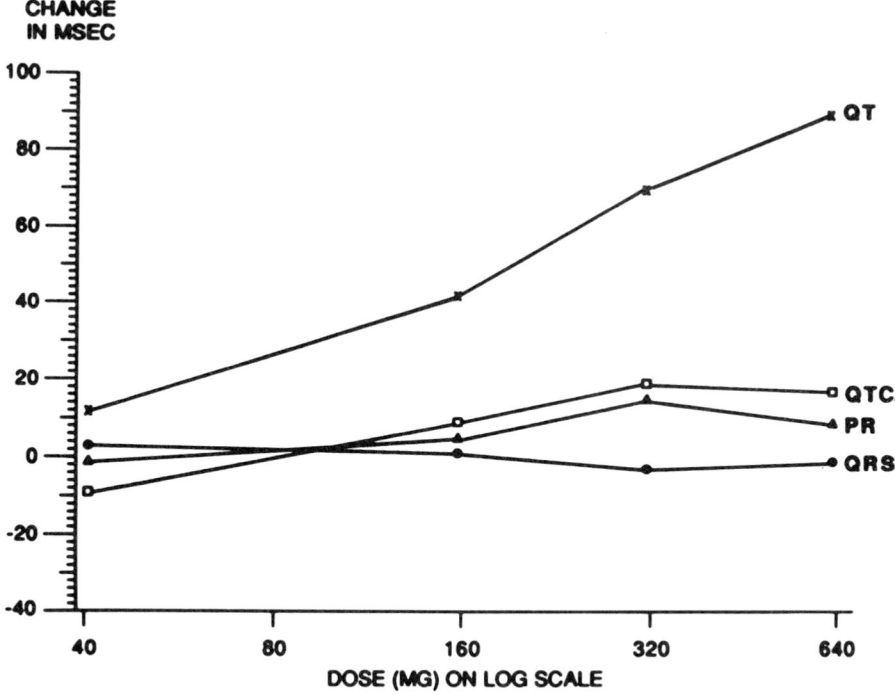

Figure 7. Changes in surface ECG after various doses of sotalol in patients treated for premature ventricular beats. Values are mean for at least 22 patients. Changes in QT intervals were statistically significant from baseline at all doses; changes in PR interval were significantly different after 160, 320, and 640 mg; changes in QTc interval were significantly different after 320 mg only. QRS intervals were not different at any dose. (Reproduced with permission from Reference 1.)

QT intervals were corrected for rate, sotalol still produced a significant increase, whereas propranolol actually produced a decrease.

d-Sotalol has clinical electrophysiological effects similar to those of dl-sotalol, except for the degree of β blockage.[58] Thus, infusions of d-sotalol (1–2 mg/kg) or dl-sotalol (1 mg/kg) increased QT and QTc intervals, and refractoriness in atrium, AV node and right ventricle whereas PR, QRS, AH and HV intervals were unchanged. Furthermore, RR intervals were more potently reduced by dl- as compared to d-sotalol.

Thus, the increase in APD produced by d- and dl-sotalol is reflected in patients by an increase in both QT and QTc intervals and no change in QRS intervals. These effects are readily differentiatable from those of standard β antagonists, which increase only the PR interval because of β adrenoceptor blocking actions on the AV node. Also, the refractory periods of both atria and ventricles are significantly increased after sotalol, this effect presumably a consequence of its ability to prolong repolarization times.

Inotropic and Hemodynamic Effects

In Vitro Effects

Sotalol and both of its isomers increased force development in canine ventricular trabecular muscle preparations stimulated at a frequency of 2 Hz.[22] An increase in force development was observed only in Purkinje strand preparations stimulated at slower frequencies. At a bath concentration of 10^{-6} M of racemic, d-, or l-sotalol, ventricular muscle mean force development was increased 20.0, 7.1, and 13.9 mg, respectively. These results are unlike those produced by other β adrenergic blockers and suggest that the inotropic effects of sotalol are related primarily to its effects on APD.

The effects of sotalol and propranolol on contractile activity have been assessed on the isolated cat papillary muscle.[59] Sotalol produced a 13% increase in force development at concentrations of 10^{-4} and 10^{-3} M, while propranolol had only negative inotropic effects at concentrations of more than 10^{-6} M. The positive inotropic effects of sotalol were maintained despite catecholamine depletion or prior α or β blockade. Propranolol caused a reduction in adenylate cyclase activity of myocardial extracts of the cat at concentrations of higher than 10^{-9} M, with an increasingly greater effect above 10^{-4} M. In contrast, sotalol produced a small (9%) but significant increase in adenylate cyclase activity at 10^{-5} M and did not produce depression until concentrations exceeding 10^{-4} were attained.

The positive inotropic effects of sotalol and its isomers are directly related to their Class III effects on APD prolongation.[1,2] It is clear that agents that increase APD, regardless of structure or mechanism, are also capable of causing positive inotropic activity.[60] Occasionally, there are reports where sotalol or its isomers do not have any positive inotropic effect in isolated cardiac tissue[20,61] but this is probably a result of blocking some β receptors activated by norepinephrine release from suprathreshold stimulating currents.[20]

In Vivo Hemodynamic Effects

Studies in anesthetized dogs indicated that intravenous doses of sotalol from 0.075 to 10 mg/kg decreased heart rate, depressed contractile force, reduced total peripheral resistance, dilated the systemic arterial bed, and reduced systolic pressure without an alteration in diastolic pressure.[10] The heart rate and contractile force changes appeared to be the result of an attenuation of normal levels of adrenergic tone because suppression was greatest following the lowest and least following the highest administered doses of sotalol. When infused at a constant slow rate of 0.31 mg/kg per minute rather than given by bolus injections, sotalol had no effect on cardiac output, mean arterial blood pressure, calculated peripheral resistance, or pulmonary resistance in the anesthetized dog, and actually increased stroke volume while decreasing heart rate.[10]

Measurements of blood flow in select vascular beds of the dog indicated that 0.14–8.7 mg sotalol administered intra-arterially increased femoral blood flow and decreased calculated peripheral resistance without altering mean arterial blood pressure.[10] Coronary flow, coronary vascular resistance, heart rate, contractile force, and mean arterial perfusion pressure were not altered subsequent to intracoronary injections of sotalol over a dose range of 0.017–4.4 mg.

In anesthetized baboons, 1, 2, or 4 mg/kg sotalol was administered orally.[62] The changes evoked by isoproterenol after sotalol administration were significantly lower for coronary flow, cardiac output, heart rate, left ventricular (LV) pressure, LV dP/dt, aortic pressure, and the rate-pressure product. In contrast, the changes in renal blood flow, stroke volume, and stroke work index were not significantly different. β-Blockade with sotalol, moreover, had no inherent effect on renal blood flow. The reduction of coronary blood flow was associated with a reduction in the rate-pressure product; that is, myocardial oxygen consumption. However, the oxygen supply-demand relationship was maintained. The recorded decrease in cardiac output was due largely to a reduction in heart rate because stroke volume and LV stroke work index were unaffected by β blockade as a result of sotalol administration.

In a comparative assessment of drug effect on renal function, intravenous administration of sotalol (3 mg/kg ± 3 mg/kg per hour), propranolol (0.3 mg/kg ± 0.3 mg/kg per hour), or nadolol (0.1 mg/kg ± 0.1 mg/kg per hour) produced no statistically significant alterations in urine flow, urine sodium excretion, or glomerular filtration rate in volume expanded in dogs anesthetized with pentobarbital.[63] At the dose administered, sotalol had no consistent effect on effective renal plasma flow, whereas propranolol significantly decreased this variable. The administration of nadolol at a higher dose (1 mg/kg ± 1 mg/kg per hour) significantly reduced urine flow,

urinary sodium excretion, and effective renal plasma flow. Over the range of doses administered, these three β blockers thus appeared to have distinct, qualitatively different effects on renal function. The relative order of negative properties was nadolol > propranolol > sotalol.

Canine models including intact anesthetized dogs,[11] an aortic shunt model,[12] and a heart-lung preparation[64] were utilized for direct comparative assessments between sotalol and propranolol on peripheral hemodynamics and cardiac function. Over a broad range of intravenous doses, sotalol (0.5–16 mg/kg), like propranolol (0.0625–2 mg/kg), decreased contractile force, heart rate, and the rate-dependent variables of myocardial function in both nonpretreated and atropine/reserpine-treated dogs anesthetized with chloralose.[11] In both groups of animals, sotalol consistently evoked more marked negative chronotropic effects than propranolol and, as a consequence, lowered calculated systolic ejection period to a greater extent. Mean arterial blood pressure, aortic flow, computed LV minute work, and LV dP/dt were depressed to equivalent degrees by both β-blocking agents in both groups of animals. The alterations in minute flow and minute work indicate that sotalol's effects appeared to be exclusively rate related because both stroke volume and stroke work remained at or above control at all drug levels. The fall in minute output and minute work variables following propranolol, in contrast, appeared to result from a composite of both rate slowing and a decrement in stroke capacity.

Left ventricular end diastolic pressure (LVEDP) remained essentially unchanged from control (in nonpretreated dogs) or was decreased below basal levels (in catecholamine depleted animals) after administration of sotalol, whereas increases in LVEDP were consistently noted after administration of propranolol. Computed peripheral resistance was increased by both agents, the change after sotalol being uniformly greater at comparable β-blocking levels in both nonpretreated and reserpine treated dogs. In terms of the determinants of oxygen utilization, these data suggested that sotalol produced a substantial depression in myocardial wall tension per minute as the primary result of a reduction of heart rate. Change in wall tension, stress, and maximum LV dP/dt, in association with a reduction of heart rate, would all tend to operate in the same direction following sotalol, that is, toward a lowering of the oxygen required to maintain an adequate level of cardiac output.

At equiactive β-blocking doses, propranolol promoted greater decreases in both right ventricular contractile force and LV dP/dt and more marked elevations in LVEDP than sotalol in a canine aortic bypass model in which aortic flow, aortic pressure, and heart rate were maintained constant.[12] In contrast, sotalol produced more profound slowing of heart rate. Propranolol evoked an essentially equivalent pattern of responses even in aortic shunt preparations using dogs in which baseline sympathetic stimulation of the heart had been removed by pretreatment with reserpine. In a similar study population, sotalol produced less compromise of myocardial performance.

Thus, in both the presence and the absence of baseline sympathetic regulation of cardiac function, for a given decrease in heart rate, propranolol caused greater depression in myocardial contractility (as interpreted from changes in LV dP/dt and LVEDP) than did sotalol (Figure 8). Comparisons of responses at equiactive β-blocking doses in reserpine pretreated shunt preparations with fixed heart rates clearly indicated that sotalol produced less nonspecific depressant effects on myocardial contractility than propranolol.

In chloralose anesthetized dogs, cumulative doses of 30 to 10,000 mg/kg intravenous of d-sotalol had no effect on blood pressure, LV pressure, LVEDP, or LV dP/dt.[65] Heart rate was slightly, but significantly reduced at doses of 3,000 and 10,000 mg/kg. Similarly, after β blockade with propranolol in anesthetized dogs, d-sotalol in doses of 1, 4, and 10 mg/kg intravenous had no effect on blood pressure, LV systolic and end-diastolic pressures, LV dP/dt, stroke volume, cardiac output, or total peripheral resistance.[66] Once again, heart rate decreased from 159 ± 9 to 133 ± 7 beats per minute after the highest dose.

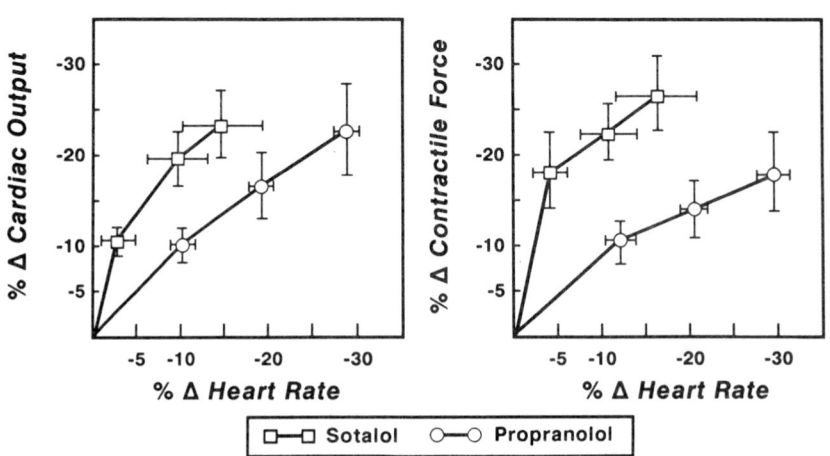

Hemodynamic Effects of Sotalol vs. Propranolol in Reserpine - Treated Atropinized Dogs

Figure 8. Percentage reductions in aortic flow (left) and contractile force (right) at the simultaneously recorded percent decreases in heart rate after sotalol (0.5, 2, and 8 mg/kg intravenously). (Reproduced with permission from Reference 11.)

In rats, after myocardial ischemia (3×4 minutes of asphyxia with intermittent 4 minutes of reoxygenation), infusion of d-sotalol (2 mg/kg) reduced LV pressure (to $58 \pm 5\%$), dP/dt (to $21 \pm 3\%$), stroke volume (to $66 \pm 6\%$), ejection fraction (to $62 \pm 7\%$), and cardiac output (to $51 \pm 6\%$). dl-Sotalol at the same dose had similar effects.[67] Whether these effects of sotalol are a species effect or a consequence of the ischemic damage is unknown.

Pharmacokinetics of Sotalol and d-Sotalol

The pharmacokinetic profile of sotalol is unique among β adrenoceptor antagonists. Unlike other agents, sotalol is virtually 100% bioavailable because it is completely absorbed and not metabolized (Table 4). Also, sotalol is very hydrophilic and does not bind to plasma proteins. In addition, sotalol does not accumulate in the brain, and consequently clinical central nervous system side effects are rare.[68,69]

Sotalol is excreted unchanged primarily by the kidneys. Since the drug is 100% bioavailable, is not metabolized, and is not bound to plasma proteins, variations in serum concentration are very small, the plasma half-life is very long (15 hours), and plasma levels are linearly related to dose. Table 4 summarizes the clinical pharmacokinetic profile of sotalol.

Electrophysiological and Antiarrhythmic Correlates of Sotalol Action: Experimental Background

Numerous experimental and clinical reports document a broad range of antiarrhythmic effects in the case of dl-sotalol. The spectrum of its effects in arrhythmias is wider than that of conventional β blockers and may exceed that of d-sotalol, being a composite of its β-blocking as well as its effects on its voltage-dependent refractory period.[70]

Ventricular Arrhythmias

In anesthetized dogs, sotalol (0.125–2 mg/kg), nadolol (0.125–2 mg/kg), atenolol (0.5–8 mg/kg), and propranolol (1–16 mg/kg) given intravenously were equally effective in increasing the electrical threshold for induc-

Table 4
Summary of Clinical Pharmacokinetic Profile of Sotalol

Absorptive rate	T$_{MAX}$ 2–3 h
Extent of absorption	>80% of dose
Extent of bioavailability	~100% of dose
Binding to plasma protein	0%
Approximate volume of distribution	1.6–2.4 L/kg
Elimination	
Renal (unchanged)	~90%
Biotransformation	0%
Approximate plasma half-life	15 (7–18) hours
Pattern of elimination kinetics	First order
Kinetic model applicable	Open two compartment
Metabolites	None detected
Steady state/dose ratio	Twofold variation
Special features	Accumulation in renal failure, kinetics not affected by liver function

From Sundquist H: Basic review and comparison of β-blocker pharmacokinetics. *Curr Ther Res* 28:385, 1980.

tion of ventricular fibrillation (VF).[71,72] Efficacy in this model, however, failed to correlate with β-blocking potency. Electrophysiologically, sotalol, atenolol, and propranolol, but not nadolol, significantly increased the myocardial ERP. Propranolol significantly increased excitation threshold and decreased myocardial conduction time, whereas neither sotalol, atenolol, nor nadolol affected either variable. Subsequent observations demonstrated that the weak β blocking d-isomers of both sotalol and propranolol were equipotent and equally effective as their respective parent racemates in increasing the VF threshold. The efficacious antifibrillatory actions of sotalol when compared with those of atenolol, nadolol, and propranolol consequently appeared to be attributable to something other than β adrenergic receptor blockade or specific alterations in the membrane properties of cardiac cells.

Other investigators[73,74] have shown that d- and dl-sotalol increase ventricular fibrillation threshold (VFT) both in normal and ischemic tissues. The lack of correlation between β adrenoceptor antagonism as well as antifibrillatory actions of sotalol with its ability to increase VFT suggests that VFT may not be a useful predictor of a drug's antiarrhythmic activity. Interestingly, both d- and dl-sotalol decrease defibrillation energy requirements in pentobarbital, enflurane, and pentanyl anesthetized dogs,[75] an effect associated with an increase in VERP.

Sotalol protected mice against the arrhythmogenic actions of methylchloroform in the Lawson test.[76] The ED50 for sotalol given intraperitoneally 30 minutes prior to methylchloroform exposure was 24 mg/kg. Comparatively, by the same route, the values for propranolol and alprenolol were 1.7 and 19 mg/kg, respectively.

Sotalol at an intravenous dose of 10 mg/kg partially protected guinea pigs anesthetized with pentobarbital from the cardiotoxic actions of ouabain.[10] Sotalol pretreatment was found to be substantially more effective in protecting urethane anesthetized guinea pigs from ouabain-induced arrhythmias when the latter was administered intermittently (3.6 mg infused during 30 seconds every 2 minutes) followed by a stabilization/equilibration interval of 90 seconds (A. Gomoll, unpublished observation). In this model, significant protection was noted following an intravenous dose of 2 mg/kg sotalol given 5 minutes prior to commencement of ouabain administration. Comparable responses in terms of preventing or delaying the appearance of ventricular flutter/ventricular fibrillation and of increasing the ouabain dose required to reduce cardiac arrest were also observed following pretreatment with d-sotalol (8 mg/kg) or l-sotalol (0.5 mg/kg). The protective effects of sotalol were uniformly associated with a decline in basal heart rate and prolongation of QT interval. The reference agents amiodarone (10 mg/kg), propranolol (0.5 mg/kg), and to a significantly lesser extent, quinidine (10 mg/kg) were also effective in delaying or preventing ouabain-induced arrhythmias. In contrast, bretylium (10 mg/kg), was ineffective and appeared to exaggerate the toxic effects of ouabain in this guinea pig model.

The runs of uni- or multifocal VT (and associated occasional ectopic premature contractions) induced by the rapid intravenous administration of epinephrine (100 mg/kg) in anesthetized dogs were significantly reduced by intravenous pretreatment with 2 mg/kg sotalol 10 minutes prior to challenge.[77] Administration of 2–5 mg/kg intravenous sotalol 3–10 minutes prior to sensitization of the myocardium by intratracheal exposure to a hydrocarbon (halothane, methylchloroform, n-hexane) and subsequent intravenous injection of epinephrine was effective in protecting dogs from VF.[77-79] A similar protective effect was observed 10 minutes after the slow (10 minute) infusion of a 3- or 6-mg total dose of sotalol in the dog heart-lung preparation subsequently exposed to a combination of aerated halothane and epinephrine injection.[80] The duration of protection against fibrillation was sustained for an interval of 90–120 minutes following a single dose of sotalol in most preparations.

Sotalol displayed only weak antiarrhythmic activity against an established ouabain-induced tachyarrhythmia in the anesthetized dog[77–79] and canine heart-lung preparation.[80] In these investigations, intravenous doses of 10, 15, 20, or 25 mg/kg, were ineffective in converting VT to normal sinus rhythm. In each case, however, sotalol administration was associated with an increase in arrhythmia cycle length; that is, slowing of the repetitive rate. A similar fall of overall heart rate, in the absence of suppression of the arrhythmia, was also noted in the canine heart-lung preparation following infusion of a 50-mg total dose of sotalol.[80]

Slow intravenous infusion (0.25 mg/kg per minute) of sotalol to maximum levels of 15 mg/kg was efficacious in suppressing ectopic ventricular tachyarrhythmias in three of five conscious dogs studied (18–24 hours after two-stage ligation of the left anterior descending [LAD] coronary artery).[78] The average intravenous converting dose in responsive animals was 5.0 mg/kg. Comparatively, quinidine was effective in 5 of 5 animals at a mean intravenous dose of 9.1 mg/kg (range 5–18 mg/kg). In another series of conscious dogs, bolus intravenous injection of 10 mg/kg sotalol failed to suppress the premature ventricular contractions (PVCs) and runs of VT recorded during an observation interval 18–24 hours after total occlusion of the LAD.[77] Sotalol did, however, produce a perceptible slowing in overall heart rate.

The antiarrhythmic efficacy of sotalol was also evaluated in dogs anesthetized with pentobarbital subjected the previous day to a two-stage ligation of the LAD coronary artery.[81] Utilization of this canine model permitted the assessment of drug effects on not only spontaneous uni- and/or multifocal ectopic ventricular arrhythmias, but also dysrhythmias associated with aberrant conduction or reentrant excitation pathways. Quantification of ectopic/total beat ratios revealed that at cumulative intravenous doses of 2, 4, and 8 mg/kg, sotalol caused statistically significant dose related slowing (22%, 30%, and 36%, respectively) of total heart rate. The number of ectopic beats, however, was not consistently influenced. As a result, the percentage of total beats that were ectopic in character increased from a control level of 72% to 96% following administration of 8 mg/kg sotalol (Figure 9). In contrast, sotalol was highly effective in preventing the induction of reentrant ventricular tachyarrhythmias (Figure 9).

The efficacy of sotalol in abolishing dysrhythmias associated with aberrant conduction or reentrant excitation pathways was evaluated after both two-stage total occlusion of the LAD coronary artery[46,81] and a transient ischemic occlusion/reperfusion maneuver of that same artery. In 7 anesthetized dog studies 18–22 hours after total occlusion of the LAD, 2 were noninducible, 1 had sustained VT, and 4 displayed VT that degenerated into VF in response to provocative stimuli.[81] After the cumulative intravenous administration of 2, 4, and 8 mg/kg sotalol, both noninducible animals remained so throughout the course of repeated programmed electrical stimulation (PES) trials. The remaining inducible animals, however, were all less responsive and/or showed a dose related decrease in the severity of the arrhythmias evoked by critically timed stimuli. These changes were associated with significant increases (27%, 44%, and 52%, respectively) in the induced VT cycling after the sequential cumulative doses of sotalol.

In a model of postmyocardial infarction arrhythmias in conscious dogs, Cobbe et al.[46] found that ventricular arrhythmias were prevented by sotalol in 11 of 19 studies (58%) compared with 1 of 14 (7%) with metoprolol, which does not lengthen the APD. The salutary effect of sotalol could be correlated with the lengthening of the refractory period of the infarct zone, whereas metoprolol had no effect on this parameter, indicating that the antiarrhythmic effect of sotalol was not mediated solely through β blockade. These findings are also consistent with the findings of Euler et al.,[73] who found that intravenous sotalol significantly increased the VFT of both normal as well as ischemic myocardium in the anesthetized rat, whereas metoprolol had no effect on the VFT in the normal myocardium and merely prevented the decrease in VFT after

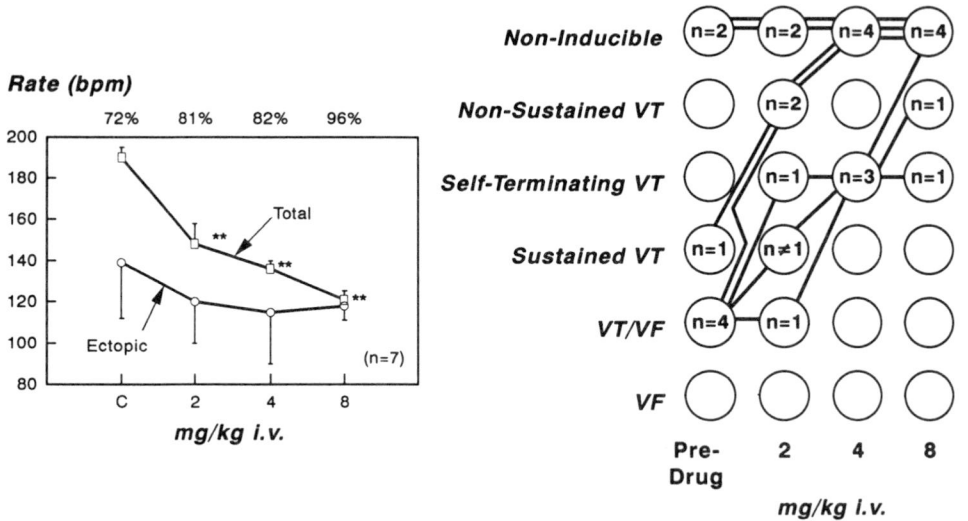

Figure 9. Top: Alterations in total heart rate and ectopic rate following the cumulative intravenous administration of 2, 4, and 8 mg/kg of sotalol in anesthetized dogs. Asterisks denote significantly different changes from control. Bottom: Ability of sotalol to reduce repetitive ventricular responses evoked by electrical stimulation. (Reproduced with permission from Reference 81.)

coronary artery occlusion. Again, these findings indicate the antifibrillatory and antiarrhythmic actions of sotalol in a variety of animal models, as emphasized by Patterson and Lucchesi.[72] The major effect appears to be mediated through the lengthening of the APD. Lynch et al.[47] recently found that 8 mg/kg of intravenous cumulative doses of the levo- as well as the dextroisomer suppressed induction of VT in their conscious canine ischemic model of sudden death in 50% of the dogs. At this dose, only the l-sotalol exerted an antiadrenergic effect such as lengthening the PR interval of the surface electrocardiogram, but both isomers produced equivalent increases of 15% to 20% in the VERP.

Culling et al.[82] found that sotalol prevented ventricular arrhythmias associated with myocardial ischemia and reperfusion in the isolated buffer perfused model of the guinea pig heart. In this preparation, ischemia was produced by reduction of flow to 10% for

30 minutes followed by reperfusion. However, the beneficial effect on the arrhythmia could not be accounted for by alterations in the measured electrophysiological parameters, such as refractoriness or the time course of the monophasic action potentials. During myocardial ischemia, sotalol has been shown to elevate myocardial pH in the canine heart,[82] and the drug's effect on its so-called Class III action is not negated by elevated extracellular potassium.[75]

Programmed electrical stimulation was also performed in conscious nonsedated dogs 4–7 days after 2-hour occlusion followed by reperfusion of LAD coronary artery.[48] During control observations, the resulting dysrhythmias consisted of nonsustained VT (n = 1), sustained VT (n = 5), and polymorphous VT degenerating into VF (n = 3). At cumulative intravenous doses of 2, 4, and 8 mg/kg, sotalol was efficacious in preventing the induction of repetitive responses in nine dogs during this subacute phase of myocardial infarction. Following administration of the highest dose, PES failed to produce reentrant ventricular arrhythmias in five animals and evoked only nonsustained VT in the remaining four. The mean increase in ventricular refractoriness (from 156 to 191 msec) recorded following 8 mg/kg sotalol prevented the induction of premature ventricular stimuli at coupling intervals previously producing ventricular arrhythmias despite the documented persistence of continuous diastolic electrical activity in the region of chronic myocardial injury.

Fatal VF occurred in 10 of 11 chloralose or pentobarbital anesthetized control (nondrug treated) dogs subjected to an acutely maintained one-stage occlusion of the LAD coronary artery.[45] The mean delay between occlusion and VF was 9 minutes with a range of intervals between 50 seconds and 19 minutes. In a second group of 10 dogs given 10 mg/kg intravenous sotalol 10 minutes prior to ligation, the typical infarction electrocardiographic patterns failed to occur in any animal. All members of the sotalol pretreatment group survived for periods of more than 30 minutes; death, when it occurred, supervened as a result of progressive AV block in most animals.

The prevention of sudden cardiac death in dogs is not related to β adrenoceptor blockade since d-sotalol was just as effective[71] as dl-sotalol (Figure 10). In addition, other β blockers such as pindolol and celiprolol were ineffective in this model.[59] Finally, Class I antiarrhythmic agents such as flecainide are not effective in reducing sudden cardiac death whereas dl-sotalol has dramatic preventive actions (Figure 11).

Application of an anodal current to the intimal surface of the circumflex coronary artery of conscious dogs previously subjected

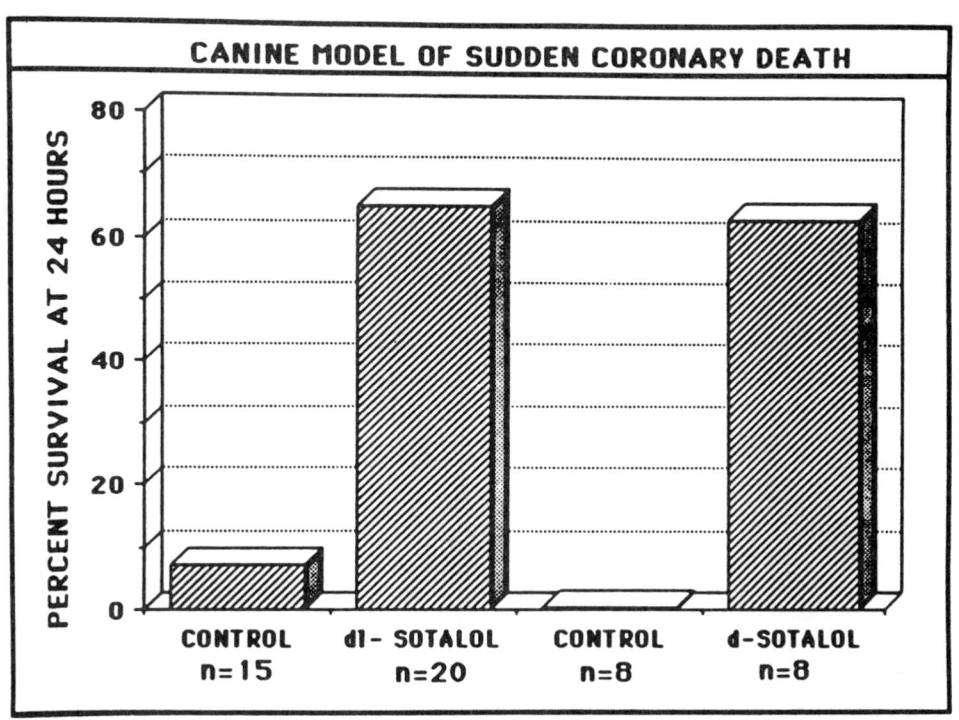

Figure 10. Effects of d- and dl-sotalol upon survival for 24 hours in a canine model of sudden coronary death. (Reproduced with permission from Reference 71.)

Conscious Canine Model of Sudden Cardiac Death

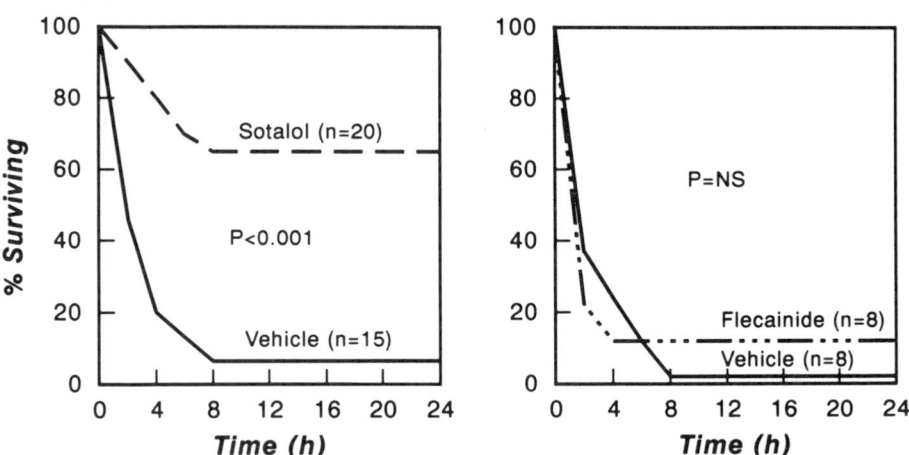

Figure 11. Comparison of the ability of dl-sotalol (left) and flecainide (right) to alter survival for 24 hours in a canine model of sudden cardiac death. (Reproduced with permission from Reference 48.)

to occlusion/reperfusion of the LAD coronary artery provoked spontaneous VF.[48] The sequence of events was analogous to that thought to occur during sudden death. In the absence of pretreatment, only 1 of 15 (7%) animals survived. Pretreatment with sotalol at intravenous doses of 2 (n = 7) or 8 (n = 13) mg/kg decreased the incidence of VF and increased survival at 24 hours to 13 of 20 (65%). Composite electrograms recorded from the anterior and posterolateral surfaces of the heart demonstrated the rapid development of activation delays over the latter area(s) with the appearance of ischemic ST segment changes. Sotalol did not alter the development of these epicardial conduction delays. These results, like others demonstrating the antiarrhythmic (and antifibrillatory) actions of sotalol, suggested that the drug produced its salutary effects by virtue of an ability to prolong the ERP of the myocardium without altering ventricular conduction velocity.

Antifibrillatory Actions in the Atria

Finally, there are data that suggest that the antifibrillation effects of dl-sotalol are not confined to ventricular tissue. For example, sotalol was highly efficacious in abolishing atrial fibrillation induced by topical application of aconitine to the right atrium.[10,78] When infused at a rate of 0.25 mg/kg per minute, sotalol fully converted 3 of 5 animals to normal sinus rhythm and provided improvement or partial protection in the remaining 2 dogs at an average total intravenous dose of 3.2 mg/kg.[78] At a slower infusion rate (50 mg/kg per minute intravenously) in another study, sotalol reduced the atrial rate, but not the ventricular rate of dogs displaying aconitine-induced atrial arrhythmias.[10] Also in this study, atrial flutter produced by electrical stimulation or the local injury stimulation technique was effectively suppressed by intravenous administration sotalol at doses of 1–10 mg/kg in anesthetized dogs.[10]

In a comparison of d-sotalol, quinidine and lidocaine, Feld et al.[83] found that d-sotalol restored sinus rhythm in 14 of 15 (93%) dogs with atrial flutter (induced by an intercaval crush and rapid atrial pacing) whereas quinidine was effective in 9 of 15 (60%) and lidocaine in 2 of 10 (20%). d-Sotalol also prevented reinduction in 8 (53%) whereas quinidine was effective in 4 (27%) and lidocaine in none. Prolongation of atrial refractoriness was the crucial determinant of both conversion and prevention of reinduction of atrial flutter.

In another dog model of atrial flutter, several Class I agents (disopyramide, flecainide, propafenone, and SC-40230) were very effective in terminating the arrhythmia as was d-sotalol. However, the Class I agents acted by markedly increasing cycle length whereas d-sotalol prolonged refractoriness.[84] Of particular interest, Bertrix et al.[85] measured the fibrillation threshold in canine ventricle and atria concurrently with the amplitude and duration of the monophasic action potential, ERP, the conduction time in the contractile fibers, and the fibrillation rate once fibrillation had been triggered. Sotalol increased the fibrillation threshold in association with an increase in the duration of the action potential and the ERP. The fibrillation rate slowed but conduction time did not change. The overall changes were more striking in the case of the atria (than in the ventricles) in which vulnerability to fibrillation had been enhanced by acetylcholine (presumably by reversing the cholinergically mediated shortening of the APD and refractoriness). Sotalol antagonized the changes induced by acetylcholine. Experimental data thus provide a compelling basis for the antiarrhythmic and antifibrillatory effects in a broad spectrum of supraventricular and ventricular arrhythmias especially in the case of dl-sotalol. The data for d-sotalol is less secure.

Clinical Antiarrhythmic Spectrum of Sotalol in Supraventricular Arrhythmias

Because sotalol is a β blocker, it is likely to be as effective as conventional β blockers in reducing atrial extrasystoles and other ectopic atrial tachycardias, in slowing sinus tachycardia, and the ventricular response in atrial flutter and fibrillation, in terminating reentrant supraventricular tachycardia and in controlling the recurrence of a proportion of such arrhythmias during prophylactic drug administration. The antifibrillatory effects of sotalol due to its Class III action is likely to make it more effective in maintaining sinus rhythm in patients with atrial fibrillation and flutter following cardioversion. The experience of Teo et al.,[86] showing a 100% response demonstrated as conversion of paroxysmal supraventricular tachycardia (PSVT) with intravenous bolus administration of sotalol indeed suggests that this might be the case. This figure appears to be unusually high however; the current trend now is in favor of adenosine as first-line therapy for its extremely high efficacy, ultrashort elimination half-life and the transient nature of its side effects.

As far as the antifibrillatory effects of sotalol in the atria are concerned, the data from a study of Brugada et al.[87] are of interest. They demonstrated that at a dose of 1.5 mg/kg intravenous sotalol significantly prolonged the right and left atrial refractory periods. The degree of prolongation was significant although they were not obtained at heart rates that may be relevant to the cycle lengths of most of the supraventricular arrhythmias encountered in clinical practice. However, preliminary observations suggests that, unlike most β blockers, intravenous sotalol will convert many patients with atrial fibrillation and flutter into sinus rhythm and maintain stability of sinus rhythm after pharmacological or electrical conversion. Orally administered sotalol is also likely to be more effective than conventional β blockers in preventing recurrences of PSVT, both with AV nodal reentry and those with accessory pathways. One might also expect sotalol to be of use in the control of atrial flutter and fibrillation in patients with Wolff-Parkinson-White syndrome. It must be pointed out, however, that in the prevention of most PSVT, drug therapy is now being superseded by electrode catheter ablation with radiofrequency energy. Thus, as far as the role of sotalol in atrial arrhythmias are concerned, the major role is likely to be in the acute and the chronic treatment of atrial flutter and fibrillation.

Atrial Flutter and Fibrillation

Sotalol has been studied both after intravenous administration to convert atrial flutter and fibrillation to sinus rhythm and in oral regimens to prevent recurrences of these arrhythmias during chronic prophylaxis. These studies have not been adequately controlled, nor have they employed techniques to study dose-response relationships.[86,88,89] There have been variable conversion rates, but a slowing of the ventricular rates have been consistent as might be expected for a β blocker.[70] The maintenance of sinus rhythm after conversion is potentially of greater practical importance.

Antman et al.[90] recently studied 74 patients with symptomatic chronic recurrent atrial fibrillation unresponsive to conventional Class I antiarrhythmic agents (1 to 5 drugs with a median of 2 drugs). The design of the study was such that the effects of stepped care treatment with propafenone, sotalol, and amiodarone was evaluated in alleviating the symptoms by controlling ventricular rate and/or conversion to sinus rhythm. Sotalol was highly effective (72% success rate) in maintaining sinus rhythm in patients with chronic atrial fibrillation previously refractory to Class Ia antiarrhythmic agents. Although at 6-month follow-up only 41% of the 74 patients were free from atrial fibrillation while receiving propafenone, a total of 72% of patients receiving sotalol remained free from atrial fibrillation.

The effects of oral sotalol in maintaining sinus rhythm after direct current conversion were recently evaluated and compared with quinidine in a large multicenter Swedish clinical trial.[91] In this study, 183 patients with chronic atrial fibrillation were randomized to receive sotalol (98 patients) or quinidine (85 patients) 2 hours after conversion to sinus rhythm with direct current conversion. Patients randomized to sotalol initially received 80 mg b.i.d. dosage for 1 week, after which, if needed, the dose could be increased to 160 mg twice daily. For patients assigned to quinidine, slow release preparation of quinidine sulphate was administered in 600 mg b.i.d. dosage. At the end of the 6-month study period, 49 of 95 (52%) patients randomized to sotalol were still in sinus rhythm compared to 38 of 79 (48%) patients receiving quinidine. Although some patients were receiving digitalis, the presence or absence of digitalis therapy did not significantly alter the success rate in the two groups of patients. At 1 month, 39 patients were receiving 80 mg of sotalol twice a day and 50 patients were receiving 160 mg twice a day. Sixty-four percent of patients on 80-mg dose and 50% of the patients receiving the 160-mg dose were in sinus rhythm at 6 months. In patients with relapse into atrial fibrillation while on treatment with sotalol and digitalis, the ventricular rate decreased from 80 to 68 beats per minute ($p < 0.03$) compared with the baseline recording before direct current conversion. In patients treated with digitalis in the quinidine group, the ventricular rate increased from 80 to 109 beats per minute ($p < 0.02$) compared to baseline. Compared to sotalol, a significantly greater number of patients receiving quinidine experienced overall adverse drug reaction as well as the need to withdraw from the study due to intolerable side effect. In patients treated with sotalol, 27 of 97 patients (28%) reported side effects compared with 43 of 86 patients (50%) in the group treated with quinidine ($p < 0.01$). The overall withdrawal rate for intolerable side effects or recurrence of atrial fibrillation was 11% for sotalol patients compared with 27% for patients treated with quinidine ($p < 0.03$). Two patients (one in each treatment group) had proarrhythmic events in the early phase of treatment, while the patients were still in the hospital. The results of this prospective clinical trial are interesting on several counts. First, the results demonstrated no significant differences between the numbers of patients maintained in sinus rhythm after 6 months of sotalol or quinidine treatment given after successful direct current cardioversion. Second, the patients treated with quinidine had a significantly greater incidence of adverse drug experience and a large percentage (27%) of them were withdrawn due to intolerable side effects of recurrence of atrial fibrillation. Finally, during recurrence of atrial fibrillation, patients treated with sotalol and digitalis maintained a slow ventricular response whereas those receiving quinidine and digitalis had an increase in their ventricular response during the recurrence. These findings clearly suggest that sotalol is not only equally effective in maintaining sinus rhythm after direct current conversion in patients with chronic atrial fibrillation, but it is also better tolerated than quinidine in the chronic treatment of these patients. These results are particularly noteworthy in view of the recent findings from meta-analysis performed by Coplen et al.[92] that indicated that in patients with atrial fibrillation, chronic therapy with quinidine is associated with increased mortality. Although not fully established, it is thought that the increased mortality is most likely secondary to the proarrhythmic effects of quinidine. In the study by Juul-Moller et al.[91] the effects of sotalol or quinidine on cardiac mortality could not be evaluated because there was no placebo group. The overall efficacy of sotalol in maintaining sinus rhythm compared to low dose amiodarone (see Chapter 34) remains unknown but is of much importance in light of the emerging data indicating a high degree of efficacy of amiodarone in this setting.

Sotalol in Paroxysmal Supraventricular Tachycardia

The effects of sotalol in a variety of PSVTs (reentrant or ectopic) have been evaluated in several studies, but controlled studies have been few. In the acute conversion of reentrant PSVTs, the precise role of the drug is uncertain as no blinded comparative studies against established therapy (eg, intravenous verapamil or adenosine) have been carried out. A recent publication[93] summarized the findings of seven open trials using intravenous sotalol (0.4–1.5 mg/kg) in the acute management of patients with PSVT. Of the 106 patients studies in these trials, 47 (46%) patients converted to

sinus rhythm. The results of electrophysiological studies in six clinical trials demonstrated that administration of intravenous sotalol (0.6 to 2.75 mg/kg) prevented reinduction of sustained PSVT in 44 of 75 (59%) patients. However, predictive accuracy of the acute response for the long-term effects of the drug remains unclear.

Manz et al.[94] studied the effects of intravenous sotalol (80 mg) in 11 patients with the Wolff-Parkinson-White syndrome and in 9 patients with AV nodal reentrant PSVT. Sotalol prolonged the ERP of the right atrium and ventricle with a delay in conduction in the AV node and bypass tracts in the anterograde as well as retrograde directions. The tachycardia rate was slowed from 182 to 153 beats per minute and the ventricular rate during atrial fibrillation slowed from 148 to 112 beats per minute. Sotalol exerted a depressant effect in all parts of the reentrant circuit including the atrium, ventricle, AV node, and bypass tracts. Thus, the data indicate that the drug is likely to be effective in preventing the rapid ventricular response to atrial fibrillation in patients with Wolff-Parkinson-White syndrome as well as in preventing reciprocating tachycardias. In a recent study[95] of 22 patients with the Wolff-Parkinson-White syndrome resistant to multiple conventional drugs, the effects of sotalol were evaluated during electrophysiological study as well as long-term prophylactic therapy. Sustained reciprocating tachycardia was rendered noninducible in 13 of 18 patients with inducible tachycardia during the electrophysiological evaluation. The anterograde as well as retrograde effective periods of accessory pathways were significantly prolonged by 20% and 28%, respectively. The long-term therapy during a follow-up period ranging from 1 to 47 months revealed a 77% success rate in controlling symptomatic tachycardia. Again, these salutary effects of the drug need to be considered in light of the emerging data on electrode catheter ablation of these arrhythmias, a technique that is highly effective in providing a cure in the majority of cases of reentrant PSVT with or without bypass tracts (see Chapter 45) although the long-term effects of the invasive procedure requires continued surveillance.

Antiarrhythmic Spectrum of Sotalol in Ventricular Arrhythmias

As in the case of supraventricular arrhythmias, the overall effects of sotalol in the entire spectrum of ventricular arrhythmias needs to be considered relative to the β-blocking properties of the drug along with its clearly demonstrated Class III actions. It might be possible to delineate the relative significance of the two actions by directly comparing the therapeutic effects of dl-sotalol with those of d-sotalol. Currently, such data are not available. The bulk of the discussion that follows deals with the efficacy of dl-sotalol.

Suppression of Premature Ventricular Contractions

In most of these studies, there was a significant decrease in PVCs in about 50% of the patients.[37,89] Anderson[96] recently reported sotalol to be effective in 59% of the patients versus 11% in placebo. Liddell et al.[97] found that 67% of patients responded to sotalol (in doses up to 640 mg/day) compared to 39% responding to procainamide in a multicenter crossover design protocol. Deedwania[98] found a higher degree of PVC suppression by sotalol compared to propranolol for the same degree of β blockade. Whether such a difference can be attributed to the Class III action of sotalol remains an attractive possibility that requires confirmation.

Impact of Sotalol in Survivors of Acute Infarction

It is now well established that β blockade given prophylactically after the index event reduces mortality at 1 year by 18% to 47% in different trials (see Chapter 28). Such an effect could not be related to the associated proper-

ties such as local anesthetic effects or cardioselectivity but could be correlated with the degrees of reduction in heart rate.[99] Although a reduction in mortality was also seen in the case of sotalol,[100] the figure of 18% did not reach statistical significance. Because of the associated Class III action of the drug, one might have expected a greater impact on mortality than that effected by conventional β blockers. The precise reason for such a discrepancy is uncertain. However, a number of factors might have contributed to the lower impact on mortality. The trial design used 60:40 randomization scheme; the dose of the drug was fixed and it is possible that a number of patients had been given potassium wasting diuretics in the early stages of the trial. Indeed, the survival curves indicated a slight excess in deaths during the early phases of the study suggesting a proarrhythmic (torsades de pointes) reaction to the drug. Finally, the patients were not selected for high risk on the basis of ambient arrhythmias in which the Class III action of the drug might have exerted a greater beneficial effect. Clearly, these are speculations and it is unlikely that a trial with sotalol in infarct survivors will be repeated. The impact of the Julian trial[100] may need to be interpreted in light of the data on sotalol in patients with VT/VF.

Sotalol in Patients With Symptomatic VT/VF and in Those With Aborted Sudden Death

The role of sotalol in treating patients with recurrent VT/VF and in those with survivors of sudden death began to be evaluated in early the 1980s.[57,101] An interest in the Class III actions of the drug stemmed from reports on the effects of amiodarone—another Class III agent—in recalcitrant VT/VF (see Chapters 30 and 34).

Two systematic unblinded studies[57,101] have provided the initial data on the efficacy of sotalol in controlling refractory VF/VF. These studies however were conducted with only double stimuli during therapy guided by PES.

Senges et al.[101] performed electrophysiological testing in 18 patients before and after administration of an intravenous 1.5 mg/kg dose of sotalol with double stimuli for VT/VF induction. In this study, sotalol prevented reinduction of the tachycardia in 12 of 18 patients (67%). The effect on inducibility was not systematically related to the lengthening of the QTc interval. Nine of these 12 patients were given oral sotalol, and 4 other patients were given another regimen. Of these 13 patients, 12 had successful long-term effects and 1 had partial response over a mean follow-up period of 16 months (range 89 to 24 months). Heart failure or sinus node dysfunction developed in 3 patients during the early months of treatment. The investigators concluded that sotalol's overall antiarrhythmic response was not typical of β blockers; they related sotalol's observed effects to its property of prolonging repolarization.

Nademanee et al.[57] found that sotalol prevented inducible VT in 43% of patients given the drug intravenously. They studied 37 patients (36 men, 1 woman; mean age 58 years, range 25 to 72 years) with clinically sustained recurrent VT/VF. None had a reversible cause of ventricular arrhythmias but all but one had coronary disease. The mean left ventricular ejection fraction (LVEF) in 23 patients was 33.0 ± 14.0%. Patients were excluded who exhibited contraindication to β blockade or evidence of decompensated cardiac failure. Two patients whose VT could not be induced at baseline were also excluded. Of the 35 patients who had undergone electrophysiological testing, 33 had inducible VT/VF. A 1.5 mg/kg intravenous dose of sotalol prevented VT/VF reinduction in 15 patients (45.5%). Twenty-five of the 33 patients (15 had positive results and 10 had negative results on electrophysiological testing) were given oral sotalol (dose range of 160–460 mg twice a day).

The clinical outcome of patients with inducible versus noninducible VT/VF were evaluates after intravenous and subsequent oral sotalol therapy. Intravenous sotalol prevented inducible VT/VF in 15 patients. Oral sotalol controlled the arrhythmias in 13 of

these patients (86.7%). Sotalol had no effect early (within the first month) in 1 patient and appeared to aggravate the condition in another. During chronic therapy (longer than 1 month), the arrhythmia recurred in 2 patients (at 8 and 8.4 months, respectively); adverse effects precluded continued use of the drug in another 2 patients. Eight patients remained arrhythmia free and had no adverse effects during a mean follow-up period of 14.5 ± 7.5 months (range 2 to 23 months). Sotalol was unable to suppress VF/VF in 18 patients. Of these, 10 were given oral sotalol; the other 8 were not treated with sotalol because they did not have significant VPCs on baseline ambulatory electrocardiographic recordings. Six of the 10 who were given oral sotalol had recurrent VF/VF and 1 had a limiting adverse effect, despite the inducible VT after intravenous sotalol. The remaining 3 patients have been free of arrhythmias (mean follow-up period 8.6 months, range 8 to 9 months). The 6 patients treated with 160 mg of oral sotalol twice a day had mean plasma levels of 2.3 ± 0.8 μg/mL. The 3 patients treated with 320 mg of oral sotalol twice a day had mean plasma levels of 3.1 ± 0.4 μg/mL.

Patients in this study were also analyzed for their response to sotalol in terms of suppression of ventricular arrhythmias documented on Holter recordings. A significant concordance for the predictive accuracy for long-term outcome between the Holter technique and the PES was found. However, no definitive conclusions regarding the relative merits of the two techniques in this regard can be made on the basis of such a small sample size.

Steinbeck et al.[102] performed programmed ventricular stimulation and ambulatory ECG monitoring during therapy with sotalol in 39 patients with inducible ventricular tachyarrhythmias (sustained VT in 31, VF in 3, and nonsustained VT in 5 patients). Oral sotalol was started at 80 mg twice a day and then gradually increased until a mean daily dose of 300 mg (range 160–480 mg) was reached. In 12 of 34 patients with inducible sustained VT/VF the arrhythmias were suppressed; all 5 patients with nonsustained VT had complete suppression during sotalol therapy. Thus, 17 of 39 patients (44%) had a favorable electrophysiological response during therapy with sotalol. Nonresponders had a higher incidence of previously ineffective drug trials. In 22 patients treated long term with sotalol the suppression of arrhythmia inducibility predicted freedom from recurrences (16 of 17 responders), whereas continued inducibility indicated drug failure (5 of 5). Unlike the observations of Nademanee et al.,[57] the results of serial Holter monitoring did not correlate with the results of electrophysiological testing.

Kienzle et al.[103] evaluated the efficacy of oral sotalol in 9 patients with sustained VT who had inducible VT while receiving quinidine or procainamide. Eight patients had coronary disease with remote myocardial infarction and 1 had cardiomyopathy. During sotalol therapy (average daily dose 600 ± 103 mg) none of the patients had inducible VT during the repeat electrophysiological study. Five of the 8 chronically treated patients had no recurrence of VT during a mean follow-up of 23 months; sudden cardiac death occurred in 1, and 2 patients had nonfatal VT recurrence. The results indicate that in patients refractory to type I agents procainamide and quinidine, sotalol is effective in suppressing serious ventricular tachyarrhythmias.

In the study by Kopelman et al.[56] the electrophysiological effects of intravenous and oral sotalol were prospectively evaluated in 16 patients with ≥ 1 episode of clinically documented sustained VT in the absence of acute myocardial infarction. All patients had ischemic heart disease, the majority (63%) had severe left ventricular dysfunction (LVEF < 30%) and most patients had drug-induced refractory VT. Nine patients received intravenous sotalol and 11 were given oral sotalol. Both intravenous and oral sotalol caused significant increases in sinus cycle length, AH interval, AV nodal refractoriness, as well as prolonged the atrial and right VERPs. Although induction of sustained VT was only prevented in 22% of patients receiving intravenous sota-

lol and 18% of those on oral sotalol, the cycle length of VT significantly increased during both forms of therapy. The slowing of VT rate was accompanied by an increase in the mean arterial blood pressure. These results suggest that even if sotalol is not effective in preventing the induction of sustained VT, it may be of therapeutic benefit by slowing the VT rate and thus preventing the associated hemodynamic consequences. Singh[104] reported the results of sotalol therapy evaluated by electrophysiological testing and ambulatory ECG recordings in 16 patients with recurrent sustained VT or nonfatal cardiac arrest. The patients were refractory to an average of 4.8 conventional antiarrhythmic agents. At baseline, sustained VT was inducible in 12 of the 14 patients tested. Treatment with oral sotalol (320–960 mg daily) completely suppressed the sustained VT in 7 patients (58%) and modified the VT response in 3 (25%) additional patients. During a mean follow-up of 19 ± 7 months, 12 of the 14 patients receiving longterm sotalol therapy remained clinically free of sustained VT. Only 1 of 14 patients suffered sudden cardiac death. No significant adverse effects were observed during therapy with sotalol.

The results of these small-scale trials have been consistent with the results of larger trials conducted in patients with life-threatening ventricular tachyarrhythmias.[105–110] In the study by Gonzalez et al.,[105] 50 patients (43 sustained VT and 7 VF) resistant to a mean of 2.8 ± 1.4 conventional antiarrhythmic drugs were treated with sotalol, and 45 underwent invasive electrophysiological testing before and after sotalol therapy. Twenty-two of the 45 patients had complete or partial response to sotalol therapy; arrhythmia could not be induced in 10 patients and was slower and hemodynamically better tolerated in 12 patients. Twenty-five patients received long-term sotalol therapy during which there was no recurrence of clinical VT in the group with noninducible arrhythmia on the drug. Thirty-seven percent of patients with inducible VT had recurrence of clinical VT or sudden death during the follow-up. Proarrhythmic effects were observed in 2 of the 4 patients with QT interval > 600 msec. Based on these findings, the investigators concluded that sotalol is an effective therapy for the subset of patients with sustained VT unresponsive to type 1A drugs. The concordance between the response during electrophysiological testing and lack of recurrence during long-term follow-up suggest that response during electrophysiological testing is highly predictive of drug efficacy in responders. The findings of this study are supported by a subsequent report by Ruder et al.[106] In this study, 65 patients with symptomatic drug refractory sustained VT or VF were treated with oral sotalol (80 to 480 mg twice a day). Although 11 patients were discontinued in the beginning due to lack of efficacy, the clinical effectiveness of long-term sotalol therapy could be evaluated in the remaining 54 patients followed for 11.5 ± 6 months. The actuarial incidence of successful sotalol therapy as 54 ± 13% at 6 months, and 47 × 13% at 12 months. In 39 patients who had repeat electrophysiological studies while receiving sotalol, the arrhythmia was noninducible in 8 (20%) patients. Exacerbation of ventricular arrhythmia was observed in 6 patients (9%), including one patient in whom there was associated hypokalemia. Their findings and conclusion were almost identical to those previously reported by Gonzalez and co-workers,[105] and confirm the effectiveness of sotalol in drug resistant, sustained ventricular tachyarrhythmias. However, it should be emphasized that none of the studies cited above were controlled or used a comparator agent.

Controlled Studies With Sotalol in VT/VF

In a recent multicenter double-blind, randomized crossover study[107] the effects of intravenous sotalol and procainamide were compared in patients with recurrent VT/VF who had inducible arrhythmia during baseline electrophysiological testing. Forty-nine patients were randomized to treatment with procainamide and 54 were assigned to receive

sotalol. Intravenous administration of procainamide prevented induction of VT/VF in 11 patients (20%), compared to 30% response rate with intravenous sotalol. This difference did not, however, reach statistical significance. A small number of these patients followed for 12 months on the effective drug showed a trend in the event rate in favor of sotalol compared to procainamide.

Perhaps the most important controlled study recently completed is the so-called Electrophysiological Versus Electrocardiographic Monitoring (ESVEM) Study in which the relative merits of the two techniques in predicting long-term drug responses in patients with symptomatic VT/VF and those surviving cardiac arrests were determined.[108] From over 2,100 patients screened, 486 patients satisfied the predetermined entry criteria. They were randomized to Holter-guided therapy (n = 244) and to PES-guided therapy (n = 242). The drug therapy tested in a randomized fashion were six Class I agents and sotalol; drug trials were positive in 14% of the PES groups and 38% in the Holter limb with the result that of the responders (n = 297), 45% eventually had their therapy selected by PES and 77% by Holter. The patients were followed for 6 years. Two important observations emerged from ESVEM. The first indicated no statistical significance between the PES and Holter monitoring in terms of arrhythmia recurrence, sudden death, cardiac or total mortality. The second finding was that sotalol was a more effective antiarrhythmic agent than Class I agents when considered individually or collectively. At 1 year, arrhythmia recurrence was found in 44% of patients given Class I agents and 21% in those given sotalol ($p < 0.0007$). A number of conclusions may be drawn from these findings. It appears that the responses demonstrated in ESVEM might be interpreted as drug specific rather than technique specific (see Chapter 47), sotalol being more effective than Class I agents because of its unique pharmacological properties, combining as it does β-blocking properties and Class III actions. However, from these studies it cannot be concluded that Class I agents are superior to no treatment or to placebo since ESVEM could not address this fundamental issue. Indeed, in the absence of a concurrent control, the same criticism may apply to the results with sotalol. Conversely, sotalol produces β blockade which in virtually all subsets of patients produces a beneficial effect on mortality (see Chapters 17 and 47). It is also noteworthy that a recent study has indicated that β blockade with metoprolol given empirically produced effects no different from therapy guided by PES in patients with inducible monomorphic VT in the setting of clinically symptomatic arrhythmias.[109] It would appear that since sotalol was significantly more effective than Class I agents in ESVEM when considered in light of the overall data on Class I agents, it will become increasingly difficult to justify the continued use of sodium channel blockers in the prophylactic treatment of VT/VF (see Chapter 47).

Potential Role of d–Sotalol as an Antiarrhythmic Agent

The precise role of d-sotalol remains to be defined. To date, the available data does not permit definitive conclusions. However, theoretical considerations permit certain tentative conclusions. For example, the fact that the drug exerts minimal β-blocking activity, it exhibits little or no negative inotropic actions. Thus, it is likely to be safer in patients with congestive heart failure dependent on sympathetic stimulation for compensation. Another important advantage of d-sotalol is the lack of so-called β blocker side effects. Similarly, the fact it produces less bradycardia (which may be due to markedly attenuated β-blocking actions and/or the direct effects on the sinus node by prolonging the APD), d-sotalol is likely to induce a lower rate of torsades de pointes. These clearly beneficial effects may need to be considered in relation to the possibility that the loss of β-blocking actions in the dextroisomer may be associated with a corresponding reduction in the overall efficacy as antifibrillatory effects in the case of ventricular arrhythmias in terms of effects of PVCs, inducibility of VT/VF, and possibility survival. These are critical issues that can be addressed only by controlled comparisons with dl-sotalol.

Adverse Reactions with Sotalol

The adverse reactions due to sotalol may be attributed to its β-blocking actions and to its propensity to lengthen repolarization. Side effects due to β blockade (fatigue, lassitude, impotence, depression, headache) are similar to those exhibited by other β antagonists. Barring the occurrence of torsades de pointes, the cardiovascular effects are predictable on the basis of the drug's propensity to block β receptors. However, uncontrolled clinical data suggests that the proclivity of the drug to induce or exacerbate congestive heart failure is less than that with conventional β blockers. It is presumed that the Class III actions of the drug tends to negate or reverse the intrinsic depressant effects of blocking the sympathetic nervous system.[37] The major cardiovascular adverse reaction is the occurrence of torsades de pointes.

Sotalol–Induced Torsades de Pointes

Although sotalol has significant antiarrhythmic effects,[57,101,110] it has been also reported to be associated with life-threatening ventricular arrhythmia. This is especially likely in the setting of renal failure, hypokalemia and bradycardia at high concentrations of the drug and also in situations when there is preexisting lengthening of the QTc interval.[111–122] Neuvonen and co-workers[118,119] have reported a correlation between the serum sotalol concentration and prolongation of the QTc interval.

Severe ventricular arrhythmias, including VT and VF, were initially reported in 5 of 6 cases of sotalol poisoning and correlated with the prolongation of the QTc interval and serum sotalol concentration.[118,119] Most other cases of torsades de pointes following sotalol therapy have also been observed with overdosage,[112,115,117,121,122] although a case was reported in the context of so-called therapeutic serum concentration, this patient was however using an additional inappropriate concomitant medication.[114] McKibbin et al.[118] reported a series of 13 patients who developed syncope and prolonged QT interval while taking therapeutic doses of sotalol. Polymorphous VT was observed in 12 patients and criteria typical of torsades of pointes were present in 10 patients. Interestingly, 12 of 13 patients in this series had been treated with a combination of sotalol and hydrochlorothiazide without adequate potassium supplementation which results in reduced serum potassium concentration. Four patients were also taking other drugs (3 on disopyramide and 2 on tricyclic antidepressants) known to cause prolongation of QT interval. The QT interval returned to normal in all patients after withdrawal of the drugs and the correction of the hypokalemia. Sotalol can induce life-threatening ventricular arrhythmias, particularly when given in combination with hydrochlorothiazide without potassium supplementation. However, when the dose of the drug is kept low and the patient's electrolyte (especially potassium) status are monitored carefully, the incidence of torsades de pointes is low.[57,101] The use of sotalol in the setting of renal failure or with concomitant therapy with drugs known to prolong the QT interval (eg, quinidine, disopyramide, phenothiazines or tri- and tetracyclic depressants) is not advisable due to greater risk of proarrhythmia and when absolutely necessary it should only be done under close medical supervision.

The risk of torsades de pointes in patients with ventricular arrhythmia has been described in several recent studies.[110,123] In the study by Kehoe et al.,[110] 236 patients with sustained ventricular tachyarrhythmias were treated acutely with sotalol and 151 received long-term oral sotalol therapy. Seven of 18 patients (7%) developed proarrhythmia, 17 during the acute phase and 1 during long-term follow-up. Eleven patients had torsades de pointes and most proarrhythmic events occurred within 7 days of therapy. From the data in 181 clinical studies which enrolled 5,856 patients, 1,288 patients with ventricular arrhythmias were examined by Soyka et al.[93] for arrhythmogenic effects. The overall incidence of proarrhythmic events in these patients was 4.3% (56 patients) and 24 of the 56 patients had torsades de pointes. Although no universal relationship was found with previously described factors such as bradycardia, hypokalemia, and long QT interval, the patients with proarrhythmic events had longer mean QTc interval at baseline as well at 1 week during therapy with sotalol. The results of available studies also indicated that the overall risk of proarrhythmic events including torsades de pointes was greater in patients with sustained ventricular tachyarrhythmias, left ventricular dysfunction, marked bradycardia, and prolonged QT interval. Because most of the proarrhythmic events occurred within the first 7 days and in general responded to reduction in dosage or discontinuation of sotalol, it is advisable that the high-risk patients be hospitalized and given sotalol therapy under close supervision and continuous ECG monitoring.

While the occurrence and the incidence of torsades de pointes complicating sotalol therapy are well documented, the precise underlying mechanisms are less clearly defined.[124] Hiromasa et al.[31] showed that in the case of d-sotalol, large concentrations of the drug induced EADs that were abolished by the administration of verapamil. The data suggested that the charge carrier for the EADs is calcium. However, it is not known whether the concomitant administration of calcium channel blockers and Class III agents may result in a lower incidence of torsades de pointes than if the latter were given alone. Day et al.[125] reported in patients surviving myocardial infarction sotalol tended to decrease the degree of spatial dispersion of repolarization. In contrast, in another subset of patients, Cui et al.[126] found that sotalol had no effect on regional dispersion of repolarization whereas amiodarone, after prolonged treatment, markedly reduced it. Clearly, further studies are needed to determine the significance of dispersion versus the development of EADs as a basis for the development of torsades de pointes in the case of various Class III agents relative to sotalol.

Conclusions

The available, expanding experimental and clinical data indicate that sotalol (recently approved by the Food and Drug Administration for the treatment of life-threatening ventricular arrhythmias) is a unique antiarrhythmic agent combining potent nonselective β-blocking properties with propensity to prolong cardiac repolarization in all myocardial fibers. The negative inotropic effect due to β blockade is attenuated by its action potential lengthening effect. Its pharmacokinetics is simple with an elimination half-life of 10–15 hours. Its major electrophysiological profile constitutes the composite effects of β blockade with prolonged repolarization. Sotalol prevents inducible VT/VF in approximately 30%–40% of patients with a higher figure for the suppression of spontaneously occurring arrhythmias documented on Holter recordings. Therapy in VT/VF can be guided by either technique although the possibility is not excluded that empiric therapy might be equally valid. Sotalol exerts a potent antifibrillatory action modulated by its antiadrenergic effects. The compound therefore exerts broad spectrum antiarrhythmic actions in supraventricular and ventricular arrhythmias. The role of the dextroisomer of the compound remains unclear but the enantiomer provides an important electropharmacological probe for the determination or the relative merits of β blockade and lengthened repolarization in the control of cardiac arrhythmias.

Acknowledgments: We gratefully acknowledge Mary Jo Biedka and Diane Gertschen for their valued assistance with this chapter. This chapter relies substantively on previous publications by the authors on similar subject published as Singh BN: Antiarrhythmic actions of dl-sotalol in ventricular and supraventricular arrhythmias. *J Cardiovasc Pharmacol* 2:S75, 1992.

References

1. Antonaccio MJ, Gomoll AW: Sotalol: pharmacological and antiarrhythmic effects. *Cardiovasc Drug Rev* 6:239, 1988.
2. Antonaccio MJ, Gomoll AW: Pharmacology, pharmacodynamics and pharmacokinetics of sotalol. *Am J Cardiol* 65:12A, 1990.
3. Blinks JR: Evaluation of the cardiac effects of several β-adrenergic blocking agents. *Ann NY Acad Sci* 139:673, 1967.
4. Kaumann AJ, Blinks JR: Comparative potencies of β-adrenergic blocking agents on isolated heart muscle. *Fed Proc* 26:401, 1967.
5. Strauss HC, Bigger JT Jr, Hoffman BF: Electrophysiological and β-receptor blocking effects of MJ 1999 on dog and rabbit cardiac tissue. *Circ Res* 26:461, 1970.
6. Reid J, Duker G, Almpen O, et al: (+)-Sotalol causes significant occupation of β-adrenoceptors at concentrations that prolong cardiac repolarization. *Naunyn-Schmiedeberg's Arch Pharmacol* 341:215, 1990.
7. Manley BS, Alexopoulos D, Robinson GJ, et al: Subsidiary Class III effects of β-blockers? A comparison of atenolol, metoprolol, nadolol, oxprenolol and sotalol. *Cardiovasc Res* 20: 705, 1986.
8. Larsen AA, Lish PM: A new bio-isostere: alkysulphonamidophenethanolamines. *Nature (Lond)* 203:1383, 1964.
9. Lish PM, Weikel JH, Dungan KW: Pharmacological toxicological properties of two new β-adrenergic receptors antagonists. *Pharmacol Exp Ther* 149:161, 1965.
10. Stanton HC, Kirchgessner T, Parmenter K: Cardiovascular pharmacology of two new β-adrenergic receptor antagonists. *J Pharmacol Exp Ther* 149:174, 1965.
11. Gomoll AW, McKinney GR: Sotalol: cardiac and hemodynamic actions in the anesthetized dog. In: A Snart (ed): *Advances in β-Adrenergic Blocking Therapy-Sotalol.* Volume 1. Amsterdam: Excerpta Medica, 1974, p. 6.
12. Gomoll AW, Braunwald E: Comparative effects of sotalol and propranolol on myocardial contractility. *Arch Intern Pharmacodyn Ther* 205: 3438, 1973.
13. Lish PM, Shelanski MV, Labudde JA, et al: Inhibition of cardiac chronotropic action of isoproterenol by sotalol (MJ 1999) in rat, dog and man. *Curr Ther Res* 9:311, 1967.
14. Gomoll AW, Bartek MJ: Comparative β-blocking activities and electrophysiologic actions of racemic sotalol and its optical isomers in anesthetized dogs. *Eur Pharmacol* 132:123, 1986.

15. Antonaccio MJ, Gomoll AW: Pharmacologic basis for the antiarrhythmic and hemodynamic effects of sotalol. *Am J Cardiol* 72:27A, 1993.

16. Singh BN, Vaughan Williams EM: A third class of antiarrhythmic action. Effects on atrial and ventricular intracellular potentials, and other pharmacological actions on cardiac muscle of MJ 1999 and AH 3474. *Br J Pharmacol* 39:675, 1970.

17. Singh BN: *Pharmacological Actions of Certain Drugs and Hormones: Focus on Studies of Antiarrhythmic Mechanisms.* Oxford, United Kingdom: Hertford College, University of Oxford; 1971. D. Phil. Thesis., p. 43.

18. Carmeliet E: Electrophysiologic and voltage clamp analysis of the effects of sotalol on isolated cardiac muscle and Purkinje fibers. *J Pharmacol Exp Ther* 232:817, 1985.

19. Cobbe SM, Manley BS: Effects of elevated extracellular potassium concentrations on the Class III antiarrhythmic action of sotalol. *Cardiovasc Res* 19:69, 1985.

20. Tande PM, Refsum H: Class III antiarrhythmic action linked with positive inotropy: effects of the d- and l-isomer of sotalol on isolated rat atria and threshold and suprathreshold stimulation. *Pharmacol Toxicol* 62:272, 1988.

21. Berger F, Borchard U, Hofner D: Effects of (+)-sotalol on repolarizing outward currents and pacemaker current in sheep cardiac Purkinje fibers. *Naunyn-Schmiedeberg's Arch Pharmacol* 340:696, 1989.

22. Lathrop DA: Electromechanical characterization of the effects of racemic sotalol and its optical isomers on isolated canine ventricular trabecular muscles and Purkinje strands. *Can J Physiol Pharmacol* 673:1506, 1985.

23. Lathrop DA, Varro A, Schwartz A: Rate-dependent electrophysiological effects of OPC-8212: comparison to sotalol. *Eur J Pharmacol* 164:487, 1989.

24. Komeichi K, Tohse N, Nakaza H, et al: Effects of N-acetylprocainamide and sotalol on ion currents in isolated guinea-pig ventricular myocytes. *Eur J Pharmacol* 187:313, 1990.

25. Varro A, Nanasi PP, Lathrop DA: Effect of sotalol on transmembrane ionic currents responsible for repolarization in cardiac ventricular myocyte from rabbit and guinea pig. *Life Sci* 49:PL-7, 1991.

26. Gwilt M, Williams RC, Higgins AJ: Effects of action potential prolongation via different cellular mechanisms on the electrophysiological properties of rat and guinea pig ventricular myocardium. *Arch Intern Pharmacodyn* 312:66, 1991.

27. Lamontagne D, Rochette L, Vermeulen M, et al: Effect of sotalol against reperfusion arrhythmias in Sprague-Dawley and Wistar rats. *Fundam Clin Pharmacol* 3:679, 1989.

28. Sanguinetti MC, Jurkiewicz NK: Two components of cardiac delayed rectifier K^+ current. *J Gen Physiol* 96:195, 1990.

29. Courtney KR, Hill BC: Possible mechanisms for d-sotalol's effects on action potential duration and conduction velocity in myocardium. *Proc West Pharmacol* 33:1, 1990.

30. Kaumann AJ, Olson CB: Temporal relation between long-lasting aftercontractions and action potentials in cat papillary muscles. *Science* 161:293, 1968.

31. Hiromasa S, Coto H, Li Z-Y, et al: Dextrorotary isomer of sotalol: electrophysiologic effects and interaction with verapamil. *Am Heart J* 116:1552, 1988.

32. Lathrop DA, Varro A: Modulation of the effects of sotalol on Purkinje strand electromechanical characteristics. *Can J Physiol Pharmacol* 67:1463, 1989.

33. Lathrop DA, Varro A: The combined electrophysiological effects of lignocaine and sotalol in canine isolated cardiac Purkinje fibers are rate-dependent. *Br J Pharmacol* 99:124, 1990.

34. Varro A, Lathrop DA: Sotalol and mexiletine: combination of rate-dependent electrophysiological effects. *J Cardiovasc Pharmacol* 16:557, 1990.

35. Berman ND, Loukides JE: A comparison of the cellular electrophysiology of mexiletine and sotalol, singly and combined in canine Purkinje fibers. *J Cardiovasc Pharmacol* 12:286, 1988.

36. Berman ND, Wang L-Y, Ahmed A: The cellular electropharmacology of mexiletine combined with sotalol in porcine papillary muscle and Purkinje fiber. I. Alteration of mexiletine-induced V_{max} depression. *Can J Cardiol* 6:416, 1990.

37. Singh BN: Historical development of the concept of controlling cardiac arrhythmias by lengthening repolarization: particular reference to sotalol. *Am J Cardiol* 65(Suppl):3A, 1990.

38. Krikler DM, Curry PVL: Torsade de pointes, an atypical ventricular tachycardia. *Br Heart J* 38:117, 1976.

39. Laakso M, Aberg A, Savola J, et al: Diseases and drugs causing prolongation of the QT interval. *Am J Cardiol* 59:862, 1987.

40. Cobbe SM, Manley BS, Alexopoulos D: Interaction of the effects of hypoxia, substrate depletion, acidosis and hyperkalemia on the Class III antiarrhythmic properties of sotalol. *Cardiovasc Res* 19:668, 1985.

41. Cobbe SM: Modification of Class III antiarrhythmic activity in abnormal myocardium. *Cardiovasc Res* 22:847, 1988.

42. Hafner D, Berger F, Borchard U, et al: Electro-

physiological characterization of the Class III activity of sotalol and its enantiomers. *Arznei-mittelforsch* 38:231, 1988.

43. Cobbe SM, Manley BS, Alexopoulos D: The influence of acute myocardial ischemia on the Class III antiarrhythmic action of sotalol. *Cardiovasc Res* 19:661, 1985.

44. Hicks MN, Cobbe SM: Attenuation of the rise in extracellular potassium concentration during myocardial ischemia by d-,l-sotalol and d-sotalol. *Cardiovasc Res* 24:404, 1990.

45. Kaumann AJ, Aramendia P: Prevention of ventricular fibrillation induced by coronary ligation. *J Pharmacol Exp Ther* 164:326, 1968.

46. Cobbe SM, Hoffman E, Ritzenhoff A, et al: Action of sotalol on potential reentrant pathways and ventricular tachyarrhythmias in conscious dogs in the late post-myocardial infarction phase. *Circulation* 68:865, 1983.

47. Lynch JL, Wilber DJ, Montgomery DG, et al: Antiarrhythmic and antifibrillatory actions of the levo- and dextrorotary isomers of sotalol. *J Cardiovasc Pharmacol* 6:1132, 1984.

48. Patterson E, Lynch JL, Lucchesi BR: Antiarrhythmic and antifibrillatory actions of the β-adrenergic antagonist, dl-sotalol. *J Pharmacol Exp Ther* 230:519, 1984.

49. Lynch JL, Coskey LA, Montgomery DG, et al: Prevention of ventricular fibrillation by dextrorotary sotalol in a conscious canine model of sudden coronary death. *Am Heart J* 109:949, 1985.

50. Weissenburger J, Davy JM, Chezalviel F, et al: Arrhythmogenic activities of antiarrhythmic drugs in conscious hypokalemic dogs with atrioventricular block: comparison between quinidine, lidocaine, flecainide, propranolol and sotalol. *J Pharmacol Exp Ther* 259:871, 1991.

51. Nattel S, Feder-Elituv R, Matthews C, et al: Concentration dependence of Class III and β-adrenergic blocking effects of sotalol in anesthetized dogs. *J Am Coll Cardiol* 13:1190, 1989.

52. Echt DS, Bert LE, Clusin WT, et al: Prolongation of human cardiac monophasic action potential by sotalol. *Am J Cardiol* 50:1082, 1982.

53. Haywood RP, Taggart P: Effect of sotalol on human atrial action potential duration and refractoriness: cycle length dependency of Class III activity. *Cardiovasc Res* 20:100, 1986.

54. Touboul P, Atallah G, Kirkonian G, et al: Clinical electrophysiology of intravenous sotalol, a β-blocking drug with Class III antiarrhythmic properties. *Am Heart J* 107:888, 1984.

55. Blomstrom-Lundquist C, Dohmal M, Hirsch I, et al: Effect of long-term treatment with metoprolol and sotalol on ventricular repolarization measured by use of transesophageal atrial pacing. *Br Heart J* 555:181, 1986.

56. Kopelman HA, Woosley RL, Lee JT, et al: The electrophysiologic effects of intravenous and oral sotalol in patients with sustained ventricular tachycardia. *Am J Cardiol* 61:1006, 1988.

57. Nademanee K, Feld G, Hendrickson J, et al: Electrophysiologic and antiarrhythmic effects of sotalol in patients with life-threatening ventricular tachyarrhythmias. *Circulation* 72:55, 1985.

58. McComb JM, McGovern B, McGowan JB, et al: Electrophysiological effects of d-sotalol in humans. *J Am Coll Cardiol* 10:211, 1987.

59. Parmley WW, Robinowitz B, Chuck L, et al: Comparative effects of sotalol and propranolol on contractility of papillary muscles and adenyl cyclase activity of myocardial extracts of cat. *J Clin Pharmacol* 12:127, 1972.

60. Baskin EP, Serik CM, Wallace AA, et al: Effects of new and potent ethanesulfonanilide Class III antiarrhythmic agents on myocardial refractoriness and contractility in isolated cardiac muscle. *J Cardiovasc Pharmacol* 18:406, 1991.

61. Li T, Carr AA, Dage RC: Effects of MDL 11,939 on action potential and contractile force in cardiac tissue: a comparison with bretylium, clofilium and sotalol. *J Cardiovasc Pharmacol* 16:917, 1990.

62. Rogers GG, Rosendorff C, Shimell CJ, et al: Effect of peroral administration of sotalol on the hemodynamics of the baboon. *J Cardiovasc Pharmacol* 4:197, 1982.

63. Hanson RC, Deitchman D, Gomoll A: Renal effects of sotalol, propranolol and nadolol in anesthetized dogs. *Fed Proc* 39:521, 1980.

64. Cho YW, Hur Cho MM, Soito S: Blockade of cardiac calorigenic effect of epinephrine by sotalol (MJ 1999). *J Pharmacol* 24:49, 1974.

65. Wallace AA, Stupienski RF III, Brookes LM, et al: Cardiac electrophysiologic and inotropic actions of new and potent methanesulfonanilide Class III antiarrhythmic agents in anesthetized dogs. *J Cardiovas Pharmacol* 18:687, 1991.

66. Mortenson E, Toude PM, Klow NE, et al: Plasma concentrations and hemodynamic effects of d-sotalol after β-blockade in dogs. *Pharmacol Toxicol* 68:420, 1991.

67. Hoffmeister HM, Muller S, Seipel L: Effects of new Class III antiarrhythmic drug d-sotalol on contractile function of postischemic myocardium. *J Cardiovas Pharmacol* 17:581, 1991.

68. Schnelle K, Klein G, Schinz A: Studies on the pharmacokinetics and pharmacodynamics of the β-adrenergic blocking agent in normal man. *J Clin Pharmacol* 19:516, 1979.

69. Sundquist H: Basic review and comparison of β-blocker pharmacokinetics. *Curr Ther Res* 28:385, 1980.

70. Singh BN: Antiarrhythmic action of dl-sotalol

in ventricular and supraventricular arrhythmic. *J Cardiovasc Pharmacol* 2:590, 1992.

71. Lucchesi B, Lynch JJ: Preclinical studies on the antifibrillatory effects of sotalol and its optical isomers. In: BN Singh (ed): *Control of Cardiac Arrhythmias by Lengthening Repolarization.* Mount Kisco, NY: Futura Publishing Company, Inc., 1988, p. 245.

72. Patterson E, Lucchesi BR: Antifibrillatory properties of the β-adrenergic receptor antagonists nadolol, sotalol, atenolol and propranolol, in the anesthetized dog. *Pharmacology* 28:121, 1984.

73. Euler DE, Scanlon PJ: Comparative effects of antiarrhythmic drugs on the ventricular fibrillation threshold. *J Cardiovasc Pharmacol* 11:291, 1988.

74. Kwan YW, Solca AM, Gwilt M, et al: Comparative antifibrillatory effects of d- and dl-sotalol in normal and ischemic ventricular muscle of the cat. *J Cardiovasc Pharmacol* 15:233, 1990.

75. Wang M, Dorian P: dl- and d-Sotalol decrease defibrillation energy requirements. *PACE* 12:1522, 1989.

76. Hermansen K: Antifibrillatory effect of some β-adrenergic receptor blocking agents determined by new test procedure in mice. *Acta Pharmacol Toxicol* 28:17, 1970.

77. Somani P, Fleming JG, Ghan GK, et al: Antagonism of epinephrine-induced cardiac arrhythmias by 4-(2-isopropylamino-1-hydroxyethyl)-methanesulfonanilide (MJ 1999). *J Pharmacol Tox Ther* 151:32, 1966.

78. Schmid JR, Hanna C: A comparison of the antiarrhythmic actions of two new synthetic compounds, iproveratril and MJ 1999, with quinidine and pronethalol. *J Pharmacol Exp Ther* 156:331, 1967.

79. Sharma PL: Mechanism of action of a new adrenergic β-receptor antagonist IIU 1999 in the prevention of halogen-adrenaline-induced and ouabain-induced ventricular tachycardia in the dog. *Ind J Med Res* 55:1357, 1967.

80. Somani P, Lum BKB: Blockade of epinephrine- and ouabain-induced cardiac arrhythmias in the dog heart-lung preparation. *J Pharmacol Exp Ther* 152:235, 1966.

81. Gomoll A: Assessment of drug effects on spontaneous and induced ventricular arrhythmias in a 24-h canine infarction model. *Arzneimittelforsch* 37:387, 1987.

82. Culling W, Penny WJ, Sheridan DJ: Effects of sotalol on arrhythmias and electrophysiology during myocardial ischemia and reperfusion. *Cardiovasc Res* 18:397, 1984.

83. Feld GK, Venkatesh N, Singh BN: Pharmacologic conversion and suppression of experimental and canine atrial flutter: differing effects of d-sotalol, quinidine, and lidocaine and significance of changes in refractoriness and conduction. *Circulation* 74:197, 1986.

84. Spinelli W, Hoffman BF: Mechanisms of termination of reentrant atrial arrhythmias by Class I and CIass III antiarrhythmic agents. *Circ Res* 65:1565, 1989.

85. Bertrix L, Timour-Chah Q, Lang J, et al: Protection against ventricular and atrial fibrillation by sotalol. *Cardiovasc Res* 20:358, 1986.

86. Teo KK, Harte M, Horgan JH: Sotalol infusion in the treatment of supraventricular tachyarrhythmias. *Chest* 87:113, 1985.

87. Brugada P, Smeets JLRM, Brugada J, Farre J: Mechanism of action of sotalol in supraventricular arrhythmias. *Cardiovasc Drugs Ther* 4:619, 1990.

88. Prakash R, Parmaley WW, Allen HN, Matloff JM: Effects of sotalol on clinical arrhythmias. *Am J Cardiol* 29:397, 1972.

89. Fogelman F, Lightman SL, Sillett RW, McNicol MW: The treatment of cardiac arrhythmias with sotalol. *Eur J Clin Pharmacol* 5:72, 1972.

90. Antman EM, Beamer AD, Cantillon C, et al: "Stepped care": antiarrhythmic therapy for refractory symptomatic atrial fibrillation (abstract). *Circulation* 78:II-62, 1988.

91. Juul-Moller S, Edvardsson N, Ahlberg NR: Sotalol versus quinidine for the maintenance of sinus rhythm after direct current conversion of atrial fibrillation. *Circulation* 82:1932, 1990.

92. Coplen SE, Antman EM, Berlin JA, et al: Efficacy and safety of quinidine therapy for maintenance of sinus rhythm after cardioversion: a meta-analysis of randomized control trials. *Circulation* 82:1108, 1990.

93. Camm AJ, Paul V: Sotalol for paroxysmal supraventricular tachycardias. *Am J Cardiol* 100:921, 1990.

94. Manz M, Kuhl AJ, Luderitz B: Sotalol dei supraventricularer tachycardie elektrophysiologische Messungen bein Wolff-Parkinson-White Syndrom und AV-Knoten-reentrytachykardie. *Kardiologie* 74:500, 1985.

95. Scott Millar RN: Efficacy of sotalol in controlling reentrant supraventricular tachycardias. *Cardiovasc Drugs Ther* 4:625, 1990.

96. Anderson JL: Effectiveness of sotalol for therapy of complex ventricular arrhythmias and comparisons with placebo and Class I antiarrhythmic drugs. *Am J Cardiol* 65:37A, 1990.

97. Lidell C, Rehnqvist N, Sjogren A, et al: Comparative efficacy of oral sotalol and procainamide in patients with chronic ventricular arrhythmias: a multicenter study. *Am Heart J* 109:970, 1985.

98. Deedwania PK: Suppressant effects of conventional β-blockers and sotalol on complex and repetitive ventricular premature complexes. *Am J Cardiol* 65:43A, 1990.

99. Kjekshus J: Importance of heart rate determin-

ing β-blocker efficacy in acute and longterm myocardial infarction interventional trials. *Am J Cardiol* 57:43F, 1986.

100. Julian DG, Jackson FS, Prescott RJ, Szekely P: Control trial of sotalol for one year after myocardial infarction. *Lancet* 1:1142, 1982.

101. Senges J, Lengfelder W, Jauernig R, et al: Electrophysiologic testing of therapy with sotalol for sustained ventricular tachycardia. *Circulation* 69:577, 1984.

102. Steinbeck G, Bach P, Haberl R: Electrophysiologic and antiarrhythmic efficacy of oral sotalol for sustained ventricular tachyarrhythmias: evaluation by programmed stimulation and ambulatory electrocardiogram. *J Am Coll Cardiol* 8:949, 1986.

103. Kienzle MG, Martin JB, Wendt DJ, et al: Enhanced efficacy of oral sotalol for sustained ventricular tachycardia refractory to type I antiarrhythmic drugs. *Am J Cardiol* 61:1012, 1988.

104. Singh S: Sotalol for refractory sustained ventricular tachycardia and non-fatal cardiac arrest. *Am J Cardiol* 62:399, 1988.

105. Gonzalez R, Scheinman MM, Herre JM, et al: Usefulness of sotalol for drug-refractory malignant ventricular arrhythmias. *J Am Coll Cardiol* 13:1435, 1988.

106. Ruder MA, Ellis T, Lebsack C, et al: Clinical experience with sotalol in patients with drug-refractory ventricular arrhythmias. *J Am Coll Cardiol* 13:145, 1989.

107. Singh BN, Kehoe R, Woosley RL, et al: Multicenter trial of sotalol compared with procainamide in the suppression of ventricular tachycardia induced by programmed electrical stimulation: a double-blind randomized study, parallel evaluation. *Am J Cardiol* (submitted for publication).

108. Mason JW for the EVSEM Investigators: A comparison of electrophysiologic testing with Holter monitoring to predict antiarrhythmic drug efficacy for ventricular tachyarrhythmias. *N Engl J Med* 329:445, 1993.

109. Steinbeck G, Andersen D, Bach P, et al: A comparison of electrophysiologically-guided antiarrhythmic therapy with β-blocker in patients with symptomatic sustained ventricular tachyarrhythmias. *N Engl J Med* 327:987, 1992.

110. Kehoe R, Zheutlin T, Dunnington C, et al: Safety and efficacy of sotalol in patients with drug-refractory sustained ventricular tachyarrhythmias. *Am J Cardiol* 65:58A, 1990.

111. Singh BN: Safety profile of bepridil determined from clinical trials in chronic stable angina in the United States. *Am J Cardiol* 69:68D, 1992.

112. Elonen E, Neuvonen PH, Tarssanen L, Kala R: Sotalol intoxication with prolonged QT interval and severe tachyarrhythmias. *Br J Med* 1:1184, 1979.

113. Kontopoulos A, Filindris A, Manoudis F, Metaxias P: Sotalol induced torsade de pointes. *Postgrad Med* 57:321, 1981.

114. Krapf R, Gertsch M: Torsades de pointes induced by sotalol despite therapeutic concentrations. *Br Med J* 290:1784, 1985.

115. Laakso M, Pentikainen PH, Lampainen E: Sotalol, prolonged Q-T interval, and ventricular tachyarrhythmias. *Ann Clin Res* 13:439, 1981.

116. Laasko M, Pentikainen PH, Pyorola K, Neuvonen PJ: Prolongation of the Q-T interval caused by sotalol-possible association with ventricular tachyarrhythmias. *Eur Heart J* 2:355, 1981.

117. Laakso M, Pentikainen PJ, Pyorala K: Sotalol and QTc interval. *Lancet* 2:1168, 1981.

118. McKibbin JK, Pocock WA, Barlow JB, et al: Sotalol hypokalemia, syncope and torsade de pointes. *Br Heart J* 51:157, 1984.

119. Neuvonen PH, Elonen E, Vuorenmass T, Laasko M: Prolonged QT interval and severe tachyarrhythmia, common features of sotalol intoxication. *Eur J Clin Pharmacol* 20:85, 1981.

120. Neuvonen PH, Elonen E, Tanskanen A, Tuomilehto J: Sotalol prolongation of the QTc interval in hypertensive patients. *Clin Pharmacol Ther* 7:25, 1982.

121. Benton P, Sheriden J, Mulcahy R: A case of sotalol poisoning. *Irish J Med Sci* 151:126, 1982.

122. Montagna M, Groppi A: Fatal sotalol poisoning. *Arch Toxicol* 43:221, 1980.

123. Soyka LF, Wirz C, Spangenburg RB: Clinical safety profile of sotalol in patients with arrhythmias. *Am J Cardiol* 65:74A, 1990.

124. Singh BN: When is QT prolongation anti-arrhythmic and when is it pro-arrhythmic? *Am J Cardiol* 63:867, 1989.

125. Day CP, McComb JM, Campbell RWF: QT dispersion: an indication of arrhythmia risk in patients with long QT intervals. *Br Heart J* 63:342, 1990.

126. Cui G, Sen L, Uppal P, et al: Comparison of QT dispersion and RR interval induced by sematilide, amiodarone and sotalol (abstract). *Circulation* 86:I-393, 1992.

Chapter 34

Amiodarone: *Pharmacological, Electrophysiological, and Clinical Profile of an Unusual Antiarrhythmic Compound*

Bramah N. Singh

As an antiarrhythmic compound, amiodarone has drawn considerable attention in the last 10 years. In fact, in the minds of most clinicians who have used the compound as the last resort drug for the control of the most recalcitrant dysrhythmias, there now is a well-entrenched impression that the drug is the most effective agent in the prophylactic control of most supraventricular as well as ventricular arrhythmias. It is somewhat paradoxical that such an impression has been engendered without the benefit of blinded controlled clinical trials. The major shortcoming of the compound in its side effect profile. However, there now is increasing appreciation that at carefully monitored lower dose regimens, the drug can be used for long periods of times without the development of limiting side effects in many patients.

No other antidysrhythmic compound has stimulated as much interest because of an unusual degree of effectiveness. The properties of amiodarone have come under further scrutiny since the report of CAST results (see Chapter 26) that emphasized the proarrhythmic reactions of Class I agents and their potential to increase mortality (see Chapter 47). Data from placebo controlled trials[1,2] are now beginning to confirm the results of systematic but uncontrolled observations that initially formed the basis for the approval of the drug for controlling life-threatening ventricular arrhythmias when conventional therapy was deemed ineffective. However, the fundamental mechanism whereby amiodarone induces its salutary effects remains puzzling and essentially unknown. For this reason, the effects of the compound on cardiac electrophysiology relative to its associated pharmacological properties are of as much theoretical as well as practical importance. Experimental and clinical data need to account for the drug's:

(1) unusually high degree of antiarrhythmic efficacy, including its potential to prolong survival;

(2) very low proclivity to induce proarrhythmic reactions despite its significant Class

From BN Singh, HJJ Wellens, M Hiraoka, (eds): *Electropharmacological Control of Cardiac Arrhythmias.* Mount Kisco, NY, Futura Publishing Company Inc., © 1994.

I properties and the marked tendency to produce QT/QTc prolongation;

(3) powerful suppressant effect on premature ventricular contractions (PVCs) with a low efficacy for the prevention of ventricular tachycardia/fibrillation (VT/VF) induced by programmed electrical stimulation (PES);

(4) striking differences between acute and chronic pharmacological and therapeutic effects not readily accounted for by differences in drug plasma, tissue, or membrane levels;

(5) exceedingly long and variable plasma elimination half-life and perhaps even longer therapeutic half-life with a slow onset and offset of electrophysiological and therapeutic actions;

(6) propensity to produce striking bradycardia without competitively blocking β adrenoceptors;

(7) electrophysiological effects closely resembling those in hypothyroidism;

(8) complex pattern of multiorgan side effects with tissue specificity.

A detailed discussion of all these features falls outside the scope of this chapter. Only those features that are particularly germane to the theme of this monograph will be discussed at some length and will be integrated into an overall perspective; others will be mentioned merely for completeness.

Pharmacological Considerations

Despite expanding knowledge from recent experimental and clinical studies, there have been few insights into the complexity of the drug's broad-based electropharmacological profile. However, it is felt that a better understanding of the drug's fundamental mode of action mediating the observed changes it produces in the cardiovascular system relative to its therapeutic efficacy might provide insights for the development of the ideal antifibrillatory compounds of the future. This chapter highlights, within a brief compass, the current state of the data on the relevant properties of the drug and points to future directions. The focus is on the electropharmacology of the compound.

As in the case of numerous antiarrhythmic agents, the overall effects of amiodarone may result from its direct as well as indirect actions.[3,4] There are differences between its acute versus its chronic actions on cardiac muscle.[4] The acute effects have been studied in in vitro systems and have included effects on isolated multicellular preparations, perfused organs, isolated multicellular preparations, and enzymatically desegregated myocytes. The data from studies in such systems are difficult to interpret and may not be germane to the chronic actions of the drug, which are of the greatest utility in clinical therapeutics. Under these circumstances, the intrinsic electrophysiological effects are modified by the associated interactions of the drug on autonomic transmitters. These interactions will be discussed at first, followed by a brief mention of the inotropic, hemodynamic, and pharmacokinetic features followed by a reasonably critical presentation of the electropharmacology of the drug. This is designed to serve as a preamble to the discussion of the evolving role of the drug in controlling cardiac arrhythmias and in shaping the development of newer antiarrhythmic and antifibrillatory compounds.

Amiodarone and Autonomic Antagonism

The antiadrenergic effect of the drug has come into sharp focus with the demonstration that rate lowering β blockers remain the only class of antiarrhythmic agent's focus that consistently reduce mortality in controlled clinical trials.[5] Amiodarone reduces heart rate almost to the same extent as most β blockers during long-term drug administration (see Chapter 31). However, the basis for the antisympathetic actions of the drug is not well understood, but like β blockers, the drug may reduce mortality in survivors of myocardial infarction. Thus, the role of the drug's antiadrenergic properties may be of importance either acting directly or by influencing myocardial ischemia.

Experimental Observations

Polster and Broekhuysen[6] compared the effects of the competitive β-antagonist propranolol in isolated rabbit atria with those of amiodarone. For propranolol, the pA_2 value was 8.33. Noncompetitive β antagonism was found in the case of amiodarone with a pD_2 value of 4.17 against isoproterenol as agonist. The drug also exhibited a noncompetitive antagonism to α receptors in rat aortic strips induced to contract by norepinephrine. For phentolamine the pA_2 value was 8.69, the pD_2 value for amiodarone being 4.06. Amiodarone had no effect on calcium permeability in this preparation, in contrast to its calcium channel blocking effect in the sinus node and cardiac muscle. Thus, the mechanisms of the peripheral and coronary vasodilator effects of the drug and those mediating the changes in the sinus node and atrioventricular (AV) nodes differ. Such a tissue specificity of action is characteristic of amiodarone in contrast to most other antiarrhythmic agents.

Charlier[7] found that in anesthetized animals, amiodarone produced bradycardia that was not influenced by β-receptor blockade. Although amiodarone in vitro decreases cholinergic receptors in the rat heart and brain,[8] in in vivo studies the drug produced bradycardia that was resistant to atropine.[9,10] On amiodarone, bradycardia develops gradually as a function of time on a constant dose,[11,12] coincident with a decrease in myocardial β adrenoceptors.[13–15] This has also been found in the case of desethylamiodarone, the principal active metabolite of amiodarone.[15] There is evidence that the effect is somewhat greater after chronic than acute amiodarone or desethylamiodarone administration. Of interest, Sharma et al.[14] found that amiodarone had no effect on α adrenoceptors but the findings have not been consistent. For example, in in vitro systems

Polster and Broekhuysen[6] found the drug to exhibit noncompetitive effects against α- and β-catecholamine receptors. In rat heart membrane preparations, Gagnol et al.[16] found amiodarone to noncompetitively antagonize the activation of adenylate cyclase by isoproterenol, glucagon, and secretin but not by sodium fluoride. Thus, the antisympathetic effects of amiodarone stem from the inhibition of the coupling of β receptors with the regulatory unit of the adenylate cyclase complex. Alternatively, it might be due to a decrease in the number of functional β receptors at the myocardial cell surface; this is consistent with the in vivo effects of amiodarone in attenuating the positive chronotropic actions of catecholamines.[16] In sum, these properties will lead to bradycardia following long-term treatment as has been demonstrated in conscious[7] or anesthetized dogs[11] and in the spontaneously beating atria of chronically treated rabbits.[9] Bacq et al.[17] found that amiodarone inhibited neurotransmitter overflow from the spleen induced by electrical stimulation of the splenic nerve, indicating that an adrenergic blocking action of the drug at high doses might contribute to the drug-induced bradycardia. As indicated elsewhere, none of these properties of the drug accounts for the degree of bradycardia it produces nor the temporal evolution of the effect as a function of time. A tenable hypothesis is one that a component of the drug-induced bradycardia may stem from a cardiospecific inhibition of thyroid hormone action.[9]

Antiadrenergic Actions in Humans

In line with the experimental observations,[9] bradycardia as a function of time in patients converted from atrial fibrillation to sinus rhythm was noted by Olsson et al.[18] and in patients with ischemic heart disease by Pritchard et al.[19] It develops in nearly all patients given the drug chronically. Sarma et al. (see Chapter 31) found that chronically administered amiodarone markedly attenuates the circadian rhythmicity of heart rate. The peak effect was reached in approximately 3 months. The precise mechanism is unclear and no single factor appears to account for the degree of heart rate reduction observed. It may be multifactorial, encompassing noncompetitive adrenergic inhibition, action potential lengthening in the sinoatrial (SA) node, calcium channel blocking effect, and possibly cardiospecific hypothyroidism. A role for an effect on the pacemaker current can also be invoked but experimental verification of such a possibility methodologically would be extremely difficult since it is an effect that is seen after long-term therapy. Heart rate reduction by amiodarone may be of importance in mediating its salutary effects in controlling ventricular arrhythmias.

Hemodynamic Effects of Amiodarone

Very little data are available on the inotropic effects of amiodarone in isolated cardiac muscle. Because the drug does block the inward calcium current, some reduction in cardiac contractility might be expected. Unlike sotalol and other Class III agents (see Chapter 30), amiodarone does not significantly lengthen the action potential duration (APD) during acute superfusion studies nor during intravenous infusion. Thus, it is unlikely to exert a positive inotropic effect by this mechanism unlike the case of pure Class III agents. Conversely, the intravenous administration of the drug does produce peripheral and coronary vasodilator effects. Therefore, as indicated previously[20] the net hemodynamic effects of the drug derives from a complex interplay of simultaneous alterations in preload, afterload, ventricular contractility, and heart rate. This may be further modified in ischemia since the drug increases coronary blood flow and exerts a cardioprotective effect. Clearly, the overall effect will also depend on the dose of the drug, rate of its infusion, and the degree of ventricular dysfunction. In 5% aqueous solutions, intravenous amiodarone (2.5–10 mg/kg) reduced heart rate and blood pressure, depressed systemic vascular resistance, and increased coronary blood flow. However, the drug did not reduce cardiac output; at the highest dose it increased the left ventricular end-diastolic pressure and reduced the left ventricular dP/dt. This pattern of effects in open chest anesthetized dogs[20,21] have also been found in humans although in human studies the intravenous formulation used contained Tween 80. This vehicle itself exerts some depressant effects on systemic hemodynamics.[22] The drug increased cardiac output and decreased the left ventricular filling pressure while decreasing systemic and coronary vascular resistance.[23]

During long-term drug administration, there is no significant fall in the left ventricular ejection fraction determined by radionuclide ventriculography even in patients with severely depressed baseline ejection fractions. In uncontrolled studies, there appears to be an increase in the left ventricular ejection fraction.[4] The drug has been used to control arrhythmias in cardiac failure in patients with markedly reduced myocardial function or even in those with manifest cardiac decompensation.[24–30] This is in line with the observation that amiodarone is well tolerated in patients with heart failure awaiting cardiac transplantation and has been safely used in a number of clinical trials in patients with heart failure.[31] Nevertheless, there are anecdotal cases in which amiodarone has aggravated cardiac failure; this may result from impaired diastolic function.[32] Conversely, several small trials in heart failure have not suggested a major depressant effect of the drug; controlled data on this issue is likely to become available from a large placebo controlled mortality study in progress in patients with heart failure[33] and in patients with depressed left ventricular ejection fraction.

Amiodarone Pharmacokinetics

Only salient features will be summarized here.[34–37] Amiodarone is well absorbed with a bioavailability between 22% and 86%, is highly protein bound, is metabolized extensively in the liver, and at least one active metabolite (desethylamiodarone) has been pharmacologically characterized. The major pathway of excretion is the biliary tract with little or no renal excretion. The elimination half-life of the drug varies between 15 and 110 days and that of the metabolite is even longer. Amiodarone is an amphophilic compound. There is reasonable linearity between plasma drug concentrations and dose of amiodarone and the plasma level of the drug in patients successfully treated with amiodarone usually range between 1.5 to 2.5 μg/mL; desethylamiodarone level rises as a function of time and may either approximate those of the parent compound or may exceed them. In experimental studies, no relationship between electrophysiological effects and serum, and tissue or sarcolemmal drug levels has been established.[15] Moreover, the differences between the acute and chronic electrophysiological effects of the drug is not accounted for by differing plasma drug levels.[36] In humans, there does not appear to be a significant correlation between plasma drug levels and drug efficacy or the incidence of adverse reactions. There is however some evidence that in the case of drug-induced organ toxicity higher tissue levels of the metabolite than those of the parent compound are found. The main pharmacokinetic features of amiodarone are listed in Table 1. Desethylamiodarone is electropharmacologically active with a similar pattern of onset and offset effects; thus, while the metabolite may contribute substantially to the overall effects of the parent compound, it does not appear to account for the delayed onset of action of amiodarone. A terminal elimination half-life of 24.8 ± 11.7 days was reported by Holt et al.[34] after a 400-mg intravenous dose in healthy volunteers. In the case of amiodarone a clear distinction needs to be made between drug elimination half-life and the drug's pharmacodynamic and therapeutic half-life. As discussed in Chapter 31, the effects on heart rate does not reach peak effects for several months and in the case of the QT/QTc, steady-state effects may not be evident for periods of a year or more. Amiodarone remains unique in having the propensity for interacting pharmacokinetically and pharmacodynamically with an extensive list of drugs which are metabolized in the liver.[15] Among others, this includes digoxin, coumadin, diphenylhydantoin, quinidine, procainamide, N-acetylprocai-

---

Table 1
Clinical Pharmacokinetic Profile of Amiodarone

Absorption rate	T_{MAX}: 2–12 h (lag time, 0.4–3 h)
Extent of absorption	Poor and slow
Bioavailability	Variable (22%–56%)
Protein binding	96.3% ± 0.6%
Volume of distribution	1.3–65.8 L/kg (acute)
Elimination	Negligible renal excretion
Biotransformation	Hepatic and intestinal
Elimination half-life	3.2–20.7 h (acute); 13.7–52.6 days (chronic)
Total body clearance	0.10–0.77 liters/min
Pattern of elimination kinetics	First order
Metabolites	Major: mono *N* desethylamiodarone;
	Minor: bis-*N* desethylamiodarone, deiodinated metabolites
Therapeutic plasma range	1–2.5 μg/mL
Dose schedule	Once daily
Special factors	Slow onset and offset of action

namide, verapamil, and to a lesser extent, propafenone and flecainide.

On Defining the Electrophysiological Profile of Amiodarone

In characterizing the electrophysiological profile of amiodarone, it must be stressed that when the drug is given intravenously to experimental animals and humans, the electrophysiological effects are much less striking than those noted after long-term administration at a constant dose over long periods. There is much evidence that amiodarone exhibits all four or five electrophysiological classes of action[15]; they are most readily demonstrated during steady-state drug administration. However, it is not clear whether such electrophysiological features stem from independent actions in terms of the molecular structure of the compound or whether they arise as a result of an overall metabolic effect the drug might produce as a function of time. The evidence is compelling for this being so at least in the case of the long-term effects of the drug on the myocardium. This issue is discussed at the end of this chapter.

Effects on the Transmembrane Potentials in Multicellular Preparations

The details of the early studies of amiodarone's complex electrophysiological actions[39] are presented in Chapter 30. In the very first study designed to elucidate the long-term effects of the drug in rabbits,[9] there was a significant slowing of the sinus rate with a striking increase in the APD in atrial and ventricular muscle (Figure 1). There was only a modest depressant effect (about 10%) on the upstroke velocity of phase 0 when the preparations were stimulated at a fixed stimulation frequency. In contrast, at the end of 6 weeks of drug administration there was a 30% increase in the APD.

Subsequent studies have greatly enlarged our understanding of the drug's electrophysiological effects in vitro. Ikeda et al.[39] confirmed the effects on the APD lengthening in atrial and ventricular muscle in rabbits in whom they also found a significant lengthening of the APD in the AV node, with lesser change in the SA node (Figure 2). Similar observations have been reported by other investigators[40] in different animal species. When the amiodarone effects were tested acutely in

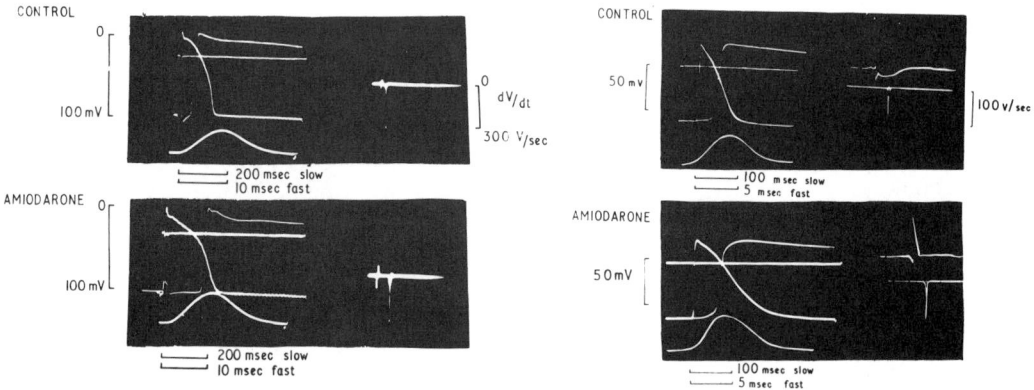

Figure 1. Effects of long-term amiodarone treatment on the transmembrane potentials in ventricular (left) and atrial (right panels) myocardium in the rabbit. In the right part of each panel, the upper trace shows 0 potential; middle trace, the action potential at slow and fast sweep speeds; and lower trace isometric tension. In the left part of each panel, $\dot{V}_{max}$ is shown. Note amiodarone lengthens the APD in ventricular as well as atrial action potential. (Reproduced with permission from Reference 12.)

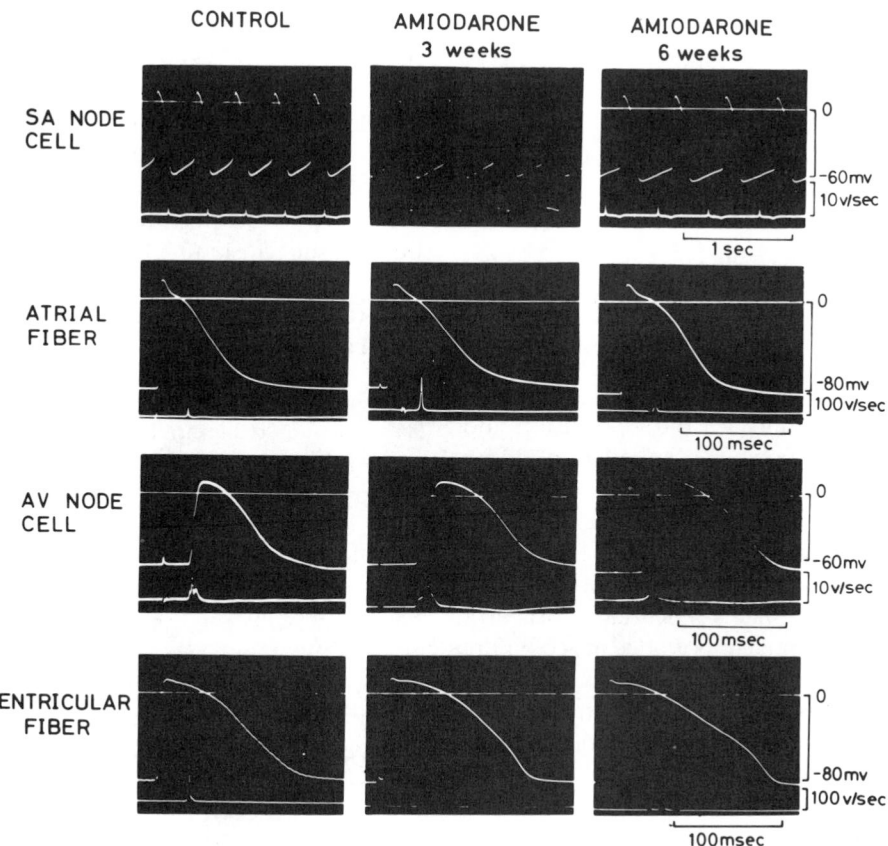

Figure 2. Effects of long-term amiodarone treatment on transmembrane action potentials in various cardiac tissues following 3 weeks and 6 weeks of drug treatment compared to those in representative controls. The upper trace in all panels represent 0 potential, middle trace shows action potentials, lower trace shows upstroke velocity of phase 0 of the action potential. Time and voltage calibrations as shown. The major feature noted is the stepwise increase in the APD in all tissues studied. The slowing of sinus frequency is due largely to the depression of phase 4 in the sinus node potential. (Reproduced with permission from Reference 39.)

superfusion studies, the effects of the drug became evident on the maximal rate of depolarization in fast channel fibers especially at fast stimulation frequencies. At these higher rates, amiodarone exhibited the typical responses of a sodium channel blocker.[40] This effect was seen in concentrations in which the effect on the APD was minimal acutely. The time constants of recovery of the sodium channel block after amiodarone are short, 0.3 to 1.6 seconds, somewhat longer than that for lidocaine (0.15 seconds) being comparable to those of tocainide and procainamide (see chapter 16).

In the rabbit SA node preparations super-

fused with amiodarone, Goupil and Lenfant[41] found significant drug-induced decreases in the action potential amplitude, the maximal diastolic potential, and the slope of phase 4. This has been confirmed by Yabek et al.[42] who found a similar effect under the action of desethylamiodarone. Of note, the acute effects of amiodarone versus those of the chronically administered drug are divergent. Thus, whereas during acute drug superfusion, there is shortening of the APD in Purkinje fibers, after long-term drug administration a prolongation in the APD occurs albeit not as markedly as it does in the ventricular muscle.[43] The initial shortening of APD may be due to the block of the sodium window current; this effect is subsequently nullified or reversed by the drug's more potent effect on blocking potassium current during long-term drug treatment.

Effects of Amiodarone on Inward and Outward Ionic Currents in Cardiac Muscle

Studies attempting to delineate these effects have been during acute superfusion studies with the drug being suspended in physiological media in conjunction with serum albumin and alcohol. Since the major clinical effects of the drug are found during long-term drug administration, the relevance of these acute effects remains uncertain. However, they are of potential importance in accounting for the electrophysiological changes that occur when the drug is given intravenously. When amiodarone was injected directly into the sinus and AV nodal arteries the drug appeared to act by inhibiting the slow channel in nodal tissues as it was not influenced by cholinergic or adrenergic blockade. Similarly, the depressant effect on AV nodal conduction and prolongation of refractoriness in humans[39] might be mediated via its antiadrenergic and calcium antagonistic actions in the SA and AV nodes. These effects are consistent with the marked decreases in sinus cycle length by the depression of phase 4 depolarization noted in the studies reported by Yabek et al.[42] as well as in those of Goupil and Lenfant.[41] The slow channel blocking action may be the basis for impaired myocardial contractility evident with the intravenous drug in high doses.[20]

Amiodarone on Inward Calcium Current

In isolated guinea pig myocytes, Nishimura et al.[45] recently confirmed that amiodarone is a potent calcium channel blocker; it reduces the inward calcium current (I_{Ca}) in a use-dependent manner with a time constant of recovery of the same order as that of recovery of $\dot{V}_{max}$ for the upstroke of the slow channel potentials in the presence of the drug.[3] This is consistent with the observations in SA preparations[41,42] and as well as those in slow channel potentials produced in Purkinje fibers by superfusion with barium.[45]

Amiodarone on Fast Sodium Current

A number of studies in isolated myocytes with the patch clamp techniques have confirmed that amiodarone is a potent blocker of the inward sodium current (I_{Ca}); it produces a use-dependent block of the current preferentially in the inactivated state.[46] The inhibitory effect of the drug on sodium channel is consistent with the rate-dependent depression of $\dot{V}_{max}$ in action potentials recorded from tissues taken from chronically amiodaronized animals[47] and with the effects of the drug on conduction intervals in humans at fast heart rates.[48]

Amiodarone Effects on the Outward Plateau Currents

In isolated guinea pig myocytes, the major effect of amiodarone is to nonselectively block the delayed rectifier K$^+$ current[49] with minor effects on the inward rectifier[49] and the ATP-sensitive K$^+$ channel.[50] While these acute effects have been well studied, there is no data on the effects of the drug on myocardial ion channels when it is administered chronically. The acute effects have not been associated with increases in APD at least of the same magnitude as seen following protracted drug. For these reasons, the relevance of acute data to the pattern of electrophysiological actions evident during long-term therapy with the compound is uncertain.[5,52]

Chronic Electrophysiological Effects of Amiodarone

The reasons for the differences between the acute and long-term effects of amiodarone especially on repolarization remains uncertain. Despite the very high concentrations of amiodarone, a finite duration of exposure of the myocardium to the drug on a long-term basis is necessary for the full expression of the electrophysiological effect. As mentioned already, the most striking effect is the consistent prolongation of the APD in atria, sinus node fibers, AV nodal fibers, and ventricular tissues. In Purkinje fibers the lengthening is less striking than that in ventricular muscle.[43] The mechanism of the stepwise increase in the APD in the case of atrial and ventricular muscle remains unclear; the delayed onset of drug action is not due to the formation of active metabolites or to the slow build-up of amiodarone itself in tissues or myocardial membranes.[15] Desethylamiodarone is active, having qualitatively the same pharmacodynamic profile, its action is not immediate[42]; its actions also exhibit a delay in onset (Figure 3) although its elimination half-life is longer than that of amiodarone.[36] Thus, long-term effects of amiodarone and its metabolite will be additive but the delay in the onset of amiodarone action cannot be attributed solely to the effects of desethylamiodarone.

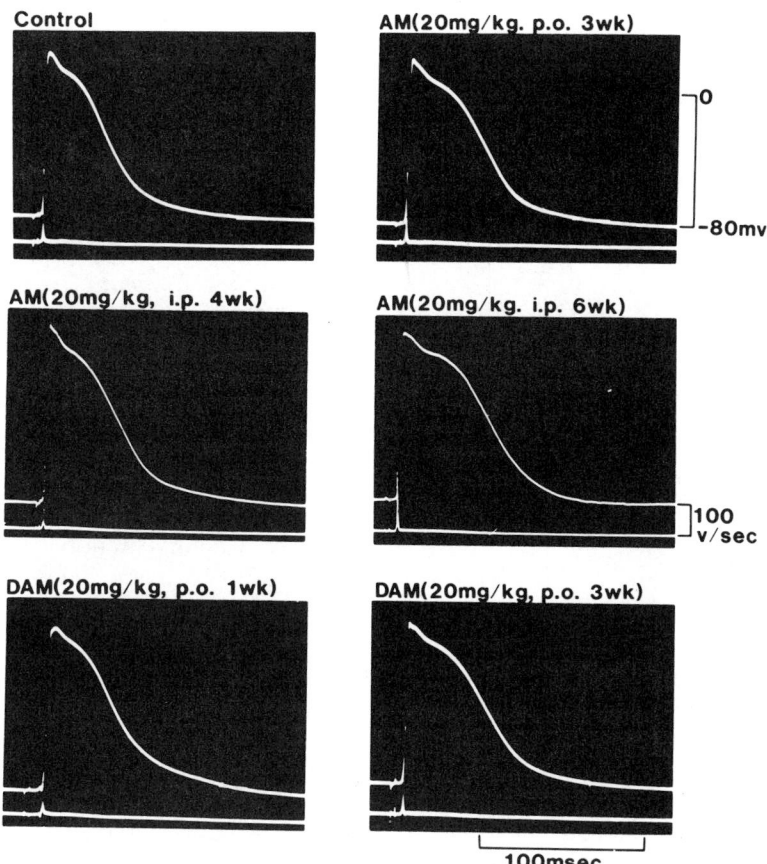

Figure 3. The effects of long-term amiodarone (AM) and desethylamiodarone (DAM) treatment on atrial transmembrane action potentials in rabbit atria. Note that the effects of AM and DAM are time dependent; the effects of DAM at 3 weeks is more pronounced on the action potential duration (APD) than it is at 1 week. (unpublished data; R. Kato and B.N. Singh)

Potential Significance of Amiodarone—Lipid Interactions

It has long been recognized that amiodarone may produce localized or generalized lipidoses.[15] It also inhibits the enzyme phospholipase[53] thereby preventing the breakdown of membrane phospholipids produced by phospholipase. Amiodarone is a complex molecule with a charge, nonpolar hydrophobic moiety, and a small hydrophilic side chain. This amphiphilic nature confers on the drug the propensity to alter lipid metabolism of the myocardium intracellularly as well as in the membrane. For example, Gross and Somani[54] reported the development of lysosomal and myelinoid inclusion bodies after long-term administration. Thus, the reduced membrane fluidity exhibited by the drug[55] are in line with the drug's effects on membrane lipids. There are other experimental data suggesting that amiodarone has effects at the level of membrane proteins. For example, the drug selectively inhibits the Na^+/K^+ adenosine triphosphatase (ATPase) of the guinea pig myocardial particulate fraction[56]; its interaction with the effects of stimulation of β-adrenergic receptors has been well defined as has been its inhibitory effects on the adenylate cyclase activity.[13]

In Vivo Electrophysiological Effects in Experimental Animals

In anesthetized animals, intravenous amiodarone in doses up to 10 mg/kg has been reported to increase the ventricular effective refractory period (ERP) by 30%[57] in the absence of a significant increase in the QTc interval as noted in another study.[20] Jaillon et al.[58] showed that in pentobarbital anesthetized animals, intravenous amiodarone (1.25–10 mg/kg) produced a dose-related decrease in heart rate and prolonged the sinus node recovery time while having no effect on His-Purkinje conduction time. There were modest increases in atrial and ventricular ERP with, as might be expected, a significant delay in AV conduction. Others[57] found similar effects in adult as well as neonatal dogs.[59] The overall observations suggest that the reported variable and modest antiarrhythmic actions of acutely administered amiodarone[60,61] may in part be due to the noncompetitive α- and β-adrenergic receptor antagonism.[6,11] The effects of the inhibitory actions on α and β receptors cannot be excluded. They may contribute substantively to the observed effects of amiodarone during intravenous injection.

Clinical Electrophysiological Effects

The effects of the drug in humans are consistent with those found in experimental animals. The changes following acute and long-term amiodarone administration on the various electrophysiological variables are shown in Figure 3. There is little or no effect on ventricular ERP in unanesthetized patients after acute intravenous drug (5 mg/kg) administration[39,60–62] despite plasma levels often exceeding 10 μg/mL.[39]

The experimental and clinical data emphasize that the maximal or steady-state effects with amiodarone in cardiac muscle do not become apparent acutely despite extremely high drug concentrations. This is reflected in the marked differences found between the effects of acute intravenous versus long-term oral drug therapy. For example, with intravenous amiodarone administration the electrophysiological effects are much less striking.[39,48,62] The main acute effect is the lengthening of AV nodal refractoriness and intranodal conduction (AH interval) time[39,57,60–62] with minimal effect on the ERPs of the atrial, ventricular, the bypass tract, or the His-Purkinje tissue when the drug is administered in a dose of 5 mg/kg body weight. There is no significant effect on the HV or QRS intervals nor the QTc duration. The acute effect on the AV node may be due to the blockade of the slow channels and/or the noncompetitive adrenergic antagonism exerted by the drug.[6,11,15] At somewhat higher doses (10 mg/kg) intravenous amiodarone has been shown to increase the ERP by 20–30 msec with some lengthening of the QRS duration at fast stimulus frequencies consistent with a use-dependent effect on fast sodium channels.[62] Despite the well-documented in vitro depressant effects of amiodarone on sinus node automaticity, intravenous amiodarone in conscious humans does not produce the expected reduction in heart rate,[39,48,62] presumably due to the opposing effects of sympathetic activation resulting from the peripheral vasodilator actions of the drug.[4]

In contrast, when administered chronically, amiodarone predictably lengthens repolarization (QTc) and refractoriness in most cardiac tissues as a function of time with little or no change in the QRS duration and a modest increase in the HV interval with a significant prolongation of the AH interval.[29,30,63,64] As far as the effects on repolarization are concerned, they are consistent with those previously noted with studies in rabbits chronically treated with amiodarone.[4,9] QTc interval in humans increases progressively on a constant dose of amiodarone,[19] reaching what appeared to be a steady-state effect at 6 to 12 months (see Chapter 31). After long-term treatment in humans there is marked increase in the effective and the functional refractory periods in most cardiac tissues (atria, ventricles, AV node, His-Purkinje system, accessory

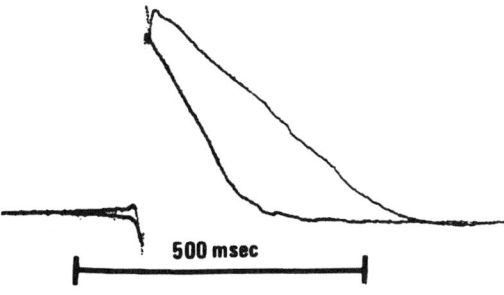

Figure 4. Superimposed human monophasic action potential recordings from the atria before (shorter action potential) and after 6 weeks of treatment with amiodarone after cardioversion. Note marked lengthening of the atrial action potential duration (APD). (Reproduced with permission from Reference 18.)

tracts of the heart) as a function of time with little or no change in the QRS duration and a modest increase in the HV interval.[48,62] The effects of 6 weeks of amiodarone treatment in human atrial tissue are shown in Figure 4. An increase in the QRS duration does, however, occur[62] as do increases in infranodal conduction (anterograde or retrograde) following fast stimulation frequencies, again reflecting effects on the fast sodium channel.[65] It is clear that the overall electrophysiological changes, which are accompanied by a progressive decrease in heart rate, are significantly greater during long-term therapy when compared with those found after acute intravenous or short-term oral administration.[15]

Antiarrhythmic and Antifibrillatory Actions of Amiodarone in Experimental Models

The antiarrhythmic effects of acute intravenous doses versus long-term oral dosing of amiodarone differ significantly. Ventricular fibrillation produced by chloroform inhalation or calcium chloride administration in mice or rats, responded poorly to intravenous amiodarone.[66] High drug doses effectively suppressed ventricular arrhythmias induced by aconitine.[66] Intravenous amiodarone was found to be effective in suppressing multifocal premature ventricular ectopic beats produced by the injection of epinephrine in anesthetized dogs and rabbits and by the injection of barium chloride in the anesthetized dogs and rabbits. Pretreatment with amiodarone of anesthetized guinea pigs has also been reported to increase the dose of intravenous infusion of ouabain required to produce VF due to glycoside intoxication.[9,12]

The antifibrillatory effects of acutely and chronically administered amiodarone are of particular significance. For instance, pretreatment of rats with amiodarone for 2 minutes to 3 weeks and studied in a Langendorff preparation led to a dose-related decrease in spontaneous heart rate with an increase in VF threshold both before as well as after coronary artery ligation.[67] The drug also reduced the number of premature ventricular ectopic beats as well as VT/VF after coronary artery ligation and after reperfusion. In this model, amiodarone prevented ischemia-induced increases in the tissue cyclic adenosine monophosphate concentration after coronary artery ligation. The study provided convincing evidence for the protective effects of the compound against increases in ventricular vulnerability in the early phases following coronary artery occlusion and against reperfusion VF. These data are consistent with those reported by Schoenfeld,[68] who found 20–50 mg/kg orally administered amiodarone had a markedly protective effect against both early as well as late fatal VF following coronary artery ligation in rats.

Findings in anesthetized dogs have been similar with amiodarone effectively preventing VF in all 10 pretreated animals given 40 mg/kg oral amiodarone for 1–4 weeks followed by coronary artery ligation in a study reported by Rosenbaum et al.[25] Chew et al.[69] found that chronic pretreatment with amiodarone for a period for 4 weeks also markedly attenuated the frequency of ventricular arrhythmias and prevented the development of VF following coronary artery ligation in conscious instrumented dogs.

Particularly noteworthy are the data[70] in a sudden death canine model produced by sequential ligation of coronary arteries. In this model (see Chapter 22), untreated animals developed VF in 90%–100% of cases, compared to 60% in acutely pretreated animals and 20% in chronically treated animals. The data emphasized the greater efficacy of chronically administered amiodarone as an antifibrillatory agent. In the same model, Class I agents had no protective effects, rate lowering β blockers and sotalol provided 60% to 65% protection, and pure Class III agents about 50% to 60%. These differences in the effects of acute versus long-term pretreatment with amiodarone and chronic amiodarone treatment compared to other pharmacological intervention attests to the unusual effectiveness of the compound's

antifibrillatory potential. The data is consistent with the clinical antifibrillatory effects of the drug in humans.

Clinical Antiarrhythmic and Antifibrillatory Effects of Amiodarone

The electropharmacological properties of amiodarone suggest that the compound should exhibit a broad spectrum of antiarrhythmic actions. The available clinical data are in line with the experimental observations. Only the major findings from the extensive and expanding literature will be summarized to allow some tentative conclusions. Again, the effects of the drug given intravenously should be distinguished from those found during oral drug administration.

Significance of Intravenous Amiodarone as an Antiarrhythmic Agent

Supraventricular Arrhythmias

Intravenously administered amiodarone (5 mg/kg) given over 5–10 minutes slows the ventricular response in atrial flutter and fibrillation in most patients. This effect is clearly due to the depressant effect of the drug on the AV node, mediated in part by its antiadrenergic effect and in part by its calcium antagonistic actions. Whether Class I actions of the drug contributes to the acute antiarrhythmic effects of the drug remains unclear. It is doubtful whether the acute AV nodal effect is of much clinical use since a very large range of simpler compounds are available for an effective slowing of ventricular response in atrial flutter and fibrillation. In long-standing cases, the compound effects a conversion only rarely, although this may occur frequently in cases of recent onset of the arrhythmia. However, the observations on this issue are of an anecdotal nature and no controlled studies are available. The intravenous drug may also slow the tachycardia cycle length in cases of reentrant supraventricular tachycardia and terminate it in a significant number by producing conduction block in the antegrade limb of the reentrant circuit.[60] Again, the clinical utility of intravenous amiodarone in this setting is of little practical value with the availability of intravenous diltiazem, verapamil, and particularly adenosine.

Ventricular Arrhythmias

A number of reports have suggested that intravenous amiodarone is often highly effective in the control of life-threatening ventricular arrhythmias resistant to other antiarrhythmic regimens given alone or in combination.[71,72] Similarly, there are reports indicating a markedly beneficial effect on mortality when given during the course of resuscitation of patients developing cardiac arrest in the hospital.[73] In neither case are there controlled studies to confirm or deny these possibilities. Clearly, controlled studies are needed to define the role of intravenous amiodarone in these clinical situations.

It should be emphasized that while intravenous loading of the drug has been advocated, there is little evidence indicating that this approach provides more rapid attainment of steady-state drug effects in the control of arrhythmias.

Antiarrhythmic and Antifibrillatory Actions of Chronically Administered Amiodarone

The major clinical utility of amiodarone as an antiarrhythmic compound is in the prophylactic control of supraventricular as well as ventricular arrhythmias. There are increasing data suggesting that the drug may be the most effective agent in this regard. The salutary effect in these cases may relate to the intrinsic action of the drug in atrial and ventricular tissue as well as in the AV node and the accessory tracts of the heart in terms of changes in conduction and refractoriness. Also of potential importance might be the suppression of supraventricular and ventricular ectopic beats that provide the trigger mechanism for the initiation of the tachyarrhythmias. The effect of the drug in producing conversion of atrial flutter and atrial fibrillation to sinus rhythm is generally attributed to the consistent lengthening of myocardial refractoriness as in the case of other drugs which also prolong repolarization (see Chapter 20). However, the "permissive" effect of the drug's Class I action is not excluded; the latter effect may contribute to marked slowing of fibrillation and flutter rates in the atria, often preceding the restoration of sinus rhythm. The slowing of the atrial rate in atrial fibrillation results in the development of atrial flutter with slowing of AV conduction. In VT, a similar effect may account for the markedly prolonged tachycardia cycle length during the recurrence of the arrhythmia during long-term treatment with the drug. In the case of amiodarone such an effect appears to be much greater than that seen with other Class III agents such as dl-sotalol, d-sotalol, and the newer pure Class III compounds. Whether the difference is accounted for by the lack of Class I properties in these agents in contrast to amiodarone's relatively potent sodium channel blocking action in the case of amiodarone requires further study.

Control of Supraventricular Arrhythmias

Atrial Flutter and Fibrillation

Oral administration of amiodarone (200–400 mg/day, often in lower doses) slows the ventricular response in atrial flutter and fibrillation at rest and with exercise; it produces conversion after a variable period in over 30% of cases and may maintain stability of sinus rhythm after chemical or electrical conversion in over 53%–79% of cases (with a mean follow-up of 27 months),[74] a figure significantly higher than that produced by most Class Ia compounds. Almost as high a percentage of stability of sinus rhythm has been reported in the case of Class Ic agents especially flecainide in control clinical trials but in patients with normal or near normal hearts.[75] It has been considered that Class Ic agents may exert a deleterious effect on mortality due to their proarrhythmic reactions in patients with heart disease. In contrast, such a caveat does not appear to be necessary in the case with amiodarone. However, the efficacy data on amiodarone have not been derived from blinded placebo controlled studies nor against comparator agents. A recent analysis of our own data in 110 patients with resistant atrial flutter and fibrillation followed for up to 10 years (mean 6 years) suggested a stability of sinus rhythm over 70%.[76] In our study, low-dose amiodarone was surprisingly well tolerated. This is supported by the data from a review of reports on the effects of amiodarone in maintaining sinus rhythm published by Middlekauff et al.[74] Their analysis suggested that low-dose amiodarone is well tolerated, is effective, and with most noncardiac side effects being dose related. They recommended the undertaking of a prospective randomized study to define the role of the drug in atrial fibrillation. Such a trial is in the planning stages under the aegis of the Veterans Affairs Cooperative Studies Section.

It should be emphasized that in cases of atrial flutter, the flutter rate is often markedly reduced if conversion to sinus rhythm has not occurred. Unlike the situation in the case of quinidine and disopyramide (anticholinergic effect), acceleration of the ventricular response does not occur, because AV conduction is depressed (antisympathetic effect) by amiodarone.

Paroxysmal Supraventricular Tachycardia

Although amiodarone has been used in the case of most types of reentrant supraven-

tricular tachycardias, including those due to AV nodal reentry and those using accessory tracts of the heart, the drug is of particular value in cases with antidromic tachycardias and in the atrial flutter and fibrillation complicating the Wolff-Parkinson-White syndrome.[77] A high rate of success can be achieved with relatively modest doses of the drug in this setting. However, drug therapy of these arrhythmias are now being superseded rapidly by radiofrequency catheter ablation wherever electrophysiological resources are available.

Ventricular Arrhythmias

The advent of amiodarone has had a major impact on the treatment of recurrent life-threatening ventricular tachyarrhythmias.[1,4,24–30] There is a remarkably good concordance between the effects of the drug in experimental arrhythmia models and those noted in clinical ventricular arrhythmias. However, as yet no stringently controlled clinical trials have been done to confirm that the drug does in fact reduce mortality by arrhythmia control in patients presenting with VT/VF. Likewise, no controlled observations have suggested that despite the fact amiodarone is a powerful Class I agent, it increases mortality in any subset of patients unlike the bulk of other Class I agents (see Chapter 27).

Premature Ventricular Contractions

In the meta-analysis of reported trials of various antiarrhythmic agents on the suppression of PVCs, Salerno et al.[78] found that amiodarone was the most potent agent in suppressing PVCs. It produced over 80% suppression of total number of PVCs in over 90% of patients. Indeed, this was superior to the effects of Class I agents including those of Class Ic compounds (Figure 5). However, as indicated both by Rosenbaum et al.[79] and Nademanee et al.,[28] a steady-state effect may not be achieved for many months. The effects on nonsustained VT in a meta-analysis study was

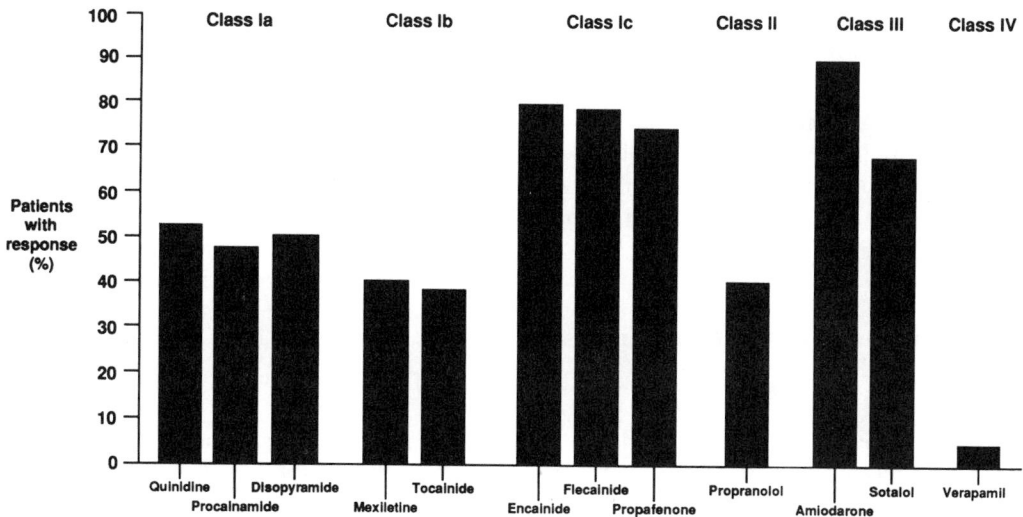

Figure 5. The comparative efficacy of various electrophysiological classes of antiarrhythmic agents in suppressing premature ventricular contractions by 80% or greater. (Based on data from Salerno et al.[78])

even more striking approaching complete suppression.[78]

The suppressant effects of arrhythmias on electrocardiographic monitoring are in sharp contrast to the overall effects on the prevention of inducibility of VT/VF by PES in patients with manifest VT/VF and in those surviving sudden death. The precise basis for this seemingly paradoxical dissociation between the effects on spontaneously occurring arrhythmias and those by PES remains unexplained (see Chapter 47).

Ventricular Tachycardia and Fibrillation and Survivors of Sudden Death

Numerous studies have shown that following the initial loading dose, a maintenance regimen of 200–400 mg/day of the drug is effective in controlling malignant arrhythmias (including those with cardiac arrest) in 60%–75% of cases in which conventional agents (especially Class I compounds) have failed[25-30]; higher figures have been reported. The data from two large studies deserve mention. The results from the two studies are con-

sistent. The first is from Herre et al.[80] They treated several hundred patients with VT/VF and cardiac arrest with amiodarone after they had been tested on an average of 2.9 drugs per patient and an effective agent was not found. At the end of 5 years of follow-up, there was 21% sudden death, ie, an average of 4% a year with a 7% incidence in the first year. In the other study reported by Weinberg et al.,[81] 469 patients were treated with amiodarone and followed for 5 years. The cumulative incidence of sudden death at 1, 2, and 5 years was 9%, 13%, and 22%, respectively and for arrhythmia recurrence was 19%, 26% and 28%, respectively. The investigators concluded that despite the side effect profile of the drug, amiodarone was an effective and reasonably well-tolerated antiarrhythmic compound. Of interest, in this series only a small number of patients who had inducible sustained VT at control electrophysiological study, became noninducible during amiodarone therapy. Clearly, these data have bearing on the continuing debate on the issue of whether long-term success of therapy can be predicted more accurately by the effects of the drug on the suppression of spontaneously occurring arrhythmias on Holter recordings or on the basis of inducible tachycardia induced by PES of the heart (see Chapter 47). The data from Weinberg et al.[81] provide further support for the belief that the failure of amiodarone to prevent ventricular induction does not necessarily preclude excellent clinical outcome.

Amiodarone in Patients at High Risk for Sudden Death

Less extensive data are available in the case of patients at high risk for sudden death. However, a relatively small study in heart failure has shown an improvement in mortality in patients with associated high-density PVCs.[82] Similarly, an uncontrolled study in hypertrophic cardiomyopathy, has indicated benefit in relation to the suppression of VT documented on Holter recordings.[83] However, the data from neither study cannot be interpreted as demonstrating a causal relationship between the suppression of PVCs and VT and the observed improvement in mortality.

Two recent clinical studies are worthy of mention as they emphasize that amiodarone in relatively low doses exerts a beneficial effect on mortality in the survivors of acute myocardial infarction. The first, designated as the BASIS study, was reported by Burkhart et al.[84] They randomized 312 survivors of acute infarction in a group given low-dose amiodarone (n = 98), no antiarrhythmic treatment (n = 100), and individualized drug therapy (n = 114). At the end of 1 year, death rate in the no treatment group was 13%, in the individualized therapy group 10%, and 5% in the case of amiodarone ($p < 0.05$ compared to no treatment group). In the other study, Ceremuzynski et al.[1] conducted a double-blind study in 305 patients given amiodarone and 308 patients given placebo and followed for 1 year. The patients enrolled were recent survivors of acute myocardial infarction who could not be given β-blockers because of specific contraindications. In this study, amiodarone reduced cardiac mortality ($p < 0.048$); there

were 21 deaths in the amiodarone group (6.9%) and 33 (10.7%) in the placebo group. Of particular interest, the low-dose amiodarone dosage was well tolerated, there being only 1 case of pulmonary toxicity out of the 305 patients followed for 12 months.

While these data provide an alternative approach to the secondary prevention in survivors of acute infarction, the issue of troublesome side effects that might develop during long-term treatment with amiodarone should be emphasized. In this regard, the observations of Pfisterer et al.[85] are of potential significance. They continued the patients from the BASIS study on a long-term study to determine whether the observed beneficial effect of the drug seen at the end of the first year might continue when the drug was discontinued. The patients were followed for a mean of 72 months (range 55–125 months). According to the Kaplan-Meier type of actuarial life-table analysis, the probability of death after 84 months was 30% for the amiodarone treated patients compared to 45% for controls. Over the entire follow-up period, the mortality rate was lower in the amiodarone group than in the concurrent controls with respect to cardiac deaths ($p = 0.047$) as well as total deaths ($p = 0.03$). The mortality reduction effected by amiodarone was essentially in the first year, there being no difference between the amiodarone and control groups when one considered survival after the discontinuation of amiodarone only. The authors concluded that the salutary effect of amiodarone outlasted the period of amiodarone administration. The sudden death and total cardiac death rates were low during the follow-up, 1.2% per year in the amiodarone group, and 4.5% per year in the control group. They suggested that treatment with amiodarone may not be necessary after the first year following myocardial infarction. The data raises the issue whether a year of continuous treatment with amiodarone leads to a long-term and favorable change in the ventricular myocardium. It is, however, important to stress the limitations of the study. The BASIS study was not a blinded trial and the patient selection cannot be excluded but the confirmation of the results by a blinded trial is likely to have major implications for the post myocardial infarction (MI) survivors.

Clinical Trials with Amiodarone in Progress with Mortality as an End Point

The perceived potential of amiodarone to curtail mortality in various subsets of patients with cardiac arrhythmias has led to the initiation of a number of controlled and blinded and unblinded clinical trials. One of these, the CASCADE Trial, which compared the effects of empirical amiodarone therapy with the PES or Holter guided therapy with Class I agents in cardiac arrest patients was recently completed.[86] The preliminary data indicated that amiodarone was superior in terms of mortality reduction as well as arrhythmia recurrence.[86]

A number of trials that deal with amiodarone on mortality are in progress in the setting of post-MI survivors. The best controlled are the Canadian Amiodarone Myocardial Infarction Trial (CAMIAT) and the European Myocardial Infarction Trial (EMTAT). The pilot component of CAMIAT indicated a favorable trend in mortality and the definitive study deals with post-MI patients with the entire spectrum of ventricular function. In contrast, EMIAT focuses on those with left ventricular ejection fraction below 40%. It is not a suppression trial.

A trial designed to test the hypothesis that the antifibrillatory effects of amiodarone will prolong survival in patients with heart failure patients with high-density PVCs is nearing completion of enrollment as a VA Co-Operative Study (CHF-STAT). This also is a placebo controlled trial. A similar trial is in progress in Argentine.

Since amiodarone is now generally perceived as constituting the best medical therapy for VT/VF and available data do not indicate a clear advantage in favor of implantable devices (ICDs), a number of trials have been initiated or planned to compare the relative merits of the two forms of therapy. The most advanced is the Canadian Implantable Device Study (CIDS) in which ICDs are being compared to empirical amiodarone therapy. The CASH trial in Germany involves a comparison of metoprolol, amiodarone (propafenone limb having been discontinued because of what appeared to be an excess mortality on the drug), and ICDs. Recently initiated is the pilot component of a study comparing best medical therapy (essentially empirical amiodarone and guided sotalol) versus ICDs in patients with VT/VF and those incurring cardiac arrest and surviving it. This study is being sponsored by the Clinical Trials Branch of the NHLBI.

Clearly, the level of interest in the role of amiodarone in reducing arrhythmia mortality is high. The outcomes of the abovementioned trials are likely to have a major impact not only in the way malignant arrhythmias will be treated in the future, but also on the development of newer antifibrillatory agents.

Side Effects Profile of Amiodarone

The available data indicate that the observed beneficial effects of the compound should be balanced against the well-known potential serious deleterious actions. Particularly important is the development of pulmonary toxicity. During the early years of therapy with amiodarone, the incidence of pulmonary toxicity was reported to be in the range of 5%–15%. With much more stringent attention dosage schedules, the incidence appears to have fallen to less than 3% and in many centers in the United States; it might be as low as 1% or lower as noted in the Polish post-MI secondary prevention trial.[1] The precise incidence of hepatoxicity, thought to be 1%, is not known. More common is the transient increase in liver enzymes. Troublesome but less serious side effects include altered thyroid state, peripheral neuropathy, central nervous system (CNS) and gastrointestinal disturbances, photosensitivity, corneal microdeposits, myopathy, and especially bluish skin pigmentation the incidence of which is unrelated to dose but increases as a function of duration of therapy. Skin changes do become increasingly common and troublesome with the increasing duration of therapy. Numerous minor side effects of the drug have been reported.

It should also be emphasized that amiodarone exhibits electrophysiological and hemodynamic interactions with a number of other cardioactive compounds but the drug's propensity to induce pharmacokinetic interactions (eg, digoxin, warfarin, quinidine, procainamide, NAPA, propafenone, flecainide, phenytoin, and sodium among others) may be associated with serious effects. Clearly, in the case of amiodarone an appropriate caution needs to be exercised that takes account of an extremely potent action and a complex side effect profile that is not readily predictable on the basis for plasma drug monitoring.

Proarrhythmic Reactions of Amiodarone

Significance of the Drug's Class I Actions

The fact that amiodarone has lower proarrhythmic reactions than Class I and other Class III agents is now generally accepted despite the lack of controlled clinical observations. Because the drug is a potent Class I agent, one might expect it to exhibit a class action in terms of aggravating cardiac arrhythmias—increasing the frequency of PVCs, converting nonsustained VT to sustained VT, and producing new cases of VT or VF. Like other Class I agents, it might be expected to increase mortality. These phenomena are rarely demonstrated in the case of the drug. An increase in mortality has not been reported although in hypertrophic cardiomyopathy, early deaths (in the first 6 months) have been attributed to amiodarone. Without the concurrent controls, it is difficult to interpret these findings

in severe cases of hypertrophic cardiomyopathy.[87] However, it is known that in some cases during the early stages of therapy with the drug more frequent episodes of VT may be seen with amiodarone. Such episodes disappear with the continued administration of amiodarone. If these are indeed cases of proarrhythmic reactions, they might represent reactions to the drug's Class I effects, being subsequently nullified or reversed by the properties of the drug that require a longer time period for full expression. In this setting the antiadrenergic and antifibrillatory effects (due to lengthened repolarization) might both be significant.

Amiodarone and Class III Actions: Occurrence of Torsades de Pointes

An unexplained feature of the drug is an unexpectedly low incidence of torsades de pointes, which appears to be a reasonably specific proarrhythmic correlate of prolonged cardiac repolarization.[88] The fact that this effect is minimal in the case of monotherapy with amiodarone over prolonged periods of time despite the prolongation of the QT intervals to 600 msec or longer and the accompanying bradycardia of 50 beats per minute or less, is in direct contrast to that seen with sotalol and newer Class III agents. When torsades de pointes occurs in the setting of amiodarone therapy, it is usually (but not invariably) seen in conjunction with therapy with other QT prolonging drugs such as quinidine or procainamide or in the context of severe electrolyte disturbances. It remains puzzling that even in heart failure the incidence of torsades de pointes during chronic amiodarone therapy is low.

Potential Electrophysiological Bases for the Low Incidence of Torsades de Pointes During Amiodarone Therapy

No clear electrophysiological basis for the difference between the effects of amiodarone and other agents that prolong the QT interval has been established relative to their differing proclivities to induce torsades. A number of features of the drug might be pertinent to this issue.

Amiodarone prevents electrically-induced early and late afterdepolarizations;[40] it prevents barium-induced EADs,[45] this may in part be related to the drug's associated Ca channel blocking effects inhibiting the propensity for EADs to develop.[45]

Unlike other Class III agents, the drug lengthens the APD more in the ventricular muscle than in the Purkinje fibers, which may be the locus of origin of early afterdepolarizations (EADs). There is data to suggest that following chronic amiodarone treatment in the dog, the APD in the ventricle may increase by 25% to 30% whereas in the Purkinje fiber, the increase is about 12%.[43] This is likely to produce a greater homogeneity of refractoriness and repolarization in the myocardium. Recent data from our laboratory indicate that amiodarone, in contrast to sotalol and sematilide (a pure Class III agent), reduces temporal (see Chapter 31) as well as spatial[89] dispersion of repolarization in humans. In the case of other Class III agents, the converse occurs in their effects on myocardial repolarization. The lengthening of the APD in Purkinje fibers on pure Class III agents is several orders of magnitude greater than that in the ventricular muscle, an effect that augments the existing heterogeneity of myocardial repolarization.

There are also differences between amiodarone and pure Class III agents in regard to the frequency-dependent effects on the APD and the ERP. Whereas most Class III agents exhibit the phenomenon of reverse use or rate dependency, amiodarone produces a parallel shift of the curve relating frequency to changes in the APD or ERP upwards and to the right.[90] In contrast, other Class III agents produce disproportionately large increases in APDs at low heart rates with an exponential increase occurring below 60 beats per minute. It is felt that this pattern of electrophysiological changes are conducive to the development of EADs and hence torsades de pointes.

The Puzzle of Amiodarone Antifibrillatory Actions

There is now little doubt about the potency of amiodarone as a broad-spectrum antiarrhythmic agent for the prophylactic control of most supraventricular and ventricular tachyarrhythmias. While the most readily measurable correlate of its antiarrhythmic action is its property to lengthen the APD in most cardiac tissues (the Class III action), this alone is unlikely to be the sole basis of the drug's unusual potency as an antiarrhythmic compound. The drug's anti-ischemic, antiadrenergic, calcium antagonistic, and its bradycardic actions cannot be ignored. Thus, barring its side effect profile, amiodarone is a desirable prototype of a broad-spectrum antifibrillatory and an antiarrhythmic compound. A precise understanding of its cellular action may therefore provide the basis for the development of the ideal agent.

On nearly all counts amiodarone differs from conventional as well as newer agents. It has a complex electrophysiological profile that is unique. It is characterized by relatively minor effects on sodium and calcium channels with a broad array of extracardiac actions; its long-term action is dominated by the marked prolongation of APD and refractoriness with a modest effect on conduction evident at fast frequencies.[47] Like β blockers, amiodarone reduces heart rate, but with a slower onset and as a function of time, reaching peak actions in 3 months (see Chapter 31). There are many features of the drug's action that suggest a metabolic basis of cellular and subcellular mode of action.

An intriguing possibility is that the drug might in part act by cardiospecifically antagonizing thyroid hormone action at a receptor level.[15,38,91–93] Amiodarone is structurally unique, resembling thyroxine (Figure 6). It is iodinated; many of its actions overlap with those of myocardial hypothyroidism.[15] Thus, the question arose whether a major component of amiodarone action is mediated via selective myocardial T_3 receptor inhibition as

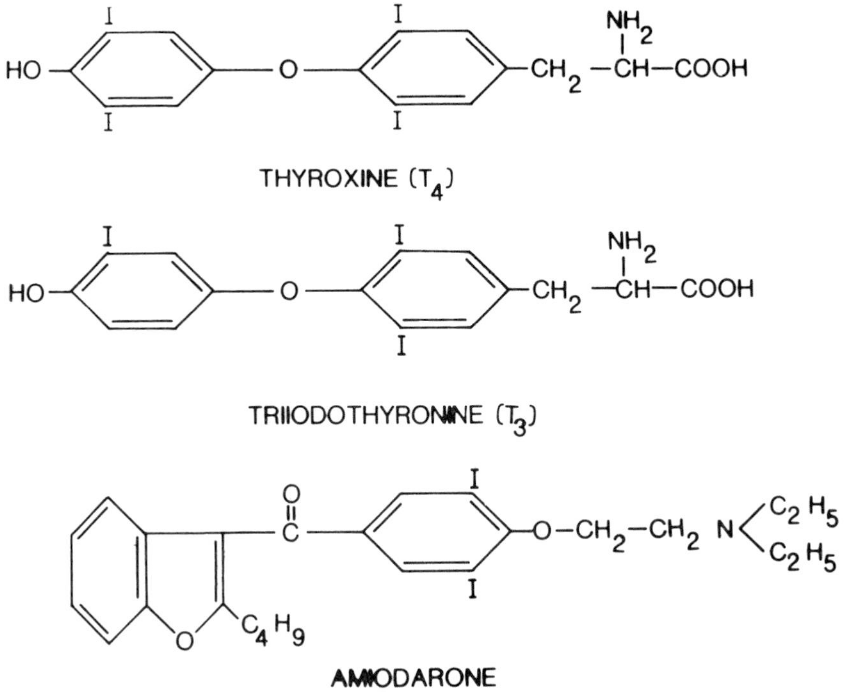

Figure 6. Structural formula of amiodarone compared to those of thyroxine and triiodothyronine. Note the structural similarities that might be relevant to the action of long-term amiodarone treatment on heart muscle.

originally suggested.[9] Now there is substantial evidence in support of this.[91] This effect is not due to the iodine contained in the amiodarone molecule; in doses equivalent to those contained in the effective dose of amiodarone, iodine alone had no effect on atrial action potentials.[9] However, the concomitant administration of amiodarone and thyroid hormone prevented the development of repolarization changes evident after amiodarone alone.[9,12] This indicated that the electrophysiological effect of amiodarone may in part be mediated by a selective T_3 block in cardiac muscle as the inhibition of the peripheral conversion of T_4 to T_3,[93,94] resulting in a decrease in T_3, an increase in reverse T_3, and a minimal increase in T_4 in the plasma due to the blockade of 5'-monodeiodinase,[94] could account for the observed electrophysiological changes. Thus, a direct inhibition of T_3 nuclear binding by amiodarone and/or its metabolite desethylam-

iodarone has been postulated to result in a hypothyroid state at a cellular level.[15]

Since the electrophysiological effects of hypothyroidism[96] on repolarization are nearly identical to those found after long-term amiodarone treatment, this phenomenon appears to exhibit cardiospecificity.[9,12] The drug generally does not produce generalized hypothyroidism.[15]

Recently, Talajic et al.[97] reported a marked attenuation of amiodarone Class III and sinus node effects in hypothyroid guinea pigs. The pattern of β-receptor density in the case of long-term amiodarone administration and in hypothyroidism also appears nearly identical.[15] In rats, the changes in heart myosin isoenzymes following long-term amiodarone treatment has been shown to be identical to those found in hypothyroidism.[98] This was confirmed by Nag et al.[99] in studies involving rat cardiac muscle cell culture in isomyosin by cardiac myocytes. Cardiac myocytes exposed to amiodarone in the absence of T_3 showed predominant V_1. When they were exposed to amiodarone in the presence of T_3, they expressed prevalent isomyosin V_3 or both V_3 and V_1 equally. Supraphysiological concentrations of T_3 counteracted amiodarone effects, showing the expression of predominant isomyosin V_1. These findings are also consistent with a direct receptor interaction between amiodarone and T_3. A competitive interaction between T_3 and amiodarone in acute studies has recently been found by Cui et al.[100] Hensley et al.[101] recently studied the effects of long-term amiodarone administration on Na^+, K^+-ATPase α-2 and β-2 expression in the rat ventricle. As in the case of hypothyroidism, the α-2 isoform was significantly depressed by amiodarone. The lack of effect on α-1 and β-1 expression in heart at 6 weeks, and lack of effect on skeletal Na^+, K^+-ATPase expression, all seen in hypothyroidism, indicated that amiodarone's actions are isoform and tissue specific.

It is of interest that in hyperthyroidism, I_{Ca} is increased, the converse in hypothyroidism[102]; the electrophysiological effects of hypothyroidism closely resembles those of long-term amiodarone administration.[15] In hyperthyroid ventricular muscle, EADs develop (blocked by verapamil) when the muscle is driven at low frequencies.[103] Finally, the rate-dependent effects on the APD in the case of hypothyroidism at least in the atria[96] are identical to those after long-term amiodarone administration.

Thus, there are compelling data suggesting that amiodarone might act fundamentally by blocking T_3. If this were the case, a number of conclusions about the properties of amiodarone can be drawn: (1) the effects of the drug on repolarization, as with hypothyroidism[96] will be homogeneous from cell to cell with little or no dispersion of refractoriness. This will minimize focal reexcitation and reentry; (2) the long refractory period with little change in conduction will be antifibrillatory action in all heart tissues; (3) since the overall myocardial effects will parallel the time course of hormone action, the net steady-state effect of the drug will have a significant latency and the pharmacological half-life of the drug will outlast the plasma half-life of the drug, there being little likelihood of a relationship between serum, tissue, or sarcolemmal drug levels and effect as shown in our laboratories[15]; (4) the attenuation of I_{Ca} in amiodaronized or hypothyroid muscle will lead to a reduced proclivity for the development of EADs and hence torsades de pointes; and (5) cardioselective hypothyroidism created by amiodarone and its own intrinsic noncompetitive antiadrenergic effect will summate to produce bradycardia and reduce oxygen consumption, properties of obvious utility in patients with coronary artery disease experiencing VT/VF. In the absence of the hypothyroid effect, the degree of observed bradycardia induced by amiodarone is unexplained. Finally, there are preliminary data from radioligand binding studies that have indicated that amiodarone and its principal metabolite, desethylamiodarone, may indeed function as thyroid hormone antagonists in different tissues. Particularly convincing is the data in the case of rat pituitary cells reported recently by Norman and Lavin.[104] Thus, an entirely novel approach to effective Class III antifibrillatory and antiarrhythmic actions might be the synthetic design of cardiospecific T_3 antagonists.

Conclusions

The mounting concerns regarding the seriousness of the proarrhythmic effects of Class I agents in the wake of data from controlled clinical trials and meta-analyses of randomized studies have provided a new impetus for the development of antifibrillatory compounds that act essentially by prolonging myocardial repolarization. Recent data allows some tentative conclusions. First, the results of β-blocker therapy in many subsets of patients emphasize the importance of adrenergic blockade as a major antiarrhythmic mechanism in its own right. This property is also an integral component of more complex molecules such as sotalol and amiodarone. Second, there is evidence that these drugs have a varying spectrum of antifibrillatory and proarrhythmic actions for a given degree of prolongation of repolarization. These differences are not readily accountable in terms of specificity of their actions for single or multiple repolarizing myocardial ion currents. Third, amiodarone stands uniquely by itself in a class only sharing with other Class III agents the property of prolonging cardiac repolarization that it does homogeneously tending to reduce dispersion of repolarization and refractoriness. In developing newer antifibrillatory agents, it is unclear whether one should focus solely on the Class III effect of amiodarone. The data suggests a need for a clear delineation of its overall electropharmacological profile including effects in terms of actions on ion channels, currents, receptors and pumps as they modulate refractoriness and conduction. This knowledge may allow the synthetic replication of compounds with amiodarone's potent antiarrhythmic and antifibrillatory actions and minimal proarrhythmic reactions, but without the drug's side effect profile.

Acknowledgments: I am much indebted to Diane Gertschen for help in the preparation of this chapter.

References

1. Ceremuzynski Y, Kleczar E, Kreminska-Pakula M, et al: Effect of amiodarone on mortality after myocardial infarction. *J Am Coll Cardiol* 20:1056, 1992.
2. Ahmed R, Singh BN: Anti-arrhythmic drugs. *Curr Opin Cardiol* 8:10, 1993.
3. Nattel S, Talajic M, Fermani B, Roya D: Amiodarone: pharmacology, clinical actions, and relationship between them. *J Cardiovasc Electrophysiol* 3:266, 1992.
4. Singh BN: Amiodarone: historical development and pharmacologic profile. *Am Heart J* 106:788, 1983.
5. Singh BN: Advantages of β-blockers versus anti-arrhythmic drugs and calcium-channel antagonists in secondary prevention in survivors of myocardial infarction. *Am J Cardiol* 66:9, 1990.
6. Polster P, Broekhuysen J: The adrenergic an-
7. Charlier R: Cardiac actions in the dog of a new antagonist of adrenergic excitation which does not produce competitive blockade of adrenoceptors. *Br J Pharmacol* 39:668, 1970.
8. Cohen-Armon M, Schreiber G, Sokolovsky M: Interaction of the anti-arrhythmic drug amiodarone with the muscarinic receptor in rat heart and brain. *J Cardiovasc Pharmacol* 6: 1148, 1984.
9. Singh BN, Vaughan Williams EM: The effect of amiodarone, a new anti-anginal drug, on cardiac muscle. *Br J Pharmacol* 39:657, 1970.
10. Kobayashi M, Godin D, Nadeau R: Acute effects of amiodarone in the isolated dog heart. *Can J Physiol Pharmacol* 61:308, 1983.
11. Charlier R, Deltour G, Baudine A, et al: Pharmacology of amiodarone, an antianginal drug with a new biological profile. *Arzneimittelforschung* 18:1408, 1968.
12. Singh BN: *Pharmacologic Actions of Certain Drugs and Hormones: Focus on Studies of Antiarrhythmic Mechanisms.* Oxford, United Kingdom: Hertford College, University of Oxford; 1971. D. Phil. Thesis.
13. Nokin P, Clinet M, Schoenfeld P: Cardiac β-receptor modulation by amiodarone. *Biochem Pharmacol* 32:2473, 1983.
14. Sharma AD, Corr PB, Sobel BE: Modulation by amiodarone of cardiac adrenergic receptors and their electrophysiologic responsiveness to catecholamines (abstract). *Circulation* 68:393, 1983.
15. Singh BN: Electropharmacology of amiodarone. In: EM Vaughan Williams, TJ Campbel (eds): *Antiarrhythmic Drugs.* Berlin, FRG: Springer-Verlag, 1988, p. 335.
16. Gagnol JP, Devos C, Clinet M, Nokin P: Amiodarone: biochemical aspects and hemodynamic effects. *Drugs* 29(Suppl 3):1, 1985.
17. Bacq ZM, Blakeley AGH, Summers RJ: The effects of amiodarone, an α and β receptor antagonist, on adrenergic transmission in the cat spleen. *Biochem Pharmacol* 25:1195, 1976.
18. Olsson B, Brorson L, Varnauskas E: Class III anti-arrhythmic action in man: observations from monophasic action potential recordings and amiodarone treatment. *Br Heart J* 35: 1255, 1973.
19. Pritchard DA, Singh BN, Hurley PJ: Effects of amiodarone on thyroid function in patients with ischemic heart disease. *Br Heart J* 37:856, 1975.
20. Singh BN, Jewitt DE, Downey JM, et al: Effects of amiodarone and L8040, novel anti-anginal and antiarrhythmic drugs on cardiac and cor-

tagonism of amiodarone. *Biochem Pharmacol* 25:131, 1976.

onary hemodynamics and on cardiac intracellular potentials. *Clin Exp Pharmacol Physiol* 3:426, 1976.

21. Petta JM, Zacheo VJ: Comparative profile of L3428 and other anti-anginal agents on cardiac hemodynamics. *J Pharmacol Exp Ther* 176:328, 1971.

22. Schwartz A, Shen E, Morady F, et al: Hemodynamic effects of intravenous amiodarone in patients with depressed left ventricular function and recurrent ventricular tachycardia. *Am Heart J* 106:848, 1983.

23. Cotè P, Bourassa MG, Delaze PR, et al: Effects of amiodarone on cardiac and coronary hemodynamics and on myocardial metabolism in patients with coronary artery disease. *Circulation* 59:1165, 1979.

24. Rosenbaum MB, Chiale PA, Haedo A, et al: Control of tachyarrhythmias associated with Wolff-Parkinson-White syndrome by amiodarone hydrochloride. *Am J Cardiol* 34:215, 1974.

25. Rosenbaum MB, Chiale PA, Halpern MS, et al: Clinical efficacy of amiodarone as an anti-arrhythmic agent. *Am J Cardiol* 38:934, 1976.

26. Mason JW: Amiodarone. *N Engl J Med* 316:455, 1987.

27. Nademanee K, Hendrickson JA, Cannom DS, et al: Control of refractory life-threatening ventricular arrhythmias by amiodarone. *Am Heart J* 101:759, 1981.

28. Nademanee K, Hendrickson J, Kannan R, Singh BN: Antiarrhythmic efficacy and electrophysiologic actions of amiodarone in patients with life-threatening ventricular arrhythmias: potent suppression of spontaneously occurring tachyarrhythmias versus inconsistent abolition of induced ventricular tachycardia. *Am Heart J* 103:950, 1982.

29. Nademanee K, Singh BN, Hendrickson J, et al: Amiodarone in refractory life-threatening ventricular arrhythmias. *Ann Intern Med* 98:577, 1983.

30. Heger JJ, Prystowsky EN, Jackman WM, et al: Amiodarone: clinical efficacy and electrophysiology during long-term therapy for recumbent ventricular tachycardias or ventricular fibrillation. *N Engl J Med* 305:539, 1981.

31. Middlekauff HR, Stevenson WG, Saxon LA, Stevenson LW: Safest anti-arrhythmic drug in advanced heart failure depends on heart failure etiology. *J Am Coll Cardiol* 19:78A, 1992.

32. Paulus WJ, Nellens P, Heyndrick GR, Andris E: Effects of long-term treatment with amiodarone on exercise hemodynamics and left ventricular relaxation in patients with hypertrophic cardiomyopathy. *Circulation* 74:544, 1986.

33. Singh S, Fletcher RD, Fisher S, et al: Congestive Heart Failure: Survival Trial of Antiarrhythmic Therapy (CHFSTAT). *Cont Clin Trials* 13:339, 1992.

34. Holt DW, Tucker GT, Jackson PR, Storey GCA: Amiodarone pharmacokinetics. *Am Heart J* 106:840, 1983.

35. Storey GCA, Adams PC, Campbell RWF, Holt HW: High performance liquid chromatographic measurement of amiodarone and desethylamiodarone in small tissue samples after enzymatic digestion. *J Clin Pathol* 36:785, 1983.

36. Kannan R, Ikeda N, Drachenberg M, et al: Serum and myocardial kinetics of amiodarone and its major metabolite desethylamiodarone in rabbits. *J Pharm Sci* 73:438, 1982.

37. Latini R, Togoni G, Kates KE: Clinical pharmacokinetics of amiodarone. *Clin Pharmacokinet* 9:136, 1984.

38. Singh BN, Venkatesh N, Nademanee K, et al: The historical development, cellular electrophysiology and clinical pharmacology of amiodarone. *Prog Cardiovasc Dis* 31:249, 1989.

39. Ikeda N, Nademanee K, Kannan R, Singh BN: Electrophysiologic effects of amiodarone: experimental and clinical observations relative to serum and tissue concentrations. *Am Heart J* 108:890, 1984.

40. Mason JW, Hondeghem LM, Katzung BG: Block of inactivated sodium channels and of depolarization induced automaticity in guinea-pig papillary muscle by amiodarone. *Circ Res* 55:277, 1984.

41. Goupil N, Lenfant J: The effects of amiodarone on the sinus node automaticity. *Eur J Pharmacol* 39:23, 1976.

42. Yabek S, Kato R, Singh BN: Acute electrophysiologic effects of amiodarone and desethylamiodarone in isolated cardiac muscle. *J Cardiovasc Pharmacol* 8:197, 1985.

43. Gallagher JD, Bianchi J, Gessman LJ: A comparison of the electrophysiologic effects of acute and chronic amiodarone administration of canine Purkinje fibers. *J Cardiovasc Pharmacol* 13:723, 1989.

44. Nishimura M, Follmer CH, Singer DH: Amiodarone blocks calcium current in single guinea-pig ventricular myocytes. *J Pharmacol Exp Ther* 251:650, 1989.

45. Takanaka C, Singh BN: Barium-induced nondriven action potentials as a model of triggered potentials from early afterdepolarization: significance of slow-channel activity and differing effects of quinidine and amiodarone. *J Am Coll Cardiol* 15:213, 1990.

46. Follmer CH, Aomine M, Yeh JZ, Singer DH:

Amiodarone-induced block of sodium-current in isolated cardiac cells. *J Pharmacol Exp Ther* 243:187, 1987.

47. Kato R, Venkatesh N, Yabek S, et al: The comparative electrophysiologic effects of desethylamiodarone and amiodarone after chronic dosing in rabbits. *Am Heart J* 115:351, 1988.

48. Morady F, DiCarlo LA, Krol RB, et al: Acute and chronic effects of amiodarone on ventricular refractoriness, intraventricular conduction and ventricular tachycardia induction. *J Am Coll Cardiol* 7(1):148, 1986.

49. Balser JR, Bennett PB, Hondeghem LM, et al: Suppression of time dependent outward current in guinea pig ventricular myocytes. *Circ Res* 69:519, 1991.

50. Colatsky TJ, Follmer CH, Starmer CF: Channel specificity in anti-arrhythmic action. Mechanism of potassium-channel block and its role in suppressing and aggravating cardiac arrhythmias. *Circulation* 82:2235, 1990.

51. Howarten RA, Goknur AB, Berkoff HA: Inhibition of ATP-sensitive potassium channels of adult rat heart cells by antiarrhythmic drugs. *Circ Res* 65:1157, 1989.

52. Vincent A, Werquin S, Caron J, et al: Effects of acute and chronic administration of acebutolol on the right ventricular effective refractory period in conscious dogs. *J Cardiovasc Dis* 21:7, 1993.

53. Shaik NA, Downar E, Butany J: Amiodarone on inhibitor of phospholipase activity: comparative study of the inhibitory effects of amiodarone, chloroquine and chlorpromazine. *Mol Cell Biochem* 76:163, 1987.

54. Gross SA, Somani P: Amiodarone-induced ultrastructural changes in the canine myocardial fibers. *Am Heart J* 112:771, 1986.

55. Chatelain P: Effects of amiodarone on lipid dynamics in erythrocyte membrane in vitro and after chronic treatment. *Arch Intern Pharmacodyn* 276:327, 1985.

56. Broekhuysen J, Charlier R, Ghislain J: Action of amiodarone on guinea-pig heart sodium and potassium activated adenosine triphosphatase. *Biochem Pharmacol* 21:2951, 1972.

57. Platou ES, Refsum H: Class III antiarrhythmic action in experimental atrial fibrillation and flutter in dogs. *J Cardiovasc Pharmacol* 4:839, 1982.

58. Jaillon P, Heckle J, Jais J-M, et al: Acute effects of intravenous prifuroline and amiodarone on canine automaticity, conduction and refractoriness. *J Cardiovasc Pharmacol* 4:486, 1982.

59. Yabek S, Kato R, Singh BN: Acute effects of amiodarone on the electrophysiologic properties of isolated neonatal and adult cardiac fibers. *J Am Coll Cardiol* 15:1109, 1985.

60. Gomes JAC, Kang PS, Hariman RJ, et al: Electrophysiologic effects and mechanisms of termination of supraventricular tachycardia by intravenous amiodarone. *Am Heart J* 107:214, 1984.

61. Hariman RJ, Gomes AC, Kang KS, El-Sherif N: Effects of intravenous amiodarone in patients with inducible repetitive ventricular responses and ventricular tachycardia. *Am Heart J* 107:1109, 1984.

62. Wellens HJJ, Brugada P, Abdollah H, Dassen WR: A comparison of the electrophysiologic effects of intravenous and oral amiodarone in the same patient. *Circulation* 69:120, 1984.

63. Waxman HL, Groh WC, Marchlinski FE, et al: Amiodarone for control of sustained ventricular tachyarrhythmias: clinical and electrophysiological effects in 51 patients. *Am J Cardiol* 50:1066, 1982.

64. Finerman WB Jr, Hamer A, Peter T: Electrophysiologic effects of chronic amiodarone therapy in patients with ventricular arrhythmias. *Am Heart J* 104:987, 1982.

65. Shenasa M, Denker S, Mahmud R, et al: Effect of amiodarone on conduction and refractoriness of the His-Purkinje system in the human heart. *J Am Coll Cardiol* 4:105, 1984.

66. Charlier R, Delaunois G, Bauthier J, et al: Recherche dans la série des benzofurannes. XL. Propriètè anti-arrhythmiques de l'amiodarone. *Cardiologia* 54:83, 1969.

67. Lubbe WF, McFadden ML, Muller CA, et al: Protective action of amiodarone against ventricular fibrillation in the isolated perfused rate heart. *Am J Cardiol* 43:553, 1978.

68. Schoenfeld P: Comparison des effets de l'amiodarone et du propranolol sur l'incidence et al sévérité des arrhythmies ventriculaires après ligature de l'artère coronarienne chez le rat anesthèsiè. *J Cardiol* 11:499, 1982.

69. Chew CYC, Collet JT, Campbell C, et al: Beneficial effects of amiodarone pretreatment on early ischemic ventricular arrhythmias relative to infarct size and regional myocardial blood flow in the conscious dog. *J Cardiovasc Pharmacol* 4:1028, 1982.

70. Patterson E, Eller BT, Abrams GD, ET AL: Ventricular fibrillation in conscious canine preparation of sudden coronary death. Prevention by short and long term amiodarone administration. *Circulation* 68:857, 1983.

71. Helmy I, Herre JM, Gee, et al: Use of intravenous amiodarone for emergency treatment of recurrent symptomatic ventricular arrhythmias. *J Am Coll Cardiol* 15:156, 1989.

72. Kadish A, Morady F: The use of amiodarone in the acute therapy of life-threatening tachyarrhythmias. *Prog Cardiovas Dis* 31:281, 1989.

73. Williams ML, Woefel A, Cascio WE, et al: Intravenous amiodarone during prolonged resuscitation from cardiac arrest. *Ann Intern Med* 110:839, 1989.

74. Middlekauff HR, Wiener I, Saxon LA, Stevenson WG: Low-dose amiodarone for atrial fibrillation: time for a prospective study? *Ann Intern Med* 116:1017, 1992.

75. Hughes MM, Trohman RG, Simmons TW, et al: Flecainide therapy in patients treated for supraventricular tachycardia with normal left ventricular ejection fraction. *Am Heart J* 123: 408, 1992.

76. Chun S, Sager P, Stevenson WG, et al: Amiodarone is highly effective in maintaining NSR in refractory atrial fibrillation/flutter. *J Am Coll Cardiol* (submitted).

77. Feld G, Nademanee K, Stevenson WG, et al: Clinical electrophysiologic effects of amiodarone in patients with atrial fibrillation complicating the Wolff-Parkinson-White syndrome. *Am Heart J* 115:102, 1988.

78. Salerno D, Gillingham KJ, Berry DA, Hodges M: A comparison of antiarrhythmic drugs for the suppression of ventricular ectopic depolarization. A meta-analysis. *Am Heart J* 120: 340, 1990.

79. Rosenbaum MB, Chiale PA, Haedo A, et al: Ten years of experience with amiodarone. *Am Heart J* 106:957, 1983.

80. Herre JM, Sauve MJ, Griffin JC, et al: Long term results of amiodarone therapy in patients with recurrent sustained ventricular tachycardia or ventricular fibrillation. *J Am Coll Cardiol* 13: 442, 1989.

81. Weinberg BA, Miles WM, Klein LS, et al: Five year follow-up of 589 patients treated with amiodarone. *Am Heart J* 125:109, 1993.

82. Dargie HJ, Cleland JGF, Leckie BJ, et al: Relation of arrhythmias and electrolyte abnormalities in survival in patients with severe chronic heart failure. *Circulation* 75(Suppl 4):98, 1990.

83. McKenna WJ, Adams RM, Poloniecki JD, et al: Long term survival with amiodarone in patients with hypertrophic cardiomyopathy and ventricular tachycardia. *Circulation* 80:II–7, 1989.

84. Burkart F, Pfisterer M, Kiowski W, et al: Effect of antiarrhythmic therapy on mortality in survivors of myocardial infarction with asymptomatic complex ventricular arrhythmias: Basel Antiarrhythmic Study of Infarct Survival (BASIS). *J Am Coll Cardiol* 16:1711, 1990.

85. Pfisterer ME, Kiowski W, Brunner H, et al: Long-term benefit of one year amiodarone treatment for persistent complex ventricular arrhythmias after myocardial infarction. *Circulation* 87:309, 1993.

86. Greene HL, Poole JE, Fellows CL, et al: Cardiac arrest in Seattle—conventional versus amiodarone drug evaluation (CASCADE): mortality results (abstract). *Circulation* 86:1656, 1992.

87. Fananapazir L, Chang AC, Epstein SE, et al: Prognostic determinants in hypertrophic cardiomyopathy. *Circulation* 86:740, 1992.

88. Singh BN: When is QT prolongation anti-arrhythmic and when is it pro-arrhythmic? *Am J Cardiol* 63:867, 1988.

89. Cui G, Sen L, Uppal P, et al: Comparison of QT dispersion and RR interval induced by sematilide, amiodarone and sotalol. *Circulation* 86:1393, 1992.

90. Anderson KP, Walker R, Dustman R, et al: Rate-related electrophysiologic effects of long-term administration of amiodarone on canine ventricular myocardium in vivo. *Circulation* 79:948, 1989.

91. Singh BN, Nademanee K: Control of arrhythmias by selective lengthening of cardiac repolarization: theoretical considerations and clinical consideration. *Am Heart J* 109:421, 1985.

92. Singh BN, Nademanee K: Amiodarone and thyroid function: clinical implications during antiarrhythmic therapy. *Am Heart J* 106(4): 857, 1983.

93. Hershman JM, Nademanee K, Sugawara M, Pekary A, et al: Thyroxine and triiodothyronine kinetics in cardiac patients taking amiodarone. *Acta Endocrin* 111:193, 1986.

94. Sogol PB, Hershman JM, Reed AW, Dillman WH: The effects of amiodarone on serum thyroid hormones and hepatic thyroxine $5'$-monodeiodination in rats. *Endocrinology* 113: 1464, 1983.

95. Latham KR, Selletti DF, Goldstein RE: Interaction of amiodarone and desethylamiodarone with solubilized nuclear thyroid hormone receptors. *J Am Coll Cardiol* 9(4):872, 1987.

96. Freedberg AS, Papp GJ, Vaughan Williams EM: The effects of altered thyroid state on atrial intracellular potentials. *J Physiol* 207:357, 1970.

97. Talajic M, Nattel S, Davies M, McCann J: Attenuation of Class III and sinus node effects of amiodarone by experimental hypothyroidism. *J Cardiovasc Pharamacol* 13:447, 1989.

98. Bagchi N, Brown TR, Schneider DS, Banerjee SK: Effect of amiodarone on rat heart isoenzymes. *Circ Res* 60:621, 1987.

99. Nag AC, Lee Mei LI, Shepherd D: Effect of amiodarone and the expression of myosin isoforms and cellular growth of cardiac muscle cells. *Circ Res* 67:51, 1990.

100. Cui G, Sen L, Singh BN: Interaction of amiodarone with T3 on Na$^+$ current in guinea pig cardiac myocytes (abstract). *J Am Coll Cardiol* 19:347, 1992.

101. Hensley CB, Bersohn MM, Sarma JSM, et al: Amiodarone decreases Na, K-ATPase α-2 and β-2 expression specifically in cardiac ventricle. *J Cell Mol Cardiol* (in press).

102. Binah O, Bernstein I, Gilat E: Effects of thyroid hormone on the action potential and membrane currents of guinea pig ventricular myocytes. *Plügers Arch* 409:214, 1970.

103. Sharp NA, Neel DS, Parsons RL: Influence of thyroid hormone levels on the electrical and mechanical properties of rabbit papillary muscle. *J Mol Cell Cardiol* 17:119, 1985.

104. Norman MF, Lavin TA: Competition of thyroid hormone action by amiodarone in rat pituitary tumor cells. *J Clin Invest* 83:306, 1989.

PART VI

Emerging Class III Compounds of Potential Clinical Utility

Chapter 35

Electrophysiological and Pharmacodynamic Profile of Sematilide HCL

Philip T. Sager
Bramah N. Singh

Ventricular arrhythmias have been pharmacologically controlled either by prolonging conduction (Class I effects) or by delaying refractoriness (Class III effects)[1-4] with or without adrenergic modulation. Refractoriness is usually increased by prolonging repolarization (ie, the action potential duration [APD]) through inhibition of outward currents or by increasing inward currents (see Chapter 3) or, alternatively, by decreasing the availability of resting sodium channels at the end of repolarization (see Chapter 16). Given the unfavorable outcome of the Cardiac Arrhythmia Suppression Trial using Class I antiarrhythmic agents,[5,6] heightened concern regarding proarrhythmic effects of Class I agents,[7,8] and the relatively high level of efficacy associated with amiodarone therapy,[9-11] there has recently been a marked interest in controlling ventricular arrhythmias with agents that exert "pure" Class III effects.

The currently available "Class III" agents, amiodarone, sotalol, and bretylium have other electrophysiological actions in addition to their ability to prolong the APD. A number of agents (eg, sematilide, dofetilide, E-4031, almokalant, ambasilide, etc.) whose sole pharmacological action is to lengthen the APD are in various stages of development (see Chapters 35–42). It has been hoped that such selective agents might afford a more effective and safer mechanism to treat ventricular arrhythmias than the currently available pharmacological approaches. At present, sematilide is perhaps the most advanced agent in its development. This chapter will review sematilide's pharmacology from results of in vitro and in vivo studies and the preliminary data from human clinical investigations.

Structure

Sematilide (N-[2(Diethylamino)ethyl]-4-[(methylsulfonyl)amino]benzamide monohydrochloride; (K1752A) (Berlex Laboratories) was specifically synthesized on the basis of structure-activity relationships of procainamide to be a specific Class III agent (Figure

From BN Singh, HJJ Wellens, M Hiraoka, (eds): *Electropharmacological Control of Cardiac Arrhythmias.* Mount Kisco, NY, Futura Publishing Company Inc., © 1994.

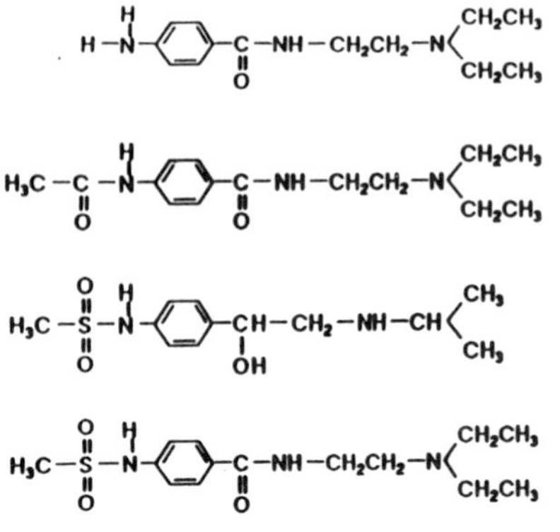

Figure 1. Chemical structure of sematilide compared to those of procainamide, N-acetyl procainamide, and sotalol.

1).[12-14] N-acetyl (as in n-acetyl procainamide) or n-sulfonyl (as in sematilide) substitutions of procainamide yield analogs with specific Class III activity. An absence of β-blocking activity for sematilide (unlike sotalol) is the result of an aldehyde instead of an alcohol moiety in the para position.

In Vitro Studies

Voltage-clamp studies in isolated ferret Purkinje fibers[15] have demonstrated that the major determinant of sematilide-induced APD prolongation is block of the delayed rectifier (I_K). A 3-μM concentration of sematilide reduced I_K by approximately 50%.[12] In addition, I_K was reduced by the same percent at the various test potentials evaluated (-30 to $+10$ mV), suggesting that sematilide's effect on the delayed rectifier is not voltage dependent.[12] A representative recording of the analysis of delayed rectifier current in isolated ferret Purkinje fibers is shown in Figure 2. Whether sematilide blocks only one (I_{Ks} or I_{Kr}) or both subtypes of I_K[16,17] has not been determined.

Studies in canine Purkinje fibers and right ventricular muscle[18] demonstrate a con-

centration-dependent (0.1–100 μM) increase in APD_{95} and effective refractory period (ERP) of these tissues during sematilide administration. The concentration producing a 20% increase (EC_{20}) in the APD_{95} was 3 μM in Purkinje tissue and 1 μM in ventricular tissue. Superimposed tracings from recordings before and after superfusion of Purkinje fibers and ventricular muscle with sematilide are shown in Figure 3. A larger change in the APD is seen in the case of Purkinje fibers than in the ventricular muscle. There was no effect on $\dot{V}_{max}$, action potential amplitude, or resting membrane potential at any of the tested concentrations. Similar electrophysiological effects were observed when $[K]_o$ was decreased from 4 μM to 2.7 μM. Thus, sematilide appears to be devoid of effects on the sodium channel. The frequency-dependent effects of sematilide on the APD in Purkinje fibers and ventricular muscle[12] demonstrated a significant attenuation of sematilide-induced APD prolongation during rapid pacing (3.3 Hz versus 1.0 Hz). This attenuation of drug-induced prolongation of repolarization at short paced cycle lengths has been termed "reverse" frequency dependence.[19,20]

The electrophysiological effects of sematilide have also been studied in isolated rabbit atrial tissue.[21] Argentieri et al.[21] demonstrated that sematilide significantly increased the sinoatrial node APD_{95} and sinus cycle length in a dose- (10–100 μM) dependent manner. The sinoatrial node APD_{95} ($EC_{20} = 15 \pm 3$ μM) increased by 34%–61% and the sinus cycle length ($EC_{20} = 54 \pm 13$ μM) by 14%–21%. In atrial muscle, sematilide increased the APD_{95} ($EC_{20} = 34 \pm 10$ μM) and ERP ($EC_{20} = 14 \pm 3$ μM) by 8%–30% and 14%–32%, respectively. Similar effects were observed on the atrioventricular (AV) node APD.

The lack of effect of sematilide on autonomic receptors was confirmed in several studies.[12] Sematilide demonstrated no interaction on norepinephrine-induced contraction of isolated renal and cardiac arteries, no binding to β or muscarinic receptors, and no effect on arachidonic acid-induced human

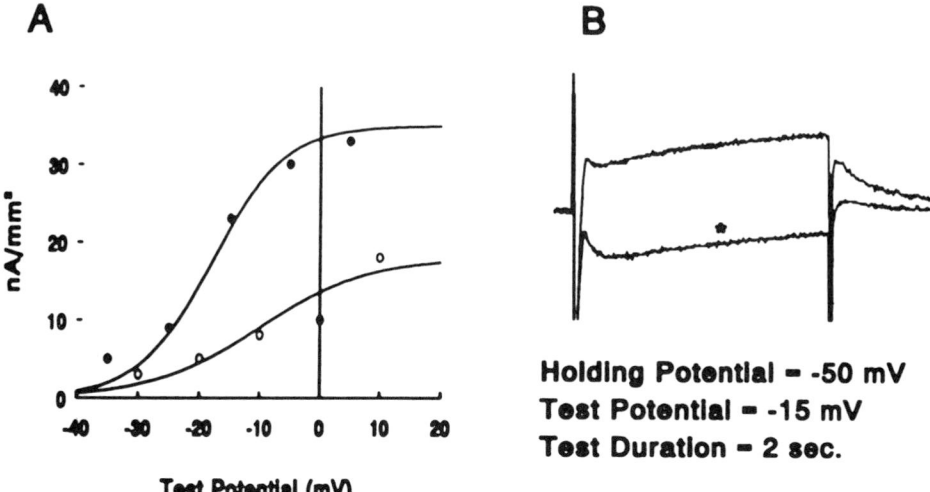

Figure 2. Analysis of delayed rectifier current in isolated ferret Purkinje fibers. Panel A shows representative delayed rectifier tail current activation curve before (closed circles) and after (open circles) exposure to 10-μM sematilide. An equal amount of block is seen at all test potentials. Panel B shows representative current tracing before and after (*) a 10-minute exposure to 10-μM sematilide. (Reproduced with permission from Reference 12.)

platelet aggregation. Thus, sematilide appears to be devoid of autonomic interactions.

In Vivo Studies

Wiggins et al.[12,22] studied sematilide's electrophysiological effects in anesthetized dogs. At all examined concentrations, sematilide (0.3–3.0 mg/kg) significantly increased the atrial ERP (15%–50%), ventricular ERP (4%–18%), the QT (9%–34%), and the QTc (9%–22%). In addition, the sinus cycle length was significantly increased (by 18%) at the highest dose level. There were no effects on AV nodal conduction, ventricular conduction, the PR interval, or the QRS interval. No deleterious effects on blood pressure, cardiac output, LV dP/dt, or coronary blood flow were observed in doses up to 100 mg/kg intravenous.[23]

Sullivan et al.[23] studied the antiarrhythmic efficacy of sematilide in a canine model 3–8 days after anterior wall myocardial infarction created by a total left anterior descending coronary artery (LAD) occlusion followed by

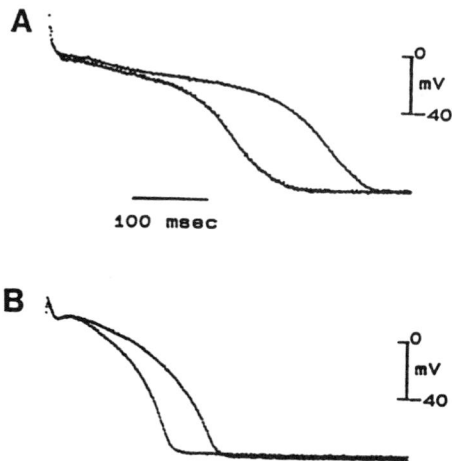

Figure 3. Representative action potentials recorded from canine Purkinje fiber (A) and ventricular muscle. Each panel shows two action potentials, a control, and the increase in action potential duration associated with exposure to 10-μM sematilide. Both preparations were recorded at a stimulus rate of 1.0 Hz. (Reproduced with permission from Reference 12.)

reperfusion. The nonsedated animals were studied using programmed ventricular stimulation (PVS). Sematilide prevented the induction of sustained ventricular tachycardia (VT) during PVS in 8 of 9 dogs after a 1 mg/kg intravenous dose and in 7 of 10 dogs after oral administration (2.5 mg/kg). No proarrhythmic responses were noted after intravenous doses of 100 mg/kg.

In a second study, also using an LAD occlusion/reperfusion canine model, Chi et al.[24] demonstrated in 10 dogs with baseline-inducible ventricular arrhythmias using PVS that sematilide suppressed arrhythmia induction in 60% of the animals. Arrhythmia suppression was correlated with increased refractoriness. In addition, when left circumflex ischemia was provoked in the same animals, 8 of 10 (80%) drug-free animals had ventricular fibrillation during the first hour of ischemia compared to only 2 of 10 (20%) receiving sematilide ($p < 0.05$). Thus, sematilide appears to significantly reduce the incidence of PVS-induced VT in an early postmyocardial infarction canine model and also reduces spontaneous arrhythmias during acute ischemia of a region distinct from the initial infarct. Sematilide was not effective in suppressing arrhythmias in dogs thought to be triggered (ouabain induced) or thought to be secondary to increased automaticity (24 hours postmyocardial infarction).[23]

Clinical Studies

Clinical Pharmacokinetics

The pharmacokinetics of sematilide were studied in six volunteers after intravenous sematilide.[25] The volume of distribution was 59 ± 5 L, total clearance was 322 ± 19 mL/min, the renal clearance was 242 ± 16 mL/min, and the mean residence time was 3.0 ± 0.1 hours. Seventy-five percent of the dose was excreted in the urine. The average absolute bioavailability (after a single oral 25-mg dose) was 47 ± 5% and was unaltered by food. Wong et al.[26] demonstrated that a 25% increase in the QTc interval is associated with a plasma concentration of approximately 2.0 μg/mL (without effects on the PR or QRS interval) and found a mean elimination half-life of 3.6 ± 0.8 hours after an intravenous infusion. However, the clearance is prolonged after repeated oral dosing and sematilide is eliminated with a β phase (5 ± 2 hours) and a γ phase (13 ± 6 hours).[27] The β phase predominated, and with every 8-hour dosing there was a 2.3 ± 0.8 fold (range 1.3–3.9) ratio of peak to trough concentrations.[27]

Electrocardiographic Effects

Dose ranging studies in 20 healthy volunteers have demonstrated a dose related effect on the QT and QTc intervals without changes in the PR or QRS intervals.[12,28] Administration of 100 mg, 150 mg, or 200 mg a day in two divided doses resulted in a maximum increase in the QTc of 12%, 18%, and 23%, respectively.

The electrocardiographic effects of sematilide were examined in a second oral dose ranging study of 48 patients with ≥ 30 premature ventricular contractions (PVCs)/h and left ventricular ejection fraction (LVEF) ≥ 20%.[28] There were no significant effects on the PR or QRS intervals. A dose of 50–150 mg was utilized every 8 hours. The QT interval was significantly increased at peak levels by 5% at the 50-mg dose and by 18% at both the 100-mg and 150-mg dose levels. Only at the 150-mg dose was the sinus cycle length significantly increased (by 11%). As expected, there was a modest reduction in PVCs with 23% of the patients having a reduction of ≥ 70% in PVCs/24 h. One patient developed new ventricular fibrillation, and one patient each developed nausea, asthenia, dizziness, and pruritis.

Antiarrhythmic Efficacy During Electrophysiological Testing

Patient Characteristics and Methods

Sematilide has been examined in a multicenter study[28] in 142 patients with malignant ventricular arrhythmias. This study enrolled patients with clinical sustained VT, ventricular fibrillation, cardiac arrest, or syncope secondary to VT. Entry criteria included inducible, sustained monomorphic VT during baseline drug-free electrophysiological study or, in cardiac arrest patients, inducible, sustained polymorphic VT or ventricular fibrillation. Exclusion criteria included patients with unstable angina pectoris, LVEF of less than 20%, Class IV untreated functional disability, myocardial infarction within the last month, serum potassium level of < 4.0 mEq/L or serum magnesium levels of < 1.5 mEq/L, or a QTc interval of > 450 msec in the drug-free state.

Patients were initially started on 75–100 mg of sematilide every 8 hours, and a repeat electrophysiological study was performed. If VT was still induced, sematilide could be increased to 125–150 mg every 8 hours, and the electrophysiological study was repeated. Patients with a creatine clearance of more than 70 mL per min were increased to 200 mg every 8 hours if VT remained inducible at the lower dose.

Electrophysiological testing was performed at twice the diastolic threshold from two right ventricular sites (right ventricular apex and the right ventricular outflow tract) at paced cycle lengths of 600, 500, and 400 msec. Up to three premature extrastimuli were given at both sites. Drug responders were defined as patients in whom ≤ 15 beats of nonsustained VT was induced during sematilide therapy. Partial drug responders were defined as patients who had more than 15 beats of nonsustained, induced VT, which lasted for less than 30 seconds and was unassociated with hemodynamic symptoms. Drug failures were defined as patients who were not drug responders.

In a subgroup of patients enrolled in this protocol, more detailed electrophysiological studies including full atrial studies with measurements of atrial refractoriness, AV nodal refractoriness, and distal conduction system properties were examined with catheters placed in the atrium, at the right ventricular

Table 1
Sematilide Hydrochloride Ventricular Tachycardia Study: Demographic Profile

Age (Mean)	61 years
Male	93%
History of myocardial infarction	77%
History of CHF	57%
Baseline LVEF	
Mean	0.37
Range	0.21 to 0.71
LVEF $\leq$30%	29%
Previous Antiarrhythmic Prescription	77%
Mean # of Drug Trials	1.8
Range	0–6
Presenting Diagnosis	
Sustained VT or syncope	84%
Cardiac arrest	16%

CHF: congenital heart failure; LVEF: left ventricular ejection fraction; VT: ventricular tachycardia.

apex, and across the tricuspid valve to measure the His-bundle electrogram.

Results of Multicenter Study in Patients with Malignant Ventricular Arrhythmias with Sematilide

This preliminary analysis of the multicenter trial includes 142 patients. Their clinical characteristics are listed in Table 1.

Electrophysiological Effects (Table 2)

Electrophysiological effects were examined at a paced cycle length of 600 msec. The atrial ERP was increased by 7% ($p < 0.05$) at a dose of 100 mg every 8 hours and by 14% ($p < 0.001$) at a dose of 150 mg every 8 hours. There were no significant effects on the AH or HV intervals at either dose. The right ventricular apex ERP was increased by 10% ($p <$

Table 2
Sematilide Multicenter HCL Ventricular Tachycardia Study:
Electrophysiology Effects (Paced Cycle Length = 600 msec)

	AERP	HV	VERP
N	24	34	36
Baseline	242 ± 33	62 ± 16	250 ± 28
SEM 100 MG q8°	256 ± 37	59 ± 14	274 ± 35
% Change	7%	−2%	10%
p-value	<.05	NS	<.001
N	30	31	33
Baseline	236 ± 26	60 ± 14	248 ± 21
SEM 150 MG q8°	268 ± 46	58 ± 11	276 ± 28
% Change	14%	−2%	12%
p-value	<.001	NS	<.001

0.001) at 100-mg dosing and by 12% ($p <$ 0.001) at 150 mg q 8 hour dosing.

Response to Premature Ventricular Stimulation (Table 3)

At the first dose level tested (75–150 mg q 8 hours), induction of sustained VT was sup-

Table 3
Sematilide HCL Multicenter Ventricular
Tachycardia Study: Suppression of
Inducible Sustained Ventricular Tachycardia
by Sematilide (N = 142)

First Dose Tested		
Dose	N	Sustained VT Suppressed
75 mg	23	3 (13%)
100 mg	58	13 (22%)
150 mg	61	17 (28%)
Nonresponders to Initial Dose		
Dose Increase	N	Sustained VT Suppressed
75 mg → 126 mg	11	2 (18%)
100 mg → 150 mg	26	5 (19%)
150 mg → 200 mg	7	0 (0%)

Overall suppression of inducible sustained VT:40 of
142 28%)

pressed in 23% of the patients. In 44 patients who did not respond to the initial dose, sematilide dosing was increased to the next dose level, and in 7 additional patients induction of sustained VT was suppressed. Thus, overall, 40 of the 144 (28%) of the patients examined had induction sustained VT suppressed by sematilide. Of these patients, 30 (21%) were full responders, and 10 (7%) were partial responders. Of note, none of the 7 patients who continued to have inducibility of sustained VT at a dose level of 150 mg q 8 hour dosing had VT suppressed after dosing was increased to 200 mg every 8 hours.

Adverse Events

There was no exacerbation of congestive heart failure in the study population, and the LVEF by equilibrium radionuclide angiography (n = 36) before and during sematilide therapy was unchanged. During the hospital course, one patient had a significant increase in runs of pause-dependent nonsustained VT of up to 7 beats (0.7%), and two patients had a significant increase in the frequency of episodes of sustained VT (1.4%). Of these latter patients, one had three episodes of sustained VT in 24 hours, and the other patient developed sustained VT that was more difficult to convert to sinus rhythm. Previously, the arrhythmia had always responded to intravenous procainamide, but following sematilide therapy the patient required direct current cardioversion. These three patients with an apparent proarrhythmic response were all successfully treated by discontinuing the medication. There were no in-hospital deaths.

Three patients (2.1%) had sematilide discontinued secondary to nonarrhythmic adverse experiences. During in-hospital dose titration, one patient developed fatigue (100 mg every 8 hours), one patient developed nausea and dizziness (100 mg every 8 hours), and one patient developed nausea and vomiting (200 mg every 8 hours). Six patients were discontinued from the protocol during hospitalization because their QT intervals reached a predefined limit of 550 msec (prior to their repeat electrophysiological study).

Effects of Sematilide on the Action Potential Duration in Humans

Sager et al.[29] have examined the frequency-dependent effects of sematilide in 10 patients with malignant ventricular arrhythmias. Monophasic action potential duration was measured during steady-state ventricular pacing at the right ventricular apex using a catheter that allowed both recording of the monophasic action potential duration and ventricular pacing at the same cardiac site. This study demonstrated that the APD_{90} was prolonged to a significantly greater extent during ventricular pacing at a cycle length of 600 msec, as compared to pacing at shorter cycle lengths (300 msec). The APD_{90} was prolonged by 15% during sematilide at a cycle length at 600 ($p = 0.01$) but by only 7% ($p = 0.06$) at a paced cycle length of 300 msec. The difference in the slopes of the curves for APD_{90} versus paced cycle length at baseline and following sematilide therapy was significantly different ($p = 0.005$) with a much steeper slope after sematilide therapy. Thus, sematilide-induced

prolongation of repolarization is attenuated during rapid ventricular pacing, which is similar to the findings in canine cardiac muscle.[12] Similar findings were also demonstrated for the right ventricular effective refractory period (VERP). Sematilide, however, had no effect on QRS duration, a measure of ventricular conduction, or the VERP/APD ratio, demonstrating that the effects of sematilide on refractoriness were essentially voltage dependent.

The predictors of suppression of inducible sustained VT during sematilide therapy have also been examined in 25 patients.[30] Suppression of inducibility was significantly correlated with relative prolongation of the VERP during sematilide therapy as compared to baseline. Fifty-five percent of drug responders had an increase in the VERP of more than 30 msec compared to none of the drug failures ($p < 0.01$). Drug response was not predicted by previous arrhythmia history, cardiac diagnosis, LVEF, left ventricular dimensions, PVC reduction, cycle length of the baseline sustained VT, or the baseline ventricular VERP. Thus, the only clinical variable (drug levels were not available) correlated with suppression of inducible VT was prolongation of refractoriness.

Sager et al.[31] have also examined the ability of isoproterenol to reverse sematilide-induced prolongation of the ventricular APD_{90} and ERP in humans. Isoproterenol (.035 μg/kg per minute) fully reversed APD_{90} prolongation following sematilide compared to baseline values. After isoproterenol, the VERP tended to be reduced to values below baseline. Thus, sematilide-induced prolongation of repolarization and refractoriness can be reversed with moderate β-adrenergic sympathetic stimulation.

Discussion

The in vitro and in vivo data indicate that sematilide's sole pharmacological action is to prolong repolarization and that it increases refractoriness by prolonging the APD. It exerts effects in both the atrium and ventricle with a modest increase in sinus cycle length, as has been noted for many of the other "pure" Class III agents under development. Also, voltage-clamp studies show that sematilide blocks the delayed rectifier, through its actions on the I_K subtypes have not been defined. Sematilide does not block sodium currents nor does it exert interactions with autonomic transmitters. Noncardiac side effects are low, dosing can be every 8 hours, and the incidence of torsades de pointes appears to be ≤5%, although the precise incidence of proarrhythmia awaits more extensive studies in different subsets of patients with cardiac disease. Overall suppression of inducibility of sustained VT was similiar to values obtained from the literature for quinidine (mean ± SD, 22 ± 9%), procainamide (23 ± 9%), and sotalol (41 ± 27%).[3] The long-term follow-up data on sematilide awaits the conclusion of current trials.

Again, as in the case of other pure Class III agents, sematilide-induced prolongation of repolarization is attenuated during rapid pacing. This "reverse" frequency dependence has been demonstrated for other agents that block outward K channels, such as dofetilide,[32] sotalol,[33,34] and quinidine,[35,36] but not amiodarone.[37,38] Some authors[19] have proposed that the reverse frequency-dependent effects of the "pure" Class III agents on repolarization may significantly limit their clinical efficacy since pharmacological effect will be attenuated at the short cycle lengths of many clinical ventricular arrhythmias. Others,[39] however, have suggested that the pure Class III agents will still prevent arrhythmias from initiating and that even small increases in repolarization may still have clinical benefit. Reverse frequency dependence of the APD has been demonstrated for sematilide in vitro and in humans using monophasic action potential recordings. The relationship of reverse frequency dependence of the APD and attenuation of sematilide-induced VERP prolongation at short cycle lengths to clinical efficacy is unclear at this time. Although sematilide has a moderate ability to suppress inducible, sustained VT during PVS, whether a higher incidence of supression of VT during electrophys-

iological study could be obtained with an agent without reverse frequency-dependent effects on repolarization is unknown. β Blockade may be of importance in the clinical use of "pure" Class III agents since the pharmacological actions of sematilide are readily reversed by β-adrenergic sympathetic stimulation. β Blockade, by accentuating bradycardia, however, may also increase the incidence of torsades de pointes. It is likely that the electrophysiological actions of other "pure" Class III agents will also be reversed during β-adrenergic stimulation. Reversal of E4031-induced APD prolongation by isoproterenol has been shown to be secondary to augmented conduction of I_{Ks} without significant effect on the rapidly activating subtype of the delayed rectifier, I_{Kr}.[17]

Conclusions

In summary, sematilide markedly prolongs repolarization in humans, is effective in suppressing the induction of sustained VT during electrophysiology study, and is well tolerated. Torsades de pointes has been associated with sematilide during short-term observations. The long-term clinical efficacy and propensity to cause proarrhythmic effects are still being evaluated. As with other pure Class III agents, the risks and benefits of the drug will require detailed studies in controlled clinical trials in patients with supraventricular and ventricular tachyarrhythmias.

References

1. Singh BN, Courtney K: On the classification of antiarrhythmic mechanisms: experimental and clinical correlations. In: DP Zipes, J Jalife (eds): *Cardiac Electrophysiology: From the Cell to the Bedside*. Philadelphia: W.B. Saunders, 1990, p. 882.
2. Singh BN, Vaughan Williams EM: A third class of antiarrhythmic action. Effects on atrial and ventricular intracellular potentials, and other pharmacologic actions on cardiac muscle, of MJ 1999 and AH 3474. *Br J Pharmacol* 29:675, 1970.
3. Nattel S: Antiarrhythmic drug classifications: a

critical appraisal of their history, present status, and clinical relevance. *Drugs* 5:672, 1991.

4. Vaughan Williams EM: A classification of antiarrhythmic actions reassessed after a decade of new drugs. *J Clin Pharmacol* 24:129, 1984.

5. Cardiac Arrhythmia Suppression Trial (CAST) Investigators: Preliminary report, effect of encainide and flecainide on ventricular tachyarrhythmias: evaluation of programmed stimulation and ambulatory electrocardiogram. *J Am Coll Cardiol* 5:949, 1986.

6. Echt DS, Liebson PR, Mitchell LB, et al: Mortality and morbidity in patients receiving encainide, flecainide, or placebo. The Cardiac Arrhythmia Suppression Trial. *N Engl J Med* 324:781, 1991.

7. Ahmed R, Singh BN: Anti-arrhythmic drugs. *Current Opin Cardiol* 8:10, 1993.

8. Morganroth J, Goin JE: Quinidine-related mortality in the short-to-medium-term treatment of ventricular arrhythmias: a meta-analysis. *Circulation* 84:1977, 1991.

9. Herre JM, Sauve MJ, Malone P, Scheinman MM: Long-term results of amiodarone therapy in patients with recurrent sustained ventricular tachycardia or ventricular fibrillation. *J Am Coll Cardiol* 12:442, 1989.

10. Nademanee K, Stevenson W, Weiss J, et al: The role of amiodarone in the survivors of sudden arrhythmic deaths. In: BN Singh (ed): *Control of Cardiac Arrhythmias by Lengthening Repolarization.* Mt. Kisco, NY: Futura Publishing Co., Inc., 1988, p.489.

11. Weinberg BA, Miles WM, Klein LS, et al: Five-year follow-up of 589 patients treated with amiodarone. *Am Heart J* 125:109, 1993.

12. Argentieri TM: Sematilide. *CV Drug Reviews* 10: 182, 1992.

13. Lumma WC, Wohl RA, Davey DD, et al: Rational design of 4-[(methylsylfonyl)amino]benzamides as Class III antiarrhythmic agents. *J Med Chem* 30:756, 1987.

14. Morgan TK, Lis R, Lumma WC: Synthesis and cardiac electrophysiologic activity of N-substituted-4-(1H-imidazol-1-yl)benzamides-new selective Class III agents. *J Med Chem* 33: 1091, 1990.

15. Argentieri TM, Carroll MS: Electrophysiologic mechanism of action of the Class III antiarrhythmic agents sematilide and clofilium. *J Molec Cell Cardiol* 22(Suppl III):S.81, 1990.

16. Sanguinetti MC, Jurkiewicz NK: Two components of cardiac delayed rectifier K$^+$ current: differential sensitivity to block by Class III antiarrhythmic agents. *J Gen Physiol* 96: 194, 1990.

17. Sanguinetti MC, Jurkiewicz NK, Scott A, Siegl PKS: Isoproterenol antagonized prolongation of refractory period by the class III antiarrhythmic agent E-4031 in guinea pig myocytes: mechanism of action *Circ Res* 68:77, 1991.

18. Sullivan ME, Argentieri TM, Stones S, et al: Electrophysiologic properties of CK-1752A, a new specific class III agent. *Cardiovasc Drugs Ther* 1:294, 1987.

19. Hondeghem LM, Snyders DJ: Class III antiarrhythmic agents have a lot of potential but a long way to go: reduced effectiveness and dangers of reverse use dependence. *Circulation* 81:686, 1990.

20. Nattel S, Zeng FD: Frequency-dependent effects of antiarrhythmic drugs on action potential duration and refractoriness of canine cardiac Purkinje fibers. *J Pharm Exp Ther* 22:283, 1984.

21. Argentieri TM, Carroll MS, Sullivan ME: Cellular electrophysiological effects of the class III antiarrhythmic agents sematilide and clofilium on rabbit atrial tissues. *J Cardiovasc Pharmacol* 18:167, 1991.

22. Wiggins J, Sullivan ME, Doroshuk CM, Reiser HJ: Antiarrhythmic and hemodynamic properties of CK-1752A, a new class III agent in experimental myocardial infarction. *Cardiovasc Drugs Ther* 1:302, 1987.

23. Sullivan ME, Argentieri TM, Reiser HJ: Electrophysiologic, antiarrhythmic and hemodynamic profile of sematilide HCl in canine cardiac tissues. *J Mol Cell Cardiol* 22:S.70, 1990.

24. Chi L, Mu D-X, Driscoll EM, Lucchesi BR: Antiarrhythmic and electrophysiologic actions of CK-3579 and sematilide in conscious canine model of sudden coronary death. *J Cardiovasc Pharmacol* 16:312, 1990.

25. Hinderling PH, Lasser T, Holyoak W, et al: Pharmacokinetics and dynamics of sematilide HCl. *Clin Pharmacol Ther* 47:193, 1990.

26. Wong W, Pavlou HN, Birgersdotter UM, et al: Pharmacology of the class III antiarrhythmic agent sematilide in patients with arrhythmias. *Am J Cardiol* 69:206, 1992.

27. Wong W, Birgersdotter UM, Turgeon J, Roden D: Steady-state pharmacokinetics and pharmacodynamics of the class III antiarrhythmic sematilide. *Circulation* 82(Suppl III): ■, 1990.

28. Data on File, Wayne, NJ: Berlex Laboratories.

29. Sager P, Antimisiaris M, Neiditch T, et al: Frequency-dependent electrophysiologic effects of sematilide, a "pure" class III antiarrhythmic agent. *Circulation* 84:II-350, 1991.

30. Sager P, Nademanee K, Antimisiaris M, et al: The antiarrhythmic role of selective prolongation of refractoriness: suppression of inducible VT with sematilide. *Circulation* 88:1072, 1993.

31. Sager P, Uppal P, Godfrey B, et al: β-adrenergic stimulation: differential electrophysiologic actions on class III agents. *Circulation* 84:I-264, 1992.

32. Tande PM, Bjornstad H, Yang T, et al: Rate-de-

pendent Class III antiarrhythmic action, negative chronotropy, and positive inotropy of a novel I_K blocking drug, UK-68,798: potent in guinea pig but no effect in rat myocardium. *J Cardio Pharm* 16:401, 1990.

33. Schmitt C, Brachmann J, Karch M, et al: Reverse use-dependent effects of sotalol demonstrated by recording monophasic action potentials of the right ventricle. *Am J Cardiol* 68:1183, 1991.

34. Strauss HC, Bigger JT, Hoffman BF: Electrophysiological and β-receptor blocking effects of MJ1999 on dog and rabbit cardiac tissue. *Circulation* 26:661, 1970.

35. Nademanee K, Stevenson WG, Weiss JN, et al: Frequency-dependent effects of quinidine on the ventricular action potential and QRS duration in humans. *Circulation* 81:790, 1990.

36. Roden DM, Hoffman BF: Action potential prolongation and induction of abnormal automaticity of low quinidine concentrations in canine Purkinje fibers: relationship to potassium and cycle length. *Circ Res* 56:857, 1985.

37. Sager P, Uppal P, Follmer C, Antimisiaris M, Pruitt C, Singh B: Frequency-dependent electrophysiologic effects of amiodarone in humans. *Circulation* 88:1063–1071, 1993.

38. Anderson KP, Walker R, Dsutoman T, et al: Rate-related electrophysiologic effects of long-term administration of amiodarone on canine ventricular myocardium in vivo. *Circulation* 79:948, 1989.

39. Colatsky TJ, Follmer CH, Starmer CF: Channel specificity in antiarrhythmic drug action: mechanism of potassium channel block and its role in suppressing and aggravating cardiac arrhythmias. *Circulation* 82:2235, 1990.

Chapter 36

E-4031

Masayasu Hiraoka
Kohei Sawada
Junichi Nitta
Hitoshi Adaniya

E-4031 (N-[4 = [[1-[2-(6-methyl-2-pyridin-yl)ethyl]-4-piperidinyl]carbonyl]phenyl] meth-anesulfonamide dihydrochloride dihydrate) is a novel compound with a structural simi-larity to sotalol (Figure 1). It has an action to prolong action potential duration without ap-preciable effects on resting potentials and up-stroke velocity.[1] The main action is believed to block the delayed outward potassium current (I_k), but its detailed mechanism is still contro-versial.[2,3] In this study to characterize its anti-arrhythmic properties, we examined electro-physiological and antiarrhythmic actions of E-4031 using various cardiac preparations.

Methods

Papillary Muscle and Purkinje Fiber Preparations

Papillary muscles and Purkinje fibers were dissected from the right ventricle of dogs and guinea pigs after the animal was anesthe-tized with sodium pentobarbital (50 mg/kg, intravenous) under artificial respiration. The preparations were then placed in the tissue bath where the Tyrode's solution was per-fused at 37°C. The composition of the Tyrode's solution (in millimoles) was: 125 NaCl, 4.0 KCl, 1.8 CaCl$_4$, 0.5 MgCl$_2$, 0.4 NaH$_2$PO$_4$, 24.6 NaHCO$_3$, and 5.5 glucose with pH adjusted to 7.3–7.4. Membrane potentials were measured by conventional microelectrode technique. Electrical stimulation of the preparations was made through bipolar silver electrodes placed at the one end of the tissues.

Isolated Ventricular Myocyte Preparations

Single ventricular myocytes from guinea pig hearts were prepared by an enzymatic dis-sociation procedure as described elsewhere.[4] Isolated cells were placed in the recording chamber set on the stage of an inverted phase contrast microscope (Diaphot TMD, Nikon, Tokyo). The temperature of the recording chamber was kept at 34–36°C. The composi-tion of the Tyrode's solution used for single myocyte experiments was (in millimoles): 144

From BN Singh, HJJ Wellens, M Hiraoka, (eds): *Electropharmacological Control of Cardiac Arrhythmias*. Mount Kisco, NY, Futura Publishing Company Inc., © 1994.

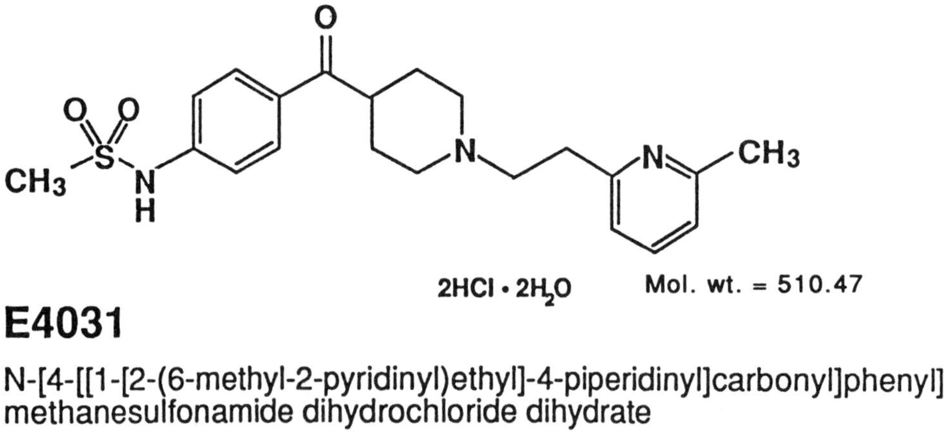

E4031

N-[4-[[1-[2-(6-methyl-2-pyridinyl)ethyl]-4-piperidinyl]carbonyl]phenyl]
methanesulfonamide dihydrochloride dihydrate

2HCl · 2H$_2$O   Mol. wt. = 510.47

Figure 1. Chemical structure of E-4031.

NaCl, 0.33 NaH$_2$PO$_4$, 4.0 KCl, 1.8 CaCl$_2$, 0.53 MgCl$_2$, 5.5 glucose, and 5.0 HEPES adjusted to pH 7.3–7.4 by addition of NaOH. The pipette solution consisted of (in millimoles): 130.0 KCl, 5.0 K$_2$ATP (Sigma Chemical Co., St Louis, MO), 5.O K$_2$ creatine phosphate (Sigma Chemical Co.), and 10.0 HEPES-KOH buffer (pH 7.2). The single pipette whole cell clamp method[5] was applied to single ventricular myocytes to record membrane potentials and currents by use of a patch clamp amplifier (Model 8900, Dagan, Minneapolis, MN) as reported previously.[4]

Arrhythmia Models

We used two types of arrhythmia models to examine antiarrhythmic effects of E-4031. The one was the model of atrial tachycardias produced in rabbit right atrial preparations.[6] Arrhythmias in this model represented macro-reentry using the atrial preferential pathways of the crista terminalis and its extension for the circulating path of impulses.

The other model was 7-day-old canine myocardial infarction, in which ventricular tachycardias (VTs) were induced by programmed electrical stimulation.[7] Ventricular tachycardias of this model were assumed to represent reentry as their mechanism, but the precise reentrant pathways were not defined.

Results

Effects of E-4031 on Action Potentials of Multicellular Preparations

Figure 2 shows effects of different concentrations of E-4031 on canine ventricular muscle (A) and Purkinje fiber (B). The concentration of E-4031 as low as 10^{-8} M caused a prolongation of action potential duration and with increasing the drug concentration the effects became prominent up to 10^{-6} M. The effects were similarly observed both in muscle and Purkinje fibers, but the latter seemed to be more sensitive to the drug than the former since the latter effect was usually seen at 10^{-8} M while the former at 5 × 10^{-8} M (n = 4). Another feature of this drug effect on action potential duration is shown in Figure 3. The drug effects were examined at different frequencies of stimulation in guinea pig papillary muscle preparations. Prolongation of action potential duration was more prominent at lower frequencies (0.5 and 1.0 Hz) than the higher ones (2.0 and 3.3 Hz) at all three concentrations tested. Therefore, the effects were frequency dependent with reversed use dependence.[8] It was also noted that the drug effects saturated at about 10^{-6} M or the higher concentration, since there were no differ-

Ventricular Muscle

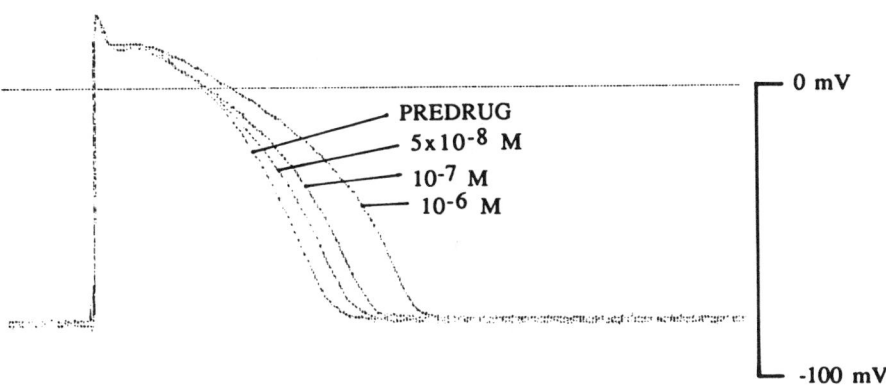

Purkinje Fibers

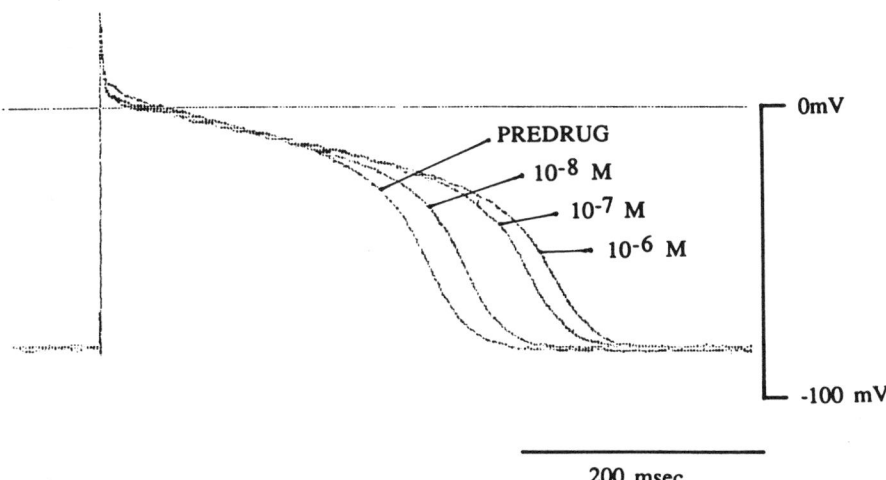

200 msec

Figure 2. Effects of various concentrations of E-4031 on action potentials of canine papillary muscle and Purkinje fiber. The drug was applied cummulatively starting from the lowest concentration after 10 minutes in each step. The frequency of stimulation was 0.1 Hz. Note that Purkinje fiber showed action potential prolongation with as low as 10^{-8} M E-4031, while papillary muscle developed a mild prolongation at 5×10^{-8} M.

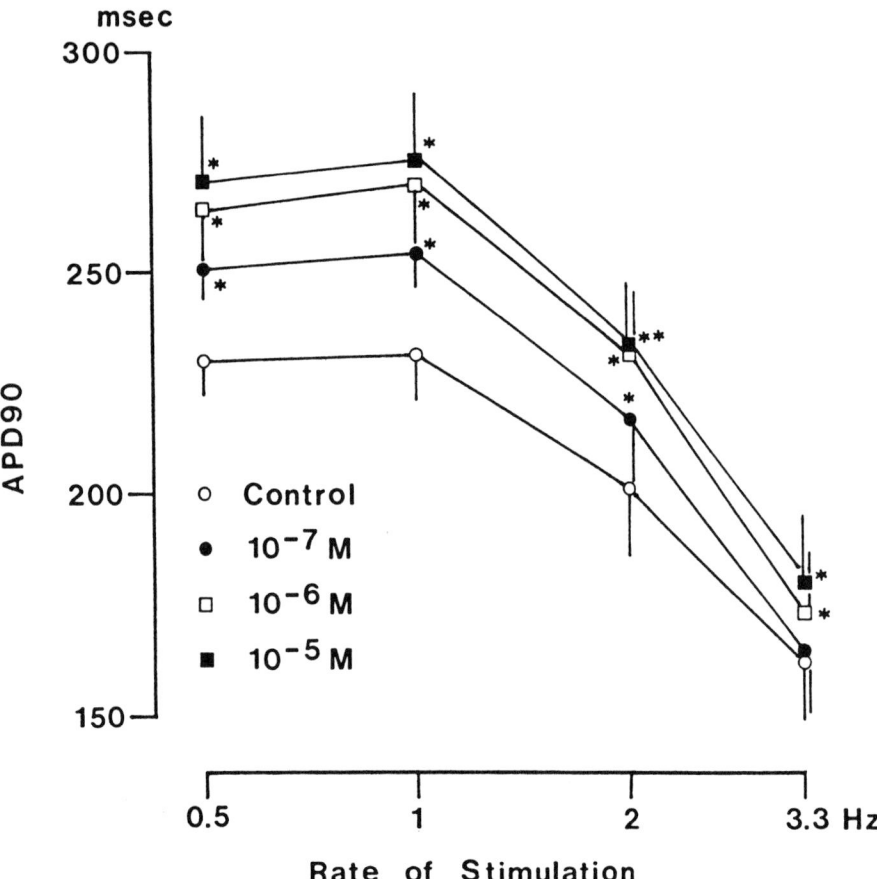

Figure 3. Effects of E-4031 on action potential duration at different stimulation rates in guinea pig papillary muscles. Results were obtained from five preparations. *: $p < 0.05$; **: $p < 0.01$ (by paired t-test). While 10^{-7} M E-4031 significantly prolonged action potential duration at the lower stimulation rates, it did not cause any change at 3.3 Hz. Although higher concentrations (10^{-6} and 10^{-5} M) prolonged action potentials at all the frequencies, effects were less prominent at 3.3 Hz than those at 0.5 or 1.0 Hz.

ences in action potential duration at concentrations between 10^{-6} M and 10^{-5} M.

Effects of E-4031 on Action Potentials and Membrane Currents of Single Ventricular Myocytes

Rate-dependent effects of E-4031 on action potential duration were also noted in single myocyte preparations. Figure 4 represents the time course of changes in action potential duration of ventricular myocyte when stimulation rate was suddenly increased from 0.2 Hz to 2.5 Hz before and during application of 5 μM E-4031. With sudden increase in stimulation rate, action potential durations in the presence and absence of E-4031 were quickly shortened with time to become nearly stable after about 4 minutes. Prolongation of action potential duration by E-4031, however, was more prominent at a slow rate than at a fast rate; namely, reverse use dependence was ap-

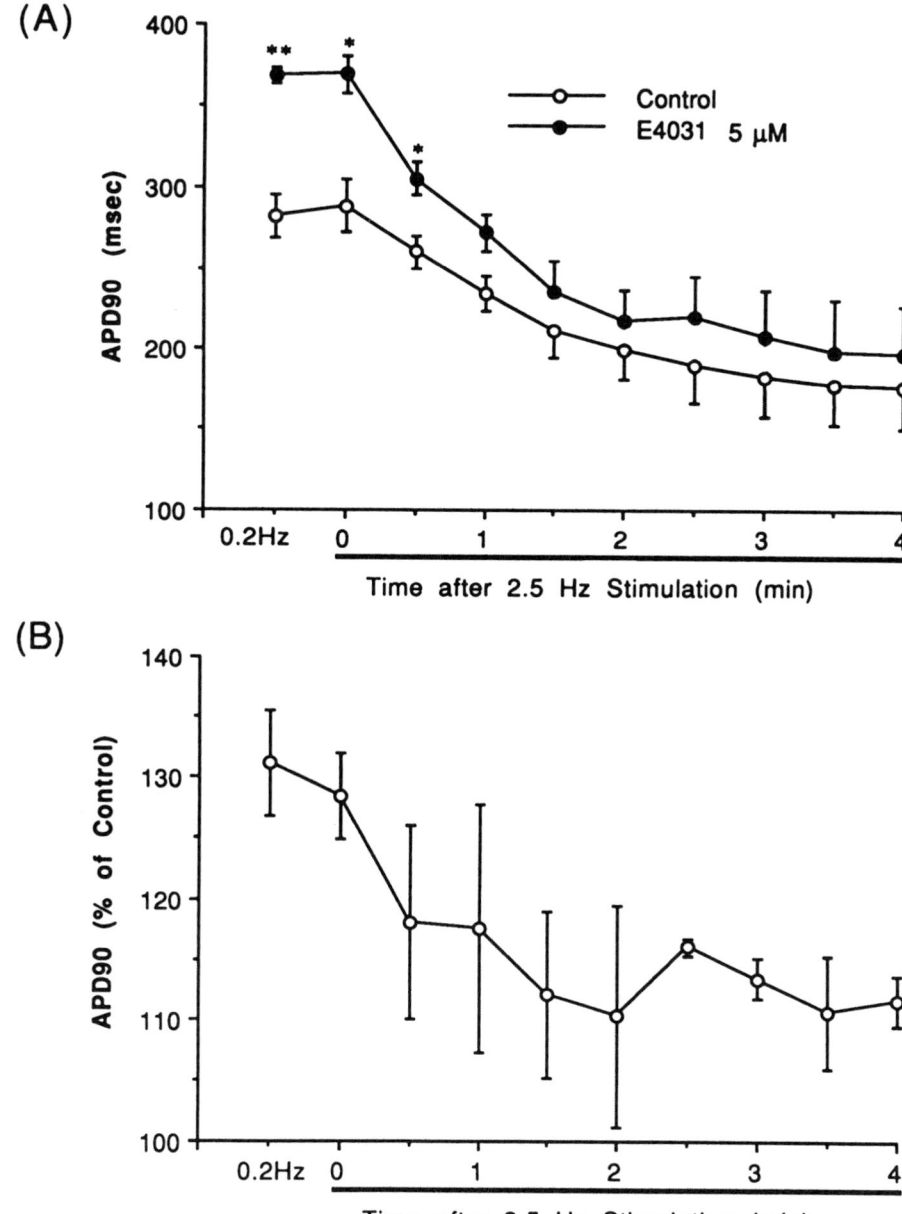

Figure 4. Effects of E-4031 on action potential duration at 90% repolarization (APD_{90}) of guinea pig single ventricular myocytes after an increase in stimulation rate. Time course of changes in APD_{90} (A) and relative APD_{90} (B) are plotted after the stimulation rate was increased from 0.2-Hz to 2.5 Hz. Values indicate mean of three experiments. Relative APD_{90} in (B) indicates percent of control APD_{90} at 0.2-Hz stimulation. Marked prolongation of APD at 0.2-Hz was gradually decreased with time after an increase in stimulation rate to 2.5 Hz.

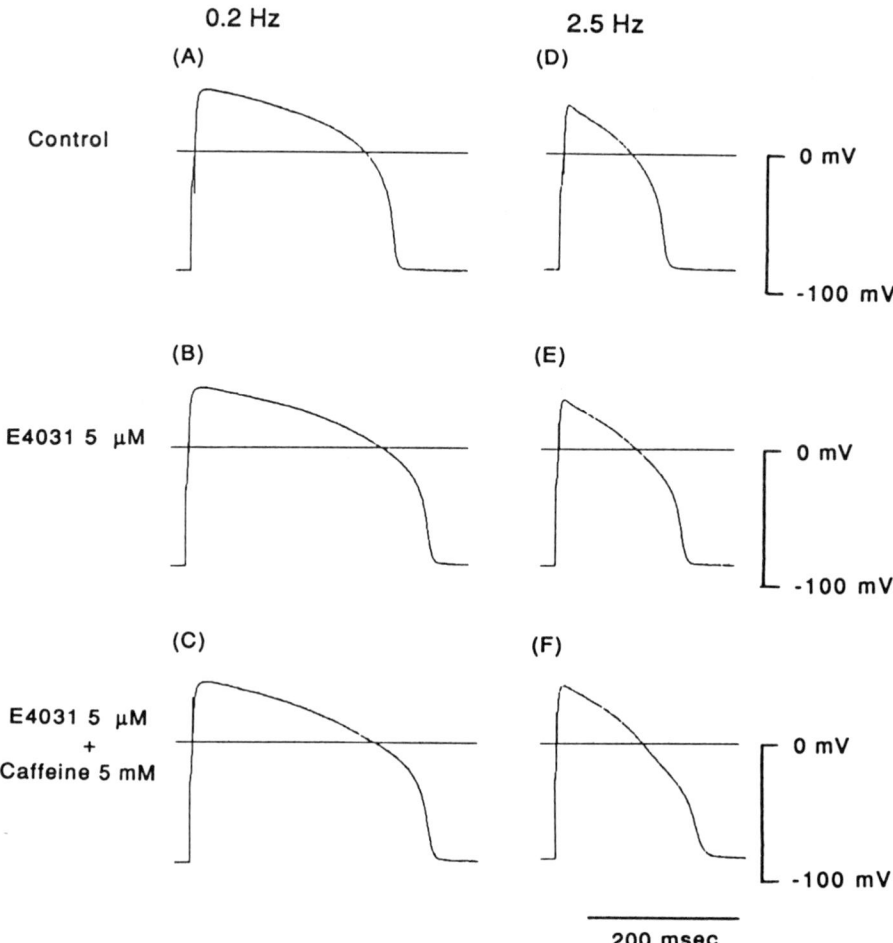

Figure 5. Effects of E-4031 and caffeine on action potentials of a guinea pig ventricular myocyte. The left raw (A,B,C) represents action potentials at 0.2-Hz stimulation and the right (D,E,F) indicates those recorded at 4 minutes after the stimulation rate was increased to 2.5 Hz. Action potential prolongation by 5-μM E-4031 was more marked at 0.2 Hz (A,B) than that at 2.5 Hz (D,E), while prolongation after addition of 5-mM caffeine was not apparent in (C) and (F). Records were obtained from a single preparation.

parent. Action potentials at slow and fast rates recorded from a single preparation are shown in Figure 5.

In our previous study, we demonstrated that one type of the transient outward current (I_{to}), which was sensitive to caffeine was activated with rapid stimulation and contributed to the repolarization phase.[9] Therefore, we tested whether or not caffeine-sensitive outward current was activated by rapid and repetitive depolarizations at the plateau level in

guinea pig ventricular myocyte, in which calcium-insensitive I_{to} was not recognizable.[10,11] Figure 6 shows one of the experimental records. Depolarizing pulses of 200-msec duration were applied from -80 mV to $+20$ mV at 2.5 Hz before and during application of 5 mM caffeine. Difference current was obtained by subtraction revealing the caffeine-sensitive current. While there was no outward current at the beginning of pulse application, rapidly activating and inactivating outward currents

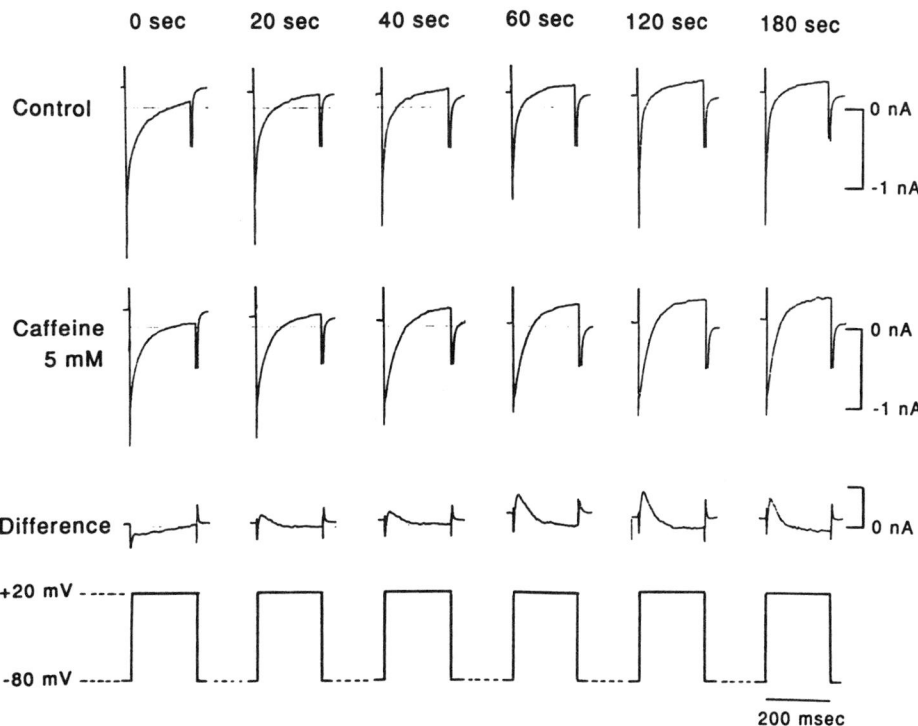

Figure 6. Activation of caffeine-sensitive transient outward current by repetitive depolarizing pulses at 2.5 Hz in a guinea pig ventricular myocyte. Voltage protocol is indicated at the bottom. Current traces at times indicated at the top after start of pulse application are presented. The top raw shows current traces in the control, the second raw represents those in 5-mM caffeine, and the third raw indicates difference currents. Difference currents demonstrate gradual development of transient outward current with time.

resembling I_{to} were developed with pulses to increase their amplitudes (n = 5). These outward currents with pulses were not inhibited by 4-mM 4-aminopyridine (n = 3; not shown) and therefore, this current component represented a caffeine-sensitive I_{to}.

To explore the role of the caffeine-sensitive I_{to} on action potential shortening after increased stimulation rate, effects of 5-mM caffeine on action potential duration was examined with the same stimulation protocol as shown in Figure 4. Figure 7A shows the results from three experiments. Caffeine partially reversed the shortening of action potential duration after increased stimulation rate and therefore the caffeine-sensitive I_{to} seemed to play a role for action potential shortening under

this conditian. However, 5-μM E-4031 did not affect the caffeine-sensitive I_{to} (Figure 7B). Effects of caffeine on action potentials at fast and slow rates are also shown in Figure 5C and 5F.

The main action of E-4031 on membrane currents seems to depress the delayed outward K^+ current (I_K). Figure 8 shows the effects of 1 μM E-4031 on depolarizing membrane current from -30 mV in the presence of 2-mM Co^{2+} to block the Ca^{2+} current and on tail current upon repolarization. E-4031 depressed the current at the end of depolarizing pulses (B) and significantly suppressed the tail current at all the test voltages (C). Figure 9 demonstrates the effects of E-4031 on activation of I_K. The analysis of the time course of the I_K activation revealed that there were two

A. Effect of Caffeine (5mM) on APD90

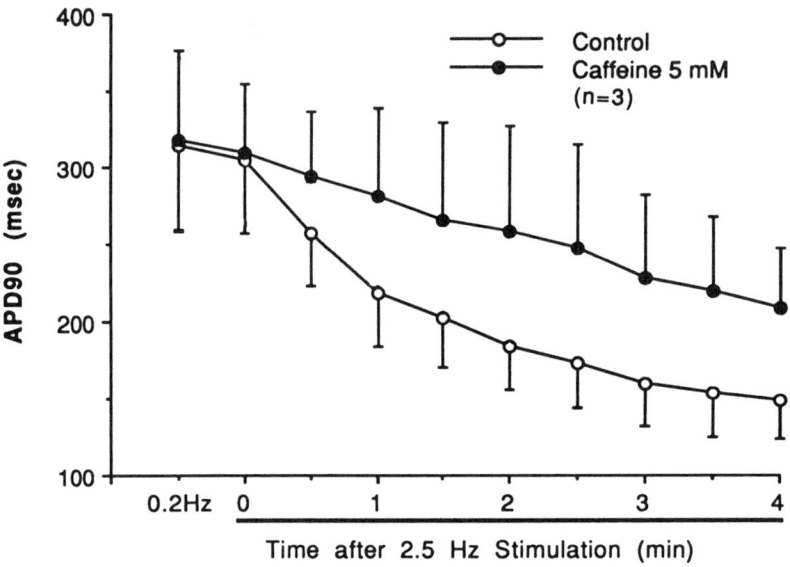

B. Effect of E4031 on Caffeine Sensitive Ito

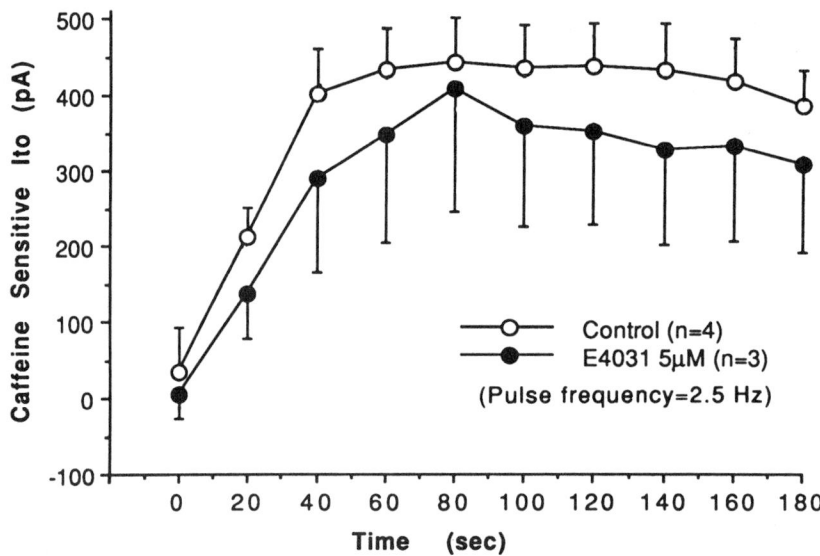

Figure 7. Effects of caffeine on APD_{90} (A) and E-4031 on caffeine-sensitive transient outward current (I_{to}) (B). Time course of changes in APD_{90} (A) and caffeine-sensitive I_{to} (B) after start of 2.5-Hz stimulation or pulse depolarization. Caffeine decreased the shortening of APD_{90} in some extent (A), while E-4031 did not affect caffeine-sensitive I_{to} (B).

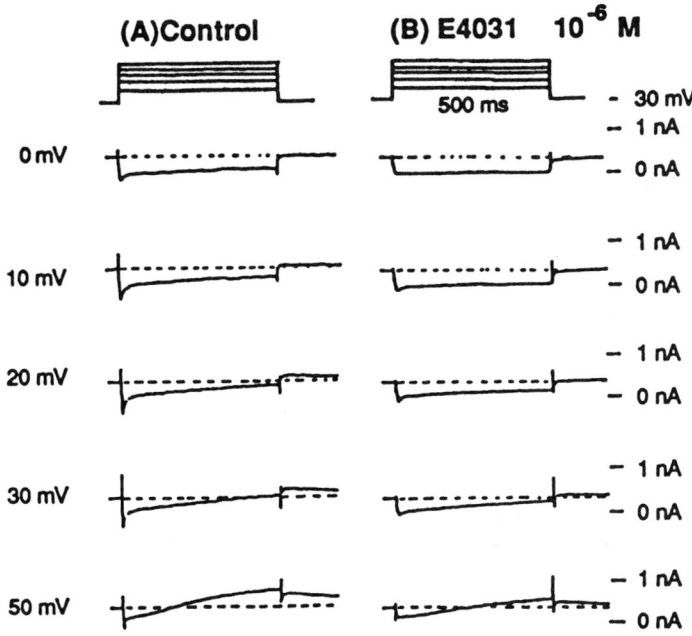

(A)Control

(B) E4031 10^{-6} M

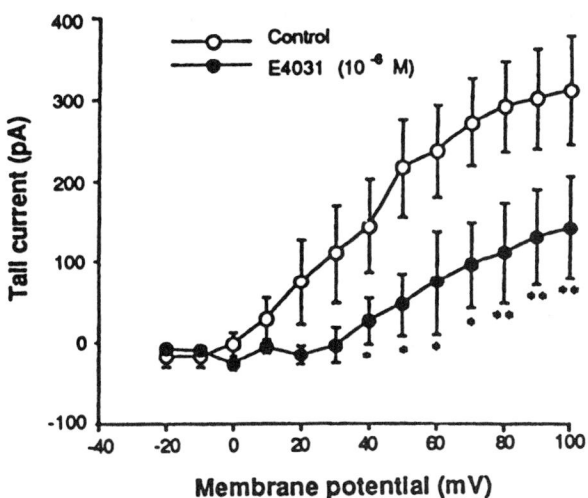

(C) Tail Current Amplitude

Figure 8. Effects of E-4031 on outward tail current in guinea pig ventricular myocytes. Depolarizing clamp pulses of 500-msec duration were applied to various test voltages indicated at the left of (A) from the holding potential at -30 mV. (A) shows current traces in the control and (B) is in the presence of 1-μM E-4031. (C) indicates the summary of four experiments on the tail current. E-4031 significantly depressed the tail current amplitude at most test voltages.

Effect of E4031 on activation of Ik

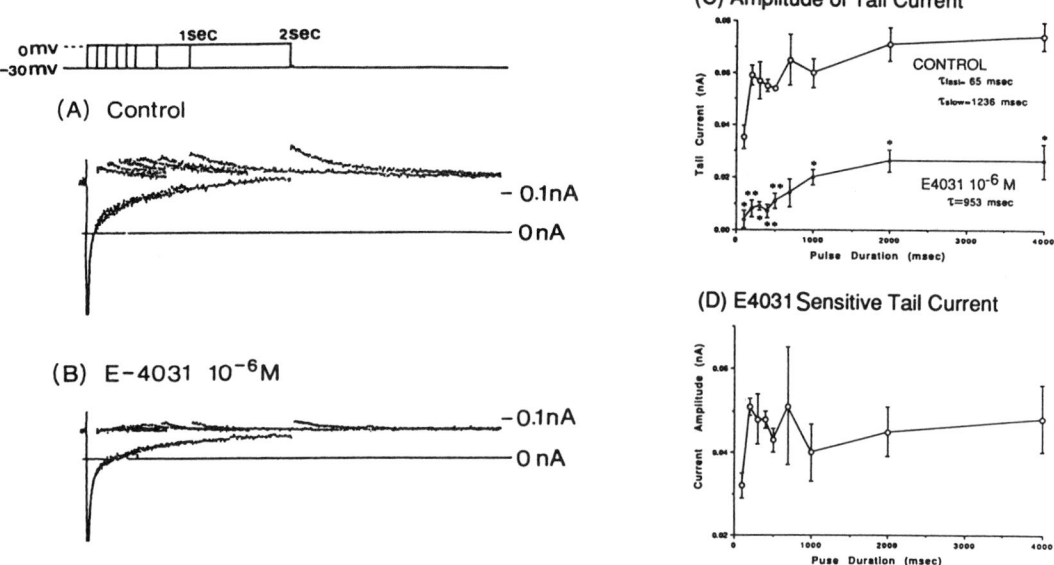

Figure 9. Effects of E-4031 on activation kinetics of delayed outward K^+ current in guinea pig ventricular myocytes. (A) and (B) indicate the envelope of the tail current of I_K in the control and in the presence of 1-μM E-4031. Voltage protocol is indicated at the top. (C) shows plots of the tail current amplitude obtained from three experiments. There were two components of the time course of analysis with fast and slow time constants. (D) represents the E-4031-sensitive tail current with prominence at shorter pulses.

components of fast and slow activating fractions.[12] The E-4031-sensitive current component seems to be a fast activating one (Figure 9C). However, if we calculated the fast and slow components of I_K by applying short (250 msec) and long (5 seconds) pulses, and the effects of E-4031 on the tail currents by respective pulses were compared, the drug had significantly stronger suppressive effect on the tail current by short pulse than the one by long pulse. Therefore, E-4031 had action to suppress predominantly the fast activating I_K, but its effect was not an exclusive one to this component showing a mild depression on the slow component as well (Figure 10).

To understand the mechanism of reverse use-dependent effect on action potential duration by this drug, we examined the state-dependent affinity of E-4031 on I_K channel. The

experimental protocol was the same as the one used by Balser et al.[13] and indicated in Figure 11A. Five-second test pulses to +60 mV were applied from the holding potential of −80 mV and were followed by repolarization to −80 mV for various durations (Ti). After various time intervals (Ti), 300-msec depolarizing pulses to +60 mV were then applied followed by repolarization to −30 mV. The amplitude of the tail current after the 300-msec pulse was compared in the presence and absence of E-4031. The relative I_K tail in the presence of E-4031 compared to that in the absence of the drug were plotted with diastolic intervals at −80 mV (Ti) (B). The relative I_K tail was decreased with prolongation of diastolic intervals (Ti). This result suggests that E-4031 has an affinity to the rested state of the I_K channel.

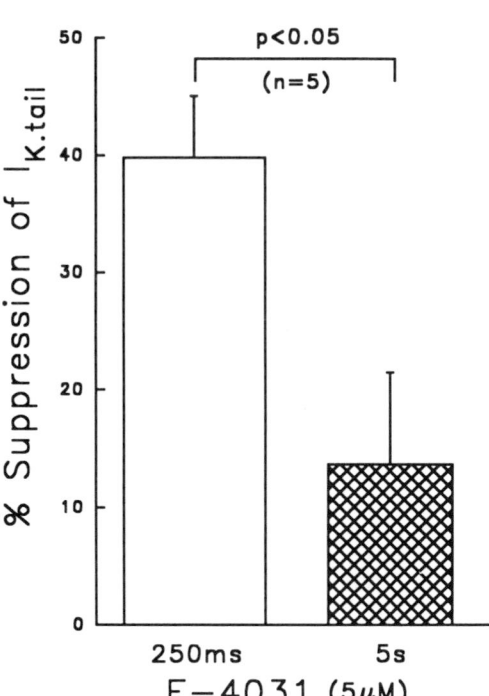

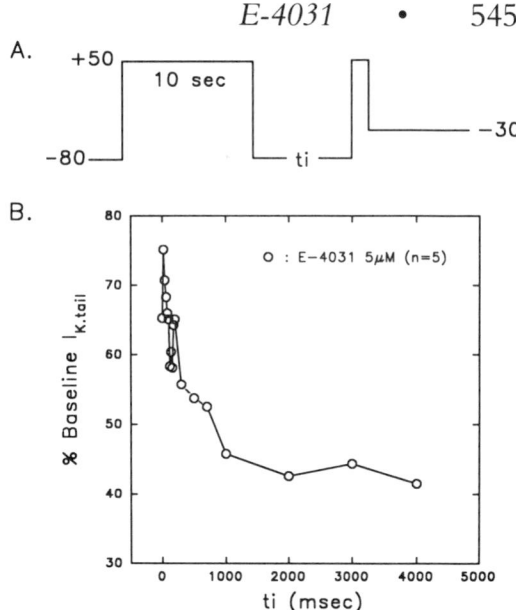

Figure 10. Effects of E-4031 on two components of I_K. The fast activating I_K was represented by the tail current amplitude induced by short 250-msec pulse and the slow activating one was by long 5-second pulse. The percent suppression compared to the control was examined by short (250 msec) and long (5 second) pulses. E-4031 exhibited stronger depression on I_K by 250-msec pulses than those by 5-second pulses.

Figure 11. Time-dependent suppression of I_K at -80 mV. Using a paired pulse protocol shown in A, effect of E-4031 on I_K was assessed as a function of time spent at -80 mV (abscissa). Magnitudes of I_K tail relative to the control before E-4031 (percent baseline $I_{K\text{-tail}}$) are plotted on the ordinate. The percent baseline $I_{k\text{-tail}}$ decreased with time at -80 mV. Values are a mean of five experiments.

Effects of E-4031 on Arrhythmia Models

Reentrant Type of Tachycardias in Rabbit Right Atrial Preparations

Antiarrhythmic effects of E-4031 on reentrant type of atrial tachycardias induced by premature stimulations were reexamined in rabbit right atrial preparation.[14] The schematic diagram of our right atrial preparations is shown in Figure 12, which contains ring-like structure of the crista terminalis and its extension surrounding the sinus node areas. When a small lesion was made to create slow conduction area on some part of the ring-like structure by cutting and premature stimuli were applied to the right atrium, regular reentrant tachycardias were easily induced.[6] In 13 of 17 preparations, premature stimulations repeatedly induced nearly regular tachycardias lasting more than 10 beats. Twelve of 13 preparations exhibited a smooth atrioventricular (AV) conduction curve without jump-up and showed activation patterns compatible with intra-atrial reentry during tachycardias, whereas a remaining preparation started tachycardia with a jump on the AV conduction curve, indicating dual AV nodal reentrant tachycardia. Application of 0.1- and 1.0-μM E-4031 completely prevented the initiation of both types of tachycardias by producing intra-atrial conduction block. One of the experimental records presenting intra-atrial reentry and prevention of its initiation by E-4031 is shown in Figure 13. The refractory period was significantly prolonged by the used concentra-

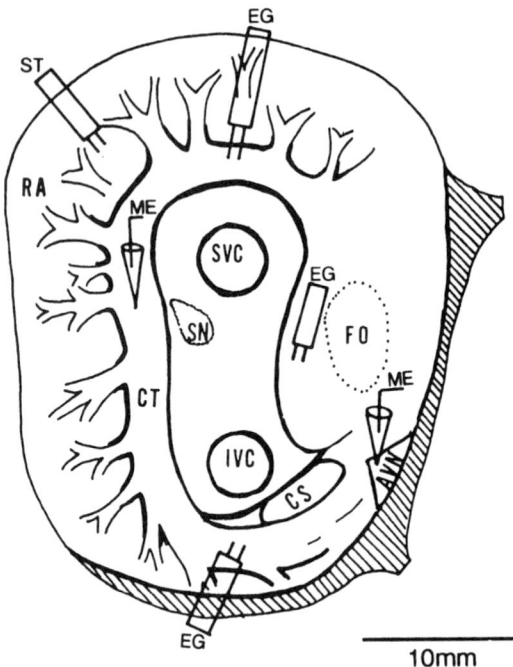

10mm

Figure 12. A schematic drawing of endocardial view of the right atrial sinus node preparation of the rabbit heart. RA: right atrium; SN: sinus node; CT: crista terminalis; SVC: superior vena cava; IVC: inferior vena cava; CS: coronary sinus; AVN: atrioventricular node; ME: microelectrode; EG: bipolar electrode; ST: stimulating electrode. (Reproduced with permission from Reference 14.)

tions of E-4031. Atrial refractory period was prolonged from 81.7 ± 19.4 msec in the control to 96.7 ± 18.6 (mean ± SD; n = 6, $p <$ 0.05) after 0.1-μM E-4031, and from 84.3 ± 16.2 in the control to 152.9 ± 71.1 msec (n = 7, $p <$ 0.05) by 1.0-μM E-4031. Similar degrees of prolongation were also noted in the refractory period of the AV node.

A Seven-Day-Old Canine Myocardial Infarction Model

Ventricular tachycardias were repeatedly induced by programmed electrical stimulation in a canine myocardial infarction model.[7] Using this model, we examined the effects of E-4031 on prevention of VT induction by programmed ventricular stimulation. In 9 of 13

dogs that underwent the coronary ligation of the left anterior descending artery and survived for 1 week after the operation, the programmed electrical stimulation repeatedly induced sustained monomorphic VT in 3 dogs and nonsustained or polymorphic VT in 2 dogs. Two dogs developed ventricular fibrillation and another two showed no arrhythmias. Application of 1-5 μg/kg per minute infusion of E-4031 after bolus injection of 10 or 50 μg/kg completely prevented induction of sustained monomorphic VT in 3 dogs and two nonsustained VT, while no effects were noted on induction of ventricular fibrillation in 2 dogs (Figure 14). No aggravation or development of new arrhythmias were recognized in any of 9 dogs by infusion of E-4031 up to 10 μg/kg per minute after a bolus injection of 100 μg/kg. All the dogs showed significant prolongation of QT intervals after infusion of E-4031.

Discussion

Our studies demonstrated that E-4031 prolonged action potential duration and refractory period without marked effects on other electrical parameters of cardiac muscles. Prolongation of action potential duration was more marked in the fast stimulation than the slow one, exhibiting reverse use dependence. E-4031 depressed the delayed outward K^+ current, especially its fast activating component, with high affinity to the rested state of the channel, which presumably explains prolongation and frequency-dependent effects on action potential duration. The drug was proven effective for prevention of macroreentry type of tachycardias in animal models of arrhythmias.

Most of the studies indicated that E-4031 prolonged action potential duration and refractory period with reverse use-dependent manner, which might relate to development of antiarrhythmic as well as proarrhythmic effects.[2,3,8] The present study also demonstrated that prolongation of action potential duration by E-4031 was decreased with increasing the stimulation rate both in multicellular and sin-

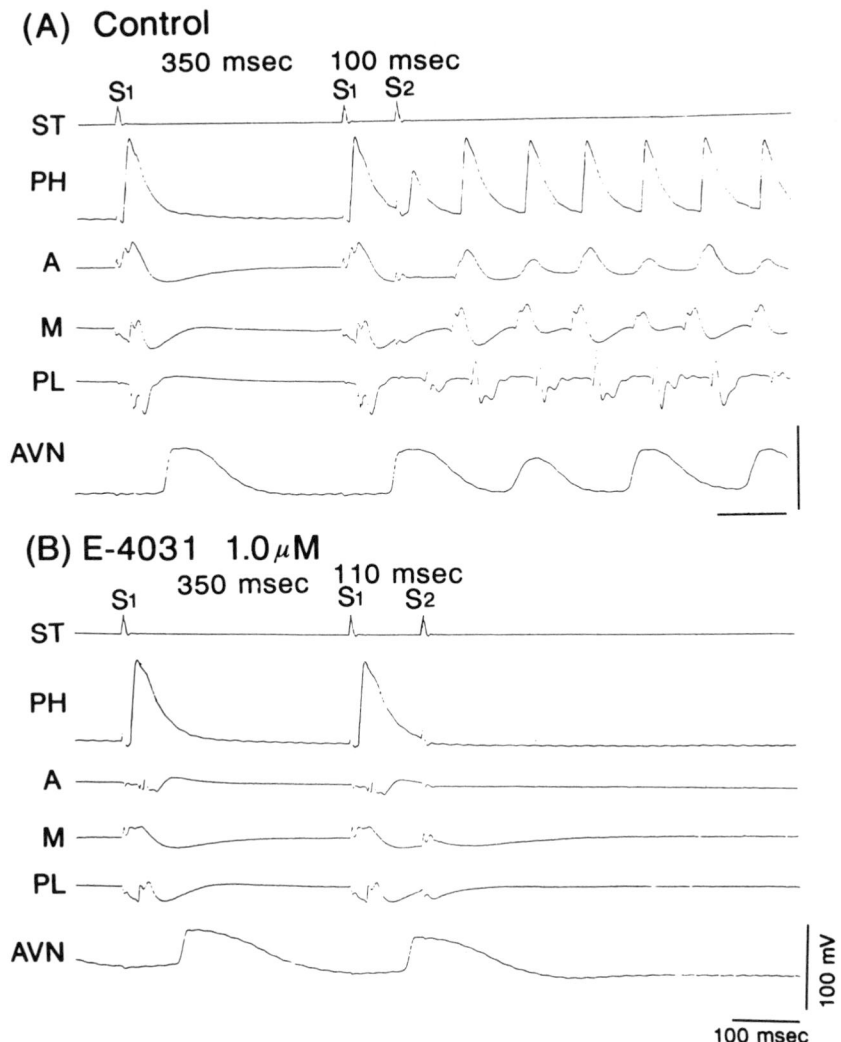

Figure 13. Effect of 1.0-μM E-4031 on intra-atrial reentry. Recording sites were from the anterior (A), middle (M), and low posterior (PL) internodal conduction routes by bipolar electrodes. Action potentials were recorded from high posterior route (PH) and atrioventricular node (AVN), respectively. The tachycardia was induced by S_2 in the control (A), but its induction was prevented by 1.0-μM E-4031 (B). (Reproduced with permission from Reference 14.)

gle cell preparations. Action potential duration in cardiac muscles generally becomes shorter with increasing stimulation rate. This effect is produced either by decreasing inward current, increasing outward current, or both.[15,16] Since the repolarization phase of action potentials is determined by multiple ionic currents, the former is mainly attributed to decreased Ca^{2+} current and the latter to in-

creased delayed outward K^+ current. Here, we demonstrated another factor to contribute to shortening of action potential duration at rapid rate of stimulation. That is activation of the caffeine-sensitive I_{to}, which was shown to be activated during rapid stimulation.[9] Although guinea pig ventricular preparations were claimed to be lacking I_{to} and the Ca^{2+}-insensitive component was actually ill-devel-

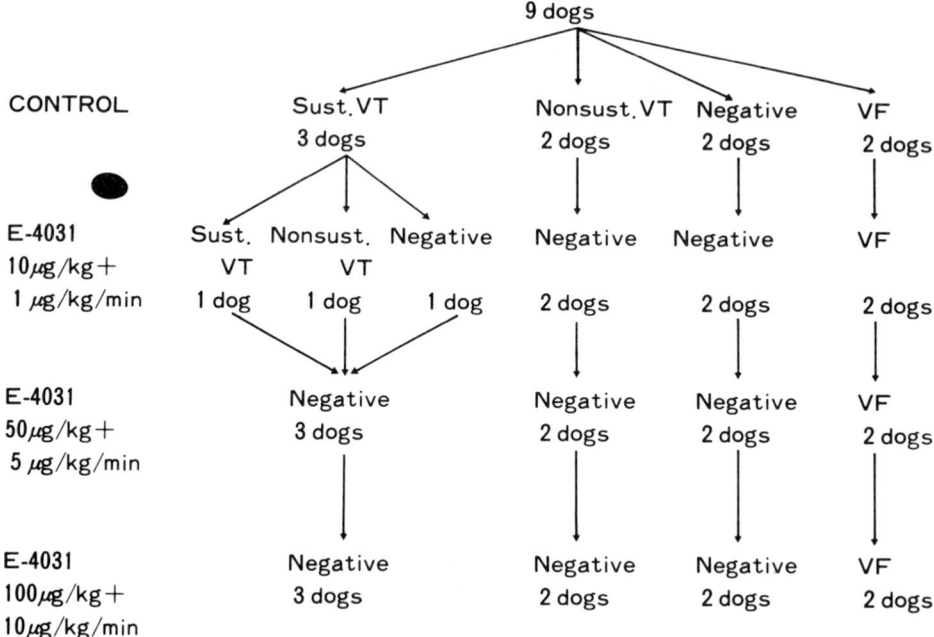

Figure 14. Results of arrhythmia induction by programmed ventricular stimulation after application of E-4031 in 7-day-old canine myocardial infarction model. Doses of E-4031 infusion are indicated on the left and the responses are presented.

oped in this preparation,[10,11] the present study is the first demonstration of the caffeine-sensitive I_{to} in guinea pigs as in rabbit ventricular myocyte. As the caffeine-sensitive I_{to} was not affected by E-4031 and it was activated only during the rapid rate of stimulation, these factors could explain a reason for less prominent prolongation of action potential duration at a fast rate than a slow rate and, therefore, contribute, at least in part, to appearance for the reverse use dependence of the effects by E-4031. Another factor to cause reverse use dependence of action potential prolongation is the effect of E-4031 on the delayed outward K^+ current, since this current seems to be the main target for the drug.[2,3] Recently, Sanguinetti and Jurkiewicz[12] reported that the delayed outward K^+ current was composed of two components with fast activating I_{Kr} and slow activating I_{Ks}, and E-4031 exclusively depressed I_{Kr}. I_{Kr} and I_{Ks} differed not only in activating and inactivating kinetics, but also voltage dependence, selectivity to K^+, and in-

ward rectification. Balser et al.[13] also pointed out that the delayed rectifier current had two components with the fast activating and slow activating one in addition to different sensitivity to La^{3+}, but they interpreted that the fast activating current contained the inactivating current component similar to I_{to}-type current and the I_{Kr}-type current. Our result disclosed that E-4031 was not an exclusive inhibitor of I_{Kr}, but it also depressed I_{Ks} to a lesser extent. Therefore, E-4031 cannot be used as a pure blocker of I_{Kr}. If one assumed that both current components were mainly carried by K^+, the drug could affect both with different sensitivities, since there was no selective and exclusive inhibitor of a single K^+ channel without effects on others in most of the K^+ channel blocking agents. We do not know the reason why different results from those reported by Sanguinetti and Jurkiewicz[12] could be obtained despite the same species of preparations used in both groups. These discrepancies are to be further studied at the single channel level with clarification of the natures of I_{Kr} and I_{Ks} and their sensitivities to E-4031.

There have been several reports describing the effectiveness of E-4031 on VTs in recent myocardial infarction models.[17-19] These results attributed its effectiveness to prolongation of refractory period in both normal and infarcted zones, thus reentrant excitation could not be induced. Our study also supported these results and extended effectiveness of E-4031 on atrial tachycardias using anatomical obstacle with macroreentry. Sustained monomorphic VTs induced in myocardial infarction in animal models and in patients are usually assumed to represent macroreentry, although an exact reentrant path is not necessarily determined.[20-23] Therefore, E-4031 can be used as an effective antiarrhythmic agent against macroreentry type of tachycardias.

Summary

E-4031 prolonged action potential duration and refractory period in atrial and ventricular preparations. These effects were prominent at the slower rate than the faster rate of stimulations revealing a reverse use dependence. Action potential prolongation by E-4031 was mainly caused by depression of delayed outward K^+ current in which the drug dominantly, but not exclusively, inhibited the fast activating component of the current. E-4031 was shown to have an affinity to the rested state of the I_K channel, which might partly explain its reverse use-dependent effects on action potential duration. Application of E-4031 suppressed induction of macroreentry type of tachycardias by programmed stimulations in right atrial preparations with anatomical obstacle and a 7-day-old canine myocardial infarction model.

References

1. Sawada K, Nomoto K, Hiraoka M: Effects of a novel class 3 antiarrhythmic agent, E-4031, on ventricular arrhythmias (abstract). *Jpn Circ J* 52:919, 1988.

2. Sawada K: Depression of the delayed outward K^+ current by a novel Class III antiarrhythmic agent, E-4031, in guinea pig single ventricular cells (abstract). *J Mol Cell Cardiol* 21:S21, 1989.

3. Sanguinetti MC, Siegel PKS, Zingaro GJ: The Class III antiarrhythmic agents, sotalol and E-4031 do not block delayed rectifier K^+ current in guinea pig or ferret ventricular cells (abstract). *J Mol Cell Cardiol* 21:S21, 1989.

4. Hirano Y, Hiraoka H: Barium-induced automatic activity in isolated ventricular myocytes from guinea-pig hearts. *J Physiol* 395:455, 1988.

5. Hamill OP, Marty A, Neher E, et al: Improved patch-clamp tehniques for high-resolution current recording from cells and cell-free membrane patches. *Pflügers Arch* 391:85, 1981.

6. Hiraoka M, Adaniya H: Function of atrial preferential conduction routes under normal and abnormal conditions. *J Electrocardiol* 16:123, 1983.

7. Nitta J, Nogami K, Aonuma H, et al: Effects of pirmenol on electrical induction of sustained ventricular tachycardia in a seven-day-old canine myocardial infarction. *J Cardiovasc Pharmacol* 17:54, 1991.

8. Hondeghem LM, Sniders DJ: Class III antiarrhythmic agents have a lot of potential, but a long way to go: reduced effectiveness and dangers of reverse use-dependence. *Circulation* 81:686, 1990.

9. Hiraoka M, Kawano S: Calcium-sensitive and -insensitive transient outward current in rabbit ventricular myocytes. *J Physiol* 410:187, 1988.

10. Josephson IR, Sanchez-Chapula J, Brown AM: Early outward current in rat single ventricular cells. *Circ Res* 54:157, 1984.

11. Hiraoka M, Kawano S: Mechanism of increased amplitude and duration of the plateau with sudden shortening of diastolic intervals in rabbit ventricular cells. *Circ Res* 60:14, 1987.

12. Sanguinetti MC, Jurkiewicz NK: Two components of cardiac delayed rectifier K^+ current. Differential sensitivity to block by Class III antiarrhythmic agents. *J Gen Physiol* 96:195, 1990.

13. Balser JR, Bennett PB, Hondeghem LM, Roden DM: Suppression of time-dependent outward current in guinea pig ventricular myocytes. Actions of quinidine and amiodarone. *Circ Res* 69:519, 1991.

14. Adaniya H, Hiraoka M: Effects of a novel Class III antiarrhythmic agent, E-4031, on reentrant tachycardias in rabbit right atrium. *J Cardiovasc Pharmacol* 15:976, 1990.

15. Carmeliet E: Repolarization and frequency in cardiac muscle. *J Physiol (Paris)* 73:903, 1977.

16. Boyett MR, Jewell BR: Analysis of the effects of changes in rate and rhythm upon electrical activity in the heart. *Prog Biophys Mol Biol* 36:1, 1980.

17. Katoh H, Ogawa S, Furuno I, et al: Electrophysiologic effects of E-4031, a Class III antiarrhythmic agent, on re-entrant ventricular arrhythmias in a canine 7-day-old myocardial infarction model. *J Pharmacol Exp Ther* 253:1077, 1990.
18. Lynch JJ, Heaney LA, Wallace AA, et al: Suppression of lethal ischemic ventricular arrhythmias by the Class III agent E-4031 in a canine model of previous myocardial infarction. *J Cardiovasc Pharmacol* 15:764, 1990.
19. Chi L, Mu D, Lucchesi BR: Electrophysiology and antiarrhythmic actions of E-4031 in the experimental animal model of sudden coronary death. *J Cardiovasc Pharmacol* 17:285, 1991.
20. Wellens HJJ, Lie KI, Duren DR: Observations on the mechanisms of ventricular tachycardia in man. *Circulation* 54:237, 1976.
21. Josephson ME, Horowitz LN, Farshidi A, Kastor JA: Recurrent sustained ventricular tachycardia. *Circulation* 57:431, 1978.
22. El-Sherif N, Scherlag BJ, Lazzara R, Hope RR: Reentrant ventricular arrhythmias in the late myocardial infarction period. 1. Conduction characteristics in the infarction zone. *Circulation* 55:686, 1977.
23. Wit AL, Allessie MA, Bonke FIM, et al: Electrophysiological mapping to determine the mechanism of experimental ventricular tachycardia initiated by premature impulses: experimental approach and initial results demonstrating reentrant excitation. *Am J Cardiol* 49:166, 1982.

Chapter 37

Evolving Experimental and Clinical Profile of Dofetilide

H.S. Rasmussen
H.W. Dalrymple
M.J. Allen
G.S. Butrous

Dofetilide (UK-68,798) is a bis(arylalkyl)amine[1] (Figure 1), which exhibits the profile of a Class III antiarrhythmic agent in in vitro and in vivo experimental models. More specifically, all of the known pharmacology of dofetilide is explicable in terms of its extreme selectivity for the rapid component of the cardiac delayed rectifier potassium current, I_{Kr}.[2] In this chapter, the pharmacological, pharmacokinetic, and emerging electrophysiological properties of the compound are discussed relative to the drug's antiarrhythmic actions demonstrated in preliminary studies.

In Vitro Electrophysiological and Pharmacodynamic Effects

Cellular Electrophysiology

In isolated canine ventricular trabeculae and Purkinje fibers, dofetilide produces concentration related increases of action potential duration (APD) at 50% and 90% repolarization and effective refractory period (ERP) without affecting conduction.[3] Purkinje fibers are slightly more sensitive and responsive than ventricular muscle (Table 1)[4], an observation that also has been made for the other Class III agents E-4031 and almokalant,[5] suggesting that it is a "class effect." At concentrations of 500 nM and 1 μM, respectively, the increases of APD in canine Purkinje fibers and ventricular myocardium appear to be attaining the "shoulder" of a sigmoid concentration effect curve,[3] thereby corroborating the data of Baskin et al.[6] from ferret papillary muscles, in which a finite maximal prolongation of APD by dofetilide is demonstrated clearly.

A number of studies demonstrate that dofetilide, at concentrations up to 1 μM, is devoid of effect on the maximum rate of depolarization (MRD) of action potentials recorded from canine Purkinje fibers,[3,4] guinea pig, canine and ferret ventricular myocardium,[3,4,7] and rabbit sinoatrial node,[8] indicating a Class III:Class I selectivity in excess of 1,000-fold.

From BN Singh, HJJ Wellens, M Hiraoka, (eds): *Electropharmacological Control of Cardiac Arrhythmias*. Mount Kisco, NY, Futura Publishing Company Inc., © 1994.

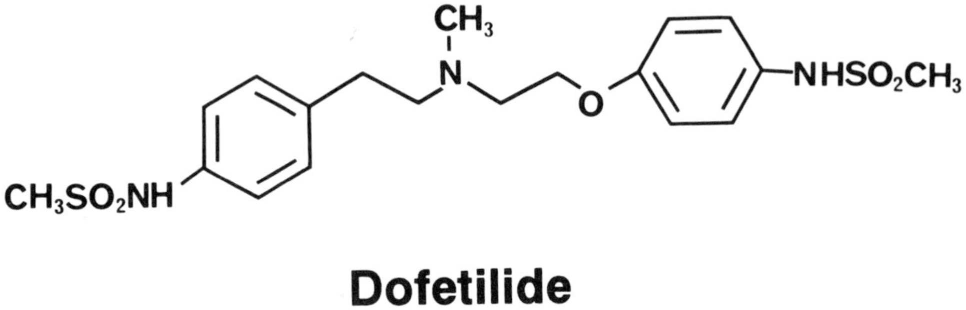

CH_3

CH_3SO_2NH — ... N(CH_3)–CH$_2$CH$_2$–O– ... –NHSO$_2$CH$_3$

Dofetilide

Figure 1. The chemical structure of dofetilide.

Moreover, the absence of effect on the rate of terminal repolarization and conservation of the APD:ERP ratio in both canine (Figures 2 and 3)[3] and guinea pig[7] ventricular muscle, and also by the maintenance of the resting membrane potential in canine myocardium and Purkinje fiber,[3,4] indicates that dofetilide does not affect the inward rectifier current, I_{K1}. Similarly, dofetilide appears not to inhibit the transient outward current, I_{to}. In canine Purkinje fibers, the slope of phase 1 repolarization is unaffected by dofetilide at a concentration of 30 nM.[4] More conclusively, dofetilide does not prolong the APD of rat papillary muscle, a preparation in which early repolarization is known to be dependent in part upon I_{to}.[9]

The electrophysiological effects of many antiarrhythmic agents are rate dependent,[10,11] and, with the exception of amiodarone,[12] agents that prolong APD have been shown to exhibit negative rate dependency.[11,13,14] This property has also been reported for dofetilide.[3,4,6,7] However, these measurements are

Table 1
Effects of Dofetilide on Cardiac Action Potentials from Canine Cardiac Tissues

	RP (mV)	APA (mV)	MRD (Vs^{-1})	APD$_{50}$ (msec)	APD$_{90}$ (msec)	ERP (msec)
			Ventricular muscle			
Predrug Dofetilide	-83 ± 1	106 ± 2	304 ± 24	140 ± 4	183 ± 2	200 ± 4
5 nM	-83 ± 1	105 ± 2	294 ± 25	$156 \pm 3^*$	$207 \pm 5^{**}$	$224 \pm 5^*$
20 nM	-83 ± 1	108 ± 2	323 ± 20	$170 \pm 5^*$	$231 \pm 11^*$	$244 \pm 10^*$
100 nM	-83 ± 1	104 ± 4	293 ± 28	$191 \pm 4^{***}$	$261 \pm 17^{**}$	$272 \pm 15^{**}$
1000 nM	-82 ± 2	107 ± 1	302 ± 20	$196 \pm 6^{***}$	$277 \pm 21^{**}$	$286 \pm 17^{**}$
			Purkinje fiber			
Predrug Dofetilide	-90 ± 1	126 ± 2	587 ± 33	201 ± 12	293 ± 19	299 ± 9
5 nM	-90 ± 1	125 ± 2	579 ± 28	$215 \pm 16^*$	$313 \pm 23^*$	$318 \pm 11^*$
20 nM	-90 ± 2	126 ± 2	604 ± 39	$260 \pm 10^{**}$	$389 \pm 22^{***}$	$394 \pm 11^{***}$
100 nM	-89 ± 2	124 ± 2	608 ± 22	$296 \pm 15^{**}$	$500 \pm 14^{***}$	$494 \pm 8^{***}$
1000 nM	-89 ± 1	125 ± 1	599 ± 23	$302 \pm 11^{***}$	$531 \pm 11^{***}$	$535 \pm 7^{**}$

Figures shown represent mean ± S.E.M. of 5 determinations of resting potential (RP), action potential amplitude (APA), maximum rate of depolarization (MRD), action potential duration at 50% (APD$_{50}$) and 90% (APD$_{90}$) repolarization, and effective refractory period (ERP).
Significance: $^* p < 0.05$, $^{**} p < 0.01$, $^{***} p < 0.001$.

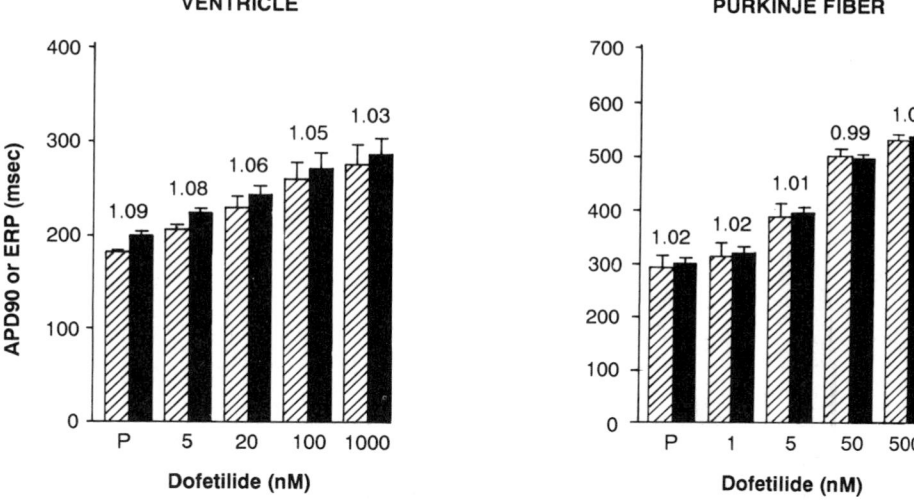

Figure 2. Influence of increasing concentrations of dofetilide on action potentials recorded from different cells from a single preparation of canine ventricular muscle (left) and Purkinje fiber (right), before and 20 minutes after superfusion with dofetilide at the final concentration indicated.

normally performed at "steady state," ie, after a number of externally applied pacing or conditioning impulses. In a more elegant study, Knilans et al.[4] demonstrated that neither the fast nor the slow time constants for restitution of APD were altered by dofetilide, and that the prolongation of APD by dofetilide is conserved following abrupt changes in diastolic intervals. This suggested that the conventional method for assessing rate dependence may be misleading, and that the conservation of prolongation of APD after an abrupt increase of rate, eg, after a premature ventricular contraction, may prevent the initiation of more malignant arrhythmias.

Early repolarization in the rat ventricular myocardium is also dependent upon a slow inward calcium current, I_{si}.[9] The complete absence of effect of dofetilide on repolarization in the rate myocardium, even at a concentration of 10 μM, indicates that the compound does not block this calcium current.[7] By virtue of its absence of effect on the rate of spontaneous phase 4 depolarization in rabbit sinoatrial node preparations, dofetilide appears to block neither the T- nor the L-type calcium currents.[8] Late repolarization in rat papillary

muscle is associated with electrogenic Na/Ca exchange.[15] The absence of effect of dofetilide on APD_{90} or ERP in rat ventricular tissue suggests that the compound does not affect Na/Ca exchange.[7]

The ionic selectivity of dofetilide in isolated tissues does not appear to be altered following maneuvers to simulate pathological conditions. In isolated guinea pig papillary muscle preparations, elevations of extracellular K^+ ($[K^+]_o$) results in reductions of the membrane diastolic potential, action potential amplitude (APA), and MRD, which are unaffected by dofetilide (10 nM); however, both APD and ERP are increased by dofetilide, despite having been shortened by the elevation of $[K^+]_o$.[16] Reduction of $[K^+]_o$ results in a hyperpolarized diastolic potential and increases of APA and MRD which, again, are unaffected by dofetilide, whereas the APD and ERP increases induced by dofetilide are comparable to those observed under normal $[K^+]_o$.[16] These results indicate that dofetilide retains both its Class III:Class I and $I_K:I_{K1}$ selectivities over a pathologically relevant range of $[K^+]_o$.

Both clofilium and sotalol have been reported to lose Class III activity under hypoxic

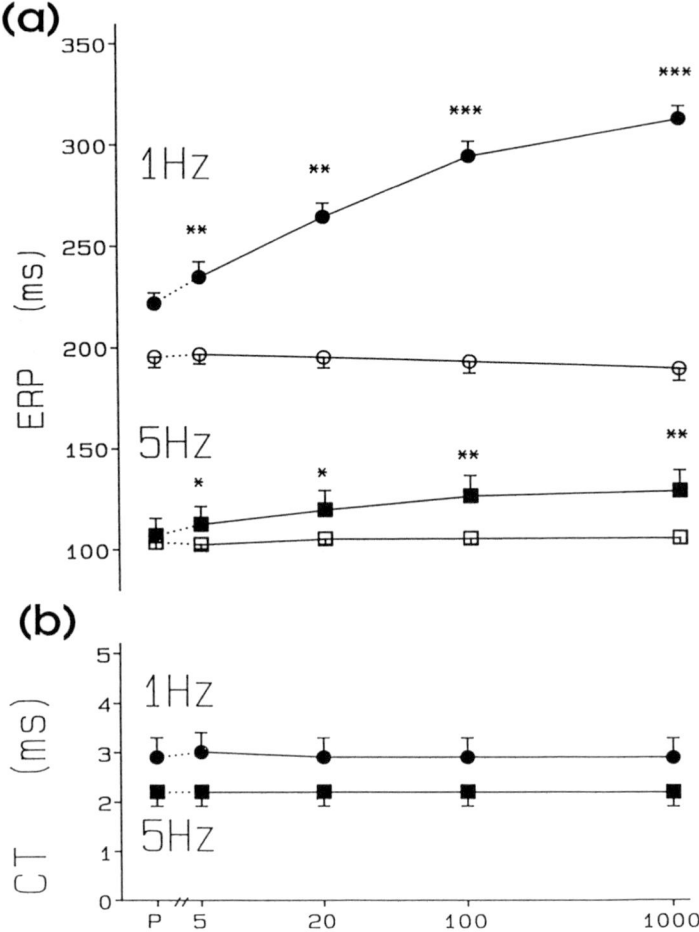

Figure 3. Effects of increasing concentrations of dofetilide (filled symbols) and vehicle (open symbols) on effective refractory period (ERP, panel a) and conduction time (CT, panel b) in isolated guinea pig papillary muscle at conduction rates of 1 Hz (circles) and 5 Hz (squares). p represents the predrug value, and points represent mean ± S.E. of five determinations; significance: $*p < 0.05$; $**p < 0.01$; $***p < 0.0001$.

conditions. In isolated guinea pig papillary muscles, in which hypoxia was induced by superfusion with O_2-free Tyrode's solution, dofetilide (100 nM) significantly reduced the magnitude of hypoxia-induced reduction of APD and contractile function.[17] The mechanism of this effect is unclear since the study was not performed under voltage-clamp conditions, but dofetilide, unlike other Class III agents like clofilium and sotalol, appears to retain Class III activity and did not demonstrate Class I activity under conditions of simulated hypoxia.

Thus, the cellular electrophysiological profile of dofetilide is that of a compound with an extreme degree of selectivity for the delayed rectifier potassium current, I_K. Estimates of the EC^{50} for dofetilide vary, but in those studies in which dofetilide has been compared directly to d-sotalol[6,7] dofetilide is between 500 and 2,000 times more potent.

In a study of guinea pig ventricular myocytes using the whole cell patch clamp technique, dofetilide (50 nM) markedly reduces, and at a concentration of 2 μM abolishes the time-dependent K^+ current reflected by the amplitude of tail currents after a series of depolarizing clamp steps (Figure 4). The duration of the clamp step in these experiments was such that I_{Kr}, and not I_{Ks}, was activated. In contrast, at more negative potentials, at which the predominant current flowing is the time-independent inward rectifier, I_{K1}, dofetilide, even at a concentration of 2 μM, does not affect the membrane current[3] (Figure 5). In studies employing the two electrode voltage-clamp technique in guinea pig ventricular myocytes,[18] the K_D for dofetilide for I_{Kr} is 3.9

nM, with a Hill coefficient of 2.0. Two thirds of the block develops with a time constant of 4.1 seconds, and the block is voltage dependent. I_{Ks} is resistant to blockade, even after enhancement of I_K by superfusion with an Na-free K-free solution.[18]

Thus, in isolated cardiac cells, dofetilide selectively attenuates I_{Kr} and expresses no effect on either I_{K1} or the inward calcium current, results that are consistent with those inferred from studies in multicellular preparations.

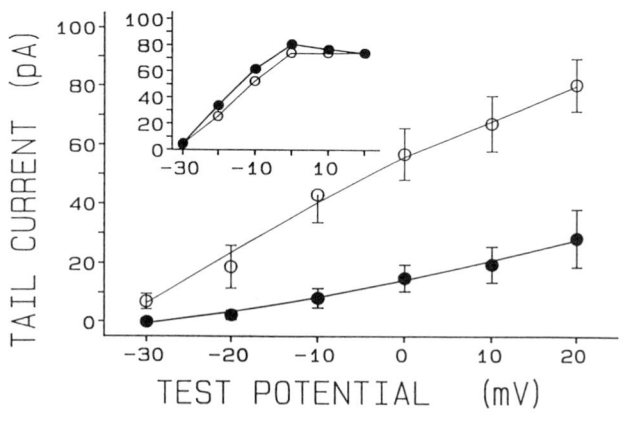

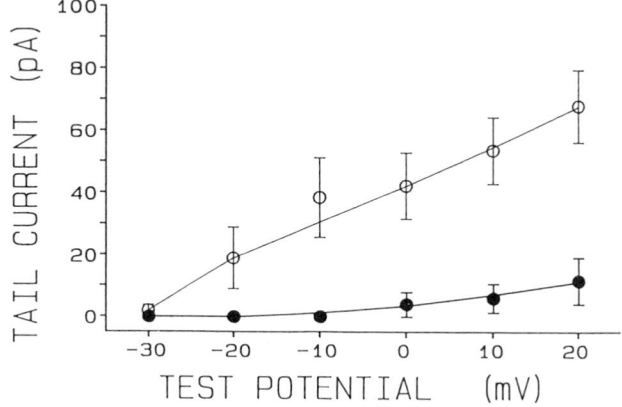

Figure 4. Effects of dofetilide at 50 nM (top panel; n = 7) and 2 μM (bottom panel; n = 5) on tail currents after depolarizing voltage-clamp steps to test potentials shown in isolated voltage-clamped guinea pig ventricular myocytes. Points represent the mean ± S.E. of the tail current amplitudes before (open circles) and after (closed circles) application of dofetilide for 3 to 5 minutes. Inset in top panel demonstrates the spontaneous variation in mean tail current amplitudes in cells not exposed to the drug before (open circles) and after a similar time period (5–7 minutes; closed circles) to that used for drug application. Each point is the mean of five determinations, and S.E. have been omitted for clarity.

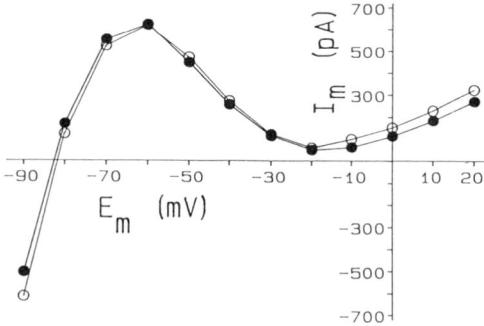

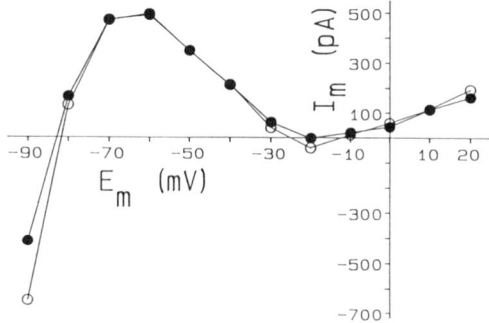

Figure 5. Current voltage relationships measured before (open circles) and after application of dofetilide (closed circles) at 50 nM (top panel; each point is mean of seven determinations) and 2 μM (bottom panel; each point is mean of five determinations). The membrane current flowing at the end of each clamp step (ie, the 500-msec isochronal membrane current) was measured.

Dofetilide and Automatic Interaction

The selectivity of dofetilide is further confirmed by radioligand binding studies in guinea pig ventricular membranes.[19] ^{3}H-dofetilide binds with relatively high affinity to an apparent single population of noninteracting sites (K_D, 23 nM, B_{max}, 150 fmol/mg protein). It is displaced from its binding site by a range of other Class III agents (Table 2A), and the rank order of potency for displacement of ^{3}H-dofetilide correlates closely to the rank order for prolongation of APD. At concentrations of up to 10 μM, dofetilide displays little affinity

for $α_1$, $α_2$, and $β$ adrenoceptors, adenosine (A_1), dopamine (D_2), 5-HT$_2$, muscarinic or opioid receptors, or dihydropyridine binding sites (Table 2B). The latter observation has been corroborated by Pong et al.[20] Although IC$_{50}$ values are quoted for binding to $α_1$ and $α_2$ adrenoceptors and muscarinic receptors, these values are all in excess of 10 μM, and when the intrinsic potency of dofetilide is taken into consideration, the compound appears to be more selective than the other Class III agents examined in this study.

Effects on Inotropic and Chronotropic Functions

Dofetilide expresses a mild negative chronotropic effect in guinea pig atrial[7,21] and Langendorff preparations[22] and rabbit sinus node preparations.[8] This effect achieves a reduction of rate of approximately 20% at 100 nM, which does not increase at concentrations up to 10 μM.[7] The negative chronotropic effect is not due to $β$ blockade,[21] thereby corroborating the findings of Greengrass et al.[19] and Pong et al.,[20] but is entirely accountable by the increase of sinoatrial APD[8] and is paralleled by increases in sinus node recovery time. The lack of effect on rate corrected sinus node recovery time indicates that spontaneous phase 4 depolarization is unaffected by dofetilide and confirms the absence of effect of the compound on the calcium channels of

Table 2A
Displacement of ^{3}H-Dofetilide by Class III Antiarrhythmic Agents in Guinea Pig Myocardial Membranes *in vitro*

| | K_i (nM) | | |
Compound	Mean	S.E.M.	n
Dofetilide	27.8	4.1	12
E-4031	107.5	11.2	6
UK-66,914	134.2	28.2	8
D-sotalol	17200.0	4500.0	5
Sematilide	33300.0	9800.0	6

Table 2B
Receptor Binding Profile of Dofetilide in Bovine Brain Tissue *in vitro*

		Activity (IC_{50}) of:	
Receptor type of sub-type	Standard agent	Standard agent	Dofetilide
Adenosine (A_1)-receptor	Cyclohexyl adenosine	23 nM	> 10 μM
α_1-adrenoceptor	Prazosin	0.2 nM	> 10 μM
α_2-adrenoceptor	Clonidine	1.5 nM	> 10 μM
β-adrenoceptor	Propranolol	25 nM	> 10 μM
Dihydropyridine site	Nitrendipine	0.6 nM	> 10 μM
Dopamine (D_2)-receptor	Spiroperidol	1.7 nM	> 10 μM
5-HT_2-receptor	Ketanserein	26 nM	> 10 μM
Muscarine-receptor	Atropine	1.6 nM	> 10 μM
Opioid-receptor	Naloxone	3.8 nM	4.5 μM

Values represent the mean ± S.E.M. of 3 experiments. IC_{50}: concentration required to displace 50% specific binding.

the sinoatrial node. A potassium current, also termed I_K, exists in sinoatrial node cells and contributes to both the pacemaker potential and repolarization.[23,24] Decay of I_K is believed to be a major controlling factor determining the rate of spontaneous depolarization,[23] and blockade of this potassium current by dofetilide would be expected to result in more rapid phase 4 depolarization.

Many pharmacological maneuvers that prolong APD have been reported to result in a positive inotropic action (for review, see reference 25). In ferret papillary muscles, dofetilide produces concentration (and thus APD) related increases in developed tension, the rate of development of tension, and the rate of relaxation without an effect on the time to peak tension and only very slightly prolonging the time to 50% relaxation.[26] Similar results were found in guinea pig papillary muscle preparations.[7] These data confirm, albeit indirectly, the absence of blockade of calcium channels by dofetilide. Thus, in contrast to Class I, Class II, and Class IV antiarrhythmic agents, dofetilide is devoid of negative inotropic activity.

Thus, the in vitro profile of dofetilide is that of a highly selective blocker of the time-dependent delayed rectifier potassium current, I_{Kr}. The compound has no discernible effect on sodium or calcium currents, nor on the other potassium channels, I_{K1} and I_{to}. By virtue of its channel selectivity, dofetilide is devoid of negative inotropic action, and its APD prolonging effect attains a finite maximum.

In Vivo Electrophysiological and Electrocardiographic Effects

As might be expected in both anesthetized and conscious dogs, dofetilide increases the QT and QTc interval and ventricular and atrial ERP without affecting indexes of conduction such as the PQ intervals or QRS duration.[27–30] The potency indicated throughout the isolated tissue such as is conserved, with clear activity following doses as low as 1 μg/kg intravenously[28] and 12.5 μg/kg orally.[27] The selectivity of dofetilide for I_{Kr} over I_{to} or Na/Ca exchange is confirmed in vivo by the absence of any effects on the ECG in rats at intravenous doses of up to 1,000 μg/kg,[31] although an intravenous dose of 5,600 μg/kg has been reported to prevent the occurrence of ventricular fibrillation (VF) following coronary artery ligation reperfusion.[32] However, the dose employed in the latter study is far in excess of that required for Class III activity in other species, in contrast to the other compounds such as d-sotalol and sematilide, which expressed antiarrhythmic activity in the rat over a dose range similar to that required to demonstrate Class III activity in other species. The absence of a disproportionate effect on the relative refractory period is consistent with a lack of effect on the inward rectifier, I_{K1}.[29] In both guinea pigs[31] and dogs,[33] the attainment of a finite maximal increase of QT interval of between 25% and 30% is, again, consistent with in vitro data and further confirms the selectivity of dofetilide in vivo.

The dispersion of ventricular repolarization induced in anesthetized dogs by rapid atrial pacing is reduced by dofetilide at the same doses required to prolong QT interval and ventricular ERP, while activation time and its dispersion were unaffected.[34] The absence of effect of dofetilide on activation confirms once more that Class I activity is not expressed in this molecule. In contrast, quinidine, at doses producing increases in repolarization time comparable to those of dofetilide did not reduce the dispersion of repolarization and actually increased the dispersion of activation,[34] reflecting a nonuniform slowing of conduction throughout the ventricles, creating a substrate prone to the induction of reentry arrhythmias.

This study also indicates that dofetilide expresses pharmacological activity at high heart rates and suggests that the negative rate dependency observed in standard in vitro preparations may possibly be misleading. This has been confirmed by Zuanetti and Corr,[30] who showed that the ventricular ERP prolongation induced by dofetilide is conserved at rapid rates.

The reduced dispersion of repolarization by dofetilide indicates an improved homogeneity of cardiac repolarization and probably underlies the elevation by intravenous dofetilide of ventricular fibrillation threshold (VFT) in anesthetized dogs, again at doses similar to those required to prolong the QT interval and ventricular ERP.[28]

Zuanetti and Corr,[30] employing a 232-electrode mapping system in dogs with stable infarcts, have demonstrated that dofetilide prevents the induction of ventricular tachycardia (VT) by lengthening the ERP in the epicardial region surrounding the infarct without affecting conduction velocity, even in the peri-infarct regions. This mechanism may also underlie the abolition of ventricular arrhythmias produced by acute microsphere-induced cardiac failure.[35] In the former study, dofetilide failed to prevent the induction of VF in dogs when this was the only arrhythmia induced. The multiple electrode mapping system confirmed that the induction of VF was dependent upon a rapid nonreentrant mechanism that was unaffected by dofetilide, and this, too, is consistent with the absence of effect of dofetilide on ionic mechanisms other than I_{Kr}.

The reduction of dispersion of repolarization may also explain the dofetilide-induced reduction of the incidence of sudden cardiac death in dogs subjected to transient myocardial posterolateral ischemia 3 to 5 days after anterior infarction.[36] Dofetilide also reduced the incidence of VT induced by programmed electrical stimulation. However, a number of animals remained inducible, although the cycle length of the induced tachycardia was significantly prolonged, perhaps reflecting the finding of Zuanetti and Corr[30] that a second dofetilide-insensitive mechanism exists. The dose employed in this study, 0.9 mg/kg 5 times daily, is vastly in excess of that employed by other authors.

Thus, the potency and selectivity of dofetilide described in vitro is conserved in vivo following both intravenous and oral administration. Intravenously, dofetilide is some 500-fold to 1,000-fold more potent than d-sotalol.

Hemodynamic Effects

Dofetilide is devoid of negative inotropic effects in vivo. In conscious dogs, intravenous dofetilide, at doses up to 100 μg/kg, consistently produces small (up to 15%) increases of various indexes of contractility (dP/dt_{max}, peak aortic flow, stroke volume), which generally correlate well with increases in the QT interval.[27] Over the same dose range, dofetilide does not impair cardiac function in pento-barbitone anesthetized dogs with normal hearts,[28] whereas at the relatively low dose of 5 μg/kg intravenously, in chloralose anesthetized dogs with normal hearts, dofetilide produces small increases of left ventricular dP/dt_{max} without affecting left ventricular end diastolic pressure or leftventricular relaxation.[29] In dogs with acute microsphere-induced cardiac failure, dofetilide, at a dose of 10 μg/kg intravenously, does not further compromise cardiac contractile function,[35] whereas it appears to cause a modest (12%) improvement in resting left ventricular contractility in dogs with ischemic hearts at an intravenous dose of 30 μg/kg.[37]

A common observation in experiments in anesthetized preparations is that dofetilide causes a slight reduction of resting heart,[28,35] which is limited to about 20%, whereas this is not seen in conscious dogs.[27] The reason for this is unclear, but dofetilide appears to be capable of reducing rapid, but not normal, resting heart rates. However, dofetilide appears not to prevent exercise-induced elevation of sinus rate in dogs with ischemic hearts undergoing exercise testing.[37]

These studies have not detected any effect of dofetilide on blood pressure. However, one study performed in rats[32] has reported an increase in blood pressure following dofetilide. However, even the lowest dose employed in this study, 600 μg/kg, is far in excess of that required for Class III activity in other species, and the effect is not dose related; the relevance of this observation remains to be determined.

Thus, the hemodynamic profile of dofetilide is concordant with that predicted from the in vitro studies. The compound expresses a mild degree of positive inotropic activity, which is correlated to its Class III activity and does not induce or aggravate cardiac depression.

Potential Proarrhythmic Activity of Dofetilide

In the studies described above, dofetilide has been examined in vitro at concentrations up to 4 orders of magnitude greater than those at which it produces discernible Class III activity (10 μM compared to 1 nM) and in vivo at doses up to 20 times the ED_{50} for QT interval prolongation.[33] No proarrhythmic activity was demonstrated. Indeed, one study performed in conscious dogs after anterior infarction employed an intravenous dose of 0.9 mg/kg (corresponding to 180 times the ED_{50} for QT interval prolongation) 5 times daily and failed to find evidence of significant proarrhythmic activity, although some of these dogs did display transient increases in ventricular ectopic activity.[36]

In 2 of 11 isolated guinea pig atria preparations, dofetilide produced afterdepolarizations at a concentration of 1 μM and a cycle length of 2,000 msec.[7] Such an effect has not been reported at this concentration or higher in vitro at a cycle length of 1,000 msec.[3] Many agents that prolong APD have been reported to elicit afterdepolarizations. However, the mechanisms by which agents such as the calcium channel agonist Bay K 8644 and the sea anemone toxin anthropleurin-A prolong the action potential are quite different from that of dofetilide, and so direct comparison with these agents may be inappropriate. Although N-acetylprocainamide[13] and clofilium,[38] both of which prolong APD by an effect on K$^+$ current(s), have been reported to induce afterdepolarizations, they do so at concentrations less than 20-fold greater than those at which they prolong APD. The concentration of dofetilide required to induce afterdepolarizations is between 500-fold and 1000-fold greater than that required to prolong APD, and so dofetilide is clearly different in this regard, in a quantitative sense, from these other agents.

The pacing rate at which this observation has been made must be borne in mind. The observation was made at a pacing cycle length of 2,000 msec in a tissue which, in vivo, beats with a cycle length of approximately 300 msec. The mechanism limited negative chronotropic effect of dofetilide has been reported to increase the spontaneous cycle length in guinea pig in vitro preparations from 382 msec to a maximum of 484 msec.[21] The cycle length of 2,000 msec employed in this part of the study is not one that is encountered naturally in that species, nor can it be induced by dofetilide. Thus, care must be taken not to overextrapolate this observation, made at a very high relative concentration of dofetilide and under conditions of bradycardia, which are more extreme than those that can be caused by dofetilide alone.

In common with many other Class III antiarrhythmic agents, dofetilide also causes an arrhythmia in rabbits that is similar to torsades de pointes VT (TdPVT).[39] However, a large number of studies of the actions of dofetilide in other species[27–31, 33–35] have indicated the absence of such an effect, even at doses substantially above the expected therapeutic range. Thus, considerable care must be exercised when attempting to extrapolate data from experimental animals to man.

Clinical Effects

Dofetilide has been administered to healthy volunteers and to patients with ischemic heart disease without arrhythmias, as well as to patients with various arrhythmias, both with and without structural heart disease. The data are, however, preliminary, and the clinical profile of this Class III agent is in the state of evolution.

Pharmacokinetics

Healthy Volunteers

Dofetilide is extensively absorbed, with a systemic bioavailability of 99% (Figure 6).[40] Mean maximal plasma concentrations (C_{max}) are achieved approximately 2 hours (range 1–4 hours) after oral administration, and the

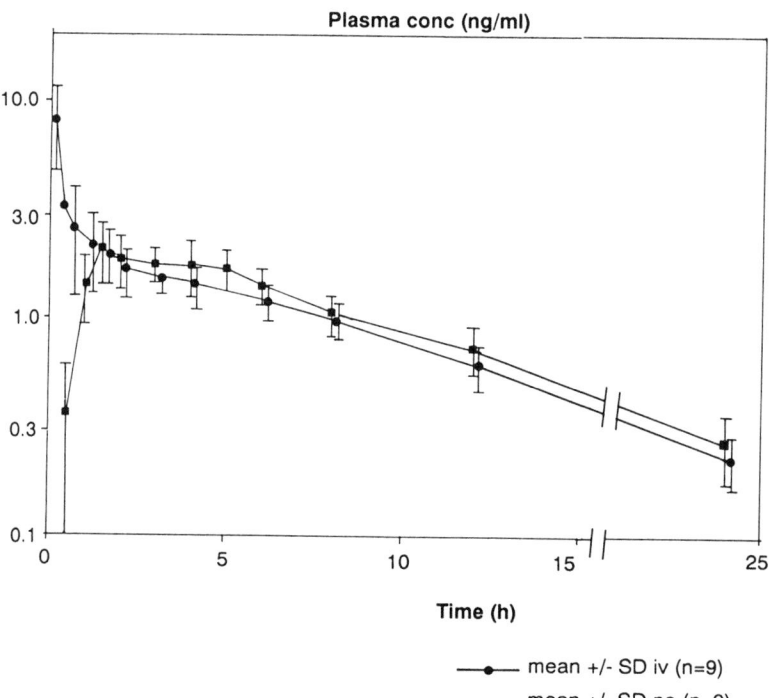

Figure 6. Mean plasma concentrations of dofetilide (ng/mL) versus time in human volunteers following single intravenous and oral doses of 0.5 mg.

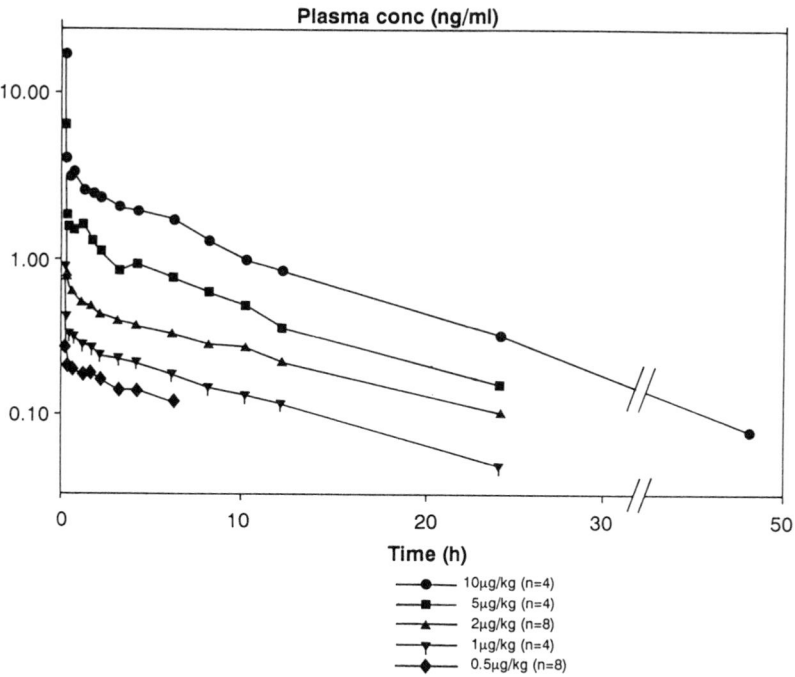

Figure 7. Mean plasma concentrations of dofetilide (ng/mL) versus time following single intravenous doses of 0.5 to 1.0 mcg/kg.

elimination half-life from plasma is about 9.5 hours (range 6–14 hours) (Figure 7).[40–42] Approximately 50% of the drug is excreted unchanged in the urine, whereas the remaining 50% is metabolized in the liver to inactive compounds. In a 10-day double blind, placebo controlled, multiple dose study, the accumulation ratio after twice daily dosing was 1.5, resulting in a peak trough plasma concentration ratio of 2.9.[43] After intravenous administration, the clearance (4.7 mL/min per kg) and volume of distribution (3.9 L/kg) are independent of dose and show low intra- and intersubject variability.[41] The dose plasma concentration relationship is linear within the dose range studied (Figure 8).[41] After oral administration, prolongation of the QTc interval was directly proportional to the plasma concentration. After intravenous administration this proportionality was delayed; that is, hysteresis was present (data on file).

The influence of food on the pharmacokinetics of dofetilide has been examined in vol-unteers. The total area under the plasma concentration time curve is not influenced by intake of food. However, the time to maximal plasma concentration is slightly delayed from the mean of 2.5 hours observed in fasting conditions to approximately 3.3 hours in the presence of food. C_{max} is independent of food (data on file).

Interaction studies with digoxin, propranolol, and warfarin have been conducted. In the digoxin interaction study, 14 volunteers received digoxin 0.25 mg once daily for 14 days. On day 8, the volunteers wcre allocated randomly to receive dofetilide (0.25 mg b.i.d.) or a placebo for the remaining 5 days. Digoxin pharmacokinetics were evaluated on days 7 and 12, and digoxin pharmacodynamics were monitored by 12-lead ECG recordings with measurements of RR, PR, QRS, and QTc intervals. No pharmacokinetic or pharmacodynamic interactions were detected.[43] The propranolol interaction study followed a similar double blind, placebo controlled design. Pro-

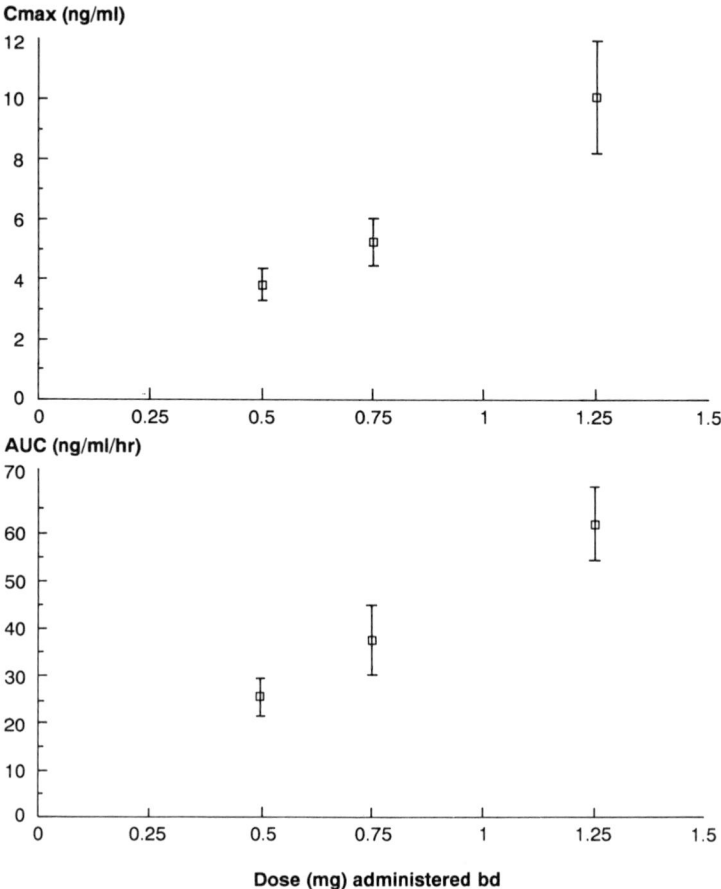

Figure 8. Maximum plasma concentrations (Cmax) and interdose area under the plasma concentration curve (AUC) versus dose at steady state (day 5) after administration of dofetilide 0.5-mg, 0.75-mg, and 1.25-mg b.i.d. Results are means ± S.E.M. from seven subjects.

pranolol pharmacokinetics were evaluated before and after 3-days treatment with dofetilide (0.25 mg b.i.d.) or a placebo added to stable background propranolol treatment. Propranolol pharmacodynamics were evaluated from exercise-induced tachycardia and 12-lead ECG recordings. Once again, no interactions were detected. In the warfarin interaction study, a single dose of warfarin was administered during double blind stable background treatment with dofetilide (0.25 mg b.i.d.) or a placebo. No pharmacokinetic or pharmacodynamic interactions were detected.

Patients

Pharmacokinetic parameters in patients with ischemic heart disease are very similar to those described in normal healthy volunteers. Sedgwick et al.[44] studied 18 patients with ischemic heart disease and stable angina pectoris, referred for a routine coronary arteriography. Five different doses of dofetilide were administered: the first 3 groups of 4 patients received dofetilide as a 10-minute intravenous infusion (1.5, 3.0, or 4.5 mcg/kg); a further 2 groups of 3 patients each received dofetilide as a 15-minute loading infusion (2/3 of total dose), followed by a 45-minute maintenance infusion (1/3 of total dose). The pharmacokinetic parameters were unaffected by the dosage regimen and were therefore combined. The mean volume of distribution was 3.9 L/kg, the mean clearance was 45 mL/min per kg, and the mean terminal elimination rate was a constant 0.078 ± 0.025 hours, corresponding to a mean elimination half-life of 9.7 ± 2.7 hours (range 4.8–13.5 hours). A linear relationship between dose and plasma concentration and between plasma concentrations and change in the QTc interval was found[44]; however, the latter correlation was only present after being corrected for hysteresis.

Pharmacodynamics

Healthy Volunteers

In all phase 1 studies, the QT interval was employed as a noninvasive measure for the influence of the drug on ventricular repolarization. Using this as an indicator of electrophysiological activity, the minimum active dose in volunteers is about 2 mcg/kg intravenously[41] and about 10 mcg/kg orally (data on file). A total daily dose of 2.5 mg, administered twice daily for a 5-day period, resulted in mean prolongations of the QTc interval of between 30 (at trough) and 100 msec (at peak), corresponding to a 10%–30% increase from baseline (unpublished data).

After intravenous administration of the compound, prolongations of the QTc interval of up to 200-msec increase from baseline have been observed.[40,41] Maximal effect is attained 10–20 minutes after completion of an intravenous infusion, indicating a rapid equilibration between plasma and ventricular myocardium. Even at the highest doses studied, there has been no evidence to suggest that dofetilide influences ECG variables other than the QTc (and QT) interval; no effects have been observed on the RR or PR intervals or the QRS width. This supports the preclinical evidence that dofetilide selectively affects repolarization without any influence on conduction time

in the myocardium (ie, exerts a highly selective Class III action).

No systematic influence of dofetilide on blood pressure or heart rate has been observed in any studies in healthy volunteers.

Patients

Intravenous administration of dofetilide to patients with ischemic heart disease[44] resulted in dose-dependent prolongations of the QTc interval. Doses of 1.5, 3.0, and 4.5 mcg/kg produced mean peak prolongations in the QTc interval at 41, 40, and 81 msec, respectively; corresponding values for uncorrected QT intervals were 36, 52, and 83 msec. All these changes were statistically significant ($p < 0.01$). Analysis of the QTc interval at 2-minute intervals from the Holter tapes revealed maximum increases of up to 130 msec at the top dose level. A comparison of plasma drug concentration and change in QTc from baseline, excluding the value at the end of the 10-minute infusion, revealed a linear correlation ($r = 0.81, p < 0.0001$).

In two invasive studies,[45,46] the effect of intravenous dofetilide on basic electrophysiological parameters of the heart has been assessed. Butrous et al.[45] studied 12 patients with supraventricular arrhythmias before and during a continuous 60-minute infusion of dofetilide. One group of 6 subjects received 10 mcg/kg over 60 minutes, whereas a second group of 6 subjects received 4 mcg/kg over 15 minutes (loading infusion), followed by 2 mcg/kg over 45 minutes (maintenance infusion). No effect of dofetilide was found at any of the dosage regimens on the RR, AH, or HV intervals or QRS width. However, significant prolongations of the QT interval and refractory periods and monophasic APD in the atria and ventricles were detected.

Sedgwick et al.[46] studied 18 patients with ischemic heart disease and stable angina pectoris in a double blind, placebo controlled study. Patients received one of two dose regimens of dofetilide or placebo as a 15-minute loading infusion, followed by a 45-minute maintenance infusion. No changes were ob-

Table 3
Influence of Dofetilide (Low Dose: 3 ± 1.5 μg/kg; High dose: 5 ± 2.5 μg/kg) and Placebo on Basic Electrophysiological Parameters in Patients with Ischemic Heart Disease

Parameter value	Predose mean ± SD	Postdose mean ± SD	Difference mean ± SD	Percent change	p
AERP 450					
Placebo	222 ± 23	228 ± 26	7 ± 8	3.0	NS
Low dose	223 ± 20	248 ± 24	25 ± 11	11.2	< 0.005
High dose	207 ± 18	225 ± 14	48 ± 16	23.4	< 0.001
VERP 450					
Placebo	242 ± 37	232 ± 11	−10 ± 32	−4.1	NS
Low dose	222 ± 24	257 ± 19	35 ± 13	15.8	0.002
High dose	225 ± 19	262 ± 23	37 ± 13	16.3	< 0.002
Sinus Cycle Length					
Placebo	807 ± 115	818 ± 111	11 ± 60	1.4	NS
Low dose	748 ± 124	771 ± 117	23 ± 24	3.1	NS
High dose	769 ± 78	839 ± 174	70 ± 111	9.1	NS
Sinus Node Recovery Time 450					
Placebo	1178 ± 233	1073 ± 175	−105 ± 136	−8.9	NS
Low dose	937 ± 189	978 ± 214	41 ± 113	4.4	NS
High dose	1061 ± 128	1100 ± 232	38 ± 146	3.6	NS
PA Interval					
Placebo	19 ± 11	25 ± 12	6 ± 15	36.4	NS
Low dose	24 ± 10	25 ± 15	1 ± 11	3.5	NS
High dose	24 ± 14	28 ± 13	4.24	17.2	NS
AH Interval					
Placebo	92 ± 23	94 ± 19	2 ± 7	2.1	NS
Low dose	80 ± 14	77 ± 15	−3 ± 8	−4.2	NS
High dose	84 ± 24	93 ± 33	9 ± 16	11.0	NS
HV Interval					
Placebo	49 ± 8	48 ± 8	−1 ± 5	−2.0	NS
Low dose	52 ± 4	49 ± 9	−3 ± 8	−4.8	NS
High dose	54 ± 6	54 ± 8	0 ± 5	0.0	NS

$AERP_{450}$: atrial effective refractory period at a drive cycle length at 450 msec; $VERP_{450}$: ventricular effective refractory period at a drive cycle length at 450 msec.

served after the administration of a placebo, whereas administration of dofetilide resulted in significant prolongations of the effective and functional refractory periods in the atria and ventricles.[38] No changes were observed in RR, PR, PA, AH, or HV intervals or sinus node recovery time. Selected data from this study are listed in Table 3.

A dose ranging study in VT patients undergoing programmed electrical stimulation has also been reported.[47] Dofetilide was studied at doses of 0.6–7.4 mcg/kg administered over 60 minutes and produced dose related increases of QT interval, right ventricular

monophasic APD, right atrial and right ventricular ERP, and RR interval without altering AH or HV intervals or QRS duration. Overall, 1 of 5 patients receiving a placebo and 7 of 15 patients receiving dofetilide became noninducible, but the small numbers of patients in every dose group preclude construction of a dose-response relationship. Again, no adverse experiences were encountered in this study.

The ability of dofetilide to convert patients with atrial fibrillation (AF) or atrial flutter (AFl) was studied in an open study of 24 patients with AF/AFl lasting less than 6 months. Mean duration of the arrhythmia prior to inclusion into the study was 42 days (range 1–150 days). Dofetilide was given intravenously during a 15-minute period; if conversion did not occur within 15 minutes after completion of the first infusion, a second infusion was given. Eight patients received 2.5 mcg/kg, followed by another 2.5 mcg/kg if required; 16 patients received 4.0 mcg/kg, followed by another 4.0 mcg/kg if required. At the lowest dose (2.5 + 2.5 mcg/kg), 4 out of 8 patients (50%) converted to normal sinus rhythm (SR) within 3 hours after completion of the second infusion. At the higher dose, 10/15 (67%) converted to SR. If the patients are subdivided independent of dose, into those with AF and those with AFl, 10 out of 18 (56%) with AF and 4 out of 5 (80%) with AFl converted to SR. No side effects were reported in this study.[48]

Safety Profile

Dofetilide has generally been very well tolerated. Side effects have been reported occasionally (eg, headache, sinus tachycardia, muscle cramps) but were usually mild and transient and occurred with similar frequencies in the placebo and the dofetilide treated groups.

One case of proarrhythmia has been reported in an intravenous/oral bioavailability study. After receiving a dose of 0.5-mg dofetilide intravenously during a 10-minute period (corresponding to 6.6 µg/kg), the volunteer developed several ventricular couplets and triplets and a short self-terminating run (5 beats) of polymorphic VT. This happened in association with an excessive prolongation of the QTc interval from 451-msec predose to 808 msec immediately postdose. The subject was asymptomatic throughout the study and did not require any treatment. Another case of self-limiting TdPVT was reported recently in an electrophysiological study in patients with VT/VF. The event occurred at the top dose of dofetilide employed in this study (15 mcg/kg intravenous).[49]

Laboratory abnormalities outside the normal range occasionally have been observed after treatment with either dofetilide or a placebo. The abnormalities have been mild and transient, and there were no indications of a causal relationship to the active drug, either in the healthy volunteer studies or in the patient studies.

Summary and Conclusions

Dofetilide is a potent and selective Class III antiarrhythmic agent, which is under development for the treatment of reentrant tachyarrhythmias, including VT, VF, AF, AFl, and paroxysmal supraventricular tachycardia. In preclinical studies, dofetilide shows the profile of an extremely selective Class III antiarrhythmic agent, increasing both ERP and APD without affecting the fast inward sodium current or calcium currents. Studies in dogs have shown that dofetilide prolongs atrial and ventricular ERP and elevates VFT in a dose-dependent manner, an effect probably attributable to reduction of dispersion of ventricular repolarization. Dofetilide does not influence conduction within the His-Purkinje system or within the myocardium nor does it impair cardiac contractility.

Dofetilide has been administered to healthy volunteers as well as to patients with ischemic heart disease and has generally been well tolerated. The few reported side effects have generally been transient and mild and occurred in placebo treated subjects as well. No clinically significant changes in laboratory safety tests have been detected. The pharmacokinetic profile of dofetilide in healthy volunteers and patients exhibits a linear dose plasma concentration relationship and a linear plasma concentration QTc relationship. The terminal plasma elimination half-life is 9–10 hours, and systemic bioavailability is in excess of 90%. Elimination is balanced, with 50% of the parent compound being excreted unchanged via the kidney and the remainder metabolized in the liver to inactive metabolites.

Pharmacodynamic data demonstrate dose- and concentration-dependent effects on myocardial repolarization, evidenced by significant prolongations in the effective and functional refractory periods, monophasic APD, and QTc interval. No effects on sinus node function, conduction parameters, or cardiac contractility have been detected in any of the clinical studies, supporting the contention that dofetilide is a highly selective Class III antiarrhythmic agent. Preliminary clinical data in AF/AFl and VT/VF patients are encouraging.

References

1. Cross PE, Arrowsmith JE, Thomas GN, et al: Selective Class III antiarrhythmic agents. 1.bis(arylalkyl)amines. *J Med Chem* 33:1151, 1990.

2. Sanguinetti MC, Jurkiewicz NK: Two components of cardiac delayed rectifier K$^+$ current. *J Gen Physiol* 96:195, 1990.

3. Gwilt M, Arrowsmith JE, Blackburn KJ, et al: UK-68,798: a novel, potent and highly selective Class III antiarrhythmic agent which blocks potassium channels in cardiac cells. *J Pharmacol Exp Ther* 256:318, 1991.

4. Knilans T, Lathrop DA, Nanasi PB, et al: Rate and concentration-dependent effects of UK-68,798, a potent new Class III antiarrhythmic agent, on canine Purkinje fibre action potential duration and $\dot{V}_{max}$. *Br J Pharmacol* 103:1568, 1991.

5. Abrahamsson C, Carlsson L, Duker G: A comparative study of three new class III drugs concerning their diverse effects on action potential duration in conducting tissue versus ventricular muscle in the rabbit heart. *J Mol Cell Cardiol* 23 (Suppl III):9, 1991.

6. Baskin E, Serik C, Wallace A, et al: Comparative effects of Class III antiarrhythmic agents on refractoriness in isolated ventricular myocardium. *FASEB J* 4:455, 1990.

7. Tande PM, Bjornstad H, Yang T, et al: Rate-dependent Class III antiarrhythmic action, negative chronotropy, and positive inotropy of a novel I$_K$ blocking drug, UK-68,798: potent in guinea-pig but no effect in rat myocardium. *J Cardiovasc Pharmacol* 16:401, 1990.

8. Montero M, Beyer T, Brachmann J, et al: Electrophysiological effects of the new Class III antiarrhythmic agent UK-68,798 in isolated rabbit sinus node and atrium. Presented at Tagung der deutschen Gesellschaft fur Herz-Kreislauf-forschung; April, 1991; and to be published in the Journal of the Society.

9. Josephson IR, Sanchez-Chapula J, Brown AM: Early outward current in rat single ventricular cells. *Circ Res* 54:157, 1984.

10. Hondeghem L, Katzung BG: Antiarrhythmic agents: the modulated receptor mechanism of action of sodium and calcium channel-blocking drugs. *Ann Rev Pharmacol Toxicol* 24:387, 1984.

11. Varro A, Nakaya Y, Elhallar V, et al: Effects of antiarrhythmic drugs on the cycle length-dependent action potential duration in dog Purkinje and ventricular muscle fibres. *J Cardiovasc Pharmacol* 8:178, 1986.

12. Anderson KP, Walker R, Dustman T, et al: Rate-related electrophysiological effects of long-term administration of amiodarone on canine ventricular myocardium in vivo. *Circulation* 79:948, 1989.

13. Dangman KH, Hoffman BF: In vivo and in vitro antiarrhythmic and arrhythmogenic effects of N-acetylprocainamide. *J Pharmacol Exp Ther* 217:851, 1987.

14. Roden DM, Hoffman BF: Action potential prolongation and induction of abnormal automaticity by low quinidine concentrations in canine Purkinje fibres. *Circ Res* 56:857, 1985.

15. Josephson IR, Sanchez-Chapula J, Brown AM: A comparison of calcium currents in rat and guinea-pig single ventricular cells. *Circ Res* 54:144, 1984.

16. Yang T, Tande PM, Lathrop DA, et al: Effect of extracellular potassium on the electrophysiological effects of UK-68,798, a Class III antiarrhythmic agent, in guinea-pig papillary muscle. *J Mol Cell Cardiol* 23 (Suppl III):111, 1991.

17. Yang T, Tande PM, Lathrop DA, et al: UK-68,798, a potent class III antiarrhythmic agent, prevents hypoxia-induced action potential shortening and negative inotropy in guinea-pig papillary muscle. *J Mol Cell Cardiol* 23 (Suppl III):10, 1991.

18. Carmeliet E: Effect of UK-68,798 on delayed K$^+$ current in cardiac myocytes. *J Mol Cell Cardiol* 23 (Suppl III):8, 1991.

19. Greengrass PM, Sanders FL, Wyllie MG: ^{3}-H-UK-68,798 (dofetilide) binds to a K$^+$-channel in guinea-pig cardiac tissue. *Fundam Clin Pharmacol* 5:408, 1991.

20. Pong SF, Kinney CM, Moorhead TJ: Receptor binding profiles of Class III antiarrhythmic agents. *FASEB J* 5:1215, 1991.

21. Yang T, Tande PM, Refsum H: Negative chronotropic effect of a novel Class III antiarrhythmic drug, UK-68,798, devoid of β-blocking action on isolated guinea-pig atria. *Br J Pharmacol* 103:1417, 1991.

22. Miller KE, Carpenter JF, Brooks RR: Beta adrenergic receptor response of guinea pig heart in the presence of Class III antiarrhythmics. *FASEB J* 5:1216, 1991.

23. Noma A, Irisawa H: Membrane currents in rabbit sinoatrial node cells studied by the double microelectrode method. *Pflügers Arch* 364:42, 1976.

24. Yanagihara K, Irisawa H: Potassium current during the pacemaker depolarisation in rabbit sinoatrial node cell. *Pflügers Arch* 388:255, 1980.

25. Platou ES, Refsum H, Hotvedt R: Class III antiarrhythmic activity linked with positive inotropy: electrophysiological and hemodynamic effects of the sea anemone polypeptide ATX II in the dog heart in situ. *J Cardiovasc Pharmacol* 8:459, 1986.

26. Serik C, Baskin E, Wiedmann R, et al: Inotropic effects of Class III antiarrhythmic agents in isolated ventricular myocardium. *FASEB J* 4:455, 1990.

27. Dalrymple HW, Butler P, Dodd MG, et al: Electrocardiographic and haemodynamic effects in conscious dogs of UK-68,798, a new Class III antiarrhythmic agent. *Eur Heart J* 10:395, 1989.

28. Gwilt M, Solca AM, Burges RA, et al: Antifibrillatory action and haemodynamic properties of UK-68,798, a new Class III antiarrhythmic agent, in anaesthetised dogs. *J Mol Cell Cardiol* 21 (Suppl II):11, 1989.

29. Stupienski R, Wallace A, Brookes L, et al: Cardiac electrophysiologic and hemodynamic effects of Class III agents in anesthetized dogs. *FASEB J* 4:A455, 1990.

30. Zuanetti G, Corr PB: Antiarrhythmic efficacy of a new Class III agent, UK-68,798, during chronic myocardial infarction: evaluation using three-dimensional mapping. *J Pharmacol Exp Ther* 256:325, 1991.

31. Beatch GN, MacLeod BA, Abraham S, et al: The in vivo electrophysiological actions of the new potassium channel blockers, tedisamil and UK-68,798. *Proc West Pharmacol Soc* 33:5, 1990.

32. Maynard AE, Carpenter JF, Decker GE, et al: Efficacy of d-sotalol, sematilide and UK-68,798 in the rat coronary artery ligation-reperfusion (CALR) model of cardiac arrhythmias. *FASEB J* 5:A1216, 1991.

33. Dalrymple HW, Butler P, Dodd MG, et al: Electrocardiographic and haemodynamic effects in conscious dogs of UK-68,798, a new Class III antiarrhythmic agent. Presented at the International Symposium on QT Prolongation and Ventricular Arrhythmias; February, 1991; Nagasaki, Japan.

34. Gwilt M, Milne AA, Solca AM, et al: UK-68,798, a potent and selective Class III antiarrhythmic agent, reduces dispersion of repolarisation in canine hearts in situ induced by rapid pacing. *Br J Pharmacol* 99:15P, 1990.

35. Yang T, Mortensen E, Bjornstad H, et al: Class III antiarrhythmic activity of UK-68,798 in acute ischemic left ventricular failure in dogs. *J Mol Cell Cardiol* 22(Suppl III):71, 1990.

36. Black SC, Chi L, Mu DX, et al: The antifibrillatory actions of UK-68,798, a class III antiarrhythmic agent. *J Pharmacol Exp Ther* 258:416, 1991.

37. Gout B, Jean J, Bril A: Effect of a Class III antiarrhythmic, UK-68,798, on cardiac function in exercise-induced ischemia in the conscious dog. *FASEB J* 5:A1215, 1991.

38. Gough WB, Hu D, El-Sherif N: Effects of clofilium on ischemic subendocardial Purkinje fibres 1 day postinfarction. *J Am Coll Cardiol* 11:431, 1988.

39. Carlsson L, Almgren O, Duker G: QTU-prolongation and torsades de pointes induced by putative Class III antiarrhythmic agents in the rabbit: etiology and interventions. *J Cardiovasc Pharmacol* 16:276, 1990.

40. Tham TCK, MacLennan BA, Harron DWG, et al: Pharmacodynamics and pharmacokinetics of the novel Class III antiarrhythmic drug UK-68,798 in man. *Br J Clin Pharmacol* 31(Suppl II): 243, 1991.

41. Gemmill JD, Howie CA, Meredith PA, et al: A dose-ranging study of UK-68,798, a novel class OIII antiarrhythmic agent in normal volunteers. *Br J Clin Pharmacol* 32:429, 1991.

42. Rasmussen HS, Allen MJ, Blackburn KJ, et al: Dofetilide: a novel class III antiarrhythmic agent. *J Cardiovasc Pharmacol* 20 (suppl 2): 96, 1992.

43. Rasmussen HS, Kleinermans D, Walker DK, et al: A double-blind, placebo controlled parallel group study of the effect of UK-68,798, a novel class III antiarrhythmic agent, on the pharmacokinetics and pharmacodynamics of digoxin. *Eur Heart J* 11 (Suppl):57, 1990.

44. Sedgwick M, Rasmussen HS, Walker D, et al: Pharmacokinetic and pharmacodynamic effects of UK-68,798, a new potential class III antiarrhythmic drug. *Br J Clin Pharmacol* 31:515, 1991.

45. Butrous GS, O'Nunain S, Ward J, et al: Clinical electrophysiologic profile of UK-68,798, a new class III antiarrhythmic agent. *PACE* 14(Suppl II):744, 1991.

46. Sedgwick M, Rasmussen HS, Cobbe SM: Clinical and electrophysiologic effects of intravenous dofetilide (UK-68,798), a new class III antiarrhythmic agent in patients with angina pectoris. *Am J Cardiol* 69:513, 1992.

47. Echt DS, Lee JT, Murray KT, et al: A randomized, double-blind, placebo-controlled study of intravenous UK-68,798 (dofetilide) in patients with inducible sustained ventricular tachycardia. *Circulation* 84 (suppl 55):714, 1991.

48. Suttorp MJ, Polak PE, van't Hof A, et al: Efficacy and safety of a new selective class III antiarrhythmic agent, dofetilide, in paroxysmal atrial fibrillation or atrial flutter. *Am J Cardiol* 69:417, 1992.

49. Thomsen P, Bashir Y, Kingma J, et al: Dofetilide in the treatment of sustained monomorphic ventricular tachycardia (VT) (abstract). *Eur Heart J* 18(Suppl):1675, 1992.

Chapter 38

Electropharmacological Profile and Antiarrhythmic Potential of Almokalant (H234/09)

Olle Almgren

The concept of a third class of antiarrhythmic action was introduced by Singh and Vaughan Williams in 1970.[1] It was defined as "prolongation of the action potential with a consequent increase of the absolute refractory period." Drugs identified as possessing a Class III mode of action were sotalol, nifenalol (INPEA), amiodarone, and bretylium, although they were all known to have other actions as well. The first drug to be developed as a selective Class III agent was clofilium,[2] but it seems not to have proceeded beyond clinical phase II evaluation. In the last few years, a large number of new chemical entities with alleged Class III action have reached the stage of clinical investigations. One of these new compounds is almokalant (H 234/09), a derivative of INPEA, a β blocker with intrinsic sympathomimetic actions and modest propensity to inhibit sodium channels. Almokalant (Figure 1), 4-3[ethyl[3-(propylsulfinyl)-propyl]amino] - 2 - hydroxy - propoxy] - ben - zonitrile, H 234/09, is an isomeric mixture of four stereoisomers, which all have very similar pharmacodynamic and pharmacokinetic properties. The base is an almost colorless, viscous liquid that is highly soluble in acids. Its pKa is 7.8 and the distribution constant, K_D, is 16 at 20°C.

Almokalant was chosen as the candidate drug in a screening program aimed at the development of a selective Class III antiarrhythmic agent. The primary screen models consisted of:

1. Prolongation of the epicardial monophasic action potential duration (MAPD) in anesthetized guinea pigs.
2. Effect on exploratory motor activity on conscious mice.
3. Effect on inotropy in isolated cat papillary muscle.

Follow-up studies were performed in anesthetized and conscious dogs to determine the drug's effect on cardiac electrophysiology, hemodynamics, central nervous system effects, and pharmacokinetics.

Chemistry

A summary of the most important steps in the synthesis screen program leading to the

From BN Singh, HJJ Wellens, M Hiraoka, (eds): *Electropharmacological Control of Cardiac Arrhythmias.* Mount Kisco, NY, Futura Publishing Company Inc., © 1994.

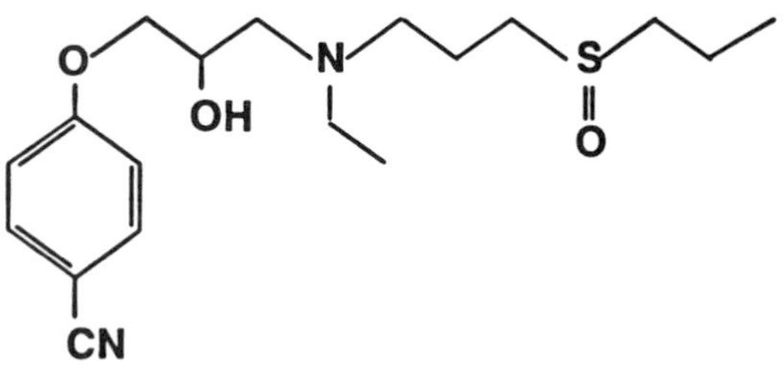

Figure 1. Structural formula of almokalant.

almokalant structure is shown in Figure 2. From a starting point in nifenalol, the work was switched over to β-blocking structures with the long side chain, and compounds with a Class III activity comparable to that of nifenalol were found. Only small changes of the molecule were needed to eliminate the β-blocking activity.

Although the nitro group was found to be the most potent parasubstituent tested, it was considered potentially toxic in this position, since it could be the target for metabolism producing toxic intermediates. For this reason it was replaced by the more stable cyano group, which was slightly less potent. Application of knowledge from the clofilium

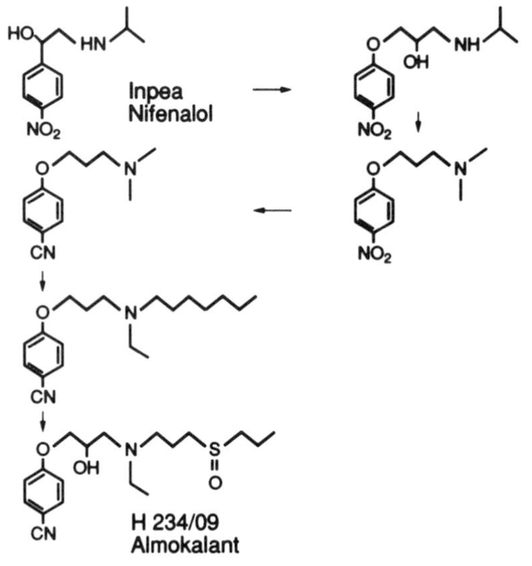

Figure 2. Steps in the synthesis screen program resulting in almokalant.

development to the end part of the side chain resulted in more potent, but also more lipophilic, structures.

Thus, the final goal was to reduce lipophilicity without the simultaneous reduction of potency. This work resulted in the introduction of the sulfoxide group in the side chain.

Pharmacology

Almokalant was found to prolong the MAPD in the anesthetized guinea pig by 10% at an intravenous dose of 10^{-7} M.[5] The intravenous dose needed in conscious mice to get a significant (20%) reduction of exploratory motor activity was 500 times higher. In the isolated cat papillary muscle, almokalant did not disclose any negative inotropic effects. Instead, there was a moderate positive inotropic effect, about 30% of the maximum response to isoproterenol. Interestingly, the EC_{50} for this positive inotropic effect in cat was about 10^{-7} M, which is similar to the EC_{50} for MAPD prolongation in the guinea pig heart in vitro. The similarity indicates that the two effects of almokalant are interrelated, and tentatively, the positive inotropic response may be interpreted as secondary to an action potential prolongation, by allowing a longer time for calcium influx that results in high intracellular calcium concentrations. Both the action potential prolongation and positive inotropic effect of almokalant have been confirmed in ex vivo experiments in human papillary muscle obtained via mitral valve surgery.[5]

Extended electrophysiological as well as hemodynamic studies were performed in anesthetized and conscious dogs.[6] Some results from a comparison with dl-sotalol in anesthetized dogs are shown in Figure 3. In summary, all the effects found were those that were expected from a pure Class III agent: prolongation of MAPD, QT interval, and ventricular as well as atrial refractoriness, and a slight positive inotropic effect. Currently no data are available relative to the effects of frequency of stimulation on the action potential duration. There were no other electrophysio-

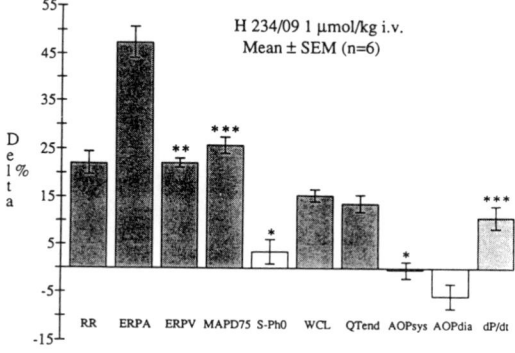

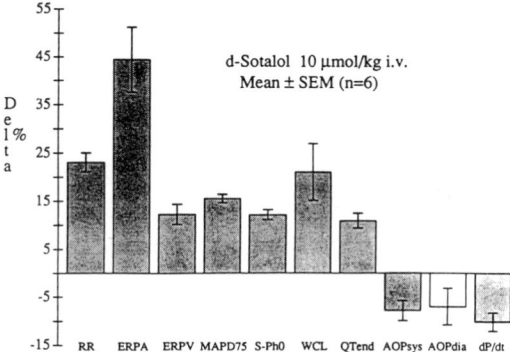

Figure 3. The change (in percent) of some electrophysiological and hemodynamic variables 30 minutes after intravenous administration of 1 μmol/kg almokalant and 10 μmol/kg d-sotalol compared to predrug control in anesthetized dogs. RR: RR interval; ERPA, ERPV: effective refractory period of the atrium and ventricle, respectively; MAPD 75: left ventricular epicardial monophasic action potential duration at 75% repolarization; S-PhD: time lag between pace stimulus in atrium and start of the monophasic action potential in left ventricle; WCL: Wenckebach cycle length; QT: QT interval measured to the end of the T wave; AOP sys: AOP dia: systolic and diastolic aortic blood pressure; dP/dt: rate of rise of left ventricular pressure. Shaded bars means statistically significant ($p < 0.05$) change from control value and asterisks (*: $p < 0.05$; **: $p < 0.001$) denominate statistically significant differences between almokalant and d-sotalol.

logical or hemodynamic effects, indicating that almokalant is a selective Class III agent. In particular, there was no effect on sinus node frequency consistent with the fact that the bulk of the β-blocking activity has been eliminated

relative to that of the parent compound (nifenalol). The mechanism mediating the effect on the action potential duration has been studied in isolated guinea pig myocytes. The interaction of almokalant with cardiac ionic currents have revealed a specific effect on the I_K current.[7] The IC_{50} for almokalant on this current was estimated 5 to 50 nm (Figure 4) and interactions with several other repolarizing or depolarizing currents at this concentration level were excluded.

It should be noted that the clinical electrophysiological effects on the drug start to be seen at plasma almokalant concentrations around 20 nmol/L and are almost maximal around 150–200 nmol/L. Since the plasma protein binding of almokalant is only about 20% (at ph 7.4, human, dog, and rat plasma), it is likely that the effect shown on I_K is responsible for the clinical electrophysiological effects. Furthermore, dog studies by Eriksson et al. (unpublished data) have demonstrated a direct relationship between plasma almokalant concentration and QT prolongation at a constant paced heart rate according to an E_{max} model.

During studies of the distribution of almokalant in rabbits a severe proarrhythmic effect in this species was detected. Conscious rabbits, receiving almokalant or any other Class III agent that was used, regularly developed a rapid ventricular tachycardia with an ECG pattern strikingly similar to described cases of torsades de pointes. Interestingly, the phenomenon was not observed in the anesthetized rabbit unless an α-receptor agonist was given simultaneously. This work led to the development and characterization of an animal model for torsades de pointes.[8]

It was also found that this exaggerated proarrhythmic effect was unique to the rabbit and was not seen in guinea pigs, dogs, rats, or mice. In the conscious rabbit, torsades de pointes already appears at low pharmacological doses of almokalant, which gives rise to a marked QT prolongation. For all tested compounds there appears to be a linear correlation between potency to prolong the QTU time and the dose needed to produce the ar-

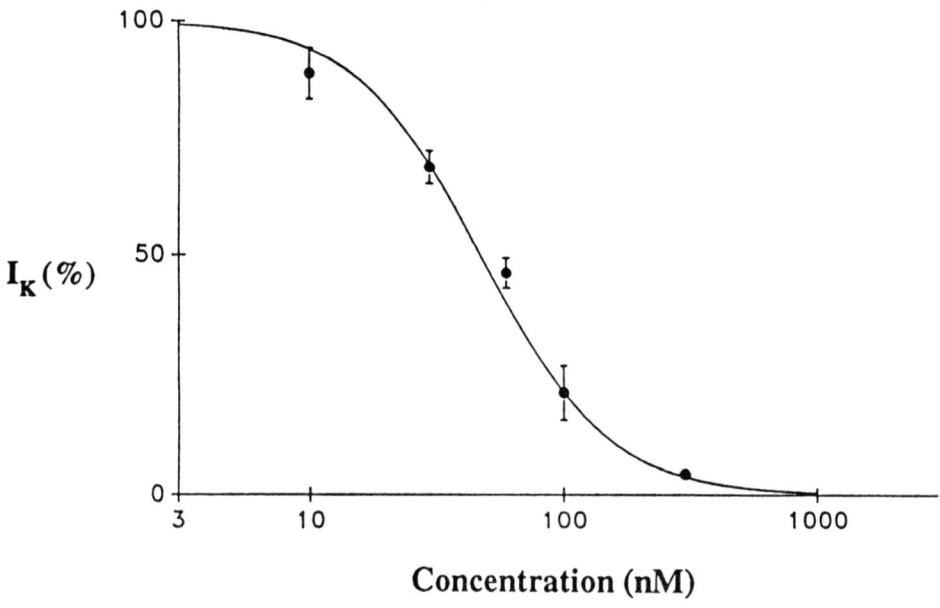

Figure 4. Effect of almokalant on the delayed rectifier (I_K) in the isolated Purkinje fiber of rabbit. (Carmeliet, personal communication)

rhythmia (Figure 5). The same finding was made in one Cynomolgus monkey in which there was already a prolonged QT time and low heart rate before receiving almokalant; after almokalant, a marked further QT prolon-

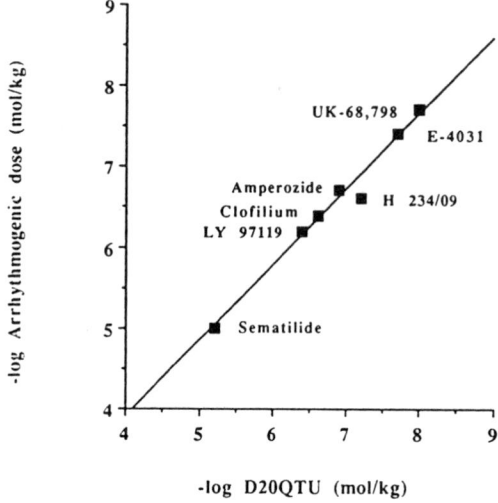

Figure 5. Correlation between proarrhythmic effect and potency for some Class III antiarrhythmic agents in the anesthetized rabbit model.

gation developed and nonsustained episodes of torsades de pointes were seen following a low intravenous dose (< 0.5 μmol/kg). The other monkeys tolerated intravenous doses up to 120 μmol/kg without any signs of arrhythmia. The data indicated that, as in the case of many QT prolonging drugs, an abnormally prolonged QT interval at baseline predisposes to the development of torsades de pointes.[9]

An interesting concept that emerged from discussions of a clinical case of torsades de pointes[10] was a possible temporary increase in the dispersion of repolarization, which is caused by a rapid infusion of drug giving rise to an initially uneven distribution of the drug within the heart. This concept was tested in the rabbit model, and it was indeed found that a fivefold difference in infusion rate of almokalant resulted in marked differences both in change of QT dispersion and of the incidence of torsades de pointes (Carlsson, unpublished data). Thus, avoiding rapid swings in plasma drug concentration may be an important safety issue in clinical trials and practice.

Pharmacokinetics

Animal pharmacokinetic studies of almokalant have revealed an oral bioavailability around 50% in both dog and rat, a relatively high volume of distribution and, in the dog, an elimination half-life in the order of 6 hours.

Toxicology

Both acute and chronic toxicity of almokalant is low. The only findings of special interest in studies of up to 1 year's chronic administration have been a selective testicular atrophy in rats comprising the germinal epithelium, but leaving other structures intact. The prostate and vesicula seminalis were unaffected, indicating that hormonal effects are not involved. Furthermore, studies have revealed that this effect occurs also with other, structurally unrelated Class III agents, such as amiodarone and dofetilide, and thus the effect appears to be related to the mechanism of action of these compounds, ie, the potassium channel blocking effect.

The atrophy has been encountered at high-dose and plasma concentration levels, about 10 times above the projected clinical levels. No atrophy has been detected in the dog studies. The fertility and teratogenicity studies revealed another mechanisms related effect of almokalant, an embryolethal effect occurring at around day 11–12 of the gestation period in rats and mice. Separate studies of almokalant and some reference compounds (d-sotalol and dofetilide) on fetal cardiac electrophysiology have shown a marked prolongation of cardiac action potentials in contrast to the lack of effect in adult rats (Abrahamsson, unpublished data). Furthermore, at higher concentrations early afterdepolarizations were seen. It is considered probable that this primary effect of the drug on the fetal cardiac electrophysiology is responsible for the fetal loss. It is noteworthy, that the plasma almokalant concentrations at which the embryolethal effect was seen is only 2–3 times higher than the projected clinically effective concentrations.

Clinical Studies

The first studies of almokalant in humans were conducted in healthy volunteers, who for safety reasons, had an esophageal pacing catheter positioned for atrial pacing. In addition to providing the possibility of performing emergency pacing, this procedure gave the added benefit of providing a means for measuring QT interval at a constant paced heart rate. Thus, a reliable analysis of the dose plasma concentration response relationship could be done. The only adverse effect recorded was a metallic taste after intravenous infusion of 9 mg over 10 minutes, which was not encountered after oral administration of up to 27 mg. The studies confirmed an oral bioavailability of about 50%, a rapid distribution phase, and an elimination half-life of 1–4 hours. The plasma drug concentration effect relationship was investigated in an invasive study in healthy volunteers that graded intravenous infusions of almokalant to predetermined pseudoequilibrium levels of 20, 50, 100, and 150 nmol/L. Several effect variables including paced QT, ventricular effective refractory periods (VERPs), and atrial effective refractory periods (AERPs) at different pacing rates were analyzed. While the effects started to appear at a concentration of 20 nmol/L, the incremental change leveled off between 100 and 150 nmol/L. Thus, the clinically effective plasma concentration range is expected to be between 50 and 200 nmol/L.

Pharmacokinetic studies in healthy volunteers have been performed. A summary of the findings is given in Table 1. The major route of metabolism of almokalant is glucoronidation, and other metabolites are of little importance. No metabolite with equal or higher Class III activity compared to almokalant has been identified.

The tolerability of intravenous almokalant and its effect on the frequency of premature ventricular contractions (PVCs) was investigated in 10 patients with frequent extrasystoles after myocardial infarction. A marked QT prolongation was seen, but no effect on

Table 1
Pharmacokinetic Parameters of Almokalant in Healthy Male Volunteers. (n = 10)

		I.V.	Oral
Dose	(μmol)	12.8	25.6
Clearance	(mL-min^{-1}kg^{-1})	12 ± 2	—
Distribution volume	(V_{ss}, l-kg^{-1})	2.6 ± 0.6	—
Elimination half-life	($t_{1/2}$, h)	2.8 ± 0.2	3.6 ± 0.5
Maximum concentration	(C_{max}, nmol/L)	—	58 ± 14
Time at C_{MAX}	(t_{max}, h)	—	0.8 ± 0.5
Oral bioavailability	(F, %)	—	51 ± 11

PQ or QRS times were recorded (Figure 6). A reduction in the frequency of PVCs or a prolongation of the coupling interval was recorded, and there was an excellent relation between the QTc prolongation and the plasma almokalant concentration. In one patient almokalant was infused at double speed, and this patient had, during the infusion, episodes of torsades de pointes that spontaneously terminated after stopping the infusion. This adverse event triggered further animal experimental work, which supported the idea that the rate of delivery is a factor of importance for the development of this proarrhythmic reaction. Clinical studies of almokalant on various arrhythmia indications are presently ongoing.

Conclusions

The early experimental and clinical data on almokalant discussed in this chapter provide the emerging profile of this compound as a Class III antiarrhythmic compound. There appears to be a reasonable concordance between its effects in experimental animals and in humans. It is not clear whether the structural differences between almokalant and the derivatives of sotalol in terms of their parasubstitution in the aromatic ring are relevant to their proarrhythmic and antiarrhythmic actions. Such potential differences may need to be explored by larger comparative clinical studies. Nevertheless, the synthesis of almokalant as a pure Class III agent provides a significant electropharmacological probe to explore the significance of structure activity relationships in the search for the ideal antifibrillatory compound for the control of ventricular and supraventricular tachyarrhythmias.

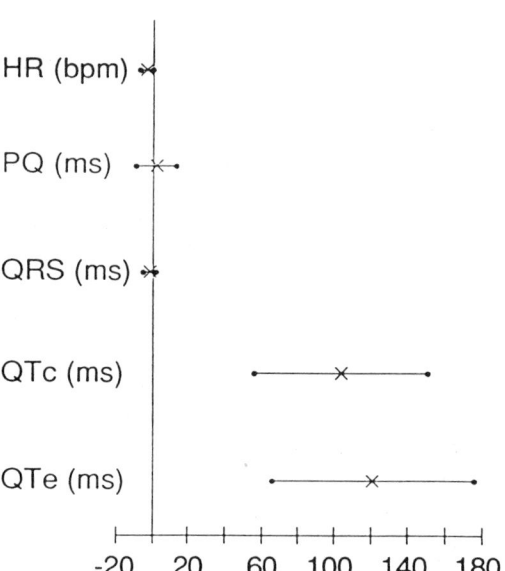

Figure 6. Effect of almokalant (12.8 μmol intravenously over 10 minutes) in patients with frequent ventricular premature beats. The 95% confidence interval for the difference between placebo and almokalant immediately after infusion is shown.

References

1. Singh BN, Vaughan Williams EM: A third class of antiarrhythmic action: effects on atrial and

ventricular intracellular potentials, and other pharmacological actions on cardiac muscle of MJ 1999 and AH 3676. *Br J Pharmacol* 39:675, 1970.

2. Steinberg MI, Michelson EL: Cardiac electrophysiologic effects of specific Class III substances. In: HS Reiser, LN Horowitz (eds): *Mechanisms and Treatment of Cardiac Arrhythmias: Relevance of Basic Studies to Clinical Management*. Baltimore, MD: Urban and Schwarzenberg, 1985, p. 263.

3. Singh BN, Vaughan Williams EM: Effects on cardiac muscle of the β blocking drugs INPEA and LB 46 in relation to their local anesthetic action on nerve. *Br J Pharmacol* 43:10, 1971.

4. Singh BN: *Pharmacologic Actions of Certain Drugs and Hormones: Focus on Studies on Antiarrhythmic Mechanisms*. Oxford, United Kingdom: Hertford College, University of Oxford; 1971. D. Phil. Thesis. p. 43.

5. Carlsson L, Abrahamsson C, Almgren O, et al: Prolonged action potential duration and positive inotrophy induced by the novel Class III antiarrhythmic agent H 234/09 (almokalant) in isolated human ventricular muscle. *J Cardiovasc Pharmacol* 18:882, 1991.

6. Duker G, Almgren O, Carlsson L: Electrophysiologic and hemodynamic effects of H 234/09 (almokalant), quinidine and (+)-sotalol in the anesthetized dog. *J Cardiovasc Pharmacol* 20:458, 1992.

7. Carmeliet E: Use-dependent block and use-dependent unblock of the delayed K^+ current by almokalant in rabbit ventricular myocytes. (personal communication).

8. Carlsson L, Almgren O, Duker G: QTU-prolongation and torsades de pointes induced by putative Class III antiarrhythmic agents in the rabbit: etiology and interventions. *J Cardiovasc Pharmacol* 16:276, 1990.

9. Singh BN: Safety profile of bepridil determined from clinical trials in chronic stable angina in the United States. *Am J Cardiol* 69:68D, 1992.

10. Wiesfeld ACP, Crijns HJGM, Tobe TJM, et al: Electrophysiologic effects and pharmacokinetics of almokalant, a new Class III antiarrhythmic, in patients with healed or healing myocardial infarcts and complex ventricular arrhythmias. *Am J Cardiol* 70:990, 1992.

Chapter 39

Electrophysiological and Pharmacodynamic Properties and Pharmacokinetics of MS-551, A New Class III Antiarrhythmic Compound

Keitaro Hashimoto
Takeo Awaji
Wu Zhenjiu

MS-551 is a new Class III antiarrhythmic drug synthesized by Mitsui Toatsu Chemicals, Inc. (Tokyo, Japan) and has been developed by Mitsui Pharmaceuticals, Inc. (Tokyo, Japan) as a compound with a potential for significant clinical utility in controlling supraventricular and ventricular tachyarrhythmias. It has all the properties of a new so-called pure Class III antiarrhythmic agent exhibiting the potential for lengthening the cardiac action potential duration (APD) and the effective refractory period (ERP), without having the property for blocking the fast sodium channel mediated conduction. The drug has been shown to have a rapid onset of action after administration in vivo and in vitro. It is undergoing intensive experimental and preliminary clinical evaluation. Several studies in experimental animals, reported in abstract form, have begun to characterize MS-551 as a Class III antiarrhythmic drug, and the results of the early clinical studies have also become available. This chapter summarizes the salient features of the emerging data on the electrophysiological profile of the drug.

Chemistry and Pharmacokinetics

Chemically, MS-551, [1,3-dimethyl-6-{2-[N-(2-hydroxyethyl)-3-(4-nitrophenyl)propyl-amino]ethylamino]-2, 4-(1H, 3H)-pyrimidinedione hydrochloride), is not a derivative of dl-sotalol, nor is it structurally similar to

The authors' studies were partly supported by a Grant-in-Aid for Scientific Research 032253103 for the Japanese Ministry of Education, Science, and Culture.
From BN Singh, HJJ Wellens, M Hiraoka, (eds): *Electropharmacological Control of Cardiac Arrhythmias.* Mount Kisco, NY, Futura Publishing Company Inc., © 1994.

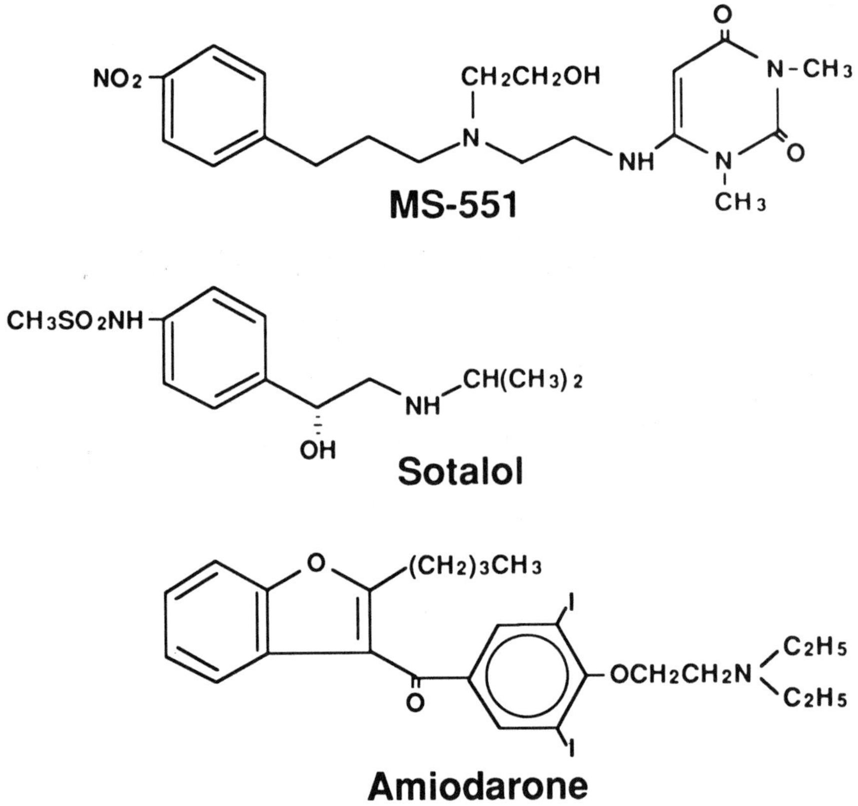

Figure 1. Chemical structure of MS-551, d-sotalol, and amiodarone. Note that the three compounds differ significantly in terms of their chemical structure. However, the drug is a potent delayed rectifier blocker and has a profile somewhat similar to that of d-sotalol.

the classical Class III drug, amiodarone. The structure of MS-551 is compared to that of sotalol and amiodarone in Figure 1. The drug clearly differs from the two prototype Class III antiarrhythmic compounds. Physicochemical data show that it is a weak base of a light yellow to yellow crystal with a molecular weight of 441.19; it is readily soluble in water and less so in ethanol, and it is almost insoluble in diethyl ether. The melting point is 171.0–174.0°C, and pKa is 7.05 (unpublished data on file with Mitsui Toatsu Pharmaceuticals, Inc.).

Only preliminary pharmacokinetic data are available both in experimental animals and in humans (unpublished data). In rats and dogs, MS-551 is well absorbed following oral administration, and the calculated oral bioavailability is about 30% in dogs. After a single oral dose, the elimination half-life was 0.34 hours in rats (10 mg/kg), and the $T_{1/2}\alpha$ and $T_{1/2}\beta$ were 2.0 and 12.6 hours in dogs (3 mg/kg), respectively. MS-551 is metabolized by the nitro group reduction, dehydroxyethylation and demethylation, which yields six identified or inferred metabolites and at least six other unidentified metabolites in the urine of beagle dogs. However, the dehydroxyethylated metabolite is as potent as MS-551 itself in pharmacological actions, but the other metabolites do not appear to have significant pharmacological activity. After oral administration of a radiolabeled compound to rats and dogs, 12% and 50% of MS-551 were found to be eliminated in the urine, and 83% and 40% of MS-551 eliminated in the feces within 7 days, respectively.

A double blind, placebo controlled, randomized phase 1 clinical study to correlate safety with the pharmacokinetics and pharmacodynamics of MS-551 was performed using single oral administration of 10, 25, 50, 100, and 150 mg (unpublished). MS-551 was readily absorbed from the gastrointestinal tract, attaining a mean maximal plasma concentration between 0.6 and 0.9 hours. The absorption of pharmacokinetics appear to be linearly related to the dose administered. The mean elimination half-life was within the range of 1.4–12.0 hours, irrespective of the dose. Oral administration after food intake altered only the T_{max} among the pharmacokinetic parameters of MS-551. Chronic administration of 100 mg MS-551 3 times daily for 7 days did not alter pharmacokinetic parameters; in the plasma, neither the peak level of about 200 ng/mL nor the trough of about 5 ng/mL changed from day 1 to the end of day 8 of chronic administration. A similar study using single intravenous administration of 0.003 to 0.4 mg/kg (unpublished) was performed. The $T_{1/2}\alpha$ and the $T_{1/2}\beta$ ranged from 3.0 to 3.6 minutes and from 1.5 to 2.1 hours, respectively. A phase II open label, single dose design study with intrapatient comparison of antiarrhythmic and cardiac electrophysiological characteristics before and after a single intravenous dose administration was completed (unpublished). Pharmacokinetic data in these patients did not differ fundamentally from those obtained in the phase 1 study.

Electrophysiological Effects of MS-551 on Isolated Cardiac Tissues

Hashimoto et al.[1,2] defined the electrophysiological effects of MS-551 in isolated cardiac tissues. The effects were compared with those of d-sotalol in canine Purkinje fibers and ventricular muscle, as well as in guinea pig atrial muscle, using the standard microelectrode technique. As shown in Figure 2, MS-551 prolonged the APD and the ERP to a similar extent in these cardiac tissues in a concen-tration-dependent manner (10^{-6}–10^{-6} M). The drug did not affect other action potential parameters, except for the $\dot{V}_{max}$ of guinea pig atrial muscle, which was depressed by 10^{-4} M MS-551. Compared to the baseline values, the extent of the prolongation of APD after 10^{-5} M of MS-551 was 36%, 27%, and 35% for canine Purkinje fibers, canine ventricular muscle, and guinea pig atrial muscle, respectively. At a tenfold higher concentration than that for MS-551, d-sotalol produced a similar APD prolongation in canine Purkinje fibers. Though MS-551 did not completely negate the APD shortening induced by high extracellular potassium (8 and 12 mM) Tyrode's solution, it prolonged the shortened APD even under these conditions. When exposed to simulated ischemic conditions in vitro (pO_2, 25–30 mmHg, pH 6.5, extracellular potassium of 8 mM, and no glucose) for 30 minutes, the APD was abruptly shortened in the first 5 minutes and thereafter gradually, until the APD shortening lasted 30 minutes. MS-551 did not prevent abrupt APD shortening but slowed the subsequent, gradual APD shortening. As for the frequency-dependent effects of MS-551, the APD prolonging action of MS-551 was enhanced at lower driving frequencies (Figure 3). Thus, the drug exhibited reverse frequency-dependent effect on repolarization characteristic of the newer Class III antiarrhythmic compounds. These data indicate that MS-551 is a "pure" Class III antiarrhythmic agent over a wide range of drug concentrations, having basically similar electrophysiological characteristics relative to those of d-sotalol; however, MS-551 was about 10 times as potent as d-sotalol in its effect on cardiac repolarization and, by inference, the ERP.

Ionic Current Correlates of Action Potential Duration Lengthening

Several cellular membrane effects of drugs can explain the prolongation of APD, and definitive answers can be obtained only by the voltage-clamp analysis. Nakaya et al.

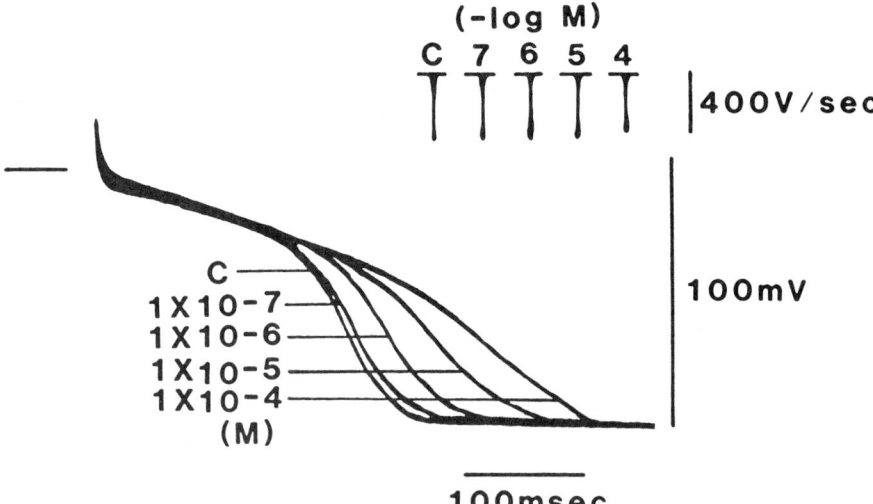

Figure 2. Effects of MS-551 on the action potential configuration of the canine Purkinje fiber. MS-551 prolonged APD without changing the V_{max} (indicated by downward direction) at the top of the panel. Not shown here is the increase in APD in the atrial and ventricular muscle by MS-551. Simultaneous recordings of the APD at Purkinje fiber ventricular muscle junction have not been made. It is, therefore, not clear whether the drug does indeed increase the APD to a differing extent in Purkinje fibers and in ventricular muscle as shown for other Class III agents (see Chapter 30).

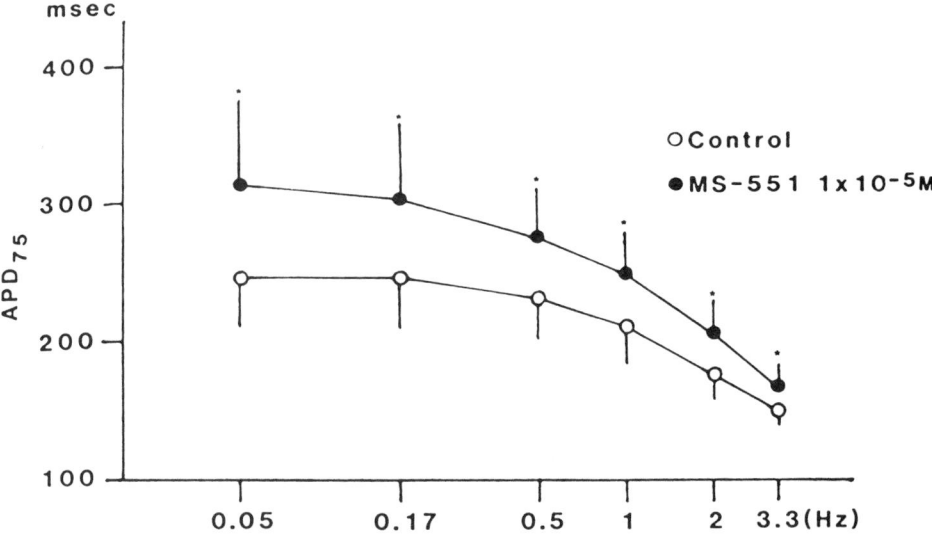

Figure 3. Frequency dependence of the effect of MS-551 on the APD in the canine Purkinje fiber at 75% repolarization time. Note that at the drug concentration studied, the effect on APD at 75% repolarization time was attenuated in an inversely proportional manner as the frequency of stimulus was increased (unpublished data on file with Mitsui Toatsu Pharmaceuticals, Inc.). This property is characteristic of all Class III agents with the exception of amiodarone (see Chapter 34).

used the rabbit ventricular cells to address this issue.[3,4] The rabbit ventricular cell was chosen as a suitable preparation for the study of MS-551 because various outward currents, including the transient outward current (I_{to}), are known to be prominent in this cell.[5] In isolated multicellular rabbit papillary muscle preparations stimulated at 0.5 Hz, MS-551 in concentrations of 3×10^{-7}–3×10^{-5} M prolonged the APD, especially at the 90% repolarization level (APD_{90}), without influencing the $\dot{V}_{max}$. MS-551 also prolonged the ERP in a concentration-dependent manner. In the collagenase treated single rabbit ventricular myocyte and under the whole-cell clamp conditions, MS-551 ($3 \times 10^{-6} - 3 \times 10^{-5}$ M) decreased the delayed rectifier potassium current (I_K) and concomitantly decreased slightly the I_{K1} and calcium current (I_{Ca}). The current-voltage relationship before and after superfusion with MS-551 (10 μM) is shown in Figure 4.

Recently, I_K has been thought to be composed of two components, namely, the low-threshold and high-threshold components.[6] It appears that MS-551 decreases mainly the low threshold I_K. These results suggest that in the rabbit ventricular cells the main Class III effect of MS-551 is to inhibit I_K. Adaniya and Hiraoka[7] also compared the effects of MS-551 with

those of d-sotalol and another newer Class III antiarrhythmic drug, E-4031. The potency of MS-551 was about one tenth that of E-4031 in prolonging the APD_{90} and ERP of rabbit ventricular cells but about 30 to 100 times more potent than d-sotalol. Iijima and Taira[8] also examined the effects of MS-551 on cardiac current systems using collagenase treated single isolated guinea pig ventricular myocytes. Under the whole cell clamp conditions, MS-551 at concentrations higher than 10^{-6} M prolonged the APD, and this effect was not blocked by tetrodotoxin. I_K recorded as tail currents on repolarization to the holding potential was decreased concomitantly with a slight decrease in the I_{K1}.

Suzuki et al.[9] examined the effects of MS-551 on delayed K currents of both the isolated guinea pig ventricular myocytes and the isolated porcine coronary vascular smooth muscle cells. In single guinea pig ventricular myocytes bathed in a solution containing 0.3-mM cadmium, tail currents recorded by the whole cell clamp technique were decreased by MS-551, as was shown by Iijima and Taira,[8] and the IC_{50} was about 10^{-6} M. In single smooth muscle cells obtained from enzymatically treated porcine coronary arteries bathed in a solution containing 0.3 mM cadmium, I_K recorded by the whole cell clamp technique

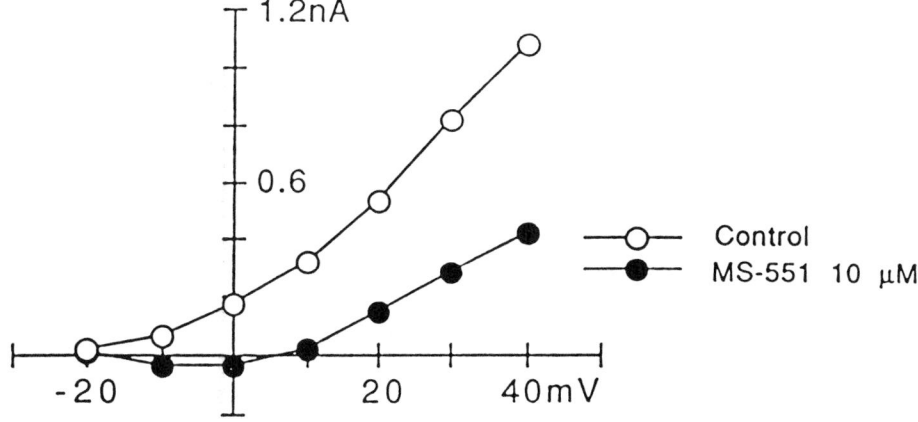

Figure 4. Current-voltage relationship of the I_K tail current before and during superfusion of an isolated guinea pig myocyte with MS-551. Note the significant blocking effect of the drug on the delayed rectifier potassium current (see text for further details).

was decreased by higher concentrations of 3 × 10^{-5}–3 × 10^{-4} M MS-551. The inhibitory effect was observed at the early phase of activation, and the effect disappeared during the long depolarizing pulse. This effect was not voltage dependent between the clamp voltages of 0 to +40 mV. There was a use-dependent development of the inhibition of the I$_K$, when the preparation was exposed to 10^{-4} M MS-551 for 10 minutes, and then the clamp pulses were introduced. Also, in the smooth muscle cells, I$_{Ca}$ did not decrease and used up to 10^{-4} M MS-551. They concluded that the effect of MS-551 on the K currents was qualitatively similar in both cardiac and smooth muscle cells, but the effects on the cardiac muscle were more potent than those on the smooth muscle cells.

In Vivo Electrophysiological Effects of MS-551

In anesthetized open chest dogs, Kamiya et al.[10] compared the hemodynamic effects of d-sotalol and MS-551 (0.1–30 mg/kg intravenous). MS-551, in a dose-dependent manner, increased both the atrial and ventricular ERPs, accompanied by an increase in the QTc (Figure 5). MS-551, 1 mg/kg intravenous, increased the atrial and ventricular ERPs 42% and 20%, respectively. However, MS-551 did not change the intranodal (AH) and intraventricular (HV) conduction times even at the highest dose studies (30 mg/kg). MS-551 was about four times more potent than d-sotalol. MS-551 also increased the left ventricular dP/dt, except at the highest dose studied, whereas d-sotalol showed a dose-dependent decrease in this parameter over the entire range of doses studied. It is also noteworthy that, although both drugs increased the QT interval, the effects on the QTc interval were all but abolished in the case of d-sotalol, but the effect persisted in the case of MS-551. Of note also, d-sotalol increased the PQ interval (suggesting residual β-blocking action in the case of the d-isomer of sotalol), and MS-551 had no effect consistent with negligible calcium

channel or sympathetic blocking effect on the atrioventricular (AV) node. Motomura et al.[11,12] used the in situ open chest dog hearts to further characterize the effects of MS-551 on the AV node. Atrioventricular conduction time (AVCT) assessed as an interval between bipolar atrial and ventricular electrograms and the ERP of the AV conduction system, obtained by programmed premature stimuli, was evaluated using an automated AV interval meter. Basal AVCT and ERP were 115 msec and 180 msec, respectively. MS-551 (3–1,000 µg/kg, intravenous) barely affected AVCT but markedly prolonged the ERP; the percent increases from each basal value were 4% in AVCT and 30% in ERP by 1 mg/kg of MS-551. They also reported that E-4031 is about 10 times more potent than MS-551, but its effect on the canine AV node was qualitatively similar. The data suggest that MS-551 may prolong the refractory period in the AV node by lengthening the APD in the AV node, although this has not been studied directly in isolated preparations.

Efficacy on Experimental Animal Arrhythmias

Kamiya et al.[13] reported the effects of MS-551 on canine ventricular arrhythmia models. They used: (1) ventricular tachycardia (VT), induced by electrical stimuli 3 to 5 days after myocardial infarction; (2) spontaneously occurring VT 24–48 hours after two-stage coronary ligation; and (3) VT induced by digitalis intoxication. Intravenous administration of MS-551 (0.1–1 mg/kg) decreased the incidence of VT or ventricular fibrillation (VF) in 10 out of 13 dogs evoked by the programmed electrical stimulation (PES) delivered to the ventricular septum. These dogs were anesthetized with pentobarbital, and myocardial infarction was surgically produced 3–5 days previously. As shown in Figure 6, oral administration of MS-551 (3 mg/kg) also decreased the incidence of VT induced by PES in 7 out of 10 conscious postinfarction dogs. These protective effects were accompanied by 7%, 17%,

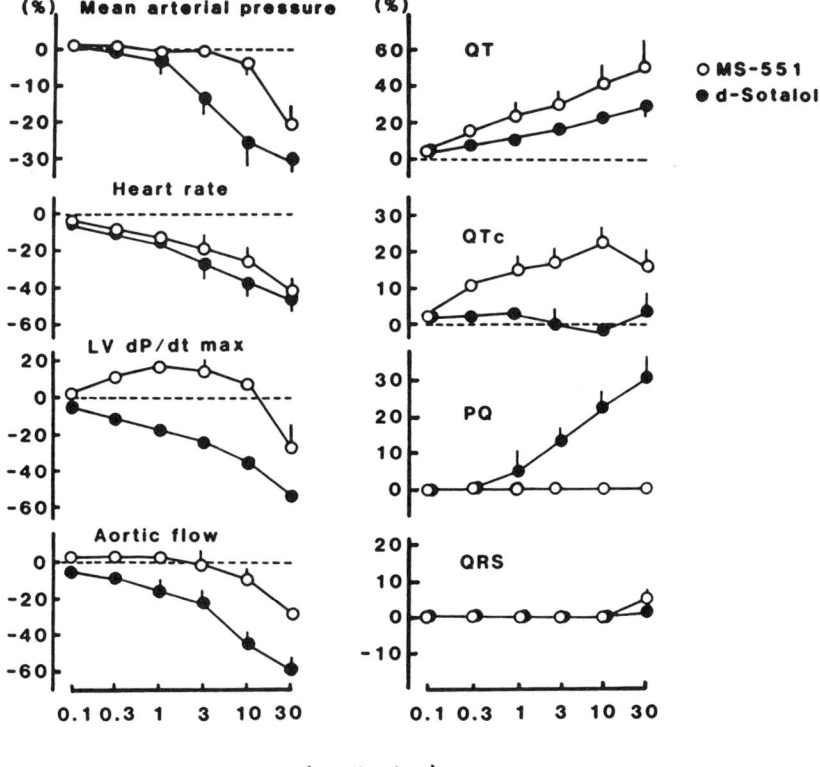

Figure 5. In situ cardiac and hemodynamic effects of MS-551 compared to those of d-sotalol in anesthetized dogs relative to the effects on electrocardiographic intervals. The drug is more potent than d-sotalol in lengthening of the QT interval with less heart rate dependency and less negative inotropic effect but, in this preparation, there appears to be a comparable bradycardic action.

and 13% increases in the ventricular ERP in cases of intravenous 0.1, 1 mg/kg, and oral 3 mg/kg MS-551. Similarly, d-sotalol (0.3–3 mg/kg intravenous and 10 mg/kg p.o.) decreased the incidence of VT evoked by PES, simultaneously accompanied by an increase in ERP. In contrast to these favorable effects, MS-551 (1 and 10 mg/kg intravenous) did not show antiarrhythmic effects on both the spontaneously occurring canine two-stage coronary ligation- and digitalis-induced arrhythmias. These results suggest that MS-551 is a relatively pure Class III antiarrhythmic drug and that MS-551 may be effective in the treatment of life-threatening reentrant tachyarrhythmias, but may not effective in those arising on the basis of enhanced automaticity.

We also examined the antiarrhythmic effects of MS-551 in other reentry-type arrhythmias and in acute coronary ligation and reperfusion arrhythmia models in beagles.[14,15] In halothane anesthetized beagles thoracotomized to expose the left anterior descending coronary artery, 30 minutes of a complete occlusion of the artery was followed by reperfusion. MS-551 was intravenously infused at a rate of 3.6 mg/kg per hour, which prolonged the QTc from 0.29 to 0.42 seconds and decreased the incidence of reperfusion VF from the 5 out of six dogs in the control group to 1 out of 6 dogs ($p < 0.05$) (Figure 7). There was no decrease in the number of ventricular ectopic beats occurring during the 30 minutes of the coronary occlusion in the MS-551

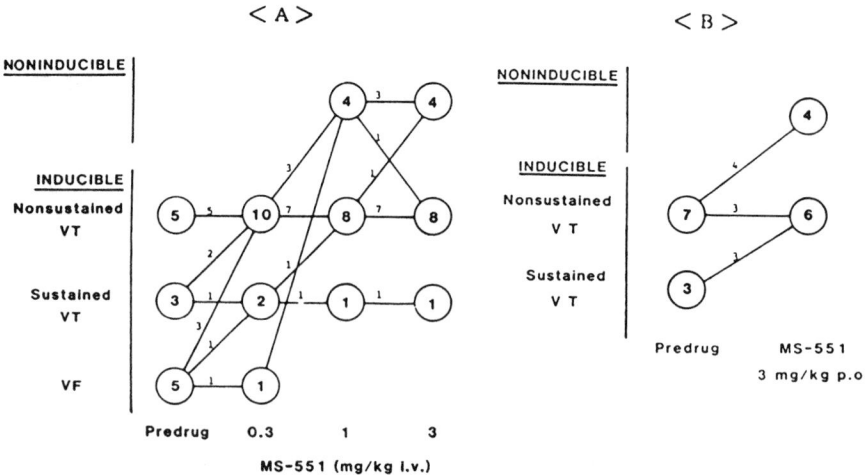

Figure 6. Antiarrhythmic effects of intravenous (left) and oral (right) administration of MS-551 on dogs with old myocardial infarction. In this model of ischemic arrhythmia, PESproduced a varying spectrum of VT and VF. Note the protective effect of MS-551 on VT and VF. See text for further details.

treated group. Similar antiarrhythmic effects were observed for another Class III drug, E-4031,[16] but we did not observe such effects in the case of d-sotalol and intravenous amiodarone groups. In the case of d-sotalol, we could show antiarrhythmic effects when we used pentobarbital anesthesia instead of halothane anesthesia (unpublished). MS-551, however, induced spontaneous ventricular ectopic beats in one out of six dogs and polymorphic VT resembling torsades des pointes in another 1 out of 6 dogs before application of a coronary occlusion. Such a proarrhythmic effect has also been observed in the E-4031 treated group.[16]

In atrial arrhythmia models, Kamiya et al.[17] studied the effects of MS-551 on atrial flutter (AF), which was reproducibly induced in the open chest anesthetized dog in which intercaval crush was surgically produced in conjunction with rapid pacing. MS-551 (0.03–0.3 mg/kg intravenous) failed to convert the AF to sinus rhythm but prolonged the cycle length of the flutter from 102 to 133 msec (30%). MS-551 (0.03–0.3 mg/kg intravenous) produced dose-dependent increases in the ERP (2%–32%) but did not change the interatrial conduction time during sinus rhythm; thus the

conversion to sinus rhythm may be mainly due to the lengthening of atrial refractoriness. Hirata et al.[18] used a canine aseptic pericarditis model and induced atrial flutter or fibrillation (AF-af) by applying extrastimuli. MS-551 (0.3 mg/kg + 0.05 mg/kg per minute) terminated the sustained AF in seven out of 10 dogs, in which sustained AF was induced, and also prevented AF induction in eight out of ten dogs. This dose of MS-551 increased ERP by 15–60 msec and decreased interatrial conduction velocity as much as 5–33 cm/sec at high rates of stimulation, ie, over 250/min. Hirata et al.[18] concluded that changes in conduction as well as those in refractoriness might mediate the antiarrhythmic effects of MS-551.

The results of these animal experiments show that MS-551 has antiarrhythmic effects on atrial and ventricular arrhythmia models in which the mechanism of generation seems to be the reentry, and this is true also for other drugs such as d-sotalol and E-4031. But at the doses exhibiting antiarrhythmic effects, MS-551 and E-4031 have the potential to induce new arrhythmias. Preliminary data reported elsewhere in this monograph (see Chapters 35 through 38 and Chapters 40 through 43) suggest that all the new pure Class III drugs might exert such proarrhythmic reactions. However, the possibility that the precise spectrum of such a potential might vary quantitatively in humans is not excluded.

Hemodynamic Actions of MS-551

Classical sodium-channel blocking Class I drugs have negative inotropic effects because they increase the cardiac transmembrane sodium concentration gradient and decrease the intracellular calcium ion concentration through the Na/Ca exchange mechanism. The resulting negative inotropic effect has been demonstrated both clinically and in experimental animals,[19–21] and this effect may contribute to the deleterious proarrhythmic effect of Class I antiarrhythmic drugs, resulting in sudden death as found in the CAST study.[22] In this respect, MS-551 and other new Class III antiarrhythmic drugs are of interest (see Chapter 30) insofar as they do not block sodium channel activity; rather, as a group instead, they share the common property of producing a positive inotropic effect. They do this by prolonging the APD increasing calcium entry, even without direct effect on the peak of the calcium currents. Kamiya et al.[10] studied the hemodynamic effects of MS-551 using in vivo canine models where intraventricular pressure was recorded using a micromanometer tipped catheter, and the ascending aortic blood flow was recorded using an electromagnetic flow probe. In pentobarbital anesthetized dogs, MS-551 (0.3–3 mg/kg intravenous) decreased the heart rate dose dependently accompanied by QTc prolongation and a slight increase in the rate of rise of the left ventricular pressure (dP/dt max). Cardiac output measured by the aortic flow did not increase but stayed constant until higher doses were used as shown in Figure 5. In contrast, d-sotalol

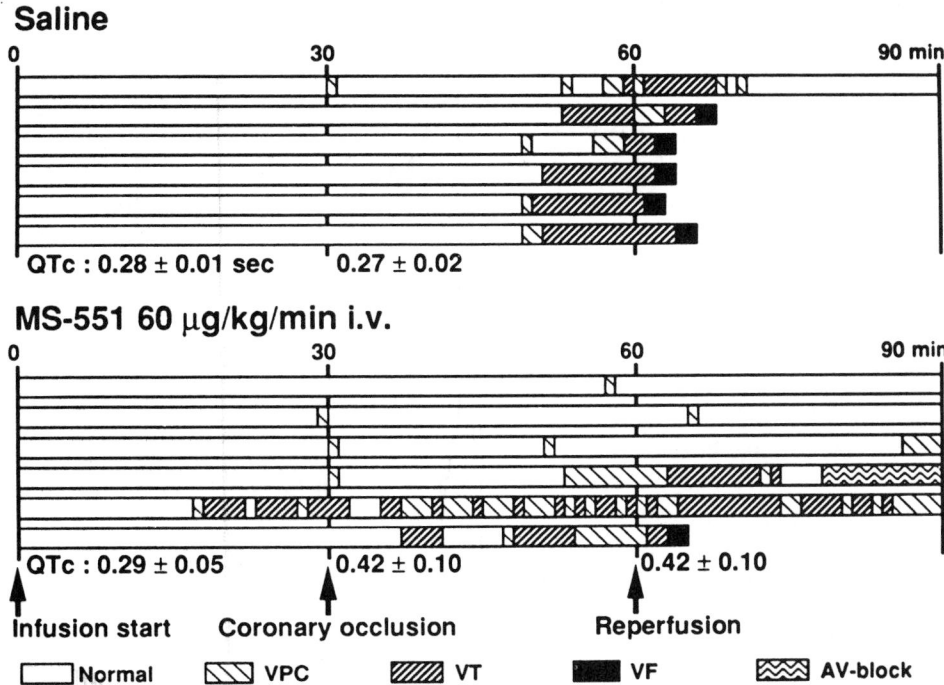

Figure 7. Effects of MS-551 on canine coronary occlusion reperfusion arrhythmias. MS-551 was infused throughout the experiment and decreased the incidence of reperfusion VF (see text).

(0.1–10 mg/kg intravenous) decreased the LV dP/dt max and the ascending aortic flow in a dose-dependent manner. It also decreased the heart rate and blood pressure as did MS-551. Thus, MS-551 might be expected to show antiarrhythmic effects without prominent negative inotropic effects.

Clinical Pharmacology

There are only a few clinical studies on MS-551 completed to date. Recently, an early phase 2 study using patients with suspected tachyarrhythmia was completed. It was an open label, single dose study examining the efficacy of intravenously administered MS-551 in patients with ventricular premature contractions (VPC) and paroxysmal atrial fibrillation (Paf) or flutter (PAF). Preliminary results in which 14 patients with VPC were given either 0.1, 0.2, or 0.3 mg/kg showed that there was a dose related increase in the number of responders, ie, 4 out of 4 patients with a marked reduction of VPC by 0.3 mg/kg dose. Similar effectiveness was observed in the Paf-PAF group of 14 patients. Both this early phase 2 and the phase 1 studies indicate that there was a dose related increase in the QTc in human subjects as predicted from animal studies. Further clinical studies in the course of the development of MS-551 involve increasing the number of entry patients into protocols and also adding electrophysiological testing.

Comments and Conclusions

The experimental and preliminary data on MS-551 reviewed herein suggest that the compound may be an effective Class III antiarrhythmic drug both in animal studies and in patients with premature ventricular contractions and AF-af. However, the clinical data are preliminary, and the drug has not been fully characterized in experimental models.

The effects of the drug are characterized by dose-dependent increases in repolarization, which is largely due to the block of the delayed rectifier potassium current with a minor effect on the inward rectifier. At high concentrations, the drug has a modest inhibitory effect on sodium and calcium currents in isolated myocytes studied by the patch clamp techniques. In terms of its overall effects on repolarization, the drug is considerably more potent than d-sotalol but exhibits a similar reverse use-dependent effect over a wide range of stimulation frequencies. There are several features of its action that are noteworthy. First, MS-551 does reduce heart rate in anesthetized animals, but the mechanism of such an effect is unexplained. One possibility might be the lengthening of the APD in the sinus node, but whether the degree of observed bradycardia in unconscious animals will be similar in conscious animals and in humans remains to be determined. Second, the drug-induced changes in the QTc interval appeared to be less dependent on heart rate than in the case of d-sotalol. Third, MS-551 appeared to exert a frankly positive inotropic effect as determined by the changes in left ventricular dP/dt in anesthetized dogs as compared to d-sotalol. This is a feature that appears to be common to all so-called pure Class III compounds. The available data suggest that the drug has an antifibrillatory as well as a profibrillatory potential, but the precise spectrum of these correlates of prolonged repolarization induced by the drug remains to be determined. The drug's clinical effects merit further investigation.

Acknowledgment: The authors thank Dr. Joji Kamiya of Mitsui Pharmaceuticals, Inc., for making available to us unpublished data, and also thank Miss Mie Yamada for preparing the manuscript.

References

1. Hashimoto K, Ishii M, Kamiya J: Cellular electrophysiological effects of MS-551, a new class III antiarrhythmic agent, in various cardiac tissues: comparison with d-sotalol (abstract). *Eur J Pharmacol* 183:1164, 1990.
2. Hashimoto K, Ishii M, Kamiya J: Electrophysio-

logical characteristics of MS-551, a class III antiarrhythmic agent using canine Purkinje fibers (abstract). *J Mol Cell Cardiol* 22:S83, 1990.

3. Nakaya H, Takeda Y, Kanno M: Effects of MS-551, a new class III antiarrhythmic agent, on action potential and membrane currents in rabbit ventricular myocytes (abstract). *Jpn J Pharmacol* 55:398P, 1991.

4. Nakaya H, Tohse N, Takeda Y, Kanno M: Effects of a new class III antiarrhythmic drug, MS-551 on action potentials and ionic currents in rabbit ventricular cells. *Br J Pharmacol* 109:157, 1993.

5. Hiraoka M, Kawano S: Calcium-sensitive and insensitive transient outward current in rabbit ventricular myocytes. *J Physiol* 410:187, 1989.

6. Sanguinetti MC, Jurkiewicz NK: Two components of cardiac delayed rectifier K^+ current. *J Gen Physiol* 96:106, 1990.

7. Adaniya H, Hiraoka M: Effects of a novel class III antiarrhythmic agent, E-4031, on reentrant tachycardias in rabbit right atrium. *J Cardiovasc Pharmacol* 15:976, 1990.

8. Iijima T, Taira N: Electropharmacological action of MS-551, a new antiarrhythmic agent, on ventricular myocytes (abstract). *Folia Pharmacol Jpn* 96:88P, 1990.

9. Suzuki M, Nagano N, Imaizumi Y, et al: Effects of an antiarrhythmic drug, MS-551, on K currents of guinea pig ventricular and porcine coronary arterial smooth muscle cells (abstract in Japanese). *Folia Pharmacol Jpn* 98:47P, 1991.

10. Kamiya J, Banno H, Yoshihara K, et al: Antiarrhythmic effect and hemodynamic properties of MS-551, a new class III antiarrhythmic agent, in anesthetized dogs (abstract). *Eur J Pharmacol* 183:1776, 1990.

11. Motomura S, Yamagishi T, Hashimoto K: Class III antiarrhythmic drugs little affect atrioventricular (AV) conduction time, but prolong effective refractory period in dog hearts (abstracts). *J Mol Cell Cardiol* 23:S24, 1991.

12. Yamagishi T, Motomura S, Hashimoto KL: Differential effects of class III antiarrhythmic drugs, AV conduction time, and on effective refractory period of the dog heart (abstract). *Jpn J Pharmacol* 55:399P, 1991.

13. Kamiya J, Ishii M, Katakami T: Antiarrhythmic effects of MS-551, a new class III antiarrhythmic agent, on canine models of ventricular arrhythmias. *Jpn J Pharmacol* 58:107, 1992.

14. Hashimoto K, Haruno A, Hirasawa A, et al: Effects of class III antiarrhythmic drugs on canine coronary occlusion-reperfusion arrhythmia (abstract). Presented at the Sixth Southeast Asian/Western Pacific Regional Meeting of Pharmacologists, Hong Kong, 1991.

15. Hirasawa A, Haruno A, Hashimoto K: Effects of class III antiarrhythmic agents on the ischemia-reperfusion arrhythmias (abstract in Japanese). *Folia Pharmacol Jpn* 96:10P, 1990.

16. Hashimoto K, Haruno A, Matsuzaki T, et al: Effects of a new class III antiarrhythmic drug (E-4031) on canine ventricular arrhythmia models. *Asia Pac J Pharmacol* 6:127, 1991.

17. Kamiya J, Hirayama M, Ishii A, et al: Antiarrhythmic effects of MS-551, a new class III antiarrhythmic agent, on experimental canine atrial flutter (abstract). *J Mol Cell Cardiol* 22:S70, 1990.

18. Hirata M, Mitsuoka T, Hirata M, et al: Effects of MS-551 (Class III) on electrically induced atrial flutter and fibrillation in the dog (abstract). *Jpn Circ J* 55 (Suppl A):200, 1992.

19. Hashimoto K, Sugiyama A, Haruno A, et al: Effects of a new antiarrhythmic drug TYB-3823 on canine ventricular arrhythmia models. *J Cardiovasc Pharmacol* 17:336, 1991.

20. Sugiyama A, Motomura S, Hashimoto K: Comparison of cardiovascular effects of a novel class IC antiarrhythmic agent, NIK-244, with those of flecainide in isolated canine heart preparations cross-circulated with a donor dog. *Jpn J Pharmacol* 56:1, 1991.

21. Sugiyama A, Motomura S, Tamura K, et al: Comparison of cardiovascular effects of pirmenol with those of disopyramide in isolated canine heart preparations cross-circulated with a donor dog. *Jpn J Pharmacol* 53:97, 1990.

22. Echt DS, Liebson PR, Mitchell B, et al: Mortality and morbidity in patients receiving encainide, flecainide, or placebo. The Cardiac Arrhythmia Suppression Trial. *N Engl J Med* 324:781, 1991.

Chapter 40

Ibutilide

John P. DiMarco
James T. VanderLugt
Kai S. Lee
J. Kenneth Gibson

Ibutilide is a new antiarrhythmic compound that was developed and is currently undergoing clinical study by the Upjohn Company. Its chemical structure is shown in Figure 1. Most studies have used a racemic mixture of both the d- and l-enantiomers. The compound has attracted considerable interest since laboratory experiments have indicated an electropharmacological profile that has features unique among agents that prolong repolarization, but it remains to be determined if these differences will be translated into enhanced clinical efficacy.

Pharmacology

The major electrophysiological effects produced by ibutilide in isolated tissues are a prolongation of the action potential duration and of the effective refractory periods (ERPs) of both atrial (Figure 2) and ventricular tissues.[1] Significant electrophysiological effects are seen in vitro at concentrations of 10^{-7} to 10^{-5} M. No significant effects are observed on

cardiac conduction or papillary muscle contraction at these concentrations. Ibutilide does not bind to α_1-, α_2-, or β-adrenergic receptors.

In isolated guinea pig myocytes, ibutilide has been noted to produce a bell-shaped dose-response curve (Figure 3) for changes in action potential duration at concentrations between 10^{-9} and 10^{-5} M.[2,3] The upstroke of the action potential and the membrane resting potential are not affected. Tetrodotoxin (0.5 to 2 μM) reverses the increase in action potential duration seen at 10^{-7} M ibutilide.[3] However, when action potential duration was prolonged by tetraethylammonium or other I_k blockers in the same preparation, ibutilide (10^{-5} M) reversed the decrease in I_k seen with the former agents. These effects on I_k were the opposite of those seen when sotalol was studied using the same protocol. Lee and co-workers[2,3] have interpreted this observation as evidence that ibutilide has a two-pronged effect on action potential duration. The initial effect seen at concentrations of about 10^{-7} M is an enhancement of an inward plateau phase current carried by Na^+.[4] At higher (10^{-5} M) concentrations, they believe ibutilide activates I_k. They

From BN Singh, HJJ Wellens, M Hiraoka, (eds): *Electropharmacological Control of Cardiac Arrhythmias.* Mount Kisco, NY, Futura Publishing Company Inc., © 1994.

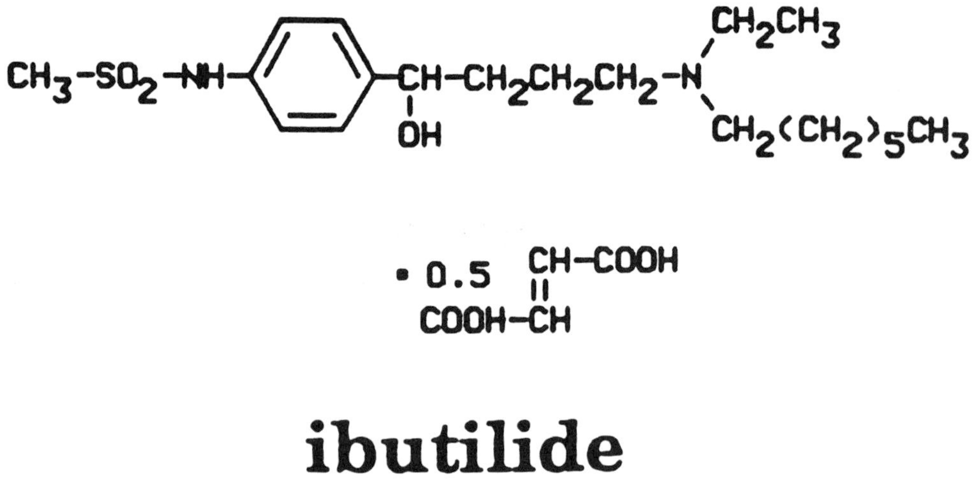

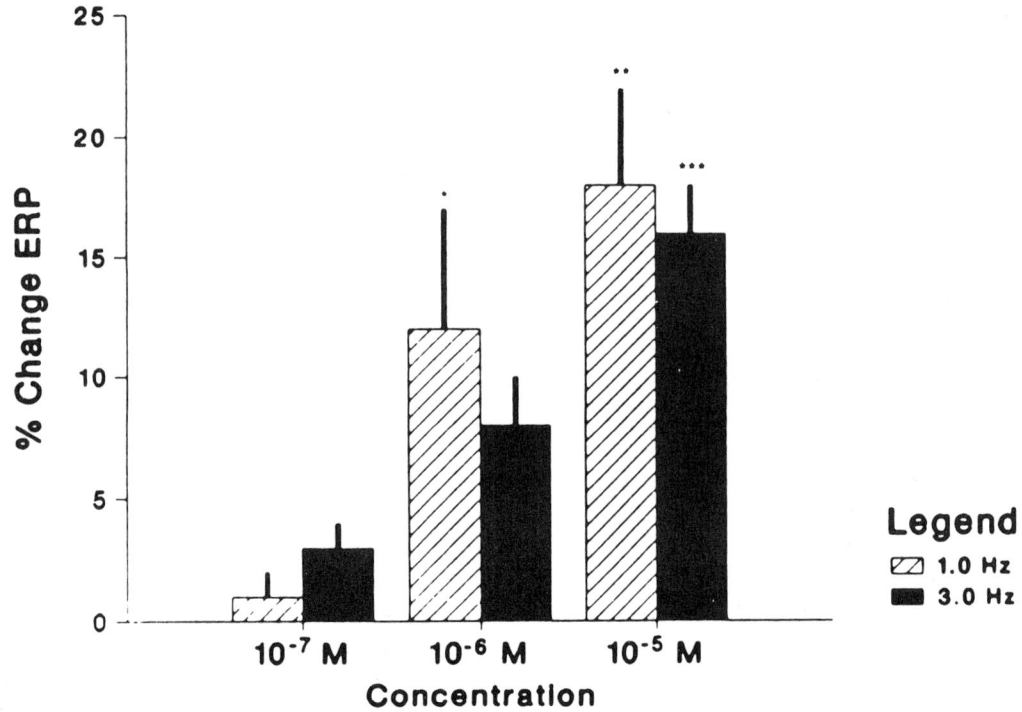

CH3-SO2-NH-
CH-CH2CH2CH2-N
OH
CH2CH3
CH2(CH2)5CH3
• 0.5 CH-COOH
COOH-CH
ibutilide

Figure 1. Chemical structure of ibutilide (N.[4 – [4-(ethylheptyl-amino)-1-hydroxybutyl]phenyl] methanesulfonamide-(E)-2-butenedioate) (U-70,226E).

25
20
15
10
5
0
% Change ERP
10-7 M
10-6 M
10-5 M
Concentration
Legend
1.0 Hz
3.0 Hz

Figure 2. Effects of 10^{-7}, 10^{-6}, and 10^{-5} M ibutilide on the effective refractory period of isolated papillary muscle at a pacing frequency of 1 Hz and a pacing frequency of 3 Hz. *$p = 0.011$ versus control.

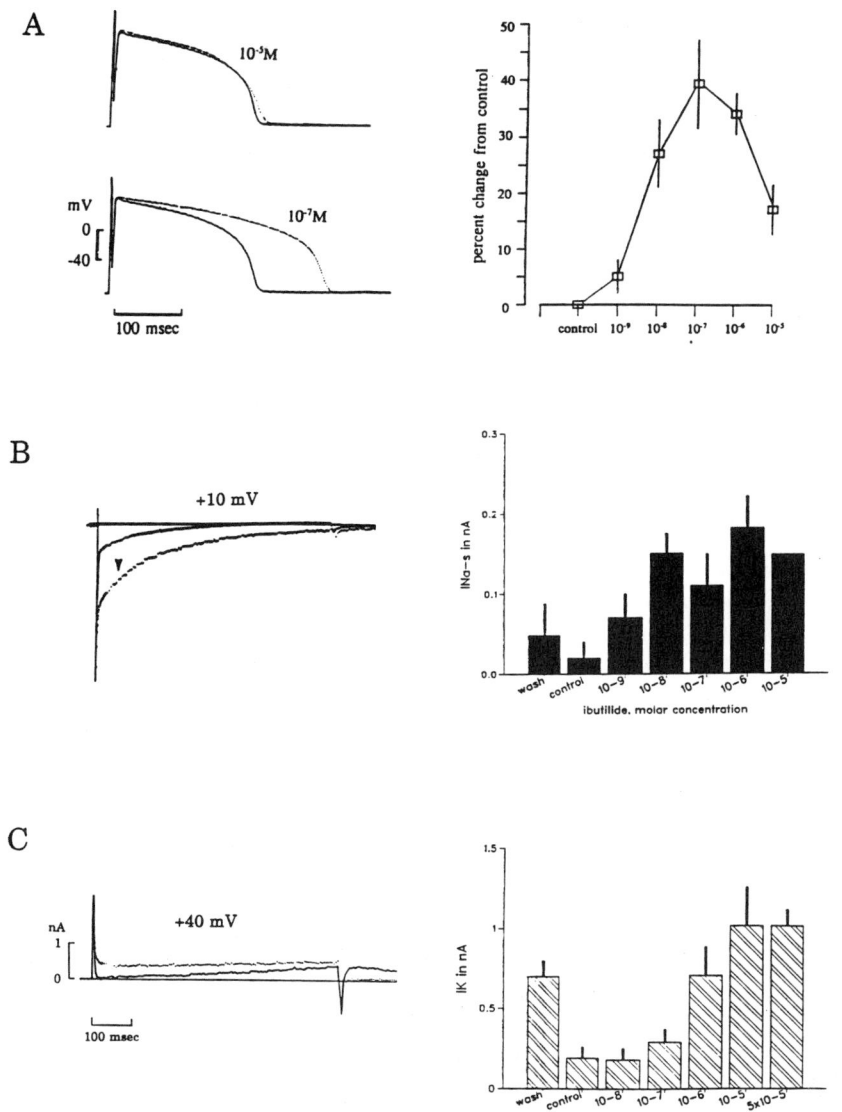

Figure 3. Effects of ibutilide on action potentials and membrane currents of single guinea pig ventricular cells. A: Left panel: action potentials before (solid trace) and after treatment (dotted trace) with 10^{-7} M and 10^{-5} M ibutilide. Right panel: bell-shaped dose-response curve of action potential duration expressed as percent of control. Microelectrodes were used for these recordings. Vertical bars are SEM of 6 cells; B: Left panel: inward currents (Na^+ and Ca^{2+}) recorded by the suction pipette method at +10 mV from a holding potential of −80 mV before (solid trace) and after (dotted trace) at 10^{-8} M ibutilide. Right panel: a dose-response of I_{Na-s} in the presence of increasing concentrations of ibutilide at +20 mV and measured at 200-msec depolarization. Vertical bars are SEM of 4 to 8 cells; and C: Left panel: outward currents (I_K) recorded at by the suction pipette method at +40 mV from a holding potential of −40 mV and measured at 600-msec depolarization before (solid trace) and after (dotted trace) 10^{-5} M ibutilide treatment; at right is an ibutilide dose-response curve of I_K at +20 mV. Vertical bars are SEM of 3 to 7 cells. Temperature: A: at 35°C; B and C: room temperature. Calibration of B applies to C.

have postulated that this dual action might be an autoregulatory phenomenon that could prevent the excessive QT prolongations that are associated with torsades de pointes.

Ibutilide has been tested in several animal models of both atrial and ventricular arrhythmias. In the canine Y-shaped atrial incision model of atrial flutter, bolus injections of ibutilide produce an increase in atrial cycle length, followed in a high percentage of animals, by termination of the arrhythmia.[5] The mean cumulative effective dose was 6 ± 1 μg/kg. The atrial ERP was increased by 44 ± 7 msec by the dose that terminated atrial flutter. Reinitiation of atrial flutter after initial conversion in this model is also inhibited by ibutilide.

Ibutilide has also been studied in several laboratory models of ventricular arrhythmias.[6] During acute coronary occlusion (30 minutes) and reperfusion (30 minutes), pretreatment with intravenous ibutilide (0.1 mg/kg) decreased spontaneous ventricular premature beats and slightly decreased the frequency of ventricular fibrillation. These actions were associated with a 15- to 30-msec increase in the ventricular ERP. Ibutilide has been shown to inhibit pacing-induced ventricular tachycardia and fibrillation in anesthetized dogs at 24 hours and 4 to 8 days after acute myocardial infarction (Figure 4). In a study that compared ibutilide with encainide and sotalol in this model, both ibutilide and sotalol were effective in preventing induction of ventricular tachycardia or ventricular fibrillation, but ibutilide was better tolerated hemodynamically. Encainide had no effect on the pacing-induced arrhythmias. In contrast, encainide, but not ibutilide or sotalol, suppressed spontaneous ventricular ectopy 24 hours after infarction (Figure 5).

A beneficial effect of ibutilide on defibrillation threshold has been reported by Wesley et al.[7] In dogs anesthetized with pentobarbital, the investigators found that there was a 22% reduction in current threshold and a 40% reduction in energy threshold for defibrillation. These effects were seen at an ibutilide dose of 0.1 mg/kg intravenously and were associated with QTc prolongation ranging from 374 ± 8 to 422 ± 10 msec. Ibutilide has not been shown to produce important hemodynamic

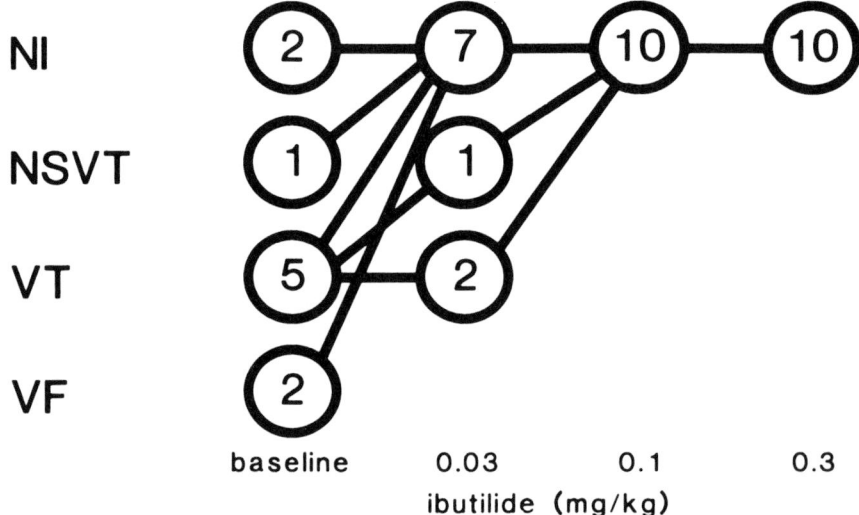

Figure 4. Effects of intravenous ibutilide on induced ventricular arrhythmias in anesthetized dogs 24 hours after acute myocardial infarction. NI: noninducible; NSVT: nonsustained ventricular tachycardia; VT: sustained ventricular tachycardia; VF: ventricular fibrillation. Number in circles indicates number of animals with that response at each dose.

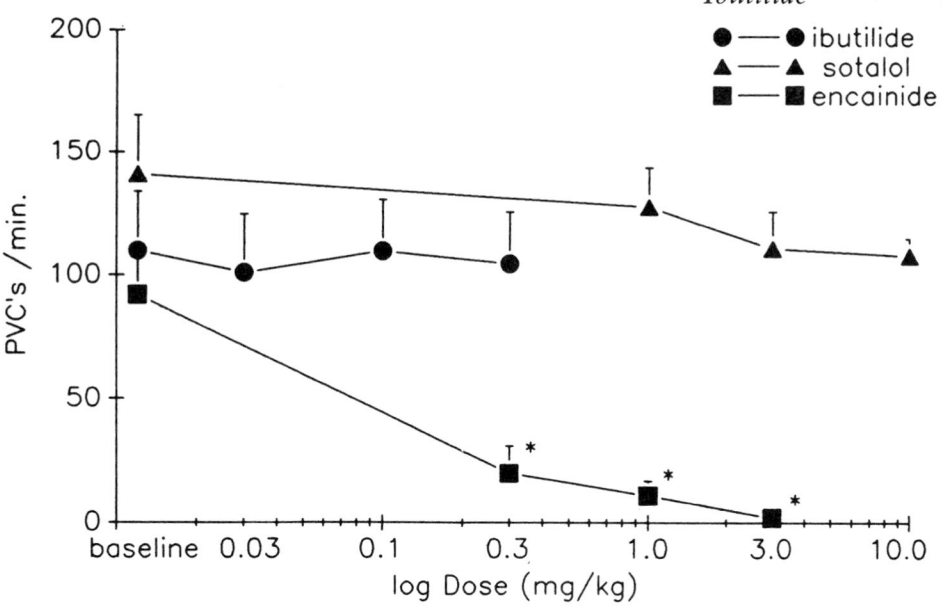

Figure 5. Effects of intravenous ibutilide, sotalol, and encainide on spontaneous ventricular premature beats in anesthetized dogs 24 hours after acute myocardial infarction. *$p < 0.05$ versus control.

changes at doses ≤3 mg/kg intravenous in anesthetized and conscious dogs.

Clinical Pharmacology

The clinical pharmacology of ibutilide in humans is still undergoing evaluation. It appears the drug is extensively metabolized in the liver. In healthy volunteers, ibutilide has a plasma clearance that approximates hepatic blood flow (approximately 30 mL/min per kilogram) and a large steady-state volume of distribution (10 to 15 L/kg). Plasma concentrations after a single infusion exhibit a triexponential decline with a terminal elimination half-life of 6 to 9 hours.[8] The metabolic fate of ibutilide and the possible activity of potential metabolites in humans have not been fully determined, but QTc interval prolongation seems to correlate well with ibutilide plasma concentrations (Figure 6). Oral administration of ibutilide does not appear practical due to presystemic elimination of oral doses. Development of an analog with similar electrophysiological activity but better oral bioavailability may be possible.

Clinical Studies

In phase 1 trials using intravenous ibutilide, dose related increases in QTc interval have been observed.[9] Mean QTc interval changes were 18% and 43% after doses of 0.01 and 0.03 mg/kg. Although ibutilide was well tolerated in these studies, one volunteer developed a run of polymorphic ventricular tachycardia after a single oral dose of 75 mg of ibutilide. No other significant side effects have been identified in volunteers.

The largest amount of clinical data on ibutilide generated to date has concerned its use for converting established atrial fibrillation and atrial flutter. In one series,[10] patients with atrial fibrillation or atrial flutter received up to three infusions of 0.005, 0.01, and 0.02 mg/kg in series to convert their arrhythmias. Patients were monitored continuously and observed for 5 minutes after each dose before going on to the next infusion. Twelve of the 15 patients converted to sinus rhythm during this protocol (Figure 7). There appeared to be a smooth dose-response relationship, but the numbers are quite small in this study.

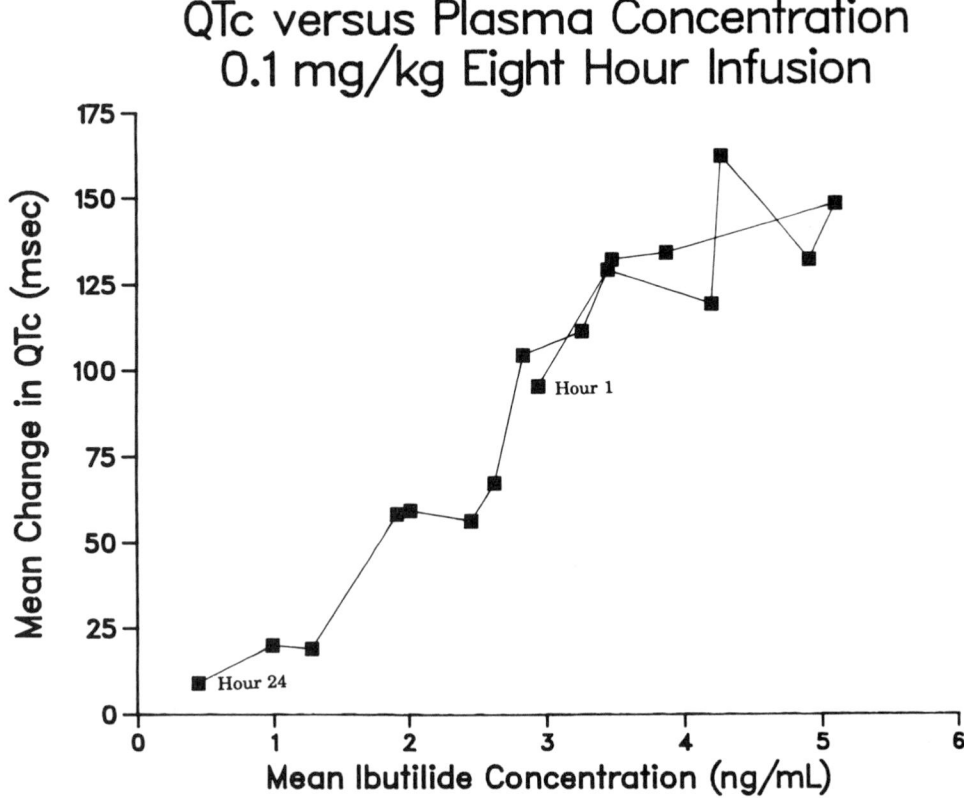

Figure 6. Effects on QTc. The relationship between plasma ibutilide concentration and QTc in a normal volunteer is shown.

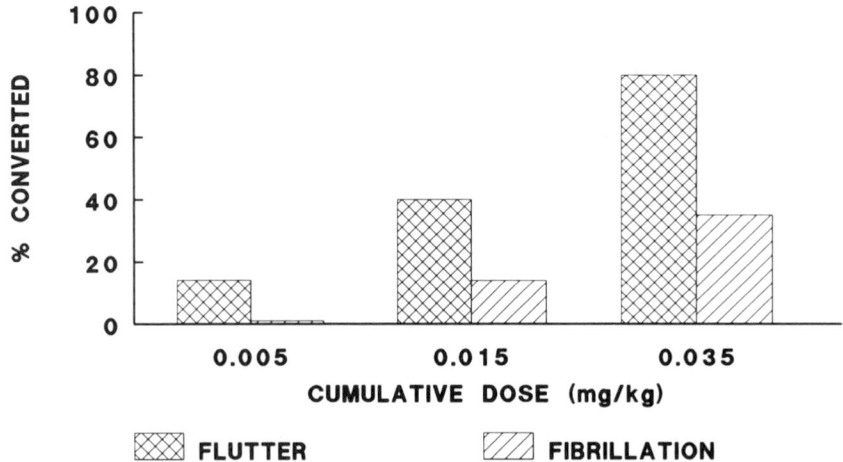

Figure 7. Conversion of atrial flutter and fibrillation by intravenous ibutilide. Patients received doses of 0.005, 0.01, and 0.02 mg/kg in a three-dose conversion protocol.

However, 2 of 15 patients in this series developed polymorphic ventricular tachycardia after receiving ibutilide. One patient converted to sinus bradycardia and then developed ventricular bigeminy that progressed to polymorphic ventricular tachycardia. The other patient developed higher grade atrioventricular block and ventricular ectopy during continued atrial flutter before an episode of sustained polymorphic tachycardia. Both patients were elderly and had advanced heart disease, but dramatic QT interval prolongation was not observed prior to these episodes. A more recent study that used single infusions of ibutilide (0.005 to 0.025 mg/kg) in atrial flutter patients has shown an overall conversion rate at the highest dose of about 40%. Further studies to determine whether single dose infusions will be superior to multiple dose protocols and to determine the optimal dosages for conversion are now underway.

Preliminary experience in patients with atrial fibrillation has also been obtained. The conversion rates are somewhat lower for atrial fibrillation than are those seen in atrial flutter (Figure 7). However, this may be due to the fact that the duration of the arrhythmias has been longer among the patients with fibrillation due to the need for anticoagulation prior to elective cardioversion in patients with established atrial fibrillation.

Only a few patients with ventricular tachycardia have received ibutilide to date, and data are too limited to permit any conclusions to be drawn. No data about the effects of ibutilide on ventricular defibrillation thresholds in humans are as yet available.

Summary

Experimental and clinical studies with drugs that prolong action potential duration are now rapidly accumulating. The largest clinical experience has been with amiodarone and sotalol, but both of these agents have electrophysiological effects in addition to simple action potential prolongation. Most of the more recently developed agents are potassium channel blockers. The laboratory studies suggesting that ibutilide produces action potential duration prolongation by a different mechanism, ie, enhancement of a plateau phase inward sodium current, raises the possibility that ibutilide may have a different spectrum of activity than many of the other drugs currently in trials. The added possibility that an enhancement of repolarizing potassium current at higher drug concentrations might be an autoregulating property of the drug that would prevent drug-induced torsades de pointes is also intriguing. However, a few episodes of polymorphic ventricular tachycardia have already been noted among 200 treated patients so it does not appear that ibutilide will be totally free of this type of proarrhythmia. Further clinical studies, including studies that directly compare the efficacy and toxicity of ibutilide to that of other agents, will be necessary to answer these questions.

Acknowledgments: The authors wish to express their appreciation to Dr. G. L. Jungbluth, Ms. Linda Wakefield, and other staff members of Upjohn Laboratories for assistance in the preparation of this chapter.

References

1. Hester JB, Gibson JK, Cimini MG, et al: N-[(.omega.-Amino-1-hydroxyalkyl]phenylmethanesulfonamide derivatives with class III antiarrhythmic activity. *J Med Chem* 43:308, 1991.
2. McKay MC, Sykes JS, Lee KS: Effects of U-70226E, a novel antiarrhythmic drug, on the action potential parameters of isolated guinea pig ventricular myocytes (abstract). *J Mol Cell Cardiol* 22(Suppl I):S15, 1990.
3. Lee EW, McKay MC, Lee KS: U-70226E, a novel class III antiarrhythmic compound activates a slow inward Na$^+$ and an outward K$^+$ current (abstract). *J Mol Cell Cardiol* 22(Suppl I):S15, 1990.
4. Lee KS: Ibutilide, a new compound with potent class III antiarrhythmic activity, activates a slow inward Na$^+$ current in guinea pig ventricular cells. *J Pharmacol Exp Ther* 262:99, 1992.
5. Buchanan LV, Turcotte UM, Gibson JK, et al: Oral efficacy of ibutilide, a new class III antiar-

rhythmic agent, in a conscious canine model of atrial flutter (abstract). *J Am Coll Cardiol* 17(Suppl A):43A, 1991.

6. Buchanan LV, Kabell G, Turcotte UM, et al: Effects of ibutilide on spontaneous and induced ventricular arrhythmias in 24-hour canine myocardial infarction: a comparative study with sotalol and encainide. *J Cardiovasc Pharmacol* 19:256, 1992.

7. Wesley RC, Farkhani F, Bautista J: Ibutilide-induced reduction in defibrillation threshold: enhanced countershock efficacy via slow inward sodium current activation (abstract). *PACE* 14: 716, 1991.

8. Jungbluth GL, VanderLugt JT, Kabell GG, et al: The pharmacokinetics and pharmacodynamics of ibutilide fumarate after intravenous infusions in healthy volunteers (abstract). *Pharm Res* 7:S-211, 1990.

9. VanderLugt JT, Gaylor SK, Wakefield LK, et al: Effects of ibutilide fumarate, a new class III antiarrhythmic agent, in man (abstract). *Clin Pharmacol Ther* 49:188, 1991.

10. DiMarco JP: Ibutilide for Atrial Arrhythmia Study Group. Cardioversion of atrial flutter by intravenous ibutilide, a new class III antiarrhythmic drug (abstract). *J Am Coll Cardiol* 17: 324A, 1991.

Chapter 41

Membrane Current Changes Responsible for the Class III Antiarrhythmic Properties of RP 58866 and its Active Enantiomer, RP 62719

Denis Escande
Sylvain Le Guern
Michel Laville
Joëlle Courteix
Laurent Pradier

Drugs that selectively prolong the normal action potential without affecting intracardiac conduction have been designated Class III antiarrhythmic agents according to the Vaughan Williams classification scheme.[1] The prolongation in cardiac refractoriness that accounts for their antiarrhythmic properties is usually due to the blockade of repolarizing K^+ currents and consequent delay in repolarization.[2] However, the currently available major representatives of this class of drugs, ie, sotalol and amiodarone, are not pure. Beside its K^+ current blocking properties,[3] sotalol is a β-receptor antagonist,[4] whereas amiodarone has an exceedingly complex mechanism of action. Amiodarone blocks both Na^{+}[5] and Ca^{2+}[6] currents, noncompetitively inhibits α- and β-catecholamine receptors,[7] and also interferes with the metabolism of thyroid hormones.[8] The need for more selective Class III drugs has thus emerged. Various molecules, particularly the dextroisomer of sotalol (which does not block β receptors) and compounds such as sematilide, risotilide, ibutilide, ambasilide, dofetilide, and E-4031, which act primarily via an inhibition of the delayed rectifier K^+ current, i_K, are currently being developed.

In this chapter, we report novel benzopyran derivatives that act to prolong cardiac action potential by selectively blocking the inward rectifying K^+ current, i_{K1}. These pure

From BN Singh, HJJ Wellens, M Hiraoka, (eds): *Electropharmacological Control of Cardiac Arrhythmias.* Mount Kisco, NY, Futura Publishing Company Inc., © 1994.

Class III compounds thus differ from sotalol and other methylsulfonamide derivatives with respect to the type of K^+ current blocked. It is anticipated that this difference may have some pharmacological and therapeutic relevance.

Methods

Cell Isolation

The method used to isolate atrial and ventricular cells from the guinea pig heart has been reported in detail elsewhere.[9,10] Single ventricular myocytes were obtained from rat hearts by a similar experimental procedure.

Solutions and Drugs

Isolated cells placed in petri dishes were continually perfused with a standard extracellular solution consisting of (in millimoles): NaCl 135, KCl 5.4, $MgCl_2$ 1.0, $CaCl_2$ 1.8, N-2-hydroxyethylpiperazine-N'-2-ethanesulfonic acid (HEPES buffer) 10, glucose 10, and pH adjusted with NaOH to 7.4. In experiments designed to explore the effect of the drugs on repolarizing K^+ currents, Ca^{2+} and Na^+ inward currents were inhibited by replacing Ca^{2+} with 2-mM $CoCl_2$ and by adding 50 μM tetrodotoxin (TTX) to the extracellular solution, respectively. Alternatively, 3-μM nitrendipine (Bayer) was used to block the L-type Ca^{2+} inward current, $i_{Ca,L}$. The pipette solution dialyzing the cell interior contained a low concentration of Mg^{2+} so that the rundown of the delayed rectifier was minimized.[11] Its composition was (in millimoles): K-aspartate 85, KCl 50, Na-pyruvate 5, $MgCl_2$ 0.3, ethylene glycol-bis(β-aminoethyl ether)-N,N,N',N'-tetraacetic acid (EGTA) 10, HEPES buffer 10, K_2-ATP 5, D-glucose 11, and pH adjusted with KOH to 7.3. Macroscopic adenosine triphosphate (ATP)-sensitive K^+ currents were induced by perfusing the cell with dinitrophenol (DNP).[12] In experiments aimed to record Ca^{2+} inward currents, K^+ currents were abolished by adding intracellular cesium and by using a K^+-free and Na^+-free extracellular

medium containing a high concentration of tetraethylammonium (TEA). In this case, the pipette medium consisted of (in millimoles): CsCl 120, TEA chloride 20, EGTA 10, HEPES buffer 10, Mg-ATP 5, cAMP 0.05, and pH adjusted to 7.3 with CsOH whereas the extracellular solution consisted of TEA chloride 140, $CaCl_2$ 5, $MgCl_2$ 1, HEPES buffer 10, D-glucose 11, and pH adjusted to 7.4 with TEA-OH.

RP 58866, ($\pm$)-[(chromanyl-4-)-2 ethyl]-1(dimethoxy-3,4phenyl)-4 piperidine, and its (S)($-$)-isomer, RP 62719 (Figure 1), were synthesized at Rhône-Poulenc Laboratories, Vitry-sur-Seine, France. Drugs dissolved in distilled water as stock solutions were introduced to the extracellular solution at the desired final concentration (0.1 to 10 μM). They were applied directly to the vicinity of the chosen cell by means of a U-shaped microtube perfusion system in which gravity is the hydrodynamic force.

Recordings and Data Analysis

Membrane potentials and ionic currents were recorded with the tight seal whole cell technique[13] by means of a patch clamp amplifier (L/M-EPC7, List Medical Electronic, Darmstadt, FRG). Experiments were conducted at 33–35°C, except if otherwise stated. Patch pipettes were pulled with a BB-CH horizontal puller from borosilicate capillary tubes (Preciver, Creteil, France) and had resistances ranging between 6 and 10 MΩ when filled with the internal solution. Liquid junction potential between the pipette and the bath solution was always corrected before the gigaΩ seal formation. Action potentials were elicited in single guinea pig ventricular myocytes by passing a current pulse through the recording patch electrode (5-msec duration, 1–5 nA amplitude, 0.5-Hz stimulation rate). Series resistance and capacitance compensations were performed. Traces were displayed on a Nicolet 3091 digital oscilloscope and on a Brush recorder (24005, Gould Inc., Cleveland, OH). Online data acquisition was achieved by means of an IBM-AT personal computer with a

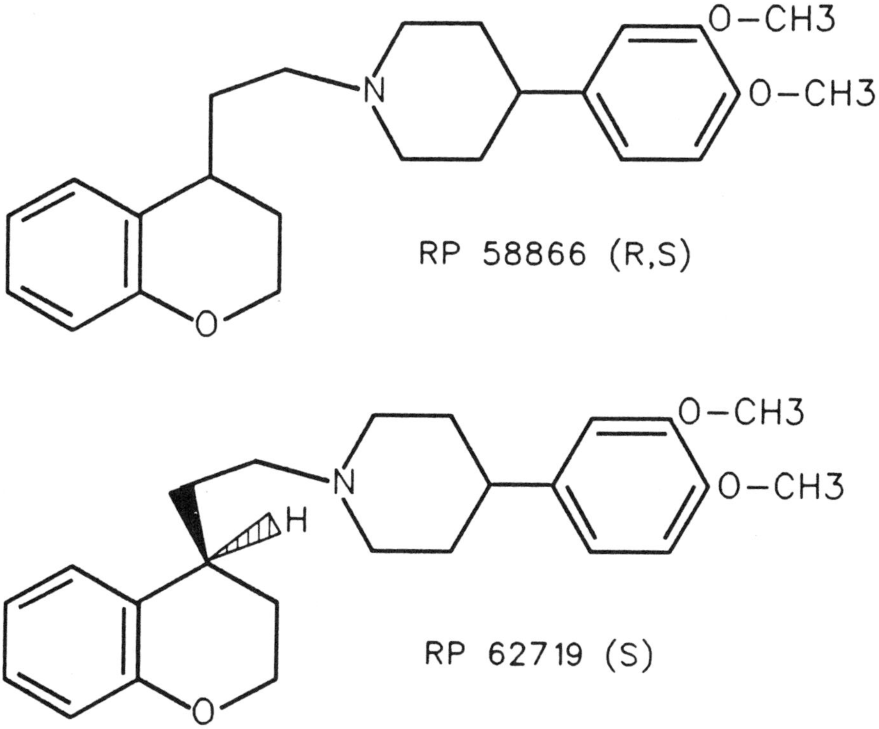

Figure 1. Chemical structure of RP 58866 and its active [(S)(−)-isomer], RP 62719 (terikalant).

TECMAR TM 40 Labmaster interface (sampling rate 0.5 to 5 kHz), which also provided the command pulses (pCLAMP software from Axon Instruments). Current records were not corrected for unspecific leak currents.

Results

RP 58866 Prolongation of Action Potentials in Single Ventricular Myocytes

We first examined the effects of RP 58866 on action potentials, which were recorded by using the current clamp mode, in single guinea pig ventricular myocytes bathed with the standard extracellular medium. As illustrated in Figure 2, RP 58866 at 3 μM augmented the normal action potential plateau duration but did not modify the plateau level or the diastolic membrane potential. On the average, the action potential duration measured at 90% repolarization was increased by 28.3 ± 5.3% (mean ± SEM of five cells) in the presence of 3-μM RP 58866. As in multicellular ventricular preparations from the same species,[14] the prolongation of the action potential plateau was clearly predominant at negative membrane potentials. Furthermore, the amount of action potential prolongation produced by 3-μM RP 58866 in isolated cells was similar to that observed in papillary muscle (+34.6 ± 3% at 37°C, n = 7).

Effects of RP 58866 on the Inward Rectifying and the Delayed Rectifier K$^+$ Currents

Outward K$^+$ currents in the presence of TTX and Co^{2+} were recorded in the voltage-clamp mode. The voltage protocol consisted of 2.5-second depolarizing pulses to +40 mV

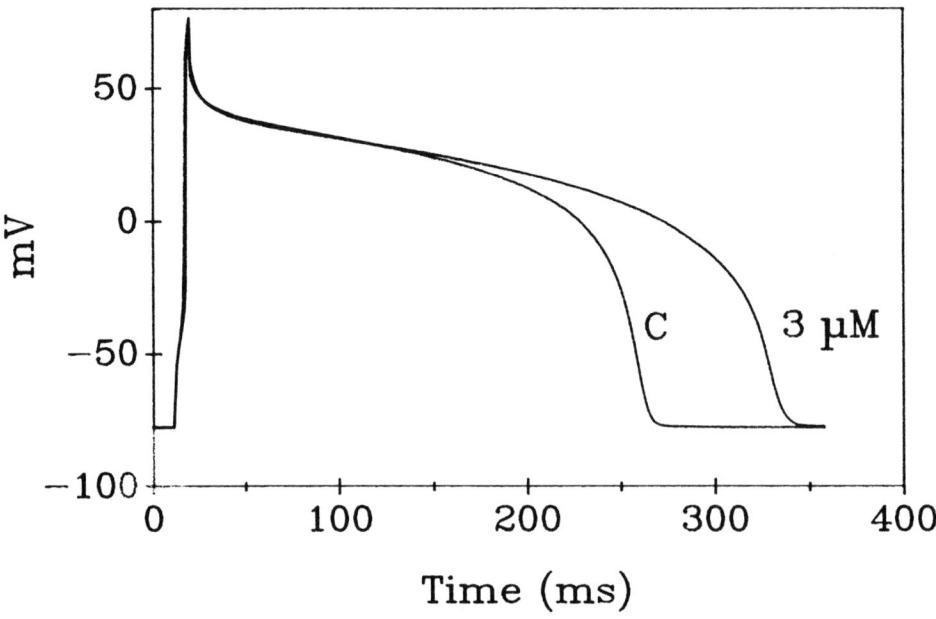

Figure 2. Superimposed action potentials recorded in the absence (C) and presence of 3-μM RP 58866 in an isolated guinea pig ventricular myocyte. Stimulation rate: 0.5 Hz.

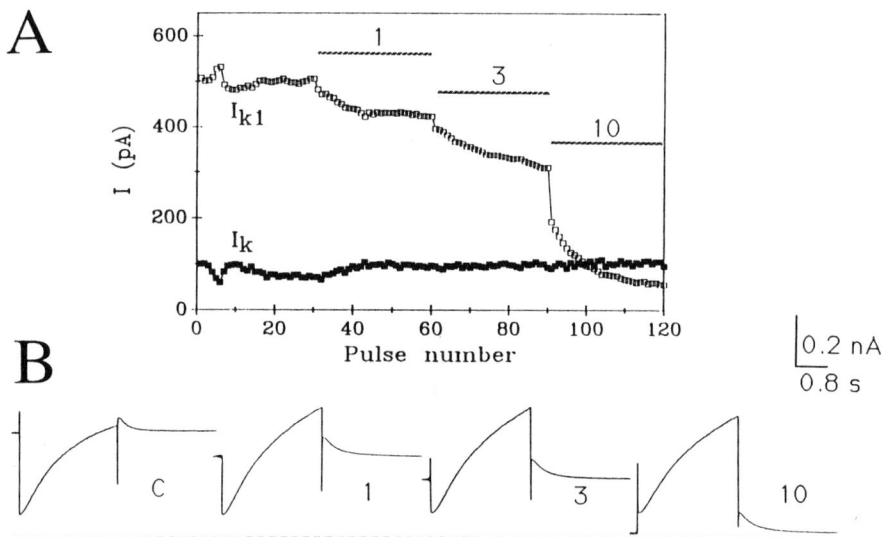

Figure 3. Effects of RP 58866 on repolarizing K$^+$ currents of guinea pig ventricular myocytes. Depolarizing pulses, 2.5-seconds in duration, were applied every 5 seconds from -40 mV to $+40$ mV. A: The amplitude of the steady current at -40 mV (mainly i_{K1}; empty symbols) and the outward current tail (i_K; filled symbols) are plotted against the pulse number. One-, 3-, and 10-μM RP 58866 were applied directly onto the cell as indicated by vertical bars; and B: Typical current traces recorded in control (C) and in the presence of increasing concentrations of RP 58866. The dotted line represents the 0 current level. Same cell as in A. Tetrodotoxin and CoCl$_2$ present throughout.

applied every 5 seconds from a holding potential of -40 mV, but did not significantly affect the amplitude of the outward current tail recorded upon repolarization. The slight increase in the outward current at the end of the pulse in Figure 3 (which was accompanied by a concomitant increase in the current tail amplitude) was probably due to the progressive dialysis of the cell with the low Mg^{2+} intracellular medium, since this phenomenon was routinely observed in the absence of the drug. The lack of effects of RP 58866 on the delayed rectifying K^+ current, i_K, is also illustrated in Figure 4 showing the voltage dependence of i_K activation determined in the presence of 1- and 10-μM RP 58866. Similar results were obtained in 12 different cells. The effects of RP 58866 on the inward rectifying K^+ current, i_{K1}, were further investigated by applying slow depolarizing voltage ramps (4.7 mV/sec)

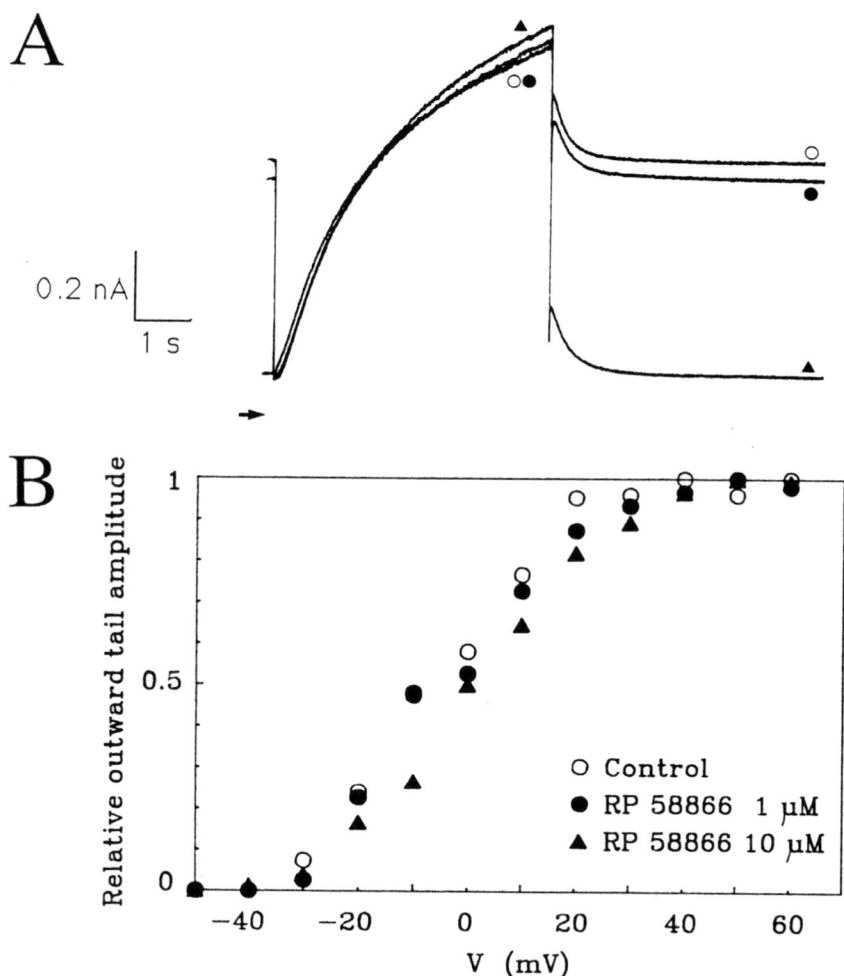

Figure 4. Effects of RP 58866 on the delayed rectifier K^+ current in guinea pig ventricular myocytes. A: Superimposed current traces recorded in response to 5-second depolarizing voltage pulses from -50 to $+60$ mV in the absence (empty circles) and presence of 1-μM (filled circles) and 10-μM (filled triangles) RP 58866. The arrow indicates the 0 current level; and B: Voltage dependence of i_K activation. The relative amplitude of the outward current tail recorded upon repolarizing the cell to -40 mV is plotted for various depolarizing pulses to the indicated voltage. Same cell as in A.

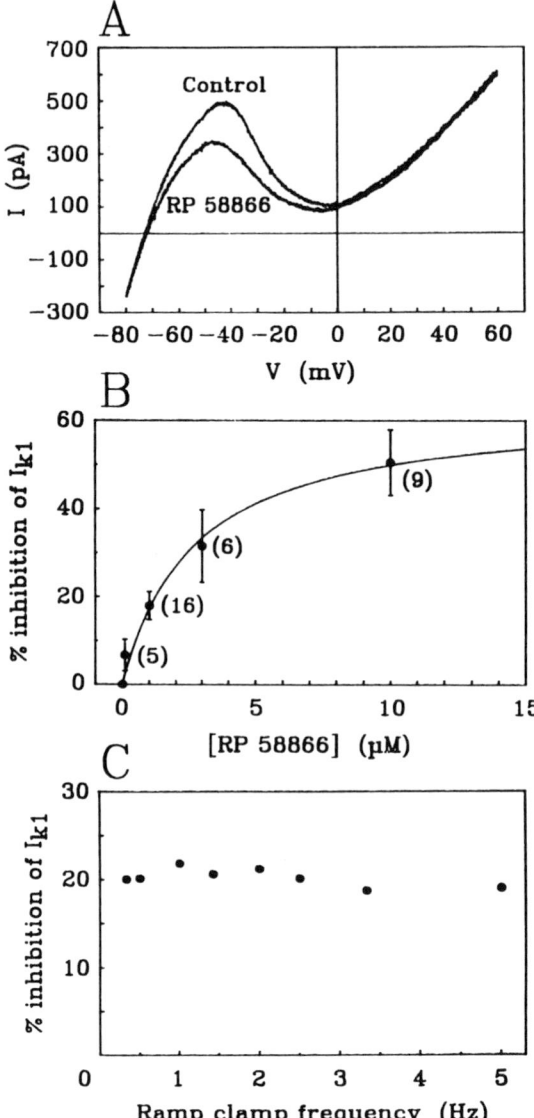

Figure 5. Effects of RP 58866 on the inward rectifier K$^+$ current, i_{K1}, in guinea pig cells. A: Current-voltage relationship for i_{K1} obtained with slow depolarizing voltage ramps in the absence and presence of 3-μM RP 58866; B: Dose-response curve for the steady current at −40 mV expressed as percent of control ± SEM. The continuous curve represents the equation: $1 - I_{RP}/I_C = 1/[1 + (K/RP)^{n_H}]$ where I_C and I_{RP} refer to the current at −40 mV in control and with various concentrations of RP 58866, $K = 9.66$ μM is the apparent dissociation constant, and $n_H = 0.67$ is the Hill coefficient. Number of cells for each data point are indicated between brackets; and C: Relative inhibition by 1-μM RP 58866 of the current at −40 mV (averaged from four different cells) determined for various ramp clamp frequencies.

from −80 mV to +60 mV. The ramp command voltage provided a direct record of the background current-voltage relationship with the current as ordinate and the command clamp as abscissa. Figure 5A shows a typical recording of the steady I-V curve in guinea pig ventricular myocytes with its characteristic prominent negative slope conductance region between −40 and 0 mV. The main effect of micromolar concentrations of RP 58866 (3 μM in Figure 5A) was to decrease reversibly the outward current in the voltage region between the reversal potential and 0 mV. This effect, which was observed in every one of the 41 cells tested, accounts for the shift of the holding current at −40 mV shown in Figure 3. Hyperpolarizing ramp clamp command from −40 mV to −120 mV were also used to investigate the effects of the molecule on the current recorded in the inward direction. At a concentration of 3 μM, RP 58866 decreased the slope conductance, g_{K1}, measured at the level of the reversal potential by 8.0 ± 1.9% (n = 6). The effects of RP 58866 on the background K^+ current were quantified by plotting the relative current at −40 mV for various concentrations (Figure 5B). The apparent dissociation constant related to the decrease of the outward current at −40 mV induced by RP 58866 was calculated by using a Hill representation of data points according to the equation: $\log [I_{RP}/(I_C\text{-}I_{RP})] = n_H \log K - n_H \log$ [RP] where I_C and I_{RP} are the current recorded in the absence and presence of various concentrations of RP 58866, respectively, K is the apparent dissociation constant and n_H is the Hill coefficient. A linear regression analysis through the points yielded a K value of 9.66 µM (r^2 = 0.999).

In five additional experiments, we used nitrendipine instead of Co^{2+} as a Ca^{2+} blocker; under both experimental conditions, the ability of RP 58866 to block the background K^+ current was of the same order of magnitude. In order to check whether the degree of blocking produced by RP 58866 depends on the stimulation rate, we used 300-

msec duration depolarizing ramps applied from −80 mV at various frequencies. It is clear from Figure 5C, which shows averaged results obtained with four different cells, that the block induced by RP 58866 was largely rate independent. In five experiments, we also explored the possibility that the effects of RP 58866 were temperature dependent. Figure 6 shows the results of a typical experiment: the holding current at −40 mV (empty squares) and the outward current tail (filled squares), are plotted against the pulse number; the initial recording was performed at 21°C, then the experimental temperature was switched to 30°C by means of a Peltier device. RP 58866 affected the background K^+ current much more strongly at 30°C than at 21°C.

Effects of RP 58866 on the Adenosine Triphosphate-Sensitive K^+ Current, $i_{K\text{-}ATP}$

In cardiac cells, ATP-sensitive K^+ channels are normally inactivated by the high-intra-

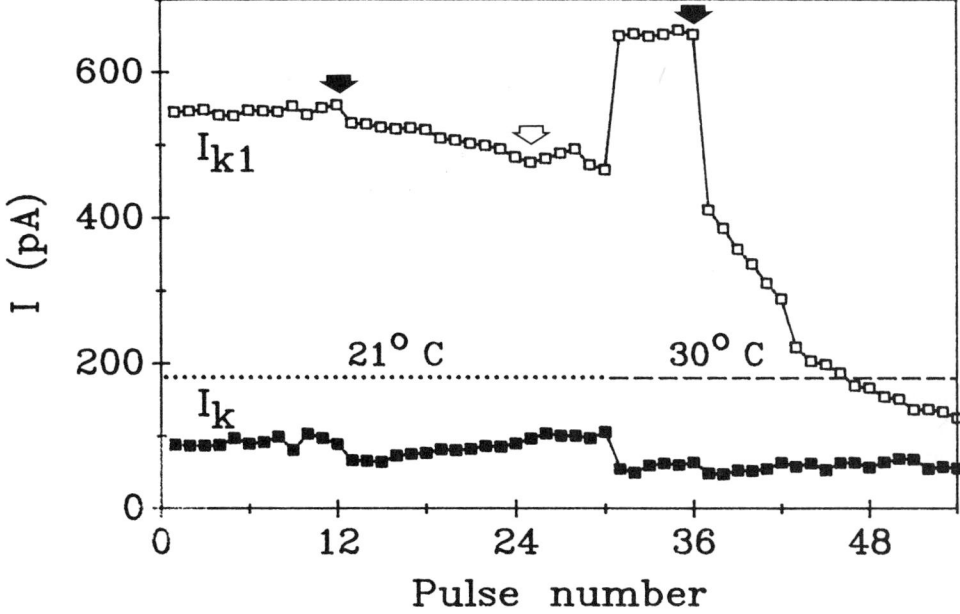

Figure 6. Temperature dependence of the effects of RP 58866 on K^+ currents. Same experimental protocol and symbols as in Figure 3A. At the time indicated by the filled arrow, a 10-µM RP 58866 containing external solution was perfused onto the cell at 21°C (left) or at 30°C (right). The empty arrow indicates return to the control solution.

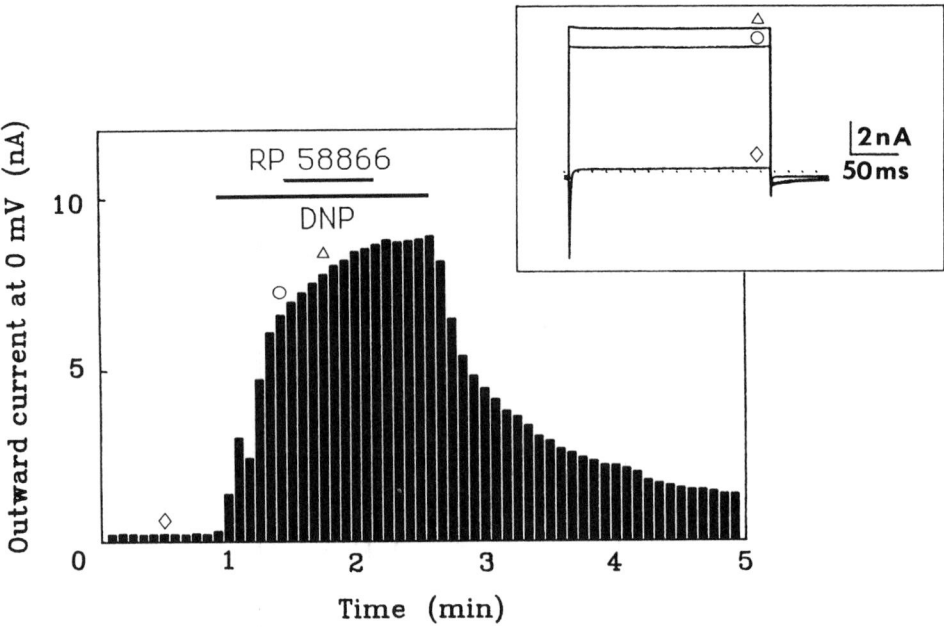

Figure 7. Effects of 10-μM RP 58866 on the dinitrophenol (DNP)-induced current. The cell membrane was clamped from −80 to 0 mV every 5 seconds. The graph represents the amplitude of the outward current at 0 mV plotted as a function of time. Dinitrophenol 0.5 mM and RP 58866 10 μM were applied as indicated by vertical bars. The inset shows corresponding current traces in control (diamond) and in the presence of DNP (circle) and of DNP plus RP 58866 (triangle).

cellular ATP concentration[15] and open under conditions of impaired cellular metabolism. In order to record macroscopic K^+-ATP currents, we used DNP, a classical uncoupler of oxidative phosphorylation, to decrease intracellular ATP and thereby activate K^+-ATP channels. We have previously shown that low concentrations of glibenclamide, a specific blocker of K^+-ATP channels, prevents the activation by DNP of a large outward current.[12] Under the same experimental conditions, RP 58866 was devoid of significant effects on the DNP-induced current (five experiments; Figure 7).

Effects of RP 58866 on the Transient Outward Current, i_{to}

The transient outward current is the main repolarizing current in the human atrium since no delayed rectifier can be recorded and

the inward rectifying current has a small amplitude.[16] Thus, it is of importance to look for the possible effects of a Class III drug on i_{to}. Because i_{to} is virtually absent from guinea pig ventricular cells, we used rat ventricular myocytes for these experiments. Figure 8 summarizes the effects of RP 58866 on the 4-aminopyridine-sensitive transient outward current that is easily observed upon depolarization of the rat myocardium.[17] At 3 to 10 μM, the drug did not modify either the I-V curve or the steady-state inactivation (n = 7; Figures 8A and 8B), but consistently increased the rate of inactivation of the current. A similar effect on the transient outward current has been reported for tedisamil, another Class III antiarrhythmic agent.[18] The results presented in Figure 8C, obtained from the same cell as in Figures 8A and 8B, show that RP 58866 also effectively blocked the inward rectifier in rat myocytes (n = 3).

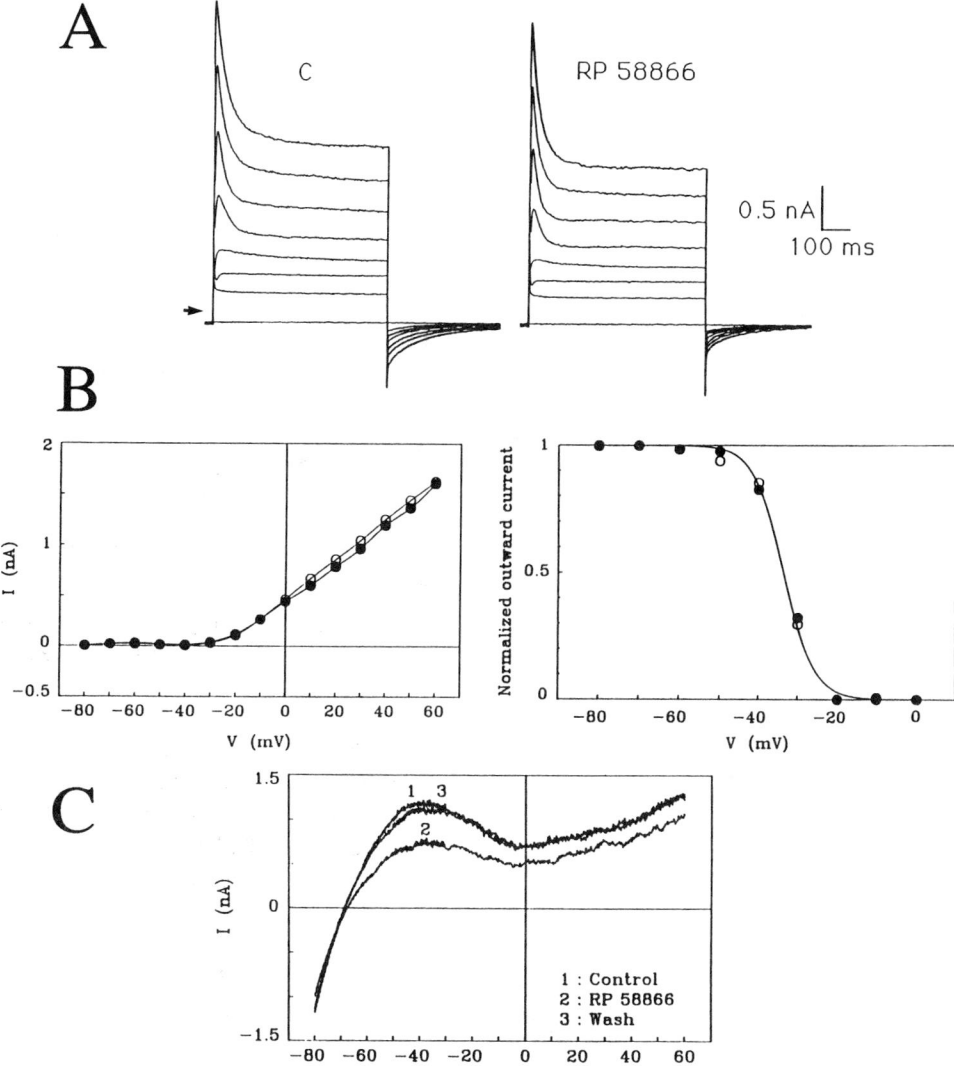

Figure 8. Effects of RP 58866 on outward K$^+$ currents in rat ventricular myocytes. A: Superimposed current traces elicited by depolarizing pulses from -80 mV to -60, -40, -20, 0, 20, 40, and 60 mV in the absence (left) and presence (right) of 10-μM RP 58866. The arrow indicates the 0 current level; B: The current-voltage relationship (left panel) and the steady-state inactivation curve (right panel) for the transient outward current determined in the absence (open symbols) and presence (filled symbols) of 10-μM RP 58866; and C: The current-voltage relationship of the inward rectifying K$^+$ current i_{K1} in rat myocytes recorded with a ramp clamp command protocol. Same cell as in A and B.

Effects of RP 58866 on the Acetylcholine-Induced Current, i_{K-ACh}

Quinidine effectively depresses the ACh-induced outward K$^+$ current in guinea pig atrial cells by blocking the muscarinic K$^+$ channel itself.[19] We thus explored whether RP 58866, like quinidine, would modify the i_{K-ACh} current. For these experiments, the standard K$^+$-aspartate internal solution was supplemented with 0.5-mM guanosine triphosphate

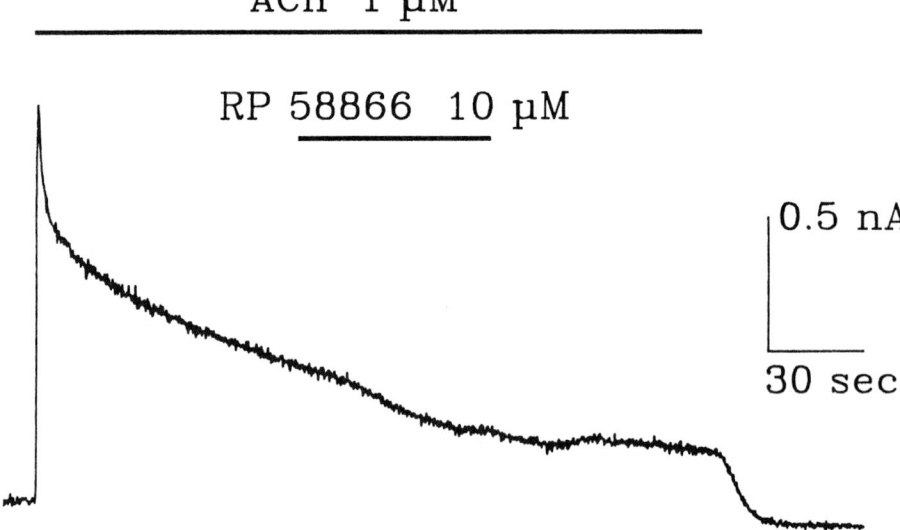

Figure 9. Effects of RP 58866 on the acetylcholine-induced outward current in guinea pig atrial myocytes. Holding potential: 0 mV. The dotted line indicates the 0 current level.

(GTP). A holding potential of 0 mV was chosen because in preliminary experiments RP 58866 was not found to affect the holding current at this voltage in atrial cells. In 18 different experiments, RP 58866 at concentrations up to 10 μM only slightly affected the acetylcholine-induced current (Figure 9).

Effects of RP 58866 on the L-Type and T-Type Ca^{2+} Currents

$i_{Ca,L}$ and $i_{Ca,T}$ were recorded in guinea pig ventricular myocytes with K$^+$ currents blocked with intracellular cesium and extracellular TEA (see *Methods*). For the purpose of recording both $i_{Ca,L}$ and $i_{Ca,T}$, a double pulse protocol was used. Concentrations of RP 58866 as high as 30 μM did not affect the current-voltage relationships of the $i_{Ca,L}$ and $i_{Ca,T}$ currents (not shown).

Enantiomeric Separation

RP 58866 is a racemic mixture containing enantiomers designated RP 62719 [(S)(-)-iso-

mer] and RP 62718 [(R)(+)-isomer]. In guinea pig papillary muscle recorded with a conventional microelectrode technique, RP 58866 and RP 62719 (terikalant) at a concentration of 3 μM prolonged the normal action potential by 34.6 ± 3% and 30.0 ± 3%, respectively. In contrast, RP 62718 at the same concentration produced a threefold lower effect. The concentration of RP 62719 prolonging the APD$_{90}$ to the same degree as RP 62718 was only 0.09 μM.[20] Therefore, RP 62719 is the eutomer and is about 150 times more potent than the inactive enantiomer, RP 62718. Although less pronounced, a difference between RP 62719 and RP 62718 was also observed when K$^+$ currents were considered. In isolated guinea pig ventricular cells, the apparent dissociation constant related to the decrease induced by RP 62719 of the outward current at -40 mV was 9.33 μM ($r^2 = 0.964$; Figure 10), ie, very similar to that of the racemate. In comparison, RP 62718 produced a twofold lower effect under similar experimental conditions. Finally, the pharmacological profile of RP 62719 with respect to the various ionic currents recorded

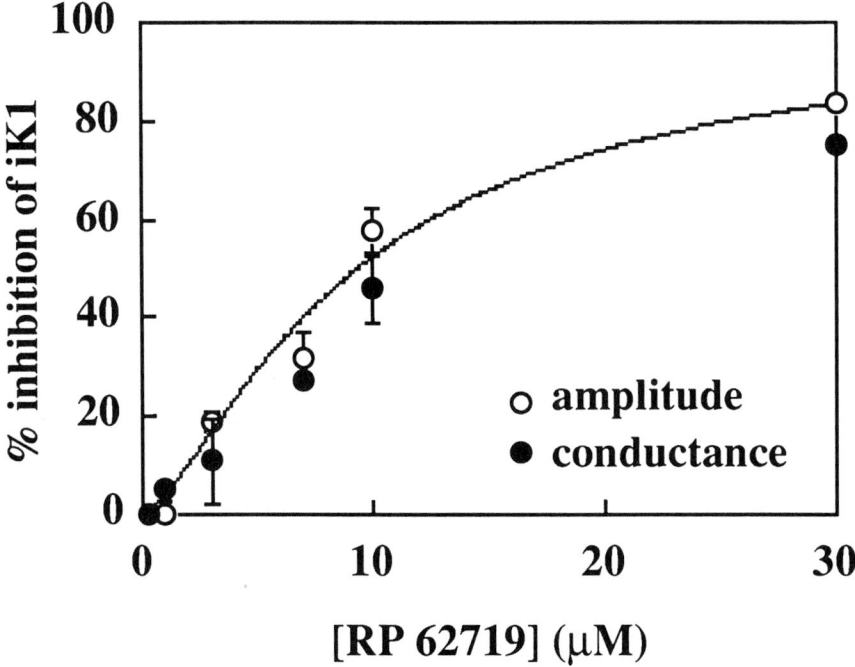

Figure 10. The dose-response curve for RP 62719: the filled symbols are the steady current at −40 mV whereas the empty symbols are the conductance of the inward rectifier, g_{K1}, measured in the inward direction. The continuous curve represents the equation: $1 - I_{RP}/I_C = 1/[1 + (K/RP)^{n_H}]$ where I_C and I_{RP} refer to the current at −40 mV recorded in control and with various concentrations of RP 62719, $K = 9.33$ μM is the apparent dissociation constant, and $n_H = 1.39$ is the Hill coefficient.

in guinea pig and rat myocytes was similar to that of RP 58866.

Discussion

From our results, we conclude that RP 58866 and its active enantiomer, RP 62719 (terikalant), act to prolong the normal cardiac action potential dose-dependently decreasing the inward rectifying K+ current, whereas these compounds remain essentially inactive on the other plateau currents that we recorded in guinea pig cardiac cells. In rat cardiac myocytes, the drugs also accelerated the inactivation of the 4-aminopyridine-sensitive transient outward current, i_{to}, thus decreasing the time during which the outward current flows through these channels. This effect, which is likely to contribute to the length-

ening of the plateau, is of importance particularly in the human atrial myocardium where i_{to} plays a key role in inducing repolarization.[16] Indeed, in this tissue, RP 58866 was found to modify the early repolarization phase and the plateau level of the action potential.[20]

After 300-msec depolarizing pulses to +40 mV, the amplitude of the delayed rectifier, i_K, at −40 mV was 10 to 20 times less than the amplitude of the inward rectifier at that voltage. Thus i_{K1} is the major outward current that governs final repolarization in guinea pig ventricular myocytes, and hence the duration of the refractory period and the electrical restitution of the ventricle. Numerous potassium channels in the heart have been identified to date, all of which modulate repolarization to a different extent depending on the physiological or physiopathological circumstances. Pharmacological inhibition of a given cardiac K^+ channel, especially of i_K, i_{K1}, or i_{to} results in less net outward current for repolarization and in a lengthening of the action potential plateau. However, depending on the type of K^+ channel blocked, the pharmacological profile and possibly the therapeutical properties of K^+ blockers may significantly differ. Most Class III antiarrhythmic agents described so far preferentially act on the delayed rectifier, i_K. This is the case for sotalol and its non-β-blocker dextroisomer,[3] for clofilium,[21] and for various methylsulfonamide derivatives such as dofetilide,[22] E-4031,[23] and risotilide.[24] With regard to the type of channel blocked, RP 58866 and its active enantiomer, terikalant, thus possess a unique profile.

The pharmacological profile of RP 58866 and RP 62719 determined both under in vitro and in vivo conditions is typical of pure Class III antiarrhythmic drugs. In anesthetized dogs, both drugs significantly prolonged the atrial, nodal, and ventricular refractory periods but did not affect the endocavitary AH, HV, and QRS intervals.[14,20] Prolongation of cardiac refractory periods was also observed in conscious dogs. Moreover, they increased the QT and QTc intervals on the surface ECG and decreased the heart rate significantly. In mongrel dogs and in Yucatan micropigs submitted to a transient ligation of the left ventricular artery, RP 58866 and RP 62719 prevented fatal ventricular arrhythmias from occurring either during the ischemic period or during reperfusion. In contrast, in this model, pretreatment of the animals with flecainide increased the incidence of fatal arrhythmias. In a chronic model of atrial fibrillation in conscious dogs,[20,25] RP 62719 administered before the induction of the atrial arrhythmia reduced the duration of the fibrillation episodes to less than 2% of the control value. Furthermore, when injected during an atrial fibrillation episode, the drug rapidly restored the normal sinus rhythm.[20] However, as is also the case for other Class III drugs,[2,26] RP 58866 and RP 62719 were devoid of significant effects against: (1) aconitine-induced arrhythmias in anesthetized rats; (2) ouabain-induced arrhythmias in anesthetized dogs; and (3) poly-morphic tachycardias occurring in conscious dogs 16 to 24 hours after a two-stage ligation of the left anterior descending artery.[27]

Electrophysiological testing of humans treated with RP 58866 led to the conclusion that the drug at a dose of 0.1 mg/kg effectively prolonged atrial and ventricular refractory periods, but did not alter the conduction properties of the myocardium. At the atrial level, prolongation of the refractory periods was largely independent of the basal stimulation rate (the same effect was also observed in conscious dogs) suggesting a favorable frequency-dependent profile of the drug. Finally, preliminary results obtained in healthy volunteers have shown that a single dose of 1.5-mg RP 62719 prolongs the QTc interval by 15.6 ± 3.0% (n = 5).

Acknowledgment: We gratefully thank Ms. Karen Pepper for her kind help with this chapter.

References

1. Vaughan Williams EM: A classification of antirhythmic actions reassessed after a decade of new drugs. *J Clin Pharmacol* 24:129, 1984.
2. Colatsky TJ, Follmer CH: K^+ channel blockers and activators in cardiac arrhythmias. *Cardiovasc Drug Rev* 7:199, 1989.
3. Carmeliet E: Electrophysiologic and voltage-clamp analysis of the effects of sotalol on isolated cardiac muscle and Purkinje fibers. *J Pharmacol Exp Ther* 232:817, 1985.
4. Singh BN, Nademanee K: Sotalol: a β blocker with unique antiarrhythmic properties. *Am Heart J* 114:121, 1987.
5. Mason JW, Hondeghem LM, Katzung BG: Amiodarone blocks inactivated cardiac sodium channels. *Pflügers Arch* 396:79, 1983.
6. Nishimura M, Follmer CH, Singer DH: Amiodarone blocks calcium current in single guinea-pig ventricular myocytes. *J Pharmacol Exp Ther* 251:650, 1989.
7. Polser P, Broeckhuysen J: The adrenergic antagonism of amiodarone. *Biochem Pharmacol* 25:131, 1976.
8. Singh BN: Amiodarone: historical development and pharmacologic profile. *Am Heart J* 106:788, 1983.
9. Baro I, Escande D: A long lasting Ca^{2+}-activated outward current in guinea-pig atrial myocytes. *Pflügers Arch* 415:63, 1989.
10. Escande D, Thuringer D, Le Guern S, et al: Po-

tassium channel openers act through an activation of ATP-sensitive K$^+$ channels in guinea-pig cardiac myocytes. *Pflügers Arch* 414:669, 1989.

11. Duchatelle-Gourdon I, Hartzell HC, Lagrutta AA: Modulation of the delayed rectifier potassium current in frog cardiomyocytes by β-adrenergic agonists and magnesium. *J Physiol (Lond)* 415:251, 1989.

12. Escande D: The pharmacology of ATP-sensitive K$^+$ channels in the heart. *Pflügers Arch* 414(Suppl I):S93, 1989.

13. Hamill OP, Marty A, Neher E, et al: Improved patch-clamp techniques for high resolution current recording from cells and cell-free membrane patches. *Pflügers Arch* 391:85, 1981.

14. Mestre M, Hardy JC, Escande D, et al: Pharmacological relevance in animal modesl of a pure class III antiarrhythmic agent. *Circulation* 80:II-139, 1989.

15. Noma A: ATP-regulated K$^+$ channels in cardiac muscle. *Nature (Lond)* 305:147, 1983.

16. Escande D, Coulombe A, Faivre JF, et al: Two types of transient outward currents in adult human atrial cells. *Am J Physiol* 252:H142, 1987.

17. Josephson IR, Sanchez-Chapula J, Brown AM: Early outward current in rat single ventricular cells. *Circ Res* 54:157, 1984.

18. Dukes ID, Morad M: Tedisamil modulates outward K$^+$ currents in rat and guinea pig ventricular myocytes. *Circulation* 80:II-517, 1989.

19. Nakajima T, Kurachi Y, Ito H, et al: Anti-cholinergic effects of quinidine, disopyramide, and procainamide is isolated atrial myocytes: mediation by different molecular mechanisms. *Circ Res* 64:297, 1989.

20. Escande D, Mestre M, Cavero I, et al: RP 58866 and its active enantiomer RP 62719 (terikalant): blockers of the inward rectifier K$^+$ current acting as pure class III antiarrhythmic agents. *J Cardiovasc Pharmacol* (in press).

21. Arena JP, Kass RS: Block of heart potassium channels by clofilium and its tertiary analogs: relationship between drug structure and type of channel blocked. *Mol Pharmacol* 34:60, 1988.

22. Dalrymple HW, Burges RA, Blackburn KJ, et al: UK-68,798 is a novel, potent and selective class III antiarrhythmic drug. *J Mol Cell Cardiol* 21:SII-11, 1989.

23. Sawada K: Depression of the delayed outward K$^+$ current by a novel class 3 antiarrhythmic agent. *J Mol Cell Cardiol* 21:SII-20, 1989.

24. Follmer CH, Poczobutt MT, Colatsky TJ: Selective block of delayed rectification (I_k) in feline ventricular myocytes by Wy-48,986, a novel class III antiarrhythmic agent. *J Mol Cell Cardiol* 21:SII-21, 1989.

25. Rensma PL, Allessie M, Lammers WJEP, et al: Length of excitation wave and susceptibility to reentrant atrial arrhythmias in normal conscious dogs. *Circ Res* 62:395, 1988.

26. Gibson JK, Kersten JA: In vivo assessment of class III agents and their antiarrhythmic activity. *Drug Dev Res* 19:173, 1990.

27. Harris AS: Delayed development of ventricular ectopic rhythms following coronary artery occlusion. *Circulation* 1:1318, 1950.

Chapter 42

Ambasilide: *A Novel Class III Antiarrhythmic Compound With a Differential Effect on Repolarization in Ventricular Muscle and Purkinje Fibers*

Christopher H. Follmer
Zhi-hao Zhang
Bramah N. Singh

Sudden cardiac death as a result of ventricular tachycardia or fibrillation is a major clinical problem in the United States, and its prevention continues to be a primary focus for drug development programs in both academia and the pharmaceutical industry.[1-4] In addition, the inability of Class I agents to reduce mortality in high-risk patients (Chapters 27 and 48) has contributed to a renewed interest in other therapeutic modalities, which include β-blockers and Class III antiarrhythmics.[5-10]

Although the concept that selectively delaying repolarization (Class III action) may be antifibrillatory is not new,[11,12] "pure" Class III agents with good bioavailability and without ancillary pharmacological effects have not been previously available. Only recently has the effort in this area by the pharmaceutical industry provided the clinical and basic scientist with interesting and increasingly selective new compounds. Of the recently developed "pure" Class III antiarrhythmic compounds under clinical investigation, most are paramethanesulphonyl substituted compounds resembling sotalol but devoid of the β-receptor blocking property.[13] In contrast, the recently developed Class III agent, ambasilide,[14,15] is chemically distinct from these compounds by being devoid of the paramethanesulphonylamide substituent and by having a bicyclic bispidine ring incorporated with the nitrogen of the carbonylamide bridge. As such, ambasilide bears a distant resemblance to the Class III antiarrhythmic, amiodarone, when one considers the possible conformations of amiodarone's butyl substituent on the benzofuran group, the carbonyl bridge, and the aromatic ring (Figure 1). Thus, ambasilide is of considerable interest on a theoretical basis because of its novel structure, but in addition, recent cellular studies suggest striking similarities

From BN Singh, HJJ Wellens, M Hiraoka, (eds): *Electropharmacological Control of Cardiac Arrhythmias.* Mount Kisco, NY, Futura Publishing Company Inc., © 1994.

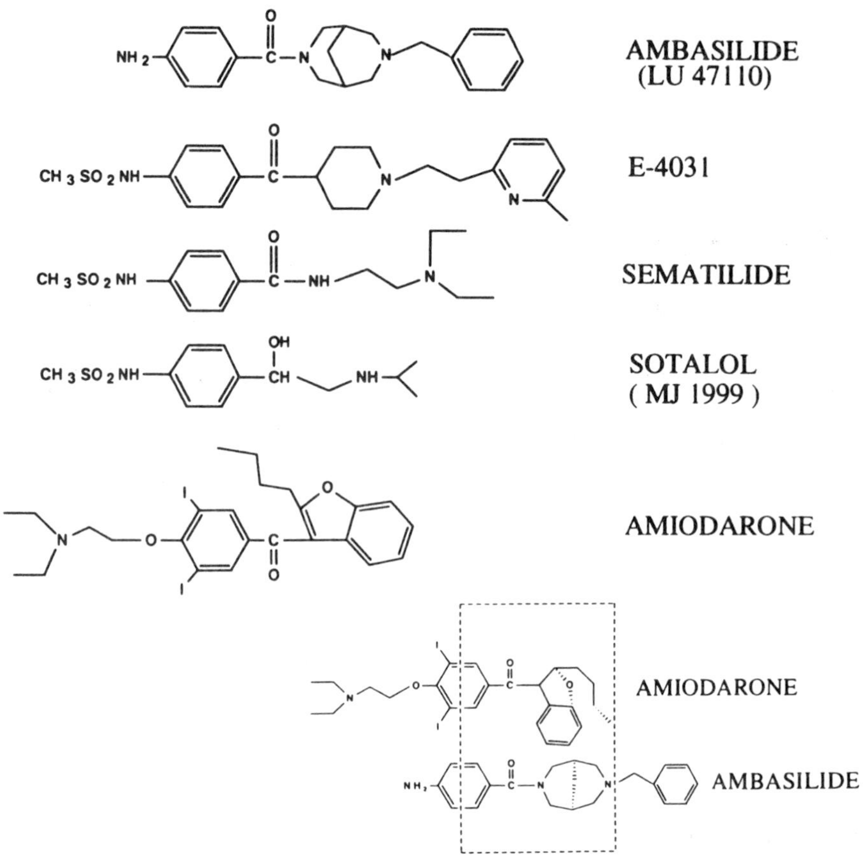

Figure 1. Structural formulas of a number of methanesulphonyl benzamide compounds that exert marked "pure" Class III actions compared to those of sotalol (a β blocker) and amiodarone (a benzofuran derivative that has noncompetitive antiadrenergic activity), both of which are regarded as prototypes of Class III agents. Structural formula of ambasilide (LU-47110) is also shown; note that ambasilide is not a methanesulphonyl benzamide, and it does not resemble sotalol. Some structural similarities between amiodarone and ambasilide can be drawn when you consider the flexibility of the butyl group attached to the benzofuran of amiodarone (inset). The butyl group of the benzofuran can be contorted to simulate a seven-member ring with an oxygen bridge (an eight-member bicyclic in total). This would compare with the nine-member bispidine ring of ambasilide. Also, the oxygen of the benzofuran and the terminal amine of ambasilide could act similarly in their ability to form hydrogen bonds or contribute spare electrons. This part of the molecule is thought to be the primary determinant of K$^+$ channel block.

between amiodarone and ambasilide in the blocking of the delayed rectifier potassium current, the absence of a frequency-dependent attenuation of the APD prolongation in the ventricular myocardium,[16] and the presence of a modest sodium channel block, which is manifest only at rapid stimulus frequencies.[14,15] In this chapter, we describe the known electrophysiological actions of the

compound essentially derived in our own cardiovascular research laboratory.

Cellular Electrophysiological Effects of Ambasilide

The data on the effects of ambasilide have been obtained from studies in multicellular preparations in cardiac muscle from several species and from isolated guinea pig myocytes.

Effects on Transmembrane Potentials

Figures 2 and 3 summarize the concentration-dependent effects of ambasilide on the transmembrane potentials of canine ventricular muscle and of Purkinje fibers constantly driven at 1 Hz.[14] In ventricular muscle, the predominant effect of ambasilide is the uniform prolongation of the action potential duration (APD) measured at both -20 mV and -80 mV (APD_{20} and APD_{80}, respectively). After exposure to 10^{-6} and 10^{-5} M ambasilide, the mean APD_{20} increase is 14% and 28%, respectively, and the APD_{80} increases about 11% and

26%, respectively. The lowest concentration of ambasilide tested (10^{-7} M) is without effect on the APD. Also, at 1 Hz, the rapid upstroke of the action potential ($\dot{V}_{max}$) is not altered by any of the concentrations under study. Thus, ambasilide shows conventional Class III behavior in the ventricular myocardium: a uniform prolongation of the APD without any effect on $\dot{V}_{max}$.

In Purkinje fibers, the results were considerably different from those described for the ventricular muscle. Although at low concentrations ambasilide increased both the APD_{20} and APD_{80} (Figure 2C), at higher concentrations the drug produced a paradoxical decrease in APD_{20} and an increase in APD_{80}. These results are reminiscent of those observed in the presence of other antiarrhythmic agents, which block both the Na^+ plateau cur-

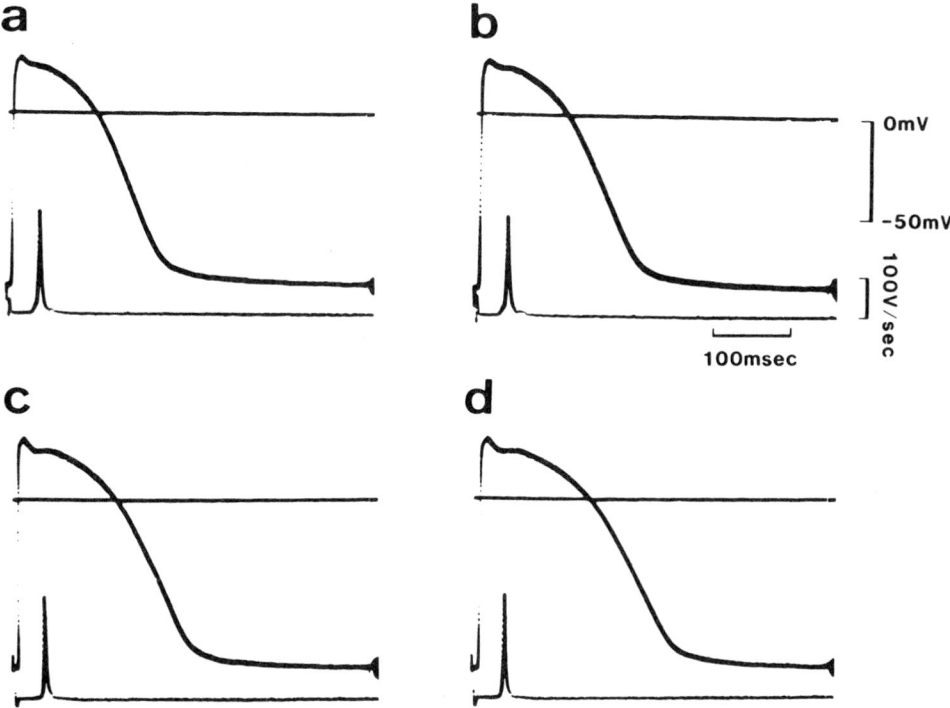

Figure 2. Effects of ambasilide on the transmembrane potential of canine Purkinje fibers. Panel (a): control voltage recording. Panels (b), (c), and (d): 10^{-7} M, 10^{-6} M, and 10^{-5} M ambasilide, respectively. The upper trace in each recording represents the membrane action potential, the middle trace is the zero potential, and the lower trace is the first derivative of the upstroke of the action potential. The preparation was constantly driven at 1 Hz. (Reproduced with permission from Reference 14.)

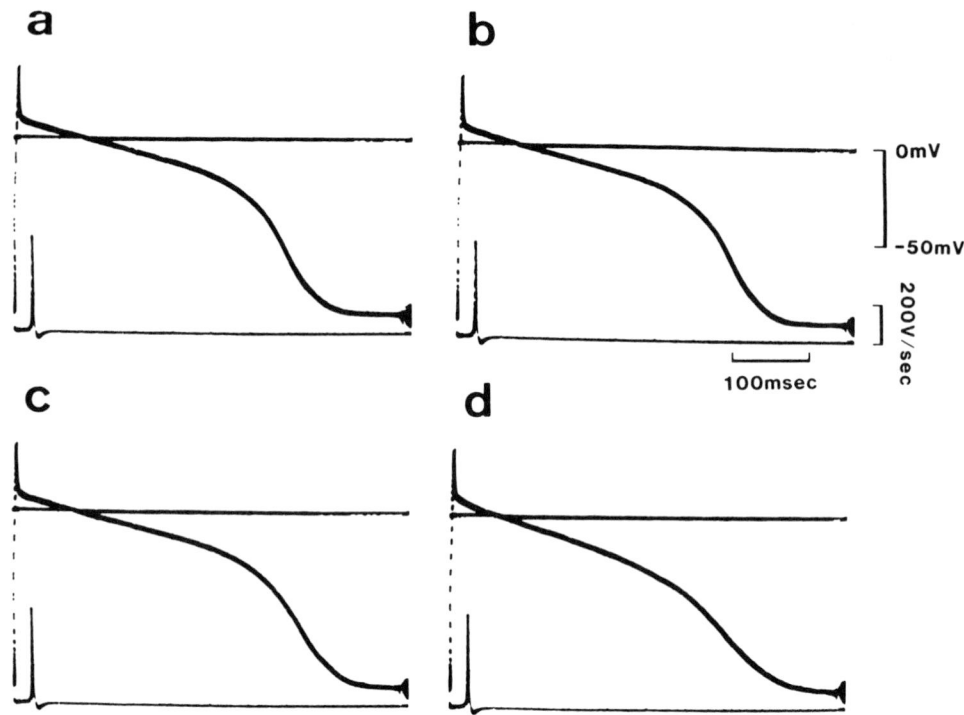

Figure 3. Effects of ambasilide on the transmembrane potential of canine ventricular muscle. Panel (a): control voltage recording. Panels (b), (c), and (d): 10^{-7} M, 10^{-6}, M, and 10^{-5} M ambasilide, respectively. The upper trace in each recording represents the membrane action potential, the middle trace is the first zero potential and the lower trace is the derivative of the upstroke of the action potential. The preparation was constantly driven at 1 Hz. (Reproduced with permission from Reference 14.)

rent and outward potassium currents.[17-20] Expressed as a percentage of controls, the changes in APD$_{80}$ induced by 10^{-5} M and 10^{-6} M ambasilide are somewhat less than those seen in the ventricle for the same two concentrations (8% and 14%, respectively). The mean values for APD$_{20}$ increase 2% at 10^{-6} M and decrease 16% after 10^{-5} M. $\dot{V}_{max}$ is unaffected by ambasilide under these conditions. Thus, in Purkinje fibers, the Class III effects of ambasilide appear to be opposed by the depression of the plateau height and duration. A similar action has been noted for several antiarrhythmic agents, and a reduction in plateau sodium current most likely underlies this effect.[18-20] The reduction in inward plateau Na$^+$ current tends to shorten the APD and diminish the Class III action by offsetting the effects of K$^+$ channel block to delay repolarization.[18]

The APD$_{20}$ decrease in the absence of any changes in $\dot{V}_{max}$ suggests that the Na$^+$ current block is modest. This is confirmed by $\dot{V}_{max}$ measurements over a wide frequency range intended to quantitate the Na$^+$ channel effects. Figure 4 summarizes the effects of ambasilide (10^{-5} M) on $\dot{V}_{max}$ in Purkinje fibers and in ventricular muscle.[14] At 1 Hz, there is no effect of ambasilide on $\dot{V}_{max}$. At 2 Hz, $\dot{V}_{max}$ is decreased by 8% and 11% in Purkinje fibers and in the ventricular muscle, respectively. Increasing the stimulus frequency still further increases the depression of $\dot{V}_{max}$. Thus, ambasilide's effects on Na$^+$ current appear to be small and primarily manifest in the reduction of the plateau duration in Purkinje fibers at fast stimulus rates. Therefore, the results are consistent with the previous observation in Purkinje fibers, noting that the plateau is more sensitive to Na$^+$ block than is $\dot{V}_{max}$.[21] In addi-

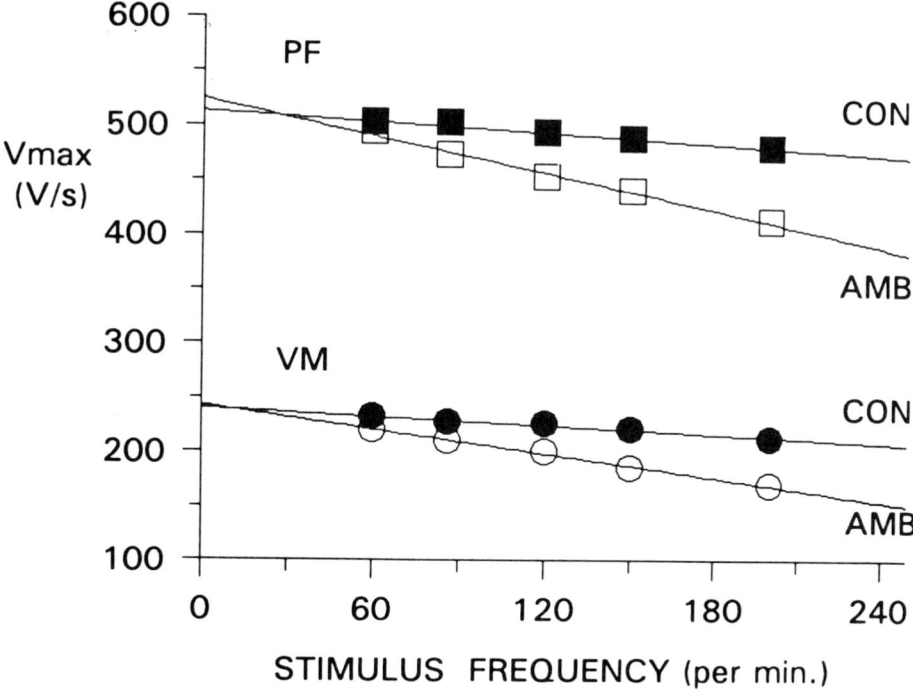

Figure 4. Frequency-dependent reduction in $\dot{V}_{max}$ by ambasilide, 10^{-5} M, in canine Purkinje fibers and ventricular muscle preparations. The mean values of $\dot{V}_{max}$ were obtained from Takanaka et al.[14] Under control conditions (CON), $\dot{V}_{max}$ was affected very little by rapid pacing. The lines describing the mean values in Purkinje fibers (PF) and ventricular muscle (VM) are the best fits to the data using linear regression (Nfit, Island Products, TX). In the presence of ambasilide (AMB), $\dot{V}_{max}$ decreased by 21% and 14% in changing the stimulus frequency from 60 to 200 per minute.

tion, one might suggest that a small degree of Na$^+$ current block may be beneficial in preventing early afterdepolarizations (EADs) secondary to excessive prolongation of the Purkinje APD.

Cycle Length Dependency of Effects on Repolarization

Recently, attention has been focused on the importance of maintaining a Class III profile at cycle lengths that more closely resemble those observed under the clinical conditions of arrhythmia.[16,22] In theory, the Class III action should be small at normal heart rates but increase substantially as the heart rate accelerates. Such a drug would prevent the induction of ventricular tachycardia (and fibrillation) by

preventing the ventricular rate from becoming life-threatening or ultimately degenerating into fibrillation. In this respect, ambasilide is of some interest because, at least in the ventricular myocardium, ambasilide uniformly prolongs the AP at slow as well as fast stimulus rates. Figure 5A summarizes the mean data of Takanaka et al.[14] and shows that ambasilide consistently prolongs the ventricular APD$_{80}$ over the entire range of stimulus frequencies tested. Represented as the mean percent change in APD from the control at each stimulus frequency, ambasilide's effects actually slightly increase at fast rates (Figure 5B). Thus, in the myocardium, ambasilide does not appear to lose its Class III profile at rates comparable to those associated with ventricular tachycardia.

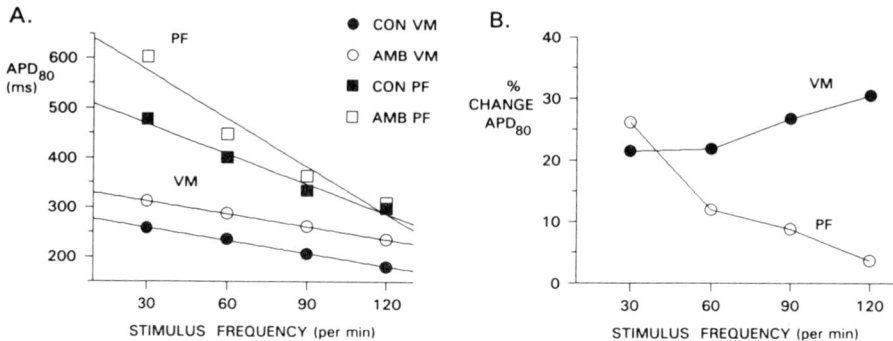

Figure 5. Frequency-dependent effects of ambasilide, 10^{-5} M, on the action potential duration in Purkinje fibers and ventricular muscle. The mean values for APD$_{80}$ were obtained from Takanaka et al.[14] The lines describing the mean values in Purkinje fibers (CON PF, AMB PF) and ventricular muscle (CON VM, AMB VM) are the best fits to the data using linear regression (Nfit, Island Products, TX). Panel A: In Purkinje fibers, rapid pacing reduced the degree of APD prolongation, whereas in the ventricular myocardium, the Class III action was unaltered by stimulus rate. Panel B: The effects of stimulus rate on APD prolongation plotted as a function of percent change. In ventricular muscle, APD prolongation actually increased at faster stimulus rates.

In contrast, the results obtained in Purkinje fibers demonstrate that the Class III action is almost completely attenuated at a stimulus frequency of 2 Hz (Figure 5A and 5B). Thus, in Purkinje fibers, ambasilide is without effect on the APD at stimulus frequencies corresponding to ventricular tachycardia. This effect is of considerable interest because it requires one to distinguish the tissue type in which APD lengthening is most desirable at fast stimulus rates. As an example, for amiodarone as well as ambasilide, the Purkinje fiber APD actually approaches the ventricular APD at fast stimulus rates. Thus, the disparity between the APD in the two tissue types decreases with increases in frequency, an action that may contribute to more homogeneous repolarization and a diminished opportunity for reentrant current flow in the presence of the drug.[23,24]

The Role of K$^+$ Channel Selectivity in Class III Agents: Effects of Ambasilide

All new Class III agents recently introduced appear to be selective blockers of the delayed outward potassium current.[22,25] More specifically, they block the inwardly rectifying (nonlinear) delayed outward current as opposed to the linear delayed outward current. The exceptions, to date, are amiodarone and clofilium, which block both the nonlinear and linear components of I$_K$.[22,26–28] Recent voltage-clamp studies indicate that with respect to K$^+$ channel block, ambasilide is more closely associated with amiodarone or clofilium than the other "pure" Class III drugs because ambasilide also blocks both components of I$_K$.[15] However, as described above, ambasilide can be further distinguished from clofilium by its Na$^+$ channel blocking actions.

Figure 6A illustrates the difference between the two types of delayed rectifiers. Most notable is the observation that the linear I$_K$ is a linear function of voltage, increasing the outward current as the membrane is depolarized. In contrast, the inwardly rectifying I$_K$ has a maximum near -40 mV and contributes increasingly smaller amounts of outward current as the membrane is depolarized. The relative contributions of each component to the action potential can be appreciated by examining Figure 6B. The computer simulation demonstrates that the linear I$_K$ essentially fol-

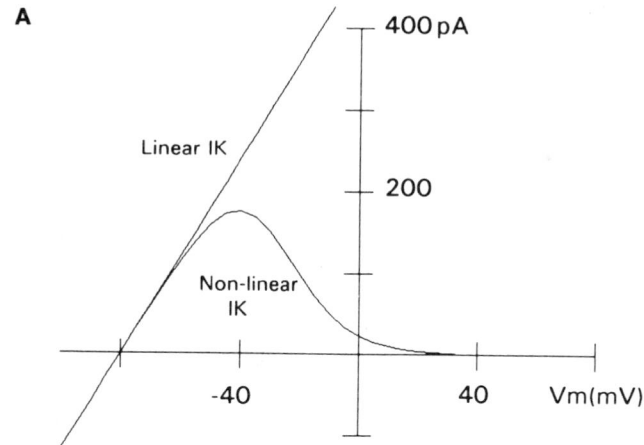

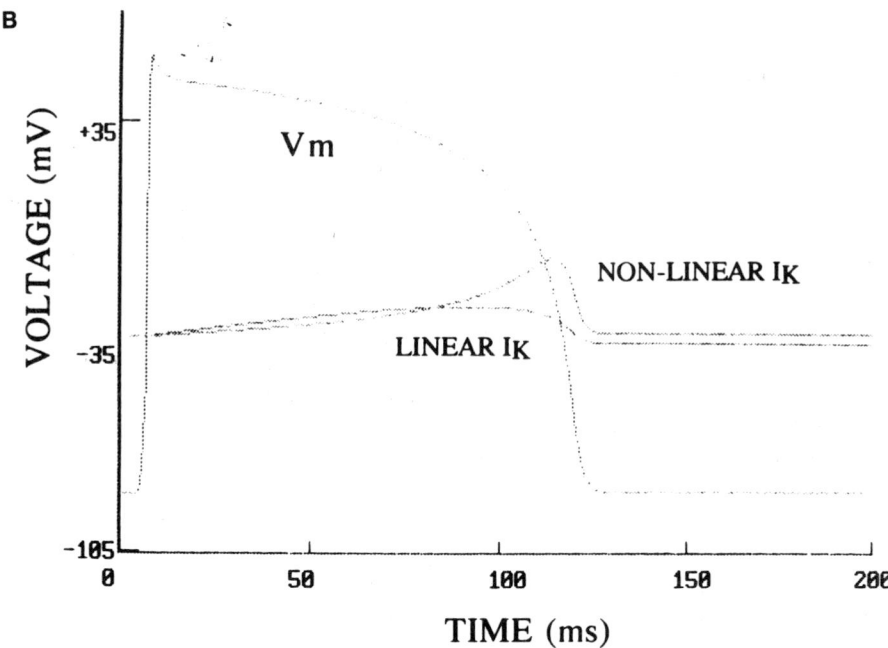

Figure 6. Fully activated current-voltage relationship for the two components of I_K in guinea pig ventricular myocytes. Panel A: The linear component represents the conventional slowly activating I_K, which is insensitive to the "pure" Class III agent, E-4031. The nonlinear component represents the rapidly activating E-4031-sensitive component. Panel B: Computer simulation of the relative contribution of the linear and nonlinear component of I_K to the repolarization process in the guinea pig ventricle. The computer model is the same as described in Courtney et al.[48] The linear component contributes primarily during the plateau, whereas the nonlinear component contributes almost entirely during phase 3 (see also Reference 30).

lows the membrane voltage, whereas the nonlinear component contributes comparatively little to repolarization during the plateau but considerably increases during phase 3 of the action potential. To date, there are no selective blockers of the linear component of I_K, but amiodarone and clofilium block both the linear and nonlinear components.[26–28] In humans, sotalol and the newer Class III agents are quite as effective as the Class III agents, which suggests that the nonlinear component plays a major role in repolarization in humans. On the other hand, the presence of a linear I_K in humans, which is similar to that described in the guinea pig[29] or chick embryo,[30] is unknown.

The two components can be further distinguished by their activation kinetics and their sensitivity to E-4031, a potent Class III agent currently under investigation.[29] An E-4031 sensitive component has a nonlinear fully activated current-voltage relationship, and it is distinguished by its relatively negative voltage threshold of activation and rapid activation kinetics. The E-4031-insensitive component is the conventional linear I_K, has an activation threshold of about 20–35 mV positive to the nonlinear component, and activates much more slowly than the nonlinear component. In this review, the effects of ambasilide on each of the two delayed rectifier currents are summarized from the work of Zhang et al.,[15] and they are compared to those obtained with E-4031.

Figure 7 shows a representative example of the time-dependent activation of I_K, and the peak tail current in a guinea pig ventricular myocyte elicited by voltage clamp steps from −40 mV to +60 mV for 200 msec and 5 seconds. For short depolarizations under control conditions, the magnitude of the time-dependent current seen on depolarization to +60 mV is the same magnitude as the peak tail current observed on repolarization to −30 mV (34 pA), despite the 90 mV difference in driving force for outward K^+ ion movement, a finding consistent with the inward rectifying properties of the rapid component.[29] In contrast, the 5-second depolarization elicited a

substantially larger outward current on depolarization than on repolarization (Figure 7B): 317 pA versus 136 pA. Thus, as noted by Sanguinetti and co-worker,[29] there appears to be two components of I_K with distinct activation kinetics: rapid and slow. Figure 7C confirms the presence of a rapidly activating nonlinear component of I_K. In the presence of E-4031 (5 μM), the peak tail current observed after a 200-msec depolarization decreases by 75%, whereas after a 5-second and depolarization the peak tail current decreases by only 39% (136 to 83 pA). In a small series of experiments, the peak tail currents decrease 65% ± 2% after a 200-msec depolarization (n = 4), whereas they decrease by 34% ± 5% after a 6.3-second depolarization.

Figure 8 shows the results from an experiment comparable to that described above, except in the presence of ambasilide. I_K is activated by a voltage step from −40 mV to +60 mV for either 200 or 2,000 msec, and tail currents were measured upon repolarization to −40 mV (Figure 8A). Under control conditions, the 200-msec depolarization step activates both a time-dependent (103 pA) and a tail current (77 pA). The time-dependent current reaches 619 pA after 2,000 msec, whereas the peak tail current increases to 219 pA. A 5-minute exposure to ambasilide (3 μM) substantially reduces both the time-dependent current and the tail current: 37% (65 pA) and 66% (26 pA), respectively. In contrast, the degree of block is similar for the time-dependent (40%, 374 pA) and the tail current (47%, 116 pA) after a 2-second depolarization. Increasing the concentration of ambasilide to 10 μM substantially increases the tail current block to 83% and 65% after the 200-msec and 2,000-msec pulse, respectively, but only modestly increases the block of the time-dependent current (54% of the control) after a 2,000-msec depolarization. After the 200-msec depolarization, the time-dependent current is unchanged. The tail current block that is most prominent after short depolarizations resembles that described for the nonlinear E-4031 sensitive component of I_K, but the block of both the tail current and the time-dependent

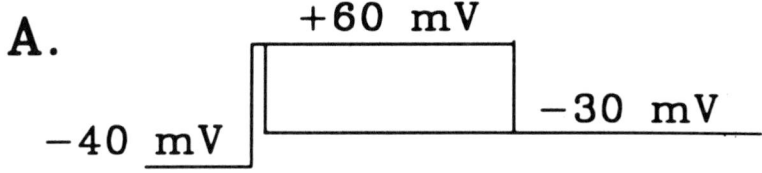

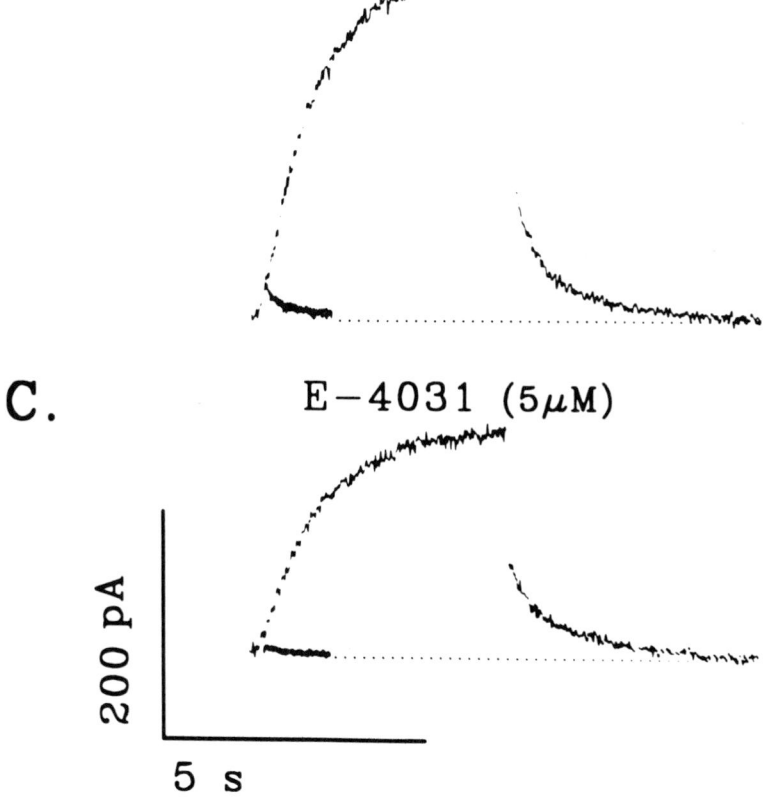

Figure 7. Effect of E-4031 on fast and slow components of I_K. Panel A: protocol to elicit slow and fast components of I_K. Voltage steps from -40 to + 60 mV for 200 msec and 5,000 msec were followed by a repolarizing step to -30 mV. Panels B and C: membrane currents before and after exposure to E-4031. The drug showed a predominant effect on the fast activating component. After the 200 msec depolarization, the tail current was nearly completely blocked.

current after long depolarizations cannot be accounted for by the magnitude of the nonlinear component alone. Ambasilide appears to block both components of I_K.

Figure 9A shows a summary of the results from a series of seven experiments. The frac-

tion of the tail current blocked by E-4031 is plotted as a function of depolarization time. The block is essentially the same for all depolarizations between 80 and 420 msec (67%), but decreases to about 34% with longer depolarizations. The results are consistent with the

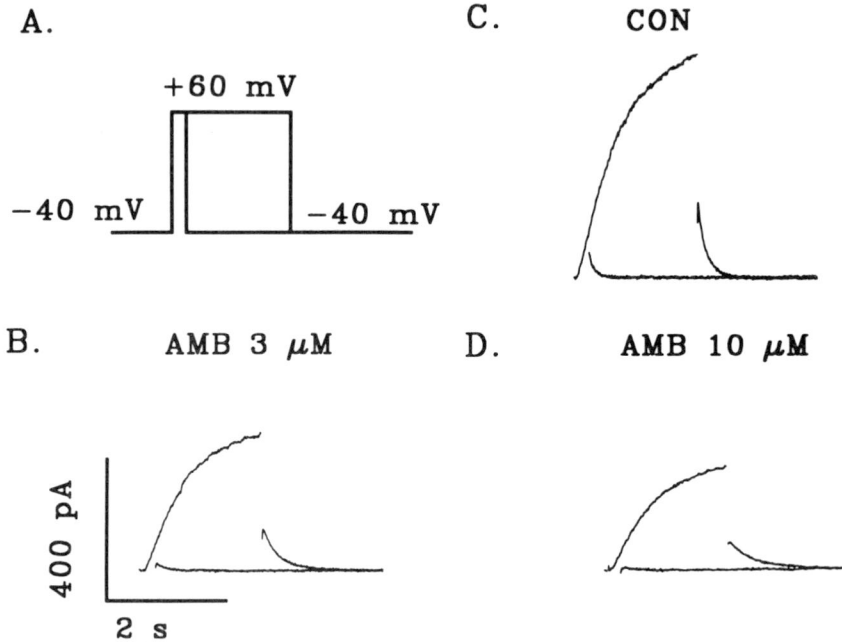

Figure 8. Concentration related block of I_K by ambasilide after 200- and 2,000-msec depolarization steps. Panel A: Protocol was used to induce the two components I_K. Panels B, C, and D: Current traces obtained before and after exposure to 3 mM and 10 mM ambasilide (AMB). AMB showed a concentration-dependent block of the two components of I_K. (Reproduced with permission from Reference 15.)

notion that the slow component (E-4031-insensitive) becomes more prominent with long step depolarizations. Figure 9B summarizes the effects of ambasilide on the tail currents as a function of pulse duration. Block by ambasilide is greatest at short depolarizations, a result similar to E-4031. However, unlike E-4031, which produces similar magnitudes of block between 200 and 420 msec, block by ambasilide decreases progressively as the pulse duration lengthens.

Block of the slow linear component of I_K by ambasilide is confirmed by showing that ambasilide (10 μM) further reduces I_K in the presence of E-4031 (5 μM). Figure 10 shows a representative example of the current traces obtained before and after exposure to ambasilide in the continued presence of E-4031. Block of the slow linear component of I^K is observed after a 2-second depolarization.

Ambasilide has no significant effect on I_{K1} or the calcium current.[15] The mean values of

I_{K1} at -110 mV are unchanged in the presence of 1 μM ambasilide. Peak calcium channel currents measured during step depolarizations from -45 mV to $+10$ mV also are unchanged by 1 μM ambasilide.[15]

Discussion

The data indicate that ambasilide's main effect is to lengthen the duration of the action potential at concentrations between 10^{-6} M and 10^{-5} M and to produce no effect on the maximal rate of depolarization when the fibers are stimulated at 1 Hz. The drug markedly prolongs repolarization (APD_{80}) in both canine ventricular muscle and in Purkinje fibers. Ambasilide exerts a differential effect on phase 2 of the action potential (APD_{20}) in ventricular muscle versus Purkinje fibers, prolonging the phase in the former and shortening it in the latter. In this regard, it is worth

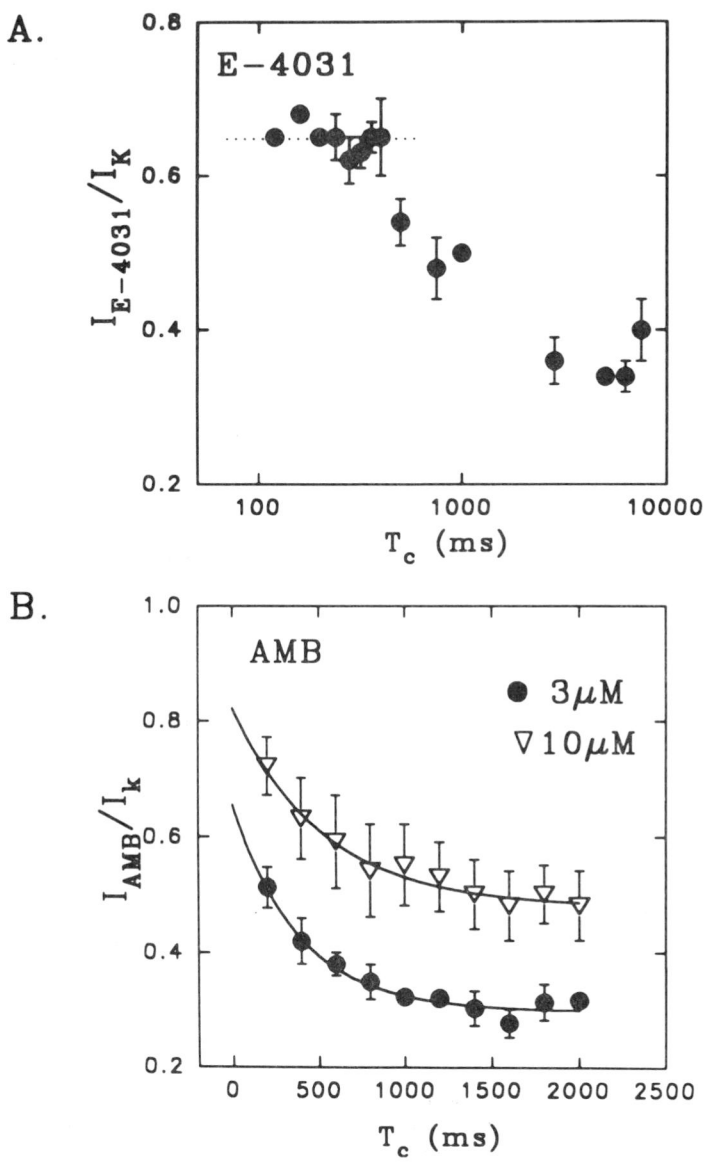

Figure 9. Fractional block of tail currents in the presence of E-4031 or ambasilide. The drug-sensitive tail currents ($I_{E\text{-}4031}$ and I_{AMB}) were normalized to the global I_K tail and plotted as a function of pulse duration. Panel A: fractional block for E-4031 5 mM (n = 7). Block was essentially the same for all depolarizations between 80 msec and 420 msec but decreased to a near steady state with longer depolarization. Panel B: Fractional block of I_K by AMB at 3 mM and 10 mM. Block by ambasilide was greatest at short depolarization and decreased progressively as the pulse duration lengthened. (Reproduced with permission from reference 15.)

A.

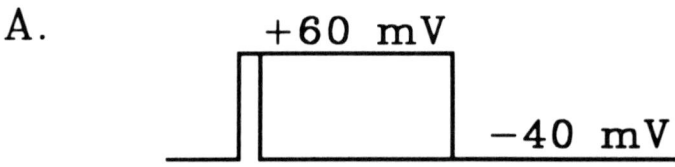

B.

E-4031

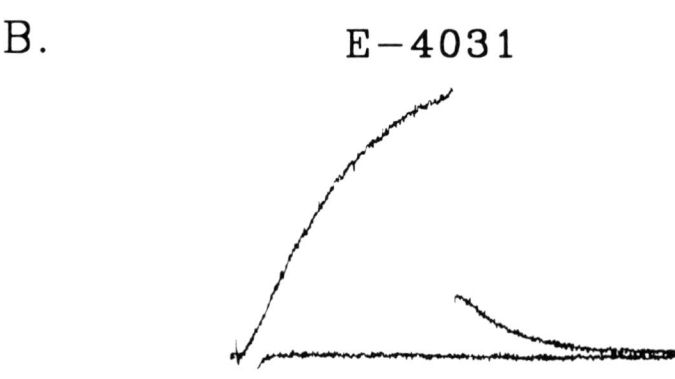

C.

E-4031+AMB

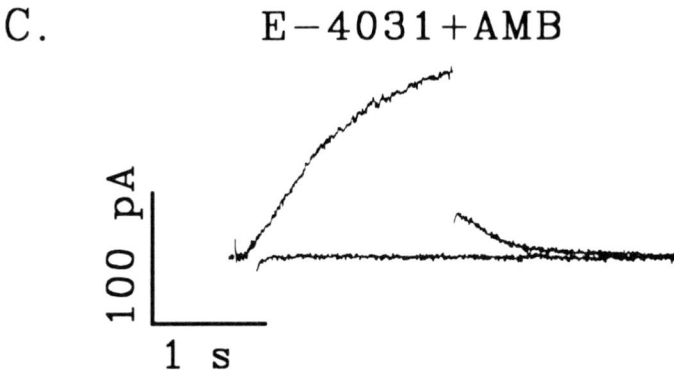

Figure 10. AMB block of the slow linear component of I_K. Panel A: protocol to elicit I_K. Panel B: I_K elicited by 200-msec and 2,000-msec depolarization steps in the continued presence of E-4031 (5 mM, 15-minute incubation period). Panel C: I_K in the presence of both E-4031 and ambasilide (AMB). In the presence of a complete block of the rapid inwardly rectifying component of I_K, AMB still blocked the I_K tail current by about 22% after the 2,000-msec depolarizing pulse. (Reproduced with permission from Reference 15.)

noting that experimental studies indicate that excessive prolongation of the APD in Purkinje fibers at low stimulation frequencies[31,32] contributes to the appearance of EADs and triggered activity, which are believed to be closely related to the development of torsade de pointes.[33-38] The initiation of EADs and triggered activity at low membrane potentials in Purkinje fibers increases the propensity for aberrant propagation to the ventricular muscle.[38-40] This is consistent with the notion that agents having the greatest proclivity to induce torsades de pointes also produce significantly greater increases in Purkinje fibers than in ventricular muscle repolarization.[31,37,38,41] Accordingly, the lack of a significant prolongation of the Purkinje-fiber APD by ambasilide in the plateau phase, particularly at higher concentrations, may reduce the probability for the development of triggered activity due to low-membrane potential EADs.

Of particular importance is the observation that ambasilide resembles amiodarone[42] insofar as its Class III action in ventricular myocardium did not vary significantly over a wide range of stimulation frequencies. Prolongation of the ventricular myocardium actually increased at faster rates, approaching the duration observed in Purkinje fibers. In both of these aspects, amiodarone and ambasilide markedly differ from other conventional and newer Class III agents. The negligible changes in $\dot{V}_{max}$ at 1 Hz suggest that ambasilide has no significant inhibitory action on fast sodium channels at normal heart rates. However, at higher stimulation frequencies, a frequency-dependent inhibition of $\dot{V}_{max}$ in both Purkinje fibers and ventricular muscle is observed. Such a frequency-dependent effect on $\dot{V}_{max}$ is commonly observed with conventional Class I drugs such as mexiletine[43] and flecainide[44]; the mechanism has been attributed to an interaction between these drugs and sodium channel receptors.[45,46] The inhibitory action on plateau sodium channels is probably important in producing the shortening of the plateau level of the action potentials in Purkinje fibers[22] and, as noted above, it may prevent, at least partially, the development of EADs and triggered activity. Whether these theoretical predictions based on studies in isolated canine myocardial tissues will be applicable directly in clinical contexts remains to be determined. To date, there is little experience with ambasilide in atrial or ventricular arrhythmias in humans.

Equally uncertain is the clinical relevance of the observations of ambasilide in isolated ventricular myocytes. In these studies, the dominant effect of ambasilide is on the delayed rectifier potassium current (I_K), which is reduced by ambasilide in a concentration related manner.[15] The drug has no significant effect on the inward rectifying potassium current (I_{K1}) nor on the slow inward calcium current (I_{Ca}). This selectivity for I_K in the guinea pig ventricular muscle is consistent with the results obtained in multicellular preparations, demonstrating that ambasilide uniformly increases ventricular muscle APD without affecting the plateau height or the resting membrane potential.

When compared with E-4031, it is apparent that ambasilide is a relatively unselective blocker of the two components of I_K, a result more closely associated with the acute actions of amiodarone,[28] rather than those of d-sotalol or many of the newer selective Class III agents.[25,47] Estimates of the EC_{50} value for block of the fast and slow components of I_K are 5.6 μM and 32 μM, respectively, assuming 1:1 drug-receptor stoichiometry.[15]

The significance of blocking the linear versus the nonlinear component of I_K may be appreciated by considering that the components will have opposite responses to changes in extracellular potassium.[29,48,49] Consider, for example, the observation that in the presence of hypokalemia (low extracellular potassium) the nonlinear component *decreases* in amplitude, while the linear component increases. The computer simulation in Figure 11 illustrates this point. Thus, the nonlinear component behaves like the inward rectifying background current (I_{K1}) by contributing less outward current to repolarization when the extracellular potassium is reduced.[29,49] One can expect, therefore, that the currently available Class III agents, as well as any agent that blocks the nonlinear component of I_K, will act synergistically with the hypokalemia-induced reduction in I_{K1} and the nonlinear I_K to prolong the cardiac APD. This idea is consistent with the observed increase in proarrhythmic events associated with Class III antiarrhythmic drugs and hypokalemia.[31,50,51]

In contrast, the linear component of I_K or any linear outward K^+ current activated

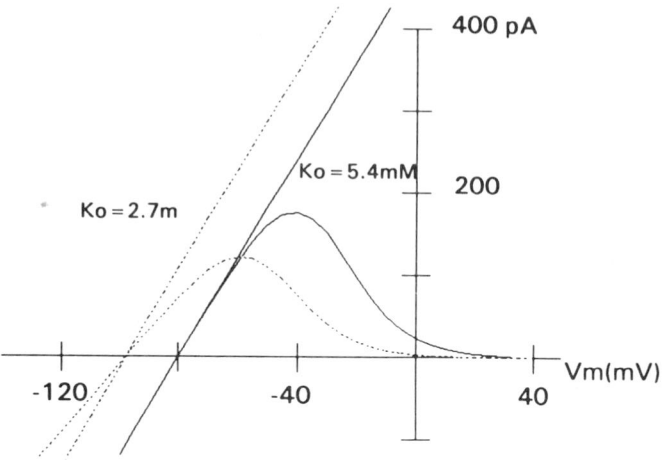

Ik_ix_Ko.gfg   30/4 pS scaled

Figure 11. Effects of external potassium (Ko) on the fully activated current-voltage relationship for the linear and nonlinear components of I_K. A reduction in external K decreases the nonlinear I_K and shifts the reversal potential toward more negative potentials. The effects are similar to that described for I_{K1}, the inward rectifying background current.[29,49] In contrast, at each potential, the linear component of I_K increases with a comparable decrease in external Ko.

during the action potential plateau (eg, I_{KATP}) will increase as a result of the increased driving force for potassium ions. This increase will tend to balance the net reduction in outward current induced by the hypokalemia. Thus, an agent that blocks only the linear component of I_K will produce APD prolongation under normal conditions but only antagonize an expected increase in the linear I_K during hypokalemia. The net effect, therefore, should be that the APD increases to the extent determined by lowering extracellular K^+ alone. This type of selectivity should yield a compound with less propensity to produce EADs, at least under conditions of hypokalemia, than the currently available agents.

The nonselective block of I_K by ambasilide is an action distinct from the newer Class III antiarrhythmics but similar to amiodarone. Selective block of the slow linear I_K may impart benefits over block of the fast nonlinear component, particularly under conditions of hypokalemia,[48] but the benefits to blocking both components is still a matter of speculation. Obviously, the electrophysiological effect will depend on the relative balance of block of each component. On the basis of the available information from studies with clofilium and amiodarone, both of which block the linear and nonlinear I_K,[22,26–28] one cannot say with certainty whether simultaneous block of both components is advantageous. On the one hand, amiodarone is a very effective antiarrhythmic agent with a low propensity to proarrhythmia.[11] On the other hand, clofilium is moderately effective and has a relatively high incidence of proarrhythmia. Thus, additional features, such as the presence and magnitude of inward current block, may play an important role. One might argue that the balance of inward and outward current block underlies the relative cardiac safety observed with amiodarone.

Recently, Hondeghem and Snyders[16]

drew attention to a potentially significant property of antiarrhythmic agents, which acted by prolonging repolarization, namely, the phenomenon of "reverse use dependence." They emphasized that, whereas agents, which acted largely by slowing fast channel mediated conduction, were more effective at fast stimulation frequencies, the so-called Class III agents such as sotalol, n-acetyl-procainamide (NAPA), and even quinidine[16] prolonged the APD_{90} in Purkinje fibers less at high stimulation frequencies and much more at low frequencies. Amiodarone does not demonstrate this behavior clinically (in the human myocardium) or in animal models following chronic administration.[16,42] Ambasilide, at least preclinical, does not exhibit "reverse use dependence" in the canine ventricular muscle. Thus, these two agents may be distinguished from "pure" Class III agents. The phenomenon of "reverse use dependence" also focuses attention on the fact that frequency-dependent APD changes are not entirely related to changes in a nonlinear quinidine-sensitive I_K. Other mechanisms governing the APD at short cycle lengths, including the block of a linear quinidine-insensitive potassium current, may play a significant role.[22,28] For example, the issue of nonspecificity of I_K block by ambasilide and amiodarone suggests that block of both components may be an electrophysiological profile, which is advantageous under certain clinical and experimental conditions. Block of inward currents, the kinetics of block, and the tissue type should also be considered because several Class I agents that appear to have a relatively high incidence of proarrhythmia exemplify those features of "reverse use dependence" considered to be desirable.[19]

Summary and Conclusions

In summary, ambasilide has a unique electrophysiological profile: it is a nonselective blocker of both components of I_K, it has no Ca^{2+} channel blocking properties, and it is a weak Na^+ channel blocker. The advantage of being devoid of Ca^{2+} channel block is uncertain and depends on whether one invokes Ca^{2+} current as a basis for the induction EADs in the presence of APD prolongation or views the absence of Ca^{2+} channel block as obviating the prospect of negative inotropy. The benefit of Na^+ channel block in the presence of K^+ channel block is also uncertain, and the potential benefits will depend on the kinetics of the drug Na^+ channel interaction in the presence of a background K^+ channel blockade: that is, whether the kinetics are flecainide-like (proarrhythmic) or amiodarone-like (antiarrhythmic) in their onset and recovery from use-dependent block.

On the basis of its electrophysiological profile, some conclusions can be reached regarding ambasilide. The drug is a newly developed Class III agent having a chemical structure and pharmacological profile distinct from the many recently developed so-called "pure" Class III agents.[22,25] Strictly speaking, however, ambasilide is not a "pure" Class III agent because it possesses weak Na^+ channel blocking properties in addition to potassium channel block, which underlies the Class III profile. Since the Na^+ channel block is seen only at rapid rates, ambasilide exhibits a conventional Class III profile at normal sinus rates. In this respect, ambasilide resembles amiodarone, but, unlike amiodarone, ambasilide has no effect on the inward calcium current,[15] and its major activity is manifest acutely. The delineation of the clinial effects of ambasilide will be of practical and theoretical importance.

References

1. Lown B: Sudden cardiac death: the major challenge confronting contemporary cardiology. *Am J Cardiol* 43:313, 1979.
2. Zipes DP: Cardiac electrophysiology: promises and contributions. *J Am Coll Cardiol* 13:1329, 1989.
3. Wellens HJJ, Brugada P: Treatment of cardiac arrhythmias: when, how and where? *J Am Coll Cardiol* 14:1417, 1989.
4. Singh BN, Courtney K: On the classification of anti-arrhythmic mechanisms: experimental

and clinical correlations. In: DP Zipes, J Jalife (eds): *Cardiac Electrophysiology: From Cell to Bedside.* Philadelphia: WB Saunders Co., 1990, p. 882.

5. Pratt CM, Francis MJ, Luck JC, et al: Analysis of ambulatory electrocardiograms in 15 patients during spontaneous ventricular fibrillation with special reference to preceding arrhythmic events. *J Am Coll Cardiol* 2:798, 1983.

6. Nikolic G, Bishop RL, Singh JB: Sudden death recorded during Holter monitoring. *Circulation* 66:218, 1982.

7. Bayes de Luna A, Coumel P, Leclerq JF: Ambulatory sudden cardiac death: mechanisms of production on the basis of data from 157 cases. *Am Heart J* 117:151, 1989.

8. The Cardiac Arrhythmia Suppression Trial (CAST) Investigators: Preliminary report: effect of encainide and flecainide on mortality in a randomized trial of arrhythmia suppression after myocardial infarction. *N Engl J Med* 321: 406, 1989.

9. Furberg CD: Effects of antiarrhythmic drugs on mortality after myocardial infarction. *Am J Cardiol* 53:32C, 1983.

10. Singh BN: Controlling cardiac arrhythmias: to delay conduction or to prolong refractoriness? (editorial) *Cardiovas Drugs Ther* 3:671, 1989.

11. Singh BN, Vaughan Williams EM: A third class of antiarrhythmic action. Effects on atrial and ventricular intracellular potentials, and other pharmacological actions on cardiac muscle, of MJ 1999 and AH 3474. *Br J Pharmacol* 39:675, 1970.

12. Singh BN, Nademanee K: Control of arrhythmias by selective lengthening of cardiac repolarization: theoretical considerations and clinical observations. *Am Heart J* 109:421, 1985.

13. Singh BN: *Control of Cardiac Arrhythmia by Lengthening Repolarization.* Mt. Kisco, NY: Futura Publishing Co., Inc., 1988, p1.

14. Takanaka C, Sarma JSM, Singh BN: Electrophysiologic effects of ambasilide (LU-47110), a new Class III antiarrhythmic agent, on isolated canine rabbit cardiac muscle. *J Cardiovasc Pharmacol* 19:290, 1992.

15. Zhang ZH, Follmer CH, Sarma JSM, et al: Effect of ambasilide, a new Class III agent, on plateau currents in isolated guinea-pig ventricular myocytes: block of delayed outward currents. *J Pharmacol Exp Ther* 263:40, 1992.

16. Hondeghem LM, Snyders DJ: Class III antiarrhythmic agents have a lot of potential but a long way to go: reduced effectiveness and dangers of reverse use dependence. *Circulation* 81:686, 1990.

17. Yabek SM, Kato R, Singh BN: Effects of amiodarone and its metabolite, desethylamiodarone,

on the electrophysiologic properties of isolated cardiac muscle. *J Cardiovasc Pharmacol* 8:197, 1986.

18. Colatsky TJ, Follmer CH: Potassium channels as targets for antiarrhythmic drug action. *Drug Dev Res* 19:129, 1990.

19. Colatsky TJ: Mechanisms of action of lidocaine and quinidine on action potential duration in rabbit cardiac Purkinje fibers. *Circ Res* 50:17, 1982.

20. Varro A, Nakaya Y, Elharrar V, Surawicz B: Effect of antiarrhythmic drugs on the cycle-length dependent action potential duration in dog Purkinje and ventricular muscle fibers. *J Cardiovasc Pharmacol* 8:178, 1986.

21. Coraboeuf E, Deroubaix E, Coulombe A: Effects of tetrodotoxin on action potentials of the conduction system in dog heart. *Am J Physiol* 236: H561, 1979.

22. Colatsky TJ, Follmer CH, Starmer CF: Channel specificity in antiarrhythmic drug action. *Circulation* 82:2235, 1990.

23. Kou WH, Nelson SD, Lynch JJ, et al: Effect of flecainide acetate on prevention of electrical induction of ventricular tachycardia and occurrence of ischemic ventricular fibrillation during the early postmyocardial infarction period: evaluation in a conscious canine model of sudden death. *J Am Coll Cardiol* 9:359, 1987.

24. Varro A, Saitoh H, Surawicz B: Effect of antiarrhythmic drugs on premature action potential duration in canine ventricular muscle fibers. *J Cardiovasc Pharmacol* 10:407, 1987.

25. Colatsky TJ, Follmer CH: Potassium channel blockers and activators in the treatment of cardiac arrhythmias. *Cardiovasc Drug Rev* 7:199, 1989.

26. Arena JP, Kass RS: Block of heart potassium channels by clofilium and its tertiary analogs: relationship between drug structure and type of channel blocked. *Mol Pharmacol* 34: 606, 1988.

27. Colatsky TJ: Modulation of cardiac repolarization currents by antiarrhythmic drugs. In: MR Rosen, MJ Janse, AL Wit (eds): *Cardiac Electrophysiology: A Textbook.* Mount Kisco, NY: Futura Publishing Co., Inc., 1990, p. 1043.

28. Balser JR, Bennett RB, Hondeghem LM, et al: Suppression of time-dependent outward current in guinea pig ventricular myocytes: actions of quinidine and amiodarone. *Circ Res* 69: 519, 1991.

29. Sanguinetti M, Jurkiewicz N: Two types of delayed rectifier K^+ currents in guinea pig ventricular myocytes. *J Gen Physiol* 96:196, 1990.

30. Shrier A, Clay JR: Repolarization currents in embryonic chick atrial heart cell aggregated. *Biophys J* 50:861, 1986.

31. Roden DM, Hoffman BF: Action potential prolongation and induction of abnormal automaticity by low quinidine concentrations in canine Purkinje fibers. *Circ Res* 56:867, 1985.

32. Nattel S, Zeng F: Frequency-dependent effects of antiarrhythmic drugs on action potential duration and refractoriness of canine cardiac Purkinje fibers. *J Pharmacol Exp Ther* 229:283, 1984.

33. Roden DM, Thompson KA, Hoffman BF, Woosley RL: Clinical features and basic mechanisms of quinidine-induced arrhythmias. *J Am Coll Cardiol* 8:73A, 1986.

34. Brachmann J, Scherlag BJ, Rosenshtraukh LV, Lazzara R: Bradycardia-dependent triggered activity: relevance to drug-induced multiform ventricular tachycardia. *Circulation* 68:846, 1983.

35. Damiano BP, Rosen MR: Effects of pacing on triggered activity induced by early afterdepolarizations. *Circulation* 69:103, 1984.

36. El-Sherif N, Zeiler RH, Craelius W, et al.: QTU prolongation and polymorphic ventricular tachycardia due to bradycardia-dependent early afterdepolarization. *Circulation* 63:286, 1988.

37. Laakso M, Pentikainen PJ, Pyorala K, Neuvonen PJ: Prolongation of the QT interval caused by sotalol-possible association with ventricular tachyarrhythmias. *Eur Heart J* 2:253, 1981.

38. Olshansky B, Martina J, Hunt S: N-acetylprocainamide causing torsades de pointes. *Am J Cardiol* 50:1439, 1982.

39. Takanaka C, Singh BH: Barium-induced nondriven action potentials as a model of triggered automaticity and early afterdepolarizations: differing effects of amiodarone and quinidine and significance of slow-channel activity. *J Am Coll Cardiol* 15:213, 1990.

40. January CT, Riddle JM, Salata JJ: A model for early afterdepolarizations: induction with Ca^{++} channel agonist Bay K 8644. *Circ Res* 62:563, 1988.

41. El-Sherif N, Craelius W, Boutjdir M, Gough WB: Early afterdepolarizations and arrhythmogenesis. *J Cardiovasc Electrophysiol* 1:145, 1990.

42. Anderson KP, Walker R, Dustman T, et al: Rate-related electrophysiologic effects of long-term administration of amiodarone on canine ventricular myocardium in vivo. *Circulation* 79:948, 1989.

43. Campbell TJ: Resting and rate-dependent depression of maximum rate of depolarization (V_{max}) in guinea pig ventricular action potentials by mexiletine, disopyramide, and encainide. *J Cardiovasc Pharmacol* 5:291, 1983.

44. Campbell TJ, Vaughan Williams EM: Voltage- and time- dependent depression of maximum rate of depolarization of guinea-pig ventricular action potential by two new antiarrhythmic drugs, flecainide and lorcainide. *Cardiovasc Res* 17:241, 1983.

45. Hondeghem LM, Katzung BG: Time- and voltage-dependent interactions of antiarrhythmic drugs with cardiac sodium channels. *Biochem Biophys Acta* 472:373, 1977.

46. Hille B: Local anesthetics: hydrophilic and hydrophobic pathways for drug-receptor reaction. *J Gen Physiol* 69:497, 1977.

47. Funck-Brentano C, Kibleur Y, Coz FL, et al: Rate dependence of sotalol-induced prolongation of ventricular repolarization during exercise in humans. *Circulation* 83:536, 1991.

48. Courtney KR, Hill BC, Follmer CH: The importance of K^+ channel rectification to cardiac repolarization. *Proc West Pharmacol Soc* 35:177, 1992.

49. Hille B, Schwarz W: Potassium channels as multi-ion pores. *J Gen Physiol* 72:409, 1978.

50. Singh BN: When is QT prolongation anti-arrhythmic and when is it pro-arrhythmic? *Am J Cardiol* 63:867, 1989.

51. Weissenberger J, Davy J-M, Chezalviel F, et al: Arrhythmogenic activities of antiarrhythmic drugs in conscious hypokalemic dogs with atrioventricular block: comparison between quinidine, lidocaine, flecainide, propranolol and sotalol. *J Pharmacol Exp Ther* 259:871, 1991.

52. Nishimura M, Follmer CH, Singer DH: Amiodarone blocks calcium current in single guinea pig ventricular myocytes. *J Pharmacol Exp Ther* 251:650, 1989.

Chapter 43

Electrophysiological and Hemodynamic Effects of WAY-123,398, a New Class III Antiarrhythmic Agent

Walter Spinelli
Issam F. Moubarak
Roderick W. Parsons
Thomas J. Colatsky

WAY-123,398 is a Class III antiarrhythmic agent that exerts its therapeutic effect by selectively prolonging repolarization in the heart. It was designed using risotilide,[1] a selective blocker of the delayed rectifier current as a template. The synthesis and structure-activity relationship of WAY-123,398 and related compounds have been described in detail.[2] This chapter reviews the basic pharmacology of WAY-123,398, and the cellular basis for its Class III activity.

Results

Cellular Electrophysiology in Canine Purkinje Fibers

WAY-123,398 prolonged action potential duration (APD) in canine Purkinje fibers in a concentration-dependent manner (Figure 1) without altering maximum diastolic potential or the maximum rate of depolarization of phase 0 ($\dot{V}_{max}$). During pacing at a basic cycle length (BCL) of 300 msec (Figure 2, top), WAY-123,398 increased APD with an EC_{20} (ie, the concentration producing a 20% increase of APD measured as the time to repolarize to -60 mV, APD_{-60}) of 0.21 ± 0.08 μM ($\bar{x}$ ± SE). For comparison, the EC_{20} for dofetilide, E-4031, and dl-sotalol were, respectively, < 0.01 mM, 0.03 ± 0.02 μM, and 38 ± 8 μM. Despite the difference in potency, WAY-123,398 was as effective as dofetilide at this cycle length. The maximum increase of APD_{-60} observed was 40 ± 7% with WAY-123,398 (3 μM) and 42% with dofetilide (0.3 μM). The large increase of APD shows that WAY-123,398 possesses a significant Class III activity at rates of pacing (200 beats per min-

---

From BN Singh, HJJ Wellens, M Hiraoka, (eds): *Electropharmacological Control of Cardiac Arrhythmias.* Mount Kisco, NY, Futura Publishing Company Inc., © 1994.

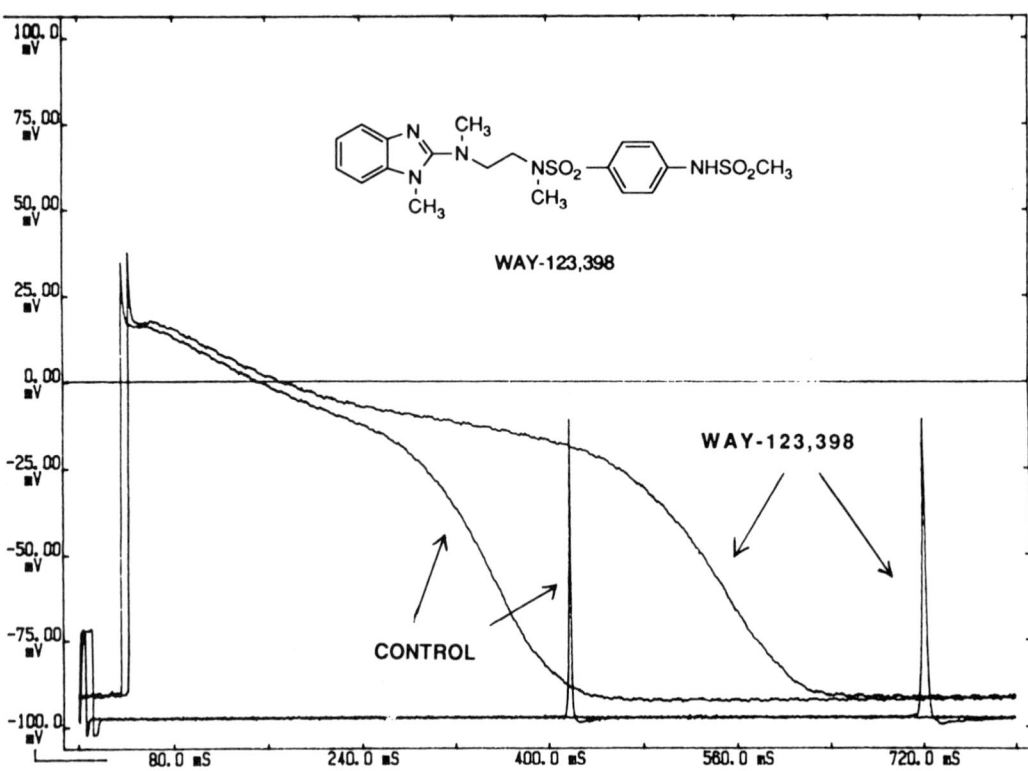

Figure 1. Effects of WAY-123,398 (3 μM) on the transmembrane potential of a canine Purkinje fiber (BCL = 1000 msec). Top trace: 0 mV reference line; middle traces: transmembrane potentials; bottom traces: calibration signals for $\dot{V}_{max}$ (200 V/sec; extreme left) and $\dot{V}_{max}$ signals. WAY-123,398 prolongs repolarization without affecting the other parameters of the action potential. (Reproduced with permission from Reference 18.)

ute) characteristic of an episode of tachycardia.

At BCL = 1,000 msec (Figure 2, bottom), a cycle length more typical of normal sinus rate, the effects of WAY-123,398 on APD appeared to saturate between 0.3 μM and 3 μM, while in contrast, dofetilide and E-4031 continued to produce additional increases in APD that were linear over the range of concentrations used. At the highest concentration, dofetilide (0.3 μM) increased APD-60 by 101% ± 15% and E-4031 (1 μM) by 100% ± 13%, which was about twice as great as the increase produced by WAY-123,398. Excessive prolongation of APD at slow rates of beating is generally regarded as an undesirable property because it might induce proarrhythmia.[3,4]

Electrophysiology and Hemodynamics in Anesthetized Dogs

The electrophysiological and hemodynamic effects of WAY-123,398 were studied in pentobarbital-anesthetized open-chest dogs following cumulative intravenous administration at doses of 0.25–10 mg/kg (Figure 3). WAY-123,398 produced dose-dependent increases in atrial and ventricular refractoriness (AERP and VERP) without affecting atrial or ventricular conduction times (ACT and VCT). During pacing at BCL = 300 msec, the dose of WAY-123,398 that increased VERP by 20% (ED_{20}) was 1.2 mg/kg, which was higher than the ED_{20} for dofetilide (0.04 mg/kg) and E-

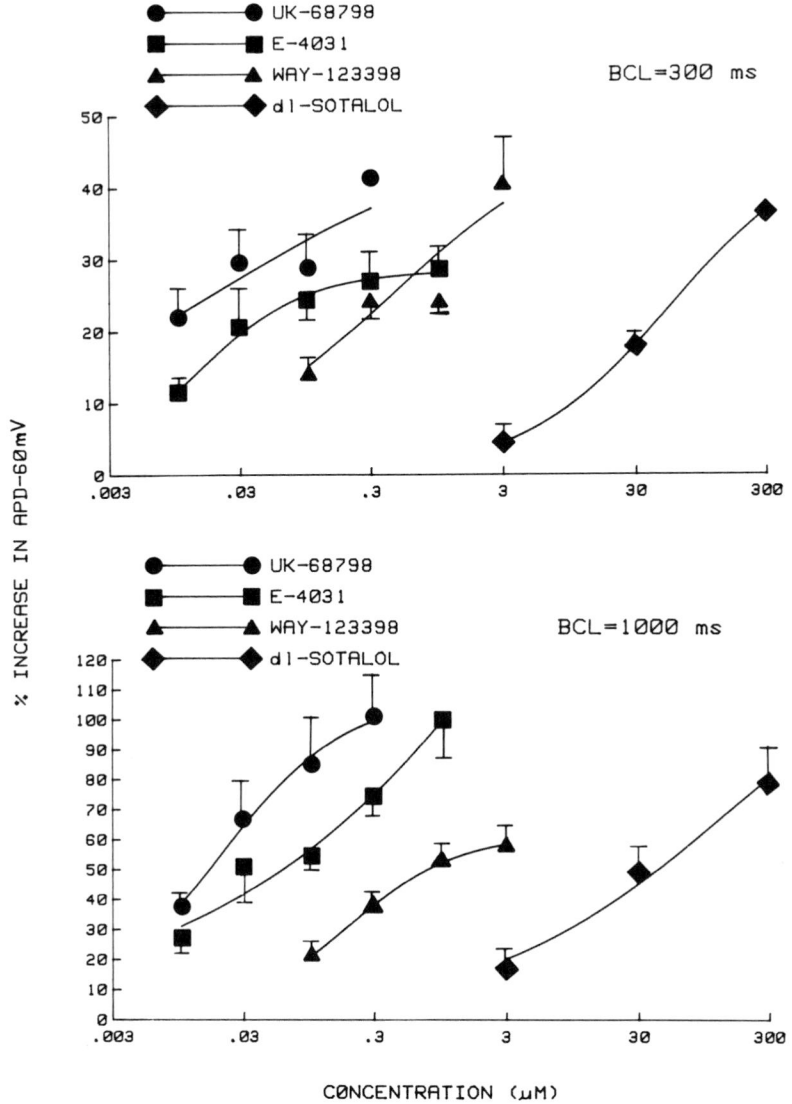

Figure 2. Concentration response curves of action potential duration (APD) prolongation during pacing at BCL = 300 msec (top figure) and 1000 msec (bottom figure). Action potential duration is measured to −60 mV (APD$_{-60}$ mV); results are expressed as percent prolongation from predrug values (reported in Tables 1 and 2). (Reproduced with permission from Reference 18.)

4031 (0.09 mg/kg), but similar to that for dl-sotalol (1.6 mg/kg). Over the range of doses used in these experiments, the prolongation of AERP produced by each agent was, in general, twice as large as that observed for VERP at the same dose. The potent effects of these compounds on atrial refractoriness suggest that WAY-123,398 and the reference com-

pounds would be highly effective against atrial arrhythmias at doses that produce little change in ventricular refractoriness.

In these experiments, WAY-123,398, E-4031, and dl-sotalol decreased heart rate and mean arterial pressure dose dependently, with dl-sotalol having the largest effect (Figure 4). Dofetilide had no significant effect on

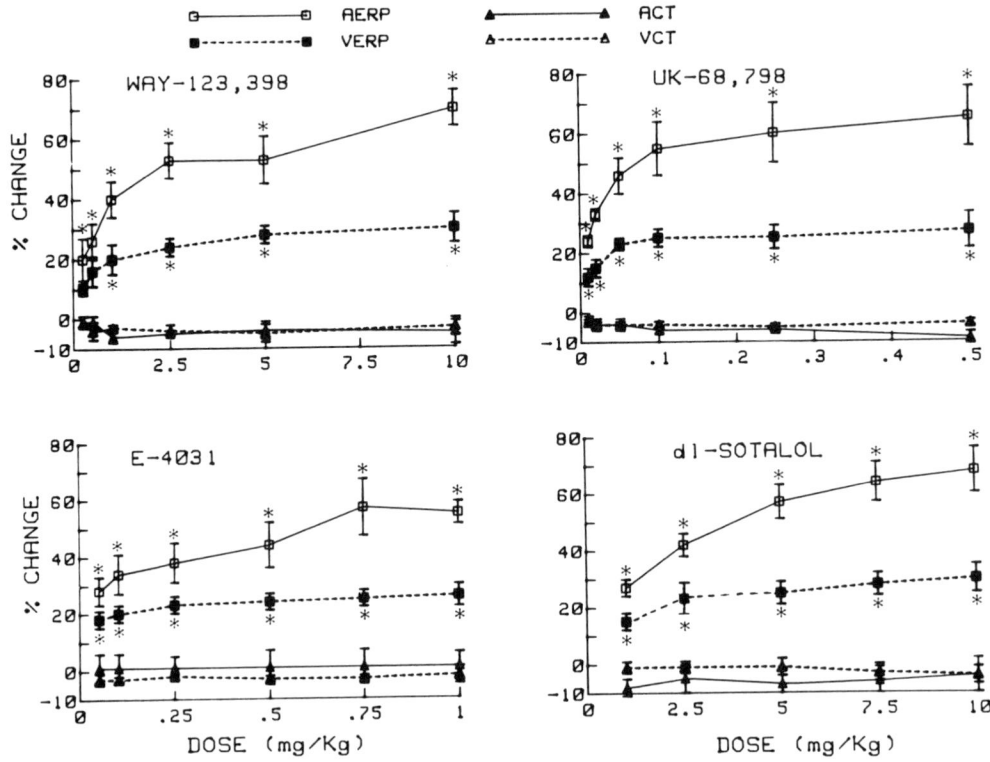

Figure 3. Effects on refractoriness and conduction times in atrial and ventricular tissue expressed as percent change from predrug. WAY-123,398 and the other compounds produced a dose-dependent increase of atrial and ventricular refractoriness (AERP and VERP) of comparable magnitude without affecting conduction times (ACT and VCT). (Reproduced with permission from Reference 6.)

mean blood pressure, although it exerted the same bradycardic action as the other compounds. While β blockade might contribute to the slowing of heart rate induced by sotalol, other mechanisms are likely to be involved for WAY-123,398, E-4031, and dofetilide, which are devoid of β-blocking activity. These mechanisms include a prolongation of the sinus node action potential due to block of the delayed rectifier current,[5] and/or a depression of phase 4 depolarization of the pacemaker cells. This latter mechanism is supported by the observation that WAY-123,398, dofetilide, and E-4031 all significantly increase sinus node recovery time.[6]

At doses producing a similar and very large increase in ventricular refractoriness (about +25%), WAY-123,398 and dofetilide

had similar hemodynamic effects, while dl-sotalol and E-4031 produced much larger decreases in heart rate and arterial pressure (Table 1). In the case of dl-sotalol, these results are likely to reflect its β-blocking action,[7] which is also likely to be responsible for the large increase in atrioventricular conduction time (A-H time) observed with every dose of dl-sotalol.[6] WAY-123,398 and dofetilide, despite the large increase in AERP, did not significantly alter the A-H time, but increased the maximum following frequency of the ventricle during atrial pacing (WCL), suggesting the existence of frequency-dependent effects on nodal refractoriness for these two compounds.[6] None of the four compounds caused a significant increase of H-V time, again indicating a lack of Class I activity.

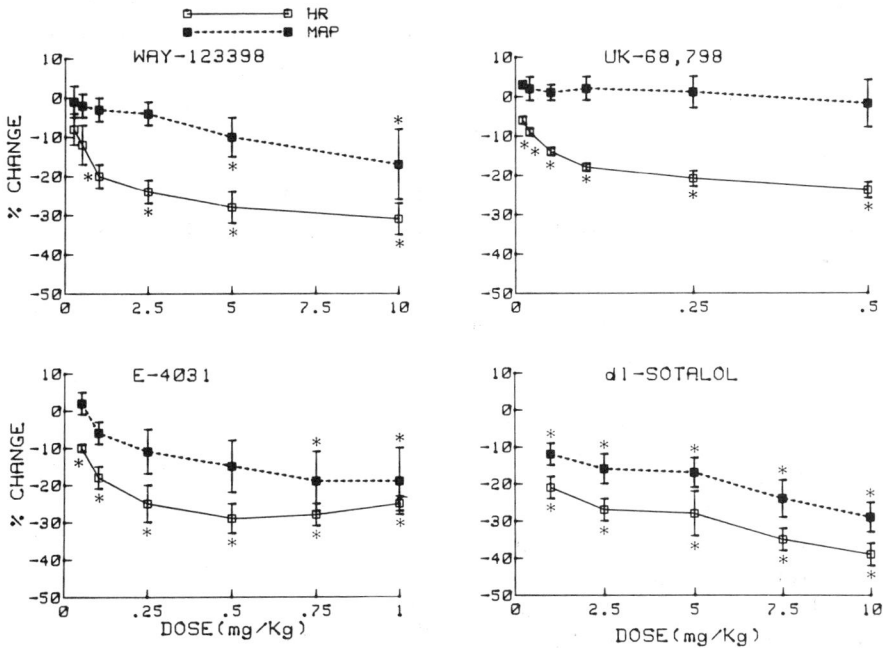

Figure 4. Effects on heart rate (HR) and mean arterial pressure (MAP) expressed as percent change from predrug. WAY-123,398 and the other compounds produced a dose-dependent decrease of HR and MAP: the decrease was largest with dl-sotalol. Unlike the other compounds, UK-69,798 did not affect HR. (Reproduced with permission from Reference 6.)

Studies of Antiarrhythmic Efficacy: Effects on Ventricular Fibrillation Threshold

The effects of WAY-123,398 on the threshold for electrical induction of ventricular fibrillation were determined to provide a measure of efficacy against a form of lethal arrhythmia most likely resulting from micro-reentry.[8,9] Ventricular fibrillation was induced during atrial pacing at a BCL = 300 msec by trains of pulses delivered to the right ventricle every 8 paced beats. The beginning of the train of pulses was timed to initiate approximately 50 msec after the peak of the R wave of the electrocardiogram. The smallest current intensity producing sustained ventricular fibrillation was defined as the ventricular fibrilla-

Table 1
Comparison of Effects on Hemodynamics *vs* Effects on Refractoriness

Compound	Dose (mg/kg)	VERP	AERP	HR	MBP	A-H	WCL
WAY-123,398	2.5	24 ± 3*	53 ± 6*	−24 ± 3*	−4 ± 3	9 ± 2	30 ± 5*
Dofetilide	0.1	25 ± 3*	55 ± 9*	−18 ± 1*	2 ± 3	4 ± 3	23 ± 5*
E-4031	0.5	24 ± 3*	44 ± 8*	−29 ± 4*	−15 ± 7*	19 ± 5*	22 ± 7*
dl-sotalol	5	25 ± 4*	57 ± 6*	−28 ± 6*	−17 ± 4*	56 ± 16*	36 ± 8*

Results are expressed as % of predrug values; x̄ ± S.E.; * $p < 0.05$ vs. predrug; VERP, AERP, and A-H times measured during pacing at BCL = 300 msec.

tion threshold (VFT). When ventricular fibrillation was induced, the heart was defibrillated within 5 seconds.[6]

The results of this study are summarized in Table 2. The doses used were selected to produce similar, large increases of VERP with each compound (Table 1). Use of higher doses of dl-sotalol was limited by hemodynamic effects that could have biased the comparison. All four compounds produced significant increases in VFT. However, administration of the Class III agents was sometimes associated with a spontaneous reversion to sinus rhythm prior to application of electric countershock. One example is shown in Figure 5A. The upper trace shows a lead II ECG tracing in a dog treated with WAY-123,398 (2.5 mg/kg). A train of stimuli delivered to the ventricle (marked by arrow) produced a run of polymorphic ventricular tachycardia/ventricular fibrillation. During the arrhythmia, the arterial pressure (lower trace) did not show any evidence of pulse pressure and rapidly approached 0. After approximately 8 seconds the arrhythmia suddenly reversed to sinus rhythm and the arterial pressure quickly recovered. This finding was observed in 2 of 6 dogs treated with WAY-123,398 and dofetilide, and 1 of 6 dogs treated with E-4031. No reversion to sinus rhythm without electrical countershock was observed after treatment with dl-sotalol or after vehicle (Figure 5B). Episodes of spontaneous reversion from electrically-induced fi-

brillation have been reported by other investigators after treatment with the Class III agents clofilium,[10] bretylium and bethanidine,[11] dofetilide,[12] and dl-sotalol.[13,14]

Additional Studies of Antiarrhythmic Efficacy

In a conscious canine model of sterile pericarditis, slow intravenous infusion of WAY-123,398 (1–2 mg/kg) produced large increases of atrial refractoriness (+40% after 2 mg/kg) without affecting atrial conduction. Flutter fibrillation was terminated in each animal (mean infused dose: 0.3 mg/kg). In a separate study, after terminating the arrhythmia, WAY-123,398 (1–2 mg/kg) prevented the reinduction of a stable flutter fibrillation for more than 30 minutes.[15]

In anesthetized cats with a healed myocardial infarction, WAY-123,398 (5 mg/kg IV) caused a significant increase in ventricular refractoriness both at baseline and after acute coronary occlusion; during ischemia, WAY-123,398 prevented the increase in dispersion of refractoriness and produced a large increase in VFT. Ventricular fibrillation induced during VFT testing was self-terminating in 4 of 8 cats; vehicle administration had no electrophysiological effects and did not terminate ventricular fibrillation.[16]

Table 2
Effects on Ventricular Fibrillation Threshold (VFT) and
Ventricular Refractory Period (VERP)

		VFT (mA)		VERP (msec)	
Treatment	N	Predrug	Treatment	Predrug	Treatment
Control	9	8 ± 1	9 ± 1	150 ± 4	143 ± 11
WAY-123,398 (2.5 mg/kg)	6	8 ± 2	24 ± 10*	165 ± 3	211 ± 9*
Dofetilide (0.1 mg/kg)	6	10 ± 1	22 ± 6*	159 ± 6	207 ± 13*
E-4031 (0.5 mg/kg)	6	12 ± 1	42 ± 9*	141 ± 2	175 ± 7*
dl-sotalol (2.5 mg/kg)	5	7 ± 2	36 ± 4*	142 ± 6	177 ± 10*

VFT and VERP measured during pacing at BCL = 300 msec.
* $p < 0.05$ vs pre-drug.

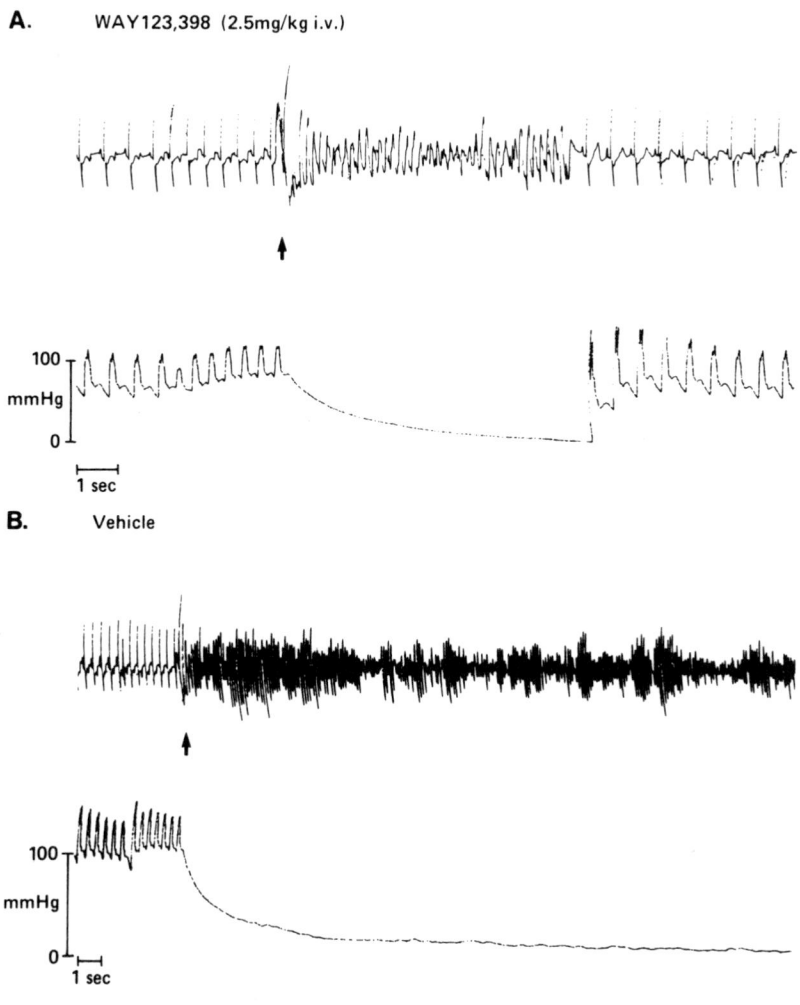

Figure 5. Restoration of sinus rhythm without electrical cardioversion by WAY-123,398 in one open-chest dog. In predrug conditions (B), electrical stimulation of the ventricle during the vulnerable period (marked by arrow) produces ventricular fibrillation (top trace: ECG) and hemodynamic collapse (bottom trace: arterial pressure). After administration of WAY-123,398 (2.5 mg/kg) (A), ventricular fibrillation terminates spontaneously after about 10 seconds with restoration of sinus rhythm. (Reproduced with permission from Reference 6.)

Proarrhythmia and Early Afterdepolarizations

Minimal proarrhythmic effects were observed with WAY-123,398 in anesthetized dogs, and consisted of occasional premature ventricular depolarizations (PVDs) observed during periods of sinus bradycardia at very high doses (higher than 7.5 mg/kg IV). In every case, the PVDs were promptly abolished when the heart was paced at a faster cycle length (300 msec). No arrhythmias occurred during normal sinus rhythm or during pacing. In normal conscious dogs, occasional PVDs were observed after high doses (higher than 10 mg/kg) following a normal sinus beat characterized by a particularly long cycle length. The results of these studies suggest that the proarrhythmic effects with WAY-123,398 are dose-dependent and occur after doses that produce a large prolongation of the QT interval and in presence of bradycardia.

It is possible that the proarrhythmia induced by WAY-123,398 is related to the production of early afterdepolarizations (EADs).[17] The induction of EADs was studied in canine Purkinje fibers perfused with normal Tyrode's solution (K_o = 4 mM) paced at long BCLs to simulate severe bradycardia. The drug concentrations used in this study were selected to produce similar increase of APD_{-60} in fibers paced at BCL = 800 msec (Figure 6, top). WAY-123,398 (0.3 μM) prolonged APD_{-60} by 55% ± 5% (SEM), dofetilide (0.03 μM) prolonged APD_{-60} by 62% ± 9% and E-4031 (0.1 μM) by 64% ± 7%. When the BCL of stimulation was increased to 1,500 and 2,500 msec, WAY-123,398 caused the least

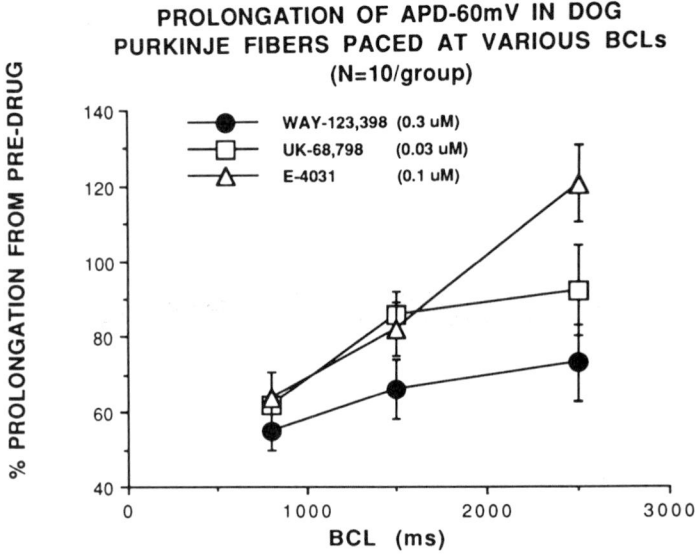

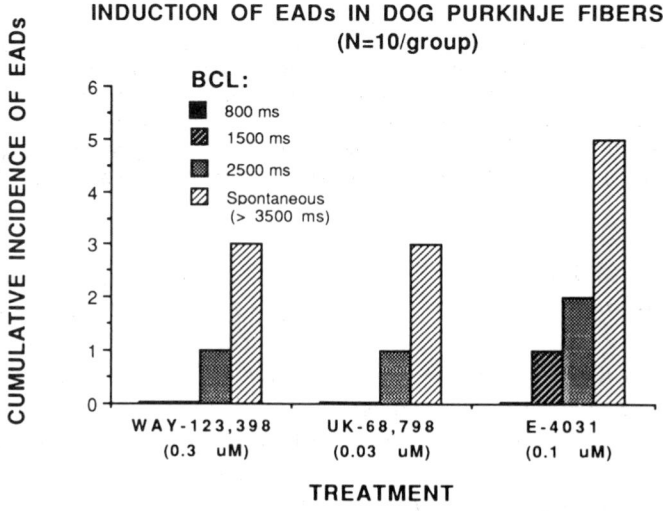

Figure 6. Top: Effects on APD_{-60} mV (expressed as percent of predrug) at various basic cycle lengths. Bottom: frequency of EADs at various basic cycle lengths.

prolongation of APD: EADs were produced in 3 fibers out of 10 and only at cycle lengths longer than 2,500 msec. Dofetilide (0.03 μM) induced EADs with the same frequency and at the same cycle lengths, while E-4031 (0.1 μM) produced EADs in 5 of 10 fibers and at shorter cycle lengths (Figure 6, bottom).

Cellular Mechanism of Action

The effects of WAY-123,398 on membrane currents were studied in cat ventricular myocytes superfused with normal Tyrode's solution (K_o = 4 mM; t = 36°C) using patch clamp techniques.[18] Under control condi-

tions, depolarizing steps more positive than −45 mV ($V_{holding}$) elicit a family of time-dependent outward currents that develop slowly over several hundred milliseconds (Figure 7). Upon repolarization to −45 mV, each outward current trace is followed by a slowly decaying outward current tail. These tail currents have been shown to represent the deactivation of the delayed rectifier K current (I_K)[19] and their peak amplitude measured in reference to holding current provides an estimate of the current activated during the depolarizing step. The cat differs from guinea pig in that the delayed rectifier current appears to consist of a single component that is sensitive to E-4031.[20] In this experiment, WAY-123,398

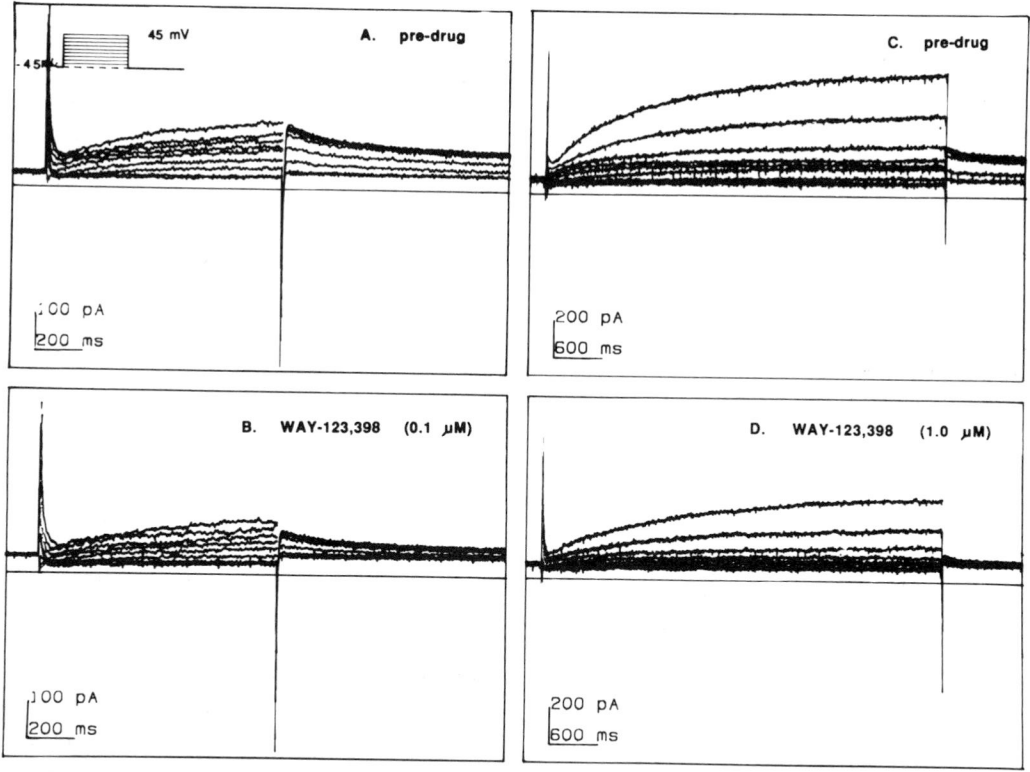

Figure 7. Effects of WAY-123,398 on the delayed rectifier K⁺ current (I_K) (voltage protocol shown above the current traces in part A). In A and B WAY-123,398 (0.1 μM) decreases the time-dependent outward currents developing during the depolarization steps and the tail currents elicited on repolarization to holding voltage. In C and D, in a different myocyte, a 10-fold higher concentration (1.0 μM) almost abolishes tail currents, but only decreases the time-dependent outward currents. Nisoldipine (300 μM) is present in Tyrode's solution to block I_{Ca-L}; I_{Na} is inactivated at Vh = −45 mV. (Reproduced with permission from Reference 18.)

(0.1 μM) caused a considerable decrease (about 50%) in the amplitude of both the time-dependent component during the depolarizing step and of the tail currents upon repolarization to holding potential (Figure 7A and 7B). In a different myocyte, tail currents following 5,000-msec long depolarizing steps are almost totally blocked by WAY-123,398 (1 μM) (Figure 7D); despite the profound effect on tail currents, the time-dependent currents are only modestly affected showing a reduction of roughly 40%. Block of the tail currents was prompt, reaching a steady state after about 5 minutes of superfusion, and was quickly reversible upon washout.

It is well known that the prolongation of APD by Class III agents is frequency dependent and decreases at faster rates of stimulation.[4] To examine the effects of different rates of depolarization on the block of tail currents by WAY-123,398, the relationship between APD and frequency of pacing was approximated by increasing the duration of depolarization steps from 200 to 500 msec as the interpulse interval was increased from 1,000 to 5,000 msec. The IC_{50} for block of tail currents was 0.085 μM at 1,000 msec and 0.11 μM at 5,000 msec. The small difference in estimated IC_{50} values at the two cycle lengths was not statistically significant ($p > 0.05$), suggesting that WAY-123,398 had similar efficacy in blocking I_K tails despite large differences in the duration and frequency of depolarization.

The effects of WAY-123,398 appeared to be selective for the delayed rectifier current, as no effects on inward rectifier (I_{K1}), transient outward (I_{to}), or L-type calcium currents were observed at 10 μM, a concentration two orders of magnitude larger than the IC_{50} for blocking I_K tails.

The relationship between frequency of depolarization and block of I_K tail currents was further examined in a separate group of experiments in which the duration of the depolarizing steps was held constant. For these experiments we used voltage steps spanning the voltage range experienced during the action potential: from a holding voltage of -90 mV, myocytes were depolarized to $+30$ mV for 250 msec and then repolarized back to

-90 mV and held at this voltage until the beginning of the next cycle. After repeating this conditioning protocol for 19 cycles the myocytes were finally repolarized to -55 mV and the amplitude of the tail current measured. By altering the residence time at -90 mV tail currents were measured in the same cell in absence of conditioning protocol and after conditioning at BCL of 400, 800, 1,500, 2,500 msec; I_{Na} and I_{Ca-L} were blocked by adding TTX (30 μM) and nisoldipine (300 nM) in Tyrode's solution. The protocol used and the results obtained from six myocytes are summarized in Figure 8. Under predrug conditions, the amplitude of the tail current (measured for this protocol in reference to 0 current) was stable over a wide range of cycle lengths, which indicates a lack of residual activation between depolarizing steps even at the shortest cycle length, and not different from the amplitude of the tail measured in the absence of conditioning steps (referred to as single step in Figure 8). After superfusion with WAY-123,398 (0.3 μM), the tail amplitude was decreased using single step by about 80 pA at every cycle length, which was similar to the amount of block observed without any conditioning step.

These results did not show any evidence of decreased block of I_K at shorter cycle lengths, a phenomenon that has been named reverse use dependence.[3] The magnitude of the drug-sensitive current blocked by WAY-123,398 (about 80 pA at 0.3 μM) compares well with the amount of block observed in previous concentration response experiments, when the size of the current was measured with reference to the holding current at -40 mV (see Figure 7 for comparison). Similar results showing a lack of reverse use dependence were also obtained in four similar experiments in which the myocytes were held at -82 mV during the conditioning protocol; -82 mV corresponds to the average reversal potential with our experimental conditions. Considering these data, it seems reasonable to suggest that the decrease of efficacy of Class III agents at a faster rate of beating might be explained by a concomitant increase of

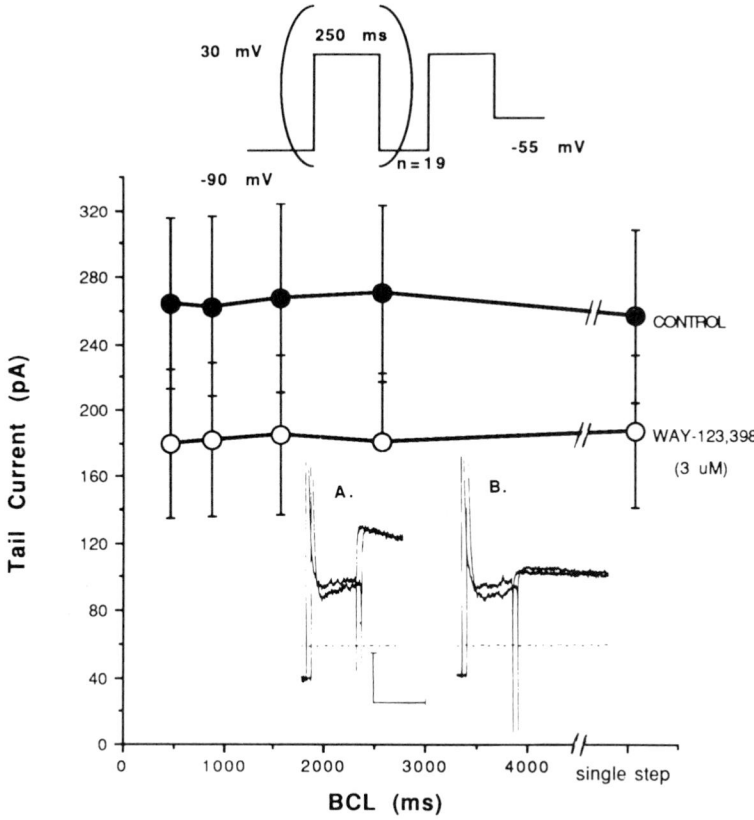

Figure 8. Effects of a train of depolarizing pulses on the block of I_K tails by WAY-123,398. Depolarizing pulses delivered at basic cycle lengths (BCLs) ranging from 400 to 2500 msec did not affect the inhibition of I_K tail. The protocol is shown on top. A: Example of tail currents after a single depolarizing step (first trace) and after a conditioning train with BCL = 400 msec (second trace). B: WAY-123,398 causes a similar block after a single step (left trace) and after a conditioning train (BCL = 400 msec). Calibration: 250 msec and 100 pA; dotted lines show 0 current level.

other repolarizing currents and not by an intrinsic "reverse use dependence" as it has been reported for quinidine, a Class I agent with significant effects on I_K channels.[21,22]

Effects on Binding to Receptor Sites

The specificity of action of WAY-123,398 was further examined by studying its effects in receptor binding assays. WAY-123,398 (10^{-9} M, 10^{-7} M, 10^{-5} M) did not affect binding to adrenergic, cholinergic, dopaminergic, and serotoninergic binding sites. No effects were observed at binding sites for amino acids, benzodiazepine, adenosine, histamine$_1$, opioid, prostanoid, phorbol ester (protein kinase C), and forskolin (adenylate cyclase) binding sites. Finally, WAY-123,398 did not have any activity at binding sites for nitrendipine (L-type Ca^{2+} channels), omegaconotoxin (N-type Ca^{2+} channels), apamin ($K_{Ca\text{-small}}$ channels), t-butylbicycloorthobenzoate (Cl^- channels).

Conclusion

The results obtained from voltage recording in Purkinje fibers and current recordings in isolated myocytes indicate that WAY-123,398 is an effective Class III agent devoid of Class I activity. Voltage-clamp studies of the mechanism of action show that WAY-123,398 selectively blocks the delayed rectifier K current (I_K) at concentrations comparable to those prolonging APD in Purkinje fibers. Studies in the whole animal have shown that WAY-123,398 prolongs refractoriness without depressing conduction, and that doses producing a very large increase of refractoriness have limited hemodynamic effects. Studies in several animal models have shown good efficacy against atrial and ventricular arrhythmias whose mechanism is thought to be reentry. It is reasonable to suggest that WAY-123,398 produces a large prolongation of refractoriness without affecting conduction and thus blocks the reentrant impulse by causing it to encounter tissue in the reentry pathway that has not yet recovered excitability. An agent with such profile of action should lack the proarrhythmic effects of Class I agents that result from excessive depression of conduction and from negative inotropic effects.[23] By increasing the duration of the plateau of the action potential, a specific Class III agent may have a limited positive inotropic effect, which could be beneficial in the treatment of arrhythmias in patients suffering from heart failure. Intravenous infusion of WAY-123,398 (5 mg/kg over 30 minutes) in anesthetized dogs produced a sustained increase of contractility which, although not statistically significant, was clear and maintained for hours after the end of the infusion.[2] This modest but sustained increase in contractility may provide further safety in the treatment of arrhythmias in patients with heart failure.

References

1. Buzby GC Jr, Colatsky TJ: Alkylsulfonamido or perfluoroalkylsulfonamido benzenesulfonamides. U.S. Patent 4,721,809, 1988.
2. Ellingboe JW, Spinelli W, Winkley MW, et al: Class III antiarrhythmic activity of novel substituted, [(4-methylsulfonyl)amido]benzamides and sulfonamides. J Med Chem 35:705, 1992.
3. Hondeghem LM, Snyders DJ: Class III antiarrhythmic agents have a lot of potential but a long way to go: reduced effectiveness and dangers of reverse use dependence. Circulation 81:686, 1990.
4. Campbell TJ: Proarrhythmic actions of antiarrhythmic drugs: a review. Aust NZ J Med 20: 275, 1990.
5. Campbell TJ: Cellular electrophysiological effects of D- and DL-sotalol in guinea-pig sino-atrial node, atrium and ventricle and human atrium: differential tissue sensitivity. Br J Pharmacol 90:593, 1987.
6. Spinelli W, Parsons RW, Colatsky TJ: Effects of WAY-123,398, a new Class III antiarrhythmic agent, on cardiac refractoriness and ventricular fibrillation threshold in anesthetized dogs: a comparison with UK-69798, E-4031 and dl-sotalol. J Cardiovasc Pharmacol 20:913, 1992.
7. Reid J, Duker G, Almgren O, Nerme V: (+)-Sotalol causes significant occupation of β-adrenoceptors at concentrations that prolong cardiac repolarization. Naunyn-Schmiedeberg's Arch Pharmacol 341:215, 1990.
8. Euler DE, Moore EN: Continuous fractionated electrical activity after stimulation of the ventricles during the vulnerable period: evidence for local reentry. Am J Cardiol 46:783, 1980.
9. Moore EN, Spear JF: Ventricular fibrillation threshold. Arch Intern Med 135:446, 1975.
10. Steinberg MI, Mallory BB: Clofilium—a new antifibrillatory agent that selectively increases cellular refractoriness. Life Sci 25:1397, 1979.
11. Bacaner MB, Clay JR, Shrier A, Brochu RM: Potassium channel blockade: a mechanism for suppressing ventricular fibrillation. Proc Natl Acad Sci USA 83:2223, 1986.
12. Gwilt M, Solca AM, Burges RA, et al: Antifibrillatory action and haemodynamic properties of UK-69798, a new Class III antiarrhythmic agent, in anesthetized dogs. J Mol Cell Cardiol 21(Suppl II):S11, 1989.
13. Patterson E, Lynch JJ, Lucchesi BR: Antiarrhythmic and antifibrillatory actions of the β adrenergic receptor antagonist, dl-sotalol. J Pharmacol Exp Ther 230:519, 1984.
14. Euler DE, Scanlon PJ: Comparative effects of antiarrhythmic drugs on the ventricular fibrillation threshold. J Cardiovasc Pharmacol 11:291, 1988.
15. Ortiz J, Igarashi M, Gonzalez X, et al: Mechanism of atrial flutter termination by WAY-123,398, a unique Class III agent. Circulation 84:II-507, 1991.
16. Rials SJ, Wu Y, Gabriel A, et al: Antifibrillatory effect of Class III drug in chronic infarction. Circulation 84:II-505, 1991.
17. Siegal MS, Spinelli W: Drug-induced early after-

depolarizations in isolated tissues. In: MR Rosen, MJ Janse, AL Wit (eds): *Cardiac Electrophysiology: A Textbook*. Mount Kisco, NY: Futura Publishing Company, Inc., 1990, p. 371.

18. Spinelli W, Moubarak IF, Parsons RW, Colatsky TJ: Cellular electrophysiology of WAY-123,398, a new Class III antiarrhythmic agent: specificity and frequency-independence of I_K block in cat ventricular myocytes. *Cardiovasc Pharmacol* 27:1580, 1993.

19. Noble D, Tsien RW: Outward membrane currents activated in the plateau range of potentials in cardiac Purkinje fibers. *J Physiol (Lond)* 200:205, 1969.

20. Follmer CH, Colatsky TJ: Block of the delayed rectifier potassium current I_K by flecainide and E-4031 in cat ventricular myocytes. *Circulation* 82:289, 1990.

21. Roden DM, Bennett PB, Snyder DK, et al: Quinidine delays I_K activation in guinea pig ventricular myocytes. *Circ Res* 62:1055, 1988.

22. Balser JR, Bennett PB, Hondeghem LM, Roden DR: Suppression of time-dependent outward current in guinea pig ventricular myocytes: actions of quinidine and amiodarone. *Circ Res* 69:519, 1991.

23. Woosley RL: Antiarrhythmic drugs. *Ann Rev Pharmacol Toxicol* 31:427, 1991.

Part VII

Nonpharmacological Approaches to Cardiac Arrhythmias

Chapter 44

Surgery for Cardiac Arrhythmias

T. Bruce Ferguson
James L. Cox

The surgical treatment of supraventricular and ventricular cardiac arrhythmias has undergone a number of dramatic changes over the past several years.[1] For certain types of reentrant supraventricular arrhythmias, surgical therapy has been supplanted by radiofrequency (RF) ablative therapy as the treatment of first choice. Those patients who now have surgery are those who have failed RF ablation or have concomitant cardiac disease processes.

At the same time, with the assistance of sophisticated computerized intraoperative mapping studies, excellent surgical results have been obtained in patients with more complex atrial arrhythmias such as ectopic tachycardias. Additionally, a new surgical cure for chronic paroyxsmal or sustained atrial flutter/fibrillation has been demonstrated to be clinically efficacious during this time. This operation, termed the Maze procedure, may well become the most frequently performed surgical procedure for the cure of supraventricular arrhythmias.

With regard to ventricular arrhythmias, the importance of multichannel computerized mapping systems has been demonstrated in the understanding and treatment of more complex monomorphic tachycardias. Furthermore, the impact of implantabel cardioverter defibrillator (ICD) therapy on reducing the operative mortality for direct surgery for ventricular arrhythmias has been demonstrated. This chapter discusses the basic principles involved in the surgical treatment of these various supraventricular and ventricular arrhythmias.

Accessory Atrioventricular Connections

Anatomy

For localization of accessory pathways responsible for reciprocating tachycardias seen in the Wolff-Parkinson-White (WPW) syndrome, the heart can be sectioned in the horizontal plane at the level of the atrioventricular (AV) groove and divided into the left free wall, the right free wall, the posterior septal and the anterior septal spaces (Figure 1). The posterior and anterior septal spaces are in fact epicardial spaces that abut onto the atrial septum posteriorly and anteriorly. The two fixed

From BN Singh, HJJ Wellens, M Hiraoka, (eds): *Electropharmacological Control of Cardiac Arrhythmias*. Mount Kisco, NY, Futura Publishing Company Inc., © 1994.

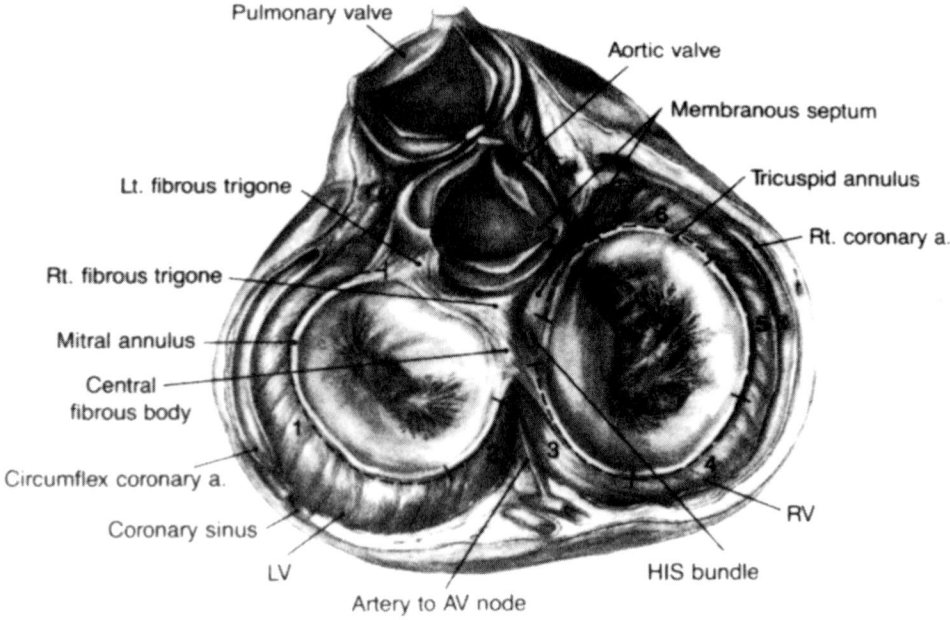

Figure 1. A superior view of the heart with the atria removed demonstrates the four anatomical areas in the horizontal plane where accessory connections can occur. These connections are not found between the left and right fibrous trigones along the area of contiguity between the mitral and aortic annuli. (Reproduced with permission from Lowe JE: Surgical treatment of the Wolff-Parkinson-White Syndrome and other supraventricular tachyarrhytmias. *J Cardiac Surg* 1:117, 1986.)

boundaries defining these spaces are the left and right fibrous trigones of the skeletal structure of the heart. Since the other boundaries are defined by adjacent anatomical landmarks, several additional subdivisions have been described to facilitate pathway localization, including the left and right paraseptal regions (Figure 2). The subdivisions have been especially helpful in defining regions for RF ablation.

However, the fibrous skeleton of the heart is not entirely horizontal. The tricuspid annulus is more apical in position than is the mitral annulus; as a result the anterior part of the central fibrous body extends into the ventricles beneath the attachment of the tricuspid valve, and the interventricular component of the membranous septum between the aortic outflow tract and the right atrium actually lies cephalad to the tricuspid annulus. For this reason RF ablation of right-sided pathways

is feasible from the atrial septum above the tricuspid valve while ablation of left-sided pathways is performed from beneath the mitral valve annulus.[2]

The AV groove between the left fibrous trigone and the right fibrous trigone (the anterior portion of the central fibrous body) lies in the horizontal plane and represents the site of continuity between the anterior leaflet of the mitral valve and the aortic valve annulus (Figure 3). This is the only area in the AV groove where atrial muscle is not in juxtaposition to ventricular muscle, and for this reason accessory AV pathways are not found between the left and right fibrous trigones.

In the vertical plane, the initial surgical experience suggested that these pathways can exist anywhere between the valve annuli and the epicardial surface of the heart (Figure 4).[3] More recently, the success of electrophysio-

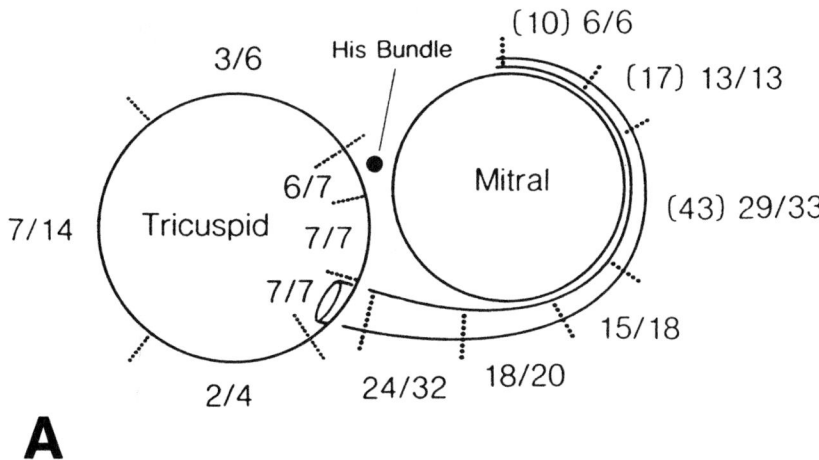

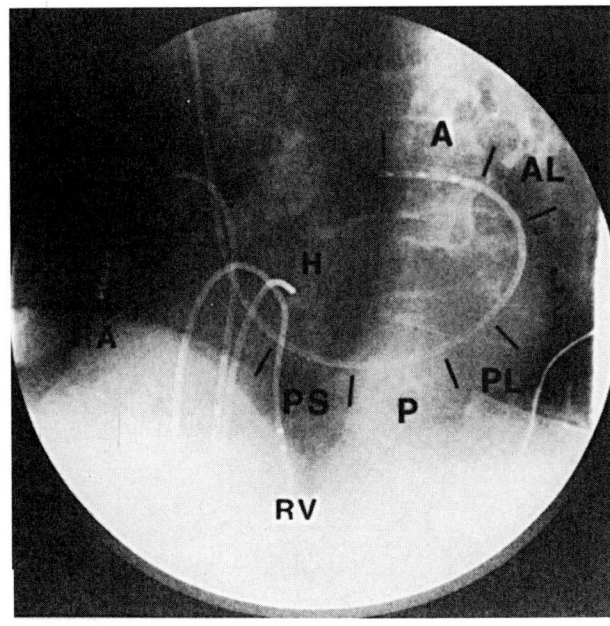

Figure 2. (A) Schematic representation of the tricuspid and mitral annuli seen fluoroscopically in (B) in the left anterior oblique projection. The numerators in (A) represent the number of recorded pathway potentials, while the denominators represent the number of pathways located in these regions; A: left anterior; AL: left anterorlateral; L: left lateral; PL: left posterolateral; P: left posterior; PS: left posteroseptal or paraseptal. (Reproduced with permission from References 2 and 7.)

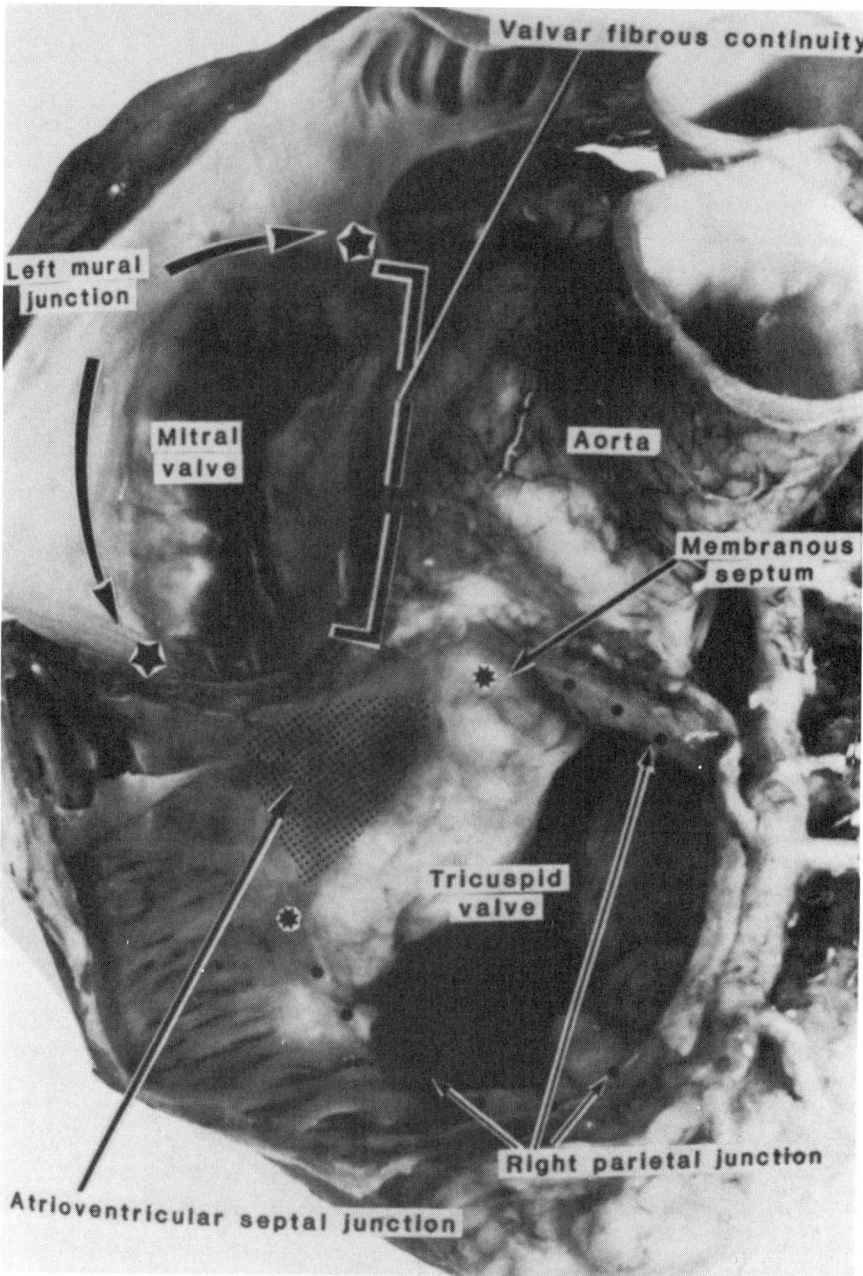

Figure 3. This dissection shows the overall structure of the atrioventricular junctions of the normal heart. Pathways may exist anywhere around the mitral or tricuspid annuli except along the mitral aortic valvar fibrous continuity. (Reproduced with permission from Anderson RH, Becker, AE: Anatomy of the conduction tissues and accessory atrioventricular connections. In: DP Zipes, J Jalife (eds): *Cardiac Electrophysiology*. Philadelphia, PA: WB Saunders, 1991, p. 240.)

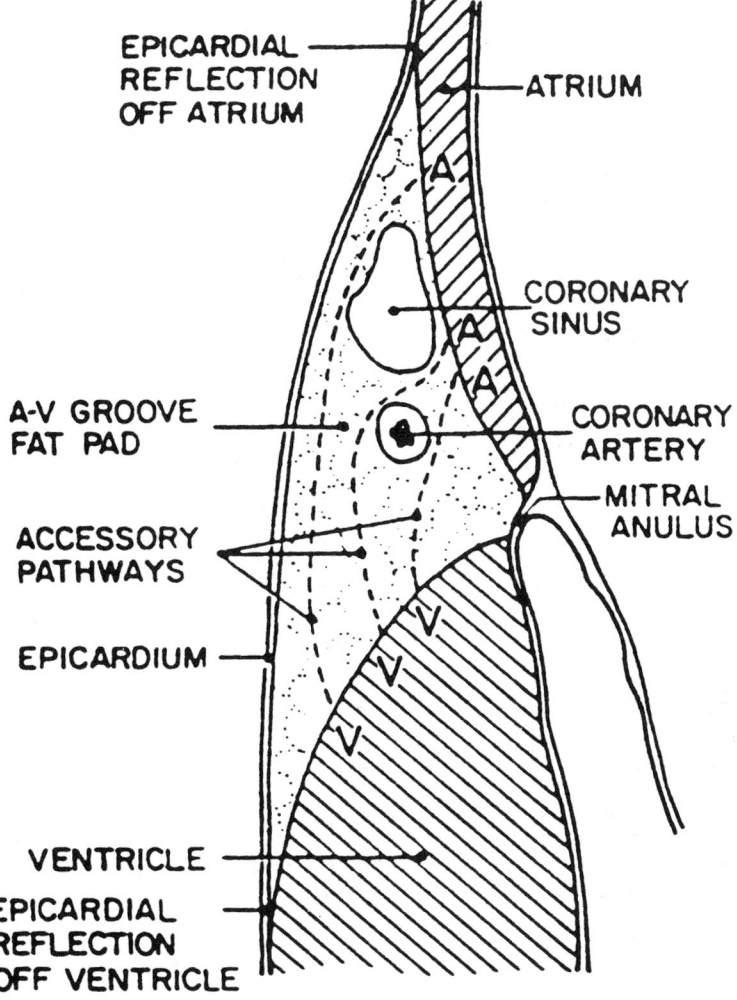

EPICARDIAL REFLECTION OFF ATRIUM

ATRIUM

CORONARY SINUS

A-V GROOVE FAT PAD

CORONARY ARTERY

MITRAL ANULUS

ACCESSORY PATHWAYS

EPICARDIUM

VENTRICLE

EPICARDIAL REFLECTION OFF VENTRICLE

Figure 4. Cross section of the left side of the heart in the vertical plane. Based on the surgical experience, pathways can be located at any depth between the valve annuli and epicardium. However, recent experience with radiofrequency ablation suggests that the majority of left-sided pathways are juxta-annular, while right-sided pathways tend to be more variable in depth. (Reproduced with permission from Reference 10.)

logical identification of the accessory pathway potentials and the results with RF ablation suggest that the majority of accessory pathways are in fact juxta-annular,[4,5] at least on the left side. Right-sided pathways appear to be more variable in location, due in part to the infolding of the right atrial and ventricular tissue (Figure 5). Posterior septal and anterior septal pathways are variable in location, as indicated by the multiple techniques that are necessary

for successful ablation. Those pathways that are not able to be ablated by the RF technique are probably disparate in location from the true annulus.

Finally, when the horizontal and vertical planes are combined, it is clear that these accessory pathways can tangentially traverse this three-dimensional space.[6,7] This conceptualization has been confirmed by intraoperative mapping in preparation for surgery (Figure 6)

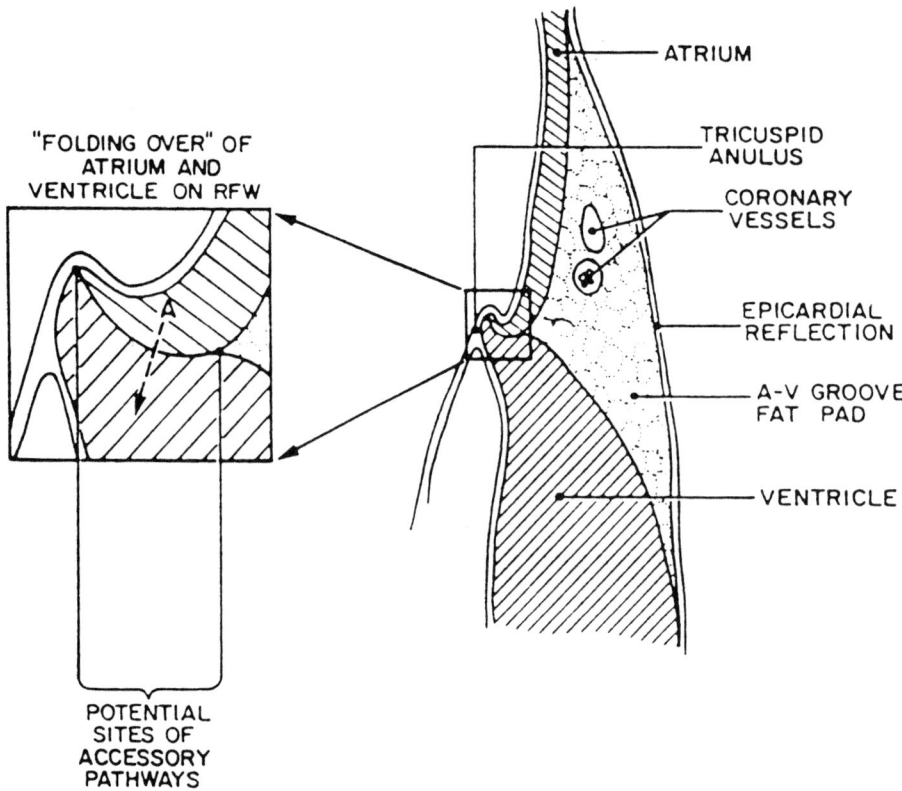

Figure 5. Folding over of the right atrium and right ventricle near the tricuspid annulus on the right free wall. Note that simple dissection of the atrioventricular (AV) groove fat pad away from this folded over tissue will not divide accessory pathways connecting the atrium and ventricle if they are near the tricuspid annulus. (Reproduced with permission from Reference 10.)

as well as by intracardiac mapping at the time of RF ablation (Figure 7).

Surgical Indications

Currently, candidates for surgical ablation of accessory pathways include patients with recurrent reciprocating tachycardia who are poorly controlled on medical therapy or have developed significant toxicity to an otherwise successful medical regimen and who: (1) have failed attempted RF ablation; or (2) have concomitant cardiac disease requiring surgical intervention.

Patients with symptomatic arrhythmias due to atrio-His, nodoventricular, and fascicu-loventricular fibers should undergo surgery if they are resistant or intolerant to medical therapy and fail RF ablation;[8] however, these procedures should probably be performed at an institution where the surgeon has extensive experience with these more complicated types of accessory connections.

The location of the pathway(s) is determined from the preoperative electrophysiological data and from intraoperative epicardial mapping; the techniques for this are described elsewhere.[9] In decreasing order of frequency, accessory pathways are located in the left free-wall, posterior septal, right free-wall, and anterior septal positions. Approximately 20% of patients in surgical series have multiple (2–4) pathways.[10]

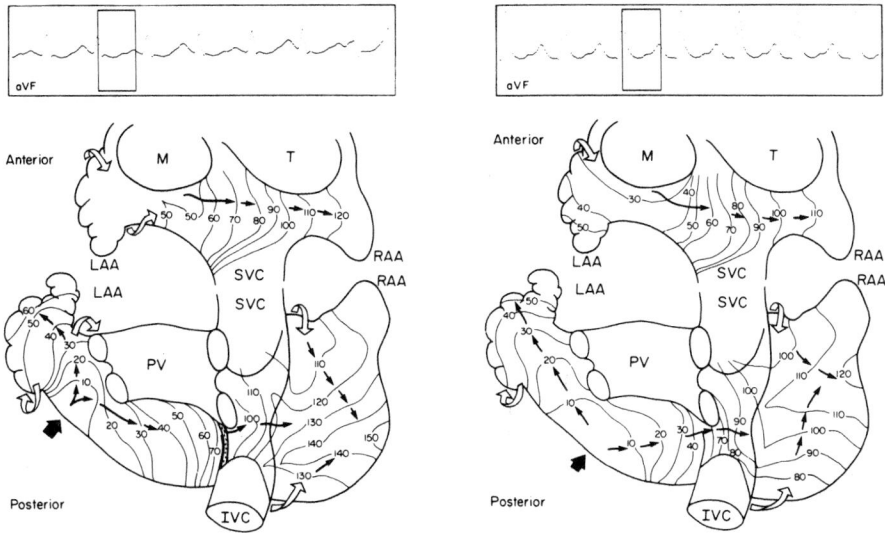

Figure 6. Atrial activation map during reciprocating tachycardias in two patients with the Wolff-Parkinson-White syndrome. The thick black arrow marks the site of atrial insertion of the accessory pathway on the posterior left atrium. Left: narrow discrete area of initial atrial activation. Right: broad band of initial activation, encompassing several centimeters of atrial tissue. LAA: left atrial appendage; SVC: superior vena cava; IVC: inferior vena cava; RAA: right atrial appendage; PV: pulmonary veins; M: mitral valve; T: tricuspid valve. (Reproduced with permission from Reference 6.)

Surgical Treatment

Two surgical approaches have been developed to divide accessory AV connections. The endocardial technique is designed to divide the ventricular end of the accessory pathway (analogous to the RF ablation techniques most commonly used),[1,10] and the epicardial technique is directed toward division of the atrial end of the pathway.[11,12]

Since 1981, we have used an endocardial technique and an anatomically based operation for division of all accessory pathways. The principles of this operative approach[3] are (1) accurate intraoperative localization of the pathway(s) to one of the four anatomical areas in the horizontal plane; (2) appreciation that the location of the pathway in the vertical plane may be variable; (3) appreciation that the endocardial dissection technique divides the ventricular insertion of the pathway and does nothing to the atrial insertion of the pathway; (4) complete dissection of the appropri-

ate anatomical space(s) in every patient regardless of the location of the pathway within that space as determined by intraoperative mapping; (5) appreciation that certain pathways may exist as broad bands and that when the ventricular insertion site is located at the junction of two anatomical areas (eg, left paraseptal region), complete dissection of both anatomical spaces should be performed; and (6) that isolation of the atrial rim of tissue above the annulus of the valve is necessary to prevent a juxta-annular pathway from retrogradely activating the atrium. The endocardial surgical dissection techniques for each of the four spaces in the horizontal plane are illustrated in Figures 8–11. The epicardial dissection techniques for pathways in these four locations have been described elsewhere.[11,12]

Surgical intervention following a failed RF ablation attempt does not seem to be more difficult or associated with increased morbidity, provided that the RF technique used places the ablation catheter below the annulus of the

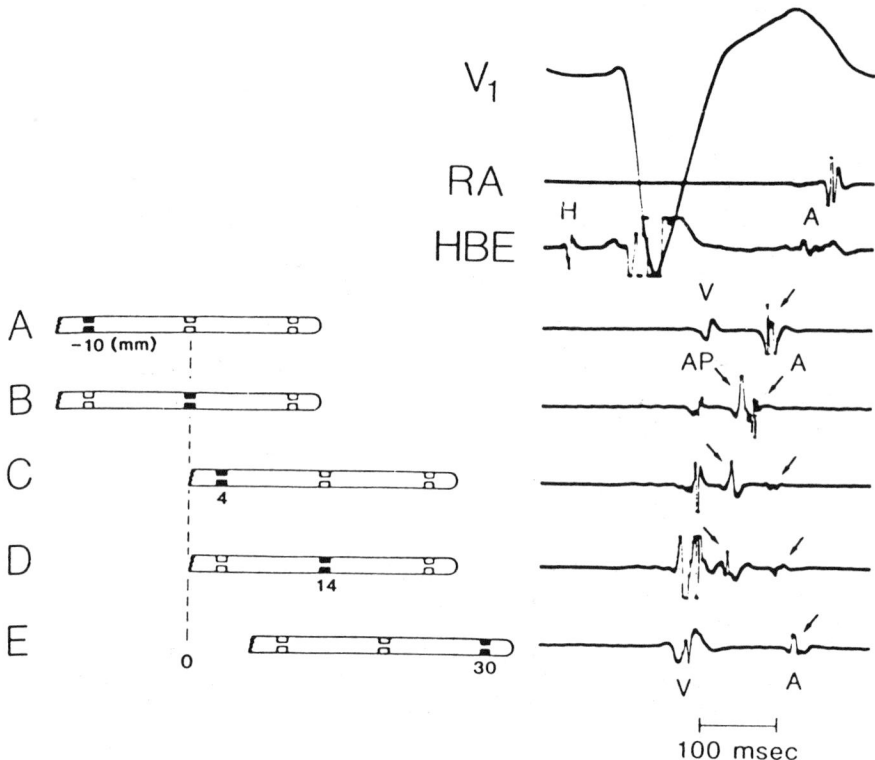

Figure 7. Composite of coronary sinus electrograms recorded during atrioventricular (AV) reentrant tachycardia demonstrating a 14-mm lateral component in the course of the accessory pathway between ventricle and atrium. RA: right atrium; HBE: His-bundle electrogram; V: ventricular potential; A: atrial potential; H: His potential; AP: accessory pathway potential; V_1: surface lead. (Reproduced with permission from Jackman W: In DG Benditt, DW Benson (eds): *Cardiac Preexcitation Syndromes.* Boston, MA: Martinus Nijhoff, 1986, p. 413.)

mitral valve and that excessive energies are not used on the right side of the heart. There appears to be a direct correlation between the total amount of energy delivered to an area and the degree of endocardial and subendocardial scarring and fibrosis that occurs. Direct RF ablation of the left atrial side of the AV groove has resulted in complete destruction of normal tissue planes and injury to circumflex coronary and coronary sinus vessels; excessive application of RF energy to the right atrial septum has likewise resulted in obliteration of normal tissue planes. Placement of a recording catheter in the coronary artery for mapping purposes has been associated with early development of severe atherosclerotic coronary disease, and RF application in the

coronary venous branches draining into the coronary sinus has been associated with perforation and tamponade. In this regard, patients with documented coronary sinus diverticuli associated with accessory pathways should probably undergo surgical ablation rather than attempted RF ablation.[8]

Surgical Results

In over 300 patients operated upon for the WPW syndrome and/or other accessory pathways since 1981, the incidence of successful surgical correction of the WPW syndrome using the techniques described is 100% with the initial operation, with an operative mortal-

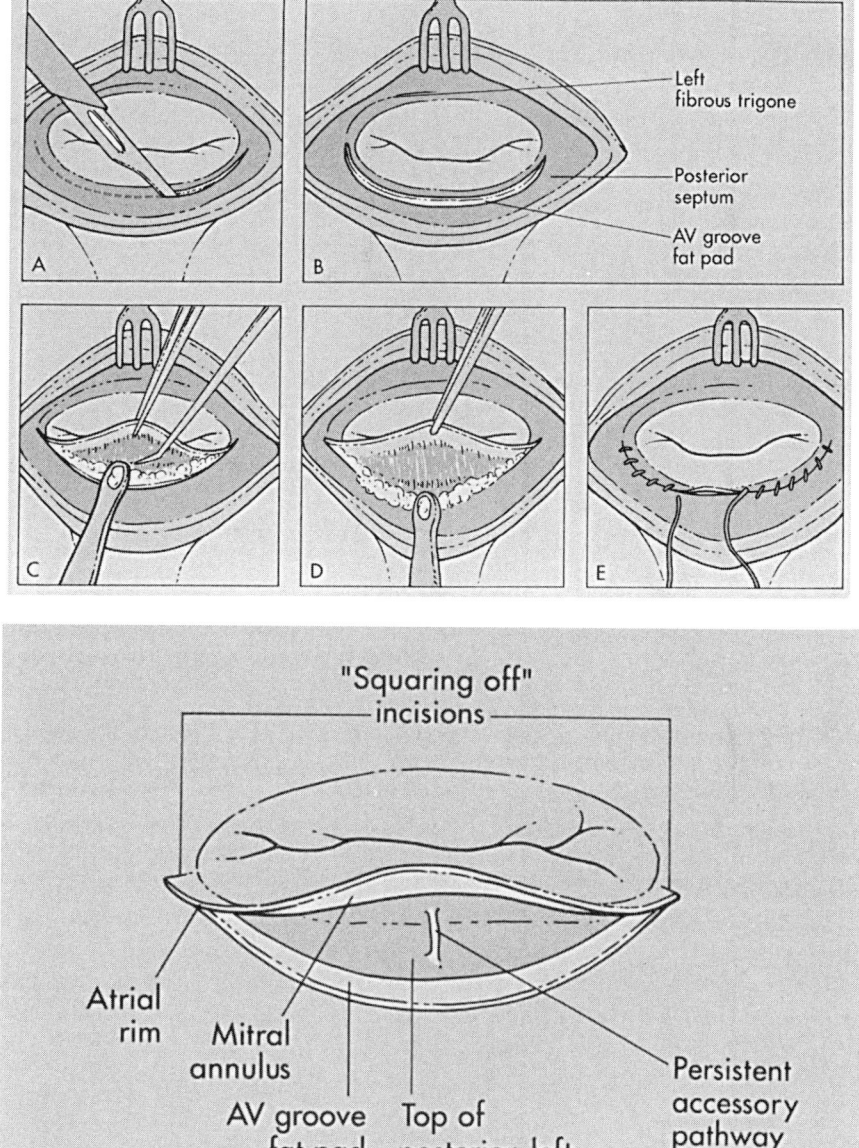

Figure 8. Top: Left free-wall endocardial dissection for the Wolff-Parkinson-White syndrome. After exposure of the mitral valve through a left atriotomy, an incision 2 mm above the posterior annulus of the valve is made (A). This incision extends from the left fibrous trigone to the posteromedial commissure of the valve (B). Using blunt dissection with a nerve hook the annulus is exposed and the posterior atrioventricular (AV) groove fat pad containing the circumflex coronary artery and coronary sinus is separated from the top of the left ventricle (C). This dissection is completed throughout the extent of the supra-annular incision out to the reflection of the epicardium off the left ventricle (D). Bottom: Appreciation that the majority of left free-wall pathways are juxta-annular resulted in addition of a "squaring-off" incision at either end of the supra-annular incision (F); this isolates juxta-annular activation to the rim of atrium above the annulus. Alternatively, a 3-mm cryolesion could be placed at either end of this incision. After isolation of the atrial rim, the supra-annular incision is closed with a multifilament suture (E, Top). (Modified with permission from Reference 1.)

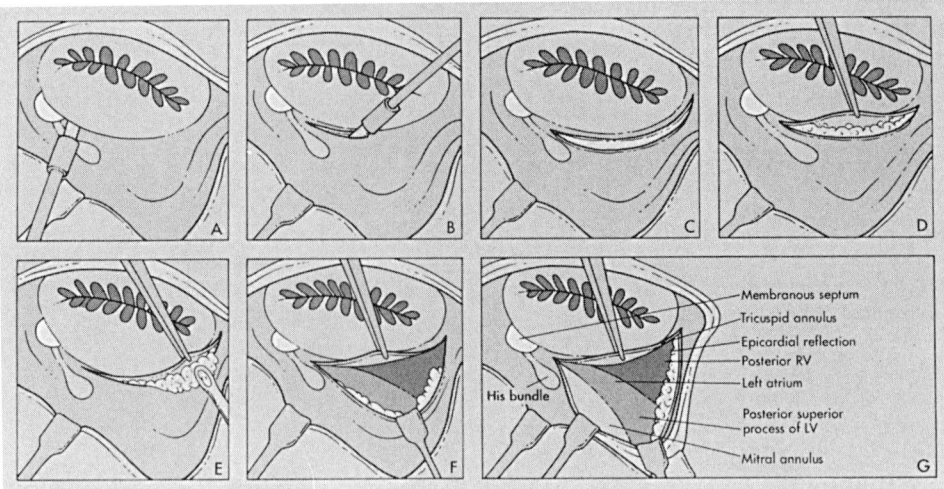

Figure 9. Endocardial dissection for surgical division of accessory pathways located in the posterior septal space. The right atrial septum is exposed in the standard fashion. Endocardial mapping, if necessary, is performed with a hand-held probe (A). A supra-annular incision is made behind the atrioventricular (AV) node-His bundle and extended out onto the right atrial free wall (B and C); this extension permits entry into the posterior septal space from behind (D). The fat pad is dissected off the top of the right ventricle and posterior septum, out to the epicardial reflection (E). The dissection is then carried medially using the mitral annulus as a guide to identify the junction of the mitral and tricuspid annuli, which is the posterior aspect of the central fibrous body (F); dissection onto the fibrous body will result in inadvertent heart block. The completed dissection is shown in panel G. (Reproduced with permission from Reference 1.)

ity for elective, uncomplicated cases of 0.5%.[1,14] Approximately 20% of patients have had multiple pathways, 13% Ebstein's anomaly, 22% congenital heart disease other than Ebstein's, 35% other arrhythmias, 60% cardiomyopathy and 6% coronary artery disease requiring concomitant revascularization. There have been no early or late recurrences following surgery using the endocardial technique described here.

Atrioventricular Nodal Reentrant Tachycardia

Anatomy

The electrophysiological substrate for both the typical and atypical forms of AV nodal reentrant tachycardia is the presence of dual AV nodal conduction pathways, one fast and one slow, through the AV node or the perino-dal tissues (Figure 12).[15] Histologic analysis of the AV nodal and perinodal tissue has not identified the anatomical correlate of the electrophysiological substrate for AV nodal reentrant tachycardia.[16] The recent experience with surgical[17] and RF ablation[18] suggests that perinodal tissue is involved, either tissue posterior to the compact node (most commonly) or tissue anterior to the node.

Surgical anatomy of the right atrial septum is critically important in the treatment of this arrhythmia (Figure 13). The AV node and His bundle are contained in the triangle of Koch, bounded superiorly by the tendon of Todaro, inferiorly by the tricuspid annulus, posteriorly by the coronary sinus, and the apex of the triangle is the atrial portion of the membranous septum. The penetrating bundle passes through the central fibrous body of the cardiac skeleton just posterior to the membranous septum; the location of the His bundle can be localized slightly more posterior

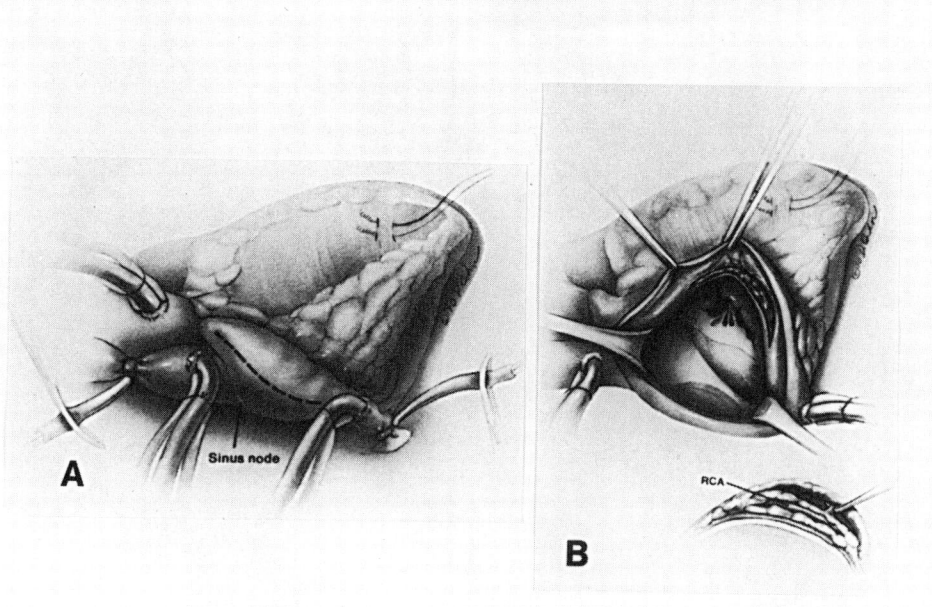

Figure 10. Right free-wall endocardial dissection for the Wolff-Parkinson-White syndrome. (A) The right atriotomy incision following bicaval cannulation and institution of cardiopulmonary bypass. This incision is made well away from the sinus node region. (B) Exposure of the right atrium. A supra-annular incision is made 2 mm above the tricuspid annulus extending from the posterior septal right free-wall junction to the pulmonary outflow tract anteriorly; the atrioventricular (AV) groove fat pad over this entire space is dissected off the right ventricular free wall out to the epicardial reflection. The supra-anular incision is "squared-off" and closed as illustrated in Figure 23. (Modified with permission from Hammon JW. In: JL Cox (ed): *Cardiac Arrhythmia Surgery. Cardiac Surgery, State of the Art Reviews.* 4:279, 1990.)

within the triangle. While the AV node is always contained within the triangle, the exact position of the node within the triangle must be considered to be variable.

Surgical Indications

Currently, the initial ablative treatment of choice is RF, and surgical intervention is reserved for failed RF ablation or when concomitant surgery is performed. However, since much of what was learned from the surgical dissection and cryoablation techniques provided the information necessary to permit successful RF ablation, a brief description of the surgical techniques is indicated.[13,17]

Patients with accessory AV connections and AV nodal reentrant tachycardia should have both entities treated at the time of the initial operation. Whether patients with WPW syndrome and dual AV nodal conduction demonstrated on electrophysiological evaluation should undergo both procedures has been a point of controversy in the past; there are no contraindications to treating both entities.[19] However, interruption of the accessory connection should be performed first so as to prevent inadvertent interruption of the AV node-His bundle during the cryosurgical procedure while AV conduction is maintained over the accessory pathway.

Surgical Treatment

The exposure for the discrete cryosurgical procedure is the same as for a posterior septal pathway dissection. During application

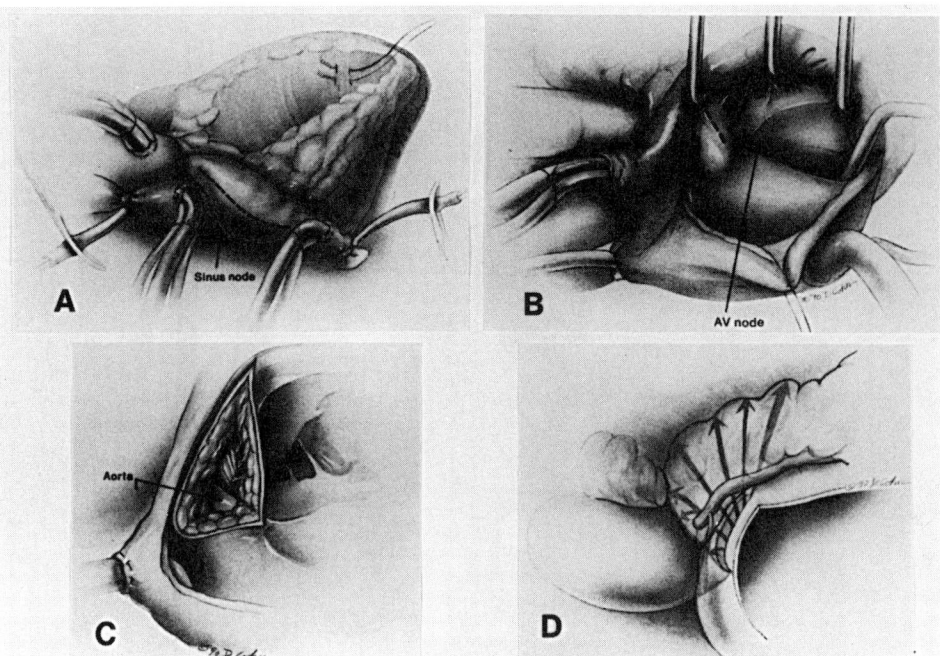

Figure 11. Endocardial anterior septal space dissection for the Wolff-Parkinson-White syndrome. (A) Exposure is obtained through the right atrium as for free-wall dissections. (B) Initial supra-annular incision is made anterior to the membranous septum after endocardial mapping confirms the location of the pathway in the anterior septal space. (C) Schematic conceptualization of the extent of the anterior septal dissection, which extends from the aorta medially to the right free-wall epicardium laterally, and out to the pulmonary outflow tract anteriorly. This dissection removes the fat pad containing the proxmial right main coronary and its branches off the anterior intraventricular septum. D: Completed dissection. (Modified with permission from Hammon JW. In: JL Cox (ed): *Cardiac Arrhythmia Surgery. Cardiac Surgery, State of the Art Reviews.* 4:279, 1990.)

of the cryolesions, the AV conduction time is monitored on a beat-to-beat basis. A nitrous oxide cryoprobe with a 3-mm tip is used to place cryolesions along the borders of the triangle of Koch, initially along the tendon of Todaro, and then along the annulus of the tricuspid valve beginning just beneath the os of the coronary sinus (Figure 14). When the cryolesion approaches the nodal tissue, the AV interval prolongs in a nearly linear fashion; impending complete heart block is heralded by a prolongation of the AV interval by 200 to 300 msec. When block occurs, cryothermia is terminated instantly and the AV interval shortens back to baseline. Used in this way the cryoprobe acts as a reversible knife. After outlining the borders of the triangle, subsequent cryolesion are placed to "fill in" the triangle of Koch

as much as possibie without causing block. Electrophysiologically, this procedure probably silently eliminates the slow pathway (regardless of whether it is anterior or posterior to the nodal tissue); the AV prolongation and heart block are produced after elimination of the alternative pathway of conduction due to proximity of the cryolesion to the remaining pathway for AV conduction. Patients with accessory nodoventricular connections and accessory atrio-His connections have been treated with this technique with excellent results.

Surgical Results

The discrete cryosurgical procedure has been performed on 37 patients at our institu-

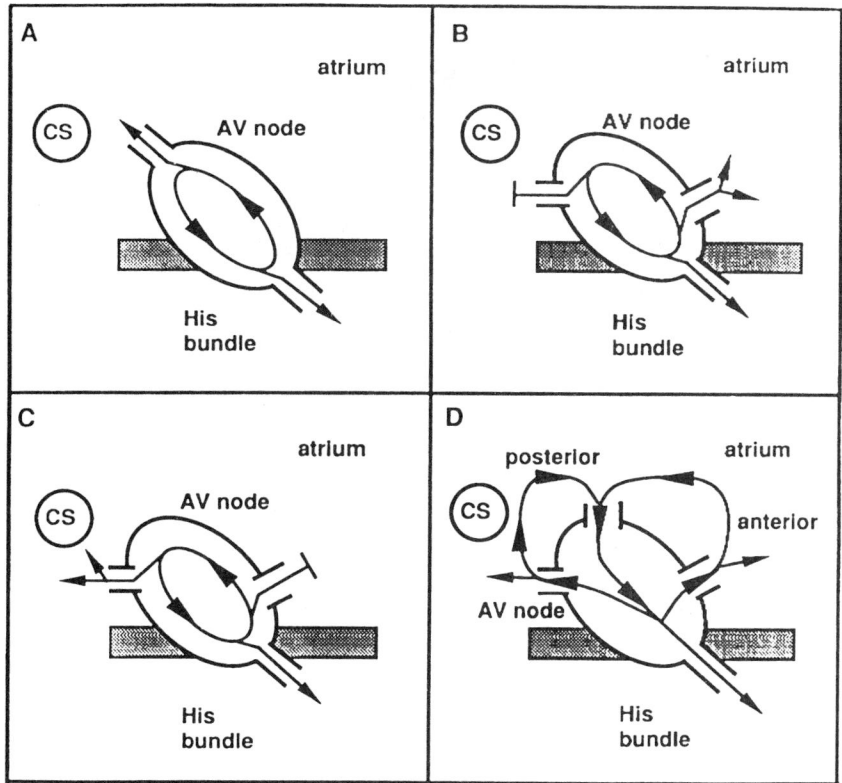

Figure 12. Possible mechanisms of atrioventricular (AV) junctional reeentrant tachycardia. (A) Commonly accepted mechanism-intranodal reentry with a common pathway of nodal tissue above and below reentrant circuit. (B) Intranodal rentry without common pathway above site of reentry. Different sequences of atrial activation may be a result of multiple atrial exits from AV node. In this case, atria are activated from anterior end of node. (C) same as (B) but with atria activated from posterior end of node. (D) Reentry using perinodal atrium as part of circuit. Multiple atrial exits form substrate for reentry. This model allows different sequences of atrial activation, ventriculoatrial intervals, and tachycardia cycle lengths and is compatible with selective surgical interruption of one circuit or the other. Two tachycardia circuits are shown, one anterior and one posterior. Multiple entry sites may be present, but for the sake of clarity only one has been depicted. CS: coronary sinus. (Reproduced with permission from Reference 21.)

tion to date. In all cases postoperative electrophysiological study has demonstrated the persistence of only a single AV conduction pathway, and the reentrant tachycardia could not be induced. There have been no instances of permanent heart block, and no late recurrences.[3]

Two other surgical techniques have been developed for this arrhythmia, both involving surgical dissection either anterior or posterior to the AV nodal tissue.[1,20,21] While effective, these techniques have been complicated by a small but finite incidence of permanent heart block, and a rather high late recurrence rate.

Ectopic or Automatic Atrial Tachycardias

Anatomy

From an anatomical point of view, ectopic or automatic atrial tachycardias can originate from foci occurring anywhere within the

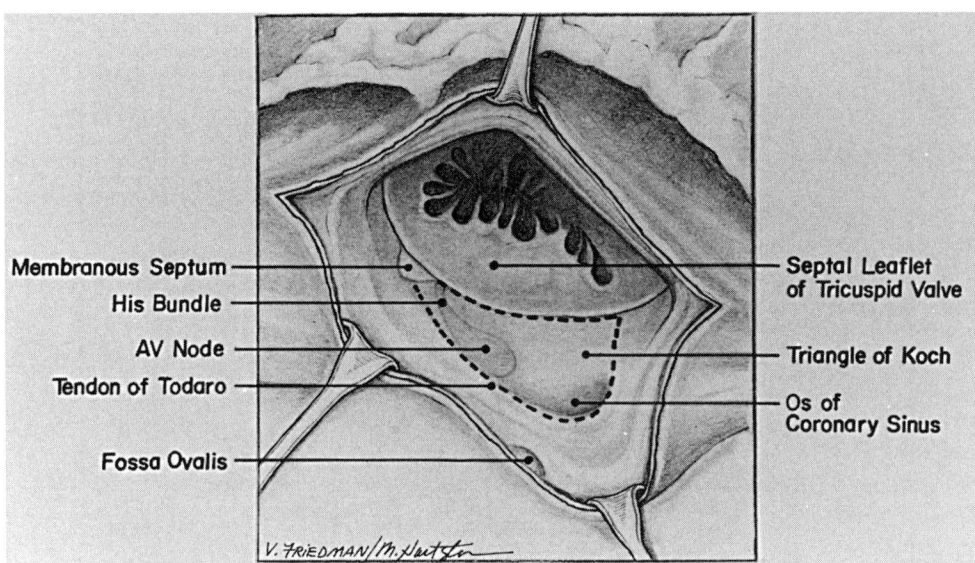

Figure 13. Surgical anatomy of the right atrial septum, including the triangle of Koch. (Reproduced with permission from Reference 10.)

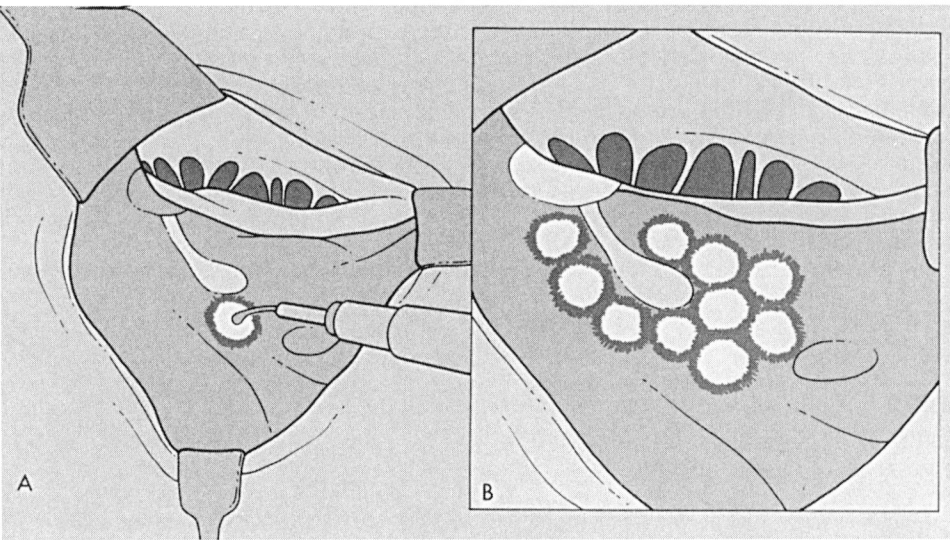

Figure 14. Discrete cryosurgical procedure for the treatment of atrioventricular (AV) node reentry tachycardia. A 3-mm cryoprobe is used to place a series of cryolesions around the periphery of the AV node (B), beginning at the os of the coronary sinus along the tendon of Todaro (A). Thus the entire perinodal tissue is cryoablated without causing permanent damage to the AV node proper or adversely affecting AV node function. (Reproduced with permission from Reference 1.)

left or right atrial tissue or atrial septum.[22] However, these occur most commonly on the right side of the heart, can be incessant, and are often markedly refractory to medical therapy. In addition, there may be multiple foci present, some of which may be latent and become manifest only at some interval following ablation of a different ectopic focus.

Surgical Indications

Accurate preoperative localization is particularly important in patients with automatic atrial tachycardias if surgical ablation of the focus is contemplated,[3] for several reasons: (1) general anesthesia frequently suppresses the ectopic focus; (2) intraoperative mapping without sophisticated computerized multipoint systems can be prohibitively difficult and time consuming; and (3) ectopic tachyarrhythmias are not inducible by standard programmed stimulation techniques.

Surgical Treatment

If the tachycardia focus can be localized, a variety of techniques have been advocated for surgical treatment including cryoablation, wide excision with pericardial patch repair, a combination of cryoablation and resection, or isolation.[3,22]

Foci on the left atrium have tended to be near the vein of Marshall and the left superior pulmonary vein; localized isolation procedures have met with limited success. In these instances, ectopic foci should be excluded from the remainder of the heart using the left atrial isolation procedure as described by Williams et al.[23] (Figure 15). Following the left atrial isolation procedure patients remain in normal sinus rhythm despite the presence of an incessant tachycardia confined to the left atrium. This therapy is preferable to the other therapeutic alternative, that of elective His-bundle ablation and pacemaker insertion.

Right atrial tachycardias are usually confined to the body of the right atrium and may be multifocal. If the arrhythmia circuit or focus

cannot be localized at surgery, then a right atrial isolation procedure that isolates the body of the right atrium while leaving the atrial pacemaker complex in continuity with the atrial septum and ventricles should be performed (Figure 16).[24]

Surgical Results

If the ectopic focus can be adequately localized in the operating room, then the operative procedures for isolation and/or ablation of the arrhythmia should be uniformly successful.[3,22] Since 1982, the left atrial isolation procedure has been performed on six patients, and the right atrial isolation procedure has been performed on three patients; there have been no adverse sequelae from these operations to date.

Our recent (1988–1991) experience with ectopic atrial tachycardias includes 14 patients, 5 of whom initially responded to medical therapy, and 9 of whom underwent map-guided surgical ablation using computerized intraoperative mapping techniques.[25] Of these 9 patients, 3 had cryoablative procedures performed, and 6 underwent some form of isolation procedure. Long-term follow-up of these 14 patients has resulted in tachycardia recurrence in 3 of 5 patients treated medically, with no recurrences in the surgically treated patients. These excellent surgical results will have to be compared to the results obtained with attempted RF ablation of these arrhythmias in the future.

Atrial Flutter and Fibrillation

Anatomy

The anatomical substrate for atrial flutter and fibrillation have been elucidated in the past several years through a combination of experimental and clinical intraoperative mapping studies. Studies by Boineau and colleagues[26,27] and Allessie and associates[28] have

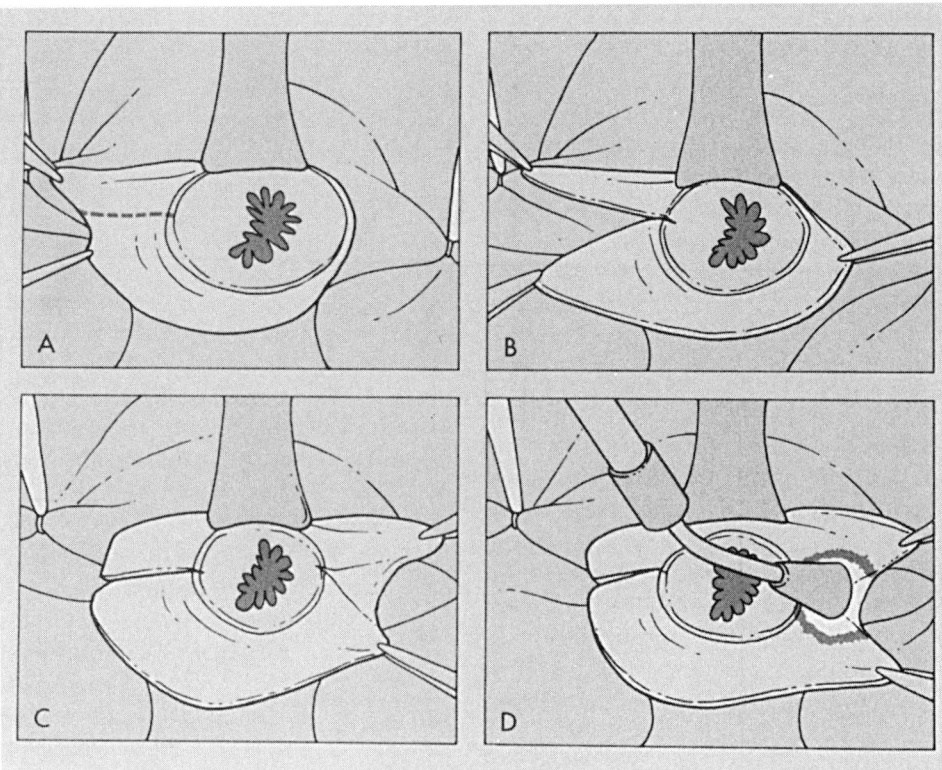

Figure 15. Left atrial isolation procedure. (A) A standard left atriotomy incison is made, and then extended anteriorly (dashed line) across Bachmann's bundle to the level of the mitral annulus just to the left of the left fibrous trigone (B). The transmural atriotomy is then extended posteriorly (C) To the level of the coronary sinus. The remaining portion of the incision is made through the endocardium extending across the mitral annulus posteriorly. The coronary sinus and atriovenrtricular (AV) groove fat pad are separated from the atrium using blunt dissection in similar fashion to endocardial dissections for left free-wall pathways and to the Maze procedure, as described below. To isolate the atrial fibers that are contained within the sinus, cryolesions are placed on the endocardial and epicardial aspects of the dissected coronary sinus at this point (D). The left atriotomy is closed with a continuous 4-0 nonabsorbable suture. (Reproduced with permission from Reference 1.)

documented that atrial flutter most likely occurs on the basis of a single macroreentrant circuit in the right atrial tissue that is dependent upon fixed anatomical obstacles (eg, the venae cavae or surgical incisions) to create areas of conduction block. Using sophisticated multipoint computerized mapping, intraoperative localization of the reentrant circuit responsible for the flutter has been possible (Figure 17).[29]

Experimental studies from our laboratory and others[30,31] have confirmed that atrial fibrillation is due to intra-atrial reentry, where multiple reentrant wavelets present in the atrium are maintained by the inhomogeneity of tissue refractoriness in atrial myocardium. This uneven refractoriness slows the activation wave front in some areas but not in other areas, resulting in uneven conduction that causes a single wave front to be dissociated into multiple reentrant waves[32] (Figure 18). No discrete anatomical structure or abnormality has been definitively associated with this arrhythmia. Further studies confirmed that as atrial size increases, the number of wave fronts during atrial fibrillation and the dura-

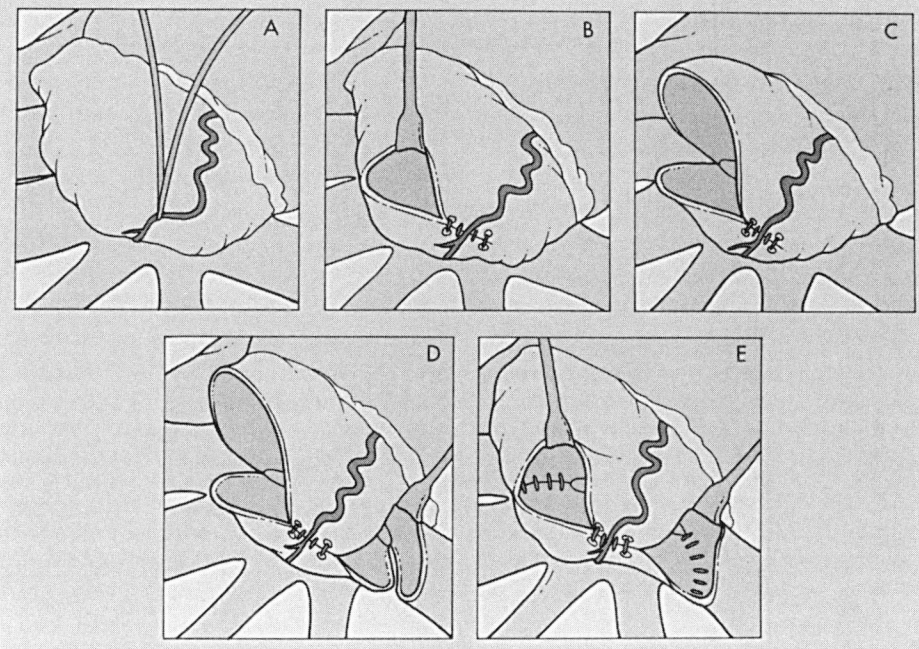

Figure 16. Right atrial isolation procedure. (A) The sinus node artery is dissected and elevated off the atrial epicardium. An incision is made beneath this artery and then closed. (B) This incision is carried anteriorly to the junction of the superior cava and the right atrial appendage, and then along the anterior limbus of the fossa ovalis to the anteromedial tricuspid valve annulus, just anterior to the membranous interatrial septum (C). Caudad extension of the atriotomy around the posterior right atrial-inferior caval junction to the posterolateral tricuspid valve annulus is performed. A cryolesion is placed at the end of this incision to ensure complete interruption of connecting atrial muscle fibers between the body of the right atrium and the remainder of the heart. (E) The incision is closed with running nonabsorbable suture. (Reproduced with permission from Reference 1.)

tion of atrial fibrillation increases. As the cycle lengths decrease and become more variable, various regions of the atria become completely dissociated from one another.

Current Medical Therapy for Atrial Flutter and Fibrillation

The goal of medical therapy for atrial fibrillation to restore the patient to sinus rhythm, and, failing that, to control the ventricular response to the rapid supraventricular arrhythmia. Quinidine has been the mainstay of conversion therapy; however, data from a number of studies suggest that only about 50%–60% of quinidine treated patients re-

main in sinus rhythm by 6–12 months.[33] Importantly, in these series almost as many patients as are successfully treated develop significant adverse reactions (30%–60%) to the drug.[34] Other type IA agents (eg, procainamide) will convert new onset atrial fibrillation in a small number of patients and probably acts to keep patients in sinus rhythm.[35] Newer agents such as propafenone and sotalol have been used with some success, but these results need confirmation by other randomized studies and should be interpreted with caution at this time. Recently, the problem with proarrhythmic effects with all these and other pharmacological agents (eg, type IC drugs) have been recognized and more clearly understood.[36–38] Cardioversion is generally

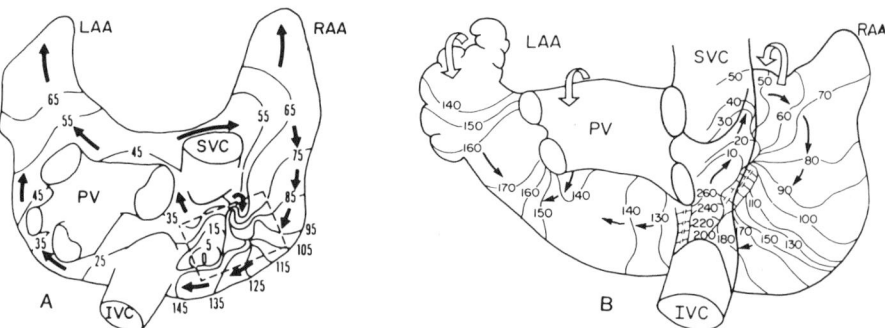

Figure 17. Atrial flutter due to right atrial reentry. (A) Experimental canine atrial flutter with a cycle length of 145 msec was produced by suture ligation (compression) of the midportion of the crista terminalis immediately lateral to the superior vena cava (SVC). Reentrant right atrial activation could be initiated by programmed stimulation only after ligation of the crista. (B) Clinical atrial flutter in a patient. The reentrant activation pattern with a cycle length of 260 msec was related to a right atrial incision previously used to close an atrial septal defect. Note similar patterns of clockwise right atrial reentry (posterior perspective) associated with block along the sulcus terminalis and passive depolarization of the left atrium. (Reproduced with permission from Reference 29.)

effective in patients if performed shortly after the onset of the fibrillation, but the efficacy decreases with the duration of the fibrillation.[39–41]

Finally, unless sinus rhythm can be maintained the only benefit to drug therapy is to control the ventricular response. In this circumstance the hemodynamic compromise associated with the fibrillation remains and, as mentioned above, anticoagulation treatment appears to reduce, but not eliminate, the risk of thromboembolism.[42]

Previous Surgical Therapies for Atrial Fibrillation

Atrial fibrillation is associated with three detrimental sequelae, namely, loss of atrial transport function, loss of a regular cardiac rhythm, and thromboembolism. In the past, when medical therapy failed to control the ventricular response associated with rapid atrial fibrillation the only therapeutic option available was to surgically ablate the His bundle and implant a VVI pacemaker. In many series, however, patients with VVI pacing and congestive heart failure experienced a 50% 3-year mortality.[43] With the efficacy of RF or di-

rect current ablation of the His bundle via the transvenous approach and implantation of a rate responsive ventricular inhibited pacemaker this has become a slightly more effective option.[44] This approach still does not address the problems of thromboembolism or loss of transport function that remain in these patients.

Defauw et al.[45] have described a corridor procedure that essentially isolates both the left and right atrial free wall from the atrial septum. There is a corridor of contiguous tissue between the sinus and AV nodes, thus permitting restoration of AV synchrony. However, this approach fails to address either the problem of loss of transport function (since both atria remain in fibrillation) or thromboembolism.

The ideal procedure for atrial fibrillation would accomplish three goals: (1) restoration of sinus rhythm; (2) restore atrial transport function; and (3) decrease or eliminate the risk of thromboembolism by eliminating passive stasis of blood in either or both atria.

Intraoperative Mapping Studies

The experimental and clinical investigations[46–51] that have been peformed over the

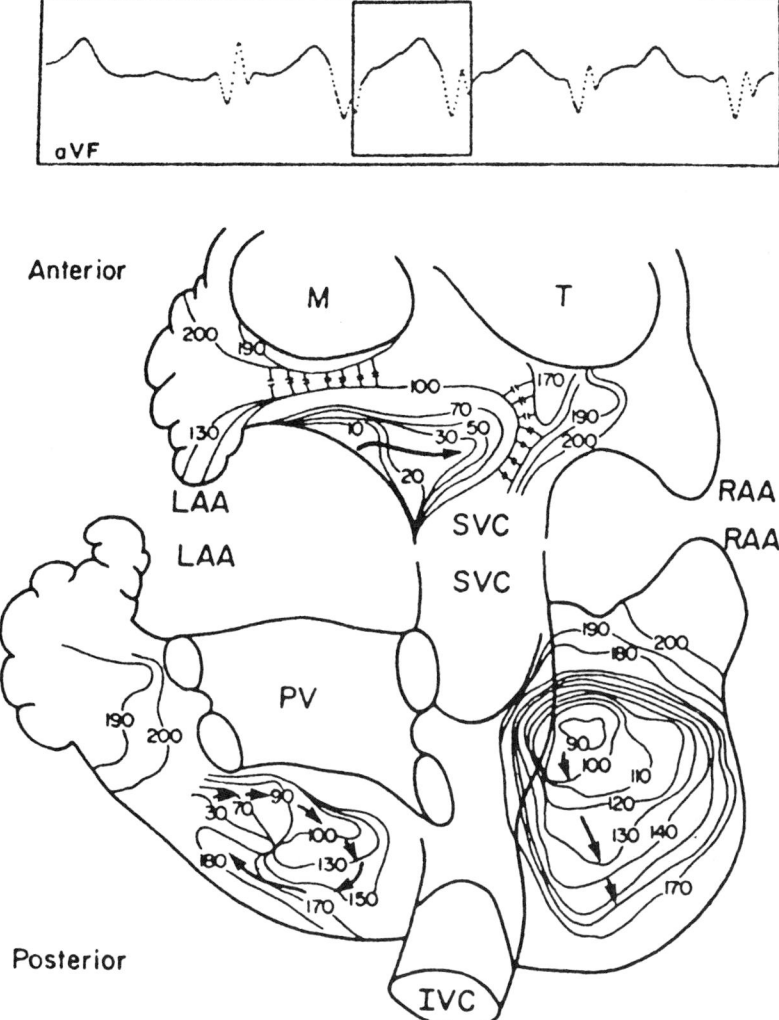

Figure 18. Human atrial fibrillation. Limb-lead aVF is shown on the top. Reentry (arrows) occurred fleetingly in the posterior left atrium but could not be conclusively demonstrated in the right atrium. The length of the window is 200 msec. Abbreviations as in Figure 6. (Reproduced with permission from Reference 30.)

past 10 years have led to the development of the Maze procedure. Using a computerized intraoperative mapping system capable of recording simultaneously 160 bipolar electrode points, the electrophysiology of human atrial fibrillation has been worked out.[47,51] Two distinct types of supraventricular arrhythmias related to fibrillation were mapped; the first was sustained atrial flutter, while the second was

actually a spectrum of arrhythmias clinically referred to as atrial fibrillation.[51]

The three electrophysiological components that determine the clinical arrhythmia of flutter or fibrillation include the reentrant circuit(s), passive atrial conduction, and AV conduction. Atrial flutter has been demonstrated to consist of a large, macroreentrant circuit that usually involves the fixed anatomical structures on the right side of the atrium: the superior and inferior venae cavae, the coronary sinus, and the annulus of the tricuspid valve. Flutter has also been demonstrated to occur in the absence of these fixed boundaries in experimental studies. The rest of the atrium was found to depolarize passively from the macroreentrant circuit (Figure 19). The clinical arrhythmias that resulted from this primary reentrant circuit were dependent primarily on the status of AV conduction and whether the passive atrial conduction is stable or variable (Figures 20-22). If all three electrophysiological components are stable, then a regular flutter wave with a regular ventricular response is seen on the electrocardiogram. If the ventricular response is variable due to varying AV conduction delay then the arrhythmia is more irregular. If passive conduction from the reentrant circuit to the atrial tissue is variable then the P wave morphology will be variable on the electrocardiogram. Surgical interruption of the circuit temporarily, but not permanently eliminated the supraventricular arrhythmia, since a different reentrant circuit has tended to form around the fixed anatomical obstacles or atrial fibrillation developed following interruption of the flutter circuit.

Atrial fibrillation was found to be a spectrum of arrhythmias consisting of multiple small macroreentrant circuits located throughout the atrial tissue (Figure 23). In its most complex form, these circuits were transient both in location and in time, with circuits migrating from one location to another and then disappearing (Figures 18 and 24). However, the clinical entity of atrial fibrillation was also found to extend as a spectrum from simple flutter to this complex form, again depending on the status of passive depolarization of the atrium and AV conduction. A single circuit with variable passive depolarization and variable AV conduction appeared clinically as atrial fibrillation (Figures 25 and 26). Importantly, it became clear than any operative procedure for atrial fibrillation could not be based upon the results of intraoperative mapping because of the transient nature and location of the circuits.

The cycle length of these circuits was variable, but was always much shorter than the cycle length of atrial flutter. In a number of patients, flutter degenerated into fibrillation, suggesting that both flutter and the various presentations of fibrillation may all be one continuous spectrum of arrhythmias.

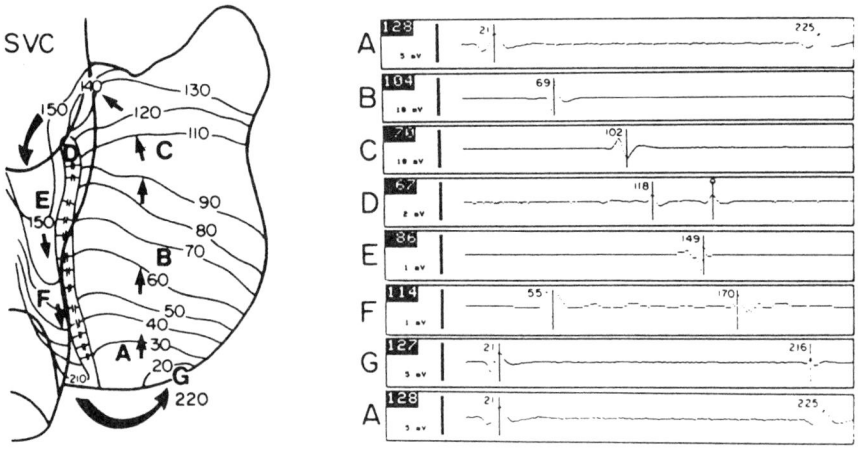

Figure 19. Human atrial flutter. The labels on the electrograms A through G (right panel) correspond to the letters on the electrophysiological map denoting the location of seven selected electrodes of the 80 electrodes covering the posterior right atrium. Note the large reentrant circuit (arrows) around an area of functional block (- ‖ -) along the crista terminalis. The numbers on the map and beside each electrogram represent the isochrones in milliseconds. (Reproduced with permission from Reference 30.)

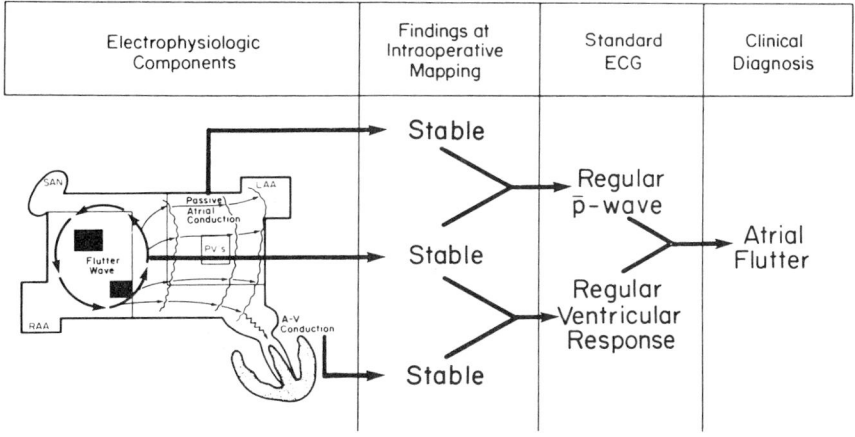

Figure 20. Electrophysiological basis of the standard electrocardiogram findings in the simplest type of atrial flutter. (Reproduced with permission from Reference 30.)

Development of the Surgical Concept of the Maze Procedure

The intraoperative mapping data acquired in humans suggested that the only effective operation would prevent the circuits from forming in the first place; that is, the space between the incisions needed to be small enough to prevent the short cycle lengths associated with the fibrillation circuits from closing back on themselves, establishing the reentrant mechanism.[52,53] In addition, the operation should permit sinus depolarization and maintain normal AV synchrony, and should restore atrial transport function; these last two characteristics theoretically would decrease or eliminate the incidence of thromboembolism.

The Maze Procedure

The complete description of the Maze procedure has been published elsewhere,[1,54,55] and is illustrated schematically in Figure 25. After completion of the Maze proce-

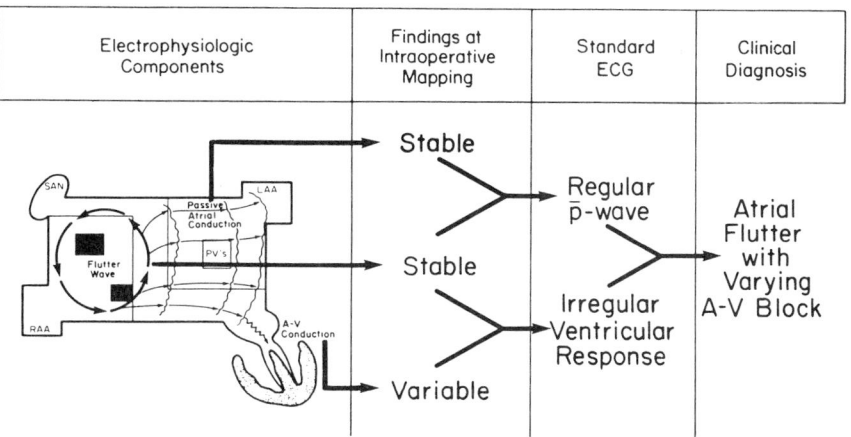

Figure 21. Electrophyisological basis of the standard electrocardiogram findings in atrial flutter with varying atrioventricular block. (Reproduced with permission from Reference 30.)

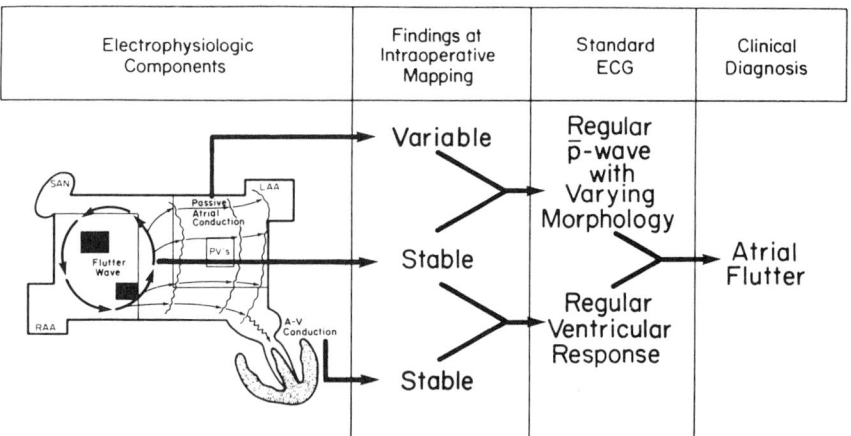

Figure 22. Electrophysiological basis of the standard electrocardiogram findings in atrial flutter in which the P wave morphology varies. (Reproduced with permission from Reference 30.)

dure, reentrant circuits cannot form because the distances between the incisions, the non-conduction fibrous skeleton of the heart, and the fixed anatomical obstacles of the right and left atrium are such that reentrant circuits cannot form; this is because the circuit becomes extinguished by one of these excisions or obstacles before a reentrant loop can be established. The only sustained conduction pathway originates from the sinus nodal area, proceeds anteriorly around the right atrial tissue, enters the atrial septum anteriorly and depolarizes the AV nodal tissue (Figure 26); this anterior atrial depolarization carries across to the anterior left atrium and then around posteriorly to depolarize the tissue beneath the pulmonary veins. Conduction down the atrial fibers contained within the coronary sinus is interrupted, however, by placement of a cryolesion on the left atrial side of the sinus (Figure 26). The remainder of the posterior atrial free walls are depolarized from the wave front exiting the atrial septum posteriorly. Thus normal AV conduction is maintained and the entire atrium is depolarized in sequential fashion after this operative procedure (Figures 25 and 26).

Surgical Results

At the time of this publication, 58 patients have undergone the Maze procedure since September 1987, with intermediate-term (> 6 months) follow-up available in 34 of these patients. The preoperative arrhythmias that the 34 patients presented with were paroxysmal fibrillation in 16, paroxysmal flutter in 2, and chronic fibrillation in 16. The duration of these arrhythmias was a mean of 6 years (range 2–13 years) in the 20 patients with paroxysmal fibrillation or flutter, 7 years (range 2–16 years) in the 9 patients with chronic fibrillation, and a total of 12 years (range 5–21 years) in the 7 patients with paroxysmal fibrillation that degenerated into chronic fibrillation; in this subset the mean duration of paroxysmal fibrillation was 9 years and the duration of chronic fibrillation was 3 years.

The indications for surgery included arrhythmia intolerance in 56% (19/34), drug intolerance in 29% (10/34), and transient ischemic attack in 15% (5/34). In approximately 40% of patients, perioperative atrial arrhythmias have occurred following the Maze procedure. Interestingly, the incidence of these arrhythmias is not significantly different from the incidence following other types of open heart surgery. The atrial arrhythmias following the Maze procedure are more difficult to diagnose due to the lack of discrete P waves on the 12-lead electrocardiogram; this makes the electrocardiogram appear as though the patient is in a junctional rhythm. The tempo-

SCHEMATIC ATRIAL ANATOMY

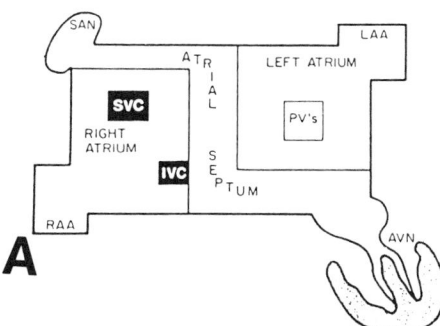

NORMAL ATRIAL ACTIVATION

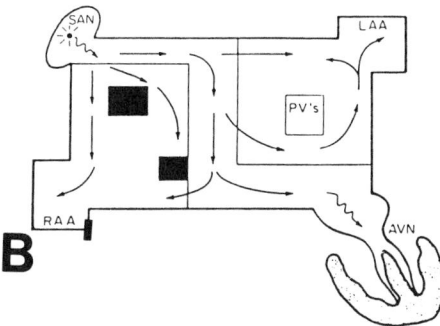

ATRIAL FIBRILLATION
(Multiple Macro-Reentrant Circuits)

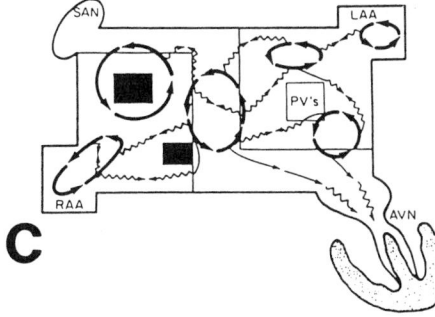

Figure 23. Schematic diagram of (A) normal atrial anatomy; (B) normal atrial activation; and (C) atrial fibrillation. The fixed obstacles on the right side of the heart are the superior vena cava (SVC) and inferior vena cava (IVC), while on the left side the fixed obstacle is the pulmonary veins (PV). Remaining structures include the right atrial (RAA) and left atrial (LAA) appendages, along with the atrial septum. In (B) normal activation begins at the sinoatrial node (SAN) to depolarize the atrio-ventricular node (AVN). The multiple macro-reentrant circuits responsible for clinical atrial fibrillation are shown in (C) superimposed on the schematic atrial anatomy. (Reproduced with permission from Reference 55.)

rary atrial pacing wires that are placed at surgery are helpful in diagnosing these arrhythmias. Most commonly a type of rapid atrial flutter is present, which responds to procainamide or encainide; these drugs lengthen the refractory period of the circuits, probably causing them to come in contact with a suture line and become extinguished. If therapy is required it is continued for 6 weeks postoperatively. These arrhythmias are truly perioperative and do not persist beyond the initial 4–6 weeks following the procedure.

All 34 patients have been cured of their atrial fibrillation by the Maze procedure; there have been no recurrences in over 4 years of follow-up. In long-term follow-up, 7 of 34 patients have been developed atrial flutter; in 1 patient this occurred spontaneously, and this has been suppressed with drug therapy. In the other 3 patients, flutter was inducible at the 6-month follow-up electrophysiological study, but has not occurred clinically and thus has not been treated.

Injury to the sinus node, probably due to devascularization of the nodal complex, has occurred in 1 patient. In the series, 9 patients had evidence of sick sinus syndrome preoperatively, and an additional 6 patients already had an endocardial pacing system in place at the time of the Maze procedure. These 16 patients required implantation or upgrade to a DDDR pacing system; in addition, four additional patients with normal intact sinus node function have required implantation of DDDR pacing systems to maintain atrial chronotropy. Thus 22 of 34 patients are in sinus rhythm postoperatively, 12 of 34 are atrially paced for chronotropic incompetence. All patients, including those requiring pacemaker implantation, have had intact AV conduction following the Maze procedure.

Documentation of restoration of atrial

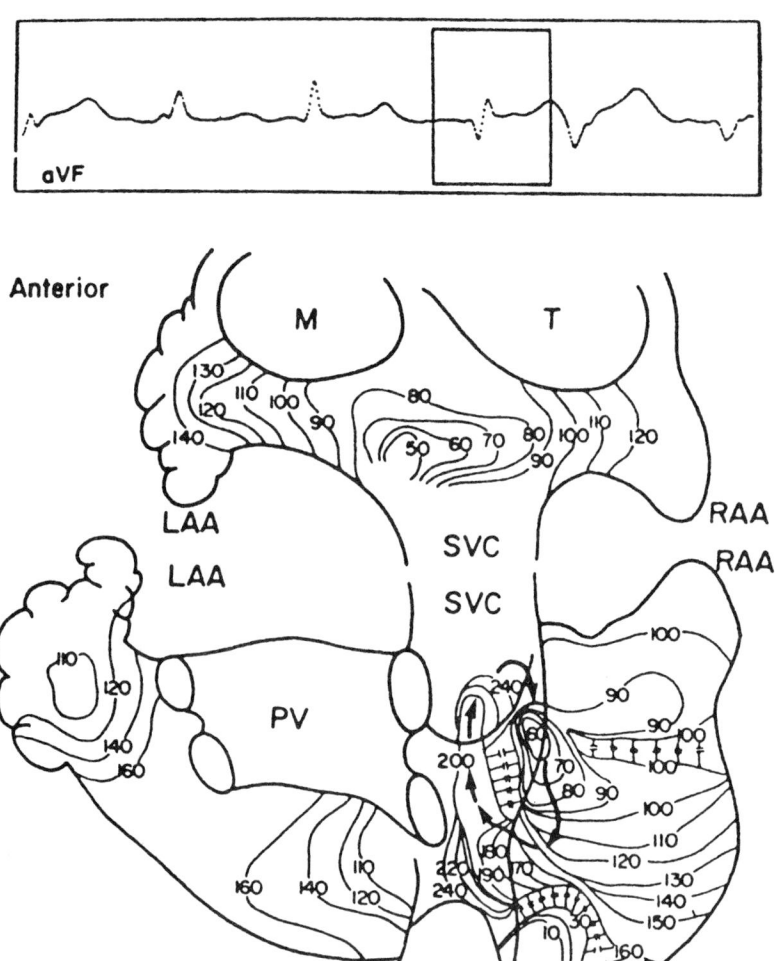

Figure 24. Human atrial fibrillation. The window (upper panel) is 200 msec in width. Note the reentrant circuit (arrows) and multiple areas of block (-‖-). The numbers on the map represent the isochrones in milliseconds. IVC: inferior vena cava; LAA: left atrial appendage; M: mitral valve; PV: pulmonary veins; RAA: right atrial appendage; SVC: superior vena cava; T: tricuspid valve. (Reproduced with permission from Reference 30.)

transport function has been demonstrated in all 34 patients by intraoperative transesophageal echocardiography following the procedure, and by dynamic magnetic resonance imaging (MRI) scan performed at the 6-month follow-up visit (Figure 27). In those patients with pacemakers, transesophageal echocardiography is performed. Atrial transport has been demonstrated even in patients who were in sustained chronic atrial fibrillation for up to 16 years preoperatively.

Finally, there are not enough patients followed for a long enough period of time to determine if the incidence of thromboembolic events is reduced in this patient population. All patients are maintained on warfarin

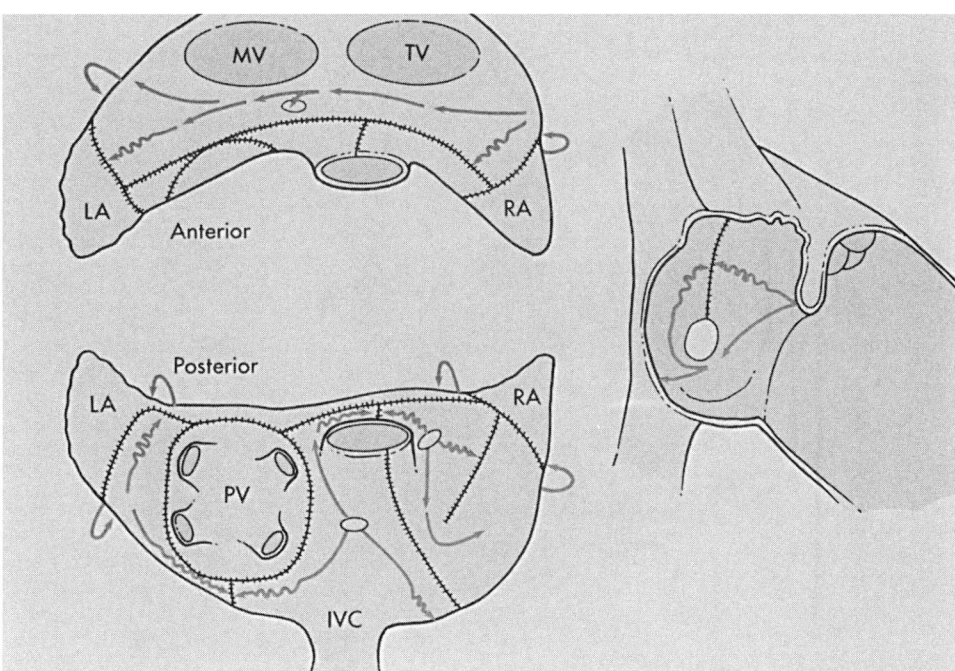

Figure 25. The Maze procedure for cure of atrial fibrillation. See text for discussion. LA: left atrial appendage; MV: mitral valve; TV: tricuspid valve; RA: right atrial appendage; PV: pulmonary veins; IVC: inferior vena cava. (Reproduced with permission from Reference 1.)

for the first 2 months postoperatively, until the suture lines heal; after that, they are maintained on aspirin and persantin therapy.

Thus far, the Maze procedure for chronic and paroyxsmal atrial fibrillation has been curative in 100% of patients. There has been no operative mortality, and the incidence of postoperative complications is similar to other types of open heart surgery. All patients have had restoration of AV synchrony, and restoration of atrial transport function has been demonstrated in all patients. Longer follow-up is needed to determine if the incidence of thromboembolic complications is reduced in these patients postoperatively.

Ventricular Tachycardia

Anatomical Principles

Ventricular tachycardia in infants and children is usually nonischemic in origin and is most often associated with a cardiomyopathy, prior surgery for congenital heart defects, and cardiac tumors.[56] In patients with diffuse cardiomyopathy due to patchy myocardial fibrosis, angiographic and hemodynamic data usually indicate some type of abnormal myocardial contractility associated with recurrent tachycardia. Ventriculography demonstrates diffuse dilatation of both ventricles. This same finding on ventriculography can also be present in cases of idiopathic ventricular tachycardia, due to repeated bouts of tachycardia; however, in this latter entity, pathological evidence of primary cardiac disease is absent. Arrhythmogenic right ventricular dysplasia (ARVD) is a congenital myopathy remarkable pathologically for transmural infiltration of adipose tissue.[57] Anatomically, this results in weakness and aneurysmal bulging of three pathological areas of the right ventricle: the infundibulum, apex, and posterior basilar region (Figure 28). Ventriculography demonstrates diffuse dilatation of the right ventricle with a significant

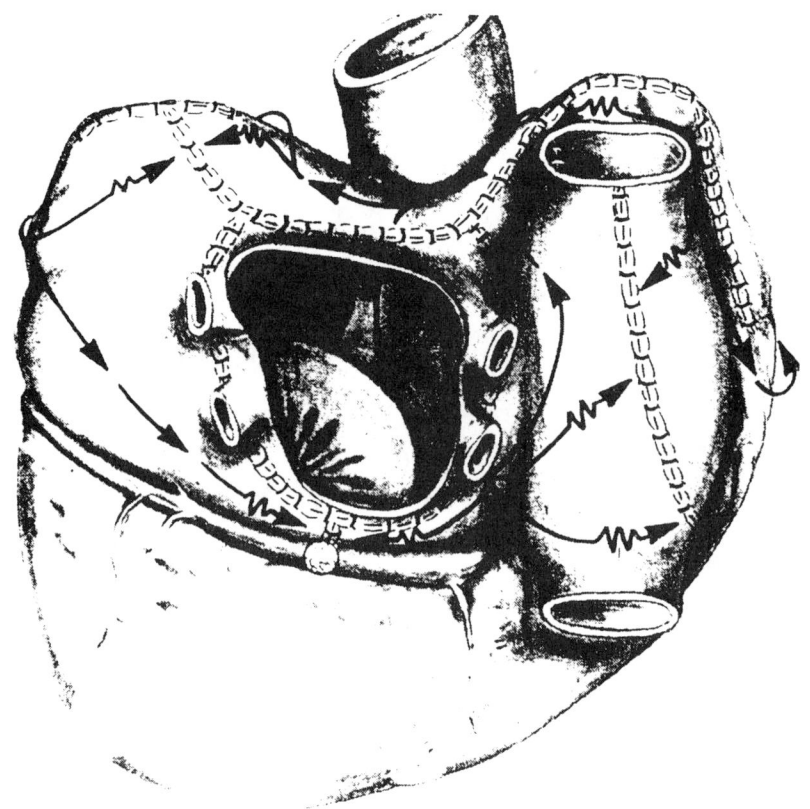

Figure 26. Propagation of a normal sinus rhythm beat following the Maze procedure. The impulse originates from the region of the sinus node and can escape from that region only by passing inferiorly and anteriorly around the base of the right atrium. The impulse continues to propagate around the anterior right atrium onto the top of the interatrial septum. There, it bifurcates into two wave fronts, one passing through the septum in an anterior-to-posterior direction to activate the posteromedial right and left atria, and the other continuing around the base of the excised left atrial appendage to activate the posterolateral left atrial wall. In this manner all atrial myocardium except the pulmonary vein orifices is activated. The activation of this atrial myocardium is fundamental to the preservation of atrial transport function postoperatively. (Reproduced with permission from Reference 52.)

reduction in contractility and marked delay in right ventricular emptying. Cardiac tumors can be localized to the left or right ventricle or septum in association with isolated arrhythmogenic tissue, or they can diffusely involve cardiac muscle and conduction tissue.[58] Localized tumors may be epicardial, intramyocardial, or on the endocardial surface of the heart. Finally, patients with congenital heart defects, especially tetralogy of Fallot, have developed ventricular arrhythmias long after the corrective procedure.[59] The occurrence of

these arrhythmias appears to be in part related to the hemodynamic result achieved with the operative procedure. Some of these arrhythmias have been shown to originate from the right ventriculotomy site.[60]

Ventricular tachyarrhythmias in adults are most commonly secondary to ischemic coronary artery disease.[61] In most patients with these arrhythmias, there is progression of acutely ischemic tissue to cell death, leaving a fibrous scar in place of the injured myocardium. The interlacing anisotropic pattern of

PATIENT
NUMBER

MITRAL
VALVE

TRICUSPID
VALVE

1

2

3

4

5

6

7

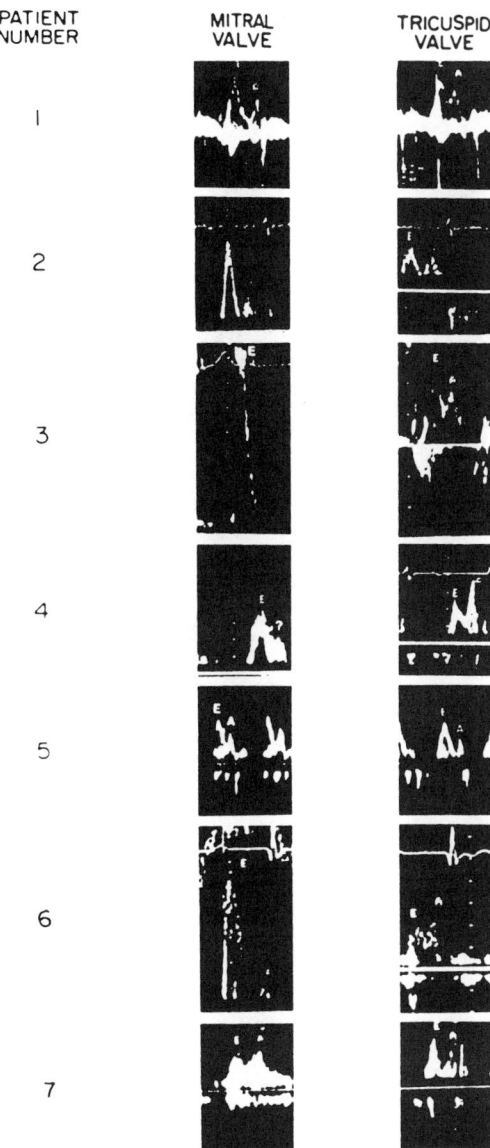

Figure 27. Doppler flow velocity spectra across the mitral and tricuspid valve in each of the seven patients showing the rapid inflow (E) and the corresponding atrial contribution (A) to filling of the ventricles. The presence of A waves documents the preservation of atrial transport function following surgical treatment of atrial fibrillation. Tracings provided courtesy of Dr. Julio E. Perez, Division of Cardiology, Washington University School of Medicine, St. Louis, Missouri. (Reproduced with permission from Reference 52.)

the remaining scar and normal myocardium may harbor local areas of slow conduction, unidirectional block, uneven refractoriness, and nonuniform repolarization, the electrophysiological substrates for the development of reentrant circuits associated with ventricular aneurysm formation.[62] Both micro- and macroreentrant circuits have been demonstrated to occur.[63] These same substrates are also produced by the application of tension and/or compression forces by the most prevalent anatomical correlate of ischemic ventricular tachycardia, that of ventricular aneurysm.[64] Most commonly these occur in the anteroapical position secondary to occlusion of flow in the left anterior descending coronary artery, but they also occur posteriorly in the distribution of the posterior descending coronary artery (Figure 29).[61]

Preoperative Evaluation

Patients with both ischemic and nonischemic ventricular tachycardias who are surgical candidates undergo complete electrophysiological, angiographic, and ventriculographic evaluation. The catheter electrophysiological study is performed: (1) to confirm that the arrhythmia is ventricular and not supraventricular in origin; (2) to demonstrate that the arrhythmia is reentrant by induction and termination with programmed electrical stimulation techniques; and (3) to identify the earliest site of origin of all morphologically distinct tachycardias using catheter mapping techniques.

Angiographic and ventriculographic evaluation is particularly helpful in the nonischemic forms of ventricular tachycardia. In patients with diffuse cardiomyopathy angiographic and hemodynamic data usually indicate abnormal myocardial contractility, and ventriculography demonstrates diffuse dilatation of both ventricles. This same finding on ventriculography can also be present in cases of idiopathic ventricular tachycardia, due to repeated bouts of tachycardia. In ARVD ventriculography demonstrates diffuse dilatation,

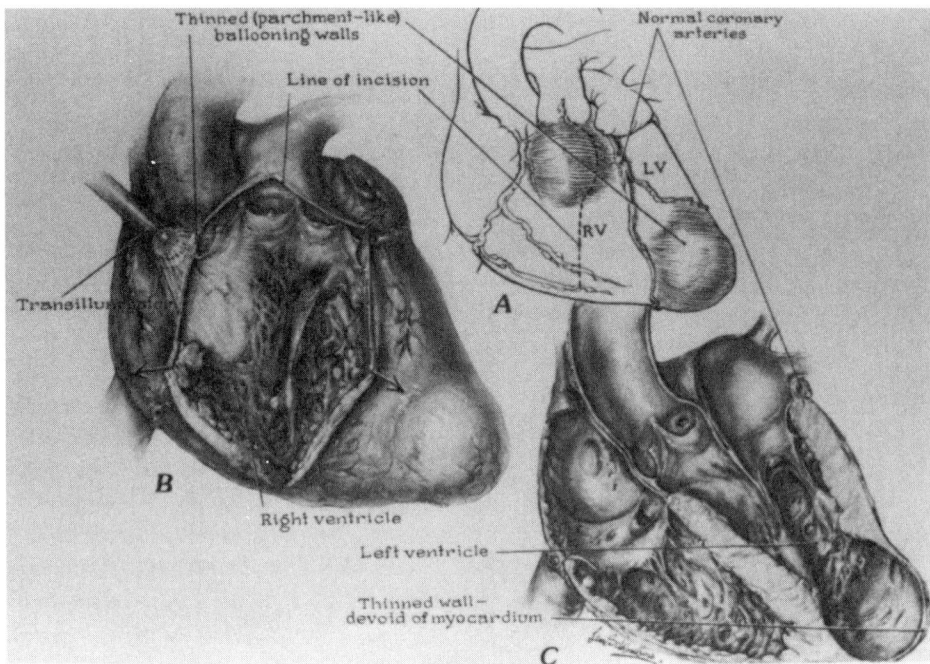

Figure 28. Arrhythmogenic ventricular dysplasia. Diagrams A–C of congenital right and left ventricular dysplasia with parchment-like thinning of the right ventricular outflow tract and left ventricular apex. (Reproduced with permission from Waller BF. *Am J Cardiol* 46:885, 1980.)

depressed contractility, and delayed emptying of the right ventricle. Frank aneurysms of the infundibulum, apex, and/or posterior basilar region are seen (Figure 28), and hypertrophic muscular bands in the infundibulum and anterior right ventricular wall result in a feathering appearance of the outflow tract.

Surgical Indications

The final decision regarding surgical therapy for ventricular tachycardias of both ischemic and nonischemic origin is based upon a variety of preoperative and clinical factors. The primary indication for surgery is refractoriness to medical therapy.

The only absolute contraindication to direct surgical intervention for ischemic ventricular tachycardia is left ventricular dysfunction so severe that the preoperative risk is judged to be prohibitive. Because most patients with ischemic heart disease and ventricular tachy-

cardia have a left ventricular aneurysm, accurate determination of the ejection fraction in these patients is often difficult and the absolute number is not an accurate predictor of operative mortality. Poor systolic function in the nonaneurysmal portion of the ventricle increases the operative risk to the patient. These patients are better served by implantation of an ICD if they meet current implant criteria.[1,56]

Nonischemic Tachycardias

Nonischemic tachycardias usually arise in the right ventricular free wall or septum and in general are extremely resistant to medical therapy.[56] Localized surgical isolation techniques are usually used for tachycardias arising in the right ventricular free wall, while multipoint map-guided cryoablative techniques are used for arrhythmias localized to the septum. In certain patients with ARVD, intraoperative mapping has suggested that the

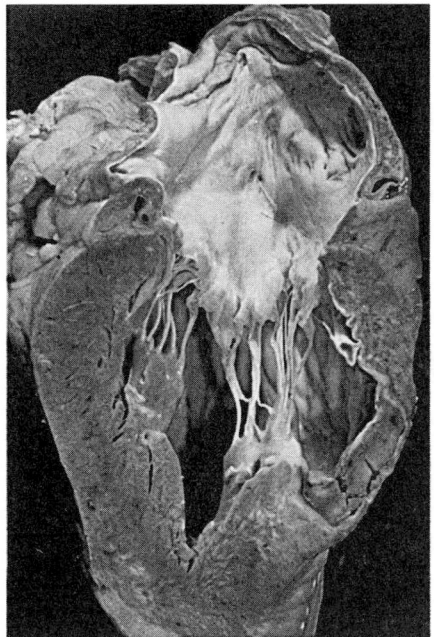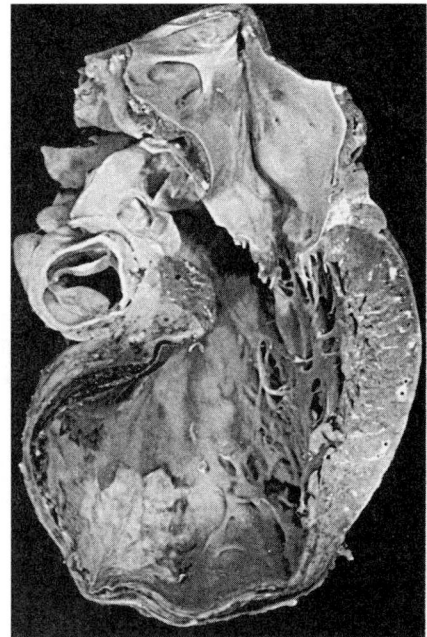

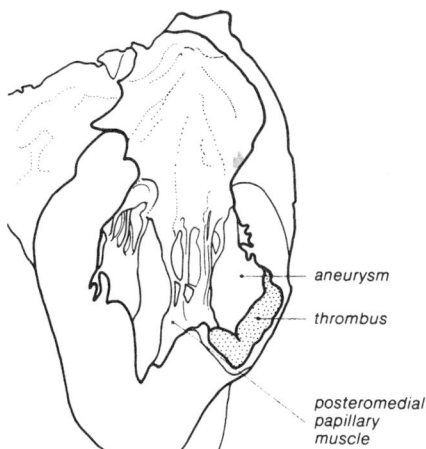

Figure 29. (A) Inferior wall aneurysm partially filled with thrombus. (B) Huge anteroseptal and apical left venrtricular (LV) aneurysm. Pump failure was the leading symptom. (Reproduced with permission from Becker AE, Anderson RH: *Cardiac Anatomy*. New York, NY: 1993.)

entire right ventricular free wall may be arrhythmogenic, giving rise to multiple morphological types of tachycardia. In the past, surgical isolation of the entire right ventricular free wall has been performed; however, postoperative right ventricular dilatation has occurred in these patients, and today cardiac transplantation in a suitable patient with this arrhythmia is the most feasibie surgical approach.[1]

Patients with ventricular tachycardia occurring in association with the long QT interval syndrome frequently have torsades de pointes as the manifestation of their tachycardia.[65] Medical therapy consists of β-adrenergic blockade, and this recently has been coupled with permanent atrial or ventricular pacing. Implantation of an ICD in those patients with a history of life-threatening arrhythmias is now recommended. In refractory cases, cardiac transplantation should be considered.

Ischemic Ventricular Tachycardia

Our current algorithm for the optimal surgical treatment of refractory ischemic ventricular tachycardia is shown in Figure 30. With this algorithm as a guide, the following points can be emphasized:[1,56]

1. Evaluation for surgical intervention should be made prior to the institution of amiodarone therapy; this is true for patients considered for either direct surgery and ICD implantation. The depressant effect of amiodarone on left ventricular function is aggravated by ischemic cardioplegic arrest in the majority of patients; moreover, complications from the pulmonary toxicity effect of the drug can significantly complicate either operative procedure.

2. For direct surgical intervention the patient should have a sufficient amount of left ventricular function remaining after aneurysmectomy to survive operative intervention. In other words, the function of the nonaneurysmal portion of the ventricle should be normal or near normal. Ejection fraction is not an ac-

curate predictor of operative mortality in patients with aneurysms.

3. If the patient has a prohibitive degree of left ventricular dysfunction, implantation of an ICD should be considered if the patient meets the standard indications for ICD therapy. Patients who do not meet these criteria should be started on amiodarone.

4. If the patient's tachycardia is uncontrolled on amiodarone or with an ICD, cardiac transplantation should be considered. If the patient is not a transplant candidate, then salvage ventricular tachycardia surgery is the only therapeutic option available.

5. If the patient's left ventricular function is acceptable for surgery, and they have sustained ventricular tachycardia that can be mapped intraoperatively, then direct surgical intervention should be undertaken.

Surgical Treatment: Direct Techniques

A number of different surgical techniques for direct surgical intervention for ventricular tachycardias have been described.[66,67] Our current technique involves intraoperative mapping using a 160-channel computerized mapping system;[68] the results of the preoperative electrophysiological study and this intraoperative map guides the surgical resection and cryoablation procedure. With the heart in the normothermic beating state, and preferably during ventricular tachycardia, the ventri-

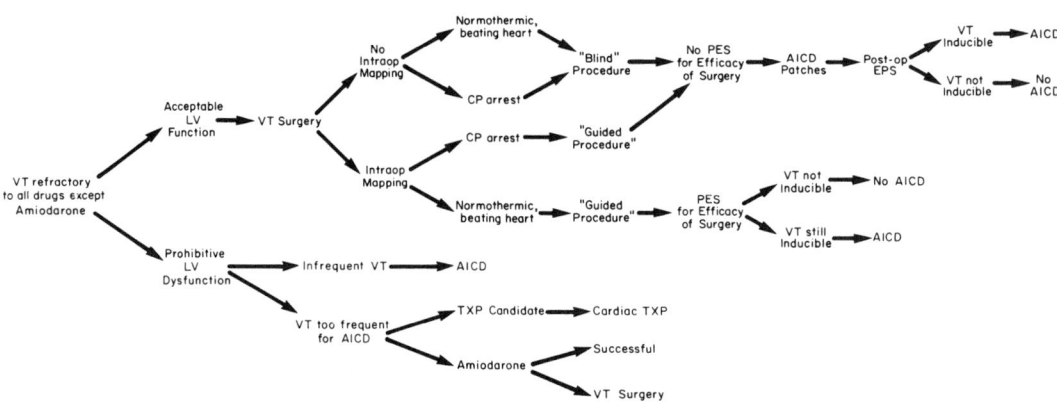

Figure 30. Algorithm for surgical treatment of ventricular tachycardia. See text for details.

cle is opened through the infarct or aneurysm and all of the associated endocardial fibrosis is resected except that which extends onto the base of the papillary muscles (Figure 31). Approximately 10% of patients will still have inducible tachycardia following resection of the endocardial fibrosis, indicating that the actual site of origin of the tachycardia in these patients is deeper in the myocardium than the visible gross border of the fibrosis. Endocardial cryolesions are then applied with a 2.5-cm nitrous oxide cryoprobe to the site(s) of origin of the tachycardia(s) as determined by the intraoperative mapping, thus ablating the myocardium deep to the visible fibrosis in case this tissue is involved in the tachycardia circuit. Resection of endocardial fibrosis ex-

tending onto the base of the papillary muscles is not performed; instead, one or more cryolesions are placed directly on the base of the involved papillary muscle, thus avoiding mitral valve replacement in these quite ill patients (Figure 32). These techniques are applicable to both anterior and posteroinferior infarct/aneurysms (Figure 33).

Programmed electrical stimulation is undertaken in an attempt to reinduce the arrhythmia. If the arrhythmia is no longer inducible there is a 98% chance that it has been permanently ablated using these techniques. If coronary artery bypass grafting or other procedures are required, they are performed after completion of the antiarrhythmic portion of the procedure.

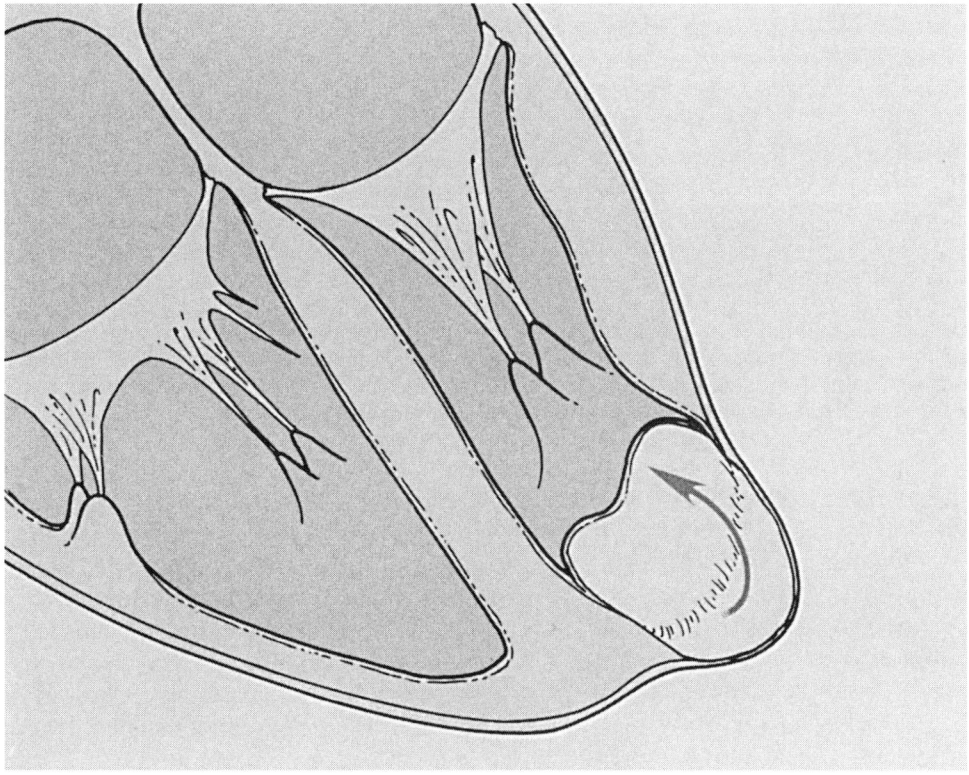

Figure 31. Diagrammatic sketch of and extended endocardial resection procedure (EERP) in an anterior ventricular aneurysm. The principle involved in this procedure is to remove all the visible endocardial scar along the septum and free wall except that at the base of the papillary muscles. Cryolesions are placed on the endocardium at the site(s) of earliest activation of the morphological types of tachycardias as determined by the preoperative and intraoperative mapping studies. (Reproduced with permission from Reference 1.)

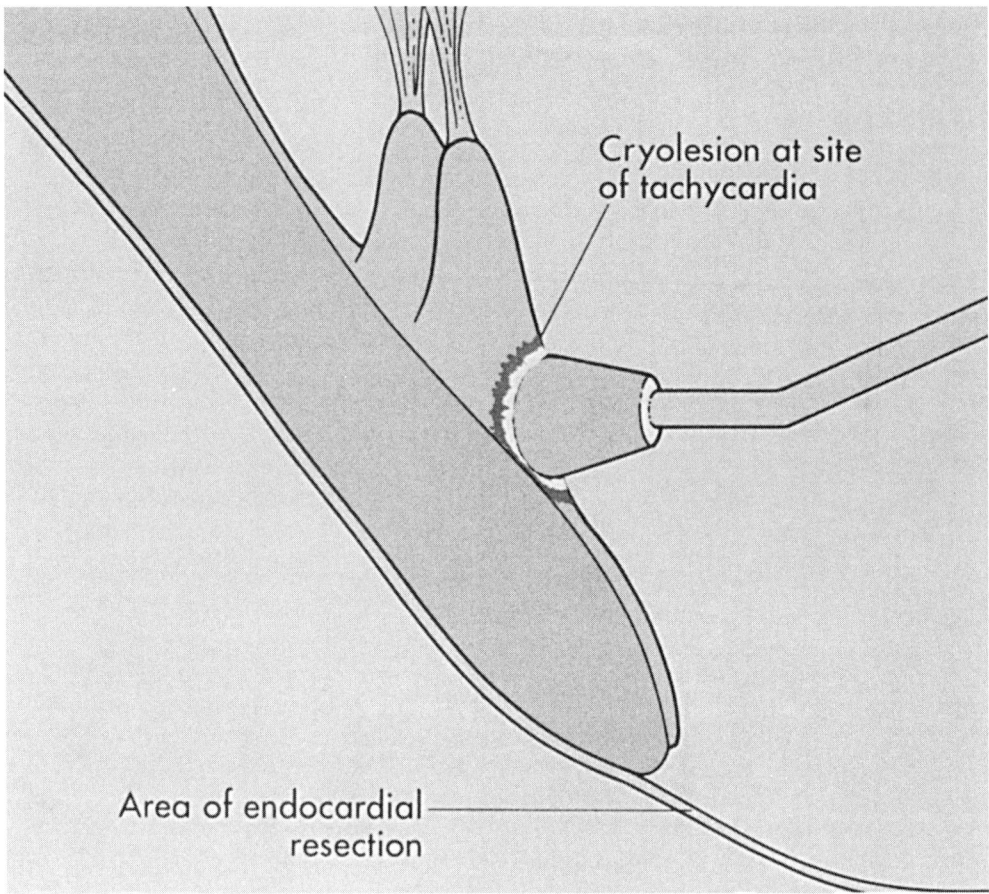

Figure 32. To obviate the necessity for mitral valve replacement due to undermining or resection of the base of the papillary muscles, cryolesions are placed on endocardial fibrosis that extends up onto the muscle base. This does not result in weakening of the tissue with resultant mitral regurgitation. (Reproduced with permission from Reference 1.)

The standard approach for ICD implantation is through a left anterior thoracotomy,[69,70] although multiple different implant techniques have been described.[71] The patches are placed in the extrapericardial position; either endocardial or epicardial rate-sensing leads are used. After demonstration of adequate sensing parameters, morphology characteristics and defibrillation thresholds the generator pocket is created below the left rectus sheath in the upper left abdominal wall. For patients requiring concomitant coronary artery bypass grafting or valve replacement a median sternotomy approach is used.

Recently, nonthoracotomy systems utilizing endocardial electrodes and a subcutaneous patch array have undergone clinical investigation;[72] while these systems are associated with higher initial defibrillation thresholds and their stability over time remains to be determined, in selected patients they will prove beneficial in the future. Algorithms to determine which patients should get which type of systems are being developed.

The following recommendations can be made as additions to the treatment algorithm outlined in Figure 30.[73]

1. If intraoperative mapping is unavailable or if the endocardial resection is performed

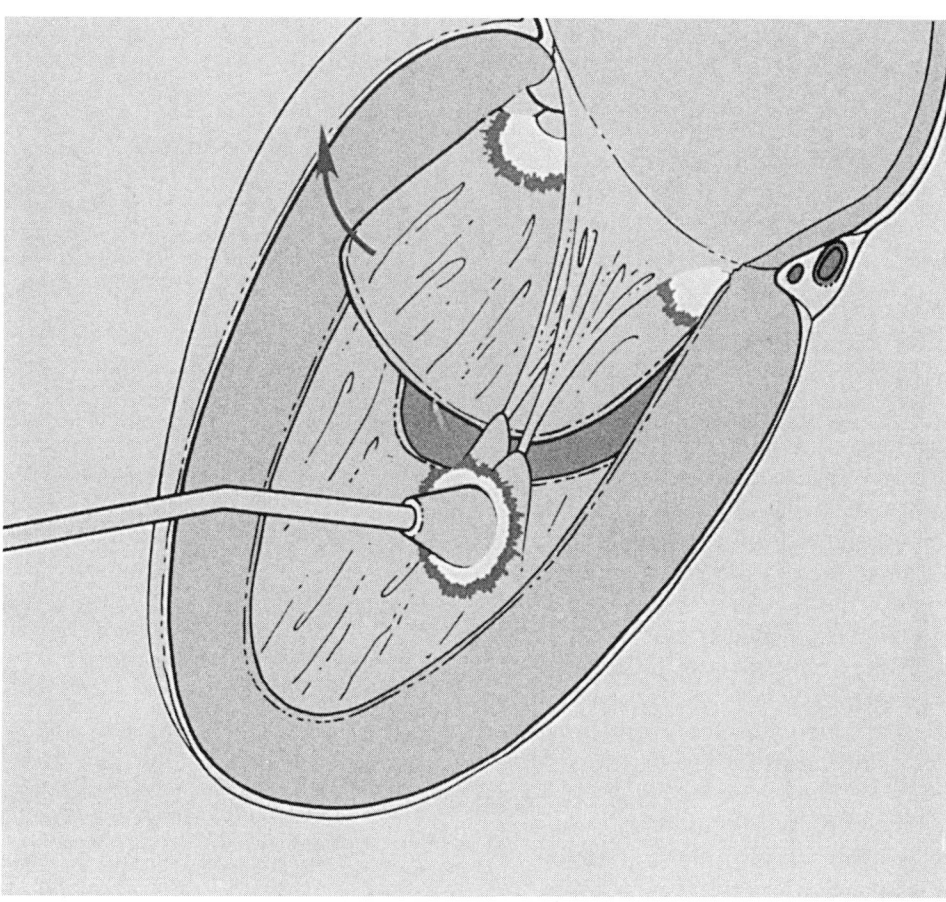

Figure 33. Extended endocardial resection with cryoablation for a posterior myocardial infarction or aneurysm. The endocardial fibrosis is dissected to within 5 mm of the aortic and mitral valve annuli. Because the site of origin of posterior tachycardias is often at the junction of the free wall and septum posteriorly at the base, cryolesions are placed at the aortic and mitral annuli. If the base of the papillary muscles is involved, cryolesions are placed as described in Figure 32. (Reproduced with permission from Reference 1.)

under cardioplegic arrest, it is appropriate to implant ICD patches in these patients at the time of the ventricular tachycardia surgery. The rationale for this recommendation is that under these circumstances, approximately 25% of patients will have inducible tachycardia following surgery. If in these patients the tachycardia is inducible at the time of a late postoperative electrophysiological study, implantation of the ICD device can be performed under local anesthesia.

2. The operative and long-term follow-up results for ventricular tachycardia surgery

argue strongly against routine implantation of the ICD device and performance of coronary bypass surgery as the primary therapeutic modality for ventricular tachycardia in patients who are otherwise candidates for a map directed, wide-resection/cryoablative procedure as described above.

3. The ICD device provides a viable therapeutic option for those patients in whom performance of ventricular tachycardia surgery has been fraught with an excessive mortality, namely, patients with extreme degrees of ventricular dysfunction. Judicious selection of

these patients for ICD implantation has been shown to reduce the operative mortality rate for patients undergoing direct procedures, while not increasing prohibitively the mortality for ICD implantation. This selection process has thereby reduced the overall operative mortality rate for ventricular tachycardia procedures.

Surgical Results: Ischemic Ventricular Tachycardias

The long-term success rate for patients who survive ventricular tachycardia surgery is 87% at 9 years in our series of patients operated on for ischemic ventricular tachycardia;[73] these data agree with the other large series published in the literature. Essentially all of this experience was gained prior to the advent of ICD therapy. The effect of the availability of ICD therapy has been to select out the less optimal candidates for direct surgery from this pool; this selection has reduced the operative mortality for direct VT surgery to 4%–5% for anterior aneurysms and 6%–7% for posterior aneurysms. Importantly, the application of ICD therapy to this group of patients who are not optimal candidates for direct surgery has not increased the operative mortality or morbidity for this procedure.[70] In follow-up, patients with ICD implants have a very low incidence of arrhythmia-related death; long-term survival is more related to underlying ventricular function.[69,70,74–76]

Summary

The surgical treatment of cardiac arrhythmias will continue to evolve as advances in: (1) understanding of the mechanisms of these arrhythmias and (2) technological developments in the areas of mapping and noninvasive diagnostic capabilites are made. As limitations with many aspects of pharmacological therapy become more apparent,[77] surgical therapies will continue to play a pivotal role in the definitive treatment of most of these supraventricular and ventricular tachyarrhythmias.

References

1. Ferguson TB Jr, Cox JL: Surgical treatment of cardiac arrhythmias. In: K Chatterjee, MD Cheitlin, J Karliner, et al. (eds): *Cardiology. An Illustrated Text/Reference*. Philadelphia, PA: Lippincott/Gower, 1991, p. 6. 185.
2. Jackman WM, Kuck K-H, Friday KJ, Lazzara R: Catheter recordings of accessory atrioventricular pathway activation. In: DP Zipes, J Jalife (eds): *Cardiac Electrophysiology*. Philadelphia, PA: W.B. Saunders and Co., 1990, p. 491.
3. Ferguson TB Jr, Cox JL: Surgical therapy for patients with supraventricular tachycardia. In: MM Scheinman (ed): *Cardiology Clinics*. Philadelphia, PA: W.B. Saunders and Co., 1990, p. 535.
4. Jackman WM, Wang X, Friday KJ, et al: Catheter ablation of accessory atrioventricular pathways (Wolff-Parkinson-White Syndrome) by radiofrequency current. *N Engl J Med* 324:1605, 1991.
5. Calkins H, Sousa J, El-Atassi R, et al: Diagnosis and cure of the Wolff-Parkinson-White Syndrome or paroxysmal supraventricular tachycardias during a single electrophysiological test. *N Engl J Med* 324:1612, 1991.
6. Canavan TE, Schuessler RB, Boineau JP, et al: Computerized global electrophysiological mapping of the atrium in patients with the Wolff-Parkinson-White Syndrome. *Ann Thorac Surg* 46:223, 1989.
7. Jackman WM, Friday KJ, Yeung-Lai-Wah JAF, et al: New catheter technique for recording left free-wall accessory atrioventricular pathway activation: identification of pathway fiber orientation. *Circulation* 78:598, 1988.
8. Ferguson TB Jr: The endocardial approach for posterior septal accessory pathways. In: JL Cox (ed): *Cardiac Arrhythmia Surgery*. Philadelphia, PA: Hanley and Belfus, 1990, p. 155.
9. Cain ME, Lindsay BD: The preoperative electrophysiologic study. In: JL Cox (ed): *Cardiac Surgery: State of the Art Reviews*. Philadelphia, PA: Hanley and Belfus, Inc., 1990, p. 1.
10. Cox JL, Ferguson TB Jr: Surgery for the Wolff-Parkinson-White syndrome: the endocardial approach. *Semin Thorac Cardiovasc Surg* 1:34, 1989.
11. Guiraudon GM, Klein GJ, Sharma AD, et al: Closed-heart technique for Wolff-Parkinson-White syndrome: further experience and potential limitations. *Ann Thorac Surg* 42:651, 1986.

12. Guiraudon GM, Klein GJ, Sharma AD, et al: Surgery for the Wolff-Parkinson-White syndrome: the epicardial approach. *Semin Thorac Cardiovasc Surg* 1:21, 1989.

13. Cox JL, Ferguson TB Jr: Surgery for atrioventricular node reentry tachycardia: the discrete cryosurgical technique. *Semin Thorac Cardiovasc Surg* 1:47, 1989.

14. Ferguson TB Jr, Cox JL: Complications related to the surgical treatment of supraventricular and ventricular cardiac arrhythmias. In: JA Waldhausen, MB Orringer (eds): *Complications in Cardiothoracic Surgery*. St. Louis, MO: Mosby Year Book, 1990.

15. Sung RJ, Huycke EC, Keung EC, et al: Atrioventricular node reentry: evidence of reentry and functional properties of fast and slow pathways. In: DP Zipes, J Jalife (eds): *Cardiac Electrophysiology*. Philadelphia, PA: W.B. Saunders and Co., 1990, p. 513.

16. Holman WL, Hackel DB, Lease JG, et al: Cryosurgical ablation of atrioventricular nodal reentry: histologic localization of the proximal common pathway. *Circulation* 77:1356, 1988.

17. Cox JL, Ferguson TB Jr, Lindsay BD, Cain ME: Peri-nodal cryosurgery for AV nodal reentrant tachycardia in 23 patients. *J Thorac Cardiovasc Surg* 99:440, 1990.

18. Leon A, El-Atassi R, Borganelli M, et al: A prospective randomized comparison of anterior and posterior approaches for radiofrequency catheter modification of AV node reentry tachycardia (abstract). *J Am Coll Cardiol* 19:145A, 1992.

19. Cox JL, Ferguson TB Jr: Surgery for dual atrioventricular node physiology in the Wolff-Parkinson-White Syndrome. *J Am Coll Cardiol* 17:1568, 1991.

20. Guiraudon GM, Klein GJ, Sharma AD, et al: Skeletonization of the atrioventricular node for AV node reentrant tachycardia: experience in 32 patients. *Ann Thorac Surg* 49:565, 1990.

21. McGuire MA, Lau K-C, Johnson DC, et al: Patients with two types of atrioventricular junctional (AV nodal) reentrant tachycardia: evidence that a common pathway of nodal tissue is not present above the reentrant circuit. *Circulation* 83:1232, 1991.

22. Lowe JE, Hendry PJ, Packer DL, Tang AS: Surgical management of chronic ectopic atrial tachycardia. *Semin Thorac Cardiovasc Surg* 1:58, 1989.

23. Williams JM, Ungerlieder GK, Lofland GK, et al: Left atrial isolation. New technique for the treatment of supraventricular arrhythmias. *J Thorac Cardiovasc Surg* 80:373, 1980.

24. Harada A, D'Agostino HJ, Schuessler RB, et al: Right atrial isolation: a new surgical treatment for supraventricular tachycardia. *J Thorac Cardiovasc Surg* 95:643, 1988.

25. Prager NA, Cox JL, Lindsay BD, et al: Long-term effectiveness of medical and surgical treatment of automatic atrial tachycardia. *J Am Coll Cardiol* (in press).

26. Boineau JP, Schuessler RB, Mooney CR, et al: Natural and evoked atrial flutter due to circus movements in dogs. *Am J Cardiol* 45:1167, 1980.

27. Boineau JP: Atrial flutter: a synthesis of concepts. *Circulation* 72:249, 1985.

28. Allessie MA, Lammers WJEP, Bonke FIM, et al: Intra-atrial reentry as a mechanism for atrial flutter by acetylcholine and rapid pacing in the dog. *Circulation* 70:123, 1984.

29. Boineau JP, Schuessler RB, Cain ME, et al: Activation mapping during normal atrial rhythms and atrial flutter. In: DP Zipes, J Jalife (eds): *Cardiac Electrophysiology*. Philadelphia, PA: W.B. Saunders and Co., 1990.

30. Cox JL, Canavan TE, Schuessler RB, et al: The surgical treatment of atrial fibrillation. II. Intraoperative electrophysiologic mapping and description of the electrophysiologic basis of atrial flutter and fibrillation. *J Thorac Cardiovasc Surg* 101:406, 1991.

31. Allessie MA, Rensma PL, Brugada J, et al: Pathophysiology of atrial fibrillation. In: DP Zipes, J Jalife (eds): *Cardiac Electrophysiology*. Philadelphia, PA: W.B. Saunders and Co., 1990, p. 548.

32. Cox JL, Schuessler RB, Boineau JP: The surgical treatment of atrial fibrillation. I. Summary of the current concepts of the mechanisms of atrial flutter and fibrillation. *J Thorac Cardiovasc Surg* 101:402, 1991.

33. Flecainide-Quinidine Research Group: Flecainide versus quinidine for treatment of chronic ventricular arrhythmias. A multicenter trial. *Circulation* 67:1117, 1983.

34. Cohen IS, Hershel J, Cohen S: Adverse reactions to quinidine in hospitalized patients. Findings based on data from Boston Collaborative Drug Surveillance Program. *Prog Cardiovasc Dis* 20:151, 1977.

35. Coumel P: Clinical approach to paroxysmal atrial fibrillation. *Clin Cardiol* 13:209, 1990.

36. Antman EM, Beamer AD, Cantillon C, et al: Therapy of refractory symptomatic atrial fibrillation and atrial flutter. A staged care approach with new antiarrhythmic drugs. *J Am Coll Cardiol* 1992.

37. Ruskin JN, McGovern B, Garan H, et al: Antiarrhythmic drugs: a possible cause of out-of-hospital cardiac arrest. *N Engl J Med* 309:1302, 1983.

38. Bauernfiend RA, Welch WJ: New hope in atrial fibrillation. *J Am Coll Cardiol* 15:708, 1990.

39. Morris JJ, Peter PH, McIntosh HD: Electrical cardioversion of atrial fibrillation. Immediate and long-term results and selection of patients. *Ann Intern Med* 65:216, 1966.

40. Lown B: Electrical reversion of cardiac arrhythmias. *Br Heart J* 38:381, 1976.

41. Radford MD, Evans DW: Long-term results of DC reversion of atrial fibrillation. *Br Heart J* 30:91, 1968.

42. Fisher CM: Embolism in atrial fibrillation. In: HE Kulbertus, SB Olsson, M Schlepper (eds): *Atrial Fibrillation*. Molndal, Sweden: AB Hassal, 1982, p. 192.

43. Alpert MA, Curtis JJ, Sanfelippo JF, et al: Comparative survival after permanent ventricular and dual chamber pacing for patients with chronic high degree atrioventricular block with and without preexistent congestive heart failure. *J Am Coll Cardiol* 7:925, 1986.

44. Scheinman MM, Morady F, Hess DS, et al: Catheter-induced ablation of the atrioventricular junction to control refractory supraventricular arrhythmias. *JAMA* 248:851, 1982.

45. Defauw JJ, Guiraudon GM, van Hemel NM, et al: Surgical therapy of paroxysmal atrial fibrillation with the "corridor" operation. *Ann Thorac Surg* 53:564, 1992.

46. Moe GK: On the multiple wavelet hypothesis of atrial fibrillation. *Arch Int Pharmacodyn Ther* 140:183, 1962.

47. Boineau JP, Schuessler RB, Mooney CR, et al: Natural and evoked atrial flutter due to circus movement in dogs. Role of abnormal atrial pathways, slow conduction, nonuniform refractory period distribution and premature beats. *Am J Cardiol* 45:1167, 1980.

48. Allessie MA, Bonke FIM, Schopman FJG: Circus movement in rabbit atrial muscle as a mechanism of tachycardia. III. The "leading circle" concept. A new mode of circus movement in cardiac tissue without the involvement of an anatomical obstacle. *Circ Res* 41:9, 1977.

49. Puech P, Grolleau R, Rebuffat G: Intraatrial mapping of atrial fibrillation in man. In: JE Kulbertus, SB Olsson, M Schlepper (eds): *Atrial Fibrillation*. Molndal, Sweden: AB Hassal, 1982, p. 94.

50. Allessie MA, Lammers WJEP, Bonke FM, et al: Experimental evaluation of Moe's multiple wavelet hypothesis of atrial fibrillation. In: DP Zipes, J Jalife (eds): *Cardiac Electrophysiology and Arrhythmias*. Orlando, FL: Grune and Stratton, 1985, p. 275.

51. Cox JL, Boineau JP, Schuessler RB, et al: Operations for atrial fibrillation. *Clin Cardiol* 14:827, 1991.

52. Cox JL, Schuessler RB, D'Agostino HJ, et al: The surgical treatment of atrial fibrillation. III. Development of a definitive surgical procedure. *J Thorac Cardiovasc Surg* 101:569, 1991.

53. Cox JL, Boineau JP, Schuessler RB, et al: Successful surgical treatment of atrial fibrillation. Review and clinical update. *JAMA* 266:1976, 1991.

54. Cox JL: The surgical treatment of atrial fibrillation. IV. Surgical technique. *J Thorac Cardiovasc Surg* 101:584, 1991.

55. Cox JL, Boineau JP, Schuessler RB, et al: A review of surgery for atrial fibrillation. *J Cardiovasc Electrophysiol* 2:541, 1991.

56. Ferguson TB Jr, Cox JL: Antiarrhythmic surgery: ventricular arrhythmias. In: LN Horowitz (ed): *Current Management of Arrhythmias*. Philadelphia, PA: B.C. Decker, 1990, p. 382.

57. Fontaine G, Fontaliran R, Linares-Cruz E, et al: The arrhythmogenic right ventricle. In: T Iwa, G Fontaine (eds): *Cardiac Arrhythmias: Recent Progress in Investigation and Management*. Amsterdam: Elsevier, 1988, p. 189.

58. Keller BB, Mehta AV, Shamszadeh J, et al: Oncocytic cardiomyopathy of infancy with Wolff-Parkinson-White syndrome and ectopic foci causing tachydysrhythmias in children. *Am Heart J* 114:782, 1987.

59. Shuman TA, Palazzo RS, Schuessler RB, et al: An experimental model based on Mustard's atrial flutter. *Surg Forum* 4190:219, 1990.

60. Horowitz LN, Vetter VL, Harken AH, Josephson ME: Electrophysiologic characteristics of sustained ventricular tachycardia occurring after repair of tetralogy of Fallot. *Am J Cardiol* 46:446, 1980.

61. Cox JL, Ferguson TB Jr: Cardiac arrhythmia surgery. In: SA Wells (ed): *Current Problems in Surgery*. 26th ed. Chicago, IL: Year Book Medical Publishers, Inc., 1989, p. 193.

62. Josephson ME, Gottlieb CD: Ventricular tachycardias associated with coronary artery disease. In: DP Zipes, J Jalife (eds): *Cardiac Electrophysiology*. Philadelphia, PA: W.B. Saunders, Inc., 1990, p. 571.

63. Branyas NB, Cain ME, Cox JL, Cassidy DM: Transmural ventricular activation during consecutive cycles of sustained ventricular tachycardia. *Am J Cardiol* 65:861, 1990.

64. Sanders R, Myerberg RJ, Gelband H: Dissimilar length-tension relations of canine ventricular muscle and false tendon: electrophysiologic alterations accompanying defamations. *J Mol Cell Cardiol* 11:209, 1979.

65. Schwartz PJ, Locati E, Priori SG, Zaza A: The long Q-T syndrome. In: DP Zipes, J Jalife (eds): *Cardiac Electrophysiology*. 1st ed. Philadelphia, PA: W.B. Saunders and Co., 1990, p. 589.

66. Hargrove WC: Surgery for ischemic ventricular tachycardia-operative techniques and long-

term results. *Semin Thorac Cardiovasc Surg* 1: 83, 1989.

67. Ostermeyer J, Kirklin JK, Borggrefe M, et al: Ten years of electrophysiologically guided direct operations for malignant ischemic ventricular tachycardia—results. *Thorac Cardiovasc Surg* 37:20, 1989.

68. Witkowski FX, Corr PB: An automated simultaneous transmural cardiac mapping system. *Am J Physiol* 247:H661, 1984.

69. Ferguson TB Jr, Lindsay BD, Ravichandran P, et al: Risk factors for implantable defibrillator therapy: the effect of ejection fraction and potential for myocardial ischemia. *J Thorac Cardiovasc Surg* (in press).

70. Ferguson TB Jr: The role of the automatic implantable cardioverter-defibrillator (AICD) in the treatment of medically-refractory ventricular arrhythmias. *Trends Cardiovasc Med* 1:131, 1991.

71. Damiano RJ: Implantable cardioverter defibrillators: current status and future directions. *J Cardiac Surg* 7:36, 1992.

72. Bardy GH, Allen MA, Mehra R, Johnson G: An effective and adaptable transvenous defibrillation system using the coronary sinus in humans. *J Am Coll Cardiol* 16:887, 1990.

73. Cox JL: Ventricular tachycardia surgery: a review of the first decade and a suggested contemporary approach. *Semin Thorac Cardiovasc Surg* 1:97, 1989.

74. Ferguson TB Jr, Cox JL: Complications related to the surgical treatment of supraventricular and ventricular cardiac arrhythmias. In: JA Waldhausen, MB Orringer (eds): *Complications in Cardiothoracic Surgery*. 1st ed. St. Louis, MO: Mosby Year Book, 1990.

75. Kim SG, Fisher JD, Choue CW, et al: Influence of left ventricular function on outcome of patients treated with implantable defibrillators. *Circulation* 85:1304, 1992.

76. Saksena S: Survival of implantable cardioverter-defibrillator recipients. *Circulation* 85:1616, 1992.

77. The Cardiac Arrhythmia Suppression Trial (CAST) Investigators: Preliminary report: effect of encainide and flecainide on mortality in a randomized trial of arrhythmia suppression after myocardial infarction. *N Engl J Med* 321: 406, 1989.

Chapter 45

The Role of Catheter Ablation in the Management of Patients with Supraventricular and Ventricular Tachycardia

Melvin M. Scheinman

Catheter ablative techniques were first introduced in 1982 for complete interruption of the atrioventricular junction in patients with drug refractory supraventricular arrhythmias.[1] The original technique was limited to the use of high-energy direct current discharges that resulted in significant barotraumatic injury, including cardiac tamponade.[2-5] Late sudden death has been reported and thought to be in part related to the widespread damage created with necrosis of the ventricular septum, producing a nidus for later development of potentially malignant ventricular arrhythmias.[6]

In 1984, Hartzler et al.[7] extended the use of catheter ablative procedures to patients with ventricular tachycardia. This procedure involved using standard techniques for ventricular tachycardia induction in the catheter laboratory. Endocardial mapping was then performed by sampling from as many endocardial sites as possible. The earliest endocardial activation relative to the surface ECG was taken as the exit point for the tachycardia focus, and high-energy direct current discharges were used in order to ablate arrhythmogenic zones.

A number of additional groups have reported the use of this technique with highly variable results. Fontaine et al.,[8] for example, reported excellent results with this technique. In contrast, others reported less favorable results.[9-11]

The most extensive report relating to catheter ablation using high-energy direct current shocks was issued by the Percutaneous Mapping and Ablation Registry.[11] The report summarized data from a voluntary worldwide registry established to assess the role of catheter ablative procedures. The results of attempted ventricular tachycardia ablation using direct current energy were summarized (Table 1) by this group.[11] Data from 164 patients with ventricular tachycardia who underwent attempted catheter ablation were reported. These patients were followed over a mean interval of 12 ± 11 months. The efficacy of this procedure for complete cure was poor (18%), but some 41% appeared to benefit

---

From BN Singh, HJJ Wellens, M Hiraoka, (eds): *Electropharmacological Control of Cardiac Arrhythmias*. Mount Kisco, NY, Futura Publishing Company Inc., © 1994.

Table 1
Results of Attempted Ventricular Tachycardia Focus Ablation in 164 Patients
(Follow-up interval = 12 ± 11 months)

Clinical response	Number of patients (% in parenthesis)
Group I: No recurrent VT Taking no antiarrhythmic drugs	30 (18%)
Group II: No recurrent VT Antiarrhythmic drug therapy required	67 (41%)
Group III: Recurrent VT or unsuccessful (includes all patients with sudden death and procedure-related death)	67 (41%)

Early Complications
Procedure-related death (11)
Hypotension (10)
Acute pulmonary edema (3)
CVA or TIA (3)
Pulmonary embolus (1)
Cardiac tamponade (2)
Pericarditis (4)
Possible myocardial infarction (1)
Syncope (1)
LV thrombus (1)
Sepsis (2)
Chest pain (2)
New arrhythmias:
  1. Sustained, new morphology VT (2)
  2. Polymorphous VT/Ventricular fibrillation (1)
  3. Second degree AV block (transient) (1)
  4. Third degree AV block (3)
  5. New SVT
  6. VF 1 hour postablation

Mortality Statistics: Total Deaths = 40 (24%)
Procedure-related deaths (11)
Death due to cardiogenic shock, possibly procedure-related (1)
Sudden cardiac death (16)
Acute MI with shock at 2 weeks (1)
Death from congestive heart failure (6)
Noncardiac deaths (5)
  1. GI bleed (1)
  2. CVA, possibly embolic (1)
  3. Suicide (1)
  4. Sepsis (1)
  5. Cancer (1)

from drug therapy after ablation. It is important to emphasize the significant early and late complications of this procedure. There were 11 procedure-related deaths that were attributed to low-out states, electromechanical dissociation, or new refractory ventricular arrhythmias.

Catheter Ablation of Supraventricular Tachyarrhythmias

A significant advance in the use of catheter ablative procedures occurred in 1987 with the introduction of the use of radiofrequency energy for control of supraventricular arrhythmias.[12,13] Radiofrequency energy was initially applied to patients with supraventricular arrhythmias who required ablation of the atrioventricular junction.[13] The subsequent introduction of steerable catheters with a large (4 mm) distal electrode made this technique more accessible for patients with other supraventricular arrhythmias.[14–16] At this point in time, catheter ablative procedures have become the treatment of choice for patients with symptomatic supraventricular arrhythmias due to atrioventricular nodal reentry or to tachycardia mediated via an accessory atrioventricular conducting pathway.[17]

The most common causes of paroxysmal supraventricular tachycardia include atrioventricular nodal reentry or tachycardia that incorporates an accessory pathway. Current ablative techniques allow for ablation of either the fast or slow atrioventricular nodal pathway. Ablation of the slow pathway has proved to be very effective and safer than attempted fast pathway ablation. Catheter ablation of accessory pathways are directed at initially defining pathway locations. Approximately 65% of pathways are left sided, and the remaining 35% of the pathways are either septal or free wall in location. Current techniques allow for ablation of these pathways in any location.

More recently these techniques have been expanded to patients with atrial tachycardia or atrial flutter. Walsh et al.[18] have recently described techniques for successful mapping and radiofrequency ablation of atrial foci. Both right and left atrial sites have been successfully mapped and ablated. These ectopic foci may occur in the atrial septum in either atrial appendage or close to the insertion of the pulmonary veins. In contrast, the critical slow area required for maintenance of atrial flutter appears to be at the base of the right atrium at the isthmus between the inferior vena cava and the septal leaflet of the tricuspid valve.[19] Successful lesions applied either posterior or apical to the coronary sinus os were most likely to result in successful ablation.

The introduction of steerable catheters as well as the use of radiofrequency energy has allowed for a wider margin of safety in application of these techniques to patients with ventricular tachycardia. In this chapter, we emphasize the technique, results, and clinical role of catheter ablative techniques for patients with ventricular tachycardia.

Catheter Ablation of Bundle Branch Reentry Tachycardia

Bundle branch reentrant tachycardia is a form of ventricular tachycardia involving the specialized intraventricular conduction system. The mechanism usually involves antegrade conduction over the right bundle branch with retrograde conduction over the left bundle.[20] The converse may be rarely observed. Bundle branch reentrant tachycardia occurs almost exclusively in patients with either severe myocardial disease or in those with significant disease of the specialized intraventricular conduction system.[20] The incidence of bundle branch reentrant tachycardia appears to be higher in patients with idiopathic cardiomyopathy compared to those with ischemic heart disease.

The salient electrophysiological features include induction of a tachycardia with left bundle branch block contour with H-V ≥ the H-V during sinus rhythm (Figure 1). In addition, variation in the H-H interval that precedes variation in the ventricular cycle length excludes ventricular tachycardia of myocardial origin. Registration of the right bundle branch potential is of paramount importance since this structure is an obligate portion of the tachycardia circuit (Figure 2).[21] During bundle branch reentrant tachycardia, the interval from the right bundle deflection to the onset of ventricular activation shortens, and this finding effectively excludes a supraventricular mechanism.

Technique for Interruption of Bundle Branch Reentrant Tachycardia

A steerable electrode catheter with a 4-mm distal electrode tip is advanced to the

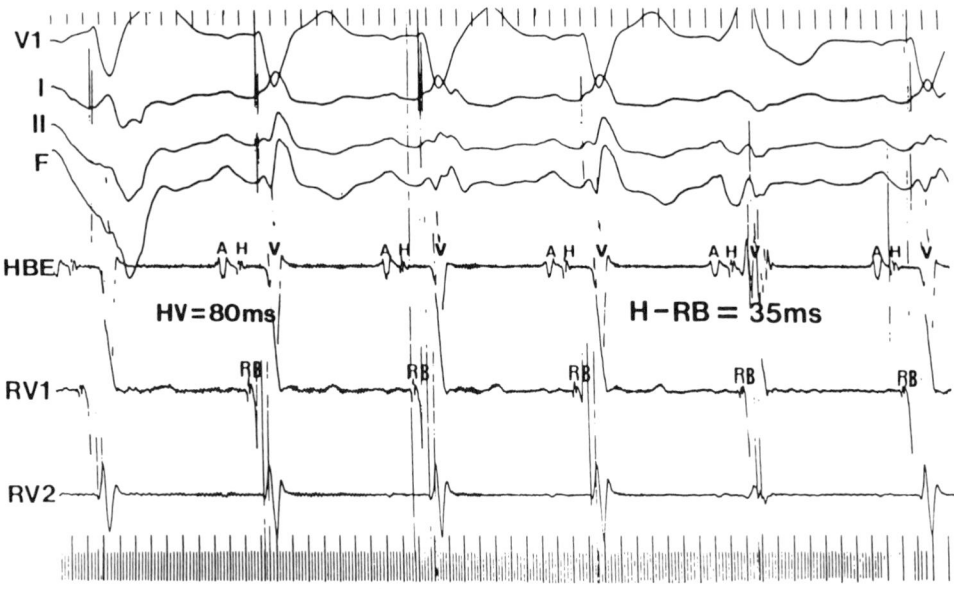

Figure 1. Baseline recordings showing simultaneous recordings of surface leads V_1, I, II, and F and intracardiac recordings from the His bundle region (HBE) and summit of the right ventricle (RV_1 and RV_2). During sinus rhythm, the surface ECG shows a left bundle branch pattern with a prolonged infranodal conduction time (HV = 80 msec). The interval from the His bundle to right bundle deflection (H-RB) is 35 msec.

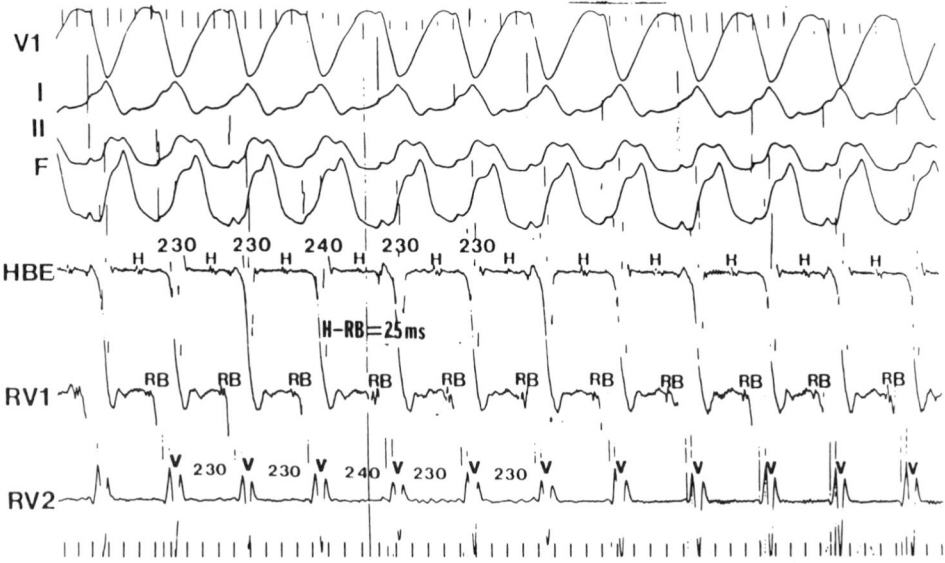

Figure 2. The tracing shows a wide complex tachycardia with atrioventricular (AV) dissociation (note dissociated P waves in lead F). A His bundle deflection (H) precedes the surface QRS recording, and the His-RB interval has decreased to 25 msec during tachycardia. The decrease in the H-RB interval excludes a supraventricular mechanism. In addition, slight changes in the H-H interval precede changes in RR interval. The latter finding excludes a myocardial source for ventricular tachycardia. These findings are diagnostic of bundle branch reentrant tachycardia. Abbreviations and format are as described in Figure 1.

usual His bundle position. The catheter is then advanced over the summit of the right ventricular septum in order to record a right bundle branch potential. Once located, a radiofrequency energy of 40 W is applied for 60 seconds in order to destroy the right bundle branch.[22] This technique is usually successful since the main right bundle branch is draped superficially over the right side of the septum. In our experience, we have found that isolated destruction of the right bundle branch does not necessarily require permanent pacemaker insertion.[23] The most important caveat in terms of appropriate management of these patients is exclusion of the presence of concomitant myocardial ventricular tachycardia, which in our experience occurs in approximately 30% of patients with bundle branch reentrant tachycardia.[23]

Patients with Right Ventricular Outflow Tract Ventricular Tachycardia

A group of patients without known heart disease, but who are afflicted with ventricular tachycardia emanating from the right ventricular outflow tract has been described.[24] In these patients, the tachycardia is often exercise- or isoproterenol-induced and shows a left bundle branch block and inferior axis pattern on surface ECG recordings (Figure 3). These tachycardias may be interrupted by either carotid sinus massage or infusions of adenosine and are thought to be cyclic adenosine monophosphate (cAMP)-dependent tachycardias.[25] The technique we use for ablation of these tachycardias involves placement of the ablation catheter into the pulmonary artery and gently withdrawing the catheter in order to map all margins of the right ventricular outlow tract. Activation mapping is of limited help since the earliest endocardial site is only 30 to 40 msec earlier than the surface recordings. The most reliable mapping technique appears to be use of the paced map with 100% concordance between paced and spontaneous ventricular tachycardia for all 12 leads (Figure 4). Once this area is identified,

then radiofrequency energy is applied as described in order to destroy the focus. The results reported, to date, appear to be quite gratifying with minimal adverse effects reported.[26]

Idiopathic Left Septal Ventricular Tachycardia

Another type of ventricular tachycardia seen in patients without apparent cardiac disease arises from the posterior inferior aspect of the left septum.[27] These tachycardias show a characteristic right bundle branch block and superior axis morphology. They appear to be reentrant in origin in that they can be readily provoked and terminated by standard pacing procedures. The unusual features of this tachycardia include the ability to induce the tachycardia from the atrium (in marked distinction from myocardial ventricular tachycardia in patients with coronary artery disease). In addition, these tachycardias are often sensitive to infusions of verapamil.[28]

Patients with this form of tachycardia may be approached with either a retrograde aortic approach or with the use of a transseptal approach. The rationale is to carefully explore the inferoposterior portion of the left side of the ventricular septum. This often requires looping the catheter against the lateral wall of the left ventricle and directing its tip toward the septum. The tachycardia is induced using standard techniques, and the septum is carefully mapped in order to detect the earliest endocardial activation site. Once the latter is found, it is confirmed using the technique of pace mapping as described above. Ablative lesions using radiofrequency energy are applied in order to destroy the reentrant circuit.

Myocardial Ventricular Tachycardia in Coronary Artery Disease

The most frequent cause of sustained ventricular tachycardia is that associated with coronary artery disease. Both canine experimental observations as well as clinical reports[29,30] support the presence of intramyo-

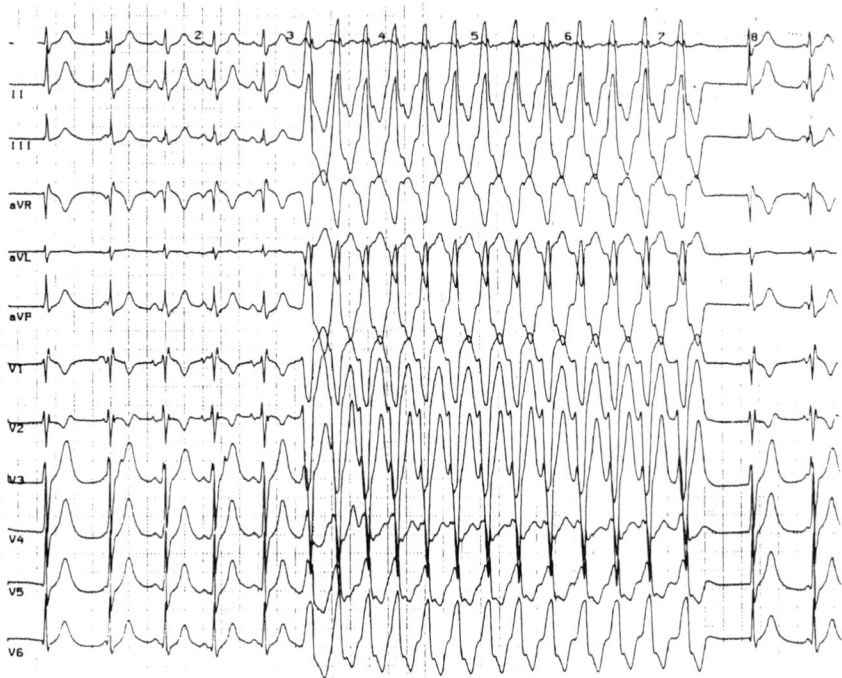

Figure 3. Baseline ECG recording from a 32-year-old female with a history of palpitations and syncope. She had no evidence of cardiac disease. The ECG pattern shows a left bundle branch block contour with superior axis.

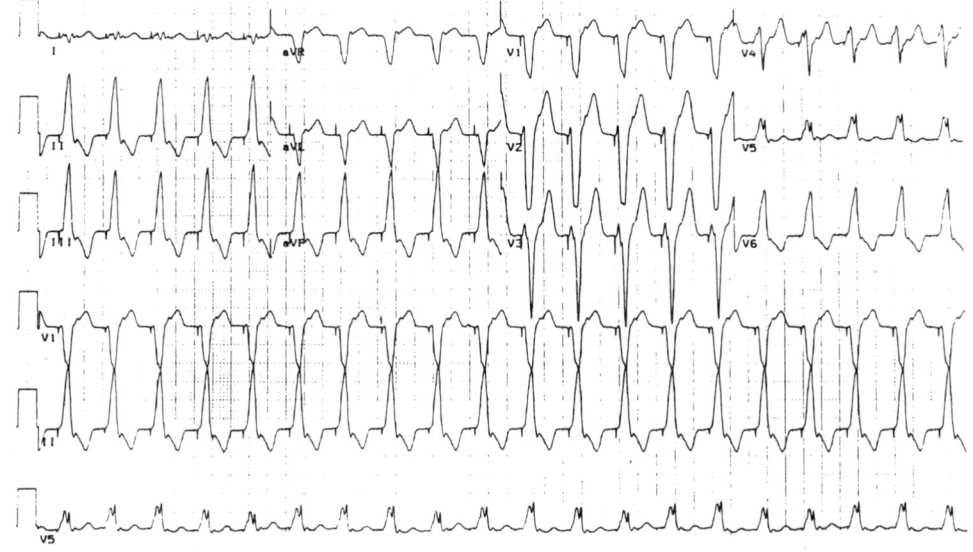

Figure 4. A 12-lead ECG obtained by pacing from the right ventricular outflow tract showing a pattern identical to that observed during spontaneous ventricular tachycardia (see Figure 3).

cardial reentry as the basis for this arrhythmia. Initial attempts to locate the ventricular tachycardia focused at cardiac catheterization involved positioning of the catheter during ventricular tachycardia in order to find the earliest endocardial potential relative to the surface complexes (Figure 5).[31] At present, newer mapping techniques have been introduced to better locate the ventricular tachycardia focus. One technique involves pace mapping as described above. In addition, entrainment mapping has been found to be effective.[32,33] This technique may be used in two ways. First, an area remote from the tachycardia is paced and the tachycardia is entrained to the paced cycle length. With termination of pacing, the putative early site again appears prior to inscription of the surface QRS.[33] Another technique, introduced by Morady et al.,[34] involves pacing

directly from the putative ventricular tachycardia site. Successful pacing from this area will show a long interval from stimulus to surface QRS, with QRS identical to that during ventricular tachycardia (Figure 6). This technique, designated as concealed entrainment, is explained by direct pacing from within the critical slow zone of the ventricular tachycardia circuit. The impulse is conducted orthodromically with an obligate delay owing to slowed conduction within the circuit itself. Others have emphasized the importance of finding early- or split-diastolic potentials during ventricular tachycardia.[35] These potentials are thought to emanate from the tachycardia circuit. Once the putative critical slow conduction zone of the reentrant circuit is identified, radiofrequency energy is applied in order to desiccate this focus (Figure 7).

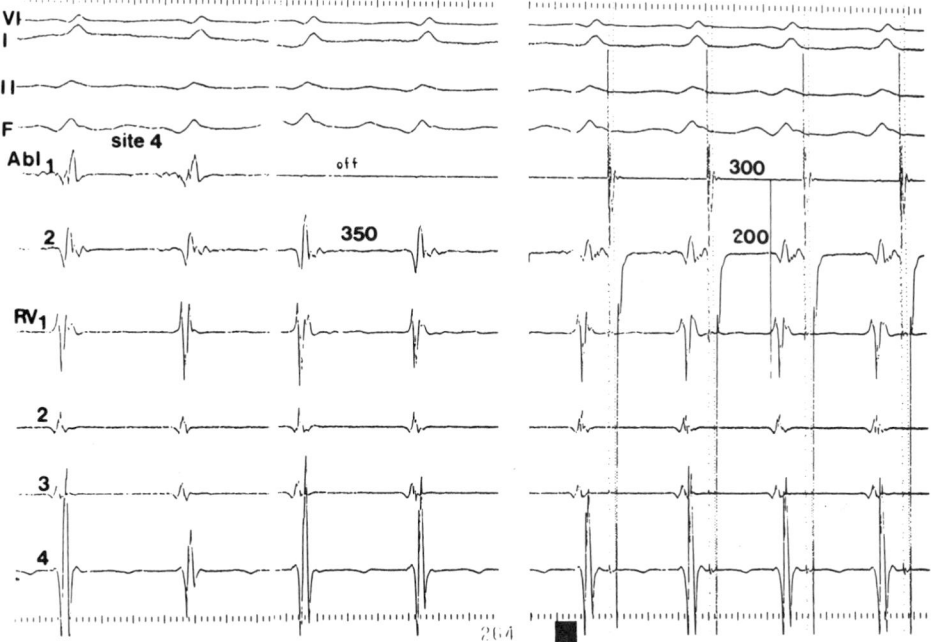

Figure 5. The left panel shows simultaneous recordings from surface leads V_1, I, II, and F, together with recordings from an ablation catheter positioned at the basal septum (Abl_1 and $_2$) and right ventricular apex ($RV_{1, 2}$) and right ventricular outflow tract ($RV_{3,4}$). This patient had a history of a prior anteroseptal myocardial infarction and recurrent episodes of ventricular tachycardia. The earliest endocardial activation site showed fractionated low amplitude potentials preceding the surface ECG recordings. Pacing from this area (right panel) resulted in entrainment of the tachycardia to the paced cycle length of 300 msec with a very long interval between the ventricular pacemaker spike and the succeeding QRS (200 msec).

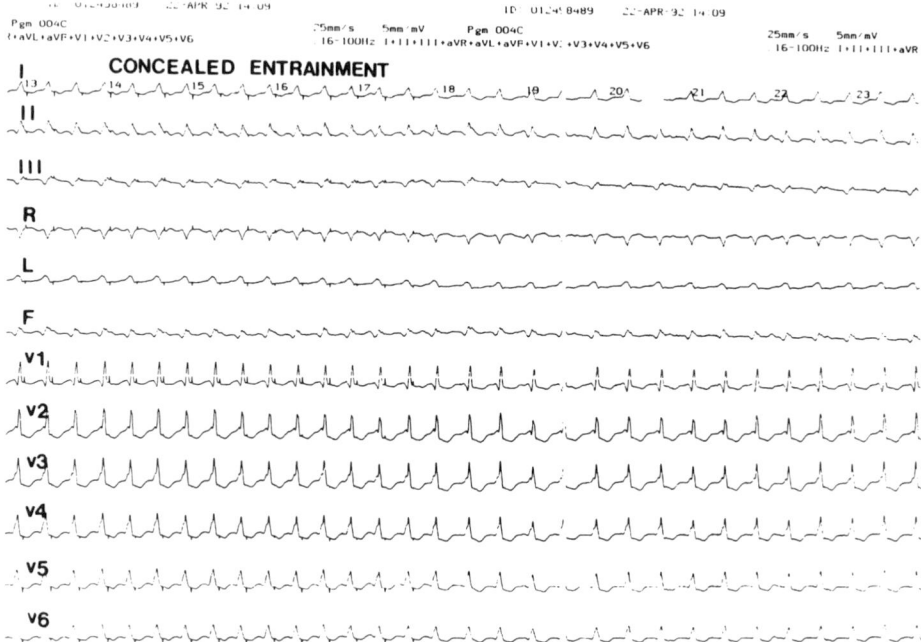

Figure 6. A 12-lead ECG recorded with pacing from the putative ventricular tachycardia focus. During overdrive pacing, there is an exact concordance between the paced complex and the spontaneous ventricular complex in all leads. After pacing is terminated, there is prompt resumption of the tachycardia, and the QRS was preceded by the early fractionated electrogram shown in Figure 5. In this patient, ventricular tachycardia could readily be initiated and terminated with pacing.

Prior reports using high-energy direct current shocks for catheter ablation have been discussed. At present, only limited reports concerning the use of radiofrequency energy for patients with ventricular tachycardia are available.[36–39] It is clear that because radiofrequency lesions can be repeatedly applied with greater safety the efficacy for this approach might exceed that reported for direct current ablation. Unfortunately, at present, no large series is available to substantiate this impression.

Summary and Conclusions

The availability of radiofrequency energy sources together with the use of newer steerable catheters has greatly altered our therapeutic approach to the management of patients with ventricular tachycardia. Although the available data are scant, use of ablative procedures has proven exceedingly safe and effective for patients with ventricular tachycardia without cardiac disease. These include patients with tachycardia emanating from the right ventricular outflow tract as well as those with left septal tachycardia. In my opinion, all symptomatic patients with these arrhythmias should undergo ablative procedures as the primary approach to therapy in order to obviate lifelong dependence on drug therapy. In addition, patients with bundle branch reentrant ventricular tachycardia often present life-threatening arrhythmias, and ablation of the right bundle branch has proved to be very safe and effective. Hence, the primary therapeutic approach for management of these patients should be catheter ablation of the right bundle branch.

In patients with myocardial ventricular

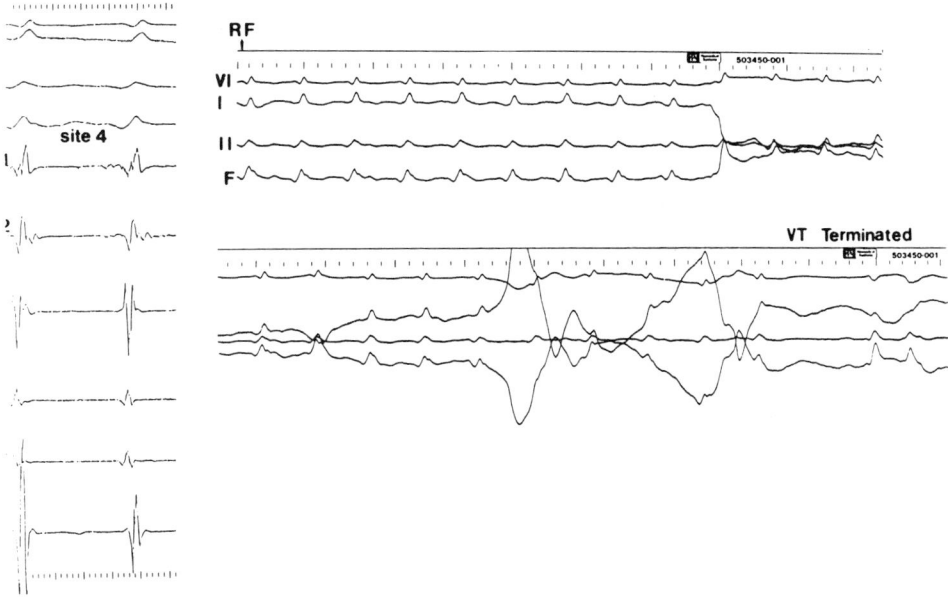

Figure 7. The left panel shows the site of the earliest endocardial activation relative to the surface recordings during ventricular tachycardia. Radiofrequency energy (RF) was applied to this area during tachycardia. Note that soon after initiation of RF energy (indicated by erratic deformation of surface ECG, top panel right), the ventricular tachycardia rate slows and finally terminates. Efforts to reinduce the tachycardia by programmed stimulation were unsuccessful. Similarly, repeat attempts to stimulate the tachycardia 4 days later were also unsuccessful.

tachycardia either due to coronary artery or myocardial disease, catheter ablation is reserved for patients with sustained, virtually incessant ventricular tachycardia of one morphology, particularly those patients who fail drug therapy and are not considered optimal candidates for surgical ablation of the ventricular tachycardia focus. Optimal candidates for surgery include those patients with well-preserved left ventricular function and single ventricular foci located in the antero-apical area and in patients who require revascularization or valve repair. Patients with virtual incessant ventricular tachycardia are not candidates for defibrillator therapy since they would be exposed to repeated shocks.

With increased experience, we feel that patients with myocardial ventricular tachycardia, particularly those with a single focus who prove refractory to drug therapy, can be considered for catheter ablative therapy. The use of radiofrequency energy has significantly di-

minished the risk and hence allows for repeated attempts at ablative therapy. Recent advances in ablative techniques have mandated that the clinician integrate use of these techniques in the management of patients with ventricular tachycardia. Future advances will in large measure depend on development of multiple electrode array catheters allowing for simultaneous recordings from multiple endocardial sites. In addition, development of newer energy sources allowing for a wider zone of myocardial ablation may be required for the successful cure of patients with myocardial ventricular tachycardia due to coronary artery disease or cardiomyopathy processes.

References

1. Scheinman MM, Morady F, Hess DS, Gonzalez R: Catheter-induced ablation of the atrioven-

tricular junction to control refractory supraventricular arrhythmias. *JAMA* 248:851, 1982.

2. Gonzalez R, Scheinman M, Margaretten W, Rubinstein M: Closed-chest electrode-catheter technique for His bundle ablation in dogs. *Am J Physiol* 241 (Heart Circ Physiol 10):H283, 1981.

3. Kempf FC Jr, Falcone RA, Iozzo RV, Josephson ME: Anatomic and hemodynamic effects of catheter-delivered ablation energies in the ventricle. *Am J Cardiol* 56:373, 1985.

4. Hauer RN, Straks W, Borst C, Robles de Medina EO: Electrical catheter ablation in the left and right ventricular wall in dogs: relation between delivered energy and histopathologic changes. *J Am Coll Cardiol* 8:637, 1986.

5. Davis JC, Finkebeiner W, Ruder MA, et al: Histologic changes and arrhythmogenicity after discharge through transseptal catheter electrode. *Circulation* 74:637, 1986.

6. Rosenqvist M, Lee MA, Moulinier L, et al: Long-term follow-up of patients after transcatheter direct current ablation of the atrioventricular junction. *J Am Coll Cardiol* 16:1467, 1990.

7. Scheinman MM, Laks MM, DiMarco J, Plumb V: Current role of catheter ablative procedures in patients with cardiac arrhythmias. A report for health professionals from the subcommittee on electrocardiography and electrophysiology, American Heart Association. *Circulation* 83:2146, 1991.

8. Fontaine G, Tonet JL, Frank R, Rougier I: Clinical experience with fulguration and antiarrhythmic therapy for the treatnent of ventricular tachycardia: long-term follow-up of 43 patients. *Chest* 95:785, 1989.

9. Morady F, Scheinman MM, DiCarlo LA, et al: Catheter ablation of ventricular tachycardia with intracardiac shocks: results in 33 patients. *Circulation* 75:1037, 1987.

10. Niwano S, Aizawa Y, Satho M, et al: Low-energy catheter electrical ablation for sustained ventricular tachycardia. *Am Heart J* 122:81, 1991.

11. Evans GT, Scheinman MM, Zipes DP, et al: The Percutaneous Cardiac Mapping and Ablation Registry: final summary of results. *PACE* 11:1621, 1988.

12. Huang SK, Bharati S, Graham AR, et al: Closed-chest catheter desiccation of the atrioventricular junction using radiofrequency energy: a new method of catheter ablation. *J Am Coll Cardiol* 9:349, 1987.

13. Langberg JJ, Chin MC, Rosenqvist M, et al: Catheter ablation of the atrioventricular junction with radiofrequency energy. *Circulation* 80:1527, 1989.

14. Jackman WM, Wang X, Friday KJ: Catheter ablation of accessory atrioventricular pathways (Wolff-Parkinson-White syndrome) by radio-

frequency current. *N Engl J Med* 324:1605, 1991.

15. Morady F, Kadish A, Calkins H, et al: Diagnosis and immediate cure of paroxysmal supraventricular tachycardia (abstract). *Circulation* 82(suppl III):III-689, 1990.

16. Kuck KH, Schluter M, Geiger M, et al: Radiofrequency current approach to successful catheter ablation of accessory pathways (abstract). *Circulation* 82(suppl III):III-689, 1990.

17. Scheinman MM: Catheter ablation: present role and projected impact on health care for patients with cardiac arrhythmias. *Circulation* 83:1489, 1991.

18. Walsh EP, Saul JP, Hulse JE, et al: Transcatheter ablation of ectopic atrial tachycardia in young patients using radiofrequency current. *Circulation* 86:1138, 1992.

19. Feld GK, Fleck RP, Chen PS, et al: Radiofrequency catheter ablation for the treatment of human type I atrial flutter: identification of a critical zone in the reentrant circuit by endocardial mapping techniques. *Circulation* 86:1233, 1992.

20. Tchou P, Jazayeri M, Denker S: Transcatheter electrical ablation of right bundle branch: a method of treating macroreentrant ventricular tachycardia attributed to bundle branch reentry. *Circulation* 78:246, 1988.

21. Chien WW, Scheinman MM, Cohen TJ, Lesh MD: Importance of recording the right bundle branch deflection in the diagnosis of His-Purkinje reentrant tachycardia. *PACE*; in press.

22. Langberg JJ, Desai J, Dullet N, Scheinman MM: Treatment of macroreentrant ventricular tachycardia with radiofrequency ablation of the right bundle branch. *Am J Cardiol* 63:1010, 1989.

23. Cohen TJ, Chien WW, Lurie KG, et al: Radiofrequency catheter ablation for treatment of bundle branch reentrant ventricular tachycardia: results and long-term follow-up. *J Am Coll Cardiol* 18:1767, 1991.

24. Klein LS, Shih HT, Hackett FK: Radiofrequency catheter ablation of ventricular tachycardia in patients without structural heart disease. *Circulation* 85:1666, 1992.

25. Lerman BB, Belardinelli L, West GA, et al: Adenosine-sensitive ventricular tachycardia: evidence suggesting cyclic AMP-mediated triggered activity. *Circulation* 74:270, 1986.

26. Coggins DL, Scheinman MM: Idiopathic right ventricular tachycardia. *J Arrhythmia Management* Fall:3, 1991.

27. Belhassen B, Shapira I, Pelleg A, et al: Idiopathic recurrent sustained ventricular tachycardia responsive to verapamil: an ECG-electrophysiologic entity. *Am Heart J* 108:1034, 1984.

28. Belhassen B, Rotmensch HH, Laniado S: Re-

sponse of recurrent sustained ventricular tachycardia to verapamil. *Br Heart J* 46:679, 1981.

29. Downar E, Harris L, Mickleborough LL, et al: Endocardial mapping of ventricular tachycardia in the intact human ventricle: evidence for reentrant mechanism. *J Am Coll Cardiol* 11: 783, 1988.

30. Kay GN, Epstein AE, Plumb VJ: Incidence of reentry with an excitable gap in ventricular tachycardia: a prospective evaluation utilizing transient entrainment. *J Am Coll Cardiol* 11: 530, 1988.

31. Josephson ME, Horowitz LN, Farshidi A, Kastor JA: Recurrent sustained ventricular tachycardia. I. Mechanism. *Circulation* 57:431, 1978.

32. Okumura K, Olshansky B, Wenthorn RW, et al: Demonstration of the presence of slow conduction during sustained ventricular tachycardia in man: use of transient entrainment of the tachycardia. *Circulation* 75:369, 1987.

33. Waldo AL, Henthorn RW: Use of transient entrainment during ventricular tachycardia to localize a critical area in the reentry circuit for ablation. *PACE* 12:231, 1989.

34. Morady F, Frank R, Kou WH, et al: Identification and catheter ablation of a zone of slow conduction in the reentrant circuit of ventricular tachycardia in humans. *J Am Coll Cardiol* 11:775, 1988.

35. Fitzgerald DM, Friday KJ, Yeung JA, et al: Electrogram patterns predicting successful catheter ablation of ventricular tachycardia. *Circulation* 77:806, 1988.

36. Gonska BD, Fleischmann C, Schaumann A, et al: Catheter ablation in recurrent ventricular tachycardia, radiofrequency energy versus direct current (abstract). *PACE* 14:686, 1991.

37. Gonska BD, Brune S, Bethge P, Kreuzer H: Radiofrequency catheter ablation in recurrent ventricular tachycardia. *Eur Heart J* 12:1257, 1991.

38. Borggrefe M, Budde T, Podczeck A, Breithardt G: Application of transvenous radiofrequency alternating current ablation in humans (abstract). *Circulation* 76(suppl IV):IV-406, 1987.

39. Kuck KH, Schluter M, Geiger M, Siebels J: Successful catheter-ablation of human ventricular tachycardia with radiofrequency current guided by an endocardial map of the area of slow conduction. *PACE* 14:1060, 1991.

Chapter 46

Implantable Defibrillators:
Implications for Antiarrhythmic Drug Therapy of Ventricular Arrhythmias

M.H. Anderson
A. John Camm

Since the first use in humans of an implantable cardioverter defibrillator (ICD) in 1980[1] the number of devices implanted annually has roughly doubled each year, and in 1992 the number of implants worldwide exceeded 10,000. Although there is evidence of the efficacy of the ICD from a considerable number of studies, no large prospective randomized controlled trial of the ICD has been published, although several such trials are in progress. Nonetheless, some data exist to allow a plausible choice of therapy between the ICD, antiarrhythmic drugs, or surgery.

In addition to the widely accepted use of the ICD in survivors of cardiac arrest several new implications in other groups of patients at high risk of sudden cardiac death are being considered. The possible use of ICD patients as a protected population for future studies of antiarrhythmic drugs has so far received little attention. The increasing numbers of patients with ICDs and the increasing sophistication of the devices may make such studies feasible within the next few years.

History

The realization that ventricular fibrillation (VF) could be treated with a transthoracic electric shock[2] and that this previously fatal arrhythmia could be reliably terminated was a major step in the development of modern cardiology without which coronary care units and invasive electrophysiology would not have evolved. However, the vast majority of sudden cardiac deaths occur outside the hospital and an obvious challenge was to find a way in which these deaths could be prevented. The idea of an ICD was first conceived in the 1960s by Michel Mirowski and the biological and engineering feasibility of such a device was demonstrated in animals in 1969.[3] The prototype version used a pressure sensing right ventricular lead to identify the loss of phasic pressure change associated with VF and delivered the defibrillating shock via electrodes on the same lead.[4] This system was shown to be capable of defibrillating dogs with 5 to 10 J.[5] At this stage the need for such

From BN Singh, HJJ Wellens, M Hiraoka, (eds): *Electropharmacological Control of Cardiac Arrhythmias.* Mount Kisco, NY, Futura Publishing Company Inc., © 1994.

a device was not widely perceived[6] and although at least one large pacemaker manufacturer was initially interested in the device its commercial viability was not certain. It was left to a small biomedical equipment company to continue the development of the device. A number of major hurdles had to be overcome before a device suitable for long-term implantation in humans could be developed. A new battery had to be developed as no existing cell was suitable,[7] and sensing and shock delivery circuits required design, miniaturization, and manufacture. These developments culminated in the first implant in a human of an automatic ICD in 1980;[8] implants in Europe began in 1983.

The early devices used a probability density function to specifically identify VF by the lack of isoelectric segments in the signal. The electrode system consisted of a spring electrode in the superior vena cava with a flexible titanium cup placed over the cardiac apex. It soon became apparent that the majority of sudden cardiac death survivors suffered from unstable ventricular tachycardias (VTs) rather than primary VF and so a bipolar right ventricular electrode was added to enable rate determination and R wave synchronization and the first ICD was introduced in 1982.

Increasingly, epicardial patch electrodes were used exclusively for shock delivery and this system was adopted by other manufacturers as they started to evaluate their own models of ICDs. However, transvenous electrode systems remained a long-term goal because of the lesser magnitude of surgery involved. If ICDs were to become smaller and implantation by a cardiologist alone was to become a practical proposition then a totally transvenous electrode system was a prerequisite. Since 1988 three manufacturers (CPI, Medtronic, and Telectronics) have been engaged in trials of transvenous electrode systems. While technical features of these systems vary, the basic approach is similar, with a subcutaneous axillary patch and two transvenous electrode surfaces mounted either on a single electrode (Endotak®, CPI, St. Paul, MN) or two separate electrodes (Transvene®, Medtronic,

Minneapolis, MN and EnGuard®, Telectronics, Englewood, CO). Several hundred Transvene and Endotak leads have been implanted and initial reports of their performance are encouraging,[9,10] although failure to meet defibrillation threshold (DFT) requirements at implant remains a problem preventing the use of transvenous systems in about 15% of patients. In a small proportion of these patients the axillary patch has been omitted giving a totally transvenous system. Currently available transvenous defibrillation systems have higher mean DFTs than systems using epicardial patches. This problem must be overcome if the dramatic reductions in defibrillator generator size that are required for prepectoral implantation are to be achieved. The most promising among the many approaches to reduce defibrillation energy requirements currently being evaluated is the use of biphasic shocks.[11] Other avenues of experimentation include modification of electrode design to achieve more even distribution of defibrillation shock field density within the myocardium.

The ICD itself has advanced dramatically simultaneously with the rapid development of electrode systems. The early first generation ICDs were capable of defibrillation/cardioversion alone. Second generation devices added provisions for bradycardia support pacing. The third generation devices, some of which are approaching market release, represent a considerable step forward. In addition to programmable defibrillation and cardioversion therapies, they offer bradycardia support and antitachycardia pacing. All models offer logging of arrhythmia events and the response to therapies delivered that can confirm correct device function and aid the recognition of inappropriate therapy delivery, for example during atrial fibrillation. In addition, some models store intracardiac electrograms from the arrhythmia, or offer transtelephonic interrogation.[12] The functions of models currently under development are summarized in Table 1. The greater range of therapies in these third generation devices may allow their use in a wider range of patients. For example, patients

Table 1
Defibrillator Features

Generation	1st	2nd	3rd
Defibrillation	+	+	+
Programmable shock output	−	+	+
Bradycardia support pacing	−	+	+
Antitachycardia Pacing	−	−	+
Low energy cardioversion	−	−	+
Holter/datalogging features	−	−	+
Electrogram storage	−	−	S
Biphasic shocks	−	−	S
Bidirectional/sequential shocks	−	−	S

+ : Present; − : Absent; S: Present on some devices only.

with hemodynamically stable VT may reasonably be treated by antitachycardia pacing, whereas repeated cardioversion therapies would be intolerable.

Thus, in the 20 years since the concept of the implantable defibrillator was born there have been rapid technical developments and it seems likely that this will continue. Over the next 5 years it is likely that we will see the increasing use of totally transvenous electrode systems, further miniaturization of the ICD generator, and a reduction in the real cost of these devices. Other foreseeable developments include improved specificity of tachycardia detection using criteria other than heart rate alone, atrial defibrillation, the availability of dual chamber devices capable of delivering the functions of a modern DDD pacemaker as well as defibrillation, and in the longer term, subthreshold pacing, tachycardia prevention pacing, and intelligent devices that are partly self-programming.

Current Role of the Implantable Cardioverter Defibrillator

As with many other new medical technologies the dramatic explosion in ICD use has occurred prior to the availability of conclusive evidence of the efficacy of the treatment. The undoubted and easily demonstrated efficacy of the ICD in experimental situations may be responsible for this. Second, there is a large volume of circumstantial data from less stringently conducted studies suggesting that the ICD is efficacious in reducing arrhythmic mortality in patients at high risk of sudden death. It is likely to be a further 2 years before results are available from the current generation of randomized controlled trials and until then the precise role of the ICD is likely to remain controversial.

The simplest sort of comparison that may be made is the historical comparison of survival data with conventional antiarrhythmic drug therapy versus that in ICD treated patients. Waller's group[13] described 258 patients who had undergone electrophysiological testing of antiarrhythmic drugs to find a suppressive drug regimen. In 104 of these no suppressive therapy was found and the majority of these patients received amiodarone therapy. Winkle and colleagues[14] described survival in 273 patients who received the ICD between 1981 and 1988. The vast majority of the patients in this study group had presented with cardiac arrest due to VT or VF, unrelated to acute ischemia or electrolyte abnormalities. Only patients in whom no suppressive antiarrhythmic drug therapy could be found at electrophsiology study received an ICD. The mean number of drug trials per patient was 3.4 (±1.8). Seventy-eight percent of these patients had coronary artery disease and the median ejection fraction was 34%. Figure 1 shows the survival curves for Waller and Winkle's groups. It shows that the ICD treated group has a clear advantage in overall survival when compared to patients who remain inducible on antiarrhythmic drugs. However, survival in patients in whom the rate of VT was slowed or VT was rendered noninducible was similar to that in the ICD group.

A second historical study by by Tordjman-Fuchs and colleagues[15] suggested improved survival free of total cardiac death at 1 and 5 years in patients treated with the ICD between

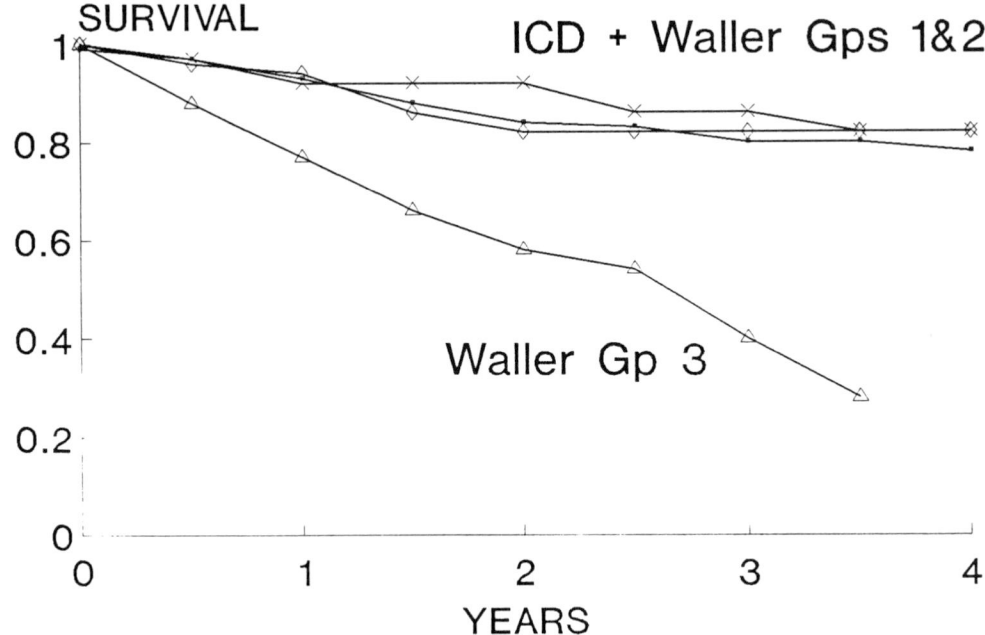

Figure 1. Total survival following implantable cardioverter defibrillator (ICD) implantation[22] compared with survival on electrophysiologically guided drug therapy.[13] The poor survival of drug nonresponders (Waller group 3[13]) is clear. The majority of ICD recipients in Winkle's study[22] would have been in this group and yet the survival in the ICD group is comparable to that in drug responders (Waller groups 1 and 2).[13]

1983 and 1988 when compared with patients treated with drug therapy patients between 1978 and 1983. This improvement occurred in spite of adverse ejection fraction and drug responsiveness in the ICD treated group. As with all historical studies, caution must be exercised in interpretating the data. For example, the control group of the CAST trial demonstrated unexpectedly low mortality when compared with previous studies in this group and similar findings have been reported for patients declining ICD implantation.[16] In the CAST study, had a randomized control group not been used the proarrhythmic effect of flecainide would not have been evident.[17]

A second approach to survival data uses ICD patients as their own controls and estimates the mortality that would have occurred had the ICD not been present. This hypothetical mortality approach was used by Gabry et al.[18] (Figure 2). They assumed that the first device discharge for ventricular tachyarrhyth-

mia prevented death. However, there are a number of serious flaws with this approach, particularly as these data were collected using first generation devices with no data logging facility. Not all episodes of untreated VT are fatal, some apparently appropriate shocks may be spurious (due to atrial fibrillation) and drug therapy in ICD patients may be discontinued leading to more frequent attacks of arrhythmia. Conversely, discontinuance of drug therapy may lead to fewer attacks of arrhythmias if the drugs were proarrhythmic and there is little doubt that some apparently spurious shocks are in fact appropriate as some patients have no symptoms associated with the initial onset of their arrhythmia.

Retrospective control studies performed in a single center may be less prone to the vagaries of geographical variation in disease and doctors. Such a study was performed by Fogoros et al.[19] on a group of 78 consecutive patients with symptomatic sustained ventricu-

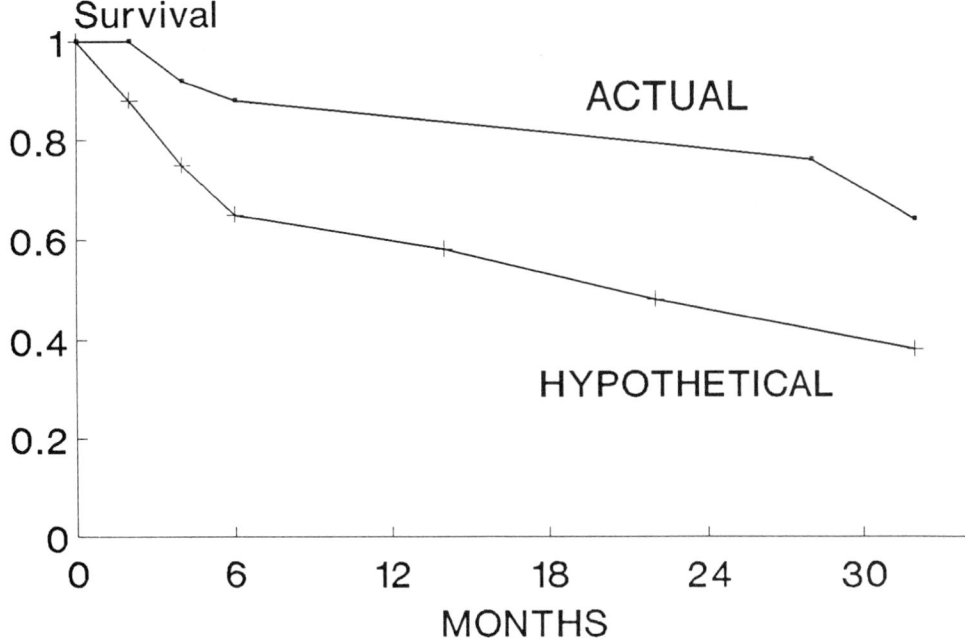

Figure 2. Hypothetical versus actual survival in 22 implantable cardioverter defibrillator (ICD) recipients calculated on the basis that the first appropriate device discharge prevents death (Data from Gabry et al.[18])

lar arrhythmias. Before February 1985 patients received treatment with the defibrillator and amiodarone if they presented with loss of consciousness (group A) and amiodarone alone if they did not lose consciousness (group C). After February 1985, when the supply of ICDs was curtailed patients in both groups were treated with amiodarone alone (group B). The survival data is shown in Figure 3. The actuarial risk of sudden death after 2 years was 0% in group A and 31% in group B. Although the groups were closely matched for factors such as ejection fraction, presenting arrhythmia, and number of drug trials their historical separation makes it difficult to rule out some unrecognized factor causing the difference in survival.

Newman[20] performed a retrospective case controlled study in the first 60 patients receiving the ICD at Moffit Hospital, San Francisco, California. Each ICD recipient was matched to two control patients for amiodarone exposure, age, ejection fraction, heart dis-

ease, and arrhythmia. During follow-up there were 12 sudden deaths in the control group and 3 in the ICD group. Overall survival in the ICD group appeared better than the controls (Figure 4) and the Cox proportional hazard model showed significantly better survival in the ICD treated group ($p < 0.05$). The apparent convergence of the survival plots at the end of the study was cause for concern, although the number of patients remaining in the groups at this stage was small.

On balance these studies suggest that the ICD probably improves overall survival when used in patients who present with cardiac arrest due to VT or VF, and in whom no effective antiarrhythmic drug therapy can be found. It seems to do so by the prevention of sudden arrhythmic death.

One dissenting opinion among the publications suggesting a dramatic reduction in sudden cardiac death in ICD recipients comes from Gross and colleagues[21] who studied 56 ICD patients and found that the cumulative

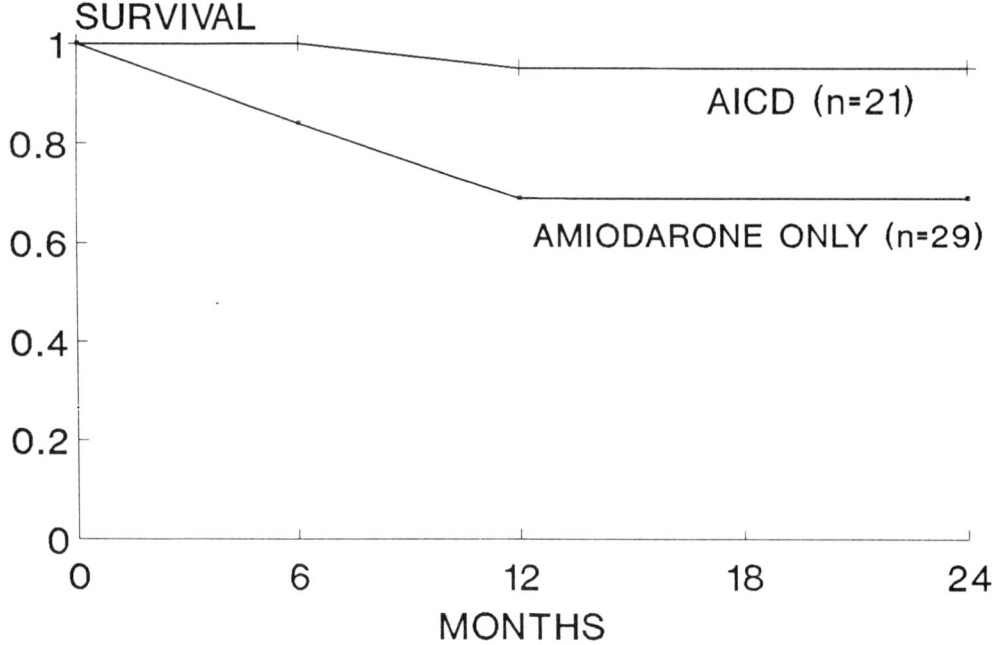

Figure 3. Retrospective control group comparison of implantable cardioverter defibrillator (ICD) survival compared with similar patients receiving amiodarone alone. (Data from Fogoros et al.[19])

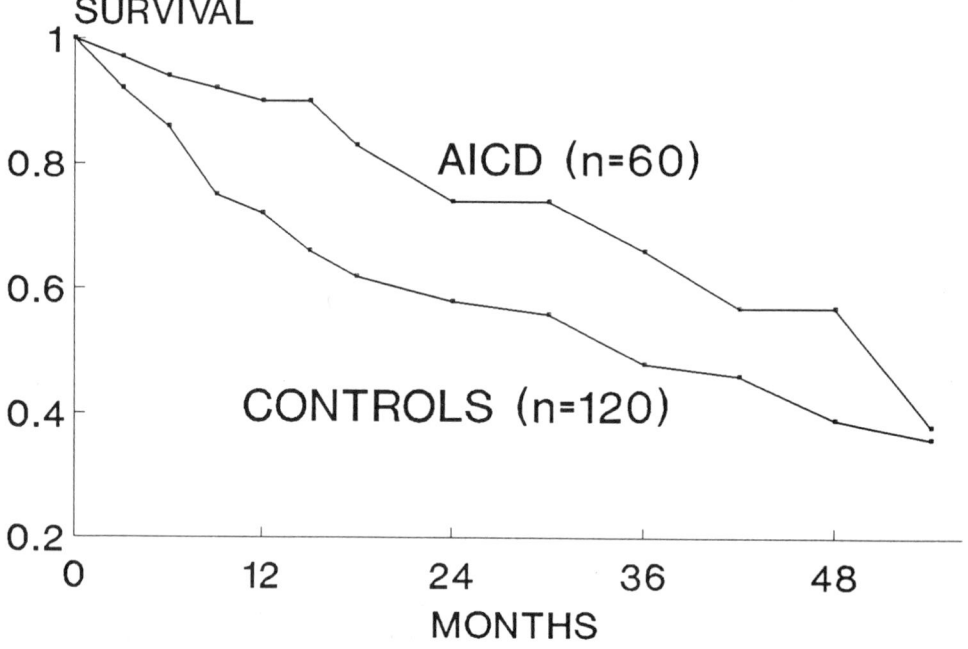

Figure 4. Matched control study of implantable cardioverter defibrillator (ICD) versus control group survival (Data from Newman et al.[20])

survival free of sudden death was 93% at 1 year, 89% at 3 years, and 75% at 5 years. Such high levels of sudden cardiac death would be of concern, but the vast majority of studies (some with much larger numbers of patients) have reported sudden cardiac death rates of the order of 1%–2% per year.[19,22,23]

There has been considerable interest in identifying factors that may predict subsequent survival in recipients of the ICD. Clearly this may help to identify groups of patients who have the most (or least) to benefit from ICD implantation. Levine and colleagues[24] have studied the factors that predict the time to first discharge and survival following ICD discharge. They identified three factors by multivariate analysis that predicted a shorter interval to first discharge. These were: (1) the combination of severe heart failure (NYHA Class II or IV) and ejection fraction of less than 25% before ICD implantation; (2) coronary artery surgery not performed at the time of ICD implantation; and (3) no β-blocker therapy after hospital discharge. Similarly they considered the factors that predicted reduced survival after first ICD discharge. Those that were significant after multivariate analysis were: (1) no coronary artery bypass surgery at the time of ICD implant; (2) first generation ICD; and (3) advanced congestive heart failure class. The authors drew attention to the very poor survival rate of patients with NYHA Class IV symptoms. Not only was their perioperative mortality high, but their survival after appropriate ICD discharge was short. In contrast, patients with NYHA Class III symptoms fared better. The fact that patients with impaired left ventricular function still benefit from ICD implantation is reinforced by Axtell and colleagues[25] who assessed survival in 68 ICD recipients with a left ventricular ejection fraction of less than 30%. Overall survival at 5 years was 60% compared with 11% projected survival (based upon appropriate utilization of ICD discharges). However, patients in NYHA Class IV were not eligible for ICD therapy in this study. The precise reason why coronary artery bypass grafting was associated with improved survival is unclear, but it may act by preventing the occurrence of new ischemic events.

Zilo et al.[26] reported that the occurrence of ICD shocks was an independent negative prognostic indicator and that the excellent prognosis of patients without shocks contributed in large part to the favorable outcome of ICD patients (Figure 5). However, other studies[27,28] have not confirmed this observation.

While there is widespread acceptance that the ICD is indicated in patients presenting with cardiac arrest and who are found to have drug refractory ventricular arrhythmias at electrophysiology study, other possible indications for the device remain controversial. Patients who survive cardiac arrest but are not found to have an inducible cardiac arrhythmia or where the induced arrhythmia is effectively suppressed by antiarrhythmic drug therapy are two groups in whom the indication for ICD implantation is unclear. While such patients have a lower incidence of sudden cardiac death than those with inducible arrhythmias not suppressed by drug therapy, the sudden death rate remains elevated.[29,30] It is possible that within these groups other factors such as left ventricular ejection fraction may usefully separate those at high and low risk of sudden death[31] and some authors have advocated ICD use as first-line therapy in cardiac arrest survivors with an ejection fraction less than 30%.[32] Given the lack of reproducibility of drug suppression at a single electrophysiology study[33] it is not surprising that this criterion alone does not perfectly separate high- and low-risk groups.

When considering ICD use in groups such as these where the annual sudden death mortality is lower the incidence of mortality and complications associated with ICD use is of greater importance in determining risk benefit (and cost efficacy) analysis of strategies. With epicardial electrode systems the mortality associated with device implantation varies widely in the published studies from 1.2% to 4.4%[34] and up to 9.8% for patients with concomitant cardiac surgery.[35] Transvenous electrode implantation appears to be associated with implant related mortalities of

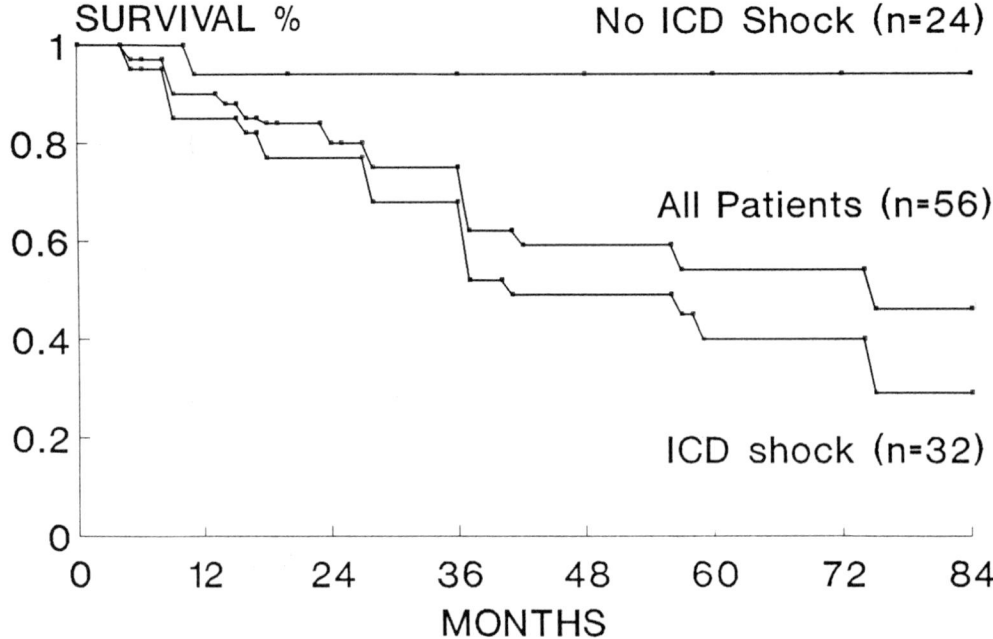

Figure 5. Implantable cardioverter defibrillator (ICD) recipient survival stratified by shock delivery. (Data from Gross et al.[21])

well below 1%[9] and such a dramatic reduction makes ICD use attractive in populations with a relatively lower incidence of sudden death.

Decision Making: Drugs Versus Implantable Cardioverter Defibrillators

When the ICD was first used in humans in 1980, it represented a daring new technology whose safety and reliability remained to be proven. For this reason it was used in patients with recurrent cardiac arrest and inducible arrhythmias resistant to conventional antiarrhythmic drug therapy. Prior to the development of the ICD there was no alternative therapy for such patients except for heart transplantation, with its inherent problems of limited and unpredictable donor supply. Because of the poor survival rate in this group when treated conventionally with empiric antiarrhythmic drug therapy, the decision to use the ICD posed few dilemmas. The primary

indication for ICD use during the first 10 years of availability has been the recognition that a patient has features that identify them as being at high risk of sudden arrhythmic cardiac death. While individual physicians may disagree about what constitutes a high risk this basic indication has been generally accepted. The use of the ICD has often been in addition to rather than in place of existing antiarrhythmic drug therapy and this has been reflected in the high percentage of ICD recipients (approximately 60%) who have remained on antiarrhythmic drug therapy.[22]

To aid the physician in the selection of patients to refer for consideration of ICD implantation and to prevent inappropriate use of the device, major international and national cardiology associations such as the American College of Cardiology, the American Heart Association,[36] the North American Society of Pacing and Electrophysiology (NASPE),[37] and the European Society of Cardiology (ESC)[38] have produced guidelines for ICD implantation. The NASPE guidelines are summarized in

Table 2
NASPE Indications for ICD Use[37]

Class I	ICD indicated (consensus)	1. Spontaneous VT/VF where EPS or Holter cannot be used to predict efficacy of other therapies 2. Recurrent VT/VF despite antiarrhythmic drug therapy or where tolerance/compliance is poor 3. Induction of VT/VF at EPS despite AAD therapy or surgical/catheter ablation in pts with spontaneous VT/VF
Class II	ICD an option (no consensus)	Recurrent syncope of undetermined etiology in a patient with VT/VF induced at EPS where AAD use is limited by inefficacy, intolerance or noncompliance
Class III	ICD not indicated	1. VT/VF ischemia/toxic/metabolic 2. Recurrent syncope without inducible arrhythmias at EPS 3. Incessant VT/VF 4. VF secondary to AF in WPW 5. Arrhythmias other than spontaneous or inducible VT/VF 6. Surgical/medical/psychiatric contraindications.

AAD: antiarrhythmic drug; EPS: electrophysiology study; VF: ventricular fibrillation; VT: ventricular tachycardia.

Table 2. While there is agreement on the general indications for ICD use there is some difference in emphasis between the guidelines of the ESC and those of the two American organizations. For example, in patients who have had an episode of VT/VF that cannot be reliably induced at electrophysiological testing, the ESC guidelines state "... an ICD may be used on an individual basis. Implantation guidelines are not clear for this group," while the NASPE guidelines state "ICD therapy is indicated, based on consensus."

One factor largely overlooked by these recommendations is the possible cost of the ICD. Kupperman and colleagues[39] used decision analysis techniques[40] along with cost information derived from the 1984 Medicare Provider Analysis and Review (MEDPAR) data file to assess cost efficacy of the ICD in comparison with conventional drug therapy. Survival figures were taken from several published studies and expert opinion was canvassed concerning resource use. An overall figure of $17,400 per life-year saved (1986 prices) was produced, but their model suggested this could fall to $7,400 per life-year by 1991 (ignoring inflation) as a result of increased defibrillator longevity and reduced

hospital stay. These figures suggested the ICD is equivalent in cost efficacy to many other medical therapies (Table 3). However, the mathematics used in this study are complex, there is difficulty in using survival data combined from several studies, and the investigators drew attention to the problem of accurately identifying the admissions on which their costs were based.

Larsen and colleagues[41] have further refined this analysis and produced a figure of $29,200 per life-year saved based on an assumption of 2-year generator life. Again, combined survival data from the literature has been used and it is noteworthy that the non-sudden mortality in the ICD group is almost half that in the group treated with amiodarone. It is unclear whether this is due to an effect of the defibrillator on the nonsudden mortality or represents an underlying difference between the two populations.

In the United Kingdom, Buxton and co-workers[42] have used a similarly complex model to assess the cost efficacy of the ICD in comparison with long-term amiodarone therapy. Their model studied a 20-year period using extrapolated survival data from a variety of studies[22,39,43] and produced a cost efficacy

Table 3
Cost Per Year of Life Saved for Various Therapies

Therapy	Cost/Life-Year (1986)
Neonatal intensive care (1,000–1,499 g)	$ 5,500
Coronary artery bypass surgery (three-vessel)	$ 7,200§
Treatment of severe hypertension (diastolic BP > 105 mm Hg) in men aged 40 years	$11,100
Implantable defibrillator	$17,400§
Treatment of mild hypertension (diastolic BP 95–104 mm Hg) in men aged 40 years	$23,200
Heart transplantation	$26,900§
Coronary artery bypass surgery (for one-vessel disease with moderately severe angina)	$44,200
Continuous ambulatory peritoneal dialysis	$57,300
Hospital haemodialysis	$59,500

All figures refer to quality-adjusted life-years except those marked §. Costs given in US dollars.
(Adapted with permission from Reference 39.)

ranging from £10,000 to £20,000 per life-year. They estimate that technical and implantation developments could reduce this as low as £6,000 per life-year.

Clearly a definitive assessment of the cost efficacy of the ICD must wait for the availability of data from prospective randomized trials such as the Dutch Prospective study[44] that are specifically designed to answer this question.

With the increasing sophistication of third generation ICDs and the availability of antitachycardia pacing and low-energy cardioversion we may be approaching a time where there is a genuine choice between the use of an antiarrhythmic drug or the ICD. The expense of the long hospital stay that may be required for electrophysiologically guided selection of antiarrhythmic drug therapy has been highlighted by O'Donoghue and colleagues.[45] They have demonstrated a 20% saving in hospital costs associated with the early implantation of the ICD instead of more extensive evaluation of antiarrhythmic drug therapy. Unfortunately the ICD as it currently exists is certainly not a "fit and forget it" device, because it requires regular follow-up checks and eventual generator replacement. Also, there are potential proarrhythmic effects and inappropriate therapy delivery particularly in

response to sinus tachycardia and atrial fibrillation.[46] Such problems are mainly related to the diagnostic nonspecificity of current ICD devices, all of which rely on heart rate as the primary diagnostic discriminator.

Thus at present there are few patients where a direct choice has to be made between antiarrhythmic drugs and the ICD. Instead, we are faced with deciding when an ICD is indicated and once the decision to use the ICD is made, whether we can limit the systematic evaluation of antiarrhythmic drug therapy. General ground rules exist to define when an ICD is indicated, but these are necessarily fairly liberal pending the availability of prospective trials of the device. The advantages and disadvantages of the ICD are summarized in Table 4.

Drugs and the Implantable Cardioverter Defibrillator

Even in patients who have received the ICD antiarrhythmic drugs may continue to play an important role, and up to 60% of patients may continue to receive such drugs after ICD implantation.[22] Although a reticence to withdraw preexisting antiarrhythmic drug

Table 4

Implantable Cardioverter Defibrillators

Advantages	Disadvantages
Minimizes risk of sudden death Programmability—allows modification of therapy to suit evolving arrhythmias	High capital expenditure Implant related mortality Does not prevent symptoms "Skill intensive"—technicians and doctors Few implanting centers Inappropriate therapies Potentially proarrhythmic Lifestyle restriction, eg, driving

Antiarrhythmic drug therapy

Advantages	Disadvantages
No capital expense Widely available When effective prevents symptoms	No "safety net" for sudden death Potentially proarrhythmic Extensive testing needed to evaluate efficacy Potentially serious side effects

therapy may be a factor, in the majority of patients such therapy is continued for good reason.

Antiarrhythmic drug therapy may be used to reduce the frequency of episodes of arrhythmia. This may improve tolerance of the ICD if the arrhythmia requires cardioversion or defibrillation, as well as extending generator longevity. Antiarrhythmic drug therapy may be effective at reducing the cycle length of VT[47] and thus rendering it more susceptible to termination by antitachycardia pacing therapy.

There has been considerable interest in the potential modulation of the DFT by antiarrhythmic drugs, particularly as quite small reductions in the DFT could considerably increase the proportion of patients in whom a transvenous defibrillation electrode system could be used. No drug in widespread clinical usage has been consistently reported to achieve a reduction in DFTs. In 1980, Tacker and colleagues[48] reported an acute reduction in DFT following administration of clofilium or bretylium. The greatest interest has surrounded the potential effect of amiodarone. Fain et al.[49] reported a reduction of DFT in

dogs following acute administration of amiodarone, but the DFT remained unchanged following chronic administration. A rise in DFT following chronic administration of amiodarone has been reported in human ICD recipients.[50] The use of sotalol at ICD implant has been reported to be associated with a reduced DFT.[51] Antiarrhythmic drugs may have other adverse effects on ICD function, including increasing pacing threshold[52] and reducing R wave amplitude and slew rate.

Antiarrhythmic drugs may have a role not only in the modulation of the therapies delivered by the ICD, but also in improving diagnostic specificity of the ICD. With the increasing availability of antitachycardia pacing, ICDs are being used increasingly to treat slower tachycardias. As current devices rely entirely on heart rate to identify arrhythmias, the risk of inappropriate triggering of therapies by sinus tachycardia or atrial fibrillation has increased.[46] β Blockers have been shown to improve separation between the rates of sinus tachycardia and VT when used in conjunction with amiodarone.[53] Thus, it seems that modulation of arrhythmias by antiarrhythmic drugs will retain an important role despite the increasing sophistication of the ICD.

Clinical Trials: Drugs Versus the Implantable Cardioverter Defibrillator

To make any further significant advance in defining the role of the ICD in the management of patients with arrhythmias, data from carefully designed randomized prospective trials is required. Many such trials are currently in progress or planned and the majority of these trials compare survival in the ICD treated group with that in a group treated with conventional electrophysiologically guided drug therapy. There has been some debate as to whether a controlled trial of the ICD in cardiac arrest survivors is ethical, given the volume of data suggesting that ICD implantation in this group is efficacious. Nonetheless, reservations about the data from historical control studies and its application to the current pattern of ICD use is likely to provide momentum for a number of controlled studies.

Controlled Trials of the Implantable Cardioverter Defibrillator in Cardiac Arrest Survivors

Several trials are in progress in this group. The Canadian Implantable Defibrillator Study (CIDS) is a randomized trial of amiodarone versus the ICD in cardiac arrest survivors. The Australasian Clinical Trial of the Automatic Implantable Defibrillator (ACTAID) is recruiting patients with VT or VF occurring late after myocardial infarction. The Cardiac Arrest Study Hamburg (CASH) is comparing ICD therapy and antiarrhythmic drug therapy in cardiac arrest survivors.

To specifically address the issue of cost efficacy of early implantation of the ICD compared with antiarrhythmic drug use in survivors of cardiac arrest due to previous myocardial infarction, the Dutch Prospective study[44]

randomizes patients to early ICD implantation or a more conventional approach of electrophysiologically guided drug therapy with catheter ablation, map guided surgery, and ICD implantation as last resorts. The study addresses important quality-of-life issues, as well as more conventional indexes of survival. The information provided by these trials should help to clarify the respective role of drugs and the ICD in such patients and should also enable a review of the cost efficacy of ICD use.

Controlled Trials of the Implantable Cardioverter Defibrillator in Patients at High Risk of Cardiac Arrest

There is increasing interest in the prophylactic use of the ICD in patients who have never suffered a cardiac arrest, but in whom a variety of risk factors are present thus identifying these patients as being at high risk of sudden cardiac death.[54,55] Patients with dilated cardiomyopathy are known to have an increased incidence of sudden cardiac death.[56] The German Dilated Cardiomyopathy study[57] is randomizing patients with dilated cardiomyopathy and no history of ventricular arrhythmias to the ICD or no antiarrhythmic therapy (this comparison has been chosen in view of the failure of any antiarrhythmic drug therapy to reduce sudden death mortality in patients with dilated cardiomyopathy). A further study to assess the more limited use of the ICD as a bridge to prevent sudden death in patients awaiting cardiac transplantation[58] (DEFIBRLAT) is also planned.

Patients with nonsustained VT, underlying coronary artery disease and impaired left ventricular function are also known to have increased mortality from sudden cardiac death.[59] Three studies are currently under way to assess mortality reduction by antiarrhythmic drug therapy or the ICD in this group. The Multicenter Unsustained Tachycardia Trial[34,54] (MUSTT) was started in 1991 to assess whether electrophysiologically guided antiarrhythmic drug prescription will reduce mortality in this group. In the active treatment group, when the inducible arrhythmia is not suppressed by antiarrhythmic drug therapy then an ICD is implanted. The Sudden Death Prevention Study (SDPS)[34,54] is based on a similar hypothesis. The Multicenter Automatic Defibrillator Implantation Trial (MADIT)[60] study takes patients inducible at baseline evaluation and still inducible on procainamide and randomizes them to ICD or conventional therapy to compare the efficacy of these two strategies.

The Coronary Artery Bypass Graft Patch (CABG Patch)[61] trial seeks to assess whether implantation of the ICD at the time of coronary artery bypass surgery will reduce late sudden death in high-risk patients. Recruitment criteria include a left ventricular ejection fraction of less than 0.36 and an abnormal signal-averaged ECG in patient requiring CABG surgery.

Anderson and co-worker[62] have considered the possible cost efficacy of the strategies proposed by the various controlled trials and finds that they are remarkably similar with a range of $60,000 to $100,000 per year of life saved. These figures are higher than those for high-risk cardiac arrest survivors (around $40,000 per life-year) reflecting a lower incidence of sudden cardiac death in these groups when compared with the higher risk groups of cardiac arrest survivors. Alterations in the relative cost of the ICD is likely to cause a dramatic reduction in these figures over the next few years.

Studies of Antiarrhythmic Drug Efficacy in Implantable Cardioverter Defibrillator Patients

With the rapid growth in the number of patients with ICDs it is possible that such patients may form population in whom to evaluate the efficacy and safety of antiarrhythmic drugs. It seems likely that ICD patients will be relatively protected from the possible proarrhythmic effects of antiarrhythmic drugs and that evaluation of antiarrhythmic drugs may

be safer in this population. In addition the arrhythmia recognition and storage facilities offered by the ICD provide a level of surveillance that is impossible to achieve with Holter or event recorders.

Such studies have only been feasible since the availability of sophisticated third generation ICDs. To be of any use in such a study the ICD must have excellent data logging of episodes and a high degree of programmability of shock and antitachycardia pacing functions. Additional features that would be of use include storage of arrhythmia electrograms, the availability of Holter functions not directly related to the delivery of therapy (for example the ability to recognize the occurrence of episodes of slow atrial fibrillation), and the availability of transtelephonic interrogation.

The performance of such studies would raise complex design issues. Identification of end points could be a source of some difficulty. The rapid intervention provided by the ICD means that spontaneously occurring arrhythmias do not have the opportunity to reach the fully developed conclusion that could have occurred in the absence of the ICD. For example, an episode of sustained monomorphic VT could be rapidly treated by the ICD with antitachycardia pacing with no sequelae. In a patient with no ICD this arrhythmia could have degenerated into VF and proved fatal. Thus, identification of an episode of "prevented sudden death" is difficult.

The potential effects of the antiarrhythmic drugs used on the performance of the ICD also have to be considered. Defibrillation thresholds and the efficacy of antitachycardia pacing must be formally assessed whenever the drug therapy is altered. Conversely, the data collected during such testing may itself be of use in evaluating the drugs concerned.

It seems likely that ICD patients will be able to evaluate antiarrhythmic drugs in future studies. However, the design of these studies will require great care if the results are to be of any use to patients who are not recipients of the ICD.

Conclusion

The progress that has been made since the early studies of defibrillation at the turn of the century[63] to the widespread use of an ICD represents dramatic technical developments. These developments have not always proceeded smoothly, but have been interspersed with periods of relative inactivity. For the ICD, intense technical developments have occurred over the last decade, but it is unlikely that such a dramatic pace of development will be maintained over the next decade. Initial enthusiasm for the device has resulted in over 20,000 implants worldwide before the availability of concrete evidence from randomized controlled trials of the device's efficacy. However, such a period of exploratory implantation may be necessary to define a framework within which more critical evaluation of the device may occur. That we are now approaching this stage is clear from the appearance over the last 3 years of a number of guidelines for selection of patients for ICD implantation and the planning and initiation of controlled trials to evaluate the use of the device in a number of scenarios.

There appears to be a clear indication for implantation of the ICD in patients who survive cardiac arrest and are found to have an inducible ventricular arrhythmia that is not suppressed by antiarrhythmic drug therapy. The ICD may also have a role in patients whose arrhythmia is suppressed or who do not have inducible arnythmias, but whose left ventricular ejection fraction is reduced. Impairment of ejection fraction per se is not a contraindication to ICD use but the presence of NYHA Class IV symptoms is associated with poor outcome after ICD implant. There are a large number of other potential roles for the ICD, but these represent an indication for the performance of randomized prospective studies rather than a license for general use.

The expense of ICD therapy remains a major factor limiting its use, particularly outside the United States. This may prove to be an illusion related to the high capital cost of the device rather than a true assessment of the cost efficacy of ICD therapy. The current generation of ICD trials should allow a more rational assessment of the cost efficacy of the device and the Dutch projective trial represents a particular advance in this field.

At present the only concrete indication for ICD use is the prevention of sudden cardiac death, but the incorporation of increasingly sophisticated antitachycardia pacing functions into third generation devices raises the question of whether an ICD may be used in place of antiarrhythmic drug therapy. Given the limitations of current devices both in terms of diagnostic specificity and therapeutic efficacy, further technical developments are likely to be necessary before a straight comparison can be made. In the majority of patients receiving an ICD, antiarrhythmic drug therapy still has something to offer.

The next decade may see less dramatic technical developments in the devices themselves, but it is likely that a wealth of information to define the role of and indications for ICD therapy will be provided.

References

1. Mirowski M, Reid PR, Mower MM, et al: Termination of malignant ventricular arrhythmias with an implantable automatic defibrillator in human beings. *N Engl J Med* 303:322, 1980.
2. Zoll PM, Linenthal AJ, Zarsky LRN: Ventricular fibrillation treatment and prevention by external electric currents. *N Engl J Med* 262:105, 1960.
3. Mirowski M, Mower M, Staewen WS, et al: Standby automatic defibrillator: an approach to prevention of sudden coronary death. *Arch Intern Med* 126:158, 1970.
4. Mower MM: Building the AICD with Michel Mirowski. *PACE* 14:928, 1991.
5. Mirowski M, Mower MM, Staewen WS, et al: Ventricular defibrillation through a single intravascular catheter electrode system (abstract). *Clin Res* 19:328, 1971.
6. Lown B, Axelrod P: Implanted standby defibrillators. *Circulation* 46:637, 1973.
7. Horning RJ, Rhoback FW: New high rate lithium/vanadium pentoxide cell for implantable medical devices. *Prog Batteries Solar Cells* 4:97, 1982.
8. Mirowski M, Reid PR, Mower MM, et al: Termi-

nation of malignant ventricular arrhythmias with an implantable automatic defibrillator in human beings. *N Engl J Med* 303:322, 1980.

9. Lindemans FW, van Binsbergen E, Connolly D: European PCD™ study patients with Transvene™ lead systems. Medtronic. Bakken Research Centre, Maastricht 1991.

10. Ehrlich S, for the ENDOTAK Investigator Group, Hospital of the Good Samaritan, Los Angeles, California: Early survival and follow-up characteristics of 151 patients undergoing transvenous cardioverter defibrillator lead system implantation (abstract). *J Am Coll Cardiol* 19:209A, 1992.

11. Marks M, Troutman C, Johnson G, Bardy GH: A prospective randomized comparison of biphasic and monophasic waveform defibrillation with a three electrode transvenous lead system in man (abstract). *Circulation* 84:II-612, 1991.

12. Anderson MH, Paul VE, Jones S, et al: Transtelephonic interrogation of implantable cardioverter-defibrillators. *PACE* (in press).

13. Waller T, Kay H, Spielman S, et al: Reduction in sudden death and total mortality by antiarrhythmic therapy evaluated by electrophysiologic drug testing: criteria of efficacy in patients with sustained ventricular tachyarrhythmias. *J Am Coll Cardiol* 10:83, 1987.

14. Winkle R, Mead H, Ruder M, et al: Long-term outcome with the automatic implantable cardioverter defibrillator. *J Am Coll Cardiol* 13:1353, 1989.

15. Tordjman-Fuchs T, Garan H, Ruskin J: Out of hospital cardiac arrest: improved long-term outcome in patients with automatic implantable cardioverter defibrillator (AICD) (abstract). *Circulation* 80:II-121, 1989.

16. Pinski S, Sgarbossa E, Alexander L, et al: Survival of patients declining defibrillator implantation (abstract). *PACE* 14:641, 1991.

17. Ruskin JN: The Cardiac Arrhythmia Suppression Trial (CAST). *N Engl J Med* 321:386, 1989.

18. Gabry MD, Brodman R, Johnston D, et al: Automatic implantable cardioverter-defibrillator: patient survival, battery longevity and shock delivery analysis. *J Am Coll Cardiol* 9:1349, 1987.

19. Fogoros RN, Fielder SB, Elson JJ: The automatic implantable cardioverter-defibrillator in drug-refractory ventricular tachyarrhythmias. *Ann Intern Med* 107:635, 1987.

20. Newman D, Sauve MJ, Herre J, et al: Survival after implantation of the cardioverter defibrillator. *Am J Cardiol* 69:899, 1992.

21. Gross J, Zilo P, Ferrick K, et al: Sudden death mortality in implantable cardioverter defibrillator patients. *PACE* 14:250, 1991.

22. Winkle RA, Mead H, Ruder MA, et al: Long-term outcome with the automatic implantable cardioverter-defibrillator. *J Am Coll Cardiol* 13:1353, 1989.

23. Winkle RA, Mead RH, Ruder MA, et al: Ten year experience with implantable defibrillators (abstract). *Circulation* 84:II-426, 1991.

24. Levine JH, Mellits ED, Baumgardner RA, et al: Predictors of first discharge and subsequent survival in patients with automatic implantable cardioverter-defibrillators. *Circulation* 84:558, 1991.

25. Axtell K, Tchou P, Akhtar M: Survival in patients with depressed left ventricular function treated by implantable cardioverter defibrillator. *PACE* 14:291, 1991.

26. Zilo P, Gross JN, Benedck M, et al: Occurrence of ICD shocks and patient survival. *PACE* 14:273, 1991.

27. Tchou P, Axtell K, Troup P, Akhtar M: Comparative survival of implantable cardioverter defibrillator patients who do and do not receive appropriate shocks (abstract). *PACE* 14:719, 1991.

28. Tchou P, Axtell K, Avitall B, Akhtar M: Benefit of automatic defibrillator implant: survival after reception of appropriate shock (abstract). *PACE* 14:719, 1991.

29. Sra J, Krebs A, Axtell K, et al: Actuarial probability of AICD shocks in sudden death survivors with no inducible ventricular tachycardia (abstract). *Circulation* 84:II-21, 1991.

30. Fogoros RN, Elson JJ, Bonnet CA, et al: Long-term outcome of survivors of cardiac arrest whose therapy is guided by electrophysiological testing. *J Am Coll Cardiol* 19:780, 1992.

31. Wilber J, Garan H, Finkelstein D, et al: Out-of-hospital cardiac arrest: use of electrophysiological testing in the prediction of long-term outcome. *N Engl J Med* 318:19, 1988.

32. Prystowsky EN: Antiarrhythmic drug therapy as an adjunct or alternative to an implantable cardioverter defibrillator. *PACE* 15:678, 1992.

33. Fogoros RN, Elson JJ, Bonnet CA, et al: Reproducibility of successful drug trials in patients with inducible sustained ventricular tachycardia. *PACE* 15:295, 1992.

34. Nisam S, Mower M, Moser S: ICD clinical update: first decade, initial 10,000 patients. *PACE* 14:255, 1991.

35. Edel T, McAlister H, Castle L, et al: Effect of combined cardiac surgery during implantable defibrillator placement on operative mortality and morbidity, late mortality and shock analysis (abstract). *PACE* 13:529, 1990.

36. Dreifus LS, Fisch C, Griffin JC, et al: Guidelines for implantation of cardiac pacemakers and antiarrhythmia devices. *J Am Coll Cardiol* 18:1, 1991.

37. Lehmann MH, Saksena S: Implantable cardioverter defibrillators in cardiovascular practice: report of the Policy Conference of the North American Society of Pacing and Electrophysiology. NASPE Policy Conference Committee. PACE 14:969, 1991.

38. A Task Force of the working groups on cardiac arrhythmias and cardiac pacing of the European Society of Cardiology. Guidelines for the use of implantable cardioverter defibrillators. Eur Heart J (in press).

39. Kupperman M, Luce BR, McGovern B, et al: An analysis of the cost effectiveness of the implantable defibrillator. Circulation 81:91, 1990.

40. Weinstein MC, Fineberg HV (eds): Clinical Decision Analysis. Philadelphia, PA: WB Saunders Co, 1980.

41. Larsen GC, Manolis AS, Sonnenberg FA, et al: Cost-effectiveness of the implantable cardioverter-defibrillator: effect of improved battery life and comparison with amiodarone therapy. J Am Coll Cardiol 19:1323, 1992.

42. Buxton MJ, O'Brien BJ, Rushby JA: Cost-effectiveness of the automatic implantable cardioverter defibrillator: a preliminary assessment. Health Economics Research Group Research Report No. 7. Brunel University. 1990.

43. Herre JM, Sauve MJ, Malone P, et al: Long-term results of amiodarone therapy in patients with recurrent sustained ventricular tachycardia or ventricular fibrillation. J Am Coll Cardiol 13: 442, 1989.

44. Wever EFD, Hauer RNW: Cost-effectiveness considerations: the Dutch prospective study of the automatic implantable cardioverter defibrillator as first-choice therapy. PACE 15:690, 1992.

45. O'Donoghue S, Platia EV, Brooks-Robinson S, Mispireta L: Automatic implantable cardioverter-defibrillator: is early implantation cost-effective? J Am Coll Cardiol 16:1258, 1990.

46. Johnson NJ, Marchlinski FE: Arrhythmias induced by device antitachycardia therapy due to diagnostic non-specificity. J Am Coll Cardiol 18:1418, 1991.

47. Prystowsky NE, Lloyd EA, Fineberg M, et al: A comparison of electrophysiologic effects of antiarrhythmic agents in humans. In: P Brugada, HJJ Wellens (eds): Cardiac Arrhythmias: Where To Go From Here? Mount Kisco, NY: Futura Publishing Company Inc., 1987, p. 495.

48. Tacker WA, Niebauer MJ, Babbs CF, et al: The effect of newer antiarrhythmic drugs on defibrillation threshold. Crit Care Med 8:177, 1980.

49. Fain ES, Lee JT, Winkle RA: Effects of acute and chronic oral amiodarone on defibrillation energy requirements. Am Heart J 114:8, 1987.

50. Guarnieri T, Levine JH, Veltri, et al: Success of chronic defibrillation and the role of antiarrhythmic drugs with the automatic implantable cardioverter/defibrillator. Am J Cardiol 60: 1061, 1987.

51. Dorian P, Feindel C, Lipton I: Usefulness of sotalol in conjunction with automatic implanted defibrillators in man (abstract). PACE 13:89, 1990.

52. Hellestrand KA, Nathan AW, Bexton RS, Camm AJ: Electrophysiological effects of flecainide acetate on sinus node function, anomalous atrioventricular connections and pacemaker thresholds. Am J Cardiol 53:30B, 1984.

53. Paul V, Bashir Y, Anderson M, et al: Antitachycardia pacing and antiarrhythmics combined: a recipe for misdiagnosis (abstract). PACE 14: 722, 1991.

54. Nisam S, Thomas A, Mower M, Hauser R: Identifying patients for prophylactic implantable cardioverter defibrillator therapy: status of prospective studies. Am Heart J 122:607, 1991.

55. Bigger JT: Future studies with the implantable cardioverter-defibrillator. PACE 14:883, 1991.

56. Packer M: Sudden unexpected death in patients with congestive heart failure: a second frontier. Circulation 72:681, 1985.

57. The German Dilated Cardiomyopathy Study Investigators: Prospective studies assessing prophylactic therapy in high risk patients: the German dilated cardiomyopathy study (GDCMS)—study design. PACE 15:697, 1992.

58. Bolling S, Deeb M, Morady F, et al: AICD: a new "bridge" to transplantation (abstract). J Am Coll Cardiol 15:223A, 1990.

59. Wilber DJ, Olshansky B, Moran JF, Scanlon PJ: Electrophysiological testing and nonsustained ventricular tachycardia. Circulation 82:350, 1990.

60. MADIT Executive Committee: Multicenter automatic defibrillator implantation trial (MADIT): design and clinical protocol. PACE 14:920, 1991.

61. Bigger JT: Future studies with the implantable cardioverter defibrillator. PACE 14:883, 1991.

62. Anderson MH, Camm AJ: Implications for present and future applications of the implantable cardioverter defibrillator resulting from the use of a simple model of cost-efficacy. Br Heart J (in press).

63. Coumel P: Historical milestones of implanted defibrillation. PACE 15:598, 1992.

Part VIII

Future Perspectives

Chapter 47

Whither Antiarrhythmic Drugs?

Bramah N. Singh

Advances in cardiac electrophysiology and electropharmacology in the last 2 decades have been truly spectacular. Such advances include an enhanced understanding of the mechanisms of arrhythmias,[1,2] their prognostic significance,[3-5] and the mechanisms of antiarrhythmic drug actions.[6,7] There have been major accomplishments in the design and refinement of implantable devices[8] for sensing and identifying arrhythmias and for their termination by pacing, cardioverting, or defibrillating (see Chapter 46). Surgical techniques for cardiac arrhythmias continue to evolve for ventricular and supraventricular tachyarrhythmias (see Chapter 44). However, the recent demonstration that numerous cardiac arrhythmias, especially those of supraventricular origin, might be amenable to cure by electrode catheter ablation (see Chapter 45) has had a major impact on the prophylactic use of antiarrhythmic drugs in the control of certain arrhythmias. Therefore, a logical question: whither antiarrhythmics? This is a question the answers to which are of immediate and practical importance to physicians, patients, developers of drugs and devices, as well as to the public and private funding agencies for health care. It is difficult to forecast the

direction in which the current train of technological advances is headed. The indications are that a very substantial number of arrhythmias will remain in which the invasive approaches, such as implantable devices and electrode catheter or surgical ablative techniques, are not readily applicable will be the sole therapy. For example, in a very large number of patients with implantable devices, concomitant drug therapy, albeit in lower doses, becomes essential. Another example is the case of atrial fibrillation. This is perhaps the most common arrhythmia now being encountered in clinical practice. The long-term stability of sinus rhythm after cardioversion of atrial fibrillation may continue to depend in large measure to pharmacological therapy. Thus, it is unlikely that drug therapy for cardiac arrhythmias will be superseded by invasive approaches. With an increasing focus on mortality as an end point during treatment of cardiac arrhythmias, data have emerged indicating the possibility that at least in the case of Class I agents, the risk-benefit ratios may not be acceptable. A major reorientation in the control of cardiac arrhythmias by drug therapy is now essential in light of the data from experimental studies, controlled clinical

Supported by the Medical Research Service of the Veterans Administration (Washington, DC) and the American Heart Association of the Greater Los Angeles Affiliate.

From BN Singh, HJJ Wellens, M Hiraoka, (eds): *Electropharmacological Control of Cardiac Arrhythmias*. Mount Kisco, NY, Futura Publishing Company Inc., © 1994.

trials of adequate sample size, and from meta-analytic studies of smaller randomized controlled clinical trials.

To develop a perspective on the changing roles of different classes of antiarrhythmic drugs (see Chapter 15), three issues will be discussed in this the final chapter of this monograph. The first issue is a critical examination of the main lines of experimental and clinical evidence that sodium channel blockers may have a greater degree of profibrillatory action than antifibrillatory action. This may be the basis for sodium channel blockers to increase rather than decrease mortality in heart disease. The phenomenon may be a "class" action. A class action effect in the converse sense might also account for the salutary effects of β blockers in postinfarct survivors. The data on β blockers may be crucial for the development of newer antifibrillatory drugs. The second aim is to discuss the issue of drug-specific versus technique-specific responses in the prediction of long-term drug therapy especially in patients with life-threatening ventricular arrhythmias. This issue has come into sharp focus with the publication of the results of the ESVEM trial.[9,10] This is relevant to the use of the Holter technique or programmed electrical stimulation (PES) of the heart in guiding antiarrhythmic therapy for asymptomatic and symptomatic ventricular arrhythmias including those with symptomatic ventricular tachycardia/fibrillation (VT/VF) and aborted sudden death. The final objective is to propose a conceptual model to account for the seemingly divergent data and views on the utility of various electrophysiological classes of agents and their choice as agents for arrhythmia mortality reduction in the setting of varying substrates of heart disease.

Cardiac Arrhythmia Suppression Trials and the Future of Class I Agents in Life-Threatening Ventricular Arrhythmias

In Chapter 26, Woosley emphasizes the profound influence of the results of the Cardiac Arrhythmia Suppression Trial (CAST),[11] which dealt with mortality as an end point in asymptomatic but serious arrhythmias. CAST drew attention to the critical importance of concurrent placebo controls and the pitfalls of using surrogate end points in clinical trials. The results of Cast II[12] further emphasized these issues. Taken together, the results indicate that Class I agents as a class may increase rather than decrease mortality in the survivors of acute infarction. The ESVEM trial[10] drew attention to the fact that in the treatment of symptomatic VT and VF, and in the survivors of cardiac arrest, sotalol was superior to Class I agents.

The results from CAST I and II and ESVEM Trials[9-12] appear to be all but the final steps in a series of experimental and clinical reports that have long suggested that agents that delay conduction may increase mortality in certain subsets of patients with cardiac disease. The data have become remarkably confluent in the last 10 years. Indeed, in a meta-analysis of randomized clinical trials with various Class I agents in infarct survivors, Furberg[13] found that Class I agents either had no effect on mortality or increased it. No agent conferred an unequivocal benefit on sudden death. The results of CAST I and II have provided a fresh impetus for a closer scrutiny of the enlarging body of clinical and experimental data.

Experimental studies have consistently indicated proarrhythmic effects of agents that delay conduction (see Chapter 23). In the Lucchesi ischemic sudden death model (see Chapter 22), flecainide, quinidine, or lidocaine all had either no protective effect or accelerated the development of VF.[14-16] Nattel et al.[17] studied the regional myocardial distribution of aprindine, a Class Ic agent, in dogs following coronary artery occlusion; myocardial drug concentrations could be correlated with arrhythmogenic effects. In humans, slowing of conduction by drugs tends to stabilize the reentrant circuit and promote the continued inducibility of VT,[18,19] which is in line with the role of slowed conduction in the genesis of VT in humans (see Chapter 12). Thus, it is not altogether unexpected that agents such as lidocaine and mexiletine[20,21] tend to produce excess mortality in infarct survivors. (The details are presented in Chapter 27). Further support for the possibility that Class I agents may increase mortality in high-risk patients is derived from reports of patients dying while wearing Holter monitors.[22–28] Many such patients were on Class I agents at the time of death. Of particular interest, in a follow-up study of post-myocardial infarction patients, the mortality rate among patients receiving antiarrhythmic agents (mostly procainamide and quinidine) reported by Rapaport and Remedios[26] was higher in the treated group compared with those who were not given antiarrhythmic agents. This is in line with the report of a meta-analysis of trials in other subsets of patients without recent myocardial infarction but with premature ventricular contractions (PVCs) given quinidine in comparison with placebo.[27]

The mortality rate has also been reported to be substantially higher in patients waiting for cardiac transplantation[28] in those who were treated with Class I agents compared both to a group that was not treated at all or to one that was treated with amiodarone. Also consistent are the findings of Ruskin et al.[29] who studied six patients on Class I agents (mostly quinidine or procainamide) who developed cardiac arrest while on antiarrhythmic therapy. When studied electrophysiologically these patients did not have inducible VT/VF when the drugs were withdrawn. A rechallenge led to inducibility in four. Perhaps of the greatest interest are the data from Hallstrom et al.[30] in the survivors of cardiac arrest. The survival rates versus antiarrhythmic drug use in 941 consecutive patients between March 1970 and March 1985 were retrospectively analyzed. Of these, 18% were treated with quinidine at least for a period of time, 17.5% with procainamide, and 39.4% received no antiarrhythmic agents; gb blockers were given to 28.3%. Unadjusted comparisons of survival estimates showed lower survival rates for patients receiving antiarrhythmic therapy independently of β-blocker therapy. The most fa-

vorable survival rate was on β blockers that were superior to no treatment and to antiarrhythmic therapy with procainamide or quinidine. Class I agents produce a variable spectrum of activity for the suppression of PVCs relative to their potencies as sodium channel blockers.[31,32] The finding that PVCs—the trigger mechanism of sudden death—represented an independent marker for the risk of sudden arrhythmic death, led to the formulation and testing of the PVC hypothesis.[3,4,33] In the event, CAST I and II data clearly indicated a striking dichotomy between PVC suppression and mortality. Meta-analytic data (see Chapter 27) indicates that none of the Class I agents are immune from a deleterious effect on mortality.[13] The data suggests that the magnitude of the adverse effect on mortality might be linked directly to the degree of slowing of conduction.[32] Therefore, paradoxical as it might seem, Class I agents with the greatest PVC suppressant effect are likely to induce the most serious life-threatening proarrhythmic potential unless their associated properties counteracts such a proclivity.

These data indicate that, given the appropriate clinical setting, slowing of myocardial conduction by Class I agents may lead to significant proarrhythmic effects that may have an adverse effect on mortality. As concluded by Hallstrom et al.[30] the use of this class of antiarrhythmic agents in patients at risk for sudden death is not only unproven, but potentially hazardous, and perhaps should be restricted to testing in randomized clinical trials. It appears to be increasingly difficult to justify their continued use in the suppression of ventricular arrhythmias.

Class I Agents in Supraventricular Arrhythmias

While the data in the high-risk subsets of patients of the effects of Class I agents is compelling in terms of their proclivity to increase mortality, there is limited data to this effect in the case of supraventricular arrhythmias. In a detailed meta-analysis of the data in about 800 patients with atrial fibrillation randomized to quinidine and placebo, Coplen et al.[35] found a mortality rate of 2.9% on quinidine and 0.8% on placebo at the end of the first year. The difference was significant ($p < 0.05$). Similar data was reported in anticoagulant studies for atrial fibrillation in patients given Class I agents compared to placebo.[36] Unexplained sudden deaths have been reported on most Class Ia agents, especially on quinidine that has long been accepted as the drug of choice for maintaining stability of sinus rhythm in patients with atrial fibrillation and flutter. The recent approval and the introduction of flecainide for the treatment of supraventricular arrhythmias[37] has broadened the use of these agents in this setting. The precise risk-benefit ratio for the use of such agents as quinidine, procainamide, and flecainide (and possibly propafenone) remains undefined, but data suggest an acceptable degree of safety in patients without demonstrable heart disease. In the case of quinidine in the setting of atrial fibrillation, further controlled studies are clearly needed especially in comparison to placebo or antifibrillatory drugs such as sotalol or amiodarone. A suggestion has been made that amiodarone might be the most effective and perhaps the safest agent at low dose for maintaining stability of sinus rhythm after cardioversion of atrial flutter and fibrillation.[38] A placebo controlled clinical trial comparing quinidine and amiodarone in this setting is clearly desirable.

Preventing Ventricular Fibrillation by Antiarrhythmic Therapy: Predicting Outcome of Therapy

Sudden death in patients with significant cardiac disease usually develops on the basis of PVCs initiating VT that deteriorates into VF.[22] Thus, in preventing sudden death from VF, drug therapy may focus on the elimination of the trigger mechanism (the PVC) or the prevention of the VT accelerating into VF (the antifibrillatory approach).

Premature Ventricular Contraction Suppression Hypothesis and Holter Guided Therapy for VT/VF

CAST and related studies focused on the elimination of the trigger mechanism. As already indicated, elimination or a statistically significant decrease in PVCs failed to predict the desired outcome in the case of flecainide, encainide, or moricizine in the case of postinfarct survivors.[11,12] This was not entirely unexpected. As a function of time, there are inevitable changes in the patient's adrenergic state, electrolyte milieu and the clinical course relative to the alterations in the substrate due to progression of the underlying disease. This is especially applicable in the case of coronary artery disease. Thus, it is inherently unlikely that the acute suppression of PVCs by a particular therapeutic regimen will provide a long-term protection against the development of VF. It is also known that major antiarrhythmic actions of drugs are often markedly attenuated by catecholamines.[39,40] Fluctuations in the adrenergic tone might be expected, directly or indirectly, to alter the net efficacy of antiarrhythmic or antifibrillatory compounds.

The results of the meta-analysis of arrhythmia trials in the survivors of acute infarction[13,34] taken in conjunction with the results from CAST,[11,12] are clearly at odds with the rationale for the continued use of the clinical end point of PVC suppression or the treatment of asymptomatic arrhythmias as realistic or desirable approaches for reducing the risk of arrhythmic death. The fact that most, if not all, Class I agents may increase mortality in this setting may simply be a reflection of a further delay in conduction they produce in the diseased substrate. The PVC suppressant effect of the various electrophysiological classes agents are shown in Figure 1. It is noted that of the Class I agents, the most potent suppressants are Class Ic agents. In CAST, they increased

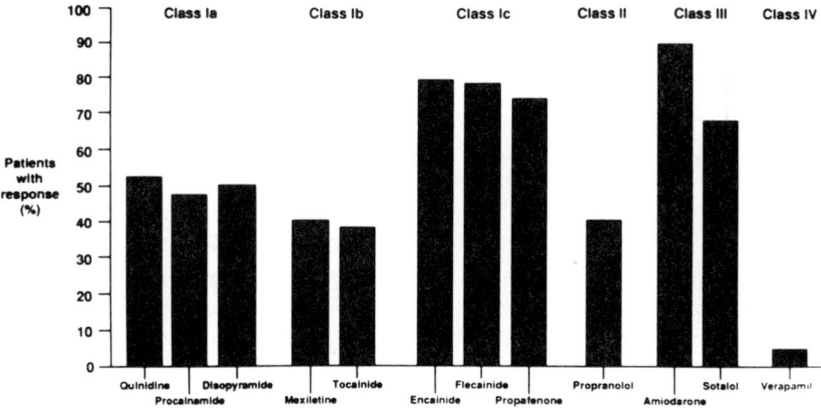

Figure 1. Effects of various electrophysiological classes of antiarrhythmic classes of agents on 80% or greater suppression of premature ventricular contractions (PVCs). The figure is based on data previously reported from meta-analytic studies by Salerno et al.[61] Note that the most potent agents are Class Ic agents and amiodarone. β Blockers produce a modest PVC suppression but they reduce mortality in a variety of subsets of patients; conversely, Class Ic agents and to a lesser extent other Class I agents exhibit a markedly greater PVC suppressant effect while they increase mortality in certain subsets of patients (see text for details).

mortality despite producing a marked suppression of PVCs. The converse is seen with β blockers. In a similar cohort of patients, β blockers reduce sudden death and total mortality while exerting only a modest PVC suppressant effect. Overall, there is little to suggest that the beneficial effect of β blockers might stem from the suppression of PVCs, whatever their frequency or complexity.[41] Thus, despite the long-entrenched belief in the lethal potential of PVCs postmyocardial infarction, the CAST and β-blocker data tend to negate the value of PVC suppression (and this may include nonsustained VT) as a valid approach to mortality reduction in any subset of patients as has been suggested previously by the PVC hypothesis. The dichotomy between PVC suppression by Class I agents and their effect on mortality (ie, adverse) in postinfarct survivors in CAST has already been emphasized (see Chapter 26). It is difficult to ignore a similar dichotomy between the suppression of Holter documented ventricular arrhythmias and mortality in patients with heart disease presenting with symptomatic VT/VF. The parallelism appears compelling especially in light of the fact that the latter subset

of patients are likely to have more advanced degrees of ventricular dysfunction with a correspondingly greater potential for proarrhythmic reactions to Class I agents.

Antiarrhythmic Therapy Guided by Programmed Electrical Stimulation

As in the case of Holter guided therapy, the validation of the PES guided technique has centered essentially on a comparison of the long-term outcome in terms of sudden death and arrhythmia recurrence in responders versus nonresponders.[42–45] The results of such a comparison rapidly came to be accepted not only as the standard approach to symptomatic sustained VTs and patients resuscitated from cardiac arrest,[45,46] but also for the approval of expanding plethora of Class I antiarrhythmic drugs (eg, encainide, flecainide, indecainide, indecainide, cibenzoline, ethmozine) by the Food and Drug Administration. However, the technique has not been validated against an independent and inherently valid control. It is thus uncertain as to how one might interpret the long-term responses to an arrhythmic agent chosen as a result of the so-called PES guided therapy. Whether the drug response might be better than that on placebo, equal to that on placebo or, as noted in the case of CAST (witness the parallelism), even more deleterious than that on placebo at least in the case of certain (Class I) antiarrhythmic compounds remains conjectural. The exact pattern of response within an electrophysiological class of agents might depend critically on the balance attained between the proarrhythmic potential of the test agent on the one hand and its antiarrhythmic or antifibrillatory effects on the other in a particular substrate. For agents used in CAST I and II, it seems inherently illogical that they might increase mortality in infarct survivors while they may decrease it in a group of patients at a higher risk for proarrhythmic actions simply because therapy in the latter were being selected on the basis of PES testing (ie, by a "technique-specific" response). Indeed, the possibility must be considered that to varying extent this may hold for most, if not all, Class I agents. This is certainly suggested by the results of meta-analysis studies.[13,34,35] A verification of this issue by controlled clinical trials might have important implications in the choice of drug therapy for VT/VF. This may also hold for nonsustained VT in which the technique of PES guided therapy is being increasingly applied.[47] In fact, the approach has led to the belief that it might be logical to treat postinfarction survivors on the basis of electrophysiological evaluation.[48] This approach is based on the belief that PES identifies asymptomatic patients at high risk for sudden death and that PES guided drug therapy prolongs survival.[43,45,46,49,50] The first assumption is clearly valid, but there are no controlled data that show that PES guided therapy, even in the case of manifest VT/VF does, in fact, increase survival. The situation may be analogous to that in CAST, in which only responders to the Class Ic agents were randomized to drug therapy versus placebo. It is likely that patients with symptomatic VT/VF in whom inducible VT/VF is preventable by drug therapy actually constitute a relatively

low-risk group when not treated. A favorable impact of drug therapy could be detected only by randomizing a large sample of such drug managed patients against a placebo group (which may well be unethical if it is subsequently shown that drug therapy guided by PES does in fact reduce mortality) or against a group receiving automatic implantable cardioverter defibrillator devices (ICDs). Again, as in the case of Holter guided responses,[51] clinical trials will need to focus not only on responders but also on nonresponders, ie, on the entire spectrum of unselected symptomatic life-threatening ventricular arrhythmias. The difficulties with the predictive accuracy of Holter versus PES guided therapy is also highlighted by the results of the so-called parallel study reported by Brugada et al.[52] as well as the substantial clinical experience with the drug amiodarone.[53-59] In this case, despite the fact that the drug prevents inducibility of VT/VF in only 8%–10% of the patients, it is effective in 60%–80% of the patients who have been found to be resistant to conventional antiarrhythmic therapy guided by PES or Holter monitoring.[53,55,57-59]

Holter Versus PES Guided Therapy in Controlling VT/VF

The inherent limitations of Holter guided therapy of VT/VF or aborted sudden death appear similar, if not identical. Arrhythmias elicited by PES and those documented by Holter monitoring over 24–48 hours might define at best the arrhythmogenic potential of a given substrate when the test is performed.

The vulnerable substrate is known to be subject to the influences of a wide variety of pathophysiological changes as a function of time. One may therefore question why a simple maneuver used under a given set of laboratory circumstances and its response to a particular pharmacological intervention at a specified instance, might accurately predict the recurrence of the arrhythmia at variable times remote in the future. It might undoubtedly provide such predictive information if the substrate were static, the environmental stimuli were not varying and, above all, drug therapy were continuous without peaks and trough serum and tissue levels, uninfluenced by the otherwise deleterious effects of the adrenergic nervous system. In clinical practice, these are conditions that are essentially impossible to meet in a consistent fashion in an individual patient at all times. Both Holter monitoring and PES have the potential to identify a group which on an effective drug during acute testing exhibits good longterm prognosis. However, this process may merely select the patients with an inherently benign prognosis in the relative sense as was clearly evident in CAST.[11] The converse is likely to hold for nonresponders.[51] It is therefore reasonable to expect that in the control of life-threatening ventricular arrhythmias, neither Holter monitoring nor electrophysiological testing coupled with acute drug responses, are unlikely to go a step beyond identifying a myocardial substrate that carries an inherently good or bad prognosis. In terms of technique specific responses, they are unlikely to differ substantially with respect to the predictive accuracy for arrhythmia recurrences, sudden death, or total cardiovascular mortality on drugs selected on the basis of their use. Conversely, by the very nature of the stimuli that operate, the two techniques will likely differ in identifying the actual numbers of patients who are responders or nonresponders to a defined intervention. The Holter guided response in a particular substrate is based on arrhythmias occurring as a result of natural environmental stimuli. The effects of such stimuli in most patients are likely to be more readily suppressible as they are responses to ordinary exigencies of daily life. In contrast, PES clearly constitutes an unnatural stimulus that is often considerably more intense and perhaps at least in some patients unphysiological; the appropriateness of the stimulus strength and its other characteristics cannot be individually matched with the patient's substrate to ensure that an elicited response is always clinically relevant. The inducible arrhythmias are likely to be predictably more severe than those recorded on Holter monitoring. They may be correspondingly more difficult to suppress pharmacologically. Thus, fewer drug responders will be identified by PES than by Holter monitoring. For example, with the exception of sotalol, various major electrophysiological classes of antiarrhythmic agents have been reported[60] to prevent inducible VT/VF in no more than 10%–20% of patients (Figure 2). In the case of Holter monitoring, the corresponding reported rate of suppression of PVCs[61] exceeding 70% is 40%–90% (Figure 1). For nonsustained VT it is 90%–100% when such arrhythmias are present under baseline conditions.[61] Because PES testing is a more stringent test, the arrhythmia recurrence rate in PES responders is likely to be lower in the short term than that in Holter guided responders. Conversely, neither technique might reliably predict sudden death or total mortality since not all arrhythmic episodes end in a fatal outcome. Moreover, antiarrhythmic agents exert profibrillatory actions and antifibrillatory actions and it is the balance between these relative to a particular substrate that is the prime determinant of mortality. CAST results indicated that the proarrhythmic reactions are not predictable from early drug responses involving Holter monitoring. Similarly, no reliable criteria involving electrophysiological testing in the laboratory to date, have been found to predict proarrhythmic effects. The incidence of arrhythmic deaths will therefore depend critically on the nature of the interaction between the substrate and the specific pharmacological regimens in use, ie, drug-specific responses irrespective of how the therapy is guided.

The notion of drug-specific responses is also supported by the β-blocker data on sudden death in the infarct survivors. β Blockers exert a modest PVC suppressant effect (Figure 1) and a weak effect on inducible VT/VF by PES (Figure 2). Yet, they decrease sudden death mortality in infarct survivors by 18%–25%;

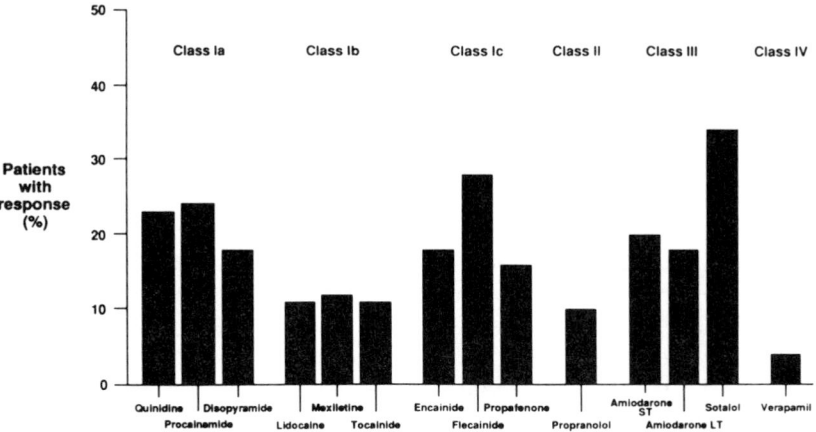

Figure 2. Effects of various electrophysiological classes of antiarrhythmic agents in preventing the inducibility of ventricular arrhythmias in patients with a history of clinical VT/VF. The figure is based on the data summarized by Nattel from the literature.[60] The figures are mean values. Overall, Class I agents are effective in 10%–20% of the patients; sotalol is about 30%; the data for the new Class III agents are sparse. Note that amiodarone, a drug that is widely accepted as the most potent antiarrhythmic agent in the control of recalcitrant VT/VF, has no greater efficacy than Class I agents when evaluated for efficacy (LT: long term; ST: short term) by the PES guided approach indicating a dichotomy between clinical response and technique guided predictive accuracy (see text for details).

[41,62] they prolong survival in the long QT interval syndromes[63] as well as in the survivors of out-of-hospital cardiac arrest.[30] Steinbeck et al.[64] randomized 115 patients with symptomatic sustained VT who also had VT inducible by PES into empirical therapy with metoprolol (n = 54) and to drugs found to be effective by serial testing (n = 61). Over a 2-year follow-up periuod, recurrent nonfatal arrhythmia occurred in 27 patients and sudden death in 27. The incidence of symptomatic arrhythmia and sudden death combined was virtually the same in the two treated groups (PES guided therapy versus metoprolol therapy, 46% versus 48%). This is another example of drug-specific response as being the critical determinant of favorable outcome of therapy in patients with life-threatening ventricular arrhythmias.

The cogency of drug-specific responses is particularly evident in the case of amiodarone. The PVC suppressant effects of various electrophysiological classes of antiarrhythmic compounds are compared to those of amiodarone

in Figure 1. If it is accepted that Class I agents tend to increase mortality while markedly suppressing PVCs while β blockers prolong survival with a relatively modest effect on PVC suppression in the same subset of patients, there does not appear to be a consistent relationship between PVC suppression and mortality is evident except in the case of amiodarone. It is known that amiodarone suppresses PVCs by over 80% in 90% of patients (Figure 1) and close to 100% in the case of nonsustained VT.[61] Thus, in the largest numbers of patients in whom the drug is used for the control of VT/VF according to the Holter criteria, it will be effective.[53] It so happens that in patients with resistant VT/VF, amiodarone that produces such vastly differing effects on inducible VT/VF and PVC suppression (Figures 1 and 2) is effective in 60%–75% of patients.[53,54,57] A beneficial effect on mortality without guided therapy is also indicated in a recent double-blind placebo controlled study in 631 survivors of acute infarction in whom β-blockers could not be used.[65] There were

33 cardiac deaths in the placebo group (10.7%) and 21 in the amiodarone group (6.9%; $p < 0.048$) at the end of the first year. Thus, both amiodarone and β-blocker data in infarct survivors data suggest that drug-specific rather than technique-specific responses are the critical determinants of the overall influence of antiarrhythmic agents on arrhythmia mortality. It is thus a tenable hypothesis that it is the unique pattern of pharmacodynamic and pharmacokinetic properties of individual agents or class of agents and the nature of their interaction with particular substrates that determine the net outcome in terms of morbidity and mortality in patients with heart disease. The outcome of recent controlled trials provide strong support for such a hypothesis.

The Significance of ESVEM Trial Outcome

ESVEM tested the relative merits of PES and Holter guided therapy in predicting long-term drug responses in patients with life-threatening ventricular arrhythmias.[9] Patients (n = 486) with VT/VF, both PES inducible and spontaneously occurring as documented on Holter recordings, were randomized to six Class I agents and sotalol.[10] The patients received in a random fashion up to six drugs until one was deemed effective by predetermined criteria in preventing the inducible VT/VF or one that suppressed arrhythmias recorded on Holter was identified. The treated patients were followed for recurrences of arrhythmia or death (cardiovascular, sudden, or total). In 108 (45%) of the 242 patients of the PES group, a drug predictive of efficacy was found compared to 188 (77%) of 244 patients in the Holter monitoring group ($p < 0.001$).

Two aspects of the results are particularly germane. First, no significant difference between the two techniques in predicting the long-term outcome in terms of arrhythmia recurrence (Figure 3), sudden death, or total cardiovascular mortality was found. These results were unexpected in view of the widely accepted view that Holter monitoring as a technique had considerably lower specificity and sensitivity then PES. Second, comparisons of sotalol (the prototype Class III agent with β-blocking property) versus Class I agents,

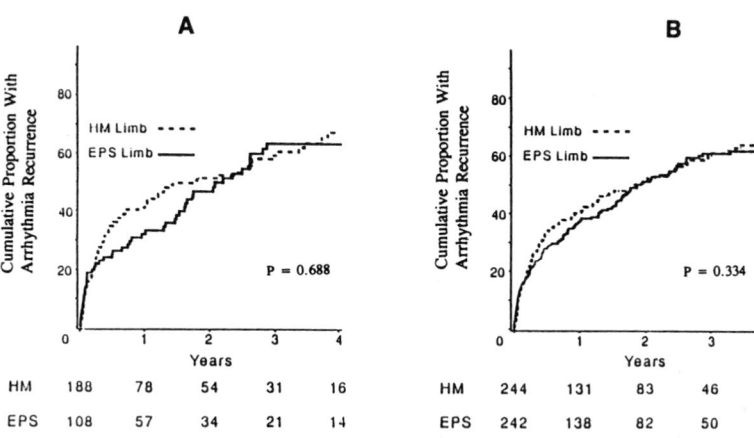

Figure 3. Actuarial probability of a recurrence of arrhythmia, according to study group, in 296 patients receiving a drug predicted to be effective (panel A) and in all 486 patients (panel B). The *p* values were determined by multivariate Cox regression. The number of patients studied initially and in each year of follow-up is shown below the graph. All these data are truncated at 4 years; the actual follow-up exceeded 6 years, and the analyses are based on the entire period of follow-up. (Reproduced with permission from Reference 9.)

collectively or individually (imipramine, quinidine, procainamide, propafenone, pirmenolol, mexiletine), with respect to arrhythmia recurrence, death from any cause, death from a cardiac cause, and that from arrhythmia[10] indicated that sotalol was significantly more effective (Figure 4). ESVEM did not use an independent control analogous to placebo. Therefore, the effects of the drugs used in the trial cannot be interpreted in absolute terms. The possibility is not excluded that in the case of some or indeed all the drugs, the mortality on drugs might have exceeded that on placebo if this could be used. However, a clear cut difference in the effects of sotalol in terms

of arrhythmia recurrence when compared to Class I agents has two implications. First, no longer does it seem appropriate to use Class I agents as first-line therapy in VT/VF. The arrhythmia recurrence rate of 21% incidence on sotalol compared to 44% for Class I agents (p < 0.0007) at 1 year is difficult to ignore. This finding is in accord with the compelling experimental and clinical data that malignant ventricular arrhythmias are more effectively controlled by prolonging refractoriness than by delaying conduction. This is especially so if the effect on refractoriness is modulated by sympathetic antagonism as in the case of sotalol and amiodarone.[41] ESVEM results further stress the significance of drug rather than technique specificity as an approach to the treatment of VT/VF and aborted sudden death.

The Relevance of the Outcome of the Cascade Study

In the Cascade Study, the effects of randomized drug therapy in survivors of cardiac arrest, when comparing empiric amiodarone administration and therapy with Class I agents guided either by Holter monitoring or PES, were determined in 228 patients.[66] The mean left ventricular ejection fraction of the group was 35% and 106 patients had prior history of congestive heart failure. Patients were followed for 6 years. In about 50 patients in each group, an implantable device (ICD) was implanted according to clinical needs. The comparative efficacy data for the two treatment limbs are of interest. The cumulative cardiac survival for all patients (comprising total cardiac mortality, resuscitated cardiac arrest, and syncopal implantable ICD shock) are shown in Figure 5; survival-free syncopal ICD shocks by therapy assignment is shown in Figure 6. For either end point, empiric amiodarone therapy was found to be significantly more effective than guided therapy with conventional (or Class I) agents. Again, as in the case of sotalol in the ESVEM trial, the superiority of amiodarone in cardiac arrest survivors com-

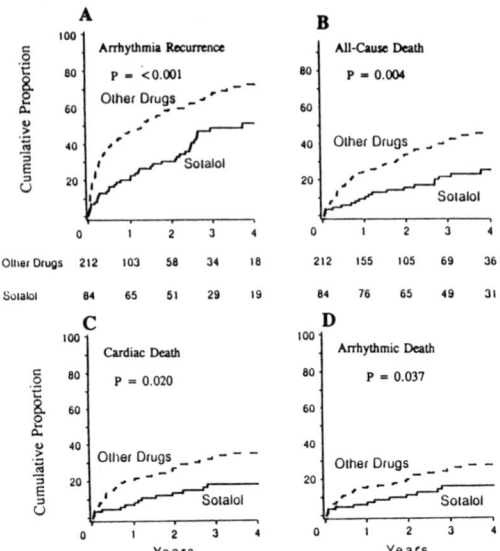

Figure 4. Comparison of sotalol with six other drugs with respect to the actuarial probability of the four end points in the patients with efficacy predictions. Cumulative percentages of patients with a recurrence of arrhythmia (panel A), death from any cause (panel B), death from a cardiac cause (panel C), and death from arrhythmia (panel D) are shown. The *p* values were determined by multivariate Cox regression. The number of patients shown in panels C and D are the same as those in panel D. The actuarial display is truncated at 4 years, but the analysis is based on the entire 6.2 years of follow-up. (Reproduced with permission from Reference 10.)

change further as the end points of clinical trials shift, as they undoubtedly should, from surrogate end points (PVCs, ambient, and inducible arrhythmias) to more direct ones such as relief of symptoms and mortality which have not been mandatory in the past for the FDA approval of antiarrhythmic agents for ventricular arrhythmias. If relief of symptoms were to be the main end point of such trials, it will be desirable that the associated impact on mortality is neutral or not significantly worse. In the case of asymptomatic arrhythmias the sole end point is clearly an improvement in mortality. The major issues in all such trials is likely to be the choice of antiarrhythmic agents with a high potential for relieving symptoms and prolonging survival. Accumulated data no longer provides strong support for the use of surrogate end points such as arrhythmias documented on Holter recordings or those induced by PES for sudden death or total mortality in antiarrhythmic drug trials. In view of the changes that have occurred during the last several years, it is likely that large clinical trials will follow individualized patterns relative to the subset of patients under investigation.

Trials in Which the Use of Placebo Has Not Posed an Ethical Dilemma

These are exemplified by the β-blocker trials in which postinfarct patients were given fixed or varying dose regimens of the test compound and compared in a double-blinded fashion to a placebo control. Because of the unequivocally positive nature of these trials, future studies with other agents will require β blockade in both treatment limbs if there are no contraindications to its use. The ongoing EMIAT and CAMIAT trials are of this kind. Mortality trials in heart failure have followed similar designs.

Trials in Which Placebo Controls Pose an Ethical Dilemma

Such trials are those in which the effects of an intervention are tested in patients with

manifest VT/VF and aborted sudden death. In the past such trials could not be carried out to determine the efficacy and safety of newer drug regimens except by the use of historical controls and by determining the outcome in responders versus nonresponders in the course of so-called guided therapy. In the case of manifest VT/VF and aborted sudden death adequately designed-controlled trials can now be undertaken by the use of implantable devices (ICDs). In such trials, ICDs may serve in lieu of the placebo arm of a randomized trial. It must be emphasized that although in themselves ICDs have not conclusively been shown to prolong survival in a controlled study,[69,70] they do overcome the ethical dilemma of doing a trial against a nontreatment (placebo) limb in patients at high risk for the recurrence of life-threatening ventricular arrhythmias. Trials involving a comparison of ICDs and best medical therapy (usually amiodarone) are currently in progress. If amiodarone is selected as representing the best medical therapy in trials of this kind, the bulk of the data suggests the use of the drug in a purely empirical manner. If amiodarone does prove as effective as ICDs in the control of VT/VF and in survivors of cardiac arrest in such trials, it would be logical and ethical to compare promising newer antifibrillatory agents versus amiodarone to determine their safety and efficacy in controlling VT/VF. Alternatively, a newer compound may be evaluated for safety and efficacy against placebo in controlled trials utilizing the implantation of ICDs in both treatment limbs. The new agent and placebo may then be randomized into the two treatment limbs. Total mortality as well as the number of episodes of VT/VF terminated by ICD may be the end points for judging antiarrhythmic efficacy.

Only stringently controlled clinical trials of this nature in unselected patients with documented VT/VF and aborted sudden death will provide the rational basis for the appropriate choice of pharmacological and nonpharmacological regimens or their combinations for making meaningful inroads into the unacceptably high continuing mortality from malignant ventricular arrhythmias.

Conclusions

For the present, as far as the pharmacological control of ventricular arrhythmias relative to mortality is concerned, some conclusions can be drawn. First, there is compelling data indicating that sodium channel blockers have the potential to increase rather than decrease mortality in patients with structural heart disease presenting with cardiac arrhythmias. This appears to be a class action. Their role as antiarrhythmic agents is likely to progressively decline and eventually be restricted to patients with minimal or no heart disease with troublesome and refractory symptomatic arrhythmias. Second, sympathetic inhibition per se (as exemplified by β blockers) or as an integral component of more complex molecules (eg, sotalol, amiodarone), is a critical feature of desirable antifibrillatory agents.[71,72] If this tenet is accepted, then pure Class III agents compared to dl-sotalol or amiodarone are likely to be less effective. This may also hold for d-sotalol. Compared to amiodarone, they are likely (and the preliminary data are in line with this presumption) to induce a higher incidence of torsades de pointes especially in case of concomitant diuretic therapy. The fact that pure Class III agents have little or no bradycardic effect and little or no effect in slowing atrioventricular nodal conduction, they will have a lower clinical utility as monotherapy in patients with ischemic heart disease which is the most common substrate for the development of VT/VF. It is improbable that the overall clinical utility of these newer compounds will prove superior to either that of sotalol or amiodarone, but more data is needed. Their overall utility may, however, be augmented in combination with β blockers or specific bradycardic agents. It is also likely that the newer agents may prove useful in converting atrial fibrillation and flutter to sinus rhythm; the preliminary data suggests that these may convert about 40% of chronic cases (of less than 12-months duration) following intravenous administration. How effective these agents might be in maintaining long-term stability of sinus rhythm is not known.

They are unlikely to be more effective than quinidine or sotalol (which are equivalent). The role of pure Class III agents in patients with VT/VF is unknown. Their beneficial effects in this setting will need to be balanced against their propensity to induce proarrhythmic reactions especially torsades de pointes. The nature of such a balance will require careful studies of individual compounds of this class relative to their electropharmacological profiles.

The evolving data on the electrophysiological effects and the antiarrhythmic and antifibrillatory actions of newer Class III agents are germane to the issue of developing such agents for therapeutic use. The preliminary data in the few compounds that have been studied thus far do not offer a cause for unrestrained enthusiasm as a concept for the effective control of ventricular or supraventricular tachyarrhythmias. The greatest promise of these agents might hold in the area of complex molecules with a diversity of electrophysiological actions as exemplified by amiodarone or relatively simpler molecules that have the added property of blunting sympathetic excitation. It might be possible to develop such molecules from considerations of structure-activity relationships that might lead to the creation of agents with augmented activity but reduced proarrhythmic potential and safer side effect profiles. In this approach, for commencing the search for the ideal antifibrillatory compound, the initial focus on a pure Class III agent nevertheless may still be a reasonable gambit.

Acknowledgments: I am grateful to Diane Gertschen for help with the preparation of this manuscript.

References

1. Wit AL, Janse MJ: Experimental models of ventricular tachycardia and fibrillation caused by ischemia and infarction. *Circulation* 85(1):142, 1992.
2. Zipes DP: Cardiac electrophysiology: promises and contributions. *J Am Coll Cardiol* 13:1329, 1989.

3. Ruberman W, Weiblatt AB, Goldberg JD: Ventricular premature beats and mortality after myocardial infarction. *N Engl J Med* 247:750, 1977.

4. Moss AJ, Davis HT, Decamilla J: Ventricular ectopic beats and their relation to sudden and non-sudden cardiac death after myocardial infarction. *Circulation* 60:998, 1979.

5. Swerdlow CD, Winkle RA, Mason JW: Determinants of survival in patients with ventricular tachyarrhythmias. *N Engl J Med* 308:1436, 1983.

6. Singh BN, Courtney K: On the classification of anti-arrhythmic mechanisms: experimental and clinical correlations. In: DP Zipes, J Jalife (eds): *Cardiac Electrophysiology: From Cell to Bedside*. Philadelphia, PA: W.B. Saunders, 1990, p. 882.

7. Singh BN (ed): *Control of Cardiac Arrhythmias by Lengthening Repolarization*. Mount Kisco, NY: Futura Publishing Company, Inc., 1988.

8. Mirowski MM, Reid PR, Watkins L, et al: Clinical treatment of life-threatening ventricular arrhythmias with automatic implantable defibrillator. *Am Med J* 102:265, 1981.

9. Mason JW, For the Electrophysiologic Study Versus Electrocardiographic Monitoring Investigators: A comparison of the electrophysiologic testing with Holter monitoring to predict antiarrhythmic efficacy for ventricular tachyarrhythmias. *N Engl J Med* 329:445, 1993.

10. Mason JW, For the Electrophysiologic Study Versus Electrocardiographic Monitoring Investigators: A comparison of seven antiarrhythmic drugs in patients with ventricular tachyarrhythmias. *N Engl J Med* 329:452, 1993.

11. The Cardiac Arrhythmia Suppression Trial (CAST) Investigators Preliminary Report: Effect of encainide and flecainide on mortality in a randomized trial of arrhythmia suppression after myocardial infarction. *N Engl J Med* 321:406, 1989.

12. Cardiac Arrhythmias Suppression Trial II Investigators: Ethmozine exerts an adverse effect on mortality in survivors of acute myocardial infarction. *N Engl J Med* 327:227, 1992.

13. Furberg CD: Effects of antiarrhythmic drugs on mortality after myocardial infarction. *Am J Cardiol* 53:32C, 1983.

14. Lynch JJ, Lucchesi BR: How are animal models best used for the study of antiarrhythmic drugs? In: DJ Hearse, AS Mouring, MJ Janse (eds): *Life-Threatening Arrhythmias During Ischemia and Infarction*. New York, NY: Raven Press, 1987, p. 169.

15. Kou WH, Nelson SD, Lynch JJ, et al: Effect of flecainide acetate of prevention of electrical induction of ventricular tachycardia and occurrence of ischemic ventricular fibrillation during the early postmyocardial infarction period. Evaluation in a conscious canine model of sudden death. *J Am Coll Cardiol* 9:359, 1987.

16. Patterson E, Lucchesi BR: Quinidine gluconate in chronic myocardial ischemic injury. Differential effects in response to programmed stimulation and acute myocardial ischemia in the dog. *Circulation* 68:111, 1983.

17. Nattel S, Pederson DH, Zipes DP: Alterations in regional myocardial distribution and arrhythmogenic effects of aprindine produced by coronary artery occlusion in the dog. *Cardiovas Res* 15:80, 1981.

18. Furukawa T, Rozanski JJ, Monroe K, et al: Efficacy of procainamide on ventricular tachycardia: relation to prolongation of refractoriness and slowing of conduction. *Am Heart J* 118:702, 1989.

19. Kus T, Dubue M, Lambert C, Shenasa M: Efficacy of propafenone in preventing ventricular tachycardia, with insights from analysis of resetting response patterns. *Am J Cardiol* 15:1229, 1990.

20. MacMahan S, Collins R, Peto R, et al: Effects of prophylactic lidocaine in suspected acute myocardial infarction. *JAMA* 20:1910, 1988.

21. IMPACT Research Group: International mexiletine and placebo anti-arrhythmic coronary trial. 1. Report on arrhythmias and other findings. *J Am Coll Cardiol* 4:1148, 1984.

22. Bayes de Luna A, Coumel P, Leclerq JR: Ambulatory sudden cardiac death: mechanisms of production on the basis of data from 157 cases. *Am Heart J* 117:151, 1989.

23. Pratt CM, Francis MJ, Luck JC, et al: Analysis of ambulatory electrocardiograms in 15 patients during spontaneous ventricular fibrillation with special reference to preceding arrhythmic events. *J Am Coll Cardiol* 2:798, 1983.

24. Nikolic G, Bishop RL, Singh JB: Sudden death recorded during Holter monitoring. *Circulation* 66:218, 1982.

25. Milner PG, Platia EV, Reid PR, et al: Ambulatory electrocardiographic recording at the time of fatal cardiac arrest. *Am J Cardiol* 56:588, 1985.

26. Rapaport E, Remedios P: The high risk patient after recovery from myocardial infarction: recognition and managements. *J Am Coll Cardiol* 1:391, 1983.

27. Morganroth J, Goin JE: Quinidine—mortality in the short-to-medium term treatment of ventricular arrhythmias. *Circulation* 84:1911, 1991.

28. Middlekauff HR, Stevenson WG, Saxon LA, Stevenson LW: Safest anti-arrhythmic drug in advanced heart failure depends on heart failure etiology. *J Am Coll Cardiol* 19:78A, 1982.

29. Ruskin J, McGovern B, DiMarco JP, Kelly E: Anti-arrhythmic drugs: a possible cause of out-of-hospital cardiac arrest. *N Engl J Med* 309:1302, 1983.

30. Hallstrom AP, Cobb LA, Yu BH, et al: An antiarrhythmic drug experience in 941 patients resuscitated from an initial cardiac arrest from 1970 and 1985. *Am J Cardiol* 68:1025, 1991.

31. Singh BN: Do anti-arrhythmic drugs work? Some reflections on the implications of the Cardiac Arrhythmia Suppression Trial. *Clin Cardiol* 13:725, 1990.

32. Singh BN: Controlling cardiac arrhythmias: to delay conduction or to prolong refractoriness? *Cardiovasc Drugs Ther* 3:671, 1990.

33. Bigger JT, Fleiss JL, Kleiger R, et al: The relationship between ventricular arrhythmias, left ventricular dysfunction, and mortality in the 2 years after myocardial infarction. *Circulation* 69:250, 1984.

34. Yusuf S, Teo KK: Approaches to sudden death: need for fundamental re-evaluation. *J Cardiovasc Electrophysiol* 2:S233, 1991.

35. Coplen SE, Antman EM, Berlin JA, et al: Efficacy and safety of quinidine therapy for the maintenance of sinus rhythm after cardioversion. A meta-analysis of randomized control trials. *Circulation* 82:1106, 1990.

36. Flaker GC, Blackshear JL, McBride R, et al: Antiarrhythmic drug therapy and cardiac mortality in atrial fibrillation. *J Am Coll Cardiol* 20:427, 1992.

37. Pritchett ELC, Wilkinson WE: Mortality in patients treated with flecainide and encainide for supraventricular arrhythmias. *Am J Cardiol* 67: 976, 1991.

38. Middlekauff HR, Wiener I, Saxon LA, Stevenson WG: Low dose amiodarone for atrial fibrillation. Time for a prospective study? *Ann Intern Med* 116:1017, 1992.

39. Jazayeri MR, Van Wyhe G, Avitall B, et al: Isoproterenol reversal of antiarrhythmic effects in patients with inducible sustained ventricular tachyarrhythmias. *J Am Coll Cardiol* 14:705, 1989.

40. Calkins H, Sousa J, El-Atassi R, et al: Reversal of antiarrhythmic drug effects of epinephrine. Quinidine versus amiodarone. *J Am Coll Cardiol* 19:347, 1991.

41. Singh BN: Advantages of beta-blockers versus antiarrhythmic agents and calcium antagonists in secondary prevention after myocardial infarction. *Am J Cardiol* 66:9C, 1990.

42. Mason JW, Winkle RA: Accuracy of ventricular tachycardia induction study for predicting long-term efficacy and inefficacy of anti-arrhythmic drugs. *N Engl J Med* 303:1073, 1990.

43. Roy D, Waxman HL, Kenzle MG, et al: Clinical characteristics and long-term follow-up in 118 survivors of cardiac arrest: relation to inducibility of electrophysiologic testing. *Am J Cardiol* 52:969, 1983.

44. Ruskin JN, DiMarco JP, Garan H: Out-of-hospital cardiac arrest electrophysiologic observations and selection of long-term antiarrhythmic therapy. *N Engl J Med* 303:607, 1980.

45. Morady F, Scheinman MM, Hess DS, et al: Electrophysiologic testing in the management of survivors of out-of-hospital cardiac arrest. *Am J Cardiol* 51:85, 1983.

46. Wilber DJ, Garan H, Finkelstein D: Out-of-hospital cardiac arrest: use of electrophysiologic testing in the prediction of long-term outcome. *N Engl J Med* 318:19, 1988.

47. Richards DAB, Byth K, Ross DR, Uther JB: What is the best predictor of spontaneous ventricular tachycardia and sudden death after myocardial infarction? *Circulation* 83:756, 1991.

48. Dennis AR, Ross DL, Cosby DV, et al: Randomized control trial of prophylactic anti-arrhythmic therapy in patients with inducible ventricular tachyarrhythmias after myocardial infarction. *Eur Heart J* 9:746, 1988.

49. Horowitz LN, Greenspan AM, Spielman SR: Usefulness of electrophysiologic testing in evaluation of amiodarone therapy for sustained ventricular tachyarrhythmias associated with coronary heart disease. *Am J Cardiol* 55:367, 1985.

50. Poole JE, Mathisen EL, Kudenchek PJ, et al: Long-term outcome in patients who survive out of hospital ventricular fibrillation and undergo electrophysiologic studies: evaluation by electrophysiology subgroups. *J Am Coll Cardiol* 16: 657, 1990.

51. Graboys TB, Lown B, Podrid PJ, DeSilva R: Long-term survival with ventricular arrhythmias treated with anti-arrhythmic drugs. *Am J Cardiol* 50:437, 1982.

52. Brugada P, Lemery R, Talajic M, et al: Treatment of ventricular tachycardia or fibrillation: first lessons from the "parallel study". In: P Brugada, HJJ Wellens (eds): *Cardiac Arrhythmias: Where to Go From Here?* Mount Kisco, NY: Futura Publishing Company, Inc., 1987, p. 457.

53. Nademanee K, Hendrickson J, Kannan R, Singh BN: Antiarrhythmic efficacy and electrophysiologic actions of amiodarone in patients with life-threatening ventricular arrhythmias: potent suppression of spontaneously occurring tachyarrhythmias versus inconsistent abolition of induced ventricular tachycardia. *Am Heart J* 103: 950, 1982.

54. Herre JM, Sauve MJ, Malone P, et al: Long-term results of amiodarone therapy in patients with recurrent sustained ventricular tachycardia or ventricular fibrillation. *J Am Coll Cardiol* 13: 442, 1989.

55. Heger JJ, Prystowsky EN, Jackman WM, et al: Amiodarone: clinical efficacy and electrophysi-

ology during long-term therapy for recumbent ventricular tachycardias or ventricular fibrillation. *N Engl J Med* 305:539, 1981.

56. Kadish AH, Marchlinski FE, Josephson ME, Buxton AE: Amiodarone: correlation of early and late electrophysiologic studies with outcome. *Am Heart J* 112:1134, 1986.

57. Nademanee K, Singh BN, Hendrickson J: Amiodarone in refractory life-threatening ventricular arrhythmias. *Ann Intern Med* 98:577, 1983.

58. Mason JW: Amiodarone. *N Engl J Med* 316:455, 1987.

59. Marchlinski FE, Buxton AE, Mittler JM, et al: Amiodarone versus amiodarone and a type IA agents for treatment of patients with rapid ventricular tachycardia. *Circulation* 74:1037, 1986.

60. Nattel S: Antiarrhythmic drug classifications: a critical appraisal of their history, present status, and clinical relevance. *Drugs* 41(5):672, 1991.

61. Salerno DM, Gillingham KJ, Berry DA, Hodges M: A comparison of antiarrhythmic drugs for the suppression of ventricular ectopic depolarization: a meta-analysis. *Am Heart J* 120:340, 1990.

62. Yusuf S, Peto R, Lewis J, et al: Beta-blockade during and after myocardial infarction: an overview of the randomized trials. *Prog Cardiovasc Dis* 27:235, 1985.

63. Schwartz PJ: Idiopathic long-QT syndrome: progress and questions. *Am Heart J* 109:399, 1985.

64. Steinbeck G, Andresen D, Bach P, et al: A comparison of the electrophysiologic-guided anti-arrhythmic therapy with beta-blocker therapy in patients with symptomatic, sustained ventricular tachyarrhythmias. *N Engl J Med* 327:987, 1992.

65. Ceremuzynski L, Krzemiska-Padula M, Kuch J, et al: The effect of amiodarone mortality after myocardial infarction. *J Am Coll Cardiol* 20:1056, 1992.

66. The CASCADE Investigators: Randomized antiarrhythmic drug therapy survivors of cardiac arrest (The CASCADE Study). *Am J Cardiol* 72:280, 1993.

67. Deedwania P, Carbajal E: Silent ischemia during life is an independent predictor of mortality in stable angina. *Circulation* 81:748, 1990.

68. Bodenheimer MM: Risk stratification in coronary artery disease. A contrary viewpoint. *Ann Intern Med* 116:927, 1992.

69. Adler SW, Remole S, Benditt DG: Impact of implantable cardioverter-defibrillators on prognosis of cardiac arrest survivors. A continuing controversy. *Circulation* 18:1348, 1993.

70. Connolly SJ, Yusuf S: Evaluations of the implantable cardioverter defibrillator in survivors of cardiac arrest: the need for randomized trials. *Am J Cardiol* 69:959, 1992.

71. Singh BN, Sarma JSM, Zhang ZH, Takanaka C: Controlling cardiac arrhythmias by lengthening repolarization: rationale from experimental findings and clinical consideration. *Ann NY Acad Sci* 664:187, 1992.

72. Singh BN: Antiarrhythmic action of DL-sotalol in ventricular and supraventricular arrhythmias. *J Cardiovasc Pharmacol* 20(2):575, 1992.

Index